DI029892

ANESTHETIC AND OBSTETRIC MANAGEMENT OF HIGH-RISK PREGNANCY

SECOND EDITION

MOORE LIBRARY

ANESTHETIC AND OBSTETRIC MANAGEMENT OF HIGH-RISK PREGNANCY

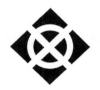

DREXEL UNIVERSITY
HEALTH SCIENCES LIBRARIES
HAHNEMANN LIBRARY

SANJAY DATTA, M.D., F.F.A.R.C.S. (ENG.)

Director of Obstetric Anesthesia
Brigham and Women's Hospital
Professor of Anaesthesia
Harvard Medical School
Boston, Massachusetts

SECOND EDITION

with 223 illustrations

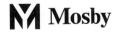 **Mosby**

St. Louis Baltimore Berlin Boston Carlsbad Chicago London Madrid
Naples New York Philadelphia Sydney Tokyo Toronto

WO
450
A5795
1996

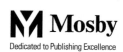 **Mosby**

Dedicated to Publishing Excellence

A Times Mirror Company

Publisher: Anne S. Patterson
Senior Editor: Laurel Craven
Senior Developmental Editor: Sandra Clark Brown
Project Manager: Linda Clarke
Senior Production Editor: Allan S. Kleinberg
Manufacturing Supervisor: Bill Winneberger
Designer: Carolyn O'Brien

SECOND EDITION

Copyright ©1996 by Mosby–Year Book, Inc.

All rights reserved. No part of this publication may be reproduced, stored in a retrieval system, or transmitted, in any form or by any means, electronic, mechanical, photocopying, recording, or otherwise, without prior written permission from the publisher.

Permission to photocopy or reproduce solely for internal or personal use is permitted for libraries or other users registered with the Copyright Clearance Center, 27 Congress Street, Salem, MA 01970, provided that the base fee of $4.00 per chapter plus $.10 per page is paid directly to the Copyright Clearance Center. This consent does not extend to other kinds of copying, such as copying for general distribution, for advertising or promotional purposes, for creating collected works, or for resale.

Printed in the United States of America
Composition by The Clarinda Company
Printing/binding by Maple-Vail

Mosby–Year Book, Inc.
11830 Westline Industrial Drive
St. Louis, MO 63146

ISBN: 0-8151-2280-2

96 97 98 99 00 / 10 9 8 7 6 5 4 3 2 1

CONTRIBUTORS

Amr E. Abouleish, M.D.
Assistant Professor of Anesthesiology
The University of Texas Medical Branch
Galveston, Texas

Ezzat I. Abouleish, M.B., Ch.B, M.D.
Professor of Anesthesiology
Professor of Obstetrics and Gynecology
Medical Director of Obstetric Anesthesia
The University of Texas Health Science Center
Houston, Texas

Lindsay S. Alger, M.D.
Professor of Obstetrics and Gynecology
Associate Director of Maternal-Fetal Medicine
Medical Director of Labor and Delivery
University of Maryland Medical Systems
Baltimore, Maryland

Angela M. Bader, M.D.
Director of Obstetric Anesthesia Research
Brigham and Women's Hospital
Assistant Professor of Anaesthesia
Harvard Medical School
Boston, Massachusetts

**Thomas F. Baskett, M.B., F.R.C.S.(C),
F.R.C.S.(Ed), F.R.C.O.G.**
Professor, Department of Obstetrics
    and Gynecology
Dalhausie University
Chief, Department of Gynecology
Halifax Infirmary
Halifax, Nova Scotia

Gerard M. Bassell, M.B., B.S.
Professor of Anesthesiology, Obstetrics
    and Gynecology
Vice-Chairman, Department of Anesthesiology
University of Kansas School of Medicine–
    Wichita
Wesley Women's Hospital
Wichita, Kansas

**Michael A. Belfort, M.D., M.B.B.C.H.,
D.A.(S.A.), M.R.C.O.G., F.R.C.S.(C),
F.S.O.G.(C)**
Assistant Professor
Division of Maternal-Fetal Medicine
Department of Obstetrics, Gynecology
    and Anesthesiology
Baylor College of Medicine
Director of Obstetric Intensive Care Unit
Houston, Texas

Richard Eaton Besinger, M.D.
Associate Professor
Division of Maternal–Fetal Medicine
Department of Obstetrics and Gynecology
Loyola University–Chicago
Maywood, Illinois

David J. Birnbach, M.D.
Director, Obstetric Anesthesiology
St. Luke's-Roosevelt Hospital Center
Assistant Professor of Anesthesiology, Obstetrics
    and Gynecology
Columbia University College of Physicians
    and Surgeons
New York, New York

Norman H. Blass, M.D.
Professor of Anesthesia
Professor of Obstetrics and Gynecology
Director–Obstetric Anesthesia
Departments of Anesthesia, Obstetrics
    and Gynecology
University of Texas Medical Branch
Galveston, Texas

William R. Camann, M.D.
Director of Obstetric Anesthesia Education
Assistant Professor of Anaesthesia
Harvard Medical School
Anesthesiologist
Brigham and Women's Hospital
Boston, Massachusetts

Harvey Carp, Ph.D., M.D.
Director of Obstetric Anesthesia
Associate Professor of Anesthesiology
 and Obstetrics and Gynecology
Oregon Health Sciences University
Portland, Oregon

Linda Chan, M.D.
Attending Perinatologist
Assistant Professor of Obstetrics, Gynecology
 and Physiology
Department of Obstetrics, Gynecology
 and Reproductive Sciences
Temple University School of Medicine
Philadelphia, Pennsylvania

Ashwin Chatwani, M.D.
Associate Professor of Obstetrics
 and Gynecology
Residency Program Director
Temple University Hospital
Philadelphia, Pennsylvania

Theodore G. Cheek, M.D.
Associate Professor of Anesthesia and Obstetrics
 and Gynecology
University of Pennsylvania Medical Center
Department of Anesthesiology
University of Pennsylvania Hospital
Philadelphia, Pennsylvania

Brian A. Clark, Ph.D., M.D.
Director, Reproductive Genetics
MetroHealth Medical Center
Assistant Professor, Department of Genetics
Assistant Professor, Department of Reproductive
 Biology
Case Western Reserve University
Cleveland, Ohio

Richard B. Clark, M.D.
Professor
Departments of Anesthesia and Obstetrics and
 Gynecology
University of Arkansas Medical Center
Little Rock, Arkansas

H. Breckenridge Collins, M.D.
Assistant Professor
Department of Obstetrics and Gynecology
University of Arkansas Medical Center
Little Rock, Arkansas

Barry C. Corke, M.B., Ch.B., F.F.A.R.C.S.
Director of Obstetric Anesthesia
Medical Center of Delaware
Christiana Hospital
Newark, Delaware

Sanjay Datta, M.D., F.F.A.R.C.S. (Eng.)
Director of Obstetric Anesthesia
Brigham and Women's Hospital
Professor of Anaesthesia
Harvard Medical School
Boston, Massachusetts

Sidney B. Effer, M.D., F.R.C.S.(C)
Assistant Professor
University of British Columbia
Perinatologist
Division of Maternal/Fetal Medicine
British Columbia Women's Hospital and Health
 Center Society
Vancouver, British Columbia

Dan Farine, M.D., F.R.C.P.(S)
Associate Professor of Obstetrics
 and Gynecology
Director of Maternal Fetal Medicine
University of Toronto
Toronto, Ontario
Canada

Bruce B. Feinberg, M.D.
Assistant Professor, Maternal–Fetal Medicine
Department of Gynecology and Reproductive
 Biology
Brigham and Women's Hospital
Harvard Medical School
Boston, Massachusetts

Larry C. Gilstrap III, M.D.
Professor of Obstetrics and Gynecology
The University of Texas
Southwestern Medical Center at Dallas
Dallas, Texas

Adam Goldstein, M.D.
Staff Anesthesiologist
United States Navy

Bernard Gonik, M.D.
Professor and Vice–Chairman
Chief, Department of Obstetrics and Gynecology
Grace Hospital
Department of Obstetrics and Gynecology
Wayne State University School of Medicine
Detroit, Michigan

Michael F. Greene, M.D.
Associate Professor of Obstetrics, Gynecology,
    and Reproductive Biology
Harvard Medical School
Director of Maternal/Fetal Medicine
Vincent Memorial Obstetrics Division
Massachusetts General Hospital
Boston, Massachusetts

Amos Grunebaum, M.D.
Director, Maternal–Fetal Medicine
Department of Obstetrics and Gynecology
St. Luke's–Roosevelt Hospital
New York, New York

Andrew P. Harris, M.D.
Associate Professor of Anesthesiology
    and Critical Care Medicine
Department of Anesthesiology and Critical
    Care Medicine
The Johns Hopkins University
    School of Medicine
Baltimore, Maryland

Barbara L. Hartwell, M.D.
Anesthesiologist
Metrowest Medical Center
Framingham, Massachusetts

Martha Ann Hauch, M.D.
Staff Anesthesiologist
Brigham and Women's Hospital
Instructor of Anaesthesia
Harvard Medical School
Boston, Massachusetts

Linda Heffner, M.D., Ph.D.
Associate Professor of Obstetrics, Gynecology
    and Reproductive Biology
Harvard Medical School
Director, Maternal–Fetal Medicine
Brigham and Women's Hospital
Boston, Massachusetts

Douglas V. Horbelt, M.D., M.A.
Professor of Obstetrics and Gynecology
Chairman, Department of Obstetrics
    and Gynecology
University of Kansas School of Medicine–
    Wichita
Wichita, Kansas

Mark D. Johnson, M.D.
Chairman, Department of Anesthesia
Director, Operating Room
Director, Post Anesthesia Care Unit
Associate Director, Intensive Care Unit
Melrose–Wakefield Hospital
Melrose, Massachusetts

Monica M. Jones, M.D.
Staff Anesthesiologist
Erlander Medical Center
Chattanooga, Tennessee

Nancy B. Kenepp, M.D.
Associate Professor of Anesthesiology
Temple University Hospital
Temple University Medical School
Philadelphia, Pennsylvania

Wesley Lee, M.D.
Clinical Assistant Professor of Obstetrics
    and Gynecology
University of Michigan
William Beaumont Hospital
Ann Arbor, Michigan

Stephen Longmire, M.D.
Associate Professor–Anesthesiology, Obstetrics,
    and Gynecology
Department of Anesthesiology
Baylor College of Medicine
Houston, Texas

Andrew M. Malinow, M.D.
Director, Obstetric Anesthesia
Associate Professor of Anesthesiology, Obstetrics
  and Gynecology
Department of Anesthesiology, Obstetrics
  and Gynecology
University of Maryland Medical Systems
Baltimore, Maryland

Ramon Martin, M.D., Ph.D.
Staff Anesthesiologist
Department of Anesthesiologist
Brigham and Women's Hospital
Instructor of Anesthesia
Harvard Medical School
Boston, Massachusetts

**Graham H. McMorland, M.B., Ch.B., D.A.,
F.R.C.P.(C)**
Professor Emeritus
Department of Anaesthesia
University of British Columbia
Vancouver, British Columbia
Canada

Bruce A. Meyer, M.D.
Assistant Professor of Obstetrics and Gynecology
Acting Director, Maternal–Fetal Medicine
Department of Obstetrics & Gynecology
Division of Maternal–Fetal Medicine
University Hospital, Stony Brook
Stony Brook, New York

**Jack Moodley, M.D.(Natal),
F.R.C.O.G.(UK)**
Professor of Obstetrics and Gynecology
Director of Medical Research Council
Pregancy Hypertension Unit
University of Natal
Durban, South Africa

Mark C. Norris, M.D.
Professor of Anesthesiology
Co-Director of Obstetrical Anesthesia
Department of Anesthesiology
Thomas Jefferson Medical College
Thomas Jefferson University
Philadelphia, Pennsylvania

Warren N. Otterson, M.D.
Professor of Obstetrics and Gynecology
School of Medicine in Shreveport
Shreveport, Louisiana

Valerie M. Parisi, M.D., M.P.H.
Professor and Chairman
University Medical Center at Stony Brook
Department of Obstetrics, Gynecology
  and Reproductive Medicine
University Medical Center at Stony Brook
School of Medicine
Stony Brook, New York

James M. Pivarnik, Ph.D.
Associate Professor
Departments of Exercise Science and Osteopathic
  Medicine
Michigan State University
East Lansing, Michigan

J. Gerald Quirk, Jr., M.D., Ph.D.
Professor and Chairman
Department of Obstetrics and Gynecology
University of Arkansas Medical Center
Little Rock, Arkansas

Dale P. Reisner, M.D.
Division of Perinatal Medicine
Department of Obstetrics and Gynecology
Swedish Hospital Medical Center
Seattle, Washington

Alfred G. Robichaux III, M.D.
Director, Division of Maternal-Fetal Medicine
Department of Obstetrics and Gynecology
Ochsner Clinic
New Orleans, Louisiana

**David Anthony Rocke, F.R.C.P. (Edin),
F.F.A.(SA)**
Professor of Anaesthesia
Chairman, Department of Anaesthesia
University of Natal
Durban, South Africa

Stephen H. Rolbin, M.D.C.M., F.R.C.P.(C)
Assistant Professor of Anaesthesia
Mount Sinai Hospital
University of Toronto
Toronto, Ontario
Canada

Francis Anthony Rosinia, M.D.
Staff Anesthesiologist
Director of Obstetric Anesthesia
Department of Anesthesiology
Ochsner Medical Foundation
New Orleans, Louisiana

Daniel H. Saltzman, M.D.
Director of Maternal & Fetal Medicine
Chief of Obstetrics
Department of Obstetrics and Gynecology
Beth Israel Medical Center
Associate Professor of
    Obstetrics and Gynecology
Albert Einstein College of Medicine
New York, New York

Philip Samuels, M.D.
Associate Professor
Department of Obstetrics and Gynecology
The Ohio State University
Columbus, Ohio

Alan C. Santos, M.D.
Associate Professor of Anesthesiology
Department of Anesthesiology
Albert Einstein College of Medicine/Montefiore
    Medical Center
Albert Einstein College of Medicine at Yeshiva
    University
Bronx, New York

Eugene Scioscia, M.D.
Residency Coordinator
Assistant Professor of Obstetrics and Gynecology
Medical College of Pennsylvania
Hahnemann Hospital
Philadelphia, Pennsylvania

John W. Seeds, M.D.
Professor and Vice Chairman
Department of Obstetrics and Gynecology
Director of Maternal/Fetal Medicine
Medical College of Virginia
Virginia Commonwealth University
Richmond, Virginia

Michael N. Skaredoff, M.D.
Chairman
Department of Anesthesiology
Provident Hospital of Cook County
Chicago, Illinois

Jonathan H. Skerman, B.D.Sc., M.Sc.D., D.Sc.
Professor of Anesthesiology
Professor of Obstetrics and Gynecology
Vice Chairman for Administration and Research
Department of Anesthesiology
School of Medicine in Shreveport
Shreveport, Louisiana

Maya S. Suresh, M.D.
Director of Obstetric Anesthesia
Associate Professor of Anesthesiology,
    Obstetrics, and Gynecology
Baylor College of Medicine
Houston, Texas

Joel William Swanson, M.D.
Coordinator, Obstetric and Gynecological
    Anesthesiology
Assistant Professor
Department of Anesthesiology
Medical College of Pennsylvania
    and Hahnemann University
Allegheny Campus
Pittsburgh, Pennsylvania

Thomas N. Tabb, M.D.
Medical Director
The Perinatal Center
Baptist Memorial Hospital East
Memphis, Tennessee

M. Mark Taslimi, M.D.
Associate Professor of Obstetrics
    and Gynecology
Division of Maternal–Fetal Medicine
University of Tennessee College of Medicine
    at Chattanooga
Chattanooga, Tennessee

Ruth E. Tuomala, M.D.
Assistant Professor of Obstetrics and Gynecology
Harvard Medical School
Director of Obstetrics and Gynecology/Infectious
    Disease
Brigham and Women's Hospital
Boston, Massachusetts

Donald H. Wallace, M.D.
Associate Professor of Anesthesiology
Department of Anesthesiology and Pain
    Management
U.T. Southwestern Medical Center at Dallas
Dallas, Texas

Frank R. Witter, M.D.
Associate Professor of Gynecology
    and Obstetrics
Medical Director of Labor and Delivery of
    The Johns Hopkins Hospital
Department of Gynecology and Obstetrics
Johns Hopkins University School of Medicine
Baltimore, Maryland

W. Desmond Writer, M.B., Ch.B.
Staff Anaesthetist
Grace Maternity Hospital
Halifax, Nova Scotia

Esther M. Yun, M.D.
Assistant Professor of Anesthesiology
Department of Anesthesiology
Albert Einstein College of Medicine/Montefiore
    Medical Center
Albert Einstein College of Medicine of Yeshiva
    University
Bronx, New York

For my wife, Gouri and daughter, Nandini, whose endless support and encouragement, continuing understanding, and valuable help made this project possible.

PREFACE

It is always gratifying to hear from one's colleagues, both inside and outside the country, positive comments about any book with which one has been involved. *Anesthetic and Obstetric Management of High-Risk Pregnancy,* particularly, gave me an enormous amount of satisfaction because of the understanding of the need for close communication between two specialties, anesthesiology and obstetrics, not only to take care of the sick parturient but also to deliver a healthy baby.

Since 1991, significant changes have taken place in the field of obstetric anesthesia as well as obstetric care. Hence, I felt a second edition was necessary in order to update the chapters. The chapters on Antepartum Hemorrhage, Neurologic and Muscular Diseases, Respiratory Changes, Orthopedic Problems, Infectious Diseases, Substance Abuse, and Fetal Distress underwent extensive revisions. The remainder of the chapters were modified where necessary. Two new chapters have been added, *Psychiatric Disease (Chapter 29)* and *Hepatic Disease (Chapter 30),* which should be of use in special situations.

The second edition now includes 32 chapters with several new authors. Like the first edition, the present edition also includes contributions from experts in the fields of obstetric anesthesia and obstetrics, both nationally and internationally. I thank all the authors for their valuable contributions and their time and effort. It is to be noted that the authors have expressed their own opinions and recommendations, which do not necessarily reflect my own views. Thus on occasion I have added an editorial footnote to the text. I also wish to thank Ms. Nancy E. Jeffery for her endless help in completing the new edition and Mr. David Baldwin for his technical assistance.

I sincerely hope this edition will further reinforce the concept of the team approach for taking care of the high-risk parturient.

Sanjay Datta

FOREWORD

Barely five years have passed since the first edition of *Anesthetic and Obstetric Management of High-Risk Pregnancy* was published. The book, conceived and edited by Sanjay Datta, was an immediate success. A second edition has become warranted, partly because of abundant new information and partly because of a near sell-out of the original text.

This second edition follows the special format of the first, namely that of collaboration between at least two specialists involved in the management of a high-risk pregnancy. Two new chapters have been added, the management of parturients with liver disorders (Chapter 30) and the management of pregnant women with psychiatric disorders (Chapter 29). Of the now 32 chapters, all but the first, Prepartum and Intrapartum Fetal Monitoring, are written by an anesthesiologist as well as by an obstetrician, sometimes by more than one. Viewing problems from both angles facilitates comprehension of pathology and risk and thus enhances a positive outcome for both mother and fetus.

The enlarged and updated information provided in this second edition makes the book a worthwhile addition to any anesthetic and obstetric library. I am confident that it will be as well received as the first.

Gertie F. Marx, M.D.
Professor of Anesthesiology
Albert Einstein College of Medicine
New York, New York

CONTENTS

1 Prepartum and Intrapartum Fetal Monitoring

Ramon Martin

When a woman presents to the Labor and Delivery Suite with contractions and the expectation of delivery, the fetus is evaluated primarily by fetal heart rate (FHR) monitoring, either electronically or with intermittent auscultation. This technique is just one of several methods to monitor the fetus from the mid first trimester through birth. As pregnancy progresses, the prenatal record contains a wealth of information not only about the parturient but also about the fetus.

The monitoring of the mother and fetus during this period of development has evolved considerably due to biochemical and technical advances, and as a result, a better understanding of the fetus has been gained. Most pregnancies proceed and end with no complications. Monitoring techniques are used not only for diagnostic purposes, thereby serving a preventive role, but they are also necessary in treatment, if the fetus should become stressed. Stress to the fetus is defined in this chapter as either hypoxia or asphyxia. This is because the supply of oxygen to the fetus is crucial. Any diminution or cessation of oxygen results in an immediate change in acid base status, affecting all organs, particularly the heart and brain. There are compensatory responses by the fetus, but fetal reserves are limited. It is therefore important to recognize the fetal response to stress, identify the cause, and treat it.

Anesthesia, as an integral part of obstetric delivery, can impact the outcome of delivery, depending on the status of the fetus. For this reason, it is important to understand the monitoring devices used, their results, and the ultimate interpretation of the underlying fetal pathophysiology, not only during labor and delivery, but also during the preceding 9 months. This chapter will review the relevant parts of fetal respiratory and cardiac physiology to define the fetal reaction to stress (i.e., asphyxia or hypoxia). The techniques and tests used during pregnancy, labor, and delivery will then be discussed.

FETAL CARDIOVASCULAR PHYSIOLOGY

Fetal gas exchange occurs via the placenta. Because the fetal lungs are nonfunctional, there are several shunts in the fetal circulation that allow oxygenated blood to pass from the placenta to the systemic circulation. Streaming or laminar blood flow keeps oxygenated and deoxygenated blood separate in the venous system and assumes great importance in preferentially supplying oxygenated blood to organs such as the heart, brain, and adrenal glands during periods of hypoxia.

Venous flow from the placenta to the fetal heart

Approximately 40% of fetal cardiac output goes to the placenta, with a similar amount returning to the right heart via the umbilical vein (Fig. 1-1). The blood in the umbilical vein has the highest oxygen saturation in the fetal circulation, so its distribution is important for the delivery of oxygen to fetal tissues. Half of the umbilical venous blood enters the ductus venosus, which connects to the inferior vena cava. The rest enters the hepatoportal venous system.[1]

Streaming, which is the separation of blood with differing oxygen saturations as it flows through a single vessel, is an important determinant of oxygen delivery to fetal tissues. This is seen when the more highly saturated umbilical venous blood passes through the ductus venosus into the inferior vena cava to meet the desaturated venous drainage from the lower trunk. In the liver, umbilical venous return is directed toward the left lobe and the portal venous return to the right lobe, so there is a marked difference in oxygen saturation (higher in the left hepatic lobe than the right).[2,3] Although both hepatic veins enter the inferior vena cava, the left hepatic vein streams preferentially with the blood flow from the ductus venosus,[3] whereas the right hepatic vein flow follows the same route as that from the abdominal vena cava.

There is preferential flow of the umbilical venous return to the left atrium because of the crista dividens, which splits the inferior vena cava blood flow into two streams. One stream includes the oxygenated blood from the umbilical vein that is directed toward the foramen ovale and into the left atrium; the other stream consists of deoxygenated

1

blood from the lower extremities and portal vein that enters the right atrium. This results in a higher oxygen saturation in the left atrium than in the right. Blood flow through the superior vena cava is also preferentially streamed along with blood flow through the coronary sinus via the tricuspid valve. The desaturated blood from the right heart is then directed toward the placenta for reoxygenation. The left heart supplies oxygenated blood for the brain.

Cardiac output. Because of intracardiac and extracardiac shunts, the two ventricles do not work in series, as in adults. Therefore, they do not have the same stroke volume. The right ventricle ejects approximately two thirds of fetal cardiac output (300 mL/kg/min), and the left ventricle ejects about one third (150 mL/kg/min). Of the right ventricular out-

put, only a small fraction (8%) flows through the pulmonary arteries. Most of the output crosses the ductus arteriosus and enters the descending aorta, allowing deoxygenated blood to return preferentially to the placenta. The left ventricular output enters the ascending aorta, and most of the output reaches the brain, upper thorax, and arms.[4-6]

This distribution of cardiac output to individual organs is shown in Table 1-1. Since flow to the organs below the diaphragm is derived from both ventricles, flow is expressed as a percent of the combined ventricles.

Myocardial function. The fetal myocardium, relative to the adult myocardium, is immature in structure, function, and sympathetic innervation. Although the length of the fetal sarcomere is the same as that in the adult,[7] the diameter of the fetal sarcomere is smaller and the proportion of noncontractile mass to the number of myofibrils is less, 30% in the fetus vs. 60% in adults.[8] Active tension generated by fetal myocardium is less than that in the adult heart at all lengths of a muscle along a length-tension curve. Passive or resting tension is higher in fetal myocardium than in the adult, suggesting lower compliance for the fetus. A study of volume loading by infusion of blood or saline solution in fetal lambs showed that the right ventricle is unable to increase stroke work or output as much as the adult.[9] Cardiac output varies directly with heart rate, so an increase in rate from 180 to 250 beats/min will increase cardiac output 15% to 20%. Conversely, a decrease in heart rate below basal levels causes a decrease in ventricular output. Histochemical staining of the sympathetic nervous system demonstrates delayed development. Compared with the adult, isolated fetal cardiac tissue has a lower response threshold to the inotropic effects of norepinephrine. This is presumed to be secondary to the incomplete de-

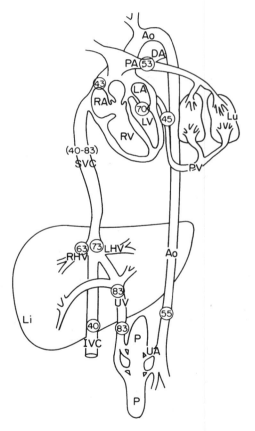

Fig. 1-1 Normal fetal circulation with major blood flow patterns and oxygen saturation values (*circled numbers* indicate percent saturation). *IVC* = inferior vena cava; *P* = placenta; *Li* = liver; *RHV* and *LHV* = right and left hepatic veins; *SVC* = superior vena cava; *RA* and *LA* = right and left atria; *RV* and *LV* = right and left ventricles; *DA* = ductus arteriosus; *PA* = pulmonary artery; *Ao* = aorta; *Lu* = lung; *DV* = ductus venosus; *PV* = pulmonary vein; *UV* = umbilical vein; *UA* = umbilical artery.

Table 1-1 Distribution of cardiac output in fetal lambs

Organ	Blood flow (ml/kg/min)	Cardiac output (%)
Heart	180	2
Brain	125	2
Upper body	25	16
Lungs	100	8
GI tract	70	5
Kidneys	150	2.5
Adrenals	200	0.1
Spleen	200	1.2
Liver	20	1.5
Lower body	25	20
Placenta	20	37

velopment of the sympathetic nervous system.[8] As a result, the fetal heart appears to operate at or near peak performance normally.

Control of the cardiovascular system

The cardiovascular system is controlled by a complex interrelationship between autoregulation, reflex effects, hormonal substrates, and the autonomic nervous system. Whereas many organs in adults are able to maintain fairly constant blood flow over a wide range of perfusion pressures, the placental circulation does not exhibit autoregulation.[10] As a result, blood flow changes directly with changes in arterial perfusion pressure. Papile et al. demonstrated in fetal lambs that the cerebral circulation does autoregulate itself.[11] The baroreflex has also been shown to exist in fetal animals. In adults it functions to stabilize heart rate and blood pressure, but in the fetus it is relatively insensitive. Marked changes in pressure are required to produce minor responses, so that the function of the baroreflex is probably minimal in utero.[12]

The chemoreceptor reflex is governed by receptors in either the carotid body or in the central nervous system (CNS) and causes hypertension and mild tachycardia with increased respiratory activity. Chemoreceptors in the aorta cause bradycardia with a slight increase in blood pressure. The former are less sensitive than the latter so that bradycardia and hypertension are seen with hypoxia because of the overriding response of the aortic chemoreceptors.

The autonomic nervous system is fully developed in the fetus, as demonstrated by the presence of receptors and an acetylcholinesterase and its responses to cholinergic or adrenergic agonists. The renin-angiotensin system is also important in regulating the normal fetal circulation and the response to hemorrhage. Angiotensin II exerts a tonic vasoconstriction on the peripheral vasculature to maintain systemic arterial blood pressure and umbilical blood flow.[13] Vasopressin, although detectable in the fetus, probably has little regulatory function. Stress, i.e., hypoxia, elicits an increase in vasopressin secretion and results in hypertension and bradycardia.[14] In the presence of decreased cardiac output, the renin-angiotensin system maintains the flow to the brain, heart, and placenta, while flow to the splanchnic bed decreases.[15] Circulating prostaglandins are present in high concentrations in the fetus[16,17] and are produced by both the placenta and fetal vasculature. Prostaglandins have diverse effects on the cardiovascular system. Infusion of PGE_1, PGE_2, PGF_2 and thromboxane constricts the umbilical-placental circulation,[18,19] whereas prostacyclin has the opposite effect. Prostaglandin E_1, PGE_2, PGI_2, and PGD_2 cause pulmonary vasodilation in the fetus and PGF_2 produces vasoconstriction.[20,21] Prostaglandins also relax smooth muscle in the ductus arteriosus, so that it remains patent in utero.[22,23]

PLACENTAL RESPIRATORY GAS EXCHANGE AND FETAL OXYGENATION

The passage of oxygen from the atmosphere to the fetus can be described in a sequence of six steps. These steps alternate bulk transport of gases with diffusion across membranes. The first three steps are primarily maternal and the last three steps are fetal (Fig. 1-2).

Transport of oxygen starts from the atmosphere to the maternal alveoli through the large airways by the respiratory muscles, in exchange for carbon dioxide. The pressure of oxygen in the alveoli is regulated by several mechanisms that respond to changes in the levels of the partial pressures of oxygen (Po_2) and carbon dioxide (Pco_2), and the pH of maternal blood. Arterial Pco_2 in the parturient is regulated at a lower level than in the nonpregnant woman, secondary to the effects of progesterone.[24]

With the second step, oxygen diffuses rapidly across the alveoli to maternal erythrocytes. The Po_2 of maternal arterial blood is slightly less than that in the alveoli because of shunting and inequality of ventilation and perfusion throughout the lung fields. In the pregnant woman, the gradient of oxygen in the arterioles and alveoli is dependent on

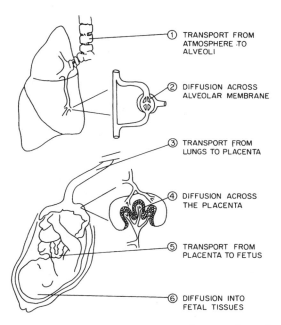

① TRANSPORT FROM ATMOSPHERE TO ALVEOLI

② DIFFUSION ACROSS ALVEOLAR MEMBRANE

③ TRANSPORT FROM LUNGS TO PLACENTA

④ DIFFUSION ACROSS THE PLACENTA

⑤ TRANSPORT FROM PLACENTA TO FETUS

⑥ DIFFUSION INTO FETAL TISSUES

Fig. 1-2 Six steps in the transport of oxygen from the atmosphere to the fetal tissues.

position and widens when going from the upright to the supine position.

Maternal blood transports oxygen to the placenta in two forms, free and bound to hemoglobin. These two forms are in a reversible equilibrium.

In the diffusion of oxygen across the placenta, the oxygen uptake by the gravid uterus is greater than that by the fetus. This is because compared with the fetus the placenta and the uterus extract oxygen and consume a relatively large fraction. In chronic sheep preparations, this has been calculated with the Fick principle: Uterine oxygen consumption is measured by the difference in oxygen content between the maternal arterial blood (A) and uterine venous blood (V). Multiplying the difference by uterine blood flow (F) yields uterine oxygen uptake:

$$(A - V)F = O_2 \text{ uptake by the gravid uterus}$$

In a sheep study the umbilical vein was observed to carry the highest concentrations of oxygenated blood delivered to the fetus, but this is low when compared with maternal Po_2. Attempts have been made to explain the low fetal Po_2 with either a concurrent or crosscurrent model of oxygen placental exchange, but the placenta is probably more complex. Nonetheless, the umbilical venous Po_2 depends on and is not higher than the venous Po_2 of the uterine circulation.[25] In addition, three other factors might contribute to the inefficiency of the exchange process:

1. *Shunting*—the diversion of blood away from the exchange surface to perfuse the myometrium and endometrium.
2. *Uneven perfusion*—differences in the ratio of maternal-fetal blood flow can vary in portions of the placenta.
3. *Oxygen diffusing capacity* is defined as the product of the quantity of oxygen transferred from maternal to fetal circulation divided by the mean Po_2 difference between maternal and fetal erythrocytes. It is the result of the permeability of the placental membrane to oxygen transport and of the reaction rate of oxygen with hemoglobin.[26]

Uterine venous Po_2, a primary factor that determines umbilical venous Po_2, is in turn influenced by a number of other factors (see Box 1-1). Chief among these are the oxygen saturation and the oxyhemoglobin dissociation curve of venous blood. The oxyhemoglobin dissociation curve is shifted by pH so that Po_2 is inversely related to pH (Bohr effect). As a result, maternal alkalosis will shift the curve to the left, decreasing oxygen delivery to the fetus. Other factors that can shift the curve

---

BOX 1-1 FACTORS THAT DETERMINE UTERINE VENOUS Po_2

Oxyhemoglobin dissociation of maternal blood
Hemoglobin structure
Temperature
Erythrocyte pH (2, 3-DPG)

Oxygen saturation in uterine venous blood
Arterial O_2 saturation
Uteroplacental blood flow
O_2 capacity
Placental and fetal O_2 consumption

---

are temperature, hemoglobinopathies and the 2,3-diphosphoglycerate (2,3-DPG) content of erythrocytes. Oxygen saturation of uterine venous blood (Sv) is a function of four variables: maternal arterial oxygen saturation (Sa), oxygen capacity of maternal blood (O_2Cap), uterine blood flow (F), and the oxygen consumption rate (Vo_2) of the gravid uterus (including placental and fetal oxygen consumption). This can be formulated as

$$Sv = Sa - Vo_2/F(O_2Cap)$$

which is an application of the Fick principle. Anemic, circulatory, or hypoxic hypoxia will decrease uterine venous saturation, leading to a decrease in fetal oxygenation.

Although umbilical vein Po_2 is less than that in the maternal circulation, there are compensatory mechanisms to ensure adequate fetal oxygenation. Fetal erythrocyte hemoglobin has a high affinity for oxygen. The rate of perfusion of fetal organs, compared with that in adults, is high in relation to their oxygen requirements. Physiologically, the low level of Po_2 in fetal arterial blood is a part of the mechanism that keeps the ductus arteriosus open and the pulmonary vascular bed constricted.

Supplemental oxygen will increase the Po_2 of maternal arterial blood, but causes only a small increase in fetal arterial Po_2. This is because of the differences in the oxyhemoglobin dissociation curves between mother and fetus (Fig. 1-3). Increasing the Fio_2 to 100% causes a rise in maternal Po_2 from 90 to 500 torr, or an increase of 1 mmol for the arterial oxygen content.[27] Because there is no change in uterine blood flow, and presumably uterine oxygen consumption rate, uterine venous oxygen content also increases 1 mmol. The resulting increase in uterine venous Po_2 is 11.5 torr. This not to say that supplemental oxygen for the mother has no effect, because it probably is more important when the fetus is hypoxic.

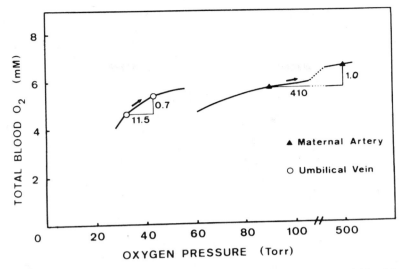

Fig. 1-3 Relationship between oxygen content and P_{O_2} in maternal and fetal blood before and after maternal inhalation of 100% oxygen.

As in the mother, carbon dioxide is one end product of fetal metabolism. Carbon dioxide from the fetus diffuses across the placenta from the umbilical circulation to the maternal side for transport to the lungs and excretion. The diffusion process requires that the P_{CO_2} of fetal blood be higher than that on the maternal side. In sheep, the umbilical venous blood is approximately 5 torr higher than that in the maternal vein. As a result, perturbations in the maternal acid base balance are quickly reflected in the fetus. Therefore, fetal respiratory alkalosis (low fetal P_{CO_2}) is secondary to a low maternal P_{CO_2}. Although fetal respiratory acidosis can be due to a high level of maternal P_{CO_2}, decreased placental perfusion resulting in inadequate gas exchange can also play a role.

FETAL HEART RATE

The average fetal heart rate decreases from 155 beats/min at 20 weeks' gestation to 144 beats/min at 30 weeks' gestation and is 140 beats/min at term. The variability is 20 beats/min in a normal fetus. The sinoatrial (SA) and the atrioventricular (AV) nodes serve as intrinsic pacemakers, with the SA node setting the rate in the normal heart. Variability of the fetal heart rate is followed either beat to beat or over a longer period, and is an important prognostic variable. Control of the fetal heart rate is the result of a number of factors, both intrinsic and extrinsic.

The parasympathetic nervous system contributes to cardiac regulation through the vagus nerve. It has endings in both the SA and AV nodes. Stimulation of the vagus nerve results in bradycardia through a direct effect on the SA node. Blocking the vagus nerve results in an increase in heart rate of approximately 20 beats/min,[28] so the vagus nerve exerts a constant influence to decrease a higher intrinsic rate. In addition, the vagus nerve transmits impulses that result in beat-to-beat variability of the fetal heart rate.[29]

The sympathetic nervous system has nerve endings throughout the myocardium at term. Stimulation of the sympathetic nerves causes release of norepinephrine and an increase in heart rate and contractility, and therefore cardiac output. If the sympathetic nerves are blocked, there is an average decrease of 10 beats/min in the fetal heart rate.

The sympathetic and parasympathetic nervous systems are modulated by other factors. Chemoreceptors located in both the peripheral nervous system and the CNS exert their primary effect on the control of respiration, but they also have an effect on the circulation. With a decrease in arterial perfusion pressure or an increase in carbon dioxide content, a reflex tachycardia develops, leading to an increase in blood pressure. Baroreceptors are located in the arch of the aorta and at the junction of the internal and external carotid arteries, and are sensitive to increases in blood pressure. When pressure rises, impulses are sent via the vagus nerve to decrease the heart rate and cardiac output.

Of the possible hormones that can contribute to heart rate control, three have an effect during periods of stress. Epinephrine and norepinephrine are secreted by the adrenal medulla during stress. Their effects are similar to those caused by sympathetic stimulation: an increase in heart rate, contractility, and blood pressure. The adrenal cortex produces aldosterone in reaction to hypotension. This increases blood volume by slowing renal sodium output, leading to water retention.

FETAL BREATHING AND BODY MOVEMENTS

Fetal breathing and body movements are important functions during fetal life. The development of skeletal and diaphragmatic muscle is dependent on these movements in utero. Fetal lung development is also dependent on diaphragmatic motion. This movement does have its cost, consuming 15% to 30% of available fetal oxygen supplies.[30] Therefore, absence of either movement or breathing can be a sign of hypoxia.[31,32]

Fetal breathing

Studies in lambs have demonstrated that breathing movements occur about 40% of the time during observation. This directly correlates with low voltage electroencephalogram activity and electroocular activity.[33] Flow in and out of the trachea to the lungs occurs in conjunction with diaphragm motion.[34] In ewes, the frequency of fetal breathing movements decreases from 39% to 7% when hypoxia is induced.[31] Gasping movements occur with asphyxia in dying fetal animal preparations.[35] Two to three days before the onset of labor, fetal breathing movements decrease.[36,37] This is thought to be secondary to the rising concentration of PGE_2, which probably plays a role in the onset of labor.[38] Infusing PGE_2[39] or inducing labor with adrenocorticotropic hormone (ACTH),[37] with a subsequent rise in PGE_2, is associated with a drop in fetal breathing movements from 40% to 15% of the time.

There are a number of other factors that can alter breathing activity in fetuses (Table 1-2). The time of day is very important, particularly during the last trimester. Two to 3 hours after a woman eats a meal, fetal breathing movements increase significantly,[45] probably secondary to the increase in maternal blood glucose. In addition, there is a

circadian rhythm. Between 1:00 A.M. and 7:00 A.M., when the mother is asleep and plasma glucose concentrations are stable, the incidence of fetal breathing movements increases. After either an oral[46] or an intravenous glucose[47] load to the mother, fetal breathing movements increase.[48] A similar pattern is seen after meals. During the last 10 weeks of pregnancy, administration of carbon dioxide (5%) to healthy pregnant women results in increased breathing movements.[49] This is thought to represent maturation in the sensitivity of the fetal respiratory center. Maternal ingestion of drugs affects fetal breathing movements. After administration of ethanol[50] and methadone,[51] there is a marked decrease in breathing movements, whereas with maternal cigarette smoking,[52] there is a transient increase in the frequency of fetal breathing activity. During the 3 days prior to the onset of spontaneous labor, fetal breathing movements decrease and are absent during active labor.[53]

Fetal body movements

Fetal body movements are considered significant when the body rolls and the extremities stretch. Isolated limb movement is not of any consequence. During the last trimester, fetal body movements occur on average 3 to 16 minutes in each hour during a 24-hour period of observation.[54] The actual or mean number of fetal body movements ranges from 20 to 50 per hour, but up to 75-minute spans of no movement have been recorded in healthy fetuses. Unlike fetal breathing movements, body movements are not influenced by maternal plasma glucose concentration[55] and maternal alcohol ingestion,[50] and they do not decrease during the last 3 days prior to onset of spontaneous labor.[56] Fetal body movements, however, are related closely to fetal heart rate accelerations. Reports show that from 91% to 99.8% of fetal movements are associated with fetal heart rate accelerations.[57]

FETAL ACID BASE PHYSIOLOGY

Fetal metabolism results in the production of carbonic and noncarbonic acids that require buffering. Carbonic acid is the hydration product of carbon dioxide, which in turn is the end product of the oxidative metabolism of glucose. Hemoglobin in the fetal erythrocyte buffers the carbonic acid and transports it to the placenta. Carbon dioxide is regenerated and diffuses quickly across the placenta. If maternal respiration and uteroplacental and umbilical blood flows are maintained, then large amounts of carbon dioxide can be eliminated rapidly. On a molar basis, the rate of fetal carbon dioxide production is basically equivalent to the oxygen consumption rate of the fetus.[58] The noncarbonic acids in the fetus include uric acid (from the

Table 1-2 Factors affecting fetal breathing movements

Drug/condition	Effect
Hypoglycemia[36]	Decrease
Glucose infusion[40]	Increase
Ethanol[41]	Decrease
Barbiturates[42]	Decrease
Diazepam[43]	Decrease
Catecholamines[36]	Increase
PGE_2[39]	Decrease
Indomethecin[44]	Increase

metabolism of non-sulfur-containing amino acids), lactate, and keto acid (from the metabolism of carbohydrates and fatty acids). These noncarbonic acids are eliminated through the maternal kidneys, after diffusing slowly across the placenta. The maternal kidney regenerates bicarbonate from the excretion of the noncarbonic acids.

There are a number of other factors that affect acid base balance in the fetus. These disrupt either the supply of oxygen or the removal of the carbonic and noncarbonic acids through the placenta. The maternal, fetal, and placental factors listed (see Box 1-2) can result in either respiratory or metabolic perturbations of fetal acid base balance. Fetal respiratory acidosis is secondary to decreased carbon dioxide elimination. This is most commonly due to a sudden decrease in placental perfusion. If flow is restored quickly, reversal of the acidosis is also rapid. Maternal hypoventilation, due to either decreased minute ventilation or V/Q mismatch, results in maternal respiratory acidosis that is reflected in the fetus. As with primary fetal respiratory acidosis, rapidly reversing the cause in the mother restores fetal acid base balance. Maternal respiratory alkalosis is caused by hyperventilation, which decreases the P_{CO_2}, increases the pH, and responds rapidly to reversal of the causes.

Fetal metabolic acidosis can be due to either primary fetal or secondary maternal metabolic acidosis. The decreased pH is from loss of bicarbonate and is usually due to chronic metabolic disorders. With prolonged fetal respiratory acidosis, due to cord compression or abruptio placentae, the accumulation of noncarbonic acids can result in a mixed respiratory-metabolic acidosis.

BOX 1-2 FACTORS THAT AFFECT FETAL ACID BASE BALANCE

Mother

Hypoxia
Hypoventilation
Altered hemoglobin
Metabolic acidosis
Decreased blood supply to placenta

Placenta

Infarction or separation
Insufficiency

Fetus

Obstruction of umbilical blood flow
Fetal anemia
Increased fixed acid production

Monitoring of acid base status in labor will be discussed in the section on fetal scalp sampling.

FETAL REACTION TO STRESS

During labor and delivery, the main causes of stress for the fetus are hypoxia and asphyxia. Fetal hypoxia is due to the mother breathing a hypoxic mixture of gases, which results in decreased oxygen tension. Asphyxia is secondary to a reduction of at least 50% in uterine blood flow. In addition to decreased oxygen tension, there is also increased carbon dioxide tension, leading to both metabolic and respiratory acidosis. With prolonged asphyxia, the fetus switches to anaerobic metabolism and produces a buildup of lactate. Metabolic acidosis subsequently develops.

The fetal responses to hypoxia or asphyxia are:

1. Bradycardia (due to increased vagal activity) with hypertension.
2. Slight decrease in ventricular output.
3. Redistribution of blood from the splanchnic bed to the heart, brain, placenta, and adrenals.[59]
4. A decrease in fetal breathing movements (from 39% to 7% of the time).
5. Terminal gasping movements with asphyxia.
6. Increased circulating catecholamine levels in fetal sheep.
7. Increased alpha-adrenergic activity.

In chronically instrumented sheep, fetal oxygen consumption drops by as much as 60% of control values with hypoxia.[60] This is accompanied by, as described above, fetal bradycardia, an increase in blood pressure, and progressive metabolic acidosis. The fetal sheep can tolerate this for approximately 1 hour; these changes are rapidly reversed with restoration of oxygenation.[61] Fetal cerebral[62] and myocardial[63] oxygen consumption have been shown to remain constant. When hypoxia is prolonged or proceeds to asphyxia, these compensatory mechanisms are lost.

The ability to reverse the effects of hypoxia or asphyxia, as quickly as possible, depends on recognition of the signs and symptoms. This is where fetal monitoring is crucial. There are a number of techniques and tests used; these will be covered in the next sections.

PERINATAL MORTALITY

According to the National Center for Health Statistics,[64] the perinatal mortality rate (PMR) is defined as the number of late fetal deaths (>28 weeks' gestation) plus early neonatal deaths (infants 0 to 6 days of age) divided by 1000 live births plus the fetal and neonatal deaths. In the United States, the PMR has declined by an average of 3% per year since 1965.[65] Over the past 6 years, fetal death rate alone has decreased 16%, and neonatal mortality has fallen 21%. Of all fetal deaths, 22% occur between the 36th and 40th week of gestation, and another 10% occur beyond the 41st week of gestation.

Congenital anomalies account for 25% of perinatal mortality and are the leading cause.[66] Premature labor and delivery was the most common event leading to death in this group. Overall, prematurity with associated respiratory distress syndrome (RDS) was the next most common cause of perinatal death. Intrauterine hypoxia and birth asphyxia account for 3% of the PMR, and placenta or cord complications accounted for 2% of the PMR. Several associated factors identified by Lammer et al.[67] were race (African-American), marital status (single), age (>34 and <20 years), parity (>5), and lack of prenatal care. Multiple gestations were associated 10% of all fetal deaths. This gives a PMR of 50/1000, which is seven times that of singleton pregnancies. Over half of all fetal deaths were associated with asphyxia or maternal causes such as pregnancy-induced hypertension (PIH) or placental abruption.

If the first step to reduce the PMR further is recognizing the causes, then the next step is prevention. A study of perinatal mortality in the Mersey region of England showed that of 309 perinatal deaths, 182, or 58.9%, were due to avoidable causes, primarily a delayed response to abnormalities of the progress of labor or fetal heart rate tracing during labor and delivery; maternal weight loss with a resulting growth-retarded fetus; and reductions in fetal movement.[68] Antepartum fetal monitoring is the means to decrease these fetal deaths. This is most useful when targeting specific groups of parturients who are at increased risk of perinatal mortality (Table 1-3).

TECHNIQUES OF FETAL ASSESSMENT
Maternal assessment of fetal activity

Having a parturient count the fetal activity over a period of time is a simple and sensitive test of fetal well-being. This test is based on the fact that from 28 weeks of gestation on, the fetus makes approximately 30 body movements each hour (about 10% of the total time), and the parturient is able to appreciate most of these.[69] While fetal movement is reassuring, lack of movement can indicate either a quiet period, which usually lasts 20 minutes (but can last as long as 75 minutes), or fetal compromise secondary to asphyxia. Factors that can decrease maternal appreciation of fetal activity are an anterior placenta, polyhydramnios, and obesity.[70]

Several studies have demonstrated that when patients reliably count fetal movements according to a set protocol, there is a significant reduction in fetal death.[71-73]

Amniocentesis

Performed before 15 weeks' gestation, early amniocentesis is an alternative to chorionic villus sampling to obtain fetal cells for diagnosis of genetic or morphologic abnormalities. Indications for amniocentesis are listed in Box 1-3. Although the success of obtaining cells is the same as for chorionic villus sampling, the disadvantages are primarily due to the withdrawal of amniotic fluid. The volume of fluid removed is a much greater proportion of the total fluid volume, and this could increase fetal loss.

After 16 weeks' gestation, midtrimester amniocentesis with ultrasound guidance is safe, with a rate of fetal loss of 0.5 to 1.0%.[74,75] The amniotic fluid is used to grow fetal cells, which in turn are used to scan for chromosomal aberrations. During the third trimester, amniocentesis is used to obtain fluid to assess fetal lung maturity.

Chorionic villus sampling

Performed between 9 and 12 weeks' gestation, chorionic villus sampling allows early determination of chromosomal abnormalities. Under ultrasound guidance, this technique is simply the aspiration of villi either through the cervix or the abdomen. Because actual tissue is obtained, results

Table 1-3 Parturients at increased risk of perinatal mortality

Maternal disease	Fetal disease
Post-dates gestation	Neonatal asphyxia
Diabetes	Perinatal death
Previous stillbirth	Perinatal death
Pregnancy-induced hypertension	Fetal distress in labor
Maternal age >35 years	Congenital anomalies
Maternal weight loss	IUGR
Premature labor	RDS

BOX 1-3 INDICATIONS FOR AMNIOCENTESIS

Maternal age of 35 years or older at delivery
History of any chromosomal abnormality in a family member
Birth of a previous child with Down syndrome or other chromosomal disorder
Parents at risk for being carriers of X-linked disorders or inborn errors of metabolism
History of recurrent spontaneous abortions
Family history of neural tube defects

from cells are available as early as 24 to 48 hours; tissue can also be analyzed for abnormalities in DNA or specific enzymatic reactions. Fetal loss was 2.3 to 2.5% in one randomized trial.[76] Limb reduction defects and oromandibular hypogenesis have been reported in a small number of infants after chorionic villus sampling,[77] but other studies[78,79] have not demonstrated any difference between the expected rates of appearance of these developmental aberrations.

Percutaneous umbilical blood sampling

Starting at 18 weeks' gestation, fetal blood can be obtained transabdominally under ultrasound guidance by needle puncture of the umbilical cord. This is useful in diagnosing a range of problems:[80]

1. Hematologic abnormalities, such as hemoglobinopathies, isoimmunization, thrombocytopenia, and coagulation factor deficiencies
2. Inborn errors of metabolism
3. Infections by viruses, bacteria, or parasites
4. Chromosomal abnormalities, especially mosaicism

The risk to the fetus is greater than with other tests, with an increase in fetal loss of 2%.[80] As a result, this test is usually reserved for situations where information cannot be obtained by other means.

Ultrasonography

Over the past two decades, ultrasound has become an important method of antepartum fetal assessment. Useful throughout gestation, ultrasound gives an accurate measurement of gestational age and provides an assessment of fetal growth as well as developmental abnormalities. It is also an important guide in the performance of amniocentesis, chorionic villus sampling, and cordocentesis. Real-time ultrasound permits a dynamic assessment of fetal well-being by following, over time, fetal breathing activity, movements, and tone.

Despite its importance as a method of fetal assessment, there is still controversy about the routine use of ultrasound in pregnancy. In Helsinki, Finland, which like many other European countries advocates routine ultrasound screening, a randomized trial showed a significant decrease in perinatal mortality in the screened group as compared with the control group.[81] This was due primarily to early detection of fetal malformations. A number of other studies have not shown a benefit from routine ultrasound screening.[82,83] A recent large-scale study of 15,151 pregnant women demonstrated no difference in adverse perinatal outcome. Subgroups of women who had either post-dates gestation or multiple pregnancies, or whose infants were small for gestational age, did not differ in perinatal outcome from the control and study populations.[84] The controversy is also fueled by the desire to contain medical costs by decreasing unnecessary testing.

During the first trimester, ultrasonography, particularly transvaginal sonography, can help determine whether a fetus is viable, when there is vaginal bleeding, or determine the presence of other processes: ectopic pregnancy, uterine anomaly, or an adnexal mass. In addition, it can provide the first measurement of fetal crown–rump length as a measure of fetal age. During the second trimester, ultrasound assessment of biparietal diameter becomes an accurate measure of gestational age.[85] From 12 to 28 weeks' gestation, the relation between biparietal diameter and gestation is linear.[86] Ultrasonic assessment of fetal growth, when continued into the third trimester, is important in diagnosing deviations from normal growth such as growth retardation, macrosomia, or developmental anomalies. Diagnoses of oligohydramnios or polyhydramnios are made by ultrasound. As mentioned previously, real-time ultrasound measures variables that are the components of the biophysical profile (amniotic fluid volume, fetal breathing, limb movement, and tone). All of these measurements can have an effect on the course of labor and delivery.

Analysis of maternal serum

Maternal serum is routinely sampled during the first trimester to assess the possibility of neural tube defects and Rh sensitization. Neural tube defects are one of the most frequent congenital abnormalities, with an incidence of 1 to 2 per 1,000 live births in the United States. Alphafetoprotein (AFP) is elevated in the fetal serum during the first trimester when the neural tube fails to close, resulting in anencephaly, meningomyelocele, or encephalocele. Alphafetoprotein passes through the placenta into the maternal serum and can be measured with a radioimmunoassay. Alphafetoprotein is also elevated in malformations of the gastrointestinal and genitourinary tracts, as well as in fetal death, decreasing the specificity of the test. Despite this, it is still used as a general screening test. With any abnormal values, ultrasonography and amniocentesis are performed for confirmation.

Rh sensitization occurs in Rh (D) negative women who are carrying a Rh positive fetus. Sensitization of the mother occurs from a prior delivery when fetal cells enter the maternal circulation and stimulate formation of maternal antibodies to fetal erythrocyte Rh antigens. With a subsequent pregnancy, the antibodies traverse the placenta and destroy fetal erythrocytes. This results in the syndrome of erythroblastosis fetalis, which is characterized by a severe hemolytic anemia that leads to edema, jaundice, and congestive heart failure. Rh titers are measured early and serially throughout the pregnancy in Rh negative mothers. Rising or elevated titers are followed up with amniocentesis.

Assessment of fetal maturity

Because fetal chronologic age does not necessarily correlate with functional maturity, particularly the pulmonary system, methods of assessing fetal maturity are important adjuncts in clinical decision making. The majority of perinatal morbidity and mortality results from complications of premature delivery. The most frequently seen complication is the respiratory distress syndrome (RDS). This disorder is due to a deficiency of a surface-active agent (surfactant) that prevents alveolar collapse during expiration. Phospholipids, produced by fetal alveolar cells, are the major component of lung surfactant and are produced in sufficient amounts by 36 weeks' gestation. The most commonly used technique measures the lecithin-sphingomyelin ratio (L/S). The concentration of lecithin, a component of surfactant, begins to rise in the amniotic fluid at 32 to 33 weeks' gestation and continues to rise until term. The concentration of sphingomyelin remains relatively constant, so that the ratio of the two provides an estimate of surfactant production that is not affected by variations in the volume of amniotic fluid. The risk of neonatal RDS when the L/S ratio is greater than 2 is less than 1%. If the ratio is less than 1.5, approximately 80% of neonates will develop RDS.

Disaturated phosphatidylcholine (SPC) is the major component of fetal pulmonary surfactant. The technique that separates SPC from lecithin in the amniotic fluid is complicated, and the results can be altered by abnormalities in amniotic fluid production and excretion (i.e., oligohydramnios or polyhydramnios). A value greater than 500 μg/dl amniotic fluid for SPC concentration is consistent with mature fetal lungs and a small risk of RDS. However, in diabetic parturients the SPC value should be 1000.

The disadvantages in measuring the L/S ratio include a long turnaround time, the use of toxic chemicals, a lack of technical expertise, and the inability to standardize the test. As a result, few hospitals are able to perform the test. Another method, the TDx fetal lung maturity test, is automated and avoids the technical involvement in sample preparation and measurement. The test relies on the fluorescence polarization of a dye added to a solution of amniotic fluid that is then compared with values on a standard curve to determine the relative concentration of surfactant and albumin. The determined values are expressed in milligrams of sur-

factant per gram of albumin. With a cutoff of 50 mg/g for maturity, the TDx test was equal in sensitivity (0.96) and more specific (0.88 vs. 0.83) when compared with the L/S ratio in one multicenter study.[87]

Biophysical profile

The biophysical profile involves evaluation of immediate biophysical activities (fetal movement, tone, breathing movements, and heart rate activity) as well as a semiquantitative assessment of amniotic fluid. The biophysical parameters reflect acute CNS activity and when present correlate positively with the lack of depression (secondary to asphyxia) of the CNS. Amniotic fluid volume represents long-term or chronic fetal compromise.

Major indications for referral for biophysical profile include suspected intrauterine growth retardation, hypertension, postdate gestation, and diabetes.

The biophysical evaluation of the fetus is done by ultrasound with the sole purpose of detecting changes in fetal activities due to asphyxia. As has been mentioned previously, changes in fetal breathing movements, heart rate, and body movements are indicators of the state of fetal oxygenation. Superimposed on these factors are the nonrandom pattern of CNS output and the sleep state, with effects that might be mistaken for hypoxia. However, extending the period of observation to find a period of normal recovery for the latter conditions helps to differentiate asphyxia from normal variants.

The scoring of the fetal biophysical profile is an assessment of five variables (Table 1-4), four of which are monitored simultaneously by ultrasound. The variables are said to be normal or abnormal and are assigned a score of 2 for normal and 0 for abnormal. The nonstress test (NST) is monitored after the biophysical evaluation. When the test score is normal, conservative therapy is indicated, with some exceptions:

1. Post-date gestation with a favorable cervix.
2. Growth-retarded fetus with mature pulmonary indices and a favorable cervix.
3. Insulin-dependent diabetic woman at 37 weeks' gestation or more with mature pulmonary indices.
4. Class A diabetic woman at term with a favorable cervix.
5. Women with medical disorders (e.g., asthma, preeclampsia, pregnancy-induced hypertension) that might pose a threat to maternal and fetal health.

Table 1-5 lists recommendations for management of biophysical profile scores.

Table 1-4 Biophysical profile scoring

Variable	Score = 2	Score = 0
Fetal breathing movements	1 episode, 30 sec duration in 30 min	Absent
Gross body movements	3 discrete body/limb movements in 30 min	<2 episodes in 30 min
Fetal tone	1 episode of extension flexion of hand limb or trunk	Absent or slow movement
Fetal heart rate	2 episodes of acceleration with fetal movement in 30 min	<2 episodes
Amniotic fluid volume	1 pocket, measuring 1 × 1 cm	No amniotic fluid or a pocket <1 × 1 cm

Table 1-5 Interpretation and management of biophysical profile score

Score	Interpretation	Recommended management
8-10	Normal infant	Repeat test in 1 week*
6	Suspect asphyxia	Repeat test in 4-6 hours†
4	Suspect asphyxia	If >36 weeks, deliver If <36 weeks, repeat in 24 hours If score <4, deliver
0-2	Strong suspicion for asphyxia	Deliver

*Repeat test twice a week if diabetic or >42 weeks' gestation.
†Deliver if oligohydramnios present.

Table 1-6 Biophysical profile and perinatal mortality

Study	No. of patients	No. of deaths	Perinatal mortality rate/1,000
Manning[88]	19,221	141	1.92
Baskett[89]	5,034	32	3.10
Platt[90]	286	4	7.0
Schiffrin[91]	158	7	12.6

Several prospective studies, summarized in Table 1-6, have shown that the majority of women studied (>97%) have normal test results and normal delivery outcome. Perinatal mortality varies inversely with the last score before delivery. In 1981 and 1985, in large groups of patients, Manning et al[92,93] found that the gross perinatal mortality rate decreased from 11.7 to 7.4 per 1,000 and the corrected value decreased from 5 to 1.9 per 1,000. In Manitoba, since the use of this testing, the stillbirth rate has decreased by 30%. A stillbirth occurring within a week of a normal test result is defined as a false negative. This ranges from 0.41 to 1.01 per 1,000 with a mean of 0.64 per 1,000.

The false negative rate, although small, directly reflects the negative predictive accuracy of the test. Manning et al[88] calculated from a study of 19,221 pregnancies a negative predictive accuracy of 99.224%, or the probability of fetal death after a normal test as 0.726 per 1,000 patients.

Because the ideal testing method would result in no false negative deaths, the biophysical profile is not perfect. The cause of the imperfection is the probability of change in the fetal status from either a chronic condition or an acute variable. While more frequent testing of all patients would decrease the false negative rate, because of the increased workload this has not been tested. The proper selection of patients requiring more vigilant monitoring (those judged to be at risk, e.g., an immature fetus with growth retardation, pre-eclampsia, diabetes, etc.) would render this more feasible.

Nonstress testing

Nonstress testing is the external detection of fetal heart rate and fetal movement in relation to uterine contractions, noting accelerations of fetal heart rate with fetal movement. These parameters are predictors of fetal outcome.

With the parturient recumbent in the semi-Fowler's position and left lateral tilt (to displace the uterus from the inferior vena cava), 20 minutes of consistent fetal heart rate tracing is followed, and a tocodynamometer is used to measure uterine contractions. Fetal movement is noted either by the mother by external palpation of the maternal abdomen or by spikes in the tocodynamometer tracing.

The test is usually interpreted as either:[94,95]

1. *Reactive*—at least two fetal movements in 20 minutes with acceleration of the fetal heart rate

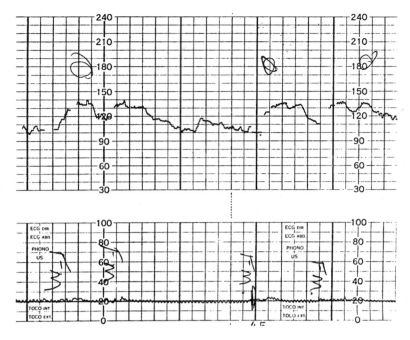

Fig. 1-4 Reactive nonstress test, characterized by accelerations in the fetal heart rate with fetal movement *(FM)*.

to at least 15 beats/min, with long-term variability of at least 10 beats/min and a baseline rate within the normal range (Fig. 1-4).

2. *Nonreactive*—no fetal movement or no acceleration of the fetal heart rate with movement, poor or no long-term variability, baseline fetal heart rate may be within or outside the normal range (Fig. 1-5).

3. *Uncertain reactivity*—fewer than two fetal movements in 20 minutes or acceleration to less than 15 beats/min, long-term variability amplitude less than 10 beats/min, baseline heart rate outside of normal limits.

Fetuses have sleep or inactive cycles that can last up to 80 minutes. The test administrator can either wait for a while or manually stimulate the infant.

A reactive test is associated with survival of the fetus for 1 or more weeks in more than 99% of cases.[94,96] A nonreactive test is associated with poor fetal outcome in 20% of cases.[97] Although the false positive rate of this technique is high (80%), further evaluation needs to be done when a nonreactive result is obtained. The next step is usually a contraction stress test (CST). Similarly, an uncertain reactive pattern needs to be followed up with either another NST or a CST.

Contraction stress test

As its name implies, the CST assesses the fetal response (heart rate pattern) to regular uterine contractions. Using the same technique as the NST, the CST requires three adequate contractions within a 10-minute period, each with a duration of 1 minute. If there are not enough spontaneous contractions, augmentation with intravenous oxytocin is indicated. Beginning at a rate of 1.0 mU/min, the infusion is increased every 15 minutes until the requisite number of contractions are obtained. It is rarely necessary to exceed 10 mU/min.

Certain clinical situations present contraindications to CSTs: prior classical cesarean section, placenta previa, and women at risk of premature labor (premature rupture of membranes, multiple gestation, incompetent cervix, and women undergoing treatment for preterm labor).

CSTs are interpreted as either:

1. *Negative*—no late decelerations and normal baseline fetal heart rate.

2. *Positive*—persistent late decelerations (even when the contractions are less frequent than 3 contractions within 10 minutes), possible absence of fetal heart rate variability.

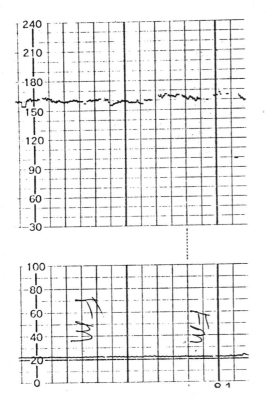

Fig. 1-5 Nonreactive nonstress test, with no accelerations in fetal heart rate with fetal movement *(FM)*.

3. *Suspicious*—intermittent late decelerations or variable decelerations, abnormal baseline fetal heart rate.
4. *Unsatisfactory*—poor quality recording or inability to achieve 3 contractions within 10 minutes.
5. *Hyperstimulation*—excessive uterine activity (contractions closer than every 2 minutes or lasting longer than 90 seconds), resulting in late decelerations or bradycardia.

A negative CST is associated with fetal survival for a week or more in 99% of cases,[94,95] whereas a positive CST is associated with poor fetal outcome in 50% of cases.[97] Like the NST, the CST also has a high false positive rate (50%), but the treatment, if delivery is elected, can be a trial of induction of labor.

Fetal heart rate patterns

The fetal heart rate pattern is characterized by its baseline between contractions and periodic changes in association with uterine contractions.[98] The baseline and periodic changes are further broken down into fetal heart rate and variability. This section will consider the baseline fetal heart rate and its variants as well as variability.

Fetal heart rate is normal from 120 to 160 beats/min between contractions (Fig. 1-6). Rates greater than 160 beats/min are described as tachycardia

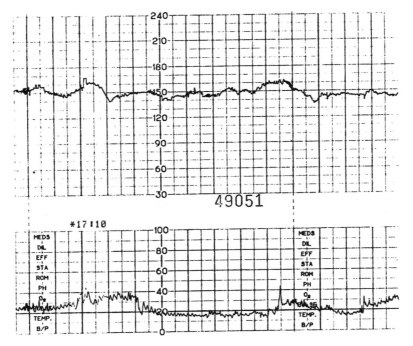

Fig. 1-6 Normal fetal heart rate pattern. The heart rate (140 beats/min) and short-term and long-term variability are normal. There are no periodic changes.

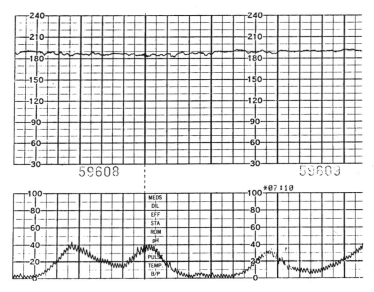

Fig. 1-7 Tachycardia. In this case there was a maternal fever secondary to chorioamnionitis.

(Fig. 1-7) and those less than 120 beats/min as bradycardia (Fig. 1-8). If the alteration in rate are less than 2 minutes in duration, they are called accelerations and decelerations.

The usual, initial response of the normal fetus to acute hypoxia or asphyxia is bradycardia. A heart rate between 100 and 120 beats/min might signify either a compensated, mild hypoxic stress, or it may be idiopathic and benign. When the heart rate falls below 60 beats/min the fetus is in distress and requires either reversal of the cause of the bradycardia or emergency delivery. Other causes of bradycardia that are nonasphyxic in origin are bradyarrhythmias, maternal drug ingestion (especially beta blockers), and hypothermia. Tachycardia is occasionally seen with fetal asphyxia or with recovery from asphyxia, but is more likely seen secondary to:

1. Maternal or fetal infection, especially chorioamnionitis.
2. Maternal ingestion of beta mimetic or parasympathetic blockers.
3. Tachyarrhythmias.
4. Prematurity.
5. Thyrotoxicosis.

Variability in the fetal heart rate tracing describes the irregularity or the difference in interval from beat to beat. If the interval between heart beats were identical, then the tracing would be smooth (Fig. 1-9). In most healthy fetuses, one notes an irregular line. This is thought to be secondary to an intact nervous pathway through the cerebral cortex, midbrain, vagus nerve, and the car-

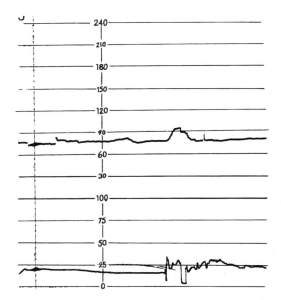

Fig. 1-8 Bradycardia, accompanied by absence of fetal heart rate variability.

diac conduction system. It is thought that when asphyxia affects the cerebrum, there is decreased neural control of the variability. This is made worse by the failure of fetal hemodynamic compensatory mechanisms to maintain cerebral oxygenation. So with normal variability, irrespective of the fetal heart rate pattern, the fetus is not suffering cerebral anoxia.

Variability is described as being either short-term or long-term. Short-term variability is the beat-to-beat difference, and it requires accurate de-

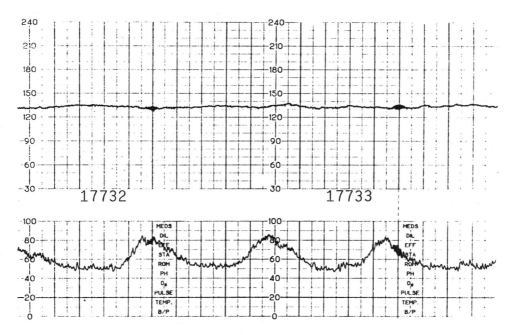

Fig. 1-9 Decreased variability of the fetal heart rate.

tection of the heart rate. Because this can only be obtained with the fetal electrocardiogram, external monitors cannot be used to describe short-term variability, which is characterized as being either present or absent. Long-term variability looks at a wider window of the fetal heart rate, between 3 to 6 minutes. It can be detected using either internal or external methods of fetal heart rate monitoring and is described by the approximate amplitude range in beats/min as:

1. *Normal*—the amplitude range is 6 beats/min or greater.
2. *Decreased*—the amplitude range is between 2 and 6 beats/min.
3. *Absent*—the amplitude range is less than 2 beats/min.
4. *Saltatory*—the amplitude is greater than 25 beats/min.

In addition to asphyxia, there are other causes of altered variability, such as anencephaly, fetal drug effect (secondary to morphine, meperidine, diazepam, and magnesium sulfate), vagal blockade (due to atropine or scopolamine), and interventricular conduction delays (complete heart block).

Periodic changes in fetal heart rate occur in association with uterine contractions. Early accelerations occur concomitantly with a uterine contraction. They have a smooth contour and are a mirror image of the contraction (Fig. 1-10). The descent of the fetal heart rate is usually never more than 20 beats/min below the baseline. The cause is pre-

sumed to be due to a vagal reflex caused by a mild hypoxia, but is not associated with fetal compromise. Late decelerations are also smooth in contour and mirror the contraction, but they begin 10 to 30 seconds after the onset of the contraction (Fig. 1-11). The depth of the decline is inversely related to the intensity of the contraction. Late decelerations have been classified as either reflex or nonreflex. Reflex late decelerations are due to maternal hypotension, which acutely decreases uterine perfusion to an otherwise healthy fetus. A uterine contraction on top of this insult further reduces oxygen flow, causing cerebral hypoxia, which then leads to the deceleration. In between contractions the fetal heart rate returns to baseline with good variability. The nonreflex late deceleration is due to prolonged hypoxia that leads to myocardial depression. Cerebral function is also depressed. This is seen with preeclampsia, intrauterine growth retardation, and prolonged repetitive late decelerations. Fetal heart rate variability is either decreased or absent.

Variable decelerations differ in duration, shape, and decrease in fetal heart rate from contraction to contraction. The abrupt onset and cessation of the deceleration is thought to be due to increased vagal firing in response to compression of either the umbilical cord (during early labor) or dural stimulation with head compression (during the second stage of labor). The vagal activity causes bradycardia, which decreases cardiac output as well as umbilical blood flow. Variable decelerations are

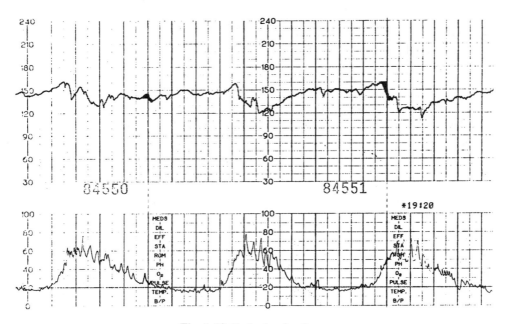

Fig. 1-10 Early decelerations.

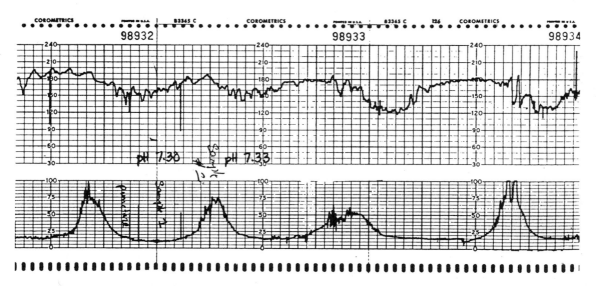

Fig. 1-11 Late decelerations, with decreased variability of the fetal heart rate between contractions.

described as severe when they fall to 60 beats/min below the baseline fetal heart rate, or last longer than 60 seconds (Fig. 1-12). Otherwise, they are classified as mild to moderate (Fig. 1-13). The normal fetus is generally able to tolerate mild to moderate variable decelerations for prolonged periods of time; however, severe variable decelerations eventually result in fetal compromise unless reversed.

Accelerations with uterine contractions represent the greater effect of sympathetic activity over the parasympathetic nervous system (Fig. 1-14). They indicate a reactive, healthy fetus and have a good prognostic significance.

The above described components of fetal heart rate comprise a normal pattern of a baseline rate of 120 to 160 beats/min, which has a variability of greater than 6 beats/min. One can see either no

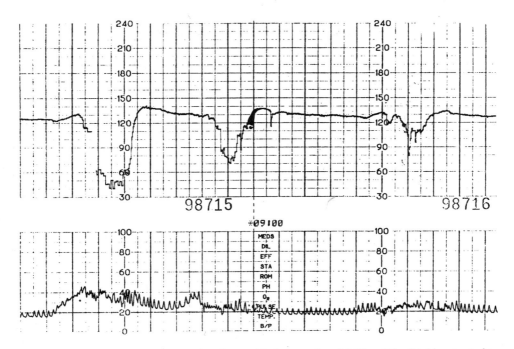

Fig. 1-12 Severe, deep variable decelerations, with decreased variability of the fetal heart rate between contractions.

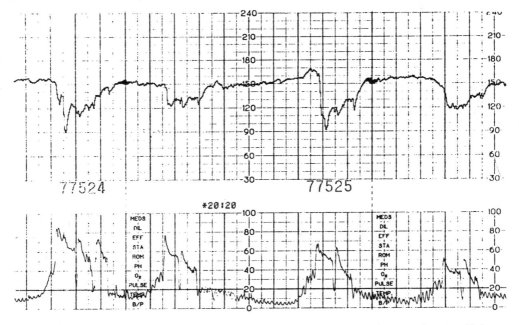

Fig. 1-13 Mild-to-moderate variable decelerations with pushing during the second stage of labor.

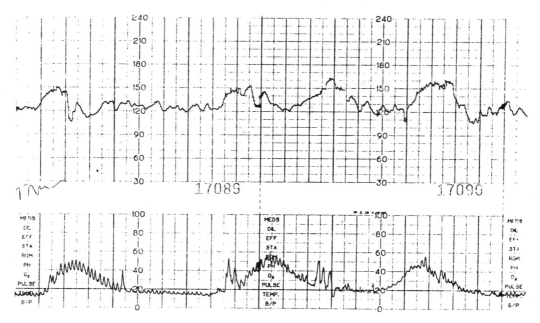

Fig. 1-14 Accelerations with uterine contractions.

decelerations, early decelerations, or accelerations with contractions. This is associated with a good fetal outcome (i.e., Apgar score >7 at 5 minutes).[98,99] Depending on the severity and duration of the stress, there are other fetal heart rate patterns seen.

The acute stress pattern is a compensatory reaction in an otherwise healthy fetus to a short-lived period of asphyxia or hypoxia. The fetal heart rate usually demonstrates bradycardia, although tachycardia is also seen, but the most important fact noted is that variability remains normal. There can be either late or variable decelerations. The fetal outcome is generally good[100] because the impact of the asphyxia is brief, with possible depression from carbon dioxide narcosis, which is rapidly reversible.

When the stress persists, bradycardia is more profound and is associated with decreased variability as well as late and/or deep variable decelerations. This is a prolonged stress pattern that indicates mounting hypoxic damage to the heart and brain, resulting in the loss of compensatory mechanisms. Unless corrected, fetal death in utero can occur.

For a growth-retarded fetus, already compromised by a placenta with marginal function, persistent asphyxia results in a sinister pattern that is characterized by absent variability. The fetal heart rate displays severe variable or late decelerations, with a smooth rather than abrupt decrease and recovery in heart rate. Persistent bradycardia without variability is also called sinister.

Effects of epidural anesthesia on fetal heart rate. The definite effects of epidural anesthesia/analgesia on maternal blood pressure and uterine smooth muscle contractility have also raised concerns about the potential effects on the fetal heart rate. In addition to local anesthetics (bupivicaine, lidocaine, and chloroprocaine), narcotics are also injected into the epidural space. A number of studies in humans[101-104] have demonstrated no deleterious effects on fetal heart rate. Studies[105-108] using Doppler velocimetry of umbilical and uterine arteries demonstrate that epidural anesthesia causes no change in the mean uterine and umbilical artery systolic-diastolic (S-D) ratios in normal parturients at term. In women with preeclampsia, epidural blockade caused a significant decrease in mean uterine artery S-D ratios without a change in the umbilical artery S-D ratio, indicating a decrease in uterine artery vasospasm. There were no changes in FHR. Alahuhta et al[109] also used M-mode echocardiography to assess fetal myocardial function. Except for an increase in right ventricular end-diastolic dimensions, there was no effect on the fetal myocardial function.

Treatment of fetal heart rate patterns. The first step in treatment is to recognize and describe an abnormal fetal heart rate pattern. Then the cause must be identified, and it should be corrected as quickly as possible. Causes and treatment of fetal heart rate patterns are presented in Table 1-7. If the pattern does not improve with these measures, then one needs to get more direct evidence of the fetal

Table 1-7 Treatment of fetal heart rate patterns

Pattern	Cause	Treatment
Bradycardia, late deceleration	Hypotension Uterine Hyperstimulation	IV fluids, ephedrine, change position Decrease oxytocin
Variable decelerations	Umbilical cord compression Head compression	Change position, amnio-infusion Continue pushing if variability good
Late deceleration	Decreased uterine blood flow	Change position, O_2 for mother
Decrease in variability	Prolonged asphyxia	Change position, O_2 for mother

status (i.e., fetal scalp sampling) or deliver the fetus immediately.

Fetal scalp sampling

Since first introduced by Saling in 1967,[110] fetal blood sampling has become the final determinant in making a diagnosis of fetal hypoxia or asphyxia. The fetal blood sample is obtained from the presenting part (scalp or buttock) during labor. The instrumentation and technique of fetal blood collecting are described in many standard textbooks. In this brief discussion, mention is made of the indications for sampling as well as the prognostic significance of values obtained.

Although a full set of blood gas determinations (pH, P_{CO_2}, and P_{O_2}) can be done on as little as 0.25 ml of blood, most institutions obtain a minimal amount of blood for pH determination. Having the pH value alone does not allow differentiation between metabolic and respiratory acidosis. Treatment of the causes of acidosis are theoretically different. Metabolic acidosis requires immediate delivery, whereas respiratory acidosis should respond to standard resuscitation. In reality, the initial resuscitative measures (oxygen for the mother, uterine displacement, intravenous fluid bolus) are generally begun immediately with any severe deceleration. If a deceleration does not respond quickly to resuscitation, the clinical situation (stage of labor, presence of meconium, estimated fetal weight, gestational age, parity) will determine whether fetal scalp sampling is needed and/or if delivery is necessary immediately.

In human newborns, there is good correlation between the pH of scalp blood taken shortly before delivery and that of umbilical cord samples. Winkler et al[111] evaluated the degree of umbilical artery acidemia with newborn morbidity. Comparing a group of 358 term infants with an umbilical artery pH < 7.20 to a matched control group, they found that only when the pH decreased to < 7.00 did the incidence of complications increase. For 23 infants with an umbilical artery pH < 7.00, the average 1- and 5-minute Apgar

Table 1-8 Correlation of fetal scalp pH and fetal heart rate pattern*

Deceleration pattern	Scalp pH
Early, mild variable	7.30 ± 0.04
Moderate variable	7.26 ± 0.04
Mild, moderate late	7.22 ± 0.06
Severe late, variable	7.14 ± 0.07

*Data from Kubli FW, Hon EW, Khazin AF, et al: *Am J Obstet Gynecol* 1969; 104:1190.

scores were significantly lower than the rest of the study and control infants. Only 2 of the 23 infants developed complications (seizures, persistent hypotonia, renal and cardiac dysfunction) secondary to asphyxia. Although both fetal scalp and umbilical artery sampling serve to indicate asphyxia, only the former allows one to alter the management of labor to either reverse the asphyxia or deliver the infant emergently.

Beard et al,[112] correlating scalp blood pH and 2-minute Apgar scores, showed that a scalp pH above 7.25 was associated with an Apgar score greater than 7 in 92% of infants. When the scalp pH was less than 7.15, the Apgar score was less than 6 in 80% of cases. Fetal heart rate decelerations have also been found to correlate with pH values (Table 1-8). This correlation is not always close, so fetal scalp sampling is used when there is any question about the fetal heart rate tracing.

There are other fetal heart rate patterns that signal the need for fetal scalp sampling in addition to persistent late decelerations:

1. Absent or decreased short-term variability, which might be due to CNS depressants given to the mother.
2. Variable decelerations when combined with reduced or absent short-term variability.
3. Severe, persistent variable decelerations.

The clinical situation also provides indications for fetal scalp sampling, especially if there is decreased variability or severe decelerations.

Pulse oximetry. Reflectance pulse oximetry is a refinement of conventional pulse oximetry, which requires transmitted light and provides a noninvasive method to assess fetal oxygenation. A study by McNamara et al[113] demonstrated in healthy parturients in labor, when the sensor was placed between the cervix and the fetal presenting part, a significant correlation between fetal oxygen saturation and umbilical vein saturation and pH as well as umbilical artery pH. The relationship of umbilical artery pH and saturation to fetal O_2 saturation was not significant. The range of the values was large: for a fetal oximetry value of 60%, the umbilical vein saturation ranged from 30 to 70% and the pH from 7.25 to 7.38. Values for fetal pulse oximetry varied from 40 to 90% when, with delivery, the umbilical vein pH was generally greater than 7.24. While there were statistical correlations, the wide range of values suggests a low specificity of the oximeter. Another study,[114] in which fetal O_2 saturation was measured after giving a parturient supplemental oxygen, found a rise in fetal O_2 saturation; however, one third of the patients were excluded because of poor signal quality. Others were excluded because of caput formation, fetal anemia, and meconium staining. Dildy et al[114] studied 73 healthy parturients in labor and was unable to obtain a reliable signal 50% of the time. These preliminary studies suggest that there are still technical problems to be overcome and as a result, the oximeter is not yet a useful clinical tool.

SUMMARY

This chapter has attempted to point out the utility of the biochemical and technical advances in monitoring the fetus throughout pregnancy. Congenital malformation, chromosomal abnormalities, and Rh sensitization are perils to fetal health and can be diagnosed in utero. With the exception of cases of Rh sensitization, the chances for treatment are limited. The major focus of this chapter has been on the oxygen supply to the fetus, because lack of oxygen quickly affects all fetal organs. It is important to note that reversal of hypoxia and asphyxia restores fetal well-being. The sooner the cause is identified and treated, the less damage there is to the fetus. Because of this, the emphasis is on fetal monitoring for early identification of asphyxia and hypoxia.

The tests described monitor the status of the fetus externally during gestation and more directly, or internally, during labor. The data provide an assessment of the condition of the fetal neurological and cardiovascular systems. Like any measurement, this assessment provides information that fits into an overall clinical picture.

REFERENCES

1. Edelstone DI, Rudolph AM, Heymann MA: Liver and ductus venosus blood flows in fetal lambs in utero. *Circ Res* 1978; 42:426.
2. Bristow J, Rudolph AM, Itskovitz J: A preparation for studying liver blood flow, oxygen consumption in the fetal lamb in utero. *J Dev Physiol* 1981; 3:255.
3. Bristow J, Rudolph AM, Itskovitz J: Hepatic oxygen and glucose metabolism in the fetal lamb. *J Clin Invest* 1983; 71:1.
4. Rudolph AM, Heymann MA: Circulatory changes during growth in the fetal lamb. *Circ Res* 1970; 26:289.
5. Peeters LLH, Sheldon RE, Jones MD Jr, et al: Blood flow to fetal organs as a function of arterial oxygen content. *Am J Obstet Gynecol* 1979; 135:637.
6. Sheldon RE, Peeters LLH, Jones MD Jr, et al: Redistribution of cardiac output and oxygen delivery in the hypoxic fetal lamb. *Am J Obstet Gynecol* 1979; 135:1071.
7. Sheldon CA, Friedman WF, Sybers HD: Scanning electron microscopy of fetal and neonatal lamb cardiac cells. *J Mol Cell Cardiol* 8:853, 1976.
8. McPherson RA, Kramer MF, Covell JW, et al: A comparison of the active stiffness of fetal and adult cardiac muscle. *Pediatr Res* 1976; 10:660.
9. Heymann MA, Rudolph AM: Effects of increasing preload on right ventricular output in fetal lambs in utero (abstract). *Circulation* 1973; 48:IV-37.
10. Berman W Jr, Goodlin RC, Heymann MA, et al: Pressure flow relationships in the umbilical and uterine circulations of the sheep. *Circ Res* 1976; 38:262.
11. Papile L, Rudolph AM, Heymann MA: Autoregulation of cerebral blood flow in the preterm fetal lamb. *Pediatr Res* 1985; 19:159.
12. Dawes GS, Johnston BM, Walker DW: Relationship of arterial pressure and heart rate in fetal newborn and adult sheep. *J Physiol* 1980; 309:405.
13. Iwamoto HS, Rudolph AM: Effects of angiotensin II on the blood flow and its distribution in fetal lambs. *Circ Res* 1982; 48:183.
14. Drummond WH, Rudolph AM, Keil LC, et al: Arginine vasopressin and prolactin after hemorrhage in the fetal lamb. *Am J Physiol* 1980; 238:E214.
15. Iwamoto HS, Rudolph AM, Keil LC, et al: Hemodynamic responses of the sheep fetus to vasopressin infusion. *Circ Res* 1979; 44:430.
16. Challis JRG, Patrick JE: The production of prostaglandins and thromboxanes in the feto-placental unit and their effects on the developing fetus. *Semin Perinatol* 1980; 4:23.
17. Mitchell MD, Flint AP, Bibby J, et al: Plasma concentration of prostaglandins during late human pregnancy: Influence of normal and preterm labor. *J Clin Endocrinol Metab* 1978; 46:947.
18. Novy MJ, Piasecki G, Jackson BT: Effect of prostaglandins E_2 and F_2 alpha on umbilical blood flow and fetal hemodynamics. *Prostaglandins* 1974; 5:543.
19. Berman W Jr, Goodlin RC, Heymann MA, et al: Effects of pharmacologic agents on umbilical blood flow in fetal lambs in utero. *Biol Neonate* 1978; 33:225.
20. Cassin S: Role of prostaglandins and thromboxanes in the control of the pulmonary circulation in the fetus and newborn. *Semin Perinatol* 1980; 4:101.
21. Cassin S: Role of prostaglandins, thromboxanes and leukotrienes in the control of the pulmonary circulation in the fetus and newborn. *Semin Perinatol* 1987; 11:53.
22. Clyman RI: Ontogeny of the ductus arteriosus response to prostaglandins and inhibitors of their synthesis. *Semin Perinatol* 1980; 4:115.

23. Clyman RI: Ductus arteriosus: Current theories of prenatal and postnatal regulation. *Semin Perinatol* 1987; 11:64.

24. Prowse CM, Gaensler EA: Respiratory and acid base changes during pregnancy. *Anesthesiology* 1965; 26:381.

25. Rankin JHG, Meschia G, Makowski EL, et al: Relationship between uterine and umbilical venous Po_2 in sheep. *Am J Physiol* 1971; 220:1688.

26. Longo LD, Hill EP, Power GG: Theoretical analysis of factors affecting placental O_2 transfer. *Am J Physiol* 1972; 222:730.

27. Meschia G: Transfer of oxygen across the placenta, in Gluck L (ed): *Intrauterine Asphyxia and the Developing Fetal Brain.* Chicago, Year Book Medical Publishers, 1977, p 109.

28. Mendez-Bauer C, Poseiro JJ, Arellano-Hernandez G, et al: Effects of atropine on the heart rate of the human fetus during labor. *Am J Obstet Gynecol* 1963; 85:1033.

29. Vapaavouri EK, Shinebourne EA, Williams RL, et al: Development of cardiovascular responses to autonomic blockade in intact fetal and neonatal lambs. *Biol Neonate* 1973; 22:1977.

30. Rurak DW, Cooper CC, Taylor SM: Fetal oxygen consumption and Po_2 during hypercapnia in pregnant sheep. *J Dev Physiol* 1986; 8:447.

31. Boddy K, Dawes GS, Fisher R, et al: Foetal respiratory movements, electrocortical and cardiovascular responses to hypoxaemia and hypercapnia in sheep. *J Physiol (Lond)* 1974; 243:599.

32. Natale R, Clewlow F, Dawes GS: Measurement of fetal forelimb movements in lambs in utero. *Am J Obstet Gynecol* 1981; 140:545.

33. Dawes GS, Fox HE, Leduc BM, et al: Respiratory movements and rapid eye movement sleep in the foetal lamb. *J Physiol (Lond)* 1972; 220:119.

34. Maloney JE, Adamson TM, Brodecky V, et al: Diaphragmatic activity and lung liquid flow in unanesthetized fetal sheep. *J Appl Physiol* 1975; 39:423.

35. Patrick JE, Dalton KJ, Dawes GS: Breathing patterns before death in fetal lambs. *Am J Obstet Gynecol* 1976; 125:73.

36. Boddy K, Dawes GS: Fetal breathing. *Br Med Bull* 1975; 31:1.

37. Patrick J, Challis JRG, Cross J, et al: The relationship between fetal breathing movements and prostaglandin E_2, during ACTH-induced labour in sheep. *J Dev Physiol* 1987; 9:287.

38. Thorburn GD, Challis JRG: Control of parturition. *Physiol Rev* 1979; 59:863.

39. Kitterman JA, Liggins GC, Fewell JE, et al: Inhibition of breathing movements in fetal sheep by prostaglandins. *J Appl Physiol* 1983; 54:687.

40. Richardson B, Hohimer AR, Mueggler P, et al: Effects of glucose concentration on fetal breathing movements and electrocortical activity in fetal lambs. *Am J Obstet Gynecol* 1982; 142:678.

41. Patrick J, Richardson B, Hasen G, et al: Effects of maternal ethanol infusion on fetal cardiovascular and brain activity in lambs. *Am J Obstet Gynecol* 1985; 151:859.

42. Boddy K, Dawes GS, Fisher RL, et al: The effects of pentobarbitone and pethidine on foetal breathing movements in sheep. *Br J Pharmacol* 1976; 57:311.

43. Piercy WN, Day MA, Neims AH, et al: Alteration of ovine fetal respiratory-like activity by diazepam, caffeine and doxapram. *Am J Obstet Gynecol* 1977; 127:43.

44. Kitterman JA, Liggins GC, Clements JA, et al: Stimulation of breathing movements in fetal sheep by inhibitors of prostaglandin synthesis. *J Dev Physiol* 1979; 1:453.

45. Patrick J, Natale R, Richardson B: Pattern of human fetal breathing activity at 34 to 35 weeks' gestational age. *Am J Obstet Gynecol* 1978; 132:507.

46. Lewis PJ, Trudinger BJ, Mangey J: Effect of maternal glucose ingestion on fetal breathing and body movements in late pregnancy. *Br J Obstet Gynecol* 1979; 85:586.

47. Boddy K, Dawes GS, Robinson JS: Intrauterine fetal breathing movements, in Gluck L (ed): *Modern Perinatal Medicine.* Chicago, Year Book Medical Publishers, 1975, p 381.

48. Natale R, Patrick J, Richardson B: Effects of maternal venous plasma glucose concentrations on fetal breathing movements. *Am J Obstet Gynecol* 1978; 132:36.

49. Ritchie K: The fetal response to changes in the composition of maternal inspired air in human pregnancy. *Semin Perinatol* 1980; 4:295.

50. McLeod W, Brien J, Carmichael L, et al: Maternal glucose injections do not alter the suppression of fetal breathing following maternal ethanol ingestion. *Am J Obstet Gynecol* 1984; 148:634.

51. Richardson B, O'Grady JP, Olsen GD: Fetal breathing movements and the response to carbon dioxide in patients on methadone maintenance. *Am J Obstet Gynecol* 1984; 150:400.

52. Thaler JS, Goodman JDS, Dawes GS: The effect of maternal smoking on fetal breathing rate and activity patterns. *Am J Obstet Gynecol* 1980; 138:282.

53. Richardson B, Natale R, Patrick J: Human fetal breathing activity during induced labor at term. *Am J Obstet Gynecol* 1979; 133:247.

54. Manning FA, Platt LD, Siopos L: Fetal movements in human pregnancies. *Obstet Gynecol* 1979; 54:699.

55. Bocking A, Adamson L, Cousin A, et al: Effects of intravenous glucose injections on human fetal breathing movements and gross fetal body movements at 38 to 40 weeks' gestational age. *Am J Obstet Gynecol* 1982; 142:606.

56. Carmichael L, Campbell K, Patrick J: Fetal breathing, gross fetal body movements and maternal and fetal heart rates before spontaneous labor at term. *Am J Obstet Gynecol* 1984; 148:675.

57. Timor-Tritsch IE, Dierker LJ, Zador I, et al: Fetal movements associated with fetal heart rate accelerations and decelerations. *Am J Obstet Gynecol* 1978; 131:276.

58. James EJ, Raye JR, Gresham EL, et al: Fetal oxygen consumption, carbon dioxide production and glucose uptake in chronic sheep preparations. *Pediatrics* 1972; 50:361.

59. Cohn HE, Piasecki GJ, Jackson BT: Cardiovascular responses to hypoxemia and acidemia in fetal lambs. *Am J Obstet Gynecol* 1974; 129:817.

60. Parer JT: The effect of acute maternal hypoxia on fetal oxygenation and the umbilical circulation in the sheep. *Eur J Obstet Gynecol Reprod Biol* 1980; 10:125.

61. Mann LI: Effects in sheep of hypoxia on levels of lactate, pyruvate and glucose in blood of mothers and fetus. *Pediatr Res* 1970; 4:46.

62. Jones MD, Sheldon RE, Peeters LL, et al: Fetal cerebral oxygen consumption at different levels of oxygenation. *J Appl Physiol* 1977; 43:1080.

63. Fisher DS, Heymann MA, Rudolph AM: Fetal myocardial oxygen and carbohydrate consumption during acutely induced hypoxemia. *Am J Physiol* 1982; 242:H657.

64. Friede A, Rochat R: Maternal mortality and perinatal mortality: Definitions, data and epidemiology, in Sachs B (ed): *Clinical Obstetrics,* PSG, Littleton, Mass., 1985, p 35.

65. Vital statistics of the United States. vol II. Mortality, 1986. U.S. Department of Health and Human Services, Public Health Services, Washington, DC, 1988.

66. CDC: Contribution of birth defects to infant mortality—United States, 1986. *MMWR* 1989; 38:633.

67. Lammer EJ, Brown LE, Anderka MT: Classification and analysis of fetal deaths in Massachusetts. *JAMA* 1989; 261:1757.

68. Mersey Region Working Party on Perinatal Mortality: Perinatal health. *Lancet* 1982; 1:491.

69. Patrick J, Campbell K, Carmichael L, et al: Patterns of gross fetal body movements over 24-hour observation intervals during the last 10 weeks of pregnancy. *Am J Obstet Gynecol* 1982; 142:363.

70. Sarokin Y, Dierker L: Fetal movement. *Clin Obstet Gynecol* 1982; 25:719.

71. Neldam S: Fetal movements as an indicator of fetal well being. *Lancet* 1980; 1:1222.

72. Rayburn W: Antepartum fetal assessment. *Clin Perinatol* 1982; 9:231.

73. Liston R, Cohen A, Mennui M: Antepartum fetal evaluation by maternal perception of fetal movement. *Obstet Gynecol* 1982; 60:424.

74. Working Party on Amniocentesis: An assessment of the hazards of amniocentesis. *Br J Obstet Gynecol* 1978; 85(suppl):12.

75. Taber A, Philip J, Madsen M, et al: Randomised, controlled trial of genetic amniocentesis of 4606 low-risk women. *Lancet* 1986; 1:1287.

76. Jackson LG, Zachary JM, Fowler SE, et al: A randomized comparison of transcervical and transabdominal chorionic villus sampling. *N Engl J Med* 1992; 327:594.

77. Burton BK, Schulz CJ, Burd LI: Limb anomalies associated with chorionic villus sampling. *Obstet Gynecol* 1992; 79:726.

78. Manni G, Ibba RM, Lai R, et al: Limb-reduction defects and chorionic villus sampling. *Lancet* 1991; 337:1091.

79. Mahoney MJ: Limb abnormalities and chorionic villus sampling. *Lancet* 1991; 337:1422.

80. Shulman LP, Elias S: Percutaneous umbilical blood sampling, fetal skin sampling and fetal liver biopsy. *Semin Perinatol* 1990; 14:56.

81. Saari-Kemppainen A, Karjalainen O, Ylostalo P, et al: Ultrasound screening and perinatal mortality: Controlled trial of systemic one-stage screening in pregnancy—The Helsinki Ultrasound Trial. *Lancet* 1990; 336:387.

82. Ewigman B, LeFevre M, Hesser J: A randomised trial of routine prenatal ultrasound. *Obstet Gynecol* 1990; 76:189.

83. Bekketeig LS, Eik-Nes SH, Jacobsen G, et al: Randomised controlled trial of ultrasonographic screening in pregnancy. *Lancet* 1984; 2:207.

84. Ewigman B, Crane JP, Frigoletto FD, et al: Effect of prenatal ultrasound screening on perinatal outcome. *N Engl J Med* 1993; 329:821.

85. Campbell S, Warsof S, Little D, et al: Routine ultrasound screening for the prediction of gestational age. *Obstet Gynecol* 1985; 65:613.

86. Kurtz A, Wapner R, Kurtz R, et al: Analysis of biparietal diameter as an accurate indicator of gestational age. *J Clin Ultrasound* 1980; 8:319.

87. Russell JC, Cooper CM, Ketchum CH, et al: Multicenter evaluation of TDx test for assessing fetal lung maturity. *Clin Chem* 1989; 35:1005.

88. Manning FA, Morrison I, Harman CR, et al: Fetal assessment by fetal BPS: Experience in 19,221 referred high-risk pregnancies. II. The false negative rate by frequency and etiology. *Am J Obstet Gynecol* 1987; 157:880.

89. Baskett TF, Allen AC, Gray JH, et al: The biophysical profile score. *Obstet Gynecol* 1987; 70:357.

90. Platt LD, Eglinton GS, Siopos L, et al: Further experience with the fetal biophysical profile score. *Obstet Gynecol* 1983; 61:480.

91. Schiffrin BS, Guntes V, Gergely RC, et al: The role of real-time scanning in antenatal fetal surveillance. *Am J Obstet Gynecol* 1981; 140:525.

92. Manning FA, Baskett TF, Morrison I, et al: Fetal biophysical profile scoring: A prospective study in 1184 high-risk patients. *Am J Obstet Gynecol* 1981; 140:289.

93. Manning FA, Morrison I, Lange IR, et al: Fetal assessment based on fetal biophysical profile scoring: Experience in 12,620 referred high-risk pregnancies. I. Perinatal mortality by frequency and etiology. *Am J Obstet Gynecol* 1985; 151:343.

94. Schiffrin BS: The rationale for antepartum fetal heart rate monitoring. *J Reprod Med* 1979; 23:213.

95. Keegan KA, Paul RH: Antepartum fetal heart rate testing. IV. The nonstress test as a primary approach. *Am J Obstet Gynecol* 1980; 136:75.

96. Evertson LR, Gauthier RJ, Collea JV: Fetal demise following negative contraction stress test. *Obstet Gynecol* 1978; 51:671.

97. Ott WJ: Antepartum biophysical evaluation of the fetus. *Perinat Neonatal* 1978; 2:11.

98. Hon EH, Quilligan EJ: The classification of fetal heart rate. *Conn Med* 1967; 31:779.

99. Schiffrin BS, Dame L: Fetal heart rate patterns: Prediction of Apgar score. *JAMA* 1972; 219:1322.

100. Krebs HB, Petres RE, Dunn LJ, et al: Intrapartum fetal heart rate monitoring. I. Classification and prognosis of fetal heart rate patterns. *Am J Obstet Gynecol* 1979; 133:762.

101. Lavin JP, Samuels SV, Miodovnik M, et al: The effects of bupivicaine and chloroprocaine as local anesthetics for epidural anesthesia of fetal heart rate monitoring parameters. *Am J Obstet Gynecol* 1981; 141:717.

102. Abboud TK, Afrasiabi A, Zhu J, et al: Bupivicaine/butorphanol/epinephrine for epidural anesthesia in obstetrics: Maternal and neonatal effects. *Reg Anesth* 1989; 14:219.

103. McLintic AJ, Danskin FH, Reid JA, et al: Effect of adrenaline on extradural anesthesia, plasma lignocaine concentrations and the feto-placental unit during elective caesarean section. *Br J Anaesth* 1991; 67:683.

104. Loftus JR, Holbrook RH, Cohen SE: Fetal heart rate after epidural lidocaine and bupivicaine for elective caesarean section. *Anesthesiology* 1991; 75:406.

105. Ramos-Santos E, Devoe LD, Wakefield ML, et al: The effects of epidural anesthesia on the Doppler velocimetry of umbilical and uterine arteries in normal and hypertensive patients during active term labor. *Obstet Gynecol* 1991; 77:20.

106. Hughes AB, Devoe LD, Wakefield ML, et al: The effects of epidural anesthesia on the Doppler velocimetry of umbilical and uterine arteries in normal term labor. *Obstet Gynecol* 1990; 75:809.

107. Lindblad A, Bernow J, Vernersson E, et al: Effects of extradural anesthesia on human fetal blood flow in utero: Comparison of three local anesthetic solutions. *Br J Anaesth* 1987; 56:1265.

108. Turner GA, Newnham JP, Johnson C, et al: Effects of extradural anesthesia on umbilical and uteroplacental arterial flow velocity waveforms. *Br J Anaesth* 1991; 67:306.

109. Alahuhta S, Rasanen J, Jouppila R, et al: Uteroplacental and fetal haemodynamics during extradural anesthesia for caesarean section. *Br J Anaesth* 1991; 66:319.

110. Saling E, Schneider D: Biochemical supervision of the foetus during labour. *J Obstet Gynaecol Br Commonw* 1967; 74:799.

111. Winkler CL, Hauth JC, Tucker JM, et al: Neonatal complications at term as related to the degree of umbilical artery acidemia. *Am J Obstet Gynecol* 1991; 164:637.

112. Beard RW, Morris ED, Clayton SE: pH of foetal capillary blood as an indication of the condition of the foetus. *J Obstet Gynaecol Br Commonw* 1967; 74:812.

113. Johnson N, McNamara H: Monitoring the fetus with a sensor covered with an irregular surface can cause scalp ulceration. *Br J Obstet Gynecol* 1993; 100:961.

114. Dildy GA, Clark SL, Loucks CA: Preliminary experience with intrapartum fetal pulse oximetry in humans. *Obstet Gynecol* 1993; 81:630.

115. Kubli FW, Hon EW, Khazin AF, et al: Observations on heart rate and pH in the human fetus during labor. *Am J Obstet Gynecol* 1969; 104:1190.

2 Genetic and Metabolic Disease

Harvey Carp and Brian A. Clark

The field of genetic diseases is one in which basic science advances are occurring at a rapid pace. Importantly, these advances are being transferred to clinical diagnosis and treatment at an almost equally rapid pace. As more women with genetic and metabolic disorders become pregnant, to deliver safe anesthetic care for mother and fetus the obstetric anesthesiologist will need to be increasingly aware of the fetal implications of prenatal genetic diagnosis as well as the maternal implications of genetic and metabolic disorders.

The first section of this chapter will concentrate on developments in fetal diagnosis. The second section will emphasize the maternal anesthetic and obstetric implications of several metabolic disorders compatible with reproduction.

PRENATAL DIAGNOSIS

The overall incidence and prevalence of birth defects and associated genetic defects are summarized in Table 2-1.

Advances in imaging and laboratory techniques permit fetal evaluation by high-resolution ultrasound; maternal blood samples; amniocentesis and chorionic villus sampling for genetic analysis; fetal blood sampling; and the use of molecular genetic techniques.

Ultrasound

The use of high-resolution, real-time ultrasound for purposes of an anomaly screen is best performed at 18 to 20 weeks after development of the major organ systems.

Ultrasound has been used successfully to detect a large number of morphologic and physiologic defects, including neural tube defects, cardiac structural and conduction defects, abdominal wall and gastrointestinal anomalies, urinary tract abnormalities, skeletal dysplasia, and intracranial abnormalities.[1]

The sensitivity of ultrasound in detecting congenital abnormalities has been reported as low as 35% in a low-risk population to as high as 99% in a high-risk population.[1]

Ultrasound has also been useful in screening for fetal chromosome abnormalities. Down syndrome

has been associated with the findings of ventriculomegaly, thickened nuchal skin, cardiac abnormalities, and echogenic bowel.

Amniocentesis

Amniocentesis is the surgical perforation of the uterus for the purpose of withdrawing amniotic fluid. For genetic diagnostic purposes it is commonly done at 15 to 16 weeks, although it has been performed as early as 12 to 14 weeks.

Extensive clinical experience has demonstrated that amniotic fluid and cultured amniotic cells can be used for genetic analysis of fetal chromosomes and fetal DNA by molecular genetic techniques, as well as for fetal biochemical and metabolic defects. Detection of metabolic errors requires that the enzyme be expressed by amniotic fluid cells. However, this requirement is not fulfilled by all genetic disorders, phenylketonuria being an example. Fortunately, this disorder can be detected by molecular techniques.[2]

Amniocentesis has the disadvantage that the test is done in the second trimester, at 16 weeks. Furthermore, all cultures may be slow and a formal karyotype analysis may take up to 3 weeks.[3] Therefore, affected pregnancies may be identified as late at 18 to 20 weeks' gestation.

Finally, extensive clinical experience using amniocentesis suggests that it is safe. Most studies suggest a fetal loss rate of 0.5% or less, depending on the indication for the procedure.[4]

Early amniocentesis at 12 to 14 weeks offers the option of an earlier result, but it is technically a more difficult procedure. It carries a higher risk of fetal loss at a time in gestation when the background fetal loss rate is higher.

Chorionic villus sampling

Chorionic villus sampling (CVS) permits earlier sampling than amniocentesis and may be performed at 8 to 12 weeks' gestation for prenatal diagnosis.[5] Although the technique can be done transcervically or transabdominally, most commonly a soft, flexible catheter is inserted transcervically under ultrasound guidance and a small sample of chorionic villi is aspirated. Unlike amniocentesis, an

Table 2-1 Incidence of congenital disorders and genetic abnormalities at birth

	% of Births
Chromosomal abnormality	0.5–1.0
Single gene disorder	1–2
Major congenital abnormality	3
Congenital abnormality with a genetic component	1.2

adequate quantity of fetal tissue can be directly obtained and direct chromosome or DNA analysis can be performed.

Both chorionic villus sampling and cultured amniotic cells offer information concerning chromosomal status, enzyme levels, and DNA status. In fact, chorionic villi are suitable material for the diagnosis of genetic defects that are currently obtained by cultured amniotic cells. However, chorionic villous sampling does not allow performance of assays that require amniotic fluid liquor (i.e., alpha-fetoprotein analysis).

CVS has now been accepted into clinical practice as a first-trimester alternative to amniocentesis, with some qualifications. Three large multicenter prospective studies have shown that the fetal loss rate from CVS may be from 0.6% to 4.6% higher than for amniocentesis. In addition, there has been further concern that CVS done before 9 weeks' gestation may be associated with the birth of infants with limb-reduction defects. This association, however, was not confirmed in the large U.S. collaborative study.[6-9]

Fetal blood sampling

Ultrasonically guided fetal blood sampling by needle or cordocentesis permits recovery of fetal blood useful for detection of genetic disorders.[10]

A specific use for this procedure is to obtain fetal blood samples for rapid chromosome analysis. Short-term lymphocyte culture permits diagnosis in 48 to 72 hours. This may be especially important late in the second trimester when amniocentesis results would be available at a time when termination is not possible. Cordocentesis may also be used to administer an intrauterine blood transfusion directly into the fetal circulation. However, the risk of fetal loss directly attributable to umbilical blood sampling is difficult to determine because this procedure is usually performed on already compromised fetuses where the background fetal loss rate is expected to be high.

Rates of fetal loss have been reported at between 1 and 5%. The role of fetal umbilical blood sampling includes karyotype analysis in cases of mosaicism at the time of amniocentesis; the diagnosis and treatment of RH disease and other fetal anemias; the diagnosis of fetal thrombocytopenia; and the diagnosis of fetal infections.

Noninvasive genetic screening tests: maternal serum alpha fetoprotein

If reliable noninvasive techniques were available, all pregnant women could be screened without risk to the mother or fetus. Currently, no such technique exists. One approach would be to recover fetal cells that are present in the maternal circulation.[11] These cells could then be used for molecular cytogenetic or DNA analysis. New techniques that suggest isolation of fetal cells from the maternal circulation and which may become clinically useful include fluorescence-activated cell sorting, magnetic-activated cell sorting, the polymerase chain reaction (PCR), and fluorescence in situ hybridization (FISH).

The use of maternal serum for screening pregnancies for fetal chromosome abnormalities or structural defects has progressed rapidly. Alpha-fetoprotein (AFP) was first noted as elevated in the serum of mothers whose babies were delivered with neural tube defects and anencephaly. It was then shown that 80% to 90% of open spina bifida and anencephaly can be detected by an elevated maternal serum alpha-fetoprotein (MSAFP).[12] However, there is considerable overlap in MSAFP levels between normal pregnancies and pregnancies characterized by an open neural tube defect. Analysis of amniotic fluid AFP by amniocentesis and sometimes high-resolution ultrasonography is the standard for confirmation of neural tube defects.

MSAFP has also been useful in screening pregnancies for chromosome abnormalities. Reduced levels of MSAFP were first reported for Down syndrome.[13] Subsequently, an association between elevated levels of maternal serum human chorionic gonadotropin (hCG) and decreased levels of unconjugated estriol (uE3) have been reported. Pregnant women are now routinely offered a "triple screen" between 15 and 20 weeks' gestation that gives a composite age and maternal serum related risk of Down syndrome. A risk greater than 1 in 270, a risk equal to that of a 35-year-old woman, is generally considered screen positive. Several prospective studies have now shown that the sensitivity of a screening test can be increased from 20% using age alone to 40% using age plus MSAFP. Sensitivity can be further increased up to 65% using age plus the triple screen. Controversy remains, however, because it is uncertain whether the triple screen can replace traditional genetic counseling and amniocentesis for women age 35 and older, and whether other aneuploidies (e.g., trisomy 18) can be detected with these three markers.

Molecular techniques for genetic diagnosis

Rapid developments in molecular biology have greatly expanded the possibilities for prenatal diagnosis. More than 600 conditions can now be diagnosed prenatally through a combination of ultrasound, chromosome analysis, biochemical testing, DNA analysis, and linkage. The techniques of molecular biology permit the direct analysis of genetic disorders in some cases, such as sickle cell anemia, or the indirect analysis of genetic disorders through linkage.

Restriction endonucleases are bacterial enzymes that cut DNA in a sequence-specific fashion. These enzymes cut DNA into different-size fragments that can be separated on a gel by electrophoresis, fragments of DNA known as *restriction fragment length polymorphisms (RFLP)*. Southern blotting is a method of transferring these DNA fragments from the gel to a membrane where they can be hybridized to specific DNA probes.[14,15] If an RFLP corresponds to a mutation site in a gene, the genetic abnormality can be diagnosed directly. If the gene causing the genetic condition has not been characterized or if the gene mutations are very heterogeneous for a condition, the mutation may be tested indirectly by linkage analysis. Polymorphisms are genetic markers that differ between individuals. When genetic abnormality is tightly linked to a known polymorphism and the family pedigree is informative, some genetic conditions can be diagnosed indirectly by their con-inheritance with a polymorphism. Duchenne muscular dystrophy is an example of a genetic disease where about 65% of the mutations are known deletions and can be tested directly. About 30% of cases must use linked DNA markers for prenatal diagnosis and carrier testing.

The expanding knowledge gained through research in molecular biology will provide the basis for future clinical approaches to genetic disorders in terms of diagnosis and perhaps treatment.

SPECIFIC METABOLIC DISORDERS: MATERNAL OBSTETRIC AND ANESTHETIC IMPLICATIONS

With improved prenatal diagnosis and medical management, more patients with genetic disease are surviving to reproductive age. However, pregnancy may still pose unique risks to mothers with certain genetic disease, as well as to their fetuses.

This section will cover several genetic metabolic disorders that are compatible with survival to reproductive age. The emphasis will be placed on maternal anesthetic and obstetric implications of these disorders. A more complete discussion of genetic syndromes and their anesthetic implications can be found in several recent reviews of this subject.[16,17]

Disorders of amino acid metabolism: phenylketonuria and homocystinuria

Although there are more than 70 known disorders of amino acid metabolism, reproductive experience is scant. Clinical manifestations of these disorders generally include mental retardation, seizures, and aminoaciduria. Acidosis, hyperammonemia, hepatic failure, and thromboembolism may also be seen. Furthermore, genetic disorders that lead to the accumulation of abnormal metabolic products may expose the fetus to toxic levels (or deficiencies) of factors in utero.

Phenylketonuria. As shown in Figure 2-1, phenylketonuria,[15] an autosomal recessive disorder of amino acid metabolism, is the result of an enzyme deficiency of phenylalanine hydroxylase with resulting phenylalanine accumulation.[18] Untreated, clinical features include mental retardation and seizures.

Obstetric implications. Treatment of this disorder by restriction of dietary phenylalanine, from birth, avoids the toxic effects of this amino acid on the developing central nervous system (CNS). Interestingly, following a period of treatment, a point in brain maturity is reached after which increased phenylalanine levels are without toxic effect.[16] However, when such individuals become pregnant, the increased maternal phenylalanine levels are still toxic to the developing fetal brain. Reinstitution of dietary phenylalanine restriction

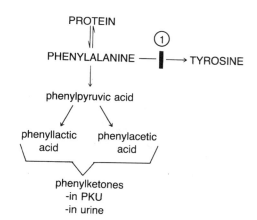

Fig. 2-1 Block of phenylalanine hydroxylase *(1)* in phenylketonuria. (Adapted from Thompson JS, Thompson MW (eds): *Genetics in Medicine,* ed 3. Philadelphia, WB Saunders, 1980.)

before pregnancy is essential to ensure fetal well-being.[18]

Anesthetic implications. There are no specific requirements for anesthetic management of these patients.

Homocystinuria. Homocystinuria,[19] another disorder of amino acid metabolism, is the result of a deficiency of cystathionine β-synthase with resultant lack of generation of precursors of collagen cross-links.[19] Manifestation of the abnormal collagen characteristic of this disease includes lens dislocation, scoliosis, mental retardation, and vascular thromboemboli. Thromboembolism can be life-threatening and probably reflects activation of the clotting cascade by homocysteine.[19]

Obstetric implications. To date, pregnancies have been reported in 15 patients with homocystinuria and have resulted in 11 spontaneous abortions, 1 hydrocephalic infant, and 3 normal infants.[20] Patients with the vitamin B_6-responsive enzyme may have better reproductive success following treatment.

Anesthetic implications. There are no specific anesthetic implications. Postoperative management is directed toward decreasing the incidence of thromboembolism in these patients.

Galactosemia

Galactosemia[21] is a disorder of carbohydrate metabolism due to an inherited autosomal recessive deficiency of galactokinase with resulting inability to convert galactose to glucose. Galactose accumulation in tissues results in mental retardation, cirrhosis of the liver, and cataracts. High levels of galactose may also decrease the release of glucose from the liver and lead to hypoglycemia. Importantly, the detrimental effects of this disease can be prevented by dietary galactose restriction.

Obstetric implications. Dietary galactose restriction during pregnancy is recommended even for heterozygotes.[22] Currently, however, reproductive experience with treated galactosemic patients is scant and has not revealed any significant obstetric problems.

Anesthetic implications. In the absence of hypoglycemia or severe hepatic dysfunction, there are no specific requirements for anesthetic management of these patients.

Wilson's disease[23]

Wilson's disease is inherited as an autosomal recessive trait characterized by deficiency of the copper transport protein ceruloplasmin. High tissue copper levels result in neurologic and hepatic dysfunction. This disease can now be treated with the copper chelator D-penicillamine, and more patients are surviving to reproductive age. Unfortunately,

penicillamine may be associated with leukopenia and thrombocytopenia.[23]

Obstetric implications. Despite the risk of penicillamine therapy, this drug should be continued throughout pregnancy to avoid rapid maternal copper reaccumulation.[23] There have been no reports of fetal injury during pregnancy in patients with treated Wilson's disease.

Anesthetic implications. Anesthetic management will be determined by the severity of preexisting neurologic or hepatic dysfunction as well as by any side effects of penicillamine therapy. This therapy may be associated with rash, fever, leukopenia, thrombocytopenia, lymphadenopathy, and proteinuria. Other complications that have been mentioned are agranulocytosis, nephrotic syndrome, systemic lupus erythematosus, severe arthralgias, and myasthenia gravis.

Porphyria[24]

Porphyria refers to a group of disease entities that result from an abnormality of porphyrin metabolism (Fig. 2-2).

Porphyria is categorized as either hepatic (acute intermittent porphyria, porphyria cutanea tarda, variegate porphyria, hereditary coproporphyria) or erythropoietic porphyria (erythropoietic porphyria and erythropoietic protoporphyria).

This section will deal with the hepatic porphyrias (mainly acute intermittent porphyria) because there is insufficient reproductive experience with the erythropoietic forms.

In the hepatic porphyrias, drugs that increase heme precursor production may overwhelm the ability of the defective enzyme to utilize the precursors. Increased levels of heme precursors are released into the circulation and may precipitate an acute attack. For example, barbiturate agents are well-known triggers of porphyria and are thought to act by inducing the increased production in the liver of the drug-metabolizing cytochrome P450 system. Since the enzymes in the P450 system require heme for catalytic activity, heme production is also stimulated. This effect results in the increased release of heme precursors that may exert neurotoxic effects and are thought to be responsible for the clinical manifestations of the disease following barbiturate administration. Heme precursors may affect neuronal function because of their structural similarity to GABA and presumed ability to block normal GABA-medicated neuronal transmission.[25] Alternatively, the indirect effects of neuronal heme deficiency may also be responsible for the clinical symptoms of porphyria.[25]

Acute intermittent porphyria, inherited as an autosomal dominant trait, is the most serious form of the hepatic porphyrias and may affect both the

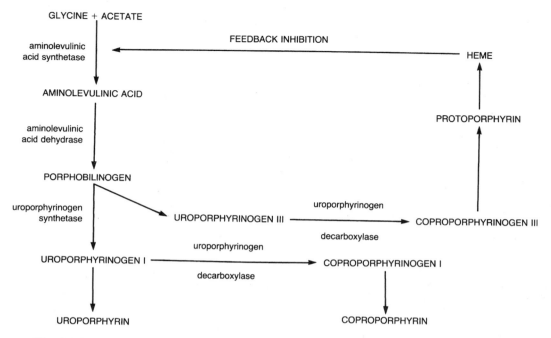

Fig. 2-2 Porphyria. The first step in the synthesis of heme is catalyzed by aminolevulinic acid synthetase and inhibited by heme. The formation of porphobilinogen is catalyzed by aminolevulinic acid dehydrase. Excess amounts of both aminolevulinic acid and porphobilinogen, as seen in acute intermittent porphyria, occur as a result of stimulation of aminolevulinic acid synthetase activity, and decreased uroporphyrinogen synthetase activity. Decreased activity of uroporphyrinogen decarboxylase can lead to an accumulation of uroporphyrin, which is believed to cause porphyria cutanea tarda. (Adapted from Stoelting RK, Dierdorf SF, McCammon RL (eds): *Anesthesia and Co-Existing Disease,* ed 2. New York, Churchill Livingstone, 1988.)

central and peripheral nervous system. Clinical manifestations include abdominal pain plus variable and often asymmetric neurologic defects. The peripheral neuropathy is mainly motor and may produce distal muscle weakness and respiratory paralysis. Cranial nerves may also be affected and may produce bulbar paralysis. In addition, autonomic nervous system dysfunction may result in labile blood pressure and the severe abdominal pain that is often the presenting sign of an acute attack of porphyria. Finally, CNS involvement may present with symptoms of seizure activity or psychosis.

Variegate porphyria and hereditary coproporhyria have a presentation similar to acute intermittent porphyria. In contrast, porphyria cutanea tarda is the only hepatic form not associated with neurologic involvement.

Obstetric implications. Women with the dominantly inherited hepatic porphyrias may be at risk for an exacerbation of their disease during pregnancy.[25,26] Interestingly, female sex hormones may stimulate heme production, and urinary excretion of heme precursors is increased during pregnancy. In one series of 55 patients, approximately half had

an acute attack during pregnancy or postpartum.[26] Fetal loss was 15% and there was one maternal death.[26] In some studies the maternal mortality following an acute attack of porphyria during pregnancy reached 20%.[25,26] However, more recent experience suggests that pregnancy may be well tolerated in many patients.

The treatment of acute porphyria is a medical emergency and requires attention to maintain adequate respiration, control seizures, and maintain normal electrolyte balance. Infusion of hematin may inhibit the enzyme delta amino acid synthetase (Fig. 2-2) and improve neurologic manifestations of this disease.[27] When clinical manifestations of porphyria occur during pregnancy, fetal loss is high.[25,26] However, in pregnancies that proceed to term there are no reported permanent effects on the newborn.

Anesthetic implications.[25,28,29] It is important to avoid drugs and conditions capable of provoking an attack of acute porphyria. In addition to drugs, volume depletion, sepsis, and hypoglycemia may also trigger an attack. More commonly, administration of drugs that stimulate porphyrin synthesis is implicated in triggering an acute attack. Classically, barbiturate drugs have been associated with acute attacks.[28,29] However, almost all anesthetic considerations are similar for variegate porphyria and hereditary coproporphyrin, as well as for acute intermittent porphyria. In contrast, porphyria cutanea tarda is not associated with drug-induced exacerbations.

Anesthetic drugs may be evaluated for their safe use in patients with porphyria on the basis of clinical reports linking their use with the development of acute symptoms. However, case reports of the uneventful administration of a drug to a few patients with porphyria does not guarantee its safety. For example, barbiturate drugs, including thiopental, are well-known triggers for acute attacks. However, even thiopental administration for anesthetic induction does not always provoke an attack, especially when administered during the latent phase of the disease.[29]

In addition to case reports, anesthetic drugs may be studied for their safety in animal models of porphyria. Drugs may be tested for their ability to increase heme production following administration to normal rats or to rats with chemically induced porphyria. However, heme metabolism in rats differs significantly from humans, and the relevance of animal data to the clinical situation is not clear.[25]

Barbiturate drugs are classically considered to be porphyrogenic and should be avoided.[29] However, a retrospective study demonstrated that the risk of triggering a porphyric reaction is low following the administration of barbiturate drugs for the induction of general anesthesia, provided the subjects were asymptomatic at the time of surgery.[29] Laboratory and clinical evidence suggests that benzodiazepine drugs (i.e., diazepam, flunitrazepam) may trigger prophyric reactions and should be avoided in patients with porphyria.[30,31] Interestingly, midazolam has been administered without complications to 14 patients with variegate porphyria.[32]

Although etomidate has been used safely in a patient with acute intermittent porphyria,[33] some authors feel this drug should be avoided in patients with porphyria.[25]

Ketamine was not found to be porphyrinogenic in rats.[34] It has been used to induce general anesthesia for cesarean delivery in an achondroplastic dwarf with intermittent porphyria.[35] Most authors would consider ketamine to be associated with an extremely low risk of triggering a porphyric attack. Therefore, ketamine would be considered an acceptable induction agent in parturients with porphyria.

The bulk of the laboratory and clinical evidence suggests that propofol is a safe anesthetic agent in patients with porphyria.[25] Propofol has been administered to patients with acute intermittent porphyria, hereditary coproporphyria, and variegate porphyria without reported porphyric reaction and in most cases without an increase in urinary porphyrin excretion.[25] Interestingly, one report describes the uneventful administrations of propofol to a patient in whom 20 out of 22 prior anesthetic agents resulted in a porphyric reaction.[36] Finally, Kantor and Rolbin[25] describe the safe administration of propofol for cesarean delivery in a parturient with acute intermittent porphyria. Although urinary porphyrins were somewhat elevated over preoperative levels, the patient remained asymptomatic.

In summary, the bulk of laboratory and clinical evidence suggests that ketamine or propofol are safe general anesthetic induction agents for cesarean delivery in parturients with porphyria. In contrast, barbiturate and benzodiazepine drugs should be avoided.

Furthermore, most authors consider that inhalation agents, narcotic drugs, muscle relaxant drugs, local anesthetic agents, and anticholinesterase drugs are not associated with a significant risk of a porphyric reaction and are safe to use in patients with porphyria.

In addition, local anesthetic agents (i.e., bupivacaine and lidocaine) are not considered to be porphyrogenic and may be safely administered. Therefore, regional anesthesia is not contraindicated in porphyria as long as the possibility of autonomic dysfunction is considered. Uncomplicated spinal anesthesia for cesarean delivery has been reported in a parturient with acute intermittent porphyria.[37]

Finally, the choice of anesthetic technique in the porphyria parturient should be guided by the same principles used to select the type of anesthesia in healthy parturients. The bulk of clinical and laboratory evidence suggests that both regional and general anesthesia may be safely administered to the parturient with porphyria. Under most conditions the authors would choose regional anesthesia as the preferred technique for labor analgesia and cesarean delivery in the parturient with porphyria.

Hemochromatosis

Hemochromatosis is an iron storage disorder related to increased deposition of iron, with resultant tissue damage in the liver, heart, pancreas, pituitary gland, and gonads.[38]

The disease is inherited as an autosomal recessive trait and is rarely clinically expressed before 20 years of age.[39] Expression of the disease may be modified by blood loss associated with menstruation and pregnancy. In fact, the disease is five to 10 times more common in males than in females.[38]

Hemochromatosis generally is expressed initially as hepatic dysfunction, leading to scarring and cirrhosis. Cardiac involvement is also common; this usually presents as congestive failure, although a variety of arrhythmias, particularly tachyarrhythmias, can occur. Diabetes mellitus also develops in the majority of patients as the result of pancreatic iron deposition. Excessive skin pigmentation, arthropathy, loss of libido, gonadal dysfunction, and adrenal insufficiency and hypothyroidism may also occur.

Treatment is designed to decrease body iron stores, and phlebotomy is generally the safest and most effective technique.[38] Iron chelating agents such as deferoxamine are generally used only when anemia is severe enough to preclude phlebotomy.[38] Early treatment may prevent or slow the development of organ failure.

Obstetric implications. Currently, reproductive experience with hemochromatosis is scant and has not revealed any significant obstetric problems. However, as more patients are being treated prior to the onset of symptoms, reproductive experience will increase.

Anesthetic implications. Anesthetic management is determined primarily by the severity of preexisting hepatic, cardiac, and endocrine dysfunction, as well as by side effects of phlebotomy or chelator therapy.

Ornithine carbamoyltransferase deficiency

Deficiency of the liver-specific urea cycle enzyme ornithine carbamoyltransferase results in an X-linked disorder of urea synthesis characterized by ammonia intoxification (i.e., coma, lethargy, cerebral edema).[40] Until recently only homozygous deficiency of this gene was thought to cause ammonia intoxication, and generally death, in the first week of life. However, a recent report[40] suggests that asymptomatic women who are carriers for a mutant form of ornithine carbamoyltransferase are at risk for development of hyperammonemic coma and death in the peripartum period. It has been estimated that at least several thousand women of childbearing age are carriers of a mutant gene and are at risk for development of hyperammonemia in the puerperium.[41] These authors[40] suggest that any woman with evidence of hyperammonemia (e.g., lethargy, stupor, seizures, coma) during the puerperium be examined for ornithine carbamoyltransferase deficiency.

A sensitive urine test is available to detect deficiencies of ornithine carbomoyltransferase in women.[42] Early detection of affected individuals could permit treatment with intravenous agents effective in lowering plasma ammonium levels.[41] Protein is usually excluded from the disk. Ammonia absorption can be decreased by the administration of lactulose. Intestinal ammonia production by bacteria can be minimized by treating with neomycin.

REFERENCES

1. Ewigman B, Crane JP, Frigoletto FD, et al, and the RADIUS Study Group: Effect of prenatal ultrasound screening on perinatal outcome. *N Engl J Med* 1993, 329:821.
2. Liasky AS, et al: Extensive restriction site polymorphism at the human phenylalanine hydroxylase locus and application in prenatal diagnosis of phenylketonuria. *Am J Hum Genet* 1985; 37:619.
3. Hsu LYF: Prenatal diagnosis of chromosome abnormalities, in Milunsky A (ed): *Genetic Disorders and the Fetus: Diagnosis, Prevention and Treatment.* New York, Plenum Press, 1986.
4. Elias S, Simpson JL: Amniocentesis, in Milunsky A (ed): *Genetic Disorders and the Fetus: Diagnosis, Prevention, and Treatment.* New York, Plenum Press, 1992.
5. Brambati B, et al: First trimester fetal diagnosis of genetic disorders: Clinical evaluation of 250 cases. *J Med Genet* 1985; 22:92.
6. Canadian collaborative chorionic villus sampling—amniocentesis clinical trial group. Multicenter randomized clinical trial or chorionic villus sampling and amniocentesis. *Lancet* 1989; 1:1.
7. Rhoads GG, Jackson LG, Schlesselman SE, et al: The safety and efficacy of chorionic villus sampling for early prenatal diagnosis of cytogenetic abnormalities. *N Engl J Med* 1989; 320:609.
8. Firth HV, Boyd PA, Chamberlain P, et al: Severe limb abnormalities after chorionic villus sampling at 55-66 days gestation. *Lancet* 1991; 337:762.
9. MRC Working Party on the Evaluation of Chorionic Villus Sampling: Medical Research Council European Trial of Chorionic Villus Sampling. *Lancet* 1991; 337:1491.
10. Hobbins JC, Grannum PA, Romero R, et al: Percutaneous umbilical blood sampling. *Am J Obstet Gynecol* 1985; 152:1.
11. Bianchi DW, Mohr A, Zickwolf GK, et al: Demonstration of fetal gene sequences in nucleated erythrocytes isolated from maternal blood. *Am J Human Genet* 1989; 45S:A252.
12. Brock DJM, Sutcliffe R: Alpha-fetoprotein in the antenatal diagnosis of anencephaly and spina bifida. *Lancet* 1972; 2:197.
13. Merkatz IR, Nitowsky HM, Macri JN, et al: An association between low maternal serum alpha-fetoprotein and fetal chromosome abnormalities. *Am J Obstet Gynecol* 1984; 148:886.
14. Kan YW, Dozy A: Antenatal diagnosis of sickle cell anemia by DNA analysis of amniotic fluid cells. *Lancet* 1978; 2:910.
15. Cooper DN, Schmidtke KJ: Diagnosis of genetic disease using recombinant DNA. *Hum Genet* 1986; 73:1.
16. Jones AEP, Pelton DA: An index of syndromes and their anesthetic implications. *Can Anaesth Soc J* 1976; 23:207.
17. Katz J, Benumof J, Kadis LB (eds): *Anesthesia and Uncommon Diseases*, ed 2, Philadelphia, WB Saunders, 1981.
18. Lenke RR, Levy HL: Maternal phenylketonuria and hyperphenylalanemia. *N Engl J Med* 1980; 303:1202.
19. Parris WCV, Quimby CW: Anesthetic considerations for the patient with homocystinuria. *Anesth Analg* 1982; 61:70.

20. Brenton DP, Cusworth DC, Biddle SA, et al: Pregnancy and homocystinuria. *Ann Clin Biochem* 1977; 14:161.

21. Nyan WL: An approach to the diagnosis of overwhelming metabolic disease in early infancy. *Curr Probl Pediatr* 1977; 7:3.

22. Donnel G, Ng WG, Oizumi J, et al: Observations on results of management of galactosemic patients, in Hsin DY (ed): *Galactosemia*. Springfield, Ill, Charles C Thomas, 1969.

23. Scheunberg IH, Sternlieb I: Pregnancy in penicillamine treated patients with Wilson's disease. *N Engl J Med* 1975; 298:1300.

24. Tschudy DP, Valsamis M, Magnussen CR, et al: Acute intermittent porphyria: Clinical and selected research aspects. *Ann Intern Med* 1975; 83:851.

25. Kantor G, Rolbin SH: Acute intermittent porphyria and Caesarean delivery. *Can J Anaesth* 1992; 39:282.

26. Short EM: Genetic disorders, in Burrow GN, Ferris TF (eds): *Medical Complications During Pregnancy*, Philadelphia, WB Saunders, 1982.

27. Watson CJ, Pierach CA, Bossenmaier I, et al: Use of hematin in acute attacks of the inducible porphyria. *Adv Intern Med* 1978; 24:265.

28. Mustojoki P, Heinonen J: General anesthesia in inducible porphyria. *Anesthesiology* 1980; 53:15.

29. Salvin SA, Christoforides C: Theiopental administration in acute intermittent porphyria without adverse effect. *Anesthesiology* 1976; 44:77.

30. Blekkenhorst GH, Harrison GG, Cook ES: Screening of certain anaesthetic agents for their ability to elicit acute porphyric phases in susceptible patients. *Br J Anaesth* 1980; 52:759.

31. Parikh PK, Moore MR: Anaesthetics in porphyria: Intravenous induction agents. *Br J Anaesth* 1975; 47:907.

32. Freedman M, Ingran HJ, Smuts JHL: Midazolam for induction of anaesthesia in patients with porphyria. *S Afr Med J* 1985; 68:212.

33. Famewo CE: Induction of anaesthesia with etomidate in a patient with acute intermittent porphyria. *Can Anaesth Soc J* 1985; 32:171.

34. Harrison GG, Moore MR, Meissner PN: Porphyrogenicity of etomidate and ketamine as continuous infusions. *Br J Anaesth* 1985; 57:420.

35. Bancroft GH, Lauria JL: Ketamine induction for cesarean section in a patient with acute intermittent porphyria and achondroplastic dwarfism. *Anesthesiology* 1983; 59:143.

36. Hughes PJ: Propofol in acute porphyrias. *Anaesthesia* 1990; 45:415.

37. McNeill MJ, Bennet A: Use of regional anesthesia in a patient with acute porphyria. *Br J Anaesth* 1990; 64:371.

38. Edward CO, Bassette ML, Bothwell TH, et al: Hereditary hemochromatosis. *N Engl J Med* 1977; 297:7.

39. Bothwell TH: *Iron Metabolism in Man*. London, Blackwell Scientific, 1979.

40. Arn PH, et al: Hyperammonemia in women with a mutation of the ornithine carbamoyltransferase locus: A cause of postpartum coma. *N Engl J Med* 1990; 322:1652.

41. Horwich AL, Fenton WA: Precarious balance of nitrogen metabolism in women with a urea-cycle defect. *N Engl J Med* 1990; 322:1668.

42. Hauser ER, et al: Allopurinol-induced orotidinuria: A test for mutations of the ornithine carbamoyltransferase locus in women. *N Engl J Med* 1990; 322:1641.

3 Fetal Congenital Abnormalities

Angela M. Bader and Linda Heffner

Advances in perinatology over the past decade have resulted in dramatic changes in the diagnosis and management of fetal abnormalities. The potential for antenatal diagnosis of a variety of congenital problems has led to the development of fetal therapeutics that may improve neonatal outcome. Perinatologists and pediatric surgeons are identifying those fetal conditions that may benefit from intrauterine therapy and those for which treatment during gestation is indicated. The identification of these fetal conditions may dictate timing and mode of delivery; in utero treatment may impact on maternal physiology. This chapter will review briefly the diagnostic and therapeutic options available for prenatal diagnosis and then address the anesthetic considerations when specific conditions are identified.

PATHOPHYSIOLOGY

Conditions affecting the fetus may be thought of broadly as either anatomic, physiologic, or both. Examples of anatomic abnormalities include neural tube defects (e.g., meningomyelocele, spina bifida), congenital heart defects (transposition of the great vessels, tetralogy of Fallot), large masses (teratomas, cystic hygromas), abdominal wall defects (gastroschisis, omphalocele), and conjoined twins. Examples of physiologic conditions include cardiac arrhythmias, immune and nonimmune hydrops, fetal Graves' disease, and intrauterine growth retardation (IUGR). Combined disorders would include multiple congenital malformations secondary to chromosomal defects and macrocrania secondary to severe hydrocephalus.

DIAGNOSIS

Currently available techniques for the detection of abnormalities are maternal serum alphafetoprotein (MSAFP) screening, ultrasound, Doppler velocimetry, chorionic villus sampling (CVS), amniocentesis, percutaneous umbilical blood sampling, and antenatal fetal heart rate monitoring. Maternal serum alphafetoprotein measurement is currently offered at 16 to 18 weeks' gestation, and both elevated and depressed concentrations require further evaluation. Disorders that may elevate

MSAFP include, but are not limited to, open neural tube defects, gastroschisis, omphalocele, cystic hygroma, and Finnish nephrosis.[1] Low MSAFP has been associated with Down syndrome and other trisomies.[2,3] The addition of maternal serum unconjugated estradiol and chorionic gonadotropin (hCG) measurements to MSAFP screening has increased the detection rate of Down syndrome.

Chorionic villus sampling is a first-trimester technique for obtaining trophoblast for use in chromosomal, enzymatic, and DNA-based assays.[4-6] Midtrimester amniocentesis is the most widely used technique to obtain fetal cells for chromosomal, DNA, or chemical study; indications include advanced maternal age, abnormal MSAFP, previous trisomy, parental chromosomal translocation sex-linked genetic disorders, and an expanding number of identifiable single gene defects. Amniocentesis also may be used in the third trimester to assay fetal lung maturity prior to anticipated delivery.

Ultrasound is used as both a primary diagnostic method and a necessary adjunct to intrauterine techniques such as CVS, amniocentesis, and percutaneous umbilical blood sampling. Examples of indications for prenatal ultrasound currently include unsure pregnancy dating, size-dates discrepancies, abnormal MSAFP, suspected polyhydramnios, suspected IUGR, and family history of congenital malformations. Many congenital malformations are diagnosed incidentally on scans obtained for another reason.

The use of routine ultrasound as a prenatal screening tool to improve perinatal outcome has not been substantiated.[7]

Ultrasound technology has recently improved, and the ability to perform Doppler velocimetry on the umbilical vasculature is now available; normative data have been established and certain abnormalities have been correlated with significant risk for fetal death.[8] Umbilical Doppler would appear useful in the management of pregnancies complicated by IUGR.

Currently limited to a few centers with the advanced ultrasound support necessary to perform the procedure, percutaneous umbilical blood sampling (PUBS) is a highly invasive but useful technique for directly accessing the fetal blood stream.[9,10] Percutaneous umbilical blood sampling can be used in midtrimester to establish risk of congenital toxoplasmosis when maternal infection is present, in the third trimester to permit rapid lymphocytic karyotyping when a lethal trisomy is suspected, and to manage isoimmunized pregnancies and those complicated by potential fetal thrombocytopenia. Percutaneous umbilical blood sampling has been suggested as a way of delivering medications that cannot cross the placenta to the fetus; this theoretical application has yet to be reported.

Once the patient is diagnosed, many options are available to deal with congenital abnormalities. Early diagnosis maximizes the range of options to include termination of the pregnancy, should that be the patient's choice. For late diagnoses and pregnancies continuing into viability, in utero treatment may be indicated. Procedures currently under investigation include urinary tract drainage procedures for obstructive uropathy, administration of cardioactive drugs for supraventricular arrhythmias, percutaneous drainage of ascites or hydrothoraces prior to delivery, and intrauterine transfusion. Infants may benefit from premature or timed delivery or from delivery by cesarean section. The anesthetic considerations at delivery are addressed individually.

OBSTETRIC AND ANESTHETIC MANAGEMENT
Cesarean delivery to prevent dystocia or traumatic injury

Cesarean delivery is sometimes indicated to prevent fetal somatic dystocia that might occur with the vaginal delivery of conjoined twins or a very large body part (see Box 3-1). Similarly, it may be necessary to prevent traumatic injury to exposed tissue, such as in neural tube defects or abdominal wall defects containing liver. Cesarean section may also be recommended for similar reasons when fetal thrombocytopenia is present, especially in the sensitized PLA 1 negative mother, as discussed in detail in Chapter 17.

In cases in which the presence of a congenital anomaly may preclude vaginal delivery, the anesthesiologist must attempt to optimize abdominal relaxation while minimizing anesthetic risk for mother and fetus. The degree of abdominal muscle relaxation provided by a spinal anesthetic or by the higher concentration of local anesthetic agents used for epidural anesthesia for cesarean section is generally adequate.

Even when a vertical incision has been performed, the presence of certain fetal malformations

---

BOX 3-1 FETAL ABNORMALITIES POTENTIALLY REQUIRING CESAREAN SECTION

Anatomic

Macrocrania
Teratoma
Conjoined twins
Cystic hygroma
Arthrogryposis multiplex congenita
Ovarian cyst
Omphalocele
Gastroschisis
Osteogenesis imperfecta types I, III, IV
Spina bifida
Cephalocele

Physiologic

Fetal distress
Thrombocytopenia
Congenital heart block
Ascites

---

such as sacral teratoma or cystic hygroma may make it difficult for the obstetrician to extract the infant. In these cases, if a regional anesthetic has been used for the cesarean delivery, additional uterine relaxation can be provided by the administration of small doses (50 mcg) of intravenous nitroglycerin.[11]

It must be remembered, however, that the use of a major regional anesthetic does not provide uterine relaxation.

Should extraction of the fetus still prove difficult and complete uterine relaxation be required, the anesthesiologist should be prepared for rapid induction of general anesthesia with thiopental, succinylcholine, endotracheal intubation, nitrous oxide, and a volatile anesthetic such as halothane, enflurane, or isoflurane to provide maximal uterine relaxation. Halothane has been traditionally used for this purpose. However, because of concerns regarding hepatotoxicity associated with the use of this agent,[12] it is no longer used by many anesthesiologists. In vitro studies on human uterine muscle have shown that equipotent concentrations of enflurane, isoflurane, and halothane depress myometrial muscle equally.[13] Therefore, either isoflurane or enflurane should be acceptable alternatives to the previously recommended halothane when maximum uterine relaxation is required.

Cesarean delivery of a fetus with some of the anomalies listed in the box may necessitate delivery through a larger vertical uterine incision than is usually used. Also, the time from uterine incision to delivery may be extended as the fetal parts are extracted. For these reasons, the anesthesiologist should be prepared for increased blood loss by establishing adequate large-bore intravenous access before the start of the procedure. Adequate preoperative volume loading with 1,500 to 2,000 ml intravenous fluids is particularly important.

Anesthetic considerations in the physiologically compromised fetus

Several specific fetal conditions may be affected by drugs normally administered during the course of obstetric anesthesia. This section will specifically address these issues for cases of fetal arrhythmias, maternal Graves' disease, fetal IUGR, and nonimmune hydrops. The issues of fetal distress, either acute or manifested by peripartum evaluations such as the nonreactive nonstress test, oxytocin challenge test, and biophysical profile, have been discussed in Chapters 1 and 29.

Fetal arrhythmias. The vast majority of antenatally diagnosed arrhythmias are supraventricular tachycardias, most commonly paroxysmal supraventricular tachycardia and, less frequently, atrial flutter and fibrillation. These rhythm abnormalities may be due to anatomic abnormalities, defects in the conduction system, or viral infection. If untreated, congestive heart failure and fetal hydrops syndrome may occur. To prevent or treat congestive heart failure, antiarrhythmic agents are administered maternally[14] because survival is improved if hydrops is not present. Prognosis is poor once hydrops has developed.[15]

Successful in utero conversion of fetal supraventricular tachycardia has been accomplished by administration of cardioactive drugs, usually digoxin or verapamil, and occasionally, quinidine, procainamide, or propranolol, to the mother.[16] Conversion presumably occurs when therapeutic concentrations of drug are obtained in the fetal circulation; this may require administration of very large doses of these drugs to the mother. Premature delivery is effected only if transplacental therapy is unsuccessful in the face of persistent or worsening hydrops fetalis.

The use of these cardiogenic medications in the presence of fetal arrhythmias has several implications for the anesthesiologist. Therapeutic levels are often what would be considered high therapeutic plasma concentrations for an adult. Maternal plasma levels must be monitored to ensure that toxic levels of digoxin are not reached. During the period in which the parturient receives nothing by mouth, digoxin is administered intravenously. Maternal plasma potassium levels should also be followed, since low potassium levels may exacerbate digoxin toxicity.

Regional anesthesia is frequently used for labor and delivery in these patients. If a parturient has been treated with beta blockers such as propranolol for fetal supraventricular tachycardia, maternal heart rate may not increase if local anesthetic is accidentally injected into an epidural vessel. Subjective symptoms should be carefully assessed to avoid inadvertent intravascular injection.

The effects of vasopressors such as ephedrine and phenylephrine, which are commonly used to treat the hypotension accompanying the induction of regional anesthesia, must also be considered. Maternal treatment with propranolol may make ephedrine therapy less effective, since the contribution of heart rate to increasing maternal blood pressure may be diminished. In these cases, larger doses of ephedrine may be required to restore maternal blood pressure. The use of a pure alpha-agonist agent such as phenylephrine may be necessary, depending upon base line heart rate.

Fetal supraventricular arrhythmias may be associated with ventricular response rates well above 200 beats/min. Maternal ephedrine administration is associated with significant increases in fetal heart rate.[17] Therefore, large doses of ephedrine may exacerbate these abnormally fast ventricular rates and cause decompensation. Although stroke volume can change in response to hemodynamic needs, fetal cardiac output is normally dependent on heart rate.[18] However, at the exacerbated fast heart rates seen with tachyarrythmias, inadequate time may be provided for ventricular filling and further deterioration may result.

Chronic fetal bradyarrhythmias are most often secondary to complete heart block, a condition with implications for both mother and fetus. Neonatal consequences vary from minimal to lethal complex structural heart disease; mothers of these infants have an increased risk of collagen vascular disease.[19] In most cases reported, patients deliver at term without intrauterine treatment. Intrapartum monitoring in these fetuses is difficult and dependent on fetal capillary blood gas measurement rather than the usual heart rate monitoring and for this reason, cesarean delivery may be unavoidable. Fetal echocardiography and umbilical Doppler assessment may be useful in some cases to avoid a cesarean section.[20]

In these cases, maternal hypotension encountered during regional anesthesia should be treated in the standard manner with ephedrine, since the ephedrine that passively crosses the placenta would not be expected to adversely affect these fetuses. Maternal administration of phenylephrine causes a reflex maternal bradycardia. Although this effect on fetal heart rate has not been reported, theoretically one may postulate that this drug may worsen the degree of fetal bradycardia and should be avoided. There is no advantage in these cases to increasing the fetal heart rate with atropine, since the fetus has chronically compensated for the persistent bradycardia. Atropine is used only for specific maternal indications, such as in cases of maternal bradycardia. Cases in which the heart block is accompanied by hydrops fetalis have not benefited from up to a 50% increase in fetal heart rate associated with maternal administration of beta agonists.[21]

Graves' disease. When maternal Graves' disease is present, even when well controlled after ablative therapy, there is a risk of fetal Graves' disease and the possibility of thyroid storm induced by delivery of the neonate. Fetuses affected by Graves' disease in utero can usually be identified by a mild fetal tachycardia (180 to 200 beats/min) and sometimes by IUGR. Patients with active maternal Graves' disease may be treated with beta blockers such as propranolol. Regional anesthesia is generally preferred for labor and delivery because the sympathetic block attenuates adrenal release of catecholamines and minimizes the hypertension and tachycardia that may be produced by the stress of delivery.[22,23] Vasopressors such as ephedrine, which may increase both fetal and maternal heart rate, should be carefully titrated; an alpha agonist such as phenylephrine may be a better choice.

The fetus may be born with a large goiter in these cases, and the anesthesiologist should ensure that personnel responsible for delivery room care of the neonate are prepared to manage neonatal respiratory obstruction.

Intrauterine growth restriction. Intrauterine growth restriction (IUGR) is an abnormality of fetal growth affecting 3% to 10% of pregnancies. Causes are diverse, including chronic uteroplacental insufficiency, congenital infection, and genetic and anatomic abnormalities, with uteroplacental insufficiency accounting for at least 50% of confirmed cases. Once diagnosed, aggressive obstetric management is indicated because those cases resulting from uteroplacental insufficiency may benefit from optimization of the intrauterine environment and timed delivery. Aggressive use of ultrasound, including Doppler velocimetry, and antepartum fetal heart rate testing are helpful. Delivery should be considered when fetal lung maturity is obtained or when acute fetal distress is present.

No literature exists specifically addressing the anesthetic considerations for the IUGR fetus. In these cases, as in all cases of suspected uteroplacental insufficiency, maintenance of optimal placental perfusion is paramount. Abrupt changes in maternal blood pressure should be avoided. Ad-

equate volume loading prior to the induction of anesthesia and prompt administration of vasopressors to treat maternal hypotension are essential. The presence of an IUGR fetus should alert the anesthesiologist to search for associated maternal conditions such as chronic hypertension, toxemia, cigarette smoking, and ilicit drug use.[24]

Fetal hydrops. Nonimmune fetal hydrops, a condition of generalized edema of fetal soft tissues in utero, with or without effusions in serous cavities and with no hematologic evidence of isoimmunization, may be caused by numerous maternal, fetal, and placental disorders. Ultrasound identification of the condition and extensive antenatal evaluation can correctly identify the cause in about 70% of cases, and in some, specific therapy can be directed to the problem.[25] Overall survival is less than 25%. In those cases in which the fetus is potentially salvageable but the hydrops still present, care must be taken at delivery to prevent generalized depression in the neonate.

As in the IUGR fetus, maintenance of optimal placental perfusion is extremely important. Maternal narcotic administration should be avoided if possible, since the respiratory status of the fetus with nonimmune hydrops may be extremely precarious and further depression could result. Regional anesthesia is preferred for labor and delivery, because this will minimize the administration of systemic agents that will transfer across the placenta. Aggressive resuscitation may be needed in the delivery room.

In some cases, the obstetrician may wish to perform percutaneous drainage of ascites or hydrothoraces before delivery to facilitate newborn resuscitation. An epidural anesthetic agent can be placed before performance of the drainage to provide maternal anesthesia during the procedure. The epidural catheter can then be used to provide analgesia for the subsequent delivery. Should the fetal status deteriorate during the drainage procedure, the epidural catheter could also be used to provide anesthesia for emergency cesarean delivery.

Fetal conditions incompatible with extrauterine life

Some fetal abnormalities are incompatible with extrauterine life. Anesthetic implications for the patient with intrauterine fetal death are discussed in Chapter 32; the following is a list of lethal malformations for which no therapeutic interventions currently exist[26]:

· Anencephaly
· Iniencephaly
· Hydranencephaly
· Alobar or semilobar holoprosencephaly

- Acrania
- Ectopia cordis
- Body stalk anomaly
- Meckel's syndrome
- Bilateral renal agenesis
- Infantile polycystic kidney disease
- Bilateral multicystic kidney disease
- Achondrogenesis
- Thanatophoric dwarfism
- Short rib—polydactyly syndromes
- Osteogenesis imperfecta, type II
- Hypophosphatasia

Extreme sensitivity to the emotional state of the parents is essential, since some families will choose aggressive therapies even if the prognosis for long-term survival is extremely poor. In these situations, appropriate consultations with the neonatologist are needed to ensure that the family is fully aware of the fetal condition and able to appropriately decide about the use of aggressive resuscitation after delivery.

After all of the information regarding the fetal condition and the options for management have been presented, a course of nonaggressive management may be chosen. Various approaches to obstetric ethics support nonaggressive management as a reasonable alternative.[27]

If a plan of nonaggressive management is selected, the anesthesiologist should make the parturient aware that her emotional and physical comfort are of paramount importance. Regional anesthesia can be used for labor and delivery. Intravenous supplementation with narcotic agents, diazepam, or midazolam can be added as required to maintain the patient's comfort. Since some of these agents will have an amnestic effect, it is important to discuss with the parturient the amount of recall that she may have of the event, and to gear use of these agents based on the patient's wishes and emotional state. Similar guidelines apply when dealing with anesthetic choices for patients undergoing destructive fetal procedures such as cephalocentesis in the case of severe hydrocephalus. General anesthesia may be desired by the patient in some of these cases and the risks and benefits should be discussed. Respect for the families' choices and concerns is essential when dealing with these issues.

REFERENCES

1. Main DM, Mennuti MT: Neural tube defects: Issues in prenatal diagnosis and counselling. *Obstet Gynecol* 1986; 67:1.
2. DiMaio MS, Baumgarten A, Greenstein RM, et al: Screening for fetal Down's syndrome in pregnancy by measuring maternal serum alpha-fetoprotein levels. *N Engl J Med* 1987; 317:342.
3. Haddow JE, Palomaki BS, Knight GJ, et al: Prenatal screening for Down's syndrome with use of maternal serum markers. *N Engl J Med* 1992; 327:588.
4. Hogge WA, Schomberg SA, Galbus MS: Chorionic villus sampling: Experience of the first 1000 cases. *Am J Obstet Gynecol* 1986; 154:1249.
5. Elias S, Simpson JL, Martin AO, et al: Chorionic villus sampling in continuing pregnancies. I. Low fetal loss rate in initial 109 cases. *Am J Obstet Gynecol* 1986; 154:1349.
6. Martin AO, Simpson JL, Rosinsky B, et al: Chorionic villus sampling in continuing pregnancies: II—Cytogenetic reliability. *Am J Obstet Gynecol* 1986; 154:1353.
7. Ewigman BG, Crane JP, Frigoletto FD, et al: Effect of prenatal ultrasound screening on perinatal outcome. *New Eng J Med* 1993; 329:821.
8. Trudinger B: Doppler ultrasound assessment of blood flow, in Creasy RK, Resnik R (eds): *Maternal-Fetal Medicine: Principles and Practice.* Philadelphia, WB Saunders, 1994, pp 243-257.
9. Hobbins JC, Grannum PA, Romero R, et al: Percutaneous umbilical blood sampling. *Am J Obstet Gynecol* 1985; 152:1.
10. Daffos F, Capella-Pavlovsky M, Forestier F: Fetal blood sampling during pregnancy with use of a needle guided by ultrasound: A study of 606 consecutive cases. *Am J Obstet Gynecol* 1985; 153:655.
11. Rolbin SH, Hew EM, Bernstein A: Uterine relaxation can be life-saving. *Can J Anaesth* 1991; 38:939.
12. Bottinger LE, Dalen E, Halen B: Halothane-induced liver damage: An analysis of the material reported to the Swedish Adverse Drug Reaction Committee 1966-1973. *Acta Anaesth Scand* 1976; 20:40.
13. Munson ES, Embro WJ: Enflurane, isoflurane and halothane and isolated human uterine muscle. *Anesthesiology* 1977; 46:11.
14. Wladimiroff JW, Stewart PA: Diagnosis and treatment of fetal tachyarrhythmias, in Maeda K (ed): *The Fetus as a Patient.* New York, Elsevier 1987, pp 335-342.
15. Klein AM, Holyman IR, Austin EM: Fetal tachycardia prior to development of hydrops. *Am J Obstet Gynecol* 1979; 134:347.
16. Kleinman CS, Copel JA, Weinstein EM, et al: In utero diagnosis and treatment of fetal SVT. *Semin Perinatol* 1985; 9:113.
17. Wright RG, Shnider SM, Levinson G, et al: The effect of maternal administration of ephedrine on fetal heart rate and variability. *Obstet Gynecol* 1981; 57:734.
18. Gilbert RD: Effects of afterload and baroreceptors on cardiac function in fetal sheep. *J Dev Physiol* 1982; 4:299.
19. Reid RL, Pancham SR, Kean WF, et al: Maternal and neonatal implications of congenital complete heart block in the fetus. *Obstet Gynecol* 1979; 54:470.
20. Kleinman CS, Copel JA, Hobbins JC: Combined echocardiographic and Doppler assessment of fetal atrioventricular block. *Br J Obstet Gynaecol* 1987; 94:967.
21. Kleinman CS, Copel JA: Fetal cardiac dysrhythmias, in Creasy RK, Resnik R (eds): *Maternal Fetal Medicine: Principles and Practice.* Philadelphia, WB Saunders, 1989, pp 344-356.
22. Bullock JL, Harris RE, Young R: Treatment of thyrotoxicosis during pregnancy with propranolol. *Am J Obstet Gynecol* 1975; 121:242.
23. Halpern SH: Anaesthesia for cesarean section in patients with uncontrolled hyperthyroidism. *Can J Anaesth* 1989; 36:454.

24. Creasy RK, Resnik R: Intrauterine growth restriction, in Creasy RK, Resnik R (eds): *Maternal-Fetal Medicine: Principles and Practice*. Philadelphia, WB Saunders, 1994, pp 558-574.

25. Holzgreve W, Holzgreve B, Curry CJR: Nonimmune hydrops fetalis: Diagnosis and management. *Semin Perinatol* 1985; 9:52.

26. Romero R, Pilu G, Jeanty P, et al (eds): *Prenatal Diagnosis of Congenital Anomalies*. Norwalk, Conn, Appleton-Lange, 1988.

27. Chervenak FA, McCollough LB: Nonaggressive obstetric management: An option for some fetal anomalies during the third trimester. *JAMA* 1989; 261:3439.

4 Intrauterine Fetal Manipulations

Barry C. Corke and *John W. Seeds*

Safe intrauterine fetal intervention or manipulation for both diagnostic and therapeutic purposes is a relatively recent development. Amniocentesis was first used for the evaluation of Rh isoimmunization in the late 1950s, and Liley first reported in 1963[1] the successful intrauterine transfusion of the fetus severely affected by Rh isoimmunization but the direct surgical intervention in the case of congenital disease has evolved only during the past decade.

Sonographically guided amniocentesis, fetoscopic visualization of the fetus, high detail dynamic image (real time) ultrasound examination of fetal anatomy, percutaneous fetal blood sampling, and intravascular intrauterine transfusion are among the fetal interventions that have become accepted for the diagnosis and treatment of fetal conditions.[2-7] Consideration of prenatal treatment or palliation of a variety of fetal conditions and malformations is closely linked to improved techniques for diagnosis.[8-19] The assumption motivating most interventions is that the earlier treatment of a progressive condition is begun, the better the outcome will be.

The medical treatment of fetal conditions has developed parallel to surgical intervention through the maternal administration of pharmacologic agents. Such agents include digitalis for the treatment of fetal supraventricular tachycardia, the suppression of congenital adrenal hyperplasia with maternally administered corticosteroids, and the acceleration of fetal lung maturity with maternal steroid administration.

Direct surgical treatment of fetal conditions other than transfusion for hemolytic disease is critically dependent on high-detail images of anatomy that have become widely available only during the past 10 years.[20] One type of surgical intervention is sonographically guided fine-needle aspiration of fluid accumulations within obstructed fetal organ systems, such as the urine from an enlarged obstructed fetal bladder, or cerebrospinal fluid from the enlarged lateral ventricle of hydrocephalus. The placement of indwelling catheters for continuous drainage of these obstructive anomalies, and the direct surgical treatment of such malformations, through open laparotomy and hysterotomy with exposure of the fetus with both obstructive uropathies and diaphragmatic hernia, has also been reported. All such interventions demand consideration of issues of safety and efficacy of both fetal and maternal analgesia or anesthesia. We will review animal models and human experience with several categories of human congenital malformations that have been targets of fetal treatment, and then we will explore appropriate anesthetic aspects of the potential procedures.

CONGENITAL DISEASE: ANIMAL MODELS AND EARLY HUMAN EXPERIENCE

Useful animal models for fetal surgical intervention have included guinea pigs, lambs, and dogs. These models have provided the experimental basis for the study of fetal intestinal obstruction, coarctation of the aorta, and diaphragmatic hernia for over half a century. More recently, sheep and primates have been used to study fetal ureteral obstruction and hydrocephalus, and have provided support for the consideration of intervention in the analogous human conditions.

Liley's first report of the treatment of severe fetal hemolytic disease described the intraperitoneal transfusion of compatible donor red cells through a needle placed percutaneously through the maternal abdomen into the fetal peritoneal cavity using fluoroscopic localization.[1] Absorption of these red cells via the thoracic duct provided effective transfusion therapy in the majority of cases. The first surgical exteriorization of the human fetus was reported by Asensio in 1966.[21] He exposed the lower limb of the human fetus through laparotomy and hysterotomy incisions, allowing cannulation of femoral vessels and complete exchange transfusion of a fetus suffering from severe hemolytic disease.[21] General anesthesia was used for this procedure. However, difficulty with maintenance of the pregnancy after the procedure associated with a low level of successful outcome compared to the Liley method resulted in abandonment of this approach.

Direct visualization of the fetus using a small fiberoptic endoscope was first described in 1974.[22] The placement of a fine needle through a side channel of the fetoscope allowed the aspiration of the first pure sample of fetal blood.[22] In addition, the direct transfusion of donor red cells was accomplished through the same needle used for the aspiration of the diagnostic sample.[23,24] Heavy maternal sedation was required for maternal comfort and also appeared to minimize fetal movement. However, the danger of producing a light plane of anesthesia without adequate protection of the maternal airway remained a serious problem. A proper method for the temporary arrest of fetal movement was not available at that time.

HIGH-DETAIL ULTRASOUND AND HUMAN FETAL THERAPY

The introduction in 1977 of dynamic image (real-time) ultrasound, allowing detailed visualization of fetal anatomy, heralded the beginning of the modern era of prenatal diagnosis of fetal conditions that might benefit from prenatal intervention.

The majority of fetal physical conditions that can benefit from direct surgical manipulation are those that result in the accumulation of fluids above the point of an obstruction. In most cases treatment is based on the assumption that failure to relieve the abnormal accumulation of fluid leads to damage of vital organs. These malformations may also produce a threat to the pregnancy itself by leading to polyhydramnios and thereby increas-ing the probability of preterm labor and/or delivery.[6,7,13,15,25-27]

Hydrocephalus was the first human fetal malformation treated in utero as a result of this kind of consideration. Narrow-gauge needle aspiration of cerebrospinal fluid from the dilated ventricles of a human fetus with severe congenital hydrocephalus using ultrasound guidance was first reported in 1981, but reaccumulation required serial procedures.[12] Needle aspiration of urine from the renal pelvis of a fetus with ureteropelvic junction obstruction was described in 1982, but experience has shown that unilateral disease rarely requires or benefits from intervention.[13] Placement of continuous diversion catheters for hydrocephalus and obstructive uropathies was described in 1982.[19] We will discuss in greater detail these types of procedures later. Percutaneous ultrasound-guided fine-needle aspiration of fetal blood from the umbilical vein followed by transfusion in the case of hemolytic disease was successfully performed by Bang et al and reported in 1982.[8] This technique has since gained wide popularity both for diagnosis and treatment of fetal hemolytic disease.[2-5,9-11]

Hydrocephalus

Isolated hydrocephalus due to aqueductal stenosis or atresia is a fetal malformation that was at one time considered a candidate for antenatal therapy (Fig. 4-1).[19] Both sheep and primate models had provided considerable evidence that prenatal treatment resulted in an arrest of progressive ventricu-

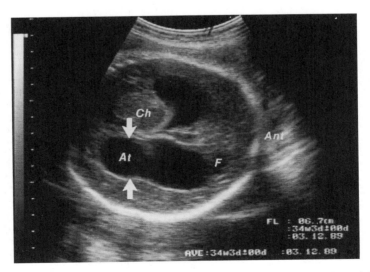

Fig. 4-1 Moderate lateral ventriculomegaly is easily seen on this occipitofrontal cranial fetal sonogram. The dark areas within the cranial outline are the dilated lateral ventricles. The anterior aspect *(Ant)* is to the right. The frontal horns *(F)* are often measured, but the atrium *(At)* of the lateral ventricle is considered the most sensitive dimension for the diagnosis *(area between arrows)*. The choroid plexus of the superior ventricle *(Chi)* is visible on this slightly off-axis view.

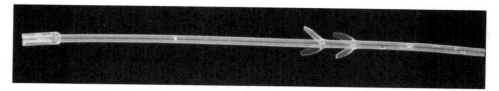

Fig. 4-2 The Denver hydrocephalus shunt was a narrow Silastic catheter similar to the catheter shown here. The thick hub to the left was to prevent migration into the head while the winglike arms to the right were to prevent passive migration out. There was a one-way valve in the hydrocephalus shunt, not shown here.

lomegaly and improved survival. Furthermore, human case series before 1982 describing the outcome for congenital hydrocephalus overt at birth reported a very poor prognosis for neurologically intact survival. Therefore, examination of the efficacy of prenatal intervention appeared appropriate.

Treatment of fetal hydrocephalus with an indwelling diversion catheter involved the sonographically guided insertion of a thin-walled cannula within a sterile field through the maternal abdominal wall into the uterus and through the fetal cranium into the dilated ventricle. The trocar was then removed and a Silastic catheter was advanced into the ventricle through the cannula as the cannula was removed, leaving the catheter lying between the ventricle and the amniotic cavity. Cerebrospinal fluid would flow through the shunt into the amniotic cavity, but amniotic fluid could not flow in the reverse direction. The Denver Hydrocephalus Shunt (Denver Biomaterials, Evergreen, Colo.) was the most frequently used device, and was designed with a one-way valve to prevent the reverse flow of amniotic fluid into the ventricle (Fig. 4-2).

Although there was initial enthusiasm for this technically feasible intervention, examination of the clinical outcomes of over 35 cases of prenatal diversion therapy of fetal hydrocephalus reported to the international registry between 1981 and 1985 indicated multiple examples of diagnostic inaccuracy and only limited clinical benefit from the treatment.[25] Although the target lesion was intended to be isolated aqueductal stenosis, the final diagnoses included instead multiple examples of related but very different diagnoses including holoprosencephaly, Dandy-Walker malformation, and others. Such diagnostic inaccuracy significantly degrades the utility of any therapeutic conclusions that might be drawn from such an experience.[25] Furthermore, significant improvement during the past decade in the neurological outcome of infants with isolated hydrocephalus overt at birth but treated for best outcome with conventional neonatal neurosurgical methods has made any potential benefit from antenatal intervention more difficult

to prove.[26,27] Therefore, since prenatal treatment of fetal hydrocephalus subjects the fetus to some considerable risks, and the benefits of such therapy are unclear, the antenatal treatment of fetal hydrocephalus has largely ceased.

Obstructive uropathies

Congenital obstructive uropathy varies from partial or complete unilateral or bilateral ureteropelvic junction, obstruction to bladder outlet, obstruction from urethral valves, urethral atresia, or cloacal plate malformations. It is estimated that half of all congenital abdominal masses are urinary tract in origin. The prognosis varies widely from very good in the case of unilateral ureteropelvic junction obstruction to very poor in the case of bilateral total obstruction or bladder outlet obstruction with severe oligohydramnios. Obstructive uropathy lends itself to prenatal diagnosis since the accumulation of urine above the point of obstruction and distention of the system is easily seen with ultrasound. Consideration of prenatal treatment is based on the assumption that progressive hydronephrosis is detrimental to fetal well-being, or that the severe oligohydramnios associated with complete obstruction contributes to pulmonary hypoplasia and significantly decreases the probability of neonatal survival.

Ureteropelvic junction obstruction. Ureteropelvic junction obstruction producing unilateral fetal hydronephrosis in the vast majority of cases is not appropriate for antenatal manipulation.[6,17,18,28] In most cases, expectant management with neonatal evaluation and treatment will result in a successful outcome of the pregnancy and even survival of the affected kidney.[28] In the majority of cases, the unilateral ureteropelvic junction obstruction results in no clinical abnormality in the pregnancy. The sonographic appearance can vary from mild dilatation of the renal pelvis to large anechoic (echo-free) masses. Complete obstruction can result in either a very dilated renal pelvis with severe caliectasis (Fig. 4-3), or in the development of a retroperitoneal urinoma. Both of these possibilities can influence bowel function and lead to

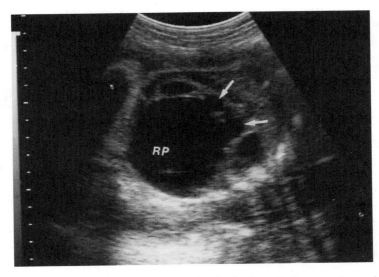

Fig. 4-3 Complete ureteropelvic junction obstruction in the fetus. In the case of complete obstruction, the renal pelvis *(RP)* can grow to extreme size, and the caliectasis *(arrows)* is severe.

polyhydramnios and preterm labor.[15] Antenatal drainage or diversion of such large masses may be of benefit in improving amniotic fluid volume equilibrium and diminishing the risk of premature delivery by decreasing the extrinsic pressure on fetal bowel.[15]

Each case must be evaluated individually for the need for treatment. Typically, these unilateral cystic masses enlarge and influence amniotic fluid dynamics until early in the third trimester, but after that their volume stabilizes or even diminishes. Therefore, consideration of antenatal treatment must take into account the gestational age as well as the clinical consequences of treatment vs. no treatment.

Bladder outlet obstruction. Fetal bladder outlet obstruction resulting in oligohydramnios associated with progressive fetal hydronephrosis before 32 weeks' gestation represents a fetal condition that might benefit from antenatal intervention (Fig. 4-4).[14,18] Not every affected fetus, however, will benefit from diversion catheterization, and careful evaluation by a team of experienced clinicians is necessary to avoid unnecessary treatment of infants with no hope of benefit.

At least three distinct causes of fetal bladder outlet obstruction are known, including posterior urethral valves, urethral atresia, and persistant cloaca or cloacal plate anomaly. The prognosis is very different for these three, even given successful prenatal diversion therapy; therefore, efforts have focused on discriminating one from the other.

Bladder outlet obstruction characterized by a very distended bladder detected between 20 and 30

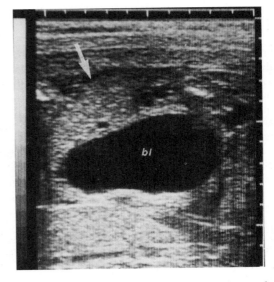

Fig. 4-4 The fetal bladder in cases of complete outlet obstruction can grow to quite a large size. The bladder *(bl)* is seen here in a fetus with posterior urethral valves. Note the severe oligohydramnios, as amniotic fluid is reduced to only a thin rim at the edge of the fetus *(arrow)*.

weeks' gestation with hydronephrosis (Fig. 4-5) and severe oligohydramnios is likely to have resulted from urethral valves and is most likely to benefit from intervention. Urethral atresia, which also produces a distended bladder and oligohydramnios, is more often detected earlier in gestation either with routine ultrasound or as a result of

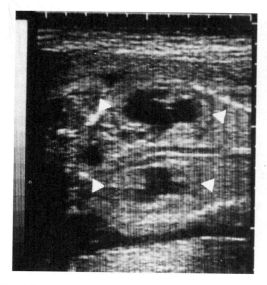

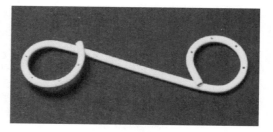

Fig. 4-6 Harrison bladder stent, a 5 Fr double pigtail catheter.

Fig. 4-5 Hydronephrosis characteristic of posterior urethral valves. The kidneys *(triangles)* are both shown, and the central caliectasis is apparent. The calices are dilated with urine that appears dark (anechoic).

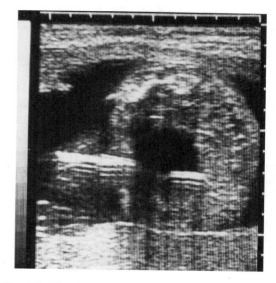

Fig. 4-7 After the removal of the cannula, the shunt can be seen extending from the dilated bladder to the amniotic cavity. The amniotic cavity was filled for purposes of placement with warmed normal saline.

an elevated maternal serum alphafetoprotein. Urethral atresia produces small echodense dysplastic kidneys instead of enlarged hydronephrotic kidneys, and prenatal intervention has little hope of improving the rather bleak prognosis. Cloacal plate anomalies produce a large fluid-filled mass in the fetal abdomen analogous to a bladder, but in contrast to the central symmetrical bladder of urethral obstruction, the mass is typically eccentric, irregular, and asymmetrical. The prognosis for infants with cloacal plate anomalies is very poor regardless of treatment.

Urinary tract interventions

Obstructive uropathy has been treated with needle aspiration as well as with indwelling diversion catheterization. Two different continuous drainage techniques have been reported; both result in the placement of a small diversion catheter between the obstructed fetal urinary tract and the sterile amniotic cavity. The Harrison bladder stent is a 5-Fr double-pigtail catheter (Fig. 4-6) loaded over a needle-trocar that is inserted percutaneously into the obstructed organ using ultrasound guidance.[18] The needle is removed as the catheter is advanced by using a sliding pusher. Difficulty is often encountered from frictional resistance between both maternal and fetal tissues and the advancing catheter. The alternative system uses a similar catheter but delivers it through the lumen of a thin-walled 13-gauge cannula advanced into the obstructed or-

gan also under ultrasound guidance (Fig. 4-7). The placement of a catheter by either method is made more difficult by severe oligohydramnios associated with the bladder obstruction. If this is considered a significant problem, warm sterile saline solution can be injected to expand the amniotic cavity, facilitating the placement of the catheter.

The potential complications of percutaneous fetal bladder catheterization include premature labor, premature rupture of membranes, and catheter displacement or malfunction. The catheters are flexible, and may be removed by fetal actions or displaced by rubbing on the uterine wall as the fetus turns. Therefore, after the placement of such a catheter, close follow-up is required to document continued functional integrity of the catheter. If catheter displacement or malfunction is detected, consideration of repeat catheterization is appropriate if the pregnancy is still sufficiently early in gestation to make delivery an unattractive option.

In 1982, the exteriorization of a fetus with bladder obstruction and bilateral hydronephrosis for surgical creation of bilateral cutaneous nephrostomies was first reported.[29] This was accomplished by laparotomy and hysterotomy as described for some earlier procedures for the treatment of fetal hemolytic disease by exchange transfusion. The exteriorization and nephrostomy procedure was technically successful, but the infant died of pulmonary hypoplasia after birth. Although it is remarkable that the pregnancy was sustained after such a significant uterine intrusion, the immediate surgical risks to the mother and the implications for subsequent obstetric care, such as the necessity for such subsequent pregnancy to be delivered by cesarean section because of the danger of uterine rupture during labor, are serious drawbacks to this technique. Furthermore, the availability of feasible and less radical methods of diverting urine, such as percutaneous catheterization, make exteriorization of the fetus for direct treatment less attractive.

Percutaneous umbilical vein blood sampling

In 1982 Bang et al[8] first described the successful ultrasonic guidance of a narrow-gauge needle to the umbilical vein within the fetal liver for aspiration and transfusion. Since that time, multiple investigators have reported the successful use of this technique for acquisition of fetal blood samples for a variety of diagnostic indications.[2-5,9-11] The use of this technique for direct fetal blood transfusions has gained wide popularity and in many centers has replaced the older intraperitoneal approach (Fig. 4-7).[10,11,16]

Other possible interventions

The precise guidance of aspiration or biopsy needles to specific fetal organs enables a wide variety of both diagnostic and therapeutic procedures.[30] The successful aspiration of fetal thoracic cysts, pleural effusions, and ascites has been reported. Fetal skin, muscle, and liver biopsies, using ultrasound-guided biopsy needles, are now possible.

ANESTHETIC MANAGEMENT

Fetal manipulation may involve painful stimuli. There is therefore a requirement to provide not only a reduction in movement but also analgesia for two patients: mother and fetus. The use of analgesic and anesthetic and neuromuscular blocking agents to facilitate the fetal manipulation reviewed in the previous section of this chapter is aimed at providing relief of maternal pain and anxiety as well as a motionless fetus, also free of pain. There is no longer any controversy whether the fetus perceives pain. It is now generally accepted that when

fetal intervention is undertaken and is potentially painful to the fetus, analgesia should be provided.[31] This knowledge has been gained from studies on the preterm infant[32] as well as from in-utero studies in animals. There is therefore a significant advantage to the presence of a fetal circulation, since maternally administered anesthetic and analgesic agents will pass to the fetus. It has been assumed that in most cases this transplacental analgesia and sedation are sufficient to block or reduce the lasting effects of the painful stimuli associated with fetal interventions. The major concern remains maternal safety, and medications should be tailored to the mother's needs with the fetus a secondary but important consideration.[33] It is not appropriate to induce significant central depression without careful attention to maternal safety. It is mandatory to use the full range of physiologic monitors when both conscious sedation and general anesthesia are administered.

Minor surgical intervention

Percutaneous placement of a needle is associated with pain; the larger the needle, the greater the pain. It is possible to minimize, but not eliminate, such pain by local infiltration of the puncture site and deeper tissues with local anesthetic. Peritoneal or uterine mural pain may not be totally blocked. Experience has demonstrated, however, that the discomfort attributed to deeper tissues is not great, and in most cases this pain is tolerable with either no analgesia or a minimum degree. In either case it is prudent to have the availability of analgesic supplementation and the appropriate degree of monitoring to ensure safety.

Major surgical intervention

Laparotomy followed by hysterotomy requires a major anesthetic technique. Adequate anesthesia for laparotomy may be provided by using a balanced endotracheal technique. Regional anesthesia may also be satisfactory but will frequently require drugs to provide supplementary sedation and analgesia. In the context of major surgical intervention, spinal and epidural analgesia will be necessary to ensure a pain-free patient who will remain still during the procedure. Hypotension, a common complication of regional anesthesia, may be hazardous to the fetus as well as to the mother. Every effort should be made to maintain maternal hemodynamic homeostasis. It should be remembered that regional anesthesia will not provide the fetus with any degree of immobilization. This factor will have to be accounted for by appropriate drug administration directly to the fetus.

Balanced endotracheal anesthesia with careful attention to the adequacy of analgesia is, in the majority of cases, the technique of choice if major operative intervention is undertaken. Initially the emphasis of the balanced technique should be with a halogenated agent such as isoflurane. The halogenated inhalation agents are very efficient uterine relaxants, and these will allow the surgeon safe access to the fetus. Use of inhalation anesthetic up to 1 MAC should be safe for the fetus.[34] At a later stage of the procedure the concentration of the inhalation agent may be reduced and the level of anesthesia maintained with the intravenous supplementation. These conclusions do not exclude the use of other techniques on an individual basis when specific advantages are anticipated.

Anxiety relief

Maternal anxiety associated with fetal surgery can have a significant impact on outcome. The anxiety may arise from concern for the seriousness of the fetal condition as well as from fear of pain and further complications from the procedure. Such anxiety varies greatly in intensity and can directly complicate the procedure. Sudden unexpected maternal movements during the procedure can lead directly to failure. Often only minimal sedation is needed to provide adequate maternal relaxation. It is unnecessary and potentially hazardous to routinely administer heavy parenteral analgesia when a lesser degree would be adequate.

Patient education remains the most reliable source of anxiety reduction. Careful informative preparation for the procedure by the operative physician can minimize the need for pharmacologic agents. A review of each step of the procedure is necessary, and if appropriate the patient may tour the operating area. A confident and informed relationship between the physician and the patient is the safest method of anxiety control. If light sedation is to be undertaken, the presence of a support person may be helpful in reducing anxiety. If adequate anxiety reduction and analgesia cannot be achieved with minimal parenteral drug administration, consideration should be given to general anesthesia, to preserve maximal airway protection as well as optimal maternal movement control.

Fetal movement

Fetal movement during antenatal intervention poses a significant risk to the fetus. When a diverting catheter for fetal obstructive uropathy is being placed, fetal movement makes appropriate placement more difficult and increases the probability of technical failure. Fetal movement at the time of percutaneous umbilical vein blood sampling could result in difficulty gaining appropriate intravenous access. Further subsequent displacement of a correctly placed needle may occur. Such technical failures require undesirable multiple needle placements, increasing the risk of catastrophic events including umbilical cord hematoma.

General anesthesia

General anesthesia provides advantages related to both mother and fetus. Adequate relief of maternal anxiety and pain can be reliably achieved. Reduction in fetal pain perception should be achieved by transplacental passage of maternal anesthetic agents. Some degree of reduced fetal movement will also occur. The maternal airway must be protected by the placement of an endotracheal tube. It should be remembered, however, that there are risks involved in the use of an endotracheal tube. The risks include aspiration during induction and esophageal intubation, as well as failed intubation. Failed intubation may lead to aspiration or hypoxia if it is not dealt with promptly. The incidence of inappropriate placement of an endotracheal tube has been significantly reduced by the use of pulse oximetry and end-tidal carbon dioxide monitoring. The use of these monitors is now part of the standard that is accepted for safe general anesthesia. Balanced general anesthesia using a combination of inhalation agents, narcotics, drugs, and neuromuscular blockers will provide adequate analgesia and amnesia. Induction of general anesthesia is frequently associated with transient hypertension secondary to an increased catecholamine release. This has the potential to interfere with the uterine circulation and hence to jeopardize the fetal oxygen supply. Fortunately this period of hypertension is usually brief and can if necessary be curtailed by adequate preparation and skillful induction. It should therefore rarely produce a significant problem. Maintenance with a halogenated anesthetic agent may be associated with maternal hypotension, this should be managed appropriately to avoid fetal oxygen deprivation. Uterine relaxation will also occur but is unlikely to be a problem during fetal surgery.

The introduction of the laryngeal mask airway (LMA) has provided an important tool in anesthetic management. With its ease of use and relative safety it might be an attractive alternative method in the management of anesthesia for short fetal surgery. The LMA avoids many of the potential problems of endotracheal placement. It establishes a reliable channel to provide oxygenation an anesthesia to the mother. Currently, however, the LMA is not recommended for use in patients with the potential of having a full stomach and therefore being at risk of aspiration. Unfortunately this group of patients includes the majority of patients undergoing fetal surgery. In the future, with its increased use and improvements in design, LMA may become a valuable asset in this field.

New anesthetic drugs are being made available. Some of these drugs have made a significant impact on anesthetic practice. Such a drug is the intravenous anesthetic agent propofol. Propofol has several properties that make it a very attractive agent for use in fetal surgery. Propofol has been used very successfully for both conscious sedation and general anesthesia. As yet the Food and Drug Administration (FDA) has not released propofol for use during pregnancy. If and when propofol is released, it should play an important role in anesthesia for fetal surgery.

Clearly the use of general anesthesia requires the presence of trained anesthetic personnel with a full operating room setting that includes the ability to monitor to an expected standard of care. This will inevitably significantly increase the cost of such procedures. For major surgery, maternal postoperative pain relief can be accomplished by using epidural morphine or intravenous patient-controlled analgesia with narcotic drugs of choice.

Maternal sedation and local anesthesia

Sedation combined with local infiltration is not adequate for major surgical interventions but will provide pain relief in the case of percutaneous needle aspiration or catheter insertion. The method is inexpensive and avoids most of the risks of major general anesthesia. The chief danger is that when sufficient sedation is administered to reduce fetal movement, a light plane of anesthesia may be produced in a patient with an unprotected airway. This leaves the patient at risk for aspiration of gastric contents. When this method is selected, any of several sedative agents may be chosen, all of which cross the placenta and can be found in fetal plasma at near maternal levels. The most commonly used drugs are the benzodiazepines, including diazepam and midazolam, and the narcotics including morphine sulfate and fentanyl.

The problem of fetal movement remains, however, even with large doses of these drugs. The temptation to repeat the doses at short intervals whenever fetal movement occurs also remains. Whenever sedation is the technique of choice, it is essential that the maternal airway be monitored by a responsible observer who is not the operator.

Local anesthesia with fetal paralysis

Since local anesthesia with minimal parenteral analgesia provides adequate pain relief for the mother in most cases, the greatest remaining problem is that of arresting fetal movement. Paralysis is a logical consideration. The intravenous injection of curare into the fetal circulation to transiently arrest fetal movement for the purpose of promoting the success of intrauterine transfusions was first reported by de Crespigney in 1983.[9] He reported 16 transfusions in four fetuses, using ultrasound-guided percutaneous venipuncture of the umbilical vein within the fetal liver. He administered 3 mg curare intravenously with great success and with no observed complications. Seeds et al reported in 1986 the first use of pancuronium bromide for the same purpose in six cases with no complications.[35] Other investigators since have confirmed the safe application of this technique for the temporary arrest of fetal movement during a variety of fetal interventions using both the intramuscular and the intravenous route of administration.[36]

Both curare and pancuronium bromide have been used with safety and effectiveness. Neither will cross the placenta in significant amounts and will therefore not lead to maternal neuromuscular blockade. Both produce effective fetal paralysis from 2 to 4 hours. The dose of drug must be adjusted depending on the route of administration, either intravenous or intramuscular.

During percutaneous fetal umbilical vein blood sampling, it may be necessary for the aspiration needle to cross the amniotic cavity. The needle is therefore at risk for displacement should fetal movement occur, and consideration of fetal paralysis is appropriate. The paralytic agent may be administered either with a separate needle injection intramuscularly into a thigh or shoulder, or the agent may be given when the needle enters the umbilical vein. Although the intramuscular route requires a second needle puncture, it offers the advantage that paralysis occurs before entry of a needle into the umbilical vein. The advantage of intravenous injection is a possible reduction in the number of needle passes, but the disadvantage is that fetal movement occurring before the paralysis could delay the acquisition of intravenous access or cause dislodgment of the needle before adequate paralysis. The dosage used in early reports for the third trimester was 3 mg curare and 0.4 to 0.6 mg pancuronium bromide.

Use of local anesthetic agents for the mother in the presence of fetal paralysis offers the advantage of maximum reduction of fetal movement with minimal maternal airway problems. Fetal paralysis may, however, require an additional needle puncture and does not provide any fetal anesthesia or analgesia. Furthermore, if as a result of a complication the fetus requires delivery, the neonate will be paralyzed and will require assisted ventila-

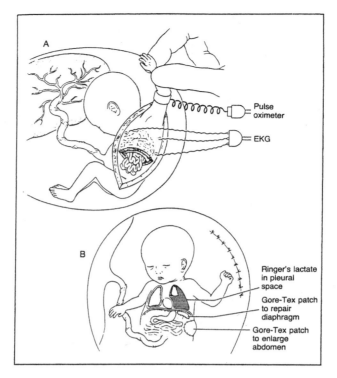

Fig. 4-8 The fetus was continuously monitored by pulse oximetry and electrocardiography (EKG). (From Harrison MR, et al: Successful repair in utero of a fetal diaphragmatic hernia after removal of herniated viscera from the left thorax. *N Engl J Med* 1990; 322(22):1582.)

tion until the paralysis is reversed. This is not a life-threatening problem for the infant if the situation is anticipated and appropriate resuscitation equipment and personnel are available.

Either light or no maternal sedation along with local anesthesia and fetal paralysis is also appropriate for percutaneous fetal umbilical vein sampling and intrauterine intravascular blood transfusion. Fetal paralysis alone may also be appropriate to optimize either magnetic resonance images or tomographic radiography.

Considerations of safety and the adequacy of a given technique must include effects on both the mother and the fetus. The use of heavy sedation is not only dangerous because of potential compromise of maternal airway but also because it does not ensure the arrest of fetal movement. General anesthesia is indicated for the rare case of major intervention or unusual anxiety unrelieved by light sedation.

Fetal monitoring

Monitoring of the fetus may be important during major surgery. This has included (1) pulse oximetry, (2) intermittent blood gas determination, and (3) fetal heart rate monitoring. Direct fetal ECG

monitoring has also been performed in a few cases[37] (Fig. 4-8).

Surgical manipulation can induce uterine contractions and thus increase uterine tone. Uterine contractions, if strong enough, can decrease the uteroplacental blood flow. Hence, uterine relaxation may be important, especially for prolonged operation. Different agents used for this purpose are:

1. Inhalation anesthetic agents
2. β-mimetic tocolytic agents such as terbutaline sulfate or ritodrine
3. Magnesium sulfate
4. Prostaglandin synthetase inhibitor (i.e., indomethacin)

Inhalation anesthetics and magnesium sulfate combinations may be an effective uterine relaxant during a major uterine manipulation, whereas β-mimetic drugs can be used in the postoperative period. Indomethacin has been used with success without fetal problems before 34 weeks' gestation.[38]

REFERENCES

1. Liley AW: Intrauterine transfusion of foetus in haemolytic disease. *Br Med J* 1963; 2:1107.

2. Daffos F, Capella-Pavlovsky M, Forestier F: Fetal blood sampling via the umbilical cord using a needle guided by ultrasound. *Prenat Diagn* 1983; 3:271.

3. Hsieh F, Chang F, Ko T, et al: Percutaneous ultrasound guided fetal blood sampling in the management of non-immune hydrops fetalis. *Am J Obstet Gynecol* 1987; 157:44.

4. Hobbins JC, Grannum PA, Romero R, et al: Percutaneous umbilical blood sampling. *Am J Obstet Gynecol* 1985; 152:1.

5. Daffos F, Capella-Pavlovsky M, Forestier F: Fetal blood sampling during pregnancy with use of a needle guided by ultrasound: A study of 606 consecutive cases. *Am J Obstet Gynecol* 1985; 153:655.

6. Vintzileos AM, Campbell WA, et al: Antenatal evaluation and management of ultrasonically detected fetal anomalies. *Obstet Gynecol* 1987; 69:640.

7. Hadlock FP, Deter RL, Carpenter R, et al: Review: Sonography of fetal urinary tract anomalies. *AJR* 1981; 137:261.

8. Bang J, Bock JE, Trolle D: Ultrasound guided fetal intravenous transfusion for severe rhesus haemolytic disease. *Br Med J [Clin Res]* 1982; 284:373.

9. de Crespigny CL, Robinson HP, Quinn M, et al: Ultrasound-guided fetal blood transfusion for severe rhesus isoimmunization. *Obstet Gynecol* 1985; 66:529.

10. Seeds JW, Bowes WA: Ultrasound-guided fetal intravascular transfusion in severe rhesus immunization. *Am J Obstet Gynecol* 1986; 154:1105.

11. Berkowitz RL, Chitkara U, Goldberg JD, et al: Intrauterine intravascular transfusions for severe red blood cell isoimmunization: Ultrasound-guided percutaneous approach. *Am J Obstet Gynecol* 1986; 155:574.

12. Birnholz JC, Frigoletto FD: Antenatal treatment of hydrocephalus. *N Engl J Med* 1981; 303:1021.

13. Kirkinen P, Jouppila P, Tuononen S: Repeated transabdominal renocenteses in a case of fetal hydronephrotic kidney. *Am J Obstet Gynecol* 1982; 142:1049.

14. Manning FA, Harman CR, Lange IR, et al: Antepartum chronic fetal vesicoamniotic shunts for obstructive uropathy: A report of two cases. *Am J Obstet Gynecol* 1983; 145:819.

15. Seeds JW, Cefalo RC, Herbert WNP, et al: Hydramnios and maternal renal failure: Relief with fetal therapy. *Obstet Gynecol* 1984; 64:26S.

16. Grannum PA, Copel JA, Plaxe SC, et al: In utero exchange transfusion by direct intravascular injection in severe erythroblastosis fetalis. *N Engl J Med* 1986; 314:1431.

17. Berkowitz RL, Glickman MG, Smith GJW, et al: Fetal urinary tract obstruction: What is the role of surgical intervention in utero? *Am J Obstet Gynecol* 1982; 144:367.

18. Harrison MR, Filly RA, Parer JT, et al: Management of the fetus with a urinary tract malformation. *JAMA* 1981; 246:635.

19. Clewell WH, Johnson ML, Meier PR, et al: A surgical approach to the treatment of fetal hydrocephalus. *N Engl J Med* 1982; 306:1320.

20. Anand KJS, Hickey PR: Pain and its effects in the human neonate and fetus. *N Engl J Med* 1987; 317:1321.

21. Asensio SH, Figuero-Longo JG, Pelegrina IA: Intrauterine exchange transfusion. *Am J Obstet Gynecol* 1966; 95:1129.

22. Hobbins JC, Mahoney MJ: In-utero diagnosis of hemoglobinopathies: Technique for obtaining pure fetal blood. *N Engl J Med* 1974; 290:1065.

23. Rodeck CH, Kemp JR, Helman CA, et al: Direct intravascular fetal blood transfusion by fetoscopy in severe rhesus isoimmunization. *Lancet* 1981; 1:625.

24. Rodeck CH, Nicolaides KH, Warsof SL, et al: The management of severe rhesus isoimmunization by fetoscopic intravascular transfusions. *Am J Obstet Gynecol* 1984; 150:769.

25. Manning FA: *International Fetal Surgery Registry.* 59 Emily St, Winnipeg, Canada, R3E OW3, May 1986.

26. Special Report of the International Fetal Surgery Registry: Catheter shunts for fetal hydronephrosis and hydrocephalus. *N Engl J Med* 1985; 315:336.

27. Chervenak FA, Duncan C, Ment LR, et al: Outcome of fetal ventriculomegaly. *Lancet* 1984; 1:179.

28. Mandell J, Kinard HW, Mittelstaedt CA, et al: Prenatal diagnosis of unilateral hydronephrosis with early postnatal reconstruction. *J Urol* 1984; 132:303.

29. Golbus MS, Harrison MR, Filly RA, et al: In utero treatment of urinary tract obstruction. *Am J Obstet Gynecol* 1982; 142:383.

30. Asher JB, Sabbagha RE, Tamura RK, et al: Fetal pulmonary cyst: Intrauterine diagnosis and management. *Am J Obstet Gynecol* 1985; 151:97.

31. Anand KJS, Brownk MJ, Cavson RC, et al: Can the human neonate mount an endocrine and metabolic response to surgery? *J Pediatr Surg* 1985; 20:41.

32. Anand KJS, Sippel WG, Aynsley-Green A: Randomized trial of fentanyl anaesthesia in preterm neonates undergoing surgery: Effects on the stress response. *Lancet* 1987; 1:243.

33. Spielman FJ, Seeds JW, Corke BC: Anaesthesia for fetal surgery. *Anaesthesia* 1984; 39:756.

34. Rosen MA: Anesthesia for fetal procedures and surgery, in Shnider SM, Gershon L (eds): *Anesthesia for Obstetrics.* Baltimore, Williams & Wilkins, 1993, pp 281-295.

35. Seeds JW, Corke BC, Spielman FJ: Prevention of fetal movement during invasive procedures with pancuronium bromide. *Am J Obstet Gynecol* 1986; 155:818.

36. Moise KJ, Carpenter RJ, Deter RL, et al: The use of fetal neuromuscular blockade during intrauterine procedures. *Am J Obstet Gynecol* 1987; 157:874.

37. Harrison MR, Adzick NS, Longaker MT, et al: Successful repair in utero of a fetal diaphragmatic hernia after removal of herniated viscera from the left thorax. *N Engl J Med* 1990; 322:1582.

38. Dudley DKL, Hardie MJ: Fetal and neonatal effects of indomethacin used as a tocolytic agent. *Am J Obstet Gynecol* 1985; 151:181.

5 The Pregnant Teenager

Monica M. Jones and M. Mark Taslimi

The pregnant teenager presents in labor with a host of potential risks that merit special attention by the anesthesiologist and the obstetrician. Pre-eclampsia, infants with a low birth weight, and inadequate prenatal care are but some of the complications that make the pregnant teenager a potentially high-risk patient.

In addition to medical problems, legal problems such as incest and rape-related pregnancies, as well as paternity and adoption concerns, may have to be addressed. This chapter addresses the problems that are frequent in a teenage pregnancy and discusses the related anesthesia considerations.

GENERAL CONSIDERATIONS
Epidemiology

In 1988, the U.S. National Center for Health Statistics reported over one million pregnancies among teenagers, of which 489,000 resulted in live births.[1]

Between 1986 and 1991, the rate of adolescent pregnancy (ages 10 to 17) in the state of Tennessee increased from 24.7 to 25.6 per thousand population. A number of these pregnancies are lost to miscarriages and voluntary abortions. In 1991 the birth rate among adolescents was 18.4 per thousand population in Tennessee (Tennessee Department of Health, 1991 Health Statistics).

Prenatal care and obstetric management

Lack of adequate prenatal care often hampers timely screening, detection, and treatment of pregnancy complications among adolescents. Inadequate prenatal care is twice as common among teenagers compared with women age 35 or older.[2] As a result, many teenagers arrive at the labor and delivery unit with inadequate documentation of both gestational age and maternal and fetal health status. Reports of screening for diabetes mellitus, chronic hypertension, underlying kidney diseases, and other organ system abnormalities may be missing, and the state of fetal growth and development in relation to gestational age may be unknown.

Low birth weight

Each year in the United States approximately 250,000 babies (7.1%) are born weighing less than 2,500 g.[3] The low birth weight (LBW) rate has been reported to be 14.5% in girls under 15 years of age, compared with 6.9% in older women.[4] In Tennessee, the highest rate of LBW (15.8%) was observed among black teenagers (Tennessee Department of Health, 1991 Health Statistics). LBW may be even more frequent among such specific populations as inner-city teenagers. The LBW rate was reported to be 26.9% among young black pregnant teens in the city of Houston.[5] To put this in perspective, one should note that only Laos, India, Sri Lanka, and Bangladesh have higher LBW rates than some pockets of inner-city populations in America.[6]

LBW babies may be preterm and/or small for gestational age, and the differentiation of the two may be impossible in the absence of early and adequate prenatal care. LBW babies, regardless of cause, are at a higher risk for intrapartum distress. Furthermore, LBW infants are nearly three times more likely to die within the first 28 days of life.[7]

Sexually transmitted diseases

Adventures in sexual activity by teenagers often lead to unwanted pregnancy and sexually transmitted diseases (STDs). When all STDs are considered together, it is possible that they represent one of the most common medical complications of pregnancy, especially in an indigent, adolescent, urban population plagued by drug abuse and prostitution.[7] In the prenatal clinics of Parkland Memorial Hospital in Dallas, Texas, gonorrhea affects 2% to 3% of all gravidas, syphilis 2% to 3%, genital herpes 1%, human immunodeficiency virus (HIV) 0.1%, and chlamydial infection 12%.[8] STDs are commonly asymptomatic in pregnant patients. Appropriate screening tests combined with diligent and universal protective measures are necessary to protect both the patient and her medical caregiver. A more ominous concern is the presence of HIV in teenagers who are pregnant. Of one million U.S. citizens who are infected with HIV, at least 80,000 are women of childbearing age.[9] In Houston, 13%

of HIV-positive pregnant patients were teenagers.[10] The rate of new infections is increasing more rapidly among women than among men, and women comprise over 11% of those infected in the United States today.

Drug abuse

Studies of legal and illegal substance exposure are difficult because of the sensitive nature of the behaviors involved. According to The National Institute of Drug Abuse, the rate of substance exposure during pregnancy in 1990 was as follows: cocaine 4.5%, marijuana 17.4%, cigarettes 27.6%, and alcohol 73%.[11] The rate of substance abuse is generally lower among teenagers compared with older women.[11,12] However, one study of adolescent mothers reported a 17% rate of cocaine use among inner-city pregnant teenagers.[13] Tobacco, alcohol, and a variety of illicit drugs have significant maternal and embryo-fetal adverse effects. Maternal risks include an increased risk of placental abruption, central nervous system damage, intracranial hemorrhage, and hepatic or renal damage. The majority of these substances cross the placenta with the affected pregnancies exhibiting growth restriction, congenital anomalies, and neonatal withdrawal syndrome.[14]

Hypertensive disorders

Pregnancy-induced hypertension (PIH) often affects nulliparous women, and adolescent pregnancies are most often nulliparous. PIH affects 5% of all pregnancies. However, Battaglia reported a 27.8% rate of PIH in 15-year old patients.[15] In another report, Duenhoelter et al showed a 35% incidence of PIH among very young patients.[16] PIH may be associated with uteroplacental insufficiency and a significantly decreased fetal tolerance to hypotension induced by regional anesthesia or supine positioning of the mother.

Cephalopelvic disproportion

Adolescents may be considered to be at increased risk for cephalopelvic disproportion (CPD). This risk has not been confirmed in current studies, although a smaller pelvic capacity is noted in patients with early menarche, and this could contribute to CPD in primiparous women younger than 15 years of age.[17]

Sexual abuse

Young victims of sexual abuse and incest typically present late in pregnancy. These patients are often reluctant to accept an examination even by female staff members. Ultrasound examination may play an important role, allowing noninvasive evaluation of these patients and their fetus. Social workers and psychologists should be involved in prenatal care. During labor such patients may be optimally managed with epidural analgesia for maximum pain relief.

Medicolegal concerns

The nature of obstetrics is complicated by difficult legal peril for both the obstetrician and the anesthesiologist. Consent must be obtained before obstetric and anesthesia care is given; this raises concerns of legal competence in adolescents.[18] In most states the age of majority to consent is 18. In some states such as Texas and Tennessee, however, a pregnant minor is considered "emancipated" and legally must sign any consent for treatment or anesthesia. If in question, the parent and adolescent could both sign the consent. Should questions arise concerning the law in other states, most hospitals have legal counsel available to address related questions.

Psychological support

Psychological support from a person close to the adolescent parturient is extremely helpful during the delivery process, whether vaginal delivery or cesarean section. Labor and its attendant pain may be extremely frightening to the young parturient, who may or may not comprehend what is occurring. This "liaison" person will frequently have the best communication established with the adolescent parturient at times when patient cooperation is needed. The support person should be chosen solely by the adolescent parturient. She may choose someone other than a family member, especially if the pregnancy resulted from sexual abuse by someone in that family. The patient should be asked in a private confidential setting whom she wishes to be or not be present.

Prenatal preparation

If prenatal care is obtained, the adolescent parturient and her support person should be encouraged to attend childbirth preparation classes. This will help educate the young parturient as to what to expect during her labor as well as to provide an opportunity to discuss mechanisms for coping with the pain.

A visit to the labor and delivery area during the prenatal preparation period will allow the young parturient to observe the area and meet the nursing staff during a nonstressful time. This is also a convenient time for the preanesthetic visit to discuss anesthesia options.

ANESTHETIC CONSIDERATIONS FOR LABOR AND VAGINAL DELIVERY ANALGESIA
Preparation

Intravenous access may be a challenge in the adolescent parturient, especially if she is mentally impaired. The use of a local anesthetic agent, or possibly EMLA cream if time allows, will facilitate catheter placement.

Parenteral analgesics

Intravenous (and, to a lesser extent, intramuscular analgesics) are the most commonly administered forms of analgesia in obstetric units. These drugs result in some degree of sedation in the parturient, and this may be helpful during early labor. However, as labor progresses and the contractions become more painful, parenteral medications relieve the pain less effectively. Narcotic administration must be carefully timed to minimize the risk of neonatal depression. The agonist-antagonist class of pain medication has become widely used because of the low degree of placental passage and therefore lessened neonatal effects.

Lumbar epidural analgesia

Epidural analgesia is frequently used in adolescent parturients because of its ability to provide profound pain relief for the first and second stages of labor. Initially, the adolescent parturient is usually hesitant in considering epidural analgesia. However, as labor progresses and the pain increases, she frequently requests additional assistance as parenteral medications provide less complete pain relief. Her support person can be helpful with positioning and coaching during placement of the block. Explaining to the patient what she can expect during placement of the epidural needle and catheter is of paramount importance in gaining her cooperation.

Since these parturients may be smaller in stature than their older counterparts, judgment must be exercised in choosing the appropriate dose of local anesthetic. Bromage noted that epidural dose requirements are linearly related to age, with the maximum dose needed at age 18½. By use of a regression equation, Bromage[19] calculated the volume per spinal segment, using 2% lidocaine, to be:

No. of milliliters (ml) per spinal segment to be blocked = 0.1063 + Age in years × 0.07531 ml

During pregnancy, the epidural dose needed is approximately two thirds of the nonpregnant dose. Therefore, the above calculated dose would need to be adjusted appropriately. No studies have been done concerning the optimal dose for a labor epidural analgesia in the pregnant adolescent who is of smaller stature.

Providing pain relief while minimizing the sensory and motor loss allows the adolescent parturient to feel the least intrusion. Initiation of the epidural analgesia with bupivacaine 0.25% and fentanyl 50 mcg followed by a low-dose continuous infusion (bupivacaine 0.125% or 0.0625% with fentanyl 1 to 2 mcg/ml at 6 to 10 ml/hour) will accomplish these goals. Maintenance of a segmental block with minimal sacral blockade will allow the adolescent parturient to sense sacral pressure and therefore also the urge to push during the second stage of labor. An additional dose of local anesthetic can then be given when sacral analgesia is needed at the time of delivery.

Epidural analgesia may be specifically indicated in the teenage parturient in rare situations. Occasionally, a young laboring patient will refuse vaginal examinations because of fear resulting from one or more episodes of sexual abuse. If perineal analgesia is established with the epidural block, these parturients usually will then allow the obstetrician to perform a vaginal examination.

ANESTHETIC CONSIDERATIONS FOR CESAREAN SECTION

The same basic anesthetic principles apply to the adolescent as to other parturients (i.e., left uterine displacement, preoperative administration of an antacid). However, a few points should be specifically considered.

Regional anesthesia (epidural or spinal) in the teenage parturient requires extensive psychological support and explanation of the events occurring (i.e., sensation of pressure intraoperatively before delivery). The presence of the adolescent parturient's support person will prove invaluable during this time period. Preoperative supplementation with intravenous sedatives, such as diphenhydramine hydrochloride (Benadryl), and intraoperative use of oxygen (70%) and nitrous oxide (30%) will help to allay the patient's apprehension. Administration of a benzodiazepine (i.e., midazolam) after delivery is also useful.

Dosing for an epidural anesthesia was discussed in the previous section. A higher concentration and volume is needed, however, for a cesarean section. As with older parturients, a sensory level between T_4 and T_6 is necessary.

Norris et al[20] investigated the effect of patient height on the level of sensory block when subarachnoid anesthesia was administered for cesarean section. He reported no difference in cephalad sensory levels in women between 4 feet 10 inches and 5 feet 8 inches in height when 15 mg of bupivacaine was administered with dextrose combined with 0.15 mg of morphine.

No correlation could be found between the level of sensory block and the factors of weight, body mass index, vertebral column length, and height. The authors suggested that, for a subarachnoid block, patient position and baricity of the anesthetic solution may be more important determinants of sensory level than patient height.

If the teenage parturient is extremely anxious, mentally impaired, or refuses a regional anesthetic, a general anesthetic may be necessary for the cesarean section. Two points in particular should be considered. First, the "usual" 250 mg induction dose of thiopental (Pentothal) may be excessive in the teenage parturient. The appropriate thiopental dose should be calculated at 3 to 4 mg/kg to minimize the risk of neonatal depression. Second, the teenage parturient may require a smaller endotracheal tube (5.0 to 6.0 mm cuffed tube). Pregnancy-induced hypertension and its accompanying laryngeal edema can further compromise the airway and affect the endotracheal tube size.

POSTANESTHESIA CARE

Postoperative pain therapy is an essential part of the management of teenage parturients. Epidural or subarachnoid opioids provide excellent analgesia following cesarean section, provided the nursing care is available for appropriate monitoring. This method is also helpful in the vaginal delivery patient who has a third- or fourth-degree perineal tear. In other vaginal delivery patients or post-cesarean section patients without a regional anesthetic, parenteral narcotic agents may be used.

Early interaction and infant bonding postpartum should be encouraged between the mother and infant. Assistance by special nurses and social workers in teaching infant care skills is needed. Coordination of social services may be necessary to monitor infant care after leaving the hospital as well as to assist in arranging child care so the teenager can continue her education postpartum.

REFERENCES

1. *Monthly Vital Statistics Report.* U.S. National Center for Health Statistics, 1990; 41(6):78.

2. Braveman P, Bennette T, Lewis C, et al: Access to prenatal care following major Medicaid eligibility expansions. *JAMA* 1993; 269:1285.
3. Frigoletto F: Diagnostic ultrasound imaging in pregnancy. U.S. Department of Health and Human Services, Public Health Services, National Institute of Health Publications No. 84667, 1986.
4. Slap G, Schwartz S: Risk factors for low birth weight to adolescent mothers. *J Adolesc Health Care* 1989; 10:267.
5. *The Health of Houston: Births, Deaths, and Other Selected Measures of Public Health,* 1982-86. City of Houston Health and Human Services Department, 1987.
6. Grant J: *The State of the World's Children 1989.* New York, Oxford University Press, 1989, pp 96.
7. Lee K, Corpuz M: Teenage pregnancy trends and impact of low birth weight and fetal, maternal, and neonatal morbidity in the U.S. *Clin Perinatol* 1988; 15:929.
8. Wendle GD: Sexually transmitted disease in pregnancy. *Semin Perinatol* 1990; 14:171.
9. Centers for Disease Control: Update: Acquired immunodeficiency syndrome. United States, 1981-1990. *MAWR* 1991; 40:357.
10. Hammill H, Murtagh C, Faro S, et al: HIV among pregnant women in Harris County, Houston, TX, surveillance 1987-88 (abstract). Presented at 1st World Congress for Infectious Diseases in Obstetrics and Gynecology, Nov. 1989, Hawaii.
11. National Institute on Drug Abuse, Rockville, Md: National household survey on drug abuse: Population estimates 1990, DHHS Pub No (ADM) 91-1732. Washington, DC, 1991, US Government Printing Office.
12. Willis G, Taslimi M: Prevalence of drug use during pregnancy in a mid-size town USA. *J Clin Pract Sexuality.* Special issue, Feb. 1994; 39.
13. Amaro H, Zuckerman B, Cabral H: Drug use among adolescent mothers: Profile of risk. *Pediatrics* 1989; 84:144.
14. Little B, Gilstrap L, Cunningham F: Social and illicit substance use during pregnancy, in Cunningham F, MacDonald P, Grant N (eds): *Williams Obstetrics Supplement No. 7, Aug 1990.* Norwalk, Appleton & Lang, 1989, pp 1-15.
15. Battaglia FC, Frazier TM, Hellegers AE: Obstetric and pediatric complications of juvenile pregnancy. *Pediatrics* 1963; 32:902.
16. Duenhoelter J, Jimenez J, Baumann, G: Pregnancy performance of patients under 15 years of age. *Obstet Gynecol* 1975; 46:49.
17. Moerman M: Growth of the birth canal in adolescent girls. *Am J Obstet Gynecol* 1982; 143:528.
18. Rhodes A: Legal issues related to adolescent pregnancy: Current concepts. *Semin Adolesc Med* 1986; 2:181.
19. Bromage PR: Age and epidural dose requirements. Segmental spread and predictability of epidural analgesia in youth and extreme age. *Br J Anaesth* 1969; 41:1016.
20. Norris MC: Patient variables and the subarachnoid spread of hyperbaric bupivacaine in the term parturient. *Anesthesiology* 1990; 72:478.

6 The Morbidly Obese Pregnant Patient

Norman H. Blass and Thomas N. Tabb

DEFINITION AND INCIDENCE

It is estimated that 34 million adults in the United States are overweight to a significant degree.[1] It is no wonder that excessive body fat has long concerned health care providers and social scientists. The magnitude of the obesity problem and its important influence on morbidity and mortality is staggering in its scope.

It is ominous that most complications of obesity appear at considerably lower degrees of overweight than the conventionally described "morbid obesity." The most important health risks of obesity are distinctly related to excess poundage with a progressive and disproportionate increase as the patient's weight rises. At a weight of 60% above standard insurance tables, there is a doubling of disease risk as compared with the general population.[2] In consideration of this fact it is important to be able to define what constitutes obesity and morbid obesity.

Utilizing the body mass index, it has been stated by the National Center for Health Statistics, that a BMI of greater than 27.3 kg/m for women indicated obesity. A BMI of greater than 40 kg/m may be defined as morbid obesity. Ten percent of pregnant women are thought to be in this category, and there is no doubt that these numbers are rising.[3]

There are several ways of defining morbid obesity. Bendexin stated that a morbidly obese individual is one who weighs twice the predicted weight for sex, age, and height as proscribed in the Metropolitan Life Assurance Company tables.[4] Garbaciak et al felt that the definition should be reserved for parturients who were 150% above ideal body weight.[5] A rather simple method of identifying this group of women is to call every pregnant patient who is 100 lb overweight as morbidly obese. It is unfortunate that the obstetrician and obstetric anesthesiologist must deal with another group of parturients who are massively obese and may be classified as "super obese." Mason defined these pregnant women as being of more than 225% of ideal weight—more than 123 kg, with a BMI of greater than 46 kg. The etiology of gross obesity is not truly known. Simply stating that the individual's caloric intake far exceeds their body's needs is superficial at best.[6]

Pathophysiology

It is unfortunate that excessive weight is not only extremely common but is a source of the development of other disease states. One series reported more than a tenfold increase in mortality from excessive body weight.[1] Obesity has been noted to be a risk factor in up to 80% of anesthetic deaths.

Morbid obesity has a direct relationship with the development of the primary alveolar hypoventilation syndrome, hypertension, cerebrovascular accidents, coronary artery disease, diabetes mellitus, congestive heart failure, gallbladder disease, and liver diseases.

It is of interest that death in an unexplained, sudden manner is several times more frequent in the grossly obese woman than in an individual of normal weight. It is well established that there is an association of obesity and fatty infiltration of the heart. Apparently, fatty infiltration of the conduction system may be the etiologic pathologic basis for the sudden death of obese women.

The Framingham heart study, done as early as 1982, revealed that obesity was an important predictor of cardiovascular disease in women.[7]

Physiologic changes of obesity

Certain physiologic changes occur in every pregnancy. In those patients with massive adipose tissue these are more pronounced and are frequently deleterious.

Cardiovascular system. From early in the first trimester, the plasma volume increases until about 32 weeks' gestation, resulting in an approximately 45% increase over nonpregnant values. There is an increase in the red blood cell mass to approximately 25% above nonpregnant values. Together, this results in a 45% rise in circulating blood volume. In the grossly overweight pregnant patient, although total blood volume is increased, when corrected for weight there is an actual decrease.[8] (As early as 1933, an association was established in the effect of obesity on cardiac function.)

Hypertension is very common in an overweight population. While it is not known whether obesity directly produces heart disease or whether the ensuing hypertension causes the cardiac problems, the incidence may be significant.

It is recognized that morbid obesity is of paramount importance in the development of obesity-hypoventilation syndrome, which leads to polycythemia and an increase in pulmonary capillary resistance. The increased strain on the right ventricle frequently leads to cor pulmonale.

Obesity leads to an increase in stroke volume and cardiac output.[9,10] Myocardial oxygen consumption must increase in an attempt to compensate for the burden of an increase in total body oxygen demand produced by the additional fat cells present. Total blood volume increases, but systemic vascular resistance remains the same or is slightly decreased. Preload increases, leading to elevation of left ventricular end-diastolic pressure and cardiac output.[4]

Pulmonary system. The massively obese parturient, with increased adipose tissue in and on the chest wall as well as intraabdominal fat pushing the diaphragm cephalad, frequently develops adverse respiratory function. This is in addition to the already altered respiration of pregnancy. There is an increase in oxygen consumption associated with pregnancy, as well as an increase in carbon dioxide production.[11] In the grossly overweight patient, oxygen consumption is increased even more, in direct proportion to the additional adipose tissue. The needs of the individual in this regard are met by hyperventilation. The normal gravida manifests an increased alveolar ventilatory pattern because of a larger tidal volume and because of a 20% reduction in residual volume. With obesity, there is a concomitant additional decrease in the function of residual capacity and expiratory reserve volume.[12]

Pregnancy plus obesity alters the posture of a woman so she frequently develops thoracolumbar lordosis and a modified thoracic curvature. Rib movement is diminished by the large and protuberant abdomen, and the patient's ability to raise the lower end of the sternum is jeopardized. The excess layers of fat on the chest wall and abdomen splint both the chest wall and the diaphragm, limiting respiratory excursion. This mechanical deficit leads to increased work in breathing, and eventually ventilatory parameters deteriorate. The large and protruding abdomen limits the movement of the rib cage and interferes with the motility of the lower end of the sternum.

The altered work in breathing is further complicated if the position of the patient is changed to lithotomy, Trendelenburg, or supine position, in which hypoxemia can and will occur. The progressive elevation of the diaphragm produced by the rising abdominal viscera aggravates this effect. Consequently, when mechanical ventilation is required, airway pressures higher than can be generated by conventional anesthesia gas machines may be needed.

Morbidly obese women have an increased metabolic need that apparently has a linear relationship to their weight. These parturients manifest elevated $\dot{V}O_2$ and carbon dioxide levels, necessitating high alveolar ventilation. As early as 1967, Alexander demonstrated that oxygen consumption increases by 100% as the weight doubles, and that carbon dioxide production rises correspondingly.[13]

Airway closure occurs more readily and often encroaches on tidal breathing in obese patients. Thus the characteristic changes, discovered during pulmonary function tests, are hypoxemia, a significant reduction in the expiratory reserve volume, maximum voluntary ventilation, and functional residual capacity. Vital capacity is only slightly depressed. Chest wall compliance is consistently reduced, but unless there is deterioration in lung parenchyma, lung compliance is only minimally affected.

These deleterious functional alterations are commonly associated with an increase in the work of breathing. As an attempt to offset this event, the grossly obese parturient changes her breathing by decreasing her tidal volume and increasing her respiratory rate.

Bedell[14] differentiated simple gross obesity and the "Pickwickian" (obesity-hypoventilation) syndrome by classifying obese individuals into three relatively distinct groups according to pulmonary function:

1. Patients with normal arterial saturation but reduced expiratory capacities.
2. Those with no lung disease having arterial hypoxemia without hypercapnia. This hypoxemia, expressed as an increased alveolar-arterial oxygen tension difference, increased significantly during anesthesia with use of mechanical ventilation and required the use of 50% inspired oxygen to maintain satisfactory saturation levels.
3. Patients who had alveolar hypoventilation with intrinsic lung disease or central nervous system lesions.
   It was stated that people with normal lungs did not have alveolar hypoventilation.

Relatively young morbidly obese patients can adjust to their hypoxemia with an increase in cardiac output and by the development of polycythemia. With the passage of time, CO_2 may be retained and somnolence may ensue. Pulmonary hypertension may occur from the increased blood volume and hypoxic vasoconstriction, and cor pulmonale develops. This obesity-hypoventilation syndrome, or "Pickwickian" syndrome, as described by Burwell et al in 1956, represents the endstage of cardiopulmonary disease for the morbidly obese individual.[15]

The Pickwickian syndrome consists of significant obesity, cardiac enlargement, polycythemia, hypoxemia, and hyperkalemia, and it occurs in about 7% to 10% of massively obese patients. There is also evidence of abnormal central control of ventilation with diminished ability to respond to the burden of hypercapnia and hypoxia. The augmented respiratory work in addition to the lessened ventilatory response to CO_2 leads to the onset of pulmonary vasoconstriction and pulmonary hypertension. Thus pulmonary vasoconstriction superimposed on the condition of obesity intensifies the circulatory abnormalities.

Hepatic/gastrointestinal system. Derangement of liver function and anatomic alterations are commonly associated with gravid obesity. Fatty accumulation in the liver is extremely common (90%). Triglyceride accumulation is usually thought to occur because of dietary indulgence in carbohydrate foods, but is most likely a result of biochemical alterations interfering with insulin metabolism.

Biotransformation of volatile anesthetic agents may differ in these pregnant women as compared with normal weight gravid patients. Halothane, at least in nonpregnant obese women, undergoes greater degradation metabolically than in nonobese women.[16] Enflurane has been shown to achieve higher free fluoride ions in the grossly overweight individual, but biotransformation of isoflurane has not been shown to be significantly different clinically than in normal-sized people.[17] Not enough data concerning desflurane or sevoflurane have been gathered to verify the amount of altered biotransformation that might occur, if any.

Pharmacokinetics has not been extensively studied in the extremely obese pregnant population, but it has been demonstrated that midazolam has a larger volume of distribution, enabling accumulation and somnolence to occur.[18] One study showed that vecuronium, as contrasted to atracurium, manifested a longer period to recovery.[19] It was postulated that obesity alters liver metabolism and clearance. Adequate oxygenation should always be maintained to prevent reductive processes from adversely affecting splanchnic function.

Pregnant patients have decreased gastric motility accompanied by a narrowing of the pressure difference between stomach and esophagus. There is an increased incidence of hiatal hernia that oc-

curs as a result of positional changes of the stomach.

There have been many studies showing that obese pregnant women have elevated gastric volumes and decreased gastric pH levels as compared with nonobese nonpregnant women. It is to be expected, therefore, that morbidly obese parturients would be at substantial risk for regurgitation and aspiration.[20]

Obstetric complications associated with gravid obesity

A definite relationship exists between obesity and the development of obstetric complications.[21] The incidence of pregnancy-induced hypertension, as well as gestational diabetes, is more frequent in the obese pregnant patient. Shoulder dystocia, macrosomia, postdate pregnancy, oxytocin induction, and augmentation are all more common. Primary cesarean section is more frequently performed in the obese parturient.[22,23] Furthermore, the morbidly obese woman, when she requires a cesarean section, has a greater risk of the surgery being emergent, with a longer time from incision to the infant's delivery time. Ordinarily there is a longer operating time with greater blood loss and an increase in postoperative infection and wound dehiscence. Increased postpartum atony with subsequent blood loss is seen with some frequency.

Many of these obstetric complications are directly related to the medical problems associated with obesity. In fact, some authors have stated that the increased risk of poor perinatal outcome is more related to the associated medical complications than to the obesity itself.[22] Diabetes, not uncommon in the obese patient, and macrosomia contribute to the increase in shoulder dystocia and cesarean section.[24] In fact, maternal weight has an independent effect on the occurrence of macrosomia.[25,26]

The distribution of the patient's fat may play a role in the risks of obesity. Krotkiewski et al[27] showed that in those patients whose fat was more centrally located and not equally distributed (the more usual situation for women), abnormal glucose tolerance tests and hypertension were more common.

Another obstetric problem in the morbidly obese patient is the difficulty with sonographic diagnosis of the fetus. Maternal weight has been found to be a good predictor for sonographic visualization of the fetus, with increasing weight making the ultrasound examination more difficult. This lack of visualization is inversely related to maternal weight and does not change with increasing gestational age or prolongation of examination time.[28]

An appropriate weight during gestation for an obese patient is unknown. A weight gain of greater than 24 lb is apparently associated with an increase in the cesarean section rate.[29] On the other hand, *low* weight gain in the morbidly obese parturient appears to produce no elevation in maternal or obstetric morbidity.[30]

Fetal and neonatal complications

There is no doubt that fetal and neonatal outcomes are related to maternal obesity. The associated medical problems, in particular hypertension and diabetes, contribute to an increase in intrauterine growth retardation, perinatal mortality, macrosomia, and neonatal admissions to the neonatal intensive care units.[22] Recently, the question has been raised concerning a possible increase in congenital anomalies in infants born to obese parturients. Waller and associates found that the children of severely obese women appear to be at greater risk for neural tube defects.[31] Further studies will have to be performed to verify the validity of this association.

OBSTETRIC AND ANESTHETIC MANAGEMENT

The obese pregnant woman is classified as a high-risk patient. Ideally, these patients should have counseling during the preconception period to fully explain the potential maternal and fetal risks and to be evaluated for medical conditions that may complicate ensuing gestation. If preconceptional or periconceptional counseling is not possible because of late entry into the prenatal care system, the initial workup should be completed at the first office visit. A detailed history should be obtained, not only to identify medical problems but to determine if any previously born infants had complicated deliveries or postnatal problems.

Careful attention must be given to the patient's cardiac and pulmonary system review in an attempt to determine if coronary artery disease or intrinsic pulmonary disease exists. A nutritionist should be consulted to evaluate the parturient's dietary habits and thus assist her in formulating a pregnancy diet to avoid excessive weight gain. A complete physical examination should be performed with special attention to the patient's cardiovascular and pulmonary status. A 12-lead ECG to evaluate ischemic heart disease and rhythm abnormalities, and a chest x-ray examination to determine heart size, should be obtained. It is important that during pregnancy the elevated diaphragm may cause a QRS shift to the left. There are other minor alterations produced by gestation and seen on the ECG that should not be construed as evidence of heart disease. However, the ECG may identify left or right ventricular dysfunction or ischemia resulting from the obesity-hypoventilation syndrome. Longstanding hypertension may be manifested by left ventricular hypertrophy.

Pulmonary status must be investigated by means of pulmonary function testing and an arterial blood gas. Preferentially, the pulmonary tests are better obtained before pregnancy, but if they have not been, then on the first prenatal visit. It would be beneficial to repeat the pulmonary function testing during the third trimester with the patient in the supine position. There is a progressive decrease in the functional residual capacity as the patient moves from the erect to the supine position. Hypoxia, if previously present, will get worse; if not present, it will develop. This is important if the obese woman must subsequently undergo a cesarean section, because this would be done in the supine position with left uterine displacement.

Certain laboratory values should be obtained, including liver function tests, blood glucose, hemoglobin and hematocrit, and serum electrolytes. Slight elevations of the transaminases may be observed in the pregnant patient.

If there are abnormalities in coagulation factors or if the rise in transaminases is greater than 30 IU, a more thorough investigation into the possibility of hepatic disease is warranted. Diabetes should be tightly controlled during pregnancy.

It would be advantageous for an anesthetic consultant to see the patient during the latter part of the second trimester. This consultant should review the patient's history and perform a physical examination, with special attention to those systems most likely to be compromised by obesity.

An important consideration during the predelivery care of the morbidly obese pregnant patient is the proper understanding of her "psychologic makeup."[32] Contrary to the popular idea that fat people are "jolly," it has been learned that these people have been misunderstood. This lack of understanding may lead to the loss of the patient's cooperation in both prenatal care and the intrapartum period.

The majority of markedly overweight patients are depressed and guilty about their eating habits and upset about their physical condition. They frequently have a distorted view of their weight and body image. For example, it is not unusual for women to significantly understate their weight and at the same time acknowledge that they are indeed overweight. The patient may smile and laugh about her condition but may be inwardly depressed about it; this can lead to a defensive state and possibly overt passive-aggressive behavior. Undoubtedly, one of the most important problems facing an anesthesiologist when dealing with a markedly obese parturient is a clear interpretation of the patient's attitude. Proper mental preparation of the gravida is a necessary part of this predelivery visit, and a cavalier approach by the physician may impair the patient's acceptance of the obstetrician and/or the anesthesiologist's plan in relation to labor or possible cesarean section.

Management of labor and delivery

Morbidly obese pregnant patients are considered a "high risk." During labor, both mother and the fetus require continual monitoring. All efforts should aim to maximize pulmonary function and minimize oxygen consumption. This requires that the parturient have noninvasive blood pressure recording. If a blood pressure cuff large enough for the patient's upper arm cannot be obtained, one should place a cuff in the region of the radial artery. This will allow trends to be followed during labor. If there is any difficulty in obtaining adequate blood pressure readings, an arterial line should be used. In fact, it would be extremely useful from the onset to place an arterial line, for both blood pressure recording and for arterial blood gas determinations. If the patient is known to be hypoxic or hypercarbic, an arterial line is necessary. Radial artery cannulation, rarely difficult to do despite the woman's size, is the preferred route.

Pulse oximetry, a simple noninvasive technique that helps determine maternal oxygen saturation, should be used routinely. Supplemental oxygen should be administered during labor.

The indications for labor induction are the same for the obese patient as for the nonobese parturient.

Obstetrical management of the delivery. It is best to avoid the lithotomy position for a vaginal delivery. The patient should be delivered from the semierect position. This helps to prevent a further decrease in the functional residual capacity and the ensuing hypoxia that is associated with the supine or lithotomy positions. Operative vaginal delivery is also performed from this position.

The indications for cesarean section are the same as for obese and normal-sized individuals. The patient either has the surgery done while on her labor bed (in the operating suite) or on a compatible operating table. Left uterine displacement is used, with the patient in approximately 10 degrees of reverse Trendelenburg position. The type of incision normally selected is the high transverse incision. Vertical midline paramedian incisions have also been used. No increase in wound complications have been found with the high transverse incision, and the patient appears better able to cough and deep breathe postoperatively, thus help-

ing to prevent atelectasis, pneumonia, and hypoxia.

After either a vaginal delivery or cesarean section, it is important that the patient ambulate as quickly as feasible, preferably during the first 24 hours postpartum. This will tend to decrease the incidence of thromboembolic phenomena, which is high in the obese gravida.

Anesthesia for labor and delivery. Labor and delivery care depends on the obstetric and physical status of the patient. While basic tenets are applicable to all situations, certain specific circumstances demand individual consideration.

Oxygen, given by nasal cannula or face mask, is advisable because of the common occurrence of hypoxemia.

Whether labor is being induced or is spontaneous, lumbar epidural analgesia should not be ruled out because of obesity. Massive size and body configuration is not a contraindication to regional anesthesia.[33] All patients who desire or are agreeable to this form of pain relief should be examined for the procedure. It is highly unusual not to be technically able to satisfactorily induce epidural analgesia.

Hood and Dewan, relating their experience with regional anesthesia, stated that "morbidly obese patients required more repeat placements of epidural catheters to achieve success."[34] They also report a much greater failure rate on the initial insertion as compared with the normal-sized individual. Certain precautions, when applied to the morbidly obese pregnant patient, may make placement of the epidural needle and catheter somewhat more easy.

While the lateral position is frequently selected for epidural placement, the sitting position is preferred for the massively obese woman. This position allows the body fat of the back and upper buttocks to fall away from the midline, not overlapping the access site for needle placement.

Most anesthesiologists pay little or no attention to the patient's labor bed when placing the epidural needle. If the head of the bed is kept elevated, there is tendency for the massive fat pads present to "lean" towards the midline and obscure the line of vision. Keeping the bed flat may help speed the placement process.

Traditionally, the standard area for epidural placement is L_2–L_3 or L_3–L_4. These sites were chosen ostensibly so as to avoid damage to the spinal cord, which in most people ends at L_1. With the advent of cervical and thoracic epidural placement for diagnostic and treatment procedures, anesthesiologists have become accustomed to this location for epidural placement. In view of this skill, consideration should be given to utilizing the low thoracic vertebral approach for labor and cesarean section epidural blocks. Blass and Abouleish,[35] in a series of what now involves 15 massively obese gravidas, selected the low thoracic epidural technique for analgesia or anesthesia. The selection of a low thoracic epidural placement was based on the following advantages:

1. Unlike the upper thoracic vertebrae, T_{10}-T_{12} vertebrae have only a slightly downward angulation and closely resemble the lumbar vertebrae.
2. Lower thoracic vertebrae may be palpable because of a frequently occurring convexity in the parturient's back when a line is drawn connecting the apices of the bilateral fat pads in the sitting position (Fig. 6-1, Blass's line).
3. With the more cephalad approach to the patient's back, the midline may be identified more easily.
4. The low thoracic approach to epidural placement avoids the excess fat that lies across the lumbar area in the morbidly obese pregnant woman.

In this study the patient's chosen weight varied from 160 to 240 kg (352 to 529 lb). In four patients, two attempts were necessary while in the remaining 11 women only one attempt was necessary. Of the 15 parturients, two required the use of a 15-cm Weiss epidural needle, while the 10-cm Weiss needle was satisfactory for the remainder of the patients. It was determined that for more effective labor analgesia the epidural catheter should be threaded in a caudad direction approximately 2 to 3 cm. Identification of the epidural space is achieved using the "loss of resistance" technique. The "hanging drop" method of epidural space confirmation rarely gives consistent results.

Once the epidural space has been successfully entered, the test dose and local anesthetic regimen to which an individual anesthesiologist is accustomed is acceptable. For labor, a segmental block of T_{10}-T_{11} with minimal motor blockade is the goal.

Placement of the epidural catheter may be performed before the actual time of dosage, ostensibly to save time. The block can be activated for the active phase of labor or after the parturient's bag of waters has been ruptured and a Pitocin infusion has begun.

After establishing initial analgesia, a continuous infusion of local anesthetic with a lipophilic narcotic drug is usually used. The continuous infusion technique is used for most patients in labor, weight notwithstanding.

The induction regimen that is most frequently chosen consists of the local anesthetic bupivacaine in a concentration of 0.125% to 0.25% to achieve initial anesthesia. The drug is given in increments

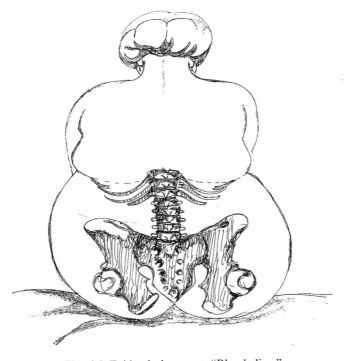

Fig. 6-1 Epidural placement: "Blass's line."

in an attempt to reach the T_{10} dermatome level. This usually requires doses of 7 to 10 ml. Sometimes it is very difficult to accurately determine the dermatome level because the massive panniculus prevents accurate measurement. The patients' expression of comfort in addition to no alteration of vital signs may have to suffice. The continuous infusion used commonly consists of 0.125% bupivacaine plus 50 µg of fentanyl or 10 to 15 µg of sufentanyl. Ordinarily, the infusion rate is 8 to 10 ml per hour, depending on the clinical condition that develops.

The patient is observed closely for a minimum of 20 minutes to ensure that no untoward side effects or complications develop. All patients who receive epidural analgesia for labor have their oxygen saturation monitored by pulse oximetry.

Once the block has been satisfactorily established, the patient should be seen regularly every 30 to 60 minutes to ensure patient safety. It would be easy to presume that with the use of low concentrations of local anesthetics the risks to the patient would be negligible. Nevertheless, catheter migration, kinking of the catheter, inadequate anesthetic level, or too high a dermatome level can occur, requiring adjustment. Furthermore, the patient deserves attention to her emotional as well as physical needs. A friendly face and attitude goes a long way to achieving good pain control.

Transcutaneous electrical nerve stimulation.
Melzack and Wall's gate theory of pain stimulated the idea that afferent nerves could be blocked by transcutaneous electrical nerve stimulation (TENS). It has been hypothesized that the stimulation of large nerve fibers would permit the small nerve fibers to be suppressed.[36] Its use has been described for the alleviation of the pain of labor in the normal-sized gravida.

In regard to the use of TENS for the relief of labor discomfort in the morbidly obese patient, our results were less than satisfactory. There were mechanical difficulties in keeping the electrodes placed on the appropriate areas because of the corpulence present as well as the perspiration and frequent chafing in the proscribed areas of the body. Not enough patients achieved adequate pain relief to warrant this method being used.

Spinal anesthesia for labor.
With the advent of the use of intrathecal lipophilic narcotic agents for labor, consideration must be given to this form of analgesia.

Many anesthesiologists are undoubtedly aware that the placement of a spinal needle in these extremely large women can be fraught with difficulties. Small-gauge pencil point spinal needles, however, can be inserted with relative ease. If accustomed to using the standard-size introducer, one would probably find it of insufficient length for

satisfactory use. However, this problem can be solved by using the epidural needle as the introducer (as with the "coaxial technique"). There are specific needles for the very large patient if the standard length of 3½ inches is too short. If desired, needles may be obtained up to 7½ inches long. On the other hand, it has been demonstrated in several studies that the incidence of postdural puncture headache is severely reduced in the morbidly obese patient. If required, a 22-gauge, 5½-inch to 7½-inch Quincke needle may be chosen with relative equanimity.

Continuous spinal anesthesia can be used in morbidly obese patients, but at the present time large-gauge catheters would have to be used. No doubt, when satisfactory small-gauge catheters become available, they will be adequate.

One statement frequently alluded to in the literature is that obesity correlates positively with the height obtained in a spinal anesthetic. Our experience coincides with that of Pitkanen,[37] who believes that if there is any relationship between the spread of spinal bupivacaine and obesity, it is clinically not significant.

Regional anesthesia for vaginal delivery.
When using a previously inserted epidural catheter for delivery, one should place the patient in a semierect position if perineal analgesia is required. The amount of local anesthetic administered to achieve satisfactory perineal analgesia is usually 8 to 10 ml, given about 10 minutes before delivery. One can use 0.25% bupivacaine, 2% chloroprocaine, or 0.375% bupivacaine. This latter dose of bupivacaine is particularly useful for forceps manipulations.

Subarachnoid blockade for vaginal delivery should be restricted to operative obstetrics (extraordinary repair, midforceps). It is probably unnecessary and unwise, however, for normal vaginal deliveries. Spinal blockade requires adequate fluid preload.

Anesthesia for cesarean section.
Obstetric literature is replete with studies asserting that morbid obesity is associated with an increase in the cesarean section rate.[21] This increase is often stated to be due to dysfunctional labor patterns, excessively large babies, and failed induction of labor.

General anesthesia for cesarean section. General anesthesia for cesarean section in the morbidly obese parturient may be divided into three major categories:

1. The elective surgical procedure
2. The urgent surgical procedure
3. The emergency surgical procedure

It may be stated that all three categories of cesarean section have certain basic similarities. In addition, certain aspects of the preoperative evaluation should be identical regardless of the urgency of the procedure. In all cases, knowledge of the parturient's respiratory and cardiac status and any potential problem with airway management should be obtained.

AIRWAY MANAGEMENT IN THE MORBIDLY OBESE PATIENT. Problems with intubation and ventilation during general anesthesia for cesarean section is more common in the extremely overweight patients. It has been reported that approximately one in every 300 to 750 intubation attempts are unsuccessful in normal obstetric women.[38] Without doubt this figure is at least reached in obese parturients.

During the preoperative evaluation, regardless of whether the procedure is emergent or elective, evaluation of the motility of the parturient's neck, its range of motion, the distance from the mentum of the chin to the substernal notch, and the amount of neck and upper thorax adipose tissue should be carefully noted. It is also useful to try to assess the potential for intubation problems by utilizing the Mallampatti classification.[39]

When one studies the body habitus of morbidly obese women and morbidly obese men, it is fortunate that the women manifest their obesity in the configuration of a pear. The head and neck are apparently smaller in relation to the progressively caudad fat deposition of these pregnant women. In the assessment of potential for difficulty in endotracheal tube placement, of no small significance is the size of the gravida's breasts and their placement when the she is in the supine position. Encroachment on the anesthesiologist's attempts to achieve the "sniffing position" frequently occurs. The short-handled laryngoscope of Datta and Briwa[40] (Fig. 6-2) is particularly useful in preventing enlarged breasts from interfering with intubation.

One should never compromise the patient's ability to maintain her airway until assured that ventilation can be satisfactorily maintained. An awake nasal or oral intubation should be considered. The use of the fiberoptic bronchoscope as an elective planned procedure rather than a choice attempted after several failed intubations makes nasal or oral intubation much more effective.

The proper technique in the use of the fiberoptic bronchoscope should be mastered in patients with normal anatomy before attempts are made in the patient with potential airway difficulties (i.e., the massively obese parturient).

The usual adult fiberoptic instrument will pass through an 8-mm (or larger) endotracheal tube. One must be aware that the normal physiologic response during gestation is for vascular engorgement, including the oronasal pharynx. This may predispose the patient to either oral or nasal bleeding when an endotracheal of this size tube is used.

The bronchoscope should be lubricated with a water-soluble jelly, because ointments with a glycol base can alter the sheath. Fogging of the lens can be decreased considerably by either using an antifogging solution or by placing the lens in warm, not hot, water, just before its use.

The most common reason for failure in the use of the bronchoscope is its use after repeated intubation attempts, which causes copious amounts of blood and secretions. This often prevents visualization and proper placement.

Before the patient is brought to the operating theater, if it is not an emergency, and regardless of whether regional or general anesthesia is contemplated, she is given ranitidine or famitidine, metoclopramide, and a clear antacid. It is preferable that no other premedication be given unless truly required.

Careful attention to these details is necessary because, as is well known, pregnant patients are considered to be at great risk for regurgitation and aspiration during general anesthesia. Furthermore, obesity aggravates this situation.

During gestation the esophageal sphincter relaxes as the pregnancy progresses, mainly because of the effect of progesterone. Hiatal hernia is fairly common during pregnancy, and it is a well-known caveat that all pregnant women are considered to have "full stomachs" for surgical procedures. Adding to the potential problem is that pregnancy and obesity both predispose to an increase in gastric volume and lowered gastric pH.

The majority of obese patients have a gastric pH of less than 2.5 and a gastric volume greater than 25 ml. It is not unusual to discover that patients scheduled for cesarean section have gastric volumes greater than 125 to 150 ml. As was previously noted, an additional hazard for the morbidly obese parturient is the not uncommon situation of difficult or impossible intubation, leading to an increase in the risk of regurgitation and aspiration.

For elective scheduled cesarean section, if the patient is in the hospital the night before surgery, she receives the histamine receptor antagonist famitidine, 150 mg at hour of sleep. Most of the scheduled patients now enter the hospital the morning of surgery; these parturients as well as those patients previously hospitalized receive 150

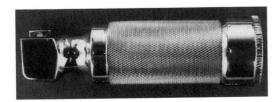

Fig. 6-2 Datta-Briwa short-handled laryngoscope.

to 300 mg of the histamine receptor antagonist per ounce one hour before surgery. In emergent situations, the H_2 receptor antagonist is omitted.

Famitidine is a satisfactory choice because of less drug interaction and less interference with liver metabolism as compared with some other H_2 receptor antagonists. It does not cross the blood-brain barrier.

Metoclopramide, 10 mg intravenously, is given preoperatively the morning of surgery in an attempt to increase both gastric emptying time and lower esophageal sphincter pressure. It is of interest that there are several studies that deal with potential troublesome side effects with this drug, but in our institution there have been no untoward effects.

All patients, elective or emergent, are given a nonparticulate matter antacid (0.3 M) in the amount of 30 ml. We use sodium citrate, which has an extremely bitter lemon taste. A new version of this product has a "grape" flavor, but it would not win any awards for palate enrichment. If the patient tries to sip this medication she will frequently gag, become nauseated, and vomit. While this may be regarded as beneficial in regard to gastric emptying, it makes the patient feel miserable and thus may interfere with induction of anesthesia. To help prevent this untoward situation the antacid is poured over ice chips. The cold liquid greatly diminishes the tendency to gag and vomit.

It is important to remember that nonparticulate antacids tend to "layer" with gastric contents; therefore the patient should be encouraged to move about to permit mixing of the gastric contents and the antacid. This technique helps lower the pH of the gastric contents.

Lowering the gastric volume and raising the pH of the stomach contents, while very useful, is not the answer to the problem of the aspiration syndrome. Despite the use of these drugs, regurgitation and aspiration can and still does occur. Prevention is best.

When the parturient is satisfactorily placed on either an oversized operating table or in her labor bed (used as a surgical table), left uterine displacement is necessary. In some of these massively overweight women there is a natural tendency for the abdomen to lie to the side.

Since hypoxemia is relatively frequent in these patients it is mandatory that preoperative oxygenation be performed. Oxygen saturation falls to about 75% of preinduction levels if one minute of apnea occurs.[41] Three or four minutes of denitrogenation should be done. If the situation is of an emergency status, four voluntary deep breaths may be efficacious.

Desaturation occurs very rapidly in the morbidly obese pregnant woman because of the decrease in the patient's functional residual capacity and the increase in her oxygen consumption. Furthermore, it has been well established that obese patients breathe at lower lung volumes and that closing capacity encroaches on tidal volume. This may lead to ventilation-perfusion problems.

As in all pregnant patients for cesarean section, induction requires the "rapid sequence" technique. The majority of these women receive sodium pentothal. There is a relative dearth of scientific work regarding the potential problems with pentothal for the induction of general anesthesia in the morbidly obese parturient. However, using 3 to 4 mg/kg per lean body weight has been successful in many patients. It is recommended that a maximum dose of 300 to 350 mg of pentothal be given.

Etomidate in a dose of 0.1 to 0.3 mg/kg may be used for those patients with cardiac problems.

Propofol has caused some difficulties when used for induction of anesthesia for cesarean section. Studies have revealed the potential for hypotension and a rather significant tendency for the mother to suffer "recall" when this drug is administered.[42]

Ketamine is occasionally used as an induction agent, particularly if the patient is hemodynamically unstable from blood loss. The customary dosage that we use is 1 mg/kg of lean body weight given intravenously. Hallucinatory activity is rarely encountered with this dosage. If the patient has known asthma, ketamine is frequently used because of its possible bronchodilatory effects. Hypertension is a relative contraindication to the choice of ketamine, as is a history of mental aberrations and hypertonicity of the uterus.

Succinylcholine, in a dose of 1 to 1.5 mg/kg, is still the drug of choice for the facilitation of intubation. In regard to the nondepolarizing muscle relaxants, there have been studies showing that obesity may alter the pharmacodynamics of the various agents. For example, obese patients required more pancuronium for maintenance of paralysis. Other studies state that if pancuronium is administered by "lean body weight" there was no difference in the obese patient. One study comparing vecuronium and atracurium revealed that while there was essentially no difference in recovery time using atracurium, vecuronium had a prolongation of action in the obese as compared with normal-sized individuals.[19] Vecuronium in a dose of 0.1 mg/kg had an apparent prolonged effect in obese patients as compared with nonobese controls. The difference has been postulated to be the result of impaired hepatic clearance in the grossly overweight. In regard to mivacurium, there has not been sufficient data established to verify the metabolism of this drug in the morbidly obese patient.

Cricoid pressure is maintained during the period of endotracheal tube placement and is not released until the cuff of the tube is inflated.

Maintenance of anesthesia consists of an FiO_2 of at least 0.5 throughout the procedure. Nitrous oxide at 50% is still used in most situations unless it is deemed necessary to use a higher FiO_2. One of the halogenated hydrocarbon volatile anesthetic agents, such as isoflurane 0.6% to 0.8%, is used in an attempt to eliminate "awareness." It also has the advantage of contributing to the anesthetic if there is prolongation between incision and the delivery of the baby. After the baby is delivered, the anesthesiologist may either continue the volatile agent for the remainder of the procedure or discontinue the drug. The inhaled anesthetic drug, if continued, will not cause atony of the uterus at this concentration, and it can contribute to the effectiveness of the anesthetic.

If the anesthesiologist deems it necessary to eliminate the halogenated hydrocarbon after the baby is born and the cord clamped, a narcotic (e.g., fentanyl, sufentanyl, alfentanyl, or morphine) may be given with the nitrous oxide for maintenance of anesthesia for the remainder of the surgical procedure.

If muscle relaxation is required after the initial use of succinylcholine for intubation, either an intermittent drip of succinylcholine or atracurium or mivacurium is chosen. A peripheral nerve stimulator should be used no matter which muscle relaxant is selected.

Regardless of the relaxant used it is probably wiser to reverse its effects with an anticholinergic such as edrophonium. Glycopyrrolate is added to prevent adverse muscarinic effects.

While it is probably preferable to extubate the parturient in the operating room, if there is any doubt as to the patient's ability to maintain adequate ventilation and oxygenation, one should continue mechanical ventilation in the postanesthesia care unit. Extubation depends on the usual criteria for termination of endotracheal intubation.

Regional anesthesia for cesarean section. Women who have satisfactory epidural analgesia for labor in most instances can have the dosage and concentration adjusted for the necessary level and density to achieve surgical anesthesia. Ideally, during labor the patient's dermatome level of anesthesia has been maintained at about a T_{10} level. A continuous infusion of low concentration of bupivacaine plus a lipophilic narcotic drug does not give the dense block needed for surgery. It becomes necessary to reach the desired T_4 to T_5 dermatome level by using a concentrated local anesthetic such as 2% lidocaine given in aliquots. Frequently, it may be logical and required to perform the surgery with the patient in her labor bed.

If the epidural anesthetic was instituted for the cesarean section, the placement of the needle and catheter should be done in the operating suite after adequate hydration (1500 to 2000 ml). Proper monitoring devices should be applied. This should include pulse oximetry, ECG leads, and a blood pressure cuff large enough to accurately measure the pressure. Commonly these patients will need direct intraarterial measurement.

Regardless of whether the epidural block was instituted for labor or whether it was placed for a cesarean section, supplemental oxygen must be administered (Figs. 6-3, 6-4).

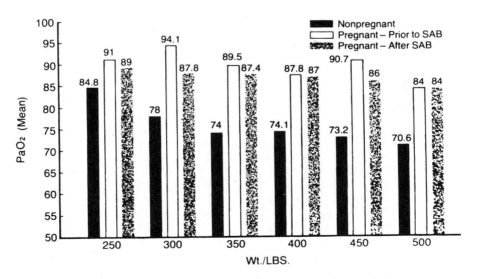

Fig. 6-3 Pao_2 levels in pregnant and nonpregnant obese patients.

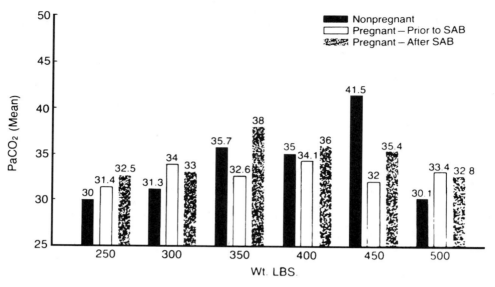

Fig. 6-4 $Paco_2$ levels in pregnant and nonpregnant obese patients.

If spinal anesthesia is selected as the anesthetic of choice, spinal bupivacaine with epinephrine and the addition of a narcotic drug such as 25 μg fentanyl or 10 μg sufentanyl is frequently selected as the spinal anesthetic agent. Epinephrine is selected, if not contraindicated, to enhance the density and effectiveness of the local anesthetic blockade. The narcotic drug is particularly useful in the prevention of untoward symptoms (such as nausea and vomiting) that occur with intraabdominal tugging on the visceral peritoneum.

The patient is maintained with head elevation and a 10- to 15-degree reverse Trendelenburg position. It should be mentioned that some of these massively obese women are so large that it is physically impossible to achieve satisfactory left uterine displacement. However, in the majority of these extremely obese patients (400 to 500 lb) there is a natural tendency for their abdomens to lie in a lateral position.

Also of note is that several studies have shown that the dosage required for satisfactory surgical anesthesia is less in the morbidly obese parturient than in the nonobese patient.[43]

Postoperative care. When the patient is brought to the postanesthesia care unit, if she has had successful regional anesthesia, oxygen by nasal cannula is administered. When general anesthesia has been used the gravida has a high-humidity face mask with an inspired oxygen of about 50% to 60%. The patient is not permitted to lie in the supine position but is placed in a semi-erect position to prevent a decrease in functional residual capacity and thus avoid hypoxia.

For those patients who remain intubated post-

operatively, the criteria for extubation are essentially the same as for any patient who remains intubated postoperatively.

Discontinuance of oxygen is based on clinical examination and maintenance of a satisfactory Pao_2 and Pco_2 level. If the aforementioned parameters are stable the oxygen is discontinued and the patient is observed for clinical or laboratory worsening of her condition for a minimum of 4 hours.

The incidence of hypoxia in the postanesthesia care unit is influenced by the type of incision made for the surgical procedure. A vertical incision made for the cesarean section leads to "splinting" postoperatively by the patient, and this frequently compromises the patient's ability to cough and to thus "bring up" secretions. All too often atelectasis is the result. The massively obese patient is a prime candidate to develop atelectasis and pulmonary dysfunction.

For postoperative pain relief in these women, the most efficacious method that helps prevent "splinting" and problems with coughing is postoperative administration of an epidural narcotic drug. It is our experience that while PCA is fairly effective in alleviating postsurgical pain, epidural narcotic usage is more effective.

For the patient who has had epidural anesthesia for her surgical delivery, our usual technique is to administer an opioid such as fentanyl (50 μg) via the catheter at the placement of the catheter. If sufentanyl is chosen, then the dose consists of 15 to 20 μg. Therefore, when the patient enters the postanesthesia care unit she frequently has residual pain relief from the previously administered lipophilic epidural narcotic. This usually will keep her comfortable for at least 2 to 3 hours. Customarily these patients are observed for 3 to 4 hours before being discharged to their rooms. Before this departure, the patient quite often receives epidural morphine in a dose of 4 to 5 mg. Experience has shown that giving more than 5 mg is unnecessary and yields no further increase in duration of pain relief or in intensity of comfort. This excess dosage may increase the incidence of side effects and complications.

The use of epidural morphine, even in the accepted dosage range, does produce side effects and complications. These include:

1. Itching, the most common complaint of patients and occurring in about 35% of postpartum women. The portion of the body that seems to be affected most frequently is the face and upper thorax. Only 7% to 10% of these patients require therapy, however. There is no doubt that relief of the pruritus without diminution of the pain relief may be difficult to achieve at times. Benadryl, administered either orally or intravenously, may be helpful in relatively mild cases, but in more severe situations a naloxone "drip" or oral naltrexone should be given.

2. Urinary retention, the true incidence of which is difficult to assess in postcesarean section patients because most have urinary bladder catheters for at least 24 hours following delivery. It has been reported, however, that 40% of patients who receive epidural morphine will manifest urinary retention.

3. Respiratory depression. As early as 1981 Rawal et al[44] demonstrated that parenterally administered narcotic drugs, more than epidural morphine sulfate, depress the voluntary response curve to carbon dioxide. Nevertheless, morbidly obese patients are more prone to respiratory difficulties that normal-sized individuals. It would be prudent to utilize apnea monitors postsurgically on obese women who have received epidural morphine for pain relief. Monitoring should be considered for about 24 hours. While this means of monitoring does not preclude the advent of respiratory depression, it serves as an instrument of care that may be useful as an alerting device for personnel caring for the parturient. Another useful tool is the pulse oximeter. When attention is paid to the patient, the risk of postoperative respiratory depression is quite rare.

Early ambulation is an extremely useful technique. It helps lower the incidence of thrombophlebitis, an occurrence not uncommon in the obese postoperative patient. There is no doubt that early ambulation lowers the morbidity rate several fold.

Patient-controlled analgesia is widely accepted as a safe technique postoperatively and is favorably accepted by cesarean section patients. Various narcotic agents such as alfentanyl, sufentanyl, fentanyl, and morphine sulfate has been used with no apparent untoward effects. When oral pain modalities are tolerated, patient-controlled analgesia should be discontinued.

REFERENCES

1. Fankel HM: Determination of body mass index. *JAMA* 1986; 255:1292.
2. Kral JG: Morbid obesity and related health risks. *Ann Intern Med* 1983; 103:1043.
3. Kleigman RM, Gross T: Perinatal problems of the obese mother and infant. *Obstet Gynecol* 1985; 66:299.
4. Bendexin HH: Marked obesity, in *Refresher Course in Anesthesiology,* 1978; vol 6, pp 1-14.
5. Garbaciak JA Jr, Richter M, Miller S, et al: Maternal weight and pregnancy complications. *Am J Obstet Gynecol* 1991; 164:1306.
6. Mason EE, Doherty C, Maher JW, et al: Super obesity and gastric reduction procedure. *Gastroenterol Clin North Am* 1987; 16:495.
7. Hubert HB, Feinlesh M, McNamera PM, et al: Obesity as an independent factor of cardiovascular disease: A 26-year follow-up of participants in the Framington Heart study. *Circulation* 1983; 67:968.
8. Blockman L, Freyschus U: Cardiovascular function in extreme obesity. *Acta Med Scand* 1973; 193:437.
9. Capeless EL, Clapp JT: Cardiovascular changes in early phase of pregnancy. *Am J Obstet Gynecol* 1989; 161:1449.
10. Clark SL, Cotton DB, Lee W, et al: Central hemodynamic assessment of normal term pregnancy. *Am J Obstet Gynecol* 1989; 161:1439.
11. Knultgen HG, Emerson K: Physiologic response to pregnancy at rest and during exercise. *J Appl Physiol* 1974; 36:549.
12. Rochester DF, Ensen Y: Current concepts in the pathogenesis of the obesity-hypoventilation syndrome. *Am J Med* 1974; 57:402.
13. Alexander JK, Pettigrove JR: Obesity and congestive heart failure. *Geriatrics* 1967; 22:101.
14. Bedell GN: Pulmonary function in obese persons. *J Clin Invest* 1955; 37:1049.
15. Burwell CS, Raben ED, Whaley RD, et al: External obesity associated with alveolar hypoventilation: A Pickwickian syndrome. *Am J Med* 1956; 21:811.
16. Bently JB, Vaughan RW, Carl RP, et al: Does evidence of reductive jalathane biotransformation correlate with hepatic binding of metabolites in obese patients? *Anesth Analg* 1981; 60:548.
17. Strube PJ: Serum fluoride levels in morbidly obese patients; enflurane compared with isoflurane anesthesia. *Anaesthesia* 1987; 42:685.
18. Greenblatt DJ: Effects of age, gender, and obesity of midazolam kinetics. *Anesthesiology* 1984; 61:27.
19. Weinstein, JA: Pharmacodynamics of vecronium and atracurium in the obese surgical patient. *Anesth Analg* 1988; 67:1149.
20. Vaughan RW, Bauer S, Wise L: Volume and pH of gastric juice in obese patients. *Anesthesiology* 1975; 43:686.

21. Abrams B, Parker J: Overweight and pregnancy complications. *Int J Obes* 1988; 12:293.
22. Perlow J, Morgan M, Montgomery D, et al: Perinatal outcome in pregnancy complicated by massive obesity. *Am J Obstet Gynecol* 1992; 167:958.
23. Naeye RL: Maternal body weight and pregnancy outcome. *Am J Clin Nutr* 1990; 273:9.
24. O'Leary JA, Leonetti HB: Shoulder dystocia: Prevention and treatment. *Am J Obstet Gynecol* 1990; 162:5.
25. Johnson SP, Kalberg BH, Vernes MW, et al: Maternal obesity and pregnancy. *Surg Gynecol Obstet* 1987; 164:431.
26. Larsen CE, Serdula MK, Sullivan KM: Macrosomia: Influence of maternal overweight among a low-income population. *Am J Obstet Gynecol* 1990; 162:490.
27. Krotkiewski M, Bjornetorp P, Sjostrom L, et al: Impact of obesity on metabolism in men and women: Importance of regional adipose tissue distribution. *J Clin Invest* 1983; 72:1150.
28. Wolfe HM, Sokol RJ, Marties SM, et al: Maternal obesity: A parenteral source of error in sonographic prenatal diagnosis. *Obstet Gynecol* 1990; 76:339.
29. Ratner RE, Hamner LH, Isada NB: Effects of "gestational" weight gain in morbidly obese women. 1. Maternal morbidity. *Am J Perinatol* 1991; 8:21.
30. Ekblad V, Grenman S: Maternal weight, weight gain during pregnancy and pregnancy outcome. *Int Fed Gynecol Obstet* 1992; 39:277.
31. Waller DK, Mills JL, Simpson JL, et al: Are obese women at higher risk for producing malformed offspring? *Am J Obstet Gynecol* 1994; 170:541.
32. Satmar-Fones G: Some psychiatric aspects of morbidly obese patients in relation to jejunoileal and gastric bypass procedures. *Can J Surg* 1984; 27:133.
33. Blass NH: Regional anesthesia in the markedly obese: Regional anesthesia in the morbidly obese. *Int J Obes* 1979; 4:20.
34. Hood DD, Devan DM: Anesthetic and obstetric outcome in markedly obese parturients. *Anesthesiology* 1993; 79:1212.
35. Blass NH, Abouleish A, Dalmeida R: Low thoracic epidural anesthesia for massively obese parturients. *Anesthesiology* 1994; 81:A1172.
36. Anderson GA: Pain control by sensory stimulation, in Bonica JJ (ed): *Advances in Pain Research and Therapy*, vol 3, New York, 1979, Raven Press.
37. Pitkänen MT: Body mass and spread of spinal anesthesia with bupivacaine. *Anesth Analg* 1987; 66:122.
38. Rocke DA, Murray WB, Rant CP, et al: Relative risk analysis of factors associated with difficult intubation in obstetric anesthesia. *Anesthesiology* 1992; 77:37.
39. Mallampatti SR, Gatt SP, Gugino LD, et al: A clinical sign to predict difficult tracheal intubation: A prospective study. *Can J Anesth* 1985; 32:429.
40. Datta S, Briwa J: Modified laryngoscope for endotracheal intubation of obese patients. *Anesth Analg* 1981; 60:120.
41. Archer GW, Marx GP: Arterial oxygen tension during apnea in parturient women. *Br J Anaesth* 1974; 46:358.
42. Dailland P, Cockshott ID, Lirzin JD, et al: Intravenous propofol during cesarean section: Placental transfer, concentrations in breast milk, and neonatal effects. A preliminary study. *Anesthesiology* 1989; 71:827.
43. Norris MC: Height, weight and the spread of subarachnoid hyperbaric bupivacaine in the term parturient. *Anesth Analg* 1988; 67:555.
44. Rawal N, Sjostrand V, Christofferson E, et al: Comparison of intramuscular and epidural morphine for postoperative analgesia in the grossly obese: Influence on postoperative ambulation and pulmonary function. *Anesth Analg* 1984; 63:583.

7 Breech Presentation, Malpresentation, Multiple Gestation

Graham H. McMorland and Sidney B. Effer

BREECH PRESENTATION

In 3% to 4% of term pregnancies the fetus presents by the breech.[1] This incidence is markedly increased by prematurity (exceeding 25% at 28 weeks' gestation) and is gradually reduced as pregnancy approaches term.[2,3] Other contributing factors to breech presentation include placenta previa, pelvic or uterine tumors, hydrocephaly, hydramnios, multiple gestation, and multiparity.

Classification

There are three types of breech presentations (Fig. 7-1):

1. *Frank Breech:* Lower extremities are flexed at the hips and extended at the knees, with the feet at the face (about 60% of all breech births).
2. *Complete Breech:* Lower limbs are flexed at both hips and knees (5% to 10% of breech births).
3. *Incomplete (Footling) Breech:* One or both hips are extended, with one or both feet below the buttocks (about 30% of breech births).

Obstetric and perinatal considerations

Individual consideration must be given to each of the following factors which, separately or combined with others, influence the plan of management:

1. Prematurity—low birth weight
2. Type of breech presentation
3. Experience of obstetric operator
4. Quality of available newborn resuscitation
5. Expertise of anesthesia personnel
6. Status of the amniotic membranes
7. Past obstetric history of the patient

Prematurity. The choice of delivery method and type of anesthesia are dictated by the category of breech and the skills and resources of the personnel and the institution, but they will vary with the gestational age of the pregnancy. The majority of published recommendations use birth weight groups (e.g., 500 to 999 g, >1500 g) and outcomes in each of these strata to base the recommendations for management. Since the obstetrician does not have accurate methods for predicting birth weight, gestational age is more useful. Some authors have published outcomes with gestations of 24 to 28 weeks,[4,5] but they have not separated these into vertex and breech. We have recently reviewed our experience (Table 7-1), and the different outcomes from previous reports may be partly due to the continued improvement in perinatal outcomes from 1977 to 1994.[4-7]

The mortality rates for births under 26 weeks are extremely high, and cesarean section does not contribute to any improvement of these high mortality rates. In the pregnancies that deliver between 24 and 25 weeks, a search for other determinants that may either further aggravate or improve outcome suggests that only birth weight has a statistically modifying effect on outcome. Neither presentation, comparing breech with vertex, nor fetal sex, comparing female with male births, show any significant, or even clinically significant, difference in mortality. However, the birth weight of babies born at 24 to 25 weeks shows a mortality rate that may be reduced from 56.3% in the lower weight group to 37.5% in babies born with birth weights below the 50th percentile of weight for gestation (Table 7-2). These observations suggest that when dealing with ultrapremature pregnancies, the use of ultrasound in the few days before birth may be of some value in predicting those babies whose survival rates are high enough to consider heroic interventions.

No consensus exists[6-11] regarding recommendations for type of delivery at varying gestational ages, but the absence of clear evidence of benefit in survival rate suggests that maternal morbidity and surgical/anesthetic risks are clear indications to recommend vaginal delivery in the following circumstances:

1. Complete and frank breech between 30 and 40 weeks' gestation, with estimated fetal weights of 1500 to 3499 g, with flexed head.

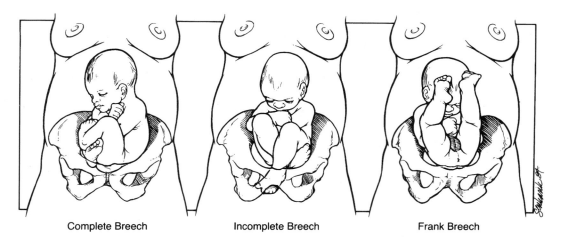

Complete Breech	Incomplete Breech	Frank Breech

Fig. 7-1 Types of breech presentation. (From Seeds JW: Malpresentations, in Gabbe SG, Niebyl JR, Simpson JL (eds): *Obstetrics: Normal and Problem Pregnancies.* New York, Churchill Livingstone, 1986, p 465. Used by permission.)

Table 7-1 Vertex and breech: 24 to 43 weeks (neonatal mortality for singleton pregnancies by gestational age and delivery mode)*

Gestation weeks	Presentation	Still births	Neonatal deaths	Survivors	NNMR%
B.C. Women's Hospital and B.C. Children's Hospital 1983-1993					
24	Vertex	18	34	38	47.2
	Breech	13	36	11	70.3
25	Vertex	9	53	78	40.5
	Breech	11	19	36	34.5
26	Vertex	15	36	86	29.5
	Breech	8	19	38	33.3
27	Vertex	4	26	125	17.2
	Breech	8	19	66	22.4
28	Vertex	8	18	161	10.1
	Breech	4	17	42	28.8
B.C. Women's Hospital 1991-1994					
29	Vertex		4	49	7.5
	Breech		3	16	15.8
30	Vertex		5	62	7.5
	Breech		5	16	23.8
31	Vertex		3	65	4.4
	Breech		1	16	5.9
32	Vertex		6	94	6.0
	Breech		4	23	14.8
33-34	Vertex		14	320	4.2
	Breech		4	43	8.5
35-36	Vertex		13	918	1.4
	Breech		2	81	2.4
37-39	Vertex		31	9465	0.3
	Breech		1	538	0.2
40-41	Vertex		16	7395	0.2
	Breech		0	122	0.0
42-43	Vertex		0	597	0.0
	Breech		0	5	0.0

*Congenital lethal anomalies are excluded.

Table 7-2 Determinants of neonatal mortality in ultrapremature (24 to 25 weeks) birth

Outcome determinants	NNMR%	OR	p	CI
Presentation				
Breech	48.9			
Vertex	42.9	0.783	0.35018	0.0619-0.1830
Sex				
Female	42.9			
Male	48.9	1.272	0.35018	0.0519-0.1712
Birth weight				
<725 g	56.3			
>724 g	37.5	2.151	0.00137	0.0770-0.2998

In ultraprematurity (24 to 25 weeks) it would appear that sex and presentation have no effect on neonatal mortality. However, when birth weight below and above the 50th percentile of weight for gestation are compared, there is a 20% difference in mortality.

Table 7-3 Gestational age and breech frequency

Weeks	Vertex	Breech	Other	Total	Breech %
20-21	37	31	5	73	42.4
22-23	61	53	15	129	41.1
24-25	95	72	12	179	40.2
26-27	179	89	16	284	31.3
28-29	235	93	12	340	27.3
30-31	290	87	25	402	21.6
32-33	491	119	6	616	19.3
34-35	912	191	12	1115	17.1
36-37	2490	427	25	2942	14.5
38-39	10,539	482	40	11,061	4.3
40-41	12,331	99	57	12,487	0.8
42-44	1646	1	18	1665	0.1
Total	29,306	1744	243	31,293	5.5
36	816	157	8	981	16.0
37	1674	290	17	1981	14.6
38	3820	289	18	4127	7.0

2. All types of breech presentation with fetal weight under 1000 g, or less than 28 weeks' gestation.

The type of anesthetic/analgesic used should allow the patient to participate in the delivery process. In our experience, conduction analgesia, when administered by a group of anesthesiologists who are skilled in obstetric anesthesia, provides optimum control and, by careful dose adjustment, allows patient participation. This type of analgesic can, at any time, be augmented with a fast-acting local anesthetic to permit obstetric intervention maneuvers and even cesarean section.

Type of breech. Gestational age is a major influence on both the type of presentation and the category of breech presentation. A review of 31,293 births at our institution has shown that there is a gradual decrease in the frequency of breech presentation from 40% at under 24 weeks to 14.6% at 37 weeks (Table 7-3). In the past, it has been recommended that version attempts should be carried out at 36 to 37 weeks, although our data suggest that 50% of all breech presentations at 37 weeks will have reverted to vertex by 38 weeks.

These observations are different from the previously reported 7% at 32 weeks[12] and may be partly explained by major changes in referral patterns of premature pregnancies for delivery at tertiary care centers. The frank breech category is present in 48% to 73% of all breech presentations,[12] but this varies greatly with gestational age. At term, 51.4% to 73.0% of all breech presentations are frank[11] (Table 7-4), whereas only 38% of breech births under 2500 g birth weight are frank in category.

The category of breech affects the risk associated with birth type (Table 7-4). The risks associ-

Table 7-4 Breech categories

	Overall proportion of breeches (%)	Risk of cord prolapse (%)	Proportion with prematurity (%)
Frank Breech	48–73	0.5	38
Complete	4.6–11.5	4–6	12
Footling*	12–38	15–18	50

*Increased with very low birth weight.
From Seeds JW: Malpresentations, in Gabbe SG, Neibyl JR, Simpson JL (eds): *Obstetrics, Normal and Problem Pregnancies.* New York, Churchill Livingstone, 1986, p 465. Used by permission.

Table 7-5 Incidence of complications seen with breech presentation

Complication	Incidence
Intrapartum fetal death	Increased 16-fold
Intrapartum asphyxia	Increased 3.8-fold
Cord prolapse	Increased 5–20-fold
Birth trauma	Increased 13-fold
Arrest of after-coming head	8.8%
Spinal cord injuries with deflexion	21%
Major anomalies	6%-18%
Prematurity	16%-33%
Hyperextension of head	5%

From Seeds JW: In Gabbe SG, Niebyl JR, Simpson JL (eds): *Obstetrics: Normal and Problem Pregnancies.* New York, Churchill Livingstone, 1986, p 473. Used by permission.

ated with vaginal delivery are cord prolapse, head entrapment, and spinal cord damage from hyperextended cervical vertebrae (Table 7-5). The footling breech carries such a high risk of cord accident that it is generally agreed that cesarean section is indicated. Current methods of continuous fetal monitoring can identify complete and frank breech. In addition, prompt management in a center staffed with skilled obstetric, anesthesia, and neonatology personnel can avoid the need for cesarean section for the benefit of the 0.5% to 6.0% of patients who suffer this complication (Table 7-4). Head entrapment is the major concern that currently cannot be predicted. It is extremely rare in complete or frank breech presentations, and with patients who are multiparous, who have normal labor progress, and who labor with intact membranes.

Experience of obstetric operator. The trend to use cesarean section for an increasing number of breech deliveries has resulted in many obstetricians completing their training with inadequate exposure to the technical skills acquired by senior colleagues. There is an increased public awareness that maternal morbidity is significantly increased by operative delivery. In addition, there is a lack of *sound* evidence that cesarean section improves fetal outcome in certain types of breech presentation. Alternatives to cesarean section, when inadequate facilities and trained personnel are the problem, include informing the patient of other facilities that do exist. In addition, large departments should provide rosters of senior consultants available to assist junior members accumulating enough cases to gain the needed expertise.

Quality of newborn resuscitation. Any obstetric facility must provide expert newborn resuscitation, even in smaller centers. Official national organizations have published approved educational packages to train and certify medical personnel to carry out resuscitation, and to certify personnel as instructors.[13] This permits small and remote centers to acquire instructors and to update staff in still smaller centers close to them. Decisions in assigning responsibility for neonatal resuscitation to the anesthesiologist, obstetrician, family physician, or any other person performing the delivery must be made by each center, based on available resources.

Quality of anesthesia services. The principle of quality anesthesia service should include the factors of constancy and prompt availability. The frequent deterrent to expert anesthesia is the sharing of surgical and obstetric anesthesia services without clearly defined personnel who are assigned to (and at all times who are free to) attend obstetric emergencies. Another limiting factor is the annual patient load of the obstetric unit. When this is too small, it inhibits the acquisition and maintenance of the necessary skills. Conduction anesthesia is the preferable technique in most situations in which an indwelling epidural catheter is already in place and known to be effective, even when emergency procedures are required. Some emergency general anesthesia will be required, such as when the after-coming head is trapped or when an emergency development requires rapid delivery in a patient without prior placement of the epidural catheter. However, even in these cases, some form of rapidly induced regional anesthesia, such as subarachnoid block, is often advisable.

Status of the amniotic membranes. The presence of ruptured membranes calls for ultrasonic assessment of residual amniotic fluid volume. Substantial lack of amniotic fluid (oligohydramnios, moderate to heavy volume) creates a high risk of cord complications and head entrapment.

Anesthetic considerations

To provide the appropriate anesthesia care, the obstetrician must communicate with the anesthesiologist when the patient is admitted to the delivery suite. The planned obstetric management must be clearly understood so the anesthesiologist can discuss the anesthesia management with both obstetrician and patient. Delivery may be by vaginal route or by cesarean section, depending on the obstetric indications or the preference of the obstetrician.[14] Cord prolapse, more commonly encountered in preterm breech presentation, may necessitate emergency cesarean section.

Labor and vaginal delivery. Ideally, the patient should meet with an anesthesiologist before going into labor. At this time, the analgesic and anesthetic alternatives can be explained; the patient's understanding and judgment will be better than when she is in active labor and perhaps distressed by painful contractions.

Sudden cord prolapse, difficulty in delivering the after-coming head, or acute fetal distress are among a number of indications for emergency administration of a general anesthetic agent or subarachnoid block. For this reason, an intravenous line must be established early in labor with a large-bore indwelling cannula. No solid food is given by mouth, and the use of oral antacids and histamine-2 antagonists is desirable. At the least, a clear antacid such as sodium citrate should be administered at the beginning of the second stage of labor. The equipment and drugs required for emergency induction of general anesthesia must be checked and be immediately available.

Epidural analgesia. Epidural analgesia for labor and delivery has been controversial in the past. Some obstetricians still believe that the second stage is prolonged by epidural analgesia and that the ability of the patient to push is inhibited. This latter effect is said to cause an increase in the number of breech extractions, with greater perinatal morbidity and mortality. However, a number of studies[2,15-18] have demonstrated that this may be the analgesic method of choice for labor and vaginal delivery in cases of breech presentation. The incidence of breech extraction is not increased by the use of epidural analgesia[18,19]; it may actually decrease because this technique provides better perineal analgesia and controlled pushing efforts.[15]

Epidural analgesia does not affect the incidence of fetal and neonatal depression in comparison with other analgesic techniques.[15-18,20] Darby and Hunter[20] reported that epidural analgesia for vaginal breech delivery was associated with 5-minute Apgar scores that were significantly higher than those following either narcotic or inhalation (nitrous oxide) analgesia. A patient with a low–birthweight breech, or a footling breech, may experience a premature urge to push if a foot or the small breech should prolapse through a partly dilated cervix. This urge can be abolished by providing perineal anesthesia via the epidural catheter. Bupivacaine, in concentrations of less than 0.25%, will not produce significant motor block, and the ability to push in the second stage can be maintained. Anesthesia for breech extraction may be produced rapidly by 2% lidocaine, carbonated lidocaine (when available), or 0.5% bupivacaine. When available, 0.5% ropivacaine can also be used.

The advantages of epidural analgesia include better pain relief than that achieved with narcotic drugs, prevention of premature bearing down, no clinically significant prolongation of labor, improved fetal status, facilitation of controlled delivery (with lessened risk of trauma), and avoidance of general anesthesia in patients whose gastric emptying has been delayed by pain and/or narcotic drugs.

Subarachnoid block. Subarachnoid block ("saddle" block) is occasionally administered for breech extraction or to prevent precipitous delivery, especially in the presence of a premature fetus. The advantages are rapid onset, good perineal relaxation, and minimal fetal drug exposure. The disadvantages are the possible excessive motor block and the possible need for hasty administration in the second stage of labor. The former concern can be addressed by the use of 1.5% lidocaine (in 7.5% dextrose solution), which will minimize the motor block and allow for somewhat more effective pushing.[20]

General anesthesia. General anesthesia is sometimes administered when the obstetrician requires uterine relaxation for intrauterine manipulation. Halothane, enflurane, and isoflurane, in anesthetic concentrations, will rapidly relax uterine muscle.[21] Frequently, the patient will be in late second-stage labor, possibly with part of the infant visible or delivered, and in a lithotomy position. Induction of general anesthesia under these circumstances is hazardous. The legs must be lowered and, after preoxygenation, a rapid-sequence induction with endotracheal intubation is performed with a reliable assistant applying cricoid pressure.

Emergency general anesthesia, with all its attendant hazards, is not always necessary to produce uterine relaxation. Amyl nitrite[22] and nitroglycerin[23,24] will both produce rapid and transient relaxation of smooth muscle. An ampule of amyl nitrite is crushed in the reservoir bag of the anesthetic machine and breathed by the patient in 100% oxygen. It has a rather unpleasant odor. Nitroglyc-

---

BOX 7-1   PREANESTHETIC PREPARATION (BREECH AND MULTIPLE BIRTH)

---

1. Start intravenous crystalloid infusion with large bore cannula.
2. Send blood for type and screen.
3. Prepare for rapid induction of general anesthesia.
4. Be prepared to resuscitate neonate.
5. Administer sodium citrate (0.3 mol/liter) 30 mL orally.
6. Monitor fetal heart continuously.

BOX 7-2   GENERAL ANESTHESIA FOR CESAREAN SECTION

---

1. Left lateral tilt: wedge under right hip, or tilt table.
2. Preoxygenate with 100% oxygen.
3. Monitor:
   a. Blood pressure every 1-2 minutes for 15 minutes and then at least every 5 minutes.
   b. ECG.
   c. Pulse oximetry.
   d. End-tidal CO_2.
4. Recheck anesthetic machine, laryngoscope, endotracheal tube cuff, suction.
5. Induction after the obstetrician is scrubbed and patient prepped and draped: thiopental 4 mg/kg and succinylcholine 1.5 mg/kg.
6. Rapid sequence intubation:
   a. No intermittent positive-pressure oxygenation by mask prior to intubation.
   b. Cricoid pressure (do not release until after endotracheal cuff is inflated).
   c. Have failed or difficult intubation drill prepared.
7. Maintenance: N_2O with 50%-60% oxygen (100% oxygen if fetus premature or distressed) until baby delivered.
8. Halothane 1%-1.5%, isoflurane 1.5%-2%, or enflurane 2% to relax uterus until delivery, then turn off or reduce to 0.5%.
9. Oxytocin infusion after delivery.
10. Muscle relaxation with succinylcholine 0.1% infusion or short-acting nondepolarizing relaxant (vecuronium, atracurium).
11. Intravenous narcotic supplement after delivery.
12. Extubate with patient on her side and after her protective reflexes have returned.

---

erin is administered intravenously. These drugs, as well as the volatile anesthetic agents, may cause rapid hypotension. Their use in hypovolemic patients must be associated with volume expansion, either with crystalloid or colloid, depending on the situation. The current practice in our institution is to administer 100 μg nitroglycerin intravenously, as a bolus. The uterus will relax in about 30 seconds, with recovery of smooth muscle tone in approximately 1 minute. In the absence of hypovolemia, this dose has not been associated with clinically significant hypotension.

Cesarean section. A prolapsed cord, or sudden severe fetal distress, demands expeditious delivery. This is usually accomplished under general anesthesia (Boxes 7-1 and 7-2), although many anesthesiologists now feel that subarachnoid block may be administered just as rapidly. Except for such acute emergency, regional anesthesia, either subarachnoid or lumbar epidural blockade (Box 7-3), has become the preferred technique. In cesarean breech deliveries, low Apgar scores were noted by Crawford[25] in 41% of general anesthesia cases and

---

BOX 7-3   EPIDURAL ANESTHESIA FOR CESAREAN SECTION

---

1. Intravenous preload with 15-20 ml/kg crystalloid solution.
2. Insert epidural catheter at L2-3 or L3-4 space.
3. Left lateral tilt: wedge under right hip or tilt table.
4. Administer oxygen via disposable plastic face mask.
5. Test dose of 3 ml 2% lidocaine with 1:200,000 epinephrine (probably a more reliable indicator of subarachnoid than intravascular placement of epidural catheter).
6. Inject local anesthetic solution through catheter in incremental doses to achieve a block to T4 dermatome. Fentanyl 75-100 μg may be added to the local anesthetic.
7. Monitor:
   a. Fetal heart until abdomen prepped.
   b. Blood pressure every 1-2 minutes for 15 minutes. Nausea is often the first indication of hypotension.
   c. ECG.
   d. Pulse oximetry is recommended.
8. Maintain verbal contact with patient. This will aid her composure and give early warning of somnolence, agitation, etc.
9. After delivery, sedative drugs may be given intravenously if necessary.
10. Be fully prepared to treat complications: hypotension, toxic reactions (cardiovascular collapse, convulsions), total spinal block.

in 7% of cases with epidural block. He also reported that the incidence of neonatal depression was increased with general anesthesia when the uterine incision to delivery time exceeded 90 seconds; this was not noted when the cesarean section was done under epidural block. This may be explained by the enhanced uteroplacental perfusion that occurs during epidural anesthesia.[26]

The premature fetus is more affected by maternally administered depressant drugs than is the term fetus,[27] particularly in the presence of fetal distress. Regional anesthesia is generally recommended in the presence of prematurity.

OTHER MALPRESENTATIONS
Obstetric considerations

Brow and face presentations. Brow and face presentations both consist of an abnormal attitude of the fetus when in a longitudinal lie. They are rare, with face presentation occurring in about one of 500 fetuses[12] and brow occurring in one of 1500.[28,29] Face presentation can be delivered vaginally in most situations and can best be managed with unhampered participation by the patient. Epidural anesthesia is helpful in those situations in which low forcep delivery is indicated.

Brow presentation is much more rare, with the frontal bone presenting. Ninety-one percent of brow presentations convert to face or occiput-posterior and delivery can be by the vaginal route. These circumstances rarely occur in a full-term or large fetus.[30] Since face and brow presentations are most often associated with prematurity, high parity, or congenitally abnormal fetuses, it is important to attempt to rule out anomalies and to carefully assess the maternal pelvis and fetal size.

Transverse lie—shoulder presentation. The cause of this malpresentation is usually any factor contributing to abnormal relaxation of maternal abdominal wall; multiple pregnancy; and factors such as placenta previa and contracted pelvis, which prevent normal accommodation of the fetus to the lower segment. The incidence is about 0.3%.[31] Delivery should be by cesarean section, except in cases of very immature pregnancies (under 26 weeks) or small fetuses proved by ultrasound to have lethal anomalies. Anesthesia is directed at providing optimal relaxation; surgically a vertical (low or classical) incision, large enough to prevent fetal trauma during delivery, may be required.[30,31]

Compound presentation. This condition is reported to occur in about one of 1000 cases,[32] but it is probably less frequent because of recent decreases in multiparity. Grandmultiparity and prematurity are the most frequent associated, or contributing, conditions.

Anesthetic considerations

Brow, shoulder, and face presentations are generally delivered by cesarean section. Either general or regional anesthesia may be administered. Cord prolapse is a common complication of shoulder presentation and usually necessitates immediate cesarean section under general anesthesia.

MULTIPLE GESTATION

The incidence of multiple gestation in the general population is about one in 90 pregnancies.[33-35] However, the recent widespread use of drugs to induce ovulation and the availability of facilities for *in vitro* fertilization have markedly increased the incidence in a growing segment of the population.[34,36] The effect of age and parity on the incidence is confined almost entirely to dizygotic twins.

Obstetric considerations

There are three major considerations in any discussion of multiple pregnancy (Fig. 7-2): diagnosis, fetal growth, and labor and delivery.

Diagnosis. The diagnosis of twins can be made with close to 100% accuracy if universal early ultrasound scanning is practiced. While physicians in the United States have not yet considered universal ultrasound for all pregnancies as being justified on a cost-benefit basis, the actual practice in our center has shown that more than 80% of all pregnant women have at least one ultrasound examination during pregnancy. Because of the high mortality rate in twins, primarily associated with prematurity, early diagnosis is mandatory. If routine ultrasound is not practiced, there should be a clear list of indications for at least one ultrasound at about 16 to 18 weeks. These indications include high parity, advanced maternal age, prior history of twins, obese patients (over 85 kg or over 20% above ideal weight for height),[37] and patients who at 18 weeks have a uterine size (symphysis-fundus height) greater than 20 cm. When the uterus is larger than expected clinically at 16 to 20 weeks' pregnancy, it is almost always due to multiple pregnancy, pronounced obesity, or short stature. All of these merit a detailed fetal scan.

Fetal growth. Multiple-pregnancy fetuses are born weighing considerably less than singleton fetuses. It has been assumed that the weight difference starts at 26 weeks and progressively increases as term approaches.[38] In data obtained from *Stats Canada,*[39] all births from 1980 to 1984 inclusive (documenting birth weights for 1.75×10^6 babies), it was apparent that the birth weight differences go back to at least 22 weeks (Table 7-6).

There are several different types of growth lag that should be identified, since their management

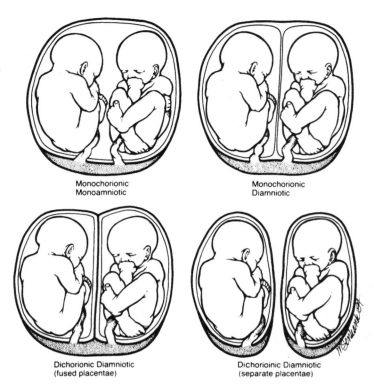

Monochorionic
Monoamniotic

Monochorionic
Diamniotic

Dichorionic Diamniotic
(fused placentae)

Dichorioinic Diamniotic
(separate placentae)

Fig. 7-2 Placentation in twin pregnancies. (From Berkowitz RL: Multiple gestations, in Gabbe SG, Niebyl JR, Simpson JL (eds): *Obstetrics: Normal and Problem Pregnancies.* New York, Churchill Livingstone, 1986, p 741. Used by permission.)

Table 7-6 Birthweight and gestation: singleton and twins

Gestation (wk)	Singleton median wt (g)	Twin median wt (g)	Weight difference (g)
22	532	438	94
24	680	615	65
26	890	803	87
28	1155	1044	111
30	1490	1400	90
32	1875	1672	203
34	2315	2040	275
36	2820	2375	445

Data from percentiles of birthweight by duration of pregnancy, Canada, except Newfoundland. 1980-1984 (singletons); 1978-1982 (twins).

differs.[40] Growth lag can occur in both twins to the same degree in each, or there can be discordant growth, with one twin more significantly affected than the other. In this latter group, growth lag may be due to placental insufficiency or twin-to-twin transfusion. To identify these abnormalities of growth, all twin pregnancies should be monitored routinely with ultrasound, at least every 4 weeks. If the growth arrest becomes evident, more frequent ultrasounds may be necessary. Ultrasound examination requests should always specify that head and abdomen diameter and circumference are required and that a description of the amniotic fluid volume should be provided. There is still considerable controversy about the difference between twins in biparietal diameter measurements and their predictive accuracy. When the predicted weight is lagging in one or both fetuses, other fetal assessment techniques and clinical judgment should guide in the decision regarding time of delivery. Nonstress tests, biophysical profile, oxytocin challenge tests, and Doppler flow studies may all be useful adjuncts to clinical assessment.

Labor and delivery controversies

The controversies and the evidence supporting individual decisions to use cesarean section or vaginal delivery are extensively reviewed by Cetrulo and Chervenak.[41,42] There appears to be general agreement that when the presenting twin is a vertex, vaginal delivery is an appropriate option. Cetrulo,[41] however, shows data that support a high cesarean section rate in all but vertex-vertex situations. When breech presentation exists in the first twin, the same decision-making process should be applied as for singleton breech.

The threshold for viability in twins is slightly higher than for the singleton fetus, and in multiple pregnancies delivering prematurely, before 27 weeks, the fetus seldom survives. Before undertaking surgical procedures with high maternal risks, careful and expert ultrasound assessment should be performed to rule out congenitally abnormal fetuses.

When making management decisions about multiple pregnancies, one of the most important considerations is that of the skills and expertise of the obstetric and anesthesia physicians and their awareness of outcomes in their own centers compared with currently published standards.

Anesthetic considerations

The anesthetic management of multiple birth is similar in many ways to that of breech delivery. Prematurity is a frequent complication of multiple birth, and the infants are therefore more sensitive to the depressant effects of narcotic drugs. The normal maternal physiologic changes in cardiocirculatory and respiratory functions are exaggerated by the larger-than-normal intrauterine mass. There is a significantly reduced functional residual capacity, an increased severity of aortocaval compression, and dyspnea. Blood loss at delivery may be excessive, and the overdistended uterus predisposes to postpartum atony. The increased incidence of pregnancy-induced hypertension will also affect anesthesia management.

The mode of delivery is largely determined by the number of fetuses. Most women with three or more fetuses will be delivered by cesarean section.[3,34,36] Other factors that affect the route of delivery include complications of pregnancy (particularly pregnancy-induced hypertension), noncephalic presentations, fetal distress, and complications of labor.

Evaluation of maternal status early in labor is essential, because anesthesia may have to be induced rapidly for complicated vaginal birth or for cesarean section. When three or more fetuses are present the anesthesiologist should preferably evaluate the patient before labor.

Labor and vaginal delivery. Before 1975, regional analgesia and anesthesia were thought to be contraindicated in multiple gestation. Prolongation of labor, an increased risk of aortocaval compression (with subsequent maternal hypotension and reduced placental perfusion), and increased need for forceps and breech delivery were the reasons given for avoiding regional analgesic techniques. Crawford[15] noted that labor is not significantly prolonged by lumbar epidural analgesia and that

the interval between the birth of the first and second twins may be shortened. The safety of this technique in multiple gestation was later confirmed by others.[43-45] In a prospective study of 200 twin deliveries, Crawford and Weaver[46] reported that in vaginal delivery with epidural analgesia, the acid-base status of the second twin was as good as, or better than, its sibling. This was not so in nonepidural deliveries. This study also reported an apparent benefit to both twins when the bearing-down reflex was abolished.

Before establishment of the epidural block, a large-bore intravenous cannula must be in place. Hypotension, associated with the increased risk of aortocaval compression, is prevented by careful prehydration and careful attention to lateral uterine displacement. A venous blood sample is drawn for type and screen. Pronounced lumbar lordosis, caused by the increased abdominal girth, and edema of the skin over the lower back will sometimes make insertion of the epidural needle difficult. Placing the parturient in a sitting position will often overcome this problem. Analgesia is provided by careful titration of low-concentration ($\leq 0.25\%$) bupivacaine or ropivacaine. Epinephrine is best avoided in patients who have had recent beta-mimetic therapy. Otherwise, 0.125% or 0.0625% bupivacaine with 1:800,000 epinephrine will provide adequate first-stage analgesia. Before delivery, or to prevent premature bearing-down through an incompletely dilated cervix, the block may be extended to the sacral segments. Anesthesia for forceps delivery or intrauterine manipulation may be rapidly induced through the epidural catheter with the use of 2% lidocaine (or carbonated lidocaine, when available), 3% 2-chloroprocaine, or 0.5% bupivacaine, with or without addition of epinephrine.

After the birth of the first twin, the overstretched uterus is usually sufficiently relaxed to allow intrauterine manipulation between contractions. If further relaxation is required, a small intravenous bolus of nitroglycerin (50 to 100 μg) will generally be adequate. Emergency administration of general anesthesia should be the exception rather than the rule.

Cesarean section. We are not aware of any studies that compare general and regional anesthesia for cesarean section in multiple pregnancy with regard to maternal safety and neonatal outcome. The choice of technique will depend on the experience and expertise of the anesthesiologist and the preferences of the patient and obstetrician. In our institution regional anesthesia (spinal or epidural) is the preferred technique.

The excessive enlargement of the uterus requires many of these patients to undergo delivery before term. The premature infant is more sensitive to the depressant effects of narcotic drugs and other general anesthetic agents. Gastric emptying may be delayed and gastric acidity may be increased because of the large uterine mass. In addition, postoperative pain is more easily controlled after regional anesthesia and the patient is more alert than after general anesthesia.

The safety of regional anesthesia in these cases has been reported.[46,47] However, the risk of hypotension is aggravated by the aortocaval compression produced by the massively enlarged uterus, compounded by the sympathetic blockade produced by the regional anesthetic. Epidural anesthesia allows for careful titration of the local anesthetic which is administered in small, incremental doses. Spinal (subarachnoid) anesthesia, which has a more rapid onset of action, is more likely to produce profound hypotension. General anesthesia is occasionally required for emergency cesarean section and for those few patients in whom regional anesthesia is contraindicated.

General anesthesia is induced with the uterus carefully displaced laterally. Preoxygenation is essential because of the rapid maternal desaturation expected after induction of anesthesia and before endotracheal intubation and ventilation of the lungs.

Regardless of the choice of anesthetic technique, a large-bore intravenous cannula must be inserted and the patient carefully prehydrated with at least 1500 ml of a dextrose-free crystalloid solution. Two or three units of blood must be crossmatched and made readily available. These patients lose more blood at cesarean section than those with a singleton gestation; they are also at greater risk of postpartum atony and severe hemorrhage. Oxytocin infusion may be required. If this does not cause contraction of the uterine muscle, prostaglandin $F_{2\alpha}$ may be injected directly into the myometrium. The contents of the vial are diluted to a concentration of 0.2 mg per milliliter. This is injected slowly, in 1- to 3-ml increments, to a total dose not exceeding 25 ml (5 mg).[48-50]

CONCLUSION

Both malpresentation and multiple gestation place parturients in a high-risk category. Thus, close interaction between the obstetrician and the anesthesiologist is essential for ideal planning of management.

REFERENCES

1. Seeds JW, Cefolo RC: Malpresentations. *Clin Obstet Gynecol* 1982; 25:145.
2. Collea JV: Current management of breech presentation. *Clin Obstet Gynecol* 1980; 23:525.
3. Pritchard JA, MacDonald PC, Grant NF: *Williams' Obstetrics,* ed 17. New York, Appleton-Century-Crofts, 1984, pp 855-866.
4. Kitchen W, Ford GW, Doyle LW, et al: Cesarean section or vaginal delivery at 24 to 28 weeks' gestation: Comparison of survival and neonatal two-year morbidity. *Obstet Gynecol* 1985; 66:149.
5. Herschel M, Kennedy JL, Kayne HL, et al: Survival of infants born at 24 to 28 weeks' gestation. *Obstet Gynecol* 1982; 60:154.
6. Effer SB, Saigal S, Rand C, et al: Effect of delivery method on outcomes in the very low birth weight breech infant: Is the improved survival related to cesarean section or other perinatal care maneuvers? *Am J Obstet Gynecol* 1983; 124:123.
7. Synnes AR, Ling EWY, Whitfield MF, et al: Perinatal outcomes of a large cohort of extremely low gestational age infants (23-28 completed weeks of gestation). *J Pediatr* 1994; 125:952.
8. Duenholter JH, Wells E, Reisch JS, et al: A paired control study of vaginal and abdominal delivery of the low birth weight breech fetus. *Obstet Gynecol* 1979; 54:310.
9. Mann LI, Gallant JM: Modern management of the breech delivery. *Am J Obstet Gynecol* 1979; 134:611.
10. Olshan AF, Shy KK, Luthy DA, et al: Cesarean birth and neonatal mortality in very low birth weight infants. *Obstet Gynecol* 1984; 64:267.
11. Main DM, Main EK, Maurer EM: Cesarean section versus vaginal delivery for the breech fetus weighing less than 1500 grams. *Am J Obstet Gynecol* 1983; 146:580.
12. Seeds JW: Malpresentation, in Gabbe SG, Niebyl JR, Simpson JL (eds): *Obstetrics: Normal and Problem Pregnancies.* New York, 1986, Churchill Livingstone, pp 464-465.
13. Bloom R, Cropley C, Drew CR: *Textbook of Neonatal Resuscitation.* American Heart Association and American Academy of Pediatrics, 1987.
14. Myers SA, Gleicher N: Brech delivery: Why the dilemma?: *Am J Obstet Gynecol* 1987; 156:6.
15. Crawford JS: An appraisal of lumbar epidural blockade in patients with a singleton fetus presenting by the breech. *J Obstet Gynaecol Br Commonw* 1974; 81:867.
16. Bowen-Simpkins P, Fergusson ILC: Lumbar epidural block and the breech presentation. *Br J Anaesth* 1974; 46:420.
17. Breeson AJ, Kovacs GT, Pickles GT, et al: Extradural analgesia: The preferred method of analgesia for vaginal breech delivery. *Br J Anaesth* 1978; 50:1227.
18. Confino E, Ismajovich B, Rudick V, et al: Extradural analgesia in the management of singleton breech delivery. *Br J Anaesth* 1985; 57:892.
19. Donnai P, Nicholas AD: Epidural analgesia, fetal monitoring and the condition of the baby at birth with breech presentation. *Br J Obstet Gynaecol* 1975; 82:360.
20. Darby S, Hunter DJ: Extradural analgesia in labour when the breech presents. *Br J Obstet Gynaecol* 1976; 83:35.
21. James FM: Anesthetic considerations for breech or twin delivery. *Clin Perinatol* 1982; 9:77.
22. Donchin Y, Evron S: Relaxation of the uterus with amyl nitrite in cases of multiple deliveries and breech presentation. *Abstracts of the 13th Annual Meeting of the Society for Obstetric Anesthesia and Perinatology,* San Diego, 1981, p 29.
23. Peng ATC, Gorman RS, Shulman SM, et al: Intravenous nitroglycerine for uterine relaxation in the postpartum patient with retained placenta (letter). *Anesthesiology* 1989; 71:172.
24. DeSimone CA, Norris MC, Leighton BL, et al: Intravenous nitroglycerine for manual extraction of a retained placenta. *Abstracts of 20th Annual Meeting of Society for Obstetric Anesthesia and Perinatology,* San Francisco, 1988, p 112.

25. Crawford JS, Davies P: Status of neonates delivered by Caesarean section. *Br J Anaesth* 1982; 54:1015.

26. Jouppila R, Jouppila P, Kuikka J, et al: Placental blood flow during Caesarean section under lumbar extradural analgesia. *Br J Anaesth* 1978; 50:275.

27. Barriere G, Sureau C: Effects of anaesthetic and analgesic drugs on labour, fetus and neonate. *Clin Obstet Gynaecol* 1982; 9:351.

28. Johnson CE: Abnormal fetal presentations. *Lancet* 1964; 84:317.

29. Meltzer RM, Sachtleben MR, Friedman EA: Brow presentation. *Am J Obstet Gynecol* 1968; 100:255.

30. Kovacs SG: Brow presentation. *Med J Aust* 1970; 2:820.

31. Cruikshank DP, White CA: Obstetric malpresentations: Twenty years' experience. *Am J Obstet Gynecol* 1973; 116:1097.

32. Breen JL, Wiesmeien E: Compound presentation: A survey of 131 patients. *Obstet Gynecol* 1968; 32:419.

33. Guttmacher AF: The incidence of multiple births in man and some of the other unipara. *Obstet Gynecol* 1953; 2:22.

34. Cetrulo CL, Ingardia CJ, Sbarra AJ: Management of multiple gestation. *Clin Obstet Gynecol* 1980; 23:533.

35. Benirschke K, Kim CK: Multiple pregnancy. *N Engl J Med* 1973; 288:1276.

36. McGillivray I: Twins and other multiple deliveries. *Clin Obstet Gynecol* 1989; 7:581.

37. Rosso P: A new chart to monitor weight gain during pregnancy. *Am J Clin Nutr* 1985; 41:552.

38. MacLennan AH: Multiple gestation: Clinical characteristics and management, in Creasy RK, Resnick R (eds): *Maternal Fetal Medicine: Principles and Practice.* Philadelphia, 1985, WB Saunders, pp 580-591.

39. *Stats Canada.* Department of Vital Statistics, National Department of Health and Welfare, Ottawa, Canada.

40. D'Alton ME, Dudley DKL: Ultrasound in the antenatal management of twin gestation. *Semin Perinatol* 1986; 10:30.

41. Cetrulo CL: The controversy of mode of delivery in twins: The intrapartum management of twin gestation (Part I). *Semin Perinatol* 1986; 10:39.

42. Chervenak FA: The controversy of mode of delivery of twins: The intrapartum management of twin gestation (Part II). *Semin Perinatol* 1986; 10:44.

43. Weeks ARL, Cheridjian VE, Mwanje DK: Lumbar epidural analgesia in labour in twin pregnancy. *Br Med J* 1977; 2:730.

44. Gullestad S, Sagen N: Epidural block in twin labour and delivery. *Acta Anaesthesiol Scand* 1977; 211:504.

45. James FM, Crawford JS, Davies P, et al: Lumbar epidural analgesia for labor and delivery of twins. *Am J Obstet Gynecol* 1977; 127:176.

46. Crawford JS, Weaver JB: Anaesthetic management of twin and breech deliveries. *Clin Obstet Gynecol* 1982; 9:291.

47. Craft JB, Levinson G, Shnider SM: Anaesthetic considerations in Caesarean section for quadruplets. *Can Anaesth Soc J* 1978; 25:236.

48. Jacobs MM, Arias F: Intramyometrial prostaglandin F_2 alpha in treatment of severe postpartum hemorrhage. *Obstet Gynecol* 1989; 55:665.

49. Bruce LS, Paul RH, Vandorsten JP: Control of postpartum uterine atony by intramyometrial prostaglandin. *Obstet Gynecol* 1982; 59(suppl):475.

50. Kamani AA, Gambling DR, Cristilaw J, et al: Anaesthetic management of patients with placenta accreta. *Can J Anaesth* 1987; 34:613.

8 Antepartum Hemorrhage

Maya S. Suresh and *Michael A. Belfort*

Most obstetric complications present as emergencies, one of which is antepartum hemorrhage. Unexpected hemorrhagic obstetric emergencies are challenging to the obstetric/anesthesia care team. Prompt, expert obstetric and anesthetic management is mandatory to ensure good maternal and fetal outcome.

MATERNAL MORTALITY

The World Health Organization defines perinatal death as the decease of any fetus weighing over 500 g. Late antepartum hemorrhage, regarded as bleeding after 22 weeks, complicates 2% to 5% of all pregnancies. Maternal mortality in the United States has decreased in recent years to less than 10 deaths per 100,000 live births.[1] Although the number of maternal deaths has decreased, a significant number of women still die each year as a result of obstetric hemorrhage. Between 1980 and 1985, antepartum or postpartum hemorrhage caused 55 (9%) of more than 600 maternal deaths.[2] The cause of maternal deaths is often related to pregnancy outcome. For example if mothers die after a live birth, antepartum hemorrhage was uncommon. Instead, leading causes of death are pulmonary embolism, pregnancy-induced hypertension, postpartum hemorrhage, and infection. Maternal death secondary to antepartum hemorrhage follows abruptio placenta and stillbirth.[3]

Physiologic changes of pregnancy and response to bleeding

The physician's prime responsibility to a bleeding pregnant patient is to institute the ABCs of resuscitation, airway, breathing, and circulation. However, some physiologic changes in the pregnant woman may impact on the diagnosis, assessment, and treatment of hemorrhage.

The circulating blood volume increases 46% (approximately 1500 ml) over the nonpregnant baseline.[4] Plasma volume and red cell mass increase disproportionately, creating a physiologic hemodilution effect. This may decrease the thromboembolism tendency that accompanies the coagulation system changes of pregnancy.

Cardiac output increases 30% to 50% during pregnancy, and 50% of this increase occurs by 8 weeks' gestation. Both stroke volume and heart rate increases. However, the former is primarily responsible for the elevated cardiac output, which reflects the larger ventricular muscle mass and end-diastolic volume.[5] The stroke volume declines toward term, but the increased heart rate prevails. Mild maternal tachycardia in the late third trimester maintains the cardiac output.[6]

There is selective regional redistribution of the physiologic increase in cardiac output during pregnancy. Uterine blood flow increases tenfold to between 500 and 800 ml/min. This represents an increase from 2% (nonpregnant) to 17% (pregnant) of total cardiac output. Renal, skin, and breast blood flow also increase significantly, but brain and liver do not.

Central hemodynamics in pregnancy have been elegantly studied by Clark et al.,[7] and their data are presented in Figure 8-1.

Central venous pressure and pulmonary capillary wedge pressure (PCWP) are not significantly changed by pregnancy. Lack of an increase in PCWP during pregnancy is the result of ventricular dilatation and reduced pulmonary vascular resistance (PVR).[7] The parturient is at higher risk for pulmonary edema from the significantly decreased gradient between colloid osmotic pressure (COP) and the PCWP.

The systemic vascular resistance (SVR) decreases approximately 21% during pregnancy because of the vasodilator effects of progesterone, estrogen, prolactin, relaxin, and prostaglandins, as well as nitric oxide. Low-resistance placental circulation may function as an "arteriovenous fistula" and further contributes to the lowered SVR. Increased circulating blood volume of the pregnant woman allows her to tolerate more blood loss than if nonpregnant. Many pregnant women do not demonstrate blood pressure or heart rate changes after moderate blood loss. Other indices such as urine output, capillary refill, and hematocrit are used to gauge blood loss.

The transcapillary refill phenomenon rapidly removes 1000 ml of blood from the circulation of a

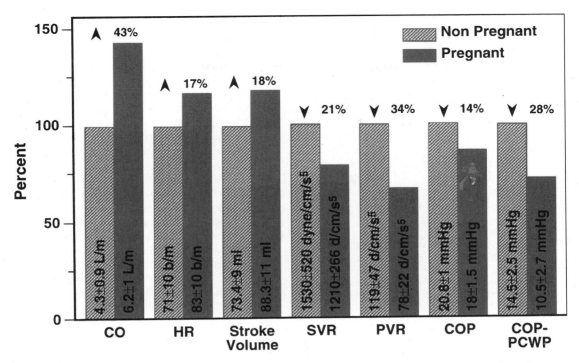

Fig. 8-1 Hemodynamic changes in pregnancy. (From Clark SL, Cotton DB, Lee W, et al: Central hemodynamic assessment of normal term pregnancy. *Am J Obstet Gynecol* 1989; 161:1439.)

pregnant woman. This occurs at cesarean section, creating immediate vasoconstriction of both arterial and venous compartments to preserve essential organ blood flow. After delivery, when the physiologic arteriovenous fistula of the uteroplacental circulation disappears, vasoconstriction occurs more effectively. While the placenta is functional, the natural vasoconstrictor response is impaired and the pregnant woman is less capable of elevating her blood pressure in emergency. Within 4 hours of a significant hemorrhage in a pregnant woman, fluid shifts occur from the interstitial space to partially correct the volume loss and reduce the degree of hypovolemia.

Although the uteroplacental circulation benefits from physiologic vasodilation of pregnancy, lack of vascular autoregulation represents a potential danger to the mother. Danger is imminent during massive blood loss if the normal vasoconstrictor response to elevate systemic vascular resistance is impeded by the arteriovenous fistula on uteroplacental circulation. Further venous compliance increases progressively throughout pregnancy, leading to decreased venous flow velocity and subsequent stasis, thus making the parturient more sensitive to autonomic blockade.[8]

Decreased colloid osmotic pressure and pulmonary vasodilation influence pulmonary edema at a lower wedge pressure during pregnancy. Pulmonary edema complicates rapid infusion of large volumes of resuscitative fluids. Therefore, caution is required in rapidly transfusing a pregnant patient. In addition to cardiovascular compensations during resuscitation, there are also respiratory system changes. The enlarging abdomen may cause pulmonary restriction and reduce the functional residual capacity (FRC). An overlap of the Critical Closing Volume and FRC occurs, as well as partial airway collapse at end-expiration. This alveolar collapse may enhance shunting within the lung and decrease the efficiency of oxygenation. Pregnant women at term increase their oxygen consumption about 17%. The fetus and placenta contribute to 7% of this increase.[9] Higher oxygen consumption makes pregnant women more susceptible to hypoxia.

Blood loss at parturition

Maternal hemorrhage after delivery is common. Delivery follows significant blood loss. Measured blood loss for parturients with no hemorrhagic diathesis or abnormal blood volume averages 500 ml and 900 ml for single and twin vaginal deliveries. Blood loss measures 900 ml for repeat cesarean section.[10] Pregnancy complications greatly exaggerate normal blood loss.

CLINICAL STAGING AND CLASSIFICATION OF HEMORRHAGE IN THE PREGNANT PATIENT

Traditional signs of hypovolemic shock in a nonpregnant subject becomes evident after 15% to 20% of total blood volume loss. A staging scheme to assess the degree of blood loss based on clinical findings is shown in Table 8-1.[11]

Practical applications of this staging scheme to the parturient is unclear for two reasons. First, as stated previously, parturients have a 35% to 40% increase in blood volume. Second, parturients tolerate considerable hemorrhage with minimal changes in cardiac output and blood pressure.

Table 8-1 Clinical staging of hemorrhagic shock by volume of blood loss

Severity of shock	Clinical findings	% Blood loss
None	None	up to 15-20
Mild	Tachycardia (<100 bpm)	20-25
	Mild hypotension	
	Peripheral vaso-constriction	
Moderate	Tachycardia (100-120 bpm)	25-35
	Hypotension (80-100 mmHg)	
	Restlessness	
	Oliguria	
Severe	Tachycardia (>120 bpm)	>35
	Hypotension (<60 mm Hg)	
	Altered consciousness	
	Anuria	

From Gonik B: Intensive care monitoring of the critically ill pregnant patient, in Creasky RK, Resnik P (eds): *Maternal-Fetal Medicine,* ed 2, Philadelphia, WB Saunders, 1989.

Table 8-2 Classification of hemorrhage in the pregnant woman

Class	Acute blood loss (ml)	% Lost
1	900	15
2	1200-1500	20-25
3	1800-2000	30-35
4	2400	40

From Baker RN: Hemorrhage in obstetrics. *Obstet Gynecol Annu* 1977; 6:295.

Hemorrhage in the parturient is classified into one of four classes, depending on the degree of blood loss,[12] as shown in Table 8-2.

The average 60-kg pregnant woman's blood volume is 6000 ml at 30 weeks' gestation. Patients with Class 1 hemorrhage rarely have acute volume deficit. With Class 2 hemorrhage, heart rate and respiratory rate increases. An increase in minute ventilation is early compensation for acute volume loss; it creates respiratory alkalemia reflected in blood gas analysis. Class 2 bleeding leads to orthostatic blood pressure changes, a positive tilt test, narrowing of pulse pressure, and decreased peripheral perfusion with prolonged capillary refill time. Pulse pressure of 30 mm Hg or less in a patient with a Class 2 bleed indicates a diastolic pressure increase (a sign of peripheral vasoconstriction) and should prompt a search for other signs of acute volume loss. Class 3 hemorrhage causes overt hypotension. In a pregnant woman, it equates to a blood loss exceeding 2000 ml, which produces tachycardia, tachypnea, and cold clammy skin. Class 4 hemorrhage results in profound shock and a nonpalpable blood pressure. This condition is an emergency and if untreated leads to circulatory arrest and death.

The hematocrit on its own is not a good indicator of blood loss. Significant changes in hematocrit after an acute blood loss may take 4 hours; complete compensation may not occur until 48 hours. Urine output is a superior indicator, and adequate urine production is a positive indicator of adequate perfusion post-hemorrhage. With acute blood loss, renal blood flow reduces and glomer-

Table 8-3 Etiology of obstetric hemorrhage

Causes	Incidence
Late pregnancy	
Abruptio placenta	1:120 deliveries
Placenta previa	1:200 deliveries
Pre-eclampsia/eclampsia	1:20 deliveries
Delivery and postpartum	
Cesarean section	1:6 deliveries
Inversion of the uterus	1:2300 deliveries
Rupture of the uterus	1:11,000 deliveries
Placenta accreta	1:7000 deliveries
Postpartum hemorrhage (including uterine atony)	1:20 deliveries
Obstetric lacerations	1:8 deliveries

Modified from American College of Obstetricians and Gynecologists: Hemorrhagic Shock. ACOG Technical Bulletin 82. Washington, DC, 1984, p 1.

ular filtration decreases. Sodium and water absorption increase, urine sodium content decreases, and urine osmolality rises. Urine sodium concentration of 20 mEq/L and urine/serum osmolar ratio >2 with urine osmolality >500 indicates reduced renal perfusion and prerenal failure.

Incidence and etiology of obstetric hemorrhage

Antepartum hemorrhage severe enough to warrant hospital admission complicates approximately 8% of all pregnancies,[13] with half of these cases occurring in the third trimester.[14] Obstetric hemorrhage is usually defined as an acute blood loss in excess of 500 mL. The more common peripartum etiologies along with their approximate incidences are shown in Table 8-3.[15]

The most common causes of third-trimester bleeding are placenta previa (22%) and abruptio placenta (31%). Thus more than 50% of patients with antepartum hemorrhage are at risk for severe, and often life-threatening, blood loss.[15] In the remaining 47% of cases, uterine rupture, local genital tract lesions, and marginal placental sinus bleeding may be responsible, but in a significant number of women no obvious source is ever determined. Given the potential for loss of both mother and fetus, all antepartum bleeding should be immediately assessed and as far as is possible a definite diagnosis should be made. This diagnosis will be important in clarifying both the immediate and the long-term therapy options.

Pathophysiology and management of hemorrhagic shock

The survival of patients with hemorrhagic shock depends on the length of time they have been in shock; many aspects of management must be performed virtually simultaneously. If possible, a team approach among the obstetric, anesthesia, and nursing personnel should be used. One algorithm for the management of hemorrhagic shock is outlined in Figure 8-2.

The two basic goals in the management of hemorrhagic shock are restoration of blood volume with adequate oxygen-carrying capacity and definitive treatment of the underlying disorder. Ideally, stabilization of the parturient should take priority before definitive therapy is begun; however, the degree of obstetric hemorrhage encountered may not allow full resuscitation to occur, especially with ongoing extensive blood loss. Based on the parturient's hemodynamic status, a minimum of diagnostic laboratory tests are required before or in conjunction with resuscitation attempts. A urinary catheter should be used routinely in these cases.

These tests include a sample of blood for type and crossmatch and hematocrit and coagulation profile. Intravenous access with one to two large-bore (14- to 16-gauge) intravenous catheters must be established. Resuscitation from hemorrhagic shock requires rapid administration of intravenous fluids to ensure the circulation of well-oxygenated blood to the brain, vital organs, and fetus. Large-bore introducer sheaths for pulmonary artery (PA) catheters can be placed percutaneously in large central veins.[16] Arterial blood gas analysis is important in hemorrhagic shock to rule out acidosis.

In addition, close monitoring of blood pressure and volume status is necessary and therefore may

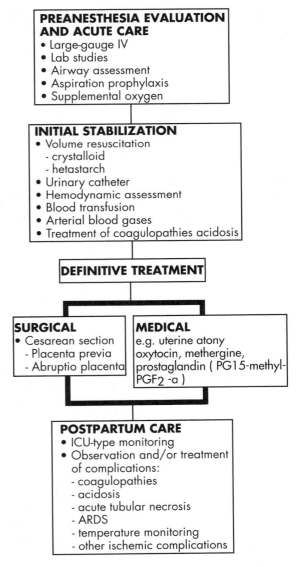

Fig. 8-2 Algorithm for management of hemorrhagic shock.

mandate the placement of arterial, central venous pressure catheters.

Rapid infusion devices using mechanical pumps may be necessary to force fluid through low-resistance tubing, thus allowing adequate resuscitation through only two intravenous catheters. Warming of intravenous fluids and keeping the parturient warm are extremely important, especially if the parturient requires several exchanges of blood volume, since hypothermia decreases the effectiveness of hemorrhagic shock resuscitation. A variety of devices are available to heat fluids and to keep the patient warm.

The priorities in resuscitation in cases of obstetric hemorrhage, in decreasing order of importance, include: restoring blood volume, hemoglobin concentration, and coagulation. The initial fluid replacement of choice should be nondextrose-containing balanced salt solution such as lactated Ringer's solutions. Proponents of crystalloid use claim that such solutions replace extracellular water more effectively than colloidal solution. Studies in nonpregnant patients show that colloidal solutions such as hydroxyethyl starch preserve intravascular volume and microcirculatory blood flow more efficiently than do crystalloids, and they increase cardiac output and oxygen delivery, as well as blood pressure, at much lower infused volume than do crystalloid solutions.[17-20] Generally accepted replacement is 3 ml of crystalloid solution per 1 ml of blood loss.[21] Crystalloid solutions may merely restore blood pressure without increasing cardiac output. A reasonable approach is to use a balanced crystalloid/colloid regimen until the point at which blood component therapy becomes necessary.

The potential for disease transmission (human immunodeficiency virus (HIV), acquired immune deficiency syndrome (AIDS), and hepatitis) by transfusion has caused the formulation of revised guidelines for transfusion of blood and blood products. The incidence of nonicteric and icteric hepatitis after multiple transfusion ranges from 3% to 10%. Recent surveys have suggested that approximately 1% of the reported cases of AIDS are associated with transfusion.[22]

AIDS antibody was positively detected in 0.04% of blood donations by Western Blot assay.[23] However, the current practice of most blood bank facilities is to routinely screen for AIDS antibodies.[24] Despite this practice, the tendency is to adopt lower thresholds for triggering replacement. In a pregnant patient a balance is required towards maintaining adequate perfusion to the fetus and maintaining adequate oxygen-carrying capacity and oxygen delivery both to the mother's vital organs as well as the fetus.

The Consensus Development Conference on Perioperative Red Cell Transfusion concluded that healthy patients tolerate a hemoglobin concentration as low as 7 g/dL.[25] Currently, in nonpregnant persons, hematocrits in the range of 18% to 22% are being accepted in patients who can tolerate such levels. There are no clear guidelines to indicate whether pregnant patients can fit in this group. Oxygen delivery is maintained with a low hematocrit as long as the patient is normovolemic. Therefore, in a *post-partum patient* in the absence of hemorrhage, the current clinical practice is to accept hematocrit in the range of 18% to 22%.

During initial resuscitation, the anesthesiologist estimates the patient's blood loss by evaluating vital signs. For losses ≤30% of pregnant blood volume, crystalloid replacement of 3 times the volume of shed blood volume will provide adequate resuscitation as long as hemorrhage is controlled. Patients with 30% of blood volume or with continuing hemorrhage not only require colloid replacement; they also require 100% oxygen to maximize oxygen delivery to the tissues until hemoglobin can be replaced.

Patients with hemorrhage ≥40% of blood volume require immediate red blood cell (RBC) transfusion along with colloid or crystalloid resuscitation fluids. Type O-negative packed cells can be safely administered to these patients without typing or crossmatch. Using standard blood bank procedures, the time required before type specific blood in excess of 10 units is available for patients needing immediate and massive transfusion is more than 20 minutes. The time taken to complete the paperwork is critical to the outcome of resuscitation of a bleeding parturient. In our institution a system exists whereby Blood Blocs and a single document make 10 to 30 units of type-specific blood ready for transfusion within 2 to 5 minutes.[26] Blocs containing units of O-positive RBCs are stored in the operating room, and 4 units of O-negative RBCs are kept in the delivery room for immediate infusion. The Blood Bloc system has proved to be a safe and effective means of rapidly providing large amounts of blood for emergency transfusions while complying with the record-keeping requirements of the American Association of Blood Banks. If transfusion is begun with type O-negative blood, it is generally recommended that after two units such transfusions continue with type O-negative blood.[27]

After initial assessment of blood loss and planned fluid replacement, the anesthesia care team monitors the patient's response to guide further fluid therapy. The goal is to obtain adequate volume replacement and optimize hemoglobin concentration to achieve and maintain a maximal oxygen consumption, a plateau in the curve of oxygen consumption versus oxygen delivery.

During active hemorrhage or before surgery, any significant coagulopathy other than disseminated intravascular coagulation (DIC) should be corrected by means of appropriate blood component therapy. Platelets and coagulation proteins as well as RBCs are contained in shed blood. Replacement of a patient's blood volume several times over leads to a coagulopathy secondary to thrombocytopenia and possibly consumption of fibrinogen and other coagulation enzymes.[28] Platelet counts <70,000/mm^3 indicate the need for immediate platelet transfusion. It is always preferable to wait for delivery of fetus and placenta and surgical hemostasis before platelet administration; otherwise, the transfused platelets will merely be lost to further hemorrhage. The two exceptions to this statement are when the patient is scheduled for surgery has a preoperative platelet count <20,000/mm^3. In the first place, hemostasis is more easily achieved when a more adequate number of platelets are available; secondary, spontaneous pulmonary hemorrhage has been reported when platelet counts are below 20,000.[29] If platelets from an Rh (D) positive donor are given to an Rh (D) negative recipient who might conceive again, immune globulin containing Rh (D) antibody should be administered promptly.[30] Fibrinogen deficiencies can be corrected with cryoprecipitate or FFP. Fresh frozen plasma may be needed concomitantly for dilutional coagulopathies; however, there is no evidence that prophylactic administration of FFP is of any benefit.[31] Fresh frozen plasma should be reserved for identifiable coagulation defects, such as PTT > 60, PT > 16, or specific factor deficiency.[31]

Shock is usually accompanied by some degree of metabolic acidosis. Usually, enhancing perfusion to vital organs and peripheral tissues corrects the acidosis. However, severe acidosis (pH < 7.2) may be corrected with sodium bicarbonate. Care must be taken to avoid hypercapnia, hypokalemia, fluid overload, and overcorrection of acidosis with administration of bicarbonate.

The type of definitive treatment (medical or surgical) necessary varies with the etiology, severity, and therapeutic response of hemorrhagic shock. Despite surgical intervention to treat the etiology of obstetric hemorrhage and blood and blood product replacement, management of ongoing hemorrhage involves uterine or hypogastric artery ligation, thus preserving fertility. However, in cases of refractory hemorrhage, a hysterectomy may be the definitive treatment.

Management and treatment of hemorrhagic shock are gauged by resolution of clinical symptoms and signs of shock, stabilization of vital signs, normalization of hemodynamic assessment, and restoration of urine output. Subsequent management is directed towards the detection and treatment of the complications of shock.

Abruptio placentae

Definition. *Abruptio placentae* is defined as the premature separation of a normally situated placenta from its attachment to the decidua basalis before the birth of the fetus. It is also called *placental abruption, accidental hemorrhage,* or *placental separation,* and is estimated to occur in 0.5% to 1.8% of all pregnancies.[32-35]

The placental separation may be complete may be partial, or it may involve only the placental margin. Complete detachment of placenta with either concealed or torrential hemorrhage can be fatal to the mother and fetus (Fig. 8-3).

A study of all births in a community indicated[32-35] that more than half of cases of maternal mortality have occurred before the 36 weeks' gestation. Maternal mortality ranged from 0% to 3.1% but may be much higher, depending on the facilities available to the physicians treating the patient. The confidential inquiry into maternal deaths in England, Scotland, Northern Ireland, and Wales (1985 to 1987) showed that maternal mortality fell from 8% in 1919 to less than 1% today. More than 50% of perinatal deaths from abruption are the result of stillbirths. Among live babies delivered after abruption, mortality (16%) occurs within 4 weeks.[36] The survival rate is strongly related to gestational age and fetal weight, and for fetuses weighing >2500 g, the survival rate is reportedly 98%.[37] Fetal mortality rate, however, increases threefold if the abruption is associated with hypertension.[38]

Incidence. Abruptio placentae occurs after the 36 weeks' gestation in 50% of cases.[39] However, less than 20% of identified placental separations occur before 32 weeks; 40% occur between 34 and 37 weeks; and 42% after 37 weeks.[40]

Pathophysiology. Contraction of the myometrium after normal delivery causes muscle retraction and compression of the open vascular channels. This mechanism is much more important than local clot formation for the control of blood loss from the uterus. In an abruption, rupture of a spiral artery results in retroplacental clot formation. Hemorrhage occurs into the decidua basalis, and blood, which would normally have perfused the placenta, is pumped into the uterine cavity at a rate that can potentially empty the maternal vascular system within minutes. The decidua basalis is dissected and a thin layer is left adherent to the myometrium. A retroplacental hematoma then forms and may expand, further separating the placenta

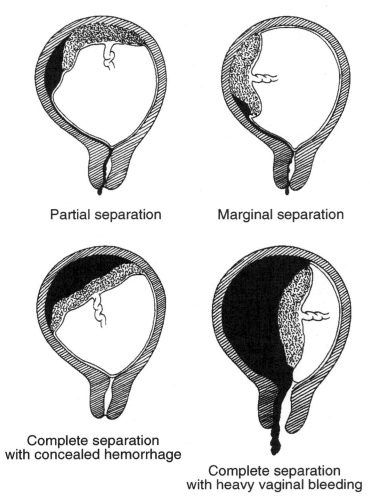

Partial separation   Marginal separation

Complete separation
with concealed hemorrhage

Complete separation
with heavy vaginal bleeding

Fig. 8-3 Various degrees of separation of normally implanted placenta. (From Scott JR: Placental previa and placental abruption, in Scott JR, DiSaia PJ, Hammond CP, et al (eds): *Danforths Obstetrics and Gynecology,* ed 7. Philadelphia, JB Lippincott, Modified and redrawn by Medical Illustration, Baylor College of Medicine.)

and involving more vessels. The uterus, distended by products of conceptions, thus is unable to contract effectively and also compress the torn vessels, and persistent retroplacental bleeding results. This process continues, leading to an ever-enlarging retroplacental hematoma and progressive loss of placental function. As long as the fetus and blood clot are present within the uterine cavity, effective myometrial contraction and retraction are prevented, impairing hemostasis at the separation site. In some cases, the maternal blood escapes into the amniotic cavity, but more frequently it tracks between the membranes and the uterine wall, ultimately escaping via the cervix. This process may take a variable amount of time, depending on the site of the placenta, the degree of separation, the adherence of the membranes, the size of the hematoma, the compliance of the uterus, and the blood pressure of the patient.

Extensive intrauterine hemorrhage may be concealed for many hours, resulting in misdiagnosis if the assessment of the severity of the case is based on the amount of visible vaginal bleeding. As intrauterine pressure increases, tissue thromboplastin and amniotic debris may be forced through open venous sinuses into the maternal circulation. The sudden entry of thromboplastin into maternal circulation explains the increased incidence of amniotic fluid embolism and disseminated intravascular coagulation seen in conjunction with abruptio placenta. The evidence of abruption in 4.5% of placentas after routine vaginal delivery suggests

Table 8-4 Clinical classification of abruptio placentae

Grade	Concealed hemorrhage	Uterine tenderness	Maternal hypotension	Coagulopathy	Fetal distress
0	No	No	No	No	No
1	No	No	No	No	No
2	Yes	Yes	No	Rare	Yes
3	Yes	Yes	Yes	Often	Death

From Page EW, King EB, Merril JA: Abruptio placentae: Dangers of delay in delivery. *Obstet Gynecol* 1954; 3:385.

that small degrees of placental abruption may be more common than is realized.[41]

Classification. A number of different classification systems have been developed for abruptio placentae. None are completely descriptive but all add to the general understanding of the condition. Only a few of the classification systems used are mentioned below.

Sonographic. Nyberg et al[42] described a sonographic classification for abruptio placentae based on the location of blood.

(a) Subchorionic: Blood clot seen between the myometrium and the membranes

(b) Retroplacental: Blood clot seen between the myometrium and the placenta

(c) Preplacental: Blood clot seen between the placenta and the amniotic cavity

Most abruptions can be classified in the first two groups, subchorionic (also referred to as marginal abruption) and retroplacental. It is believed that there are significant differences between these two types of abruption in terms of etiology, presentation, and severity. Marginal abruptions are thought to result from tears in marginal placental veins and are regarded as "low pressure" abruptions.[43-45] The bleeding seen in a marginal abruption is usually associated with dissection of the placental membranes from the myometrial wall, rather than with separation of the placenta from the myometrium.[42] This results in a blood collection that is frequently separate from the placenta, both sonographically and pathologically. The clinical symptoms are usually mild and thus may result in failure to make an early diagnosis.[45] Retroplacental abruption is thought to result from rupture of spiral arteries producing a "high pressure" bleed.

Ultrasound examination has been reported to be of little use in the diagnosis of clinically suspected abruption, probably as result of a lack of collection of blood because of free passage through the cervix.[45] Others feel that ultrasound is useful to exclude placenta previa[46] and to assess the age of the blood clot.[42] Acute hemorrhage is hyperechoic or isoechoic relative to the placenta, while an older blood clot (>2 weeks) is almost sonolucent. An

acute abruption may occasionally be seen as a discrete collection of blood between the placenta and myometrium, but more often than not the blood dissects into the placenta or myometrium and is difficult to recognize sonographically. In these cases the placenta may appear to be heterogenously thickened.[42,47-49] In addition, there may be rounding of the placental margins and intraplacental sonolucencies. The normal placenta should not measure more than 5 cm in thickness, so that a placenta with a thickness of 8 to 9 cm should raise the suspicion of an abruption, especially in an appropriate clinical scenario.[48]

Pathologic. Fox classified placental abruption from a pathologic perspective. Blood from an abruptio placentae can be found[41]:

1. *Under the membranes,* concealed as a subchorionic bleed
2. *At the cervix,* presenting as obvious vaginal bleeding
3. *In the amniotic cavity,* after rupture of the membranes
4. *Under the placenta,* leading to an increasing concealed retroplacental clot
5. *In the myometrium,* infiltrating between the muscle fibers and ultimately producing a Couvelaire uterus in severe cases

Clinical. Page et al[50] classified abruption into four grades, based on the degree of maternal and fetal morbidity (Table 8-4).

Clinical diagnosis. The classic signs and symptoms of abruptio placentae include abdominal pain, hemorrhage (revealed [20% to 35%] or concealed [65% to 80%])[39,51] uterine irritability/tetany and tenderness, coagulopathy, and fetal distress/death. Hurd et al[47] identified a number of important signs and symptoms of abruptio placentae (Fig. 8-4).

Characteristics of bleeding from placental separation is dark and nonclotting; however, sudden separation is arterial-looking, massive, and life-threatening. The shed blood is almost always a mixture of fetal and maternal blood, and for this reason the fetal condition frequently mirrors the degree of blood loss, whether it is revealed or con-

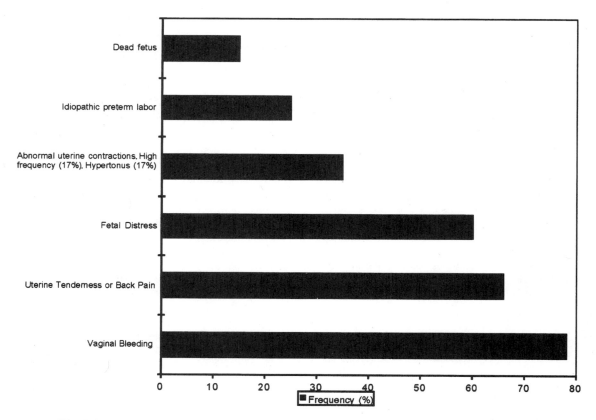

Fig. 8-4 Prevalence of signs and symptoms of placental abruption. (From Hurd WW, Miodovnik M, Hertzberg V, et al: Selective management of abruptio placenta: A prospectus study. *Obstet Gynecol* 1983; 61:467.)

cealed. By the time a fetus dies after an abruption there has been a very significant bleed (usually >2.5 L) and coagulopathy is a very real risk (35%).[51,52] Coagulopathy and maternal hypovolemic shock should be anticipated and prepared for whenever fetal demise occurs in association with abruption. Given the association between hypertension and abruption, the clinician should not be fooled by an apparently "normal" blood pressure (which may be the result of hypovolemia in a patient with chronic hypertension or preeclampsia). All available clinical signs, particularly heart rate, urine output, and respiratory rate, should be considered in the diagnosis.

Differential diagnosis. In cases in which there is obvious vaginal bleeding, the differential diagnosis must include marginal sinus rupture, placenta previa, genital tract trauma/lesions, vasa previa, cervicitis, vulva or vaginal varicosities, and hematuria.

In those patients in whom pain is the major presenting feature and there is no visible bleeding, the differential diagnosis should include acute appendicitis, ovarian cyst complications (hemorrhage,

torsion, rupture), pyelonephritis, fibroid degeneration, retroplacental hemorrhage, uterine rupture, hematoma of the rectus sheath, chorioamnionitis, medical causes of acute abdominal pain (diabetes, syphilis, sickle cell disease, porphyria, herpes zoster, myocardial infarction, pneumonia), and orthopedic causes such as lumbar or sacral strain.

Grading of abruptio placentae. The clinical grading system for placental abruption is shown in Box 8-1.

Risk factors. The associated risk factors in abruptio placentae include hypertensive disorders, low-lying placenta or placenta previa, fibroids, trauma, cocaine abuse, cigarette smoking, increased parity and age, physical work and stress, and a history of a previous abruption.[53] There is some evidence that age is not an independent risk factor, but abruption is more associated with higher parity.[14]

Hypertension. Women with mild preeclampsia do not have an increased incidence of abruption. However, parturients with chronic hypertension and superimposed preeclampsia (10%) or those with severe preeclampsia (2.3%) or eclampsia

---

BOX 8-1 CLINICAL GRADING SYSTEM FOR PLACENTAL ABRUPTION

---

0 Asymptomatic. Only diagnosed when a small retroplacental clot is noted.

I Vaginal bleeding with or without uterine tetany. No sign of maternal shock or fetal distress.

II External vaginal bleeding may or may not be present. No signs of maternal shock. Fetal distress is present.

III External vaginal bleeding may or may not be present. There is pronounced uterine tetany associated with constant abdominal pain. Maternal shock and fetal demise are present. Coagulopathy may be present.

From Knuppel AR, Drukker JE: Bleeding in late pregnancy: Antepartum bleeding, in Hayashi RH, Castillo MS (eds): *High Risk Pregnancy: A Team Approach,* Philadelphia, WB Saunders, 1986.

(23.6%) have an increased incidence of retroplacental abruption. A number of studies, however, did not find any evidence of placental abruption with hypertension.[14,33,34,54]

Trauma. Blunt trauma, particularly as a result of automobile accidents, is a definite risk for placental abruption.[55] This risk may be exacerbated by lap seat belts. Auto deceleration after collision flattens the uterus against the abdominal wall; this produces an opposite tearing force between the elastic uterine muscle and the unelastic placenta. The placenta separates from the uterine wall. Occult abruptio placentae follows maternal trauma with placental abruption, causing pain and bleeding. Abruption is also known to follow sudden decompression of the uterus; it may occasionally result from rupture of the membranes in cases of polyhydramnios.

Recreational cocaine use. A definite and increasingly seen risk factor for abruption is cocaine abuse during pregnancy.[56] Cocaine causes placental vasoconstriction, decreased blood flow to the fetus, and increased uterine contractility.[57] In a comparison of cocaine and methadone users, a significant difference in the complication rate during labor and delivery was noted, with a 17.3% abruption rate among cocaine users and a 1.3% abruption rate in methadone users.[57] With more common use of cocaine, an increased incidence should be expected during pregnancy. The prevalence of cocaine abuse during pregnancy in an indigent population is 9.8%.[58] The exact impact on the incidence of abruption is still unknown.

Physical work and stress. Schwartz[59] reported the outcome of 49 pregnancies in female physicians, which included 27 residents or fellows. Six (12%) developed acute or chronic abruptio placentae. Therefore, Schwartz concluded that long, stressful work hours are possible risk factors.

Cigarette smoking. Cigarette smoking has been shown to increase the incidence of placental abruption, usually in the form of marginal abruption. Naeye[54] noted an incidence of 1.69% in nonsmokers, 2.46% in smokers, and 1.87% in smokers who had stopped. Microscopic evaluation demonstrated evidence of decidual necrosis at the edge of the placenta.

Folic acid deficiency. It has been suggested that a diet poor in folic acid may result in an increased incidence of placental separation.[14] Large, prospective studies[60,61] have failed to confirm this, however, and confidence in this theory is unsubstantiated at present.

Obstetric management. Major factors in the obstetric management of abruptio placentae are the severity of the abruption as determined by the presence or absence of hypotension and coagulopathy, the gestational age, and the condition of the fetus.

Making the decision to allow vaginal delivery or to proceed with cesarean section in cases in which the fetus is still alive has been facilitated by the advent of electronic fetal monitoring. In most situations, consideration of maternal hemodynamic and coagulation status, coupled with fetal well-being and expected time to delivery, will guide clinical decision making.

Cesarean section is reserved for usual obstetric indications, as well as for severe hemorrhage or worsening coagulopathy developing at a time remote from expected delivery. Judicious use of abdominal delivery may well increase the chances of a viable fetus and reduce the degree of coagulation deficit.[38] Abdella et al showed that 75% of fetal deaths occurred more than 90 minutes after hospital admission,[38] and suggested that immediate action is imperative with a live fetus. As long as the fetus is not distressed, cesarean section should be reserved for situations in which bleeding is heavy and cervical dilation is not advanced. The physician should balance the risks of surgery for the mother against the risks of continued labor for the mother and fetus. With stable maternal hemodynamics in active labor with no fetal distress, a vaginal delivery can be pursued. Continuous electronic fetal monitoring is essential. Blood products should be available, and the fetal membranes should be ruptured and an intrauterine pressure catheter should be in place with preparations for emergency cesarean section should it be necessary. Oxytocin augmentation is not contraindicated if the patient is not already in strong labor. Vaginal delivery should be imminent within 6 to 8 hours, but additional time should be allowed if the patient is hemodynamically stable and there is no progression of the coagulopathy. Labor frequently progresses more rapidly in patients with abruption.[14]

However, in a small percentage of cases there is a paradoxical diminution in uterine activity that tends to total uterine atony refractory to stimulation with oxytocin.[62] In such situations, serious consideration of a ruptured uterus should be entertained, particularly if there are fetal heart rate abnormalities; cesarean section should be performed with appropriate preparation (see below). In those cases in which vaginal delivery is anticipated, operative vaginal delivery with forceps or vacuum extractor is not contraindicated and should be used to shorten the second stage of labor.

Vaginal delivery should be attempted in cases of severe abruption associated with fetal demise, coagulopathy, following appropriate component replacement and oxytocic augmentation as required. Major resuscitation measures for the patient with a dead fetus and disseminated intravascular coagulation (DIC) are often necessary. Volume resuscitation with blood and blood products is outlined in the following section.

There are, however, certain cases in which the uterus appears resistant to augmentation and labor does not progress despite maternal resuscitation and correction of the coagulopathy. In these cases, infusion of aprotinin has been reported to be of use.[62] The application of a bone screw to the fetal cranium (after decompression of the fetal head) followed by traction on the fetal skull has also been reported to effect vaginal delivery in those cases with protracted or arrested labor curves; this avoids potentially life-threatening surgery in cases complicated by DIC.[63] Despite the emotionally disagreeable nature of an operation that is destructive to the fetus, the technique and instrument described by Belfort and Moore[63] allow vaginal delivery in a situation in which surgery represents a very real additional risk to the mother's life.

If uterine atony and hemorrhage persist despite medical therapy with oxytocin, methergine, and 15-methyl prostaglandin $PGF_{2\alpha}$, surgical intervention is mandated. Clark et al[65] believe that hypogastric artery ligation should be reserved for stable patients of low parity who strongly desire further childbearing, as they found a high complication rate and a low success rate with hypogastric artery ligation in obtaining control of uterine hemorrhage.[64,65] Montgomery,[66] however, noted that hypogastric artery ligation is a safe alternative to hysterectomy if it is performed early, before the patient becomes hypotensive or coagulopathic.[66] Percutaneous transcatheter hypogastric artery embolization may be considered in certain select situations, even when bleeding is associated with DIC.[67] O'Leary[68] has popularized a technique of mass ligation of the ascending uterine arteries and veins as a method of avoiding hysterectomy.[68] The technique was noted to be successful in 255 of 265 cases of hemorrhage after cesarean hysterectomy; as a last resort, it is clearly indicated for profound intractable hemorrhage if the patient is unstable, multiparous, and does not desire future childbearing.

Anesthetic management. Hemodynamics and volume status of the mother influences anesthetic management in abruptio placentae. Initial evaluation and treatment emphasize eliminating hypovolemia and assessing the magnitude of blood loss from hematologic and coagulation profile laboratory studies. Patient preparation includes large-bore intravenous catheters, aspiration prophylaxis, left uterine displacement, and supplementary oxygen. Urinary output monitoring via an indwelling catheter is important.

Evaluation. Overt hypotension and tachycardia are signs of dangerous hypovolemia that cannot be ignored. Normal vital signs can be misleading. *Normal or even hypertensive blood pressure does not preclude imminently dangerous hypovolemia.* Hypertension, either pregnancy-induced or chronic, is associated with abruption of the placenta. Serious hemorrhage and hypovolemia result in blood pressure drop to normotensive levels. This normotensive reading creates false security and delays identification of compromised vital organs. The pulse rate may be equally misleading.[29,69]

Some parturients who bleed appreciably have normal blood pressure and pulse rate when in the recumbent position. If sitting, they are hypotensive and/or develop tachycardia. There are several reasons to maintain caution when applying and interpreting the tilt test in a parturient. The tilt test is needless and potentially dangerous for parturients who are hypotensive when recumbent. In parturients with an epidural block who subsequently develop abruption, sympathetic blockade exaggerates the hypotension in the sitting position. The hypervolemic parturient may lose excessive blood before demonstrating orthostatic hypotension.

Monitoring and fluid management. Negative circulatory effects of hemorrhage endanger the mother and compromise the placenta's ability to sustain the fetus. Maternal hypotension and hypovolemia is assessed and corrected by guidance from invasive blood pressure and central venous pressure (CVP) monitoring. Urine output below 30 ml/hr, despite adequate volume replacement, merits placing a CVP catheter.

Central venous pressure monitoring is mandatory to guide fluid resuscitation and transfusion. A review of 36 patients with severe abruptio placentae[70] had CVP monitoring in 17 (50%). Average hemoglobin concentration 24 hours postpartum was 11 g/dl compared with 8 g/dl in the unmonitored group. Further, the monitored group had greater urine output. Significant coagulopathy or DIC precludes the cannulation of subclavian or internal jugular venous sites. In these circumstances, antecubital fossa is preferable, since bleeding from this area can be controlled by pressure and dangerous hemorrhage avoided.

Absolute level of CVP is less important than response of CVP to volume infusion. The fluid challenge test helps in the diagnostic assessment of volume replacement. The hemodynamic pressures are measured before and after an intravenous fluid challenge of 10 to 20 ml/min is administered for 10 to 15 minutes. An increase >5 cm/H_2O in CVP or an increase >7 mm Hg in pulmonary capillary pressure is significant. An elevation or significant increase in pressures indicates cardiac failure or excessive volume replacement.[71]

Serious hemorrhage treatment demands prompt, adequate refilling of the intravascular compartment. Two general guidelines determine the amounts/kinds of fluids needed to combat hypovolemia: (1) Lactated Ringer's solution and blood and blood product replacement should be adequate to maintain the urine output at 0.5 to 1 ml/kg/hr, and (2) the hematocrit should be at least 30%.

Czer and Shoemaker[72] provide support for their recommendation that hematocrit be raised and kept at 30%. In their series of 94 critically ill postoperative patients, mortality rates were lower with hematocrit values maintained at 27% to 33%. However, this guideline is applicable only in the critically ill postoperative patient. In a healthy parturient who has sustained acute obstetric hemorrhage and is adequately volume resuscitated, current concerns of HIV infection and hepatitis transmission may allow a lower hematocrit to be accepted.

Anesthesia for vaginal/cesarean delivery. Vaginal delivery is possible only in mild abruption with no fetal distress, uteroplacental insufficiency, hypovolemia, or coagulopathy. Avoiding misuse of anesthetic drugs or techniques that exaggerate hypotension protects maternal and fetal safety. Therefore, parturients presenting with acute fetal distress, hypovolemia, and coagulopathy are excluded from regional anesthesia. Without these complications, a continuous epidural analgesia technique is used for labor and vaginal or cesarean delivery. Close attention to hemodynamics and fetal effects is always maintained.

Most cases of severe abruption with acute fetal distress require abdominal delivery. General endotracheal anesthesia with rapid sequence induction and cricoid pressure is recommended. Ketamine (0.75 to 1 mg/kg) is the optimum induction agent if uterine tone is normal or decreased. Theoretically, larger doses of ketamine in case of abruption can increase uterine tone and further compromise a stressed fetus. However, a study proves 2 mg/kg ketamine increased uterine tone only in the first trimester. There were no effects on uterine tone at term.[73] Etomidate (0.3 mg/kg) is used if uterine tone is increased or if hemodynamic instability exists.[74] Uterine relaxation with inhalation anesthetic agents helps increase placental perfusion. Low doses of inhalational anesthetic agents also maintain circulatory hemostasis and allows for administration of high FIO_2. Cesarean section with general anesthesia, supplemented by a halogenated agent, increases the risk for blood loss.[75] Although under normal clinical circumstances this is not significant, it may be pertinent in a bleeding parturient.

Complications. The most important sequelae of severe abruption in the postpartum period are uterine atony, postpartum hemorrhage, coagulopathy with DIC, acute renal failure, postpartum hemorrhage, pituitary necrosis or Sheehan's syndrome, anemia, rhesus sensitization and infection, in utero fetal death, newborn depression, or requiring intense resuscitation are major risks to the fetus.

Uterine atony. The uterus, including the Couvelaire uterus, contracts promptly after placental delivery.[76] A Couvelaire uterus does not unequivocally indicate hysterectomy. However, it may become necessary if uterine hemorrhage is not speedily controlled. The obstetric/anesthesia care teams must manage a postpartum hemorrhage resulting from abruption. If excessive bleeding occurs via vagina following vaginal delivery without vaginal or cervical laceration, the uterine fundus is poorly contracted. Exploring the uterine cavity eliminates retained placenta, retained blood clot, and disruption of the uterine wall. Initial management includes bimanual fundal massage and administration of oxytocin 20 to 30 U/L by rapid intravenous rate via direct intramyometrial injection. Intramuscular methylergonovine maleate (methergine) 0.2 mg is effective. Methergine should be avoided in patients with antepartum hypertension, preeclampsia, or connective tissue disorders. In these patients, severe vasoconstriction can precipitate a hypertensive crisis.

Prostaglandin derivatives are effective in treating postpartum uterine atony if other modalities fail. Intramyometrial administration of $PGF_{2\alpha}$ is superior to both intravenous or intramuscular injection.[77] Prostaglandin $F_{2\alpha}$ produces increased oxytocin levels via the Ferguson reflex and enhances release of oxytocin from the pituitary. Uterine atony unresponsive to conventional therapy is successfully controlled with 15-methyl analogue of prostaglandin $F_{2\alpha}$ (carboprost, hemabate). Intramyometrial administration is preferable to peripheral intramuscular injection, especially in patients in shock with compromised circulation.[78] Use of prostaglandins is not recommended in patients with pulmonary bronchospastic disease. Further, pronounced transient arterial desaturation secondary to intrapulmonary shunting occurs with 15-methyl prostaglandin $F_{2\alpha}$ administered for severe postpartum hemorrhage due to uterine atony.[79] Drugs, dosages, and side effects are shown in Table 8-5.

Postpartum hemorrhage. Clinically, postpartum hemorrhage is the loss of 500 ml of blood after delivery. Its incidence doubles if patients have abruption, and it increases eightfold if DIC simultaneously occurs.[80] The increased incidence in DIC is thought to result from a combination of poor myometrial contractility resulting from extravasation of blood into muscle, the inhibitory effect of the fibrin degradation products (FDP), and overdistention of the uterus. Uterine atony and hemorrhage invariably happens if FDP is elevated, since this product causes uterine relaxation and inhibits the action of oxytocin.[81] This situation demands replacement of blood and blood products and correction of DIC.

Nelson and Suresh[82] demonstrated that isolated uterine vasculature of pregnant patients with obstetric hemorrhage had impaired reactivity to multiple vasoconstrictors. Their results suggested that obstetric hemorrhage involves in part a lack of constrictor reactivity of the uterine vasculature.

Massive and rapid blood transfusion restores depleted blood volume, maintains tissue perfusion, and prevents renal failure. However, coagulopathy of massive transfusion, intrauterine retroplacental fibrinogen consumption, and hemodilution of rapid volume replacement worsen the bleeding disorder. The anesthesia care team must correct all causes for the bleeding disorder, including the coagulopathy (see section on DIC).

Coagulopathy

CONSUMPTIVE COAGULOPATHY. Differentiating a consumptive coagulopathy from a dilutional coagulopathy is difficult. Placental abruption is the most common cause of consumptive coagulopathy in pregnancy. Disseminated intravascular coagulation (DIC) complicates approximately 10% of all abruptions but is more common in those cases in which fetal death has occurred.[29] Overt hypofibrinogenemia (less than 150 mg/dL), elevated levels of FDP, and variable decreases in other coagulation factors occur in 30% of women with placental abruption that is severe enough to kill the fetus. Such coagulation defects may not be common in those cases in which there is fetal survival. The major mechanisms for consumptive coagulopathy are DIC and, to a lesser degree, retroplacental bleeding.

DIC, which produces a dramatic decline in coagulation factors and platelets, occurs because of retroplacental consumption of fibrinogen or from

Table 8-5 Pharmacologic agents useful for controlling uterine atony

Agent	Dose	Route	Side effects
Oxytocin (Pitocin)	10-20 units	IV drip, IM, intramyometral (multiple sites)	Hypotension: decreased SVR, MAP; resultant increased HR, CO Anti-diuretic activity: hyponatremia, oliguria, water intoxication Uterine hypertonicity: decreased uterine blood flow, uterine rupture
Ergonovine (Ergotrate) and methylergonovine (Methergine)	0.2 mg	IM	Arterial and venous vasoconstriction: hypertension, increased CVP and SVR, pulmonary edema, seizures, cerebral edema, intracerebral hemorrhage, cardiac arrest
Prostaglandin 15 Methyl $F_{2\alpha}$ Hemabate	0.25 mg 0.25 mg diluted in 10 cc saline	IM, intramyometrial (multiple sites)	Decreased SVR, MAP: increased CO, HR, unchanged PVR

the release of an unidentified thrombogenic substance into the circulation. The thrombogenic substance, thought to be thromboplastin, triggers extrinsic coagulation pathway activation. Thrombin converts fibrinogen to fibrin and initiates intravascular clotting. DIC ends in consumption of Factors I, II, V, and VIII, and platelets. Thrombi and fibrin are reportedly deposited in the microcirculation, thus interrupting blood flow to vital organs. The fibrinolytic system activates to lyse the excessive fibrin almost simultaneously; this is termed secondary fibrinolysis.

Retroplacental consumption of clotting factors also causes DIC by deposition of substantial fibrin in the uterine cavity. This process stimulates the secondary activation of circulating plasminogen to plasmin, which enzymatically destroys circulating fibrinogen. Thromboplastin release into the maternal circulation from a retroplacental clot is a possible cause of consumption of coagulation factors and platelets. DIC develops rapidly in the obstetric population. Development is accentuated with placental abruption or amniotic fluid embolism. Laboratory evidence of prolonged PT and PTT, hypofibrinogenemia, thrombocytopenia, and elevated fibrin degredation products (FDP) confirms DIC. The half-life of FDP is long (5 to 7 hours), and it is not useful for following the clinical course of DIC. Another test for DIC assesses antithrombin III (AIII) levels, which are lower in most patients with DIC.[83] The patient, in addition to uterine bleeding, also bleeds from intravenous sites, the gastrointestinal tract, and subcutaneous tissues. Letsky has classified the severity of DIC is classified into three stages[84]:

- *Stage I:* Low-grade, compensated DIC has elevated levels of FDPs and increased levels of soluble fibrin complexes.
- *Stage II:* Uncomplicated, and no hemostatic failure, the added findings beside Stage I features are decrease in fibrinogen levels, platelet count, and Factors V and VII.
- *Stage III:* Established, with hemostatic failure; has extremely low platelet count with elevated FDPs.

Stage I and II DIC occur in mild and moderate abruption; Stage III happens in severe abruption.

For patients with suspected abruptio placentae, measurement of clotting parameters and FDP is important. A simple observation test in delivery or emergency room gives immediate assessment for acute situations. This test requires 5 ml maternal venous blood drawn into a clean glass tube, shaken gently, and allowed to stand. If a clot does not form within six minutes, or the clot is lysed within one hour, a clotting defect is present. The fibrinogen level is <100 mg/100 dL when clots fail to form in 30 minutes. Severe hypofibringenemia is also noted in abruptio placenta associated with fetal death.[51] Cryoprecipitate is indicated (Box 8-2) if fibrinogen levels decrease below 100 mg/dL (normally 100 mg/dL is required for adequate hemostasis) and if active bleeding is present. Not all patients with fibrinogen levels below 100 mg/dL will bleed from hypofibrinogenemia. The presence of hypofibrinogenemia and active hemorrhage is a definite indication for the administration of cryoprecipitate. Hypofibrinogenemia rapidly corrects itself postpartum and hence, despite low levels, cryoprecipatate need not be given in the absence of hemorrhage.

Treatment requires prompt blood transfusion, replacing clotting factors, and delivering products of conception.

DILUTIONAL COAGULOPATHY. Massive transfusion can be defined as the transfusion of 10 or more units of blood or an amount greater than one blood volume. As blood is stored, it develops inherent storage-related problems that are responsible for complications associated with massive transfusion. During storage, the pH drops, potassium increases, 2-3 diphosphoglycerate decreases, Factors V and VIII degrade, platelets are lost, and red cells lyse.

Dilutional coagulopathy causes hemorrhagic diathesis in patients receiving multiple units of blood. Storage temperatures of 4° C damage platelets. They are trapped and absorbed by the reticuloendothelial system. Total platelet activity lessens to 50% to 70% of original *in vivo* activity after 6 hours. After 24 or 48 hours, platelet activity reduces to 10% or 5% of normal. Infusions of mul-

---

BOX 8-2 CRYOPRECIPITATE

Cryoprecipitate contains:
  Fibrinogen
  Factor VIII
  von Willebrand factor
  Factor XIII
  Resuspended 15-25 mL plasma
  One bag of cryoprecipitate contains 300 mg fibrinogen. In adults who have a plasma volume of 40 mL/kg, 1.4 bags of cryoprecipitate per 10 kg body weight raise the fibrinogen level to approximately 100 mg/dL. Therefore, a 70-kg patient requires 10 bags of cryoprecipitate.

The fibrinogen level of 100 mg/dL safely produces hemostatis. A fibrinogen level of 200 mg/dL prevents further bleeding. The dose of cryoprecipitate varies: 10 to 20 bags for an adult. Cryoprecipitate, frozen and stored at 19° C, is thawed in 30 to 40 minutes at 37° C.

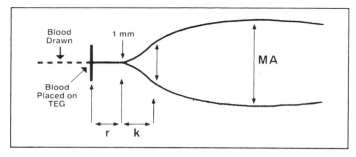

r time (min) = reaction time or time to initial fibrin formation

k time (min) = rapid fibrin build-up and crosslinking

MA (mm) = maximum amplitude of the TEG trace -- a measure
          of maximum clot strength and dependent on the
          concentration of fibrinogen, platelet numbers and function

Fig. 8-5 Schematic diagram of thromboelastography (TEG).

Table 8-6 Correlation between platelet count and incidence of bleeding

Platelet count (cells/mm³)	Total number of patients	Number of patients bleeding
>100,000	21	0
75,000-100,000	14	3
50,000-75,000	11	7
<50,000	5	5

Data from Miller RD, Robbins TO, Toug MJ, et al: Coagulation defects associated with massive blood transfusions. *Ann Surg* 1971; 174:794.

tiple units of stored blood (>24 hours) dilutes the patient's available platelet pool.

Platelet count rarely decreases to predicted lows from dilution alone.[85-87] Platelets are released into the circulation from the spleen and bone marrow, and some nonfunctional platelets exist. Prophylactic platelet administration during massive transfusion has no benefit. The practice of giving platelets to treat laboratory evidence should be discouraged.[88] Platelet therapy is needed when the platelet count is below 50,000 to 75,000/mm³. A bleeding problem may exist with the combination of dilutional thrombocytopenia and DIC. Patients with acutely induced thrombocytopenia develop a hemorrhagic diathesis at a much higher platelet count than patients with chronically induced thrombocytopenia. Adequate hemostasis from a surgical incision or trauma requires a higher platelet count to plug the holes in damaged capillaries. Platelet count reasonably and accurately indicates when a potential bleeding problem from dilutional thrombocytopenia may occur (Table 8-6).

Each platelet concentrate increases platelet count 10,000 to 12,000/mm³ in a 70-kg patient. Two to three units of fresh frozen plasma will generally increase Factors II, VII, IX, and X to levels adequate for proper coagulation.

INTRAOPERATIVE MONITORING OF COAGULOPATHY. If a coagulopathy is suspected, the diagnosis should be confirmed with laboratory data including prothrombin time, activated partial thromoboplastin time, platelet count, fibrin split products, and thromboelastography, if available. The bleeding time evaluates the integrity of the whole-blood hemostatic system, and it may be useful for determining the adequacy of platelet function. However, in anesthetized patients, the bleeding time is difficult to perform and hypothermia can affect its accuracy. Recently, several reviews have pointed out that the bleeding time is an unreliable test for bleeding.

The thromboelastogram (TEG) is a whole-blood viscoelastic test giving information about the platelet function. The maximum amplitude of the tracing is affected by the quality and quantity of platelets; hence, a decreased maximum amplitude suggests a functional platelet disorder. Variables measured by the TEG and the common abnormalities that can be distinguished by means of TEG are shown in Figures 8-5 and 8-6.

Fresh frozen plasma contains all the clotting factors except platelets. Most of the factors are stable in stored blood with two exceptions, Factors V, and VIII. Factors V and VIII are not stable in stored blood, and they decrease to 15% and 50% of normal after 21 days. Packed RBCs have even fewer coagulation factors. Consequently, FFP is recommended in the following cases:

Variable	Measures	Abnormality		Example
r reaction time	thromboplastin generation via the intrinsic pathway	↑r	Factor deficiency Heparin Severe thrombocytopenia	**Factor deficiency** 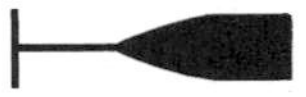
α angle of divergence	rate of clot formation	↓α	Hypofibrinogenemia Thrombocytopenia Thrombocytopathy	**Hypofibrinogenemia** 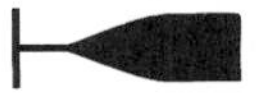
ma maximum amplitude	maximum clot strength/elasticity	↓ma	Thrombocytopenia Thrombocytopathy Hypofibrinogenemia Factor XIII deficiency	**Thrombocytopenia** 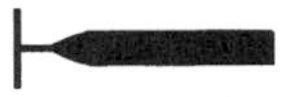
ma + 30	clot retraction after 30 minutes	↓ma+30	Fibrinolysis	**Fibrinolysis** 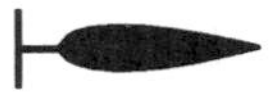

r = 21-30 mm
α = 30-41
ma = 45-54 mm
ma + 30 = minimal reduction

Fig. 8-6 Typical thromboelastogram (TEG) pattern and variables measured, normal values, and examples of some abnormal tracings. (From Faust RJ: Functional platelet disorders, in Faust RJ: *Anesthesiology Review,* ed 2, New York, Churchill Livingstone, 1994.)

· A generalized bleeding that cannot be controlled with surgical hemostasis or cautery.
· A partial thromboplastin time at least ≥1.5 times control.
· A deficient Factor V and VIII based on laboratory evidence.

However, Factors V and VIII rarely decrease below those levels required for hemostasis.

The overall increased use of FFP prompted the National Institute of Health (NIH) in 1985 to conduct a consensus conference on this issue.[89] The conference concluded that there was little or no data for the administration of FFP as part of the therapy following massive transfusion. Despite the NIH statement, component blood therapy, especially FFP, continues to be used.[89]

Acute renal failure. The overall incidence of renal failure in abruptio placentae is 1.2% to 8.9%. Acute renal failure occurs in severe abruption with and without DIC. It is believed to be secondary to hypotension and hemorrhagic shock (prerenal), microvascular clotting and fibrin deposition in periglomeroular arterioles, and myoglobinuria alone or in combination.[90,91] Some degree of renal ischemia occurs in 10% of patients with severe hemorrhage. Renal failure may manifest as transient oliguria or anemia accompanied by renal tubular or cortical necrosis. Renal cortical necrosis has been reported in cases of placental abruption; the probable cause

is severe intrarenal vasospasm from massive hemorrhage. Renal failure is reversible in most cases (acute tubular necrosis) but may be associated with varying degrees of long-term failure if cortical necrosis exists. The key to preventing acute renal failure is aggressive blood, fluid, and volume resuscitation to prevent hypovolemic shock and renal ischemia.[92] Monitoring of volume status is important in these patients to ensure adequate circulating volume without precipitating pulmonary edema. In some situations, especially when there is DIC present, noninvasive cardiac monitoring with echocardiography is very useful. Myocardial performance and ventricular filling pressures can be determined[93] and fluid management decisions can be made in lieu of PA catheter monitoring. If echocardiography is not freely available, invasive monitoring of some sort (CVP catheter, PA pressure catheter) is advisable. Diuretic agents should be used only under exceptional circumstances and with caution.

Urine output should be monitored closely postoperatively. Persistent low urine output signals the onset of renal failure after hypovolemia is corrected. If oliguria persists despite a CVP reading of 7 cm H_2O, then placement of a PA catheter may be considered, especially in a patient who has severe preeclampsia with placental abruption. A PA catheter allows preload and afterload assessment along with cardiac output and other variables.

These patients may require inotropic support or the administration of low-dose (2.5 μg/kg/min) dopamine.

Pituitary necrosis or Sheehan's syndrome. Any patient with severe hemorrhage or shock may develop hypopituitarism or Sheehan's syndrome as a result of avascular necrosis of the pituitary gland. This usually involves the anterior pituitary, resulting in failure of lactation, amenorrhea, and features of hypothyroidism and adrenocortical insufficiency. It is suggested that any pregnant patient who has had a severe hemorrhage accompanied by hypovolemic shock be followed from an endocrine standpoint for at least 12 months.[80]

Fetal compromise and death. Hypoxia and anemia are major risks to the fetus. The infant often needs aggressive, effective, and immediate resuscitation at delivery. Administering blood from the fetal surface of the placenta with a heparinized syringe corrects neonatal hypovolemia.

Pritchard and Brekken[51] noted that between 1956 and 1965 the incidence of abruption resulting in fetal death was 1 in 433 deliveries (0.2%). They estimated that at least 2 L of blood must be lost in order to result in fetal death. In 38% of the patients, the fibrinogen level was below 150 mg/100 ml and in 28% below 100 mg/100 ml.[51]

Anemia and infection. Anemia and infection are commonly encountered during the postpartum period in patients who have experienced severe abruptio placentae,[76] and anticipation and early intervention are important.

Risk of recurrence. The risk of a recurrent abruption after a single prior episode is variously reported as ranging from 8.3% to 16.7%.[51] After two previous abruptions this risk increases to 25%. Pritchard[53] noted that in those cases in which the abruption had been severe enough to kill the fetus, 7% of patients had an abruption with their next pregnancy. Of all subsequent pregnancies of women who have had an abruption, 30% will fail to result in a living child.[14]

A favorable outcome for baby, and more importantly, the mother, depends on early diagnosis of abruptio placentae and active treatment. It is satisfactorily managed only by a complete obstetric perinatal team with immediate availability of blood transfusion and anesthesia services.

Placenta previa

Definition and incidence. Placenta previa is defined as implantation of the placenta in the lower uterine segment in advance of the fetal presenting part. The placenta is normally placed in the body of the uterus and away from the cervical internal os. If the placenta obstructs the descent of the fetus, there is the potential for maternal hemorrhage as the fetus impacts it and separates it from the decidual plate. There are a number of different classifications for placenta previa, most of which depend on a description of the placenta in relation to the internal os. This may, however, be confusing since there is a potentially changing relationship between the location of placenta and the uterus during the third trimester and particularly during labor. Thus, most grading systems pertain to the antepartum period.

Grading of placenta previa. The grading system generally accepted in the United States is shown in Table 8-7.

The degree of placenta previa does not necessarily predict outcome; all degrees (with the possible exception of low-lying placenta) should be regarded as potentially capable of causing life-threatening hemorrhage. The four variations of placenta previa are shown in Figure 8-7.

Incidence. The incidence of placenta previa varies from 0.1% to 1.0% of third-trimester preg-

Table 8-7 Grading placenta previa

Grade	Description
I	**Low-lying placenta:** The placenta is implanted in the lower uterine segment but does not encroach on the internal cervical os. Differentiating between a low-lying and a marginal placenta previa can be difficult.
II	**Marginal placenta previa:** The internal cervical os is only just encroached on by the placenta. The placental edge may be palpated by the examining finger. Some authorities feel that even if the placental edge is within 2 cm of the internal cervical os, the term marginal placenta previa is still appropriate.
III	**Partial placenta previa (approximately 30%):** Internal os is partially covered by the placenta.
IV	**Total or complete placenta previa (approximately 40%):** Internal os is completely covered by placenta. When the placenta is concentrically implanted about the internal os, the term central placenta previa is applicable.

From Wilson RJ: Bleeding during late pregnancy, in Wilson RJ, Carrington ER, Ledger WJ (eds): *Obstetrics and Gynecology* St. Louis, Mosby, 1983.

nancies and maternal mortality can reach 0.9%.[94] The ratio of placenta previa in nulliparas (1/1500) as opposed to multiparas (1/20 in grand multiparas) indicates that the condition is largely a problem of parous women.[95] The risk of placenta previa recurring in a subsequent pregnancy is about 12 times the incidence of a first occurrence.

Most studies of the statistics of placenta previa pertain to symptomatic cases, and no data on asymptomatic placenta previa are currently available. There is evidence that the incidence of total placenta previa in the early second trimester may be as high as 5% (in a population of women undergoing genetic amniocentesis).[96] In 90% of these women the placenta previa appears to resolve and the patients remain asymptomatic. Interestingly, however, is that despite apparent resolution of the problem in patients with early trimester placenta previa, there is a higher rate of other complications, including antepartum hemorrhage, abruptio placentae, intrauterine growth retardation, preterm labor, and increased perinatal mortality. It has been reported that as many as 45% of women with "resolved" placenta previa have complicated pregnancies; this places them in a high-risk group.[97]

There are two potential patterns of placental growth after early central placental implantation, centripetal (resulting in complete placenta previa) and unidirectional (toward the more vascularized fundal region). The unidirectional growth may be the cause of the "resolution" as the placenta favors the more vascularized fundal region of the uterus rather than the more fibrous lower segment. Evidence for this mode of growth is provided by the eccentric placement of the cord insertion on the placental plate (eccentric, marginal, or even in some cases velamentous). The insertion point of the cord in the membranes marks the original placental location. A fundal placenta in the second trimester is evidence that there will not be placenta previa at term.

Etiology. Multiparity and the mother's advancing age are risk factors for placenta previa. A strong factor in the development of placenta previa is defective vascularization of the decidua caused by previous inflammatory or atrophic changes. The association between increasing parity and placenta previa suggests that damage of the endometrium by a prior pregnancy may be an etiologic factor. The endometrium underlying the implantation site may be rendered less available for subsequent implantation, causing future pregnancies to implant in the lower uterine segment by a process of elimination. This effect is clearly seen with previous term pregnancies but is also present in cases of multiple early pregnancy terminations.

Clark et al[98] assessed the relationship between increasing numbers of previous cesarean sections and the subsequent development of placenta previa and placenta accreta. The risk of placenta previa was 0.26% with an unscarred uterus, and the incidence increased linearly with the number of prior cesarean sections (up to 10% with four or more cesarean sections).[98]

The risk of recurrent placenta previa is between 4% to 8%.[99] The risk of placenta accreta with placenta previa and one previous cesarean section is 24%; this risk increases to 67% with placenta previa and four or more previous cesarean sections (Fig. 8-8).[98] Poorly developed decidua in the lower uterine segment results in an abnormally firm at-

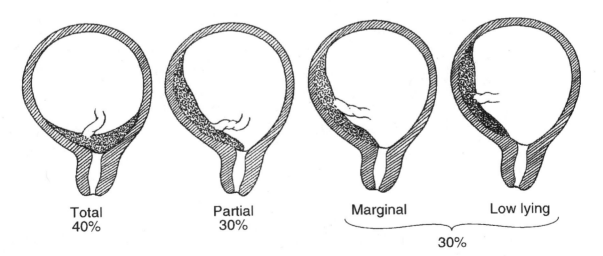

Fig. 8-7 Four variations of placenta previa. (Illustration copyright 1995 Baylor College of Medicine.)

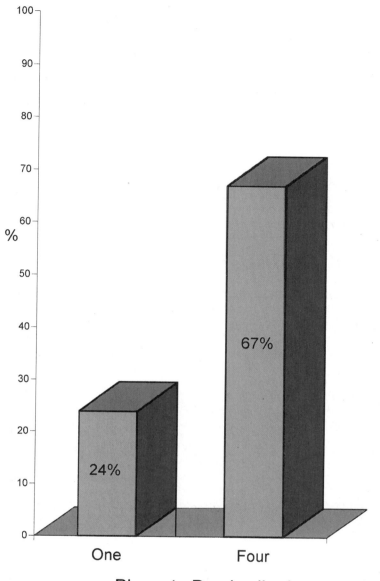

Fig. 8-8 Incidence of placenta accreta after prior cesarean section.

tachment of the placenta and an increased risk of placenta accreta.

Signs and symptoms. The most characteristic event in placenta previa, painless hemorrhage, does not usually appear until near the end of the second trimester or during the third trimester. Patients with vaginal bleeding in the third trimester are assumed to have placenta previa until diagnosed otherwise. The peak incidence of presentation is at 34 weeks' gestation,[29] and more than 50% of cases have already presented before 36 weeks. Only 2% of patients with placenta previa will present with bleeding after 40 weeks.[100] In about 30% of cases, however, bleeding occurs before 30 weeks.[101] The distinction of painless bleeding may in some cases be confusing since approximately 10% of cases of placenta previa are associated with placental separation and symptoms and signs suggestive of abruption.[95] In as many as 25% of cases there are signs of labor, with or without rupture of the membranes.[95] In 25% of cases placenta previa may present only in labor,[102] and these patients usually have a marginal placenta previa. Bleeding results from tearing of the placenta and its attachments to the decidua. The lower uterine segment contracts very poorly and therefore is unable to compress the spiral arteries. Bleeding thus continues unabated and may persist despite delivery of the fetus and removal of the placenta. The bleeding may present after an obvious inciting cause such as a vaginal examination, sexual intercourse, vaginal trauma, or onset of labor. The earlier the bleeding occurs, the more likely it is that the precipitating factor is intercourse and the greater the possibility that the placenta covers the internal os.

The obstetric management of placenta previa depends on anterior or posterior position of the placenta, degree of bleeding, presence or absence of fetal distress, fetal gestational age, fetal maturity, and the degree of previa.

Diagnosis. Clinically, the diagnosis of placenta previa is supported by palpation of a relaxed uterus. The presenting part is usually in the upper uterine segment because of the presence of the placenta in the lower uterine segment. An abnormal presentation is very common, with the fetus being in breech or transverse position in 33% of cases.[102,103] In those fetuses with a cephalic presentation, the presenting part is frequently high above the pelvic brim and difficult to palpate, especially when there is an anterior placenta previa.

Although clinical findings are important, the definitive diagnosis is made by ultrasound examination. With transabdominal ultrasound and a full maternal urinary bladder the accuracy of the diagnosis approaches 93% to 97%.[96,97] The 3% to 7% of incorrect diagnoses are usually from failure to scan the lateral aspects of the uterus or from urinary bladder distention, which causes apposition of the anterior and posterior walls of the lower uterine segment.[104] Thus, before assigning a diagnosis in a case in which there is suspected incomplete placenta previa with an anterior placenta, it is advisable to scan the patient after asking the patient to partially empty her bladder. Other causes for misdiagnosis include uterine fibroids, myometrial contractions, blood clots, late placental migration, and posterior placental location with the fetal head obscuring the placental edge.[105] Transvaginal ultrasound has recently become popular and has been shown to be safe in the diagnosis and management of patients with placenta previa despite the theoretical risk of probe-induced trauma. The transvaginal approach allows superior definition of the lower uterine segment and the placental anatomic relationship, and it has been reported to be 100% sensitive.[106] Even so, false-positive and false-negative results have been reported with the transvaginal approach. The two ultrasound approaches should be used to complement each other. The initial scan should be transabdominal; only in cases in which the diagnosis is still uncertain should the transvaginal route be used.

Ultrasound examination can be used to follow the pregnancy and determine whether the previa is "resolving" or remaining. In addition, fetal growth and fetal Doppler ratios can be assessed because in some cases intrauterine growth retardation may become an issue.[107]

Magnetic resonance imaging (MRI) has been used to diagnose placenta previa. It provides excellent magnetic resolution of the soft tissues and in particular the cervical placental interface.[108] The cost of the MRI study does not justify its routine use, however, and it should be reserved for only those cases in which ultrasound is nondiagnostic. Only in rare circumstances is a definitive diagnosis made using a "double-setup" examination. The only indication for such an examination is when ultrasound and/or MRI studies are inconclusive or when a patient presents with ongoing, but not life-threatening, bleeding in labor. Under these circumstances a digital vaginal examination in an operating room may be indicated with very specific precautions (see Double Set-Up in Anesthesia Management). Using double set-up, with all prerequisites accomplished, the vaginal fornices should be initially explored very gently (using the ultrasound information, if available, to further direct the examining finger to the regions of interest). If the fetal presenting part can be clearly felt in all four quadrants, vaginal delivery is usually feasible and the membranes can be ruptured. If there is any bogginess suggestive of placenta previa, the procedure should be abandoned and abdominal delivery performed. Digital exploration of the cervical canal is not advised because of the danger of precipitating severe hemorrhage.

Obstetric management. Most patients with placenta previa are diagnosed after the onset of painless vaginal bleeding in the late second and early third trimester, or by ultrasound examination at an even earlier gestation. The initial management of any life-threatening bleeding should be directed toward stabilizing the patient. Therefore, patients with active vaginal bleeding should be hospitalized immediately and appropriate resuscitative efforts begun. Large-bore intravenous access should be established, volume expansion must be started, and arrangements for blood products should be made. Fetal heart rate monitoring is also important during this phase of the management. Once the mother has been stabilized, more detailed ultrasound examination can be used to confirm the diagnosis. Until such time as placenta previa is excluded, vaginal examination should be avoided. In modern obstetrics, most patients who have had prenatal care will have had at least one ultrasound examination. Information as to the placement of the placenta should be specifically asked for during the initial assessment.

In general, the diagnosis of placenta previa equates to delivery by cesarean section. There are some situations in which vaginal delivery may be considered. These include minor degrees of previa (Grades I and II with an anterior placenta) and an engaged fetal head. In such patients vaginal delivery is possible since the descending fetal head compresses the placenta against the bony pelvis anteriorly. Delivery can be delayed until 39 weeks, and there are no contraindications to amniotomy or Pitocin augmentation. In cases of Grade III or IV placenta previa, the mandated route of delivery is cesarean section.

Elective cesarean delivery is preferred since emergency surgery has an adverse effect on the perinatal outcome, independent of gestational age.[29] Cotton et al[103] reported that 27.7% of neonates born after emergency cesarean section were anemic as compared with 2.9% of neonates delivered electively. In cases of complete placenta previa where the gestational age is thought to be greater than 37 weeks, we advise that the patient undergo an amniocentesis (if safe and possible) and that elective cesarean section should be performed once fetal maturity is confirmed. In the case of a patient who is unwilling to consent to amniocentesis and who is not bleeding, it may be reasonable to wait until 39 weeks (per ACOG recommendation for elective surgery) and perform an elective cesarean section at that time. The patient should understand the potential risk to herself and her fetus by waiting the additional 2 weeks. Reliance on a menstrual history may be misleading because up to 30% of patients with placenta previa have a bleed in the first trimester that may be mistaken as a menstrual bleed, with resultant underestimation of the gestational age.

Perinatal mortality associated with placenta previa is most strongly linked to the gestational age of the fetus at the time of delivery[101,103] and to a lesser extent to the degree of maternal hemorrhage and hypotension. Given the modern critical care and blood banking facilities now available, it is possible to safely prolong a pregnancy to attain fetal maturity. The expectant approach was popularized by Macafee[109] and Johnson et al,[110] who based their management on the belief that most episodes of bleeding in placenta previa are self-limiting and not fatal to mother or fetus as long as there has not been any precipitating trauma to the placenta (sexual intercourse, vaginal examination, progressive cervical dilatation).[111,112] A further potential advantage to delaying delivery is the possibility that there may be some resolution of the problem as gestation progresses, allowing, in some situations, vaginal delivery as opposed to cesarean section. As a result of expectant management and the availability of sophisticated surgical services and support, the maternal mortality rate has fallen from approximately 25% to less than 1%, and the total perinatal mortality rate has fallen from approximately 60% to under 10%. Despite improved neonatal facilities, however, the great majority (73%) of perinatal deaths in cases of placenta previa are still due to 20% of these patients being delivered before 32 weeks.[103]

The management of placenta previa in the last four decades has changed rather dramatically, and today many of the previously taught absolute contraindications[109] to prolonging pregnancy are felt to be relative contraindications. Cases in which there has been heavy vaginal bleeding, even to the point of maternal hypovolemia requiring blood transfusion, have been managed expectantly with good maternal and fetal outcome. Cotton et al[103] reported a series of patients in which 20% of patients lost more than 500 ml of blood. Of these patients half were managed expectantly, and a gain of approximately 2 weeks was accomplished without adverse outcome. In this study, 25% of the expectantly managed patients required blood transfusion, and in 66% of all patients delivery was significantly delayed. As a general rule, the patient should be transfused to a hematocrit of 30% or greater to optimize maternal and fetal oxygen consumption and to provide a reserve in the event of further heavy bleeding. This is not a hard and fast rule; depending on maternal and family wishes and the presence or absence of cardiovascular signs, transfusion strategies may be individualized.

Continuous reassessment as to the risk-benefit ratio of aggressive expectant management is required. The patient should be delivered as soon as fetal maturity is reached or maternal condition demands. The duration of prolongation required is a function of the patient's condition, the neonatal facilities available, and the preparedness of the obstetrician and hospital to undertake emergency cesarean delivery. Each team should assess its particular situation before arriving at an optimum delivery date. In a high-risk situation with excellent neonatal facilities, it may not be as pressing to delay delivery as it is in a hospital without neonatal ICU capabilities. Neonatal survival on our service approaches 100% at 28 weeks[113] (Fig. 8-9).

We would be unwilling to persevere with repeated blood transfusions and aggressive expectant management in such a situation. In a situation in which neonatal survival is considerably less at this gestational age, the obstetrician and patient

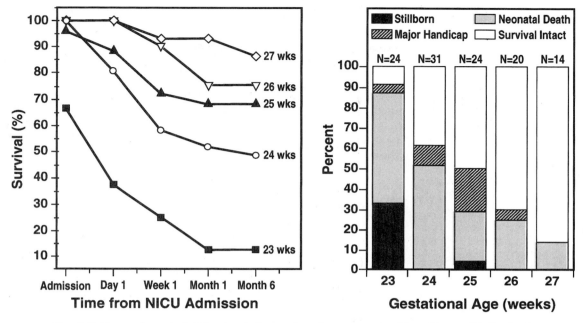

Fig. 8-9 Neonatal survival following delivery after placenta previa. (From Kramer W, Saade G, Goodrum LL, et al: Neonatal outcome after aggressive perinatal management of the very premature infant. *Am J Obstet Gynecol* 1995; 172:417.)

may understandably elect to continue aggressive expectant management. Corticosteroids are recommended in accordance with the NIH Consensus opinion.[114] We advocate the use of betamethesone, 12 mg q 24 hours for the first two doses, followed by weekly steroid injections up to 34 weeks. Expectant management does not result in a defined cutoff point for benefit, but rather demonstrates a gradual increase in the incidence of deliveries as pregnancy progresses.[115] The probability is that a pregnancy will be maintained for 1, 2, 4, or more weeks in relation to the number of weeks already attained (Fig. 8-10). This highlights the point that the further along a pregnancy, the less the potential gain possible in terms of increased maturity.

Tocolytic therapy. The use of tocolytic agents in the management of placenta previa is controversial.[115-117] Patients with placenta previa experience ruptured membranes, spontaneous labor, or some complications prompting delivery before 37 weeks. Using tocolytics after 21 weeks produces perinatal mortality of 41 per 1000 patients. Uterine contractions are a physical sign of abruption that coexists with placenta previa not treated with tocolytics.[117] The combination of tocolytics confuses the clinical picture by causing maternal tachycardia and palpitations, which indicates hypovolemia. The presence or absence of hypovolemia influences the intervention threshold, and some obstetricians deliver early believing there

was an abruption. Conversely, some ignore an abruption, interpreting the clinical signs as being a result of the tocolytic. The decision to use tocolytics must be determined by the obstetricians within each institution, taking into account their particular management style and convictions. A positive decision to use a tocolytic leads to the choice of agent.[118] Magnesium sulfate compared with ritodrine, based on studies of cardiovascular stability during hemorrhage in ewes, worsens the maternal hypotensive and fetal-acid base responses to hemorrhage.[118] Hypermagnesemia attenuates maternal compensatory response to hemorrhage. Many factors influence the choice of tocolytic because no controlled trials objectively assess advantages and disadvantages of any one tocolytic in managing placenta previa. If β-mimetics are used when maternal hypovolemia exists, serious maternal hypotension may result; this may be resistant to treatment with ephedrine and crystalloid administration. Administration of calcium chloride (10 mg/kg) slightly increases maternal cardiac output but does not substantially improve maternal mean arterial pressure, uterine blood flow, or fetal oxygenation.[119] In Baylor College of Medicine in Houston, both terbutaline and $MgSO_4$ have been used with good effect. $MgSO_4$ is favored as a first-line agent for long-term use.

Hospitalization. Home bed rest versus hospital confinement is controversial. Some recommend

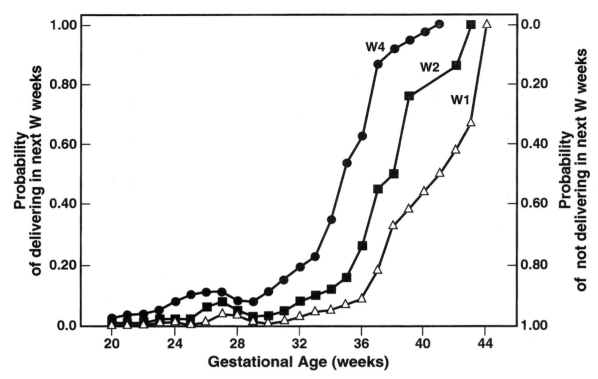

Fig. 8-10 Graph showing the probability that pregnancy in a patient with placenta previa can be maintained for some time longer (1, 2, or 4 weeks). The fetus of 32 weeks has an 80% chance of remaining in utero for 4 weeks; the fetus at 36 weeks, however, has only a 50% chance of gaining 2 additional weeks of gestation. (From Brenner WE, Edelman DA, Hendricks CH: Characteristics of patients with placenta previa and results of "expectant management." *Am J Obstet Gynecol* 1978; 132:180.)

hospitalization for placenta previa patients in fully equipped maternity hospitals from diagnosis until delivery.[109] This approach is challenged when selected patients go home as part of their expectant management.[102,103,120] Home management under appropriate surveillance is acceptable. A minimum of 72 hours of hospitalization before delivery is advised. Approximately 30% of the patients require delivery within this period.[103] Outpatient management is considered if the patient is motivated, clearly understands the gravity of her condition with necessary restrictions on her lifestyle, and is able to get to the hospital within 15 minutes. Cotton et al[103] report no differences in perinatal and mortality rates between patients managed at home and those managed in the hospital. Hospitalization sometimes reduces maternal and perinatal mortality.[121] A religious group that avoided obstetric care reports only one intrapartum maternal death from placenta previa occurred in a group of 355 women managed at home.[122]

Monitoring for pregnancy complicated by placenta previa includes fetal growth determination by ultrasound every 4 to 5 weeks and weekly antenatal assessment after 28 weeks. Two units of crossmatched blood are available for patients with atypical blood types, numerous or atypical antibodies, or designated donors. If the patient is hemodynamically stable, not bleeding, and not anemic (hematocrit greater than 35%), autologous blood donation may be an option.

Surgical considerations. The choice of abdominal incision should be dictated by the clinical situation. In the case of multiple previous surgeries, we advise a vertical skin incision. The type of uterine incision to be made should be decided on at the time of surgery. If there is well-formed lower uterine segment, a posterior placenta (or anterior placenta that is below or just above the bladder reflection), and a fetal lie that is longitudinal, a transverse incision is acceptable. In most other situations, a vertical incision (either a low vertical or a classical) that avoids the placenta as far as possible is usually recommended. There are some who believe that vertical incisions should be avoided because of the long-term implications. Scott[123] believes that it is preferable to convert a transverse incision to a J- or U-shaped incision as needed, rather than to begin with a vertical incision. In most situations where a tubal ligation is planned, we would use the vertical incision liberally, whereas in a primigravid patient who desires future fertility (or in a situation where future deliveries may be in a facility without adequate surgical backup), we would tend to use the transverse incision if at all possible.

The presence of an anterior placenta implanted in the lower segment is not an absolute contraindication to a transverse lower uterine segment incision. In this situation the surgeon has two choices: (1) deliver the fetus through the placenta, or (2) make the incision above the placental edge. Both techniques can result in excessive blood loss if the surgeon is inexperienced and takes too much time in exposing the fetus. If the fetus is to be born through the placenta, the surgeon should be ready to tear through the placenta rather than incise it, and he or she should be experienced in locating and delivering the fetal head. Although Myerscough[124] advises against this method of delivery, in our experience transplacental delivery has not been associated with any more perinatal morbidity than in attempting to avoid the placenta. Prolonged manipulation of a partially separated placenta, no matter what the uterine incision or delivery method, will result in fetal anoxia and blood loss. In most cases of anterior placenta previa there is an anticipated blood loss of more than 1500 ml, and for this reason at least 2 units of crossmatched blood should be available in the operating room. The intraoperative use of cell-saver devices that wash and reuse blood from the operative site is discouraged because of the risk of DIC from placental and amniotic thromboplastins.

Severe postpartum bleeding may occur after delivery of the placenta because the lower uterine segment contracts poorly. Bleeding from the placental implantation site is common and may be controlled by hemostatic sutures, manual compression, and medical therapy as described above in the section on abruptio placentae. If bleeding remains uncontrolled, surgical options such as bilateral uterine artery ligation, bilateral hypogastric artery ligation, or hysterectomy may need to be exercised. The recent development of the argon beam coagulator (Kline Medical, Houston, Texas), a specialized diathermy device that carries the electrical charge to the tissue in a beam of argon gas, avoids mechanical contact with the bleeding sinuses and may help to control hemorrhage from the implantation site. There are no published data on its use in placenta previa, but this technology may offer promise.

One of the major dangers of placenta previa, particularly in association with prior cesarean section, is placenta accreta. This results from the thin, poorly formed decidua in the lower segment, which is easily breeched by the placenta. Placenta accreta and its more severe forms, placenta increta and percreta, are very serious complications of placenta previa. Five of the six maternal deaths noted in Hibbard's series were directly related to placenta accreta.[120] In this situation, attempting to preserve the uterus is often folly and leads to massive blood loss and its attendant complications. The surgeon must assess the situation quickly and decisively, and if needed, a hysterectomy should be undertaken expeditiously. Undue delay leads to excessive blood loss, massive transfusion and volume replacement, dilutional coagulopathy, DIC, and hypothermia, all of which compound an already desperate state. In these cases, early administration of RBCs, FFP, blood products, and platelets, as well as aggressive temperature control, can prevent the onset of coagulopathy and multiple organ dysfunction. In those cases in which the placenta has invaded through the placenta into contiguous tissue, more heroic efforts may be required, including resecting of the tissue if accessible,[125] packing of the abdomen, and arterial embolization under fluoroscopic control.

Anesthetic management. Anesthetic management of placenta previa should take into consideration three different scenarios:

1. Double set-up for vaginal delivery/cesarean section
2. Cesarean section in hemodynamically stable patients
3. Cesarean section in an actively bleeding and hemodynamically unstable patients

Double set-up. Rarely is a definitive diagnosis of placenta previa made under "double set-up." Double set-up entails simultaneously preparing for immediate cesarean section and making available general anesthesia with crossmatched blood. Cervical examination can cause torrential hemorrhage, which mandates immediate delivery. *Consequently, the examination is safer when executed in the operating room.*

Ultrasonography and MRI has made the use of "double set-up" for diagnosing placenta previa obsolete. The remaining indication for double set-up is inconclusive ultrasonographic evidence and active labor with ongoing but not life-threatening uterine bleeding. These conditions warrant the digital vaginal examination, which yields valuable information without jeopardizing the mother or the fetus.

Preparation includes the presence of qualified anesthesia personnel, a scrub technician, instruments, experienced operating team, and a neonatologist, in addition to the obstetrician examining the patient.

Volume resuscitation preparation includes having two or more large-bore intravenous lines and four units of typed and cross-matched blood. The placement of arterial and CVP catheters depends on the patient's hemodynamic status. Monitoring CVP contributes to hemodynamic evaluation.

Parturients who have vaginal examination under double set-up conditions are prepared in the same way as cesarean section patients. Preparation for general anesthesia includes administering oral clear antacid 30 to 45 minutes before examination.

During preoxygenation an assistant is available and ready to provide cricoid pressure. With left uterine displacement, the patient is prepped and draped for cesarean section and placed in a lithotomy position. An obstetrician is ready to perform immediate cesarean section if bleeding starts, while another obstetrician performs the vaginal examination.

Cesarean section is standard procedure if the diagnosis of placenta previa is confirmed.

Hemodynamically stable patient. Anesthetic management for cesarean section in confirmed placenta previa depends on the presence or absence of active bleeding. Either regional or general anesthesia is acceptable in the patient who bled several weeks prior to delivery and is normovolemic. Adequate preparation requires the placement of two large-bore intravenous catheters. In addition, at least two to four units of crossmatched blood must be present in the operating room before proceeding with surgery.

General anesthesia is favored in patients with placenta previa undergoing cesarean section with active bleeding. These patients are at risk for excessive intraoperative blood loss for three reasons. First, the placenta may be located anteriorly; so the obstetrician incises through the placenta. Second, after delivery, the distended lower uterine sement does not contract as well as the fundus. Third, placenta previa patients with previous cesarean sections have added risk for placenta accreta. All factors precipitate extensive postpartum bleeding. Regional anesthesia for cesarean section in placenta previa patients decreases blood loss, lowers incidence of hysterectomy, and has better neonatal outcome.[126] However, hypotension induced by epidural anesthesia in the parturient results in decreased placental perfusion.[118] As stated previously, patients with placenta previa on $MgSO_4$ tocolytic therapy may have exaggerated hypotension. In hypermagnesemic gravid ewes, ephedrine and phenylephrine provided similar restoration of maternal mean arterial pressure; ephedrine was superior to phenylephrine in restoring uterine blood flow during anesthesia-induced hypotension.[127]

Actively bleeding/hemodynamically unstable patient. Copious bleeding and hemorrhagic shock make resuscitating the mother extremely difficult. Completely correcting blood loss before surgery is not always possible because bleeding continues until the placenta is removed. Evaluation of the patient, surgical preparation, aspiration prophylaxis, monitoring, and volume resuscitation should proceed as previously outlined. Preparations for volume resuscitation and induction of anesthesia should proceed simultaneously.

Induction of general anesthesia is preceded with left uterine displacement and preoxygenation (denitrogenation). Using a rapid sequence technique and utilizing cricoid pressure, anesthesia is induced either with 0.5 to 1.0 mg/kg of ketamine or 0.3 mg/kg etomidate. Ketamine produces sympathetic nervous system stimulation and blood pressure maintenance. Etomidate is associated with minimal cardiac depression and is safe in obstetrics.[74] Sodium pentothal or propofol are not the induction agents of choice in a hypovolemic patient. General anesthetic administration may further reduce placental blood flow and fetal oxygenation. Rapid infusion of crystalloid, hetastarch, colloid, and RBCs help restore circulatory volume status.

Some patients may arrive in the operating room hypotensive and moribund. In such cases establishing an airway precedes anesthesia induction. Patients in severe hemorrhagic shock with a maximally stimulated sympathetic system will have a direct myocardial depressant effect from ketamine thus causing further hypotension; therefore, ketamine is avoided. Immediate surgical intervention rectifies blood loss.

Selection of maintenance agents depends on the degree of cardiovascular compromise. Halogenated agents administered during balanced general anesthesia cause uterine muscle relaxation[128] and increase blood loss during cesarean section.[75] However, the loss is not clinically significant since the patients did not require transfusion.[75] In a bleeding patient, it is prudent to eliminate halogenated agents and uterine relaxants. Anesthesia maintenance is achieved with oxygen, small doses of short-acting narcotics, and nitrous oxide as tolerated.

Delivery of the fetus and removal of the placenta minimize the threat to the mother. If bleeding continues from the atonic lower uterine segment, oxytocin, methergine 15-methyl prostaglandin $F_{2\alpha}$, may be necessary to establish uterine tone. As assessed by blood pressure, CVP measurements, and urine output, adequate resuscitation normalizes the blood volume. The neonate also requires intensive resuscitation at birth if asphyxiated, acidotic, and/or hypovolemic.

Disseminated intravascular coagulation characteristic of consumptive coagulopathy is common with severe abruptio placentae but rare with placenta previa. Dilutional thrombocytopenia follows massive transfusions.

Placenta accreta/percreta/increta

A patient with placenta previa or otherwise identified as high risk for placenta accreta is scheduled for elective cesarean hysterectomy to avoid complications after vaginal delivery.

If undetected before delivery, placenta accreta is usually diagnosed if there is unusual adherence and difficulty in placental delivery. Placenta accreta removal results in catastrophic hemorrhage, particularly as the raw myometrium is exposed. The reported average antepartum blood loss is 477 ml.[129] Read reported the average delivery and immediate postpartum blood loss was 3846 ml and 4716 ml, respectively, in those with concurrent previas and 2639 ml in the new previa group. Average blood transfusion was 7.8 units.[129] Clark et al[98] reported an average of 3.5 L in patients having cesarean hysterectomy.[98]

Management in lesser degrees of placenta accreta may involve curettage followed by oversewing of the bleeding placental bed. However, conservative management of accreta and temporizing measures for bleeding include manually cross-clamping the abdominal aorta by compressing the aorta against the vertebral column, thereby reducing the pulse pressure and heavy bleeding at the surgical site. Other measures include intramyometrial injection transabdominally or transvaginally of 15-methyl $PGF_{2\alpha}$ oxytocic agents. Direct intramyometrial injection of 15-methyl $F_{2\alpha}$ has been shown to be superior to ergot preparations in causing immediate uterine and vascular contraction, resulting in decreased bleeding without severe side effects. Ultimately, one may perform a bilateral hypogastric artery ligation and, if that is unsuccessful, an abdominal hysterectomy.

Placenta percreta is a subtype of placenta accreta. Placenta percreta causes intraperitoneal or intravesical bleeding. This is a life-threatening event and characteristically mimics a concealed placental abruption or uterine rupture. Placenta percreta is commonly diagnosed after delivery, since any attempt for manual removal is impossible. It is associated with severe bleeding, shock, or acute inversion of the uterus. Hysterectomy is the treatment of choice since it causes the least morbidity and mortality. Maternal mortality ranges from 67% with conservative management to 2% with prompt hysterectomy, antibiotics, and adequate blood transfusions.

Pregnant women with acute abdominal pain, internal bleeding, previous uterine surgery, and a history of Asherman's syndrome should be suspected of having placenta percreta.[130] These patients are at high risk for hemorrhage, sepsis, and DIC.

The various uteroplacental relationships found in accreta, percreta, and increta are shown in Fig. 8-11.

Anesthetic management. The anesthesiologist with a bleeding, hypovolemic, and unstable patient has two priorities. They are (1) evaluating the airway/oxygen administration and (2) establishing vascular access with large-bore intravenous catheters for volume resuscitation. Blood is typed and crossmatched. Transfusion of Type O-negative or crossmatched blood must be initiated immediately and the patient transferred to the operating room.

With a functioning epidural anesthetic in situ the anesthetic can be continued provided hemodynamic stability remains. Whereas in a patient with no anesthetic on board, should sudden hemodynamic instability develop, the anesthesia care team should proceed with a general anesthesia as described previously.

The development of intraoperative bleeding diathesis can worsen complications markedly. There are no published recommendations for dealing with an epidural catheter in obstetric patients who develop coagulopathy. The anesthesiologist is faced with the dilemma of whether to remove an epidural catheter in a parturient with coagulopathy. Sprung et al[131] make the following recommendations:

1. If there is no evidence of intraspinal bleeding, the catheter must be removed as early as possible because of the potential for intravascular catheter migration and initiation of bleeding.
2. If bleeding is present around the catheter insertion site and possibly in the epidural/subarachnoid space, the catheter must be left in place.
3. Frequent assessment of neurologic status is important until the underlying cause of the coagulopathy is treated and the bleeding is resolved.
4. If intraspinal hematoma leading to neurologic deficit occurs, *immediate neurologic consultation and decompression surgery is needed.*

Elective cesarean hysterectomy in suspected placenta accreta. Preparation of the patient for elective cesarean hysterectomy involves two large-bore intravenous catheters, an arterial catheter, CVP, warming devices, and a minimum of four

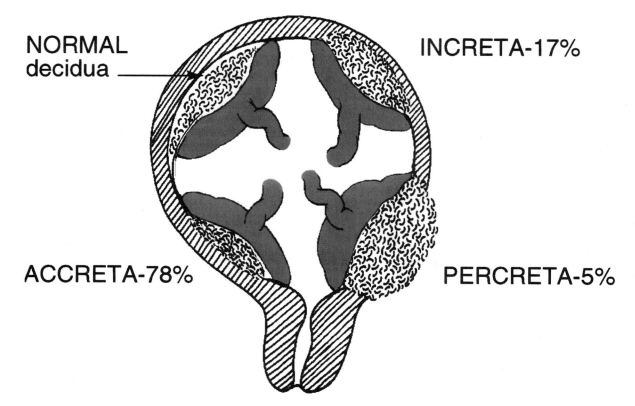

Fig. 8-11 Various uteroplacental relationships found in accreta, percreta, and increta.

units of crossmatched blood in the operating room. In addition, the blood bank is notified that more blood may be required. Anesthesia choice for elective cesarean hysterectomy is controversial.[132-134] Between 1972 and 1984, 7 (28%) out of 25 patients required intraoperative general anesthesia. The causes were patient discomfort and/or inadequate operating conditions.[133] Three reasons precipitate inadequate epidural anesthesia. First, operative time for cesarean hysterectomy is twice that required for cesarean section only. This predisposes the patient to fatigue and restlessness. Second, intraperitoneal manipulation, dissection, and traction is excessive for cesarean hysterectomy, compared with cesarean section only. The main surgical manipulation results in pain, nausea, and vomiting. Third, "the engorged edematous vasculature requires careful dissection facilitated by a quiet operative field," contrary to the previous study.[133] A subsequent, prospective, multiinstitutional study of cesarean hysterectomy[134] showed that the epidural anesthesia provided optimum anesthesia and that none of the cesarean hysterectomy patients required general anesthesia.[134]

Anesthesia determination for cesarean hysterec-tomy depends on the following factors: (1) evaluation of the patient's airway, (2) preferences of the patient and the anesthesiologist, (3) skills and experience of the obstetrician, and (4) availability of manpower.

One can proceed with either general or regional anesthesia in a patient who seems to have an easily intubatable airway. Failed intubation and pulmonary aspiration of gastric contents continue to be leading causes of maternal morbidity from anesthesia. ACOG Committee Opinion[135] states that the risk of these complications can be reduced by careful antepartum assessment and by greater use of regional anesthesia when possible. Committee opinion is valuable and applicable in most situations; however, this sort of reasoning in the case of a patient with difficult airway applied to a patient who is at risk for major hemorrhage may be dangerous. Further, massive fluid resuscitation produces airway edema, making an airway that was easily intubatable into a difficult airway. Furthermore, if the airway is questionable or difficult, the airway must be secured with the patient awake and the use of a fiberscope. An airway established before surgery is preferred in a case with potential for serious hemorrhage. Once the airway is secured, other problems such as hemorrhage and massive volume resuscitation can be managed.

Patients scheduled for cesarean section at high risk for massive hemorrhage receive a general anesthetic. Conversion from regional anesthesia to general anesthesia occurs if unabated bleeding continues.

Choice of anesthetic technique also depends on manpower availability to render help in a situation of hemorrhagic crisis. Securing an airway and simultaneously being involved in massive volume resuscitation can be a tenuous situation without adequate manpower.

The anesthesiologist and obstetrician constantly communicate to determine anticipated risks and extent of bleeding. Securing hemostasis requires special obstetric skills coupled with expert anesthetia techniques. Patients with placenta percreta are not only at high risk for extensive hemorrhage but also for sepsis and DIC.

Postoperative management after cesarean hysterectomy involves a close, ICU type of monitoring initially postpartum. Monitoring includes assessment of serial hematocrit assessment, coagulation profile, hemodynamics, volume status, urine output, ventilatory status, and core temperature.

Vasa previa

Vasa previa is uncommon and has a very high rate of fetal mortality. It is the velamentous insertion of the cord in the lower uterine segment. The umbilical vessels run through the membranes between the fetal presenting part and the cervix. The vessels are unsupported and very vulnerable to tearing or occlusion during labor. Fetal loss is very high, since late diagnosis makes intervention effective. Vaginal bleeding that occurs immediately after membrane rupture and is associated with immediate fetal heart rate abnormalities foreshadows vasa previa. The only choice is immediate cesarean section to save the fetus.

Uterine rupture

Spontaneous rupture of the gravid uterus still carries significant maternal and fetal mortality. The incidence is approximately 1 in 2000 deliveries, with a 9.7% maternal mortality rate and a rate of fetal wastage of 56%.[136] Uterine rupture may be spontaneous, secondary to trauma, or it may result from rupture of a previous uterine scar. Prolonged or obstructed labor is thought to be the predominant causative factor for spontaneous rupture.[137] Conditions associated with uterine rupture include use of oxytocin, cephalopelvic disproportion, grand multiparity, trauma, external and internal podalic version, and abruption.[136] Dehiscence of a previous cesarean section scar, with extension, is probably the most frequent etiology of uterine rupture in modern obstetrics.[136,137]

The most common clinical presentation is vaginal bleeding, shock, and lower abdominal pain.[136] In some instances, the area to which the fetal heart tones were initially localized is noted to have shifted. Sometimes, acute bradycardia or sudden profound fetal distress is noted. In cases of catastrophic rupture and fetal demise, inability to detect fetal heart tones may occur concomitantly with acute abdominal pain, hypotension, vaginal bleeding, appearance of frank blood in the urinary catheter (indicative of anterior rupture into the bladder), and retraction of the fetal presenting part (indicative of fetal expulsion into the abdomen).[136]

Treatment of uterine rupture should be individualized. Abdominal hysterectomy is no longer advocated in all cases. If the fetus is still undelivered or if uterine bleeding is believed to be secondary to a uterine or cervical defect, immediate laparotomy is indicated. If a defect is found at the time of postpartum examination after a vaginal birth after cesarean section (VBAC), but no bleeding is noted and the patient is hemodynamically stable, close observation is warranted, with resort to laparotomy only if the patient shows signs of decompensation.

VAGINAL BIRTH AFTER CESAREAN SECTION

The most important point in management of VBAC is the adequacy of an obstetric facility with the ability to perform emergency cesarean sections within 30 minutes of the decision. Skilled and efficient staff members must be available on site during labor. It is also important that the obstetrician in charge is capable of deciding on the necessity for and safety of midforceps delivery.

Anesthetic management

Potential uterine rupture is still the major consideration in the anesthetic management of this type of trial of labor. Previous cesarean section is considered by some to be a contraindication to epidural analgesia during labor.[138,139] The major concerns about epidural analgesia safety are threefold. First is the probability that an epidural block will mask pain of uterine scar separation and delay the diagnosis of ruptured uterus. Second, epidural analgesia can blunt the sympathetic responses associated with ruptured uterus (i.e., maternal tachycardia) and prevent the diagnosis of ruptured uterus. The third theoretical hazard, sympathectomy induced by an epidural block, can alter the response to hemorrhage. The sympathetic paralysis prevents compensatory vasoconstriction if severe hemor-

Table 8-8 Epidural use in trials of labor*†

Year	Author	TOL	VBAC	Epidurals	%‡
1980	Carlsson	119	105	77	65
1982	Meir	207	175	19	9
1982	Demianczuk	92	50	41	45
1983	Uppington	222	171	71	32
1983	Martin	162	101	27	17
1984	Flamm	230	181	73	32
1984	Graham	242	166	83	34
1984	MacKenzie	143	108	94	66
1984	Ruddick	115	102	115	100
1984	Nielsen	160	150	47	29
Total		1,692	1,159	647	38

*From Flamm BL: Vaginal birth after cesarean section: Controversies old and new. *Clin Obstet Gynecol* 1985; 28:735.
†TOL = trial of labor; VBAC = vaginal birth after cesarean section.
‡% of TOL patients given epidural anesthesia for pain relief during labor.

rhage occurs after uterine rupture. Furthermore, hypotension caused by the epidural anesthesia can be confused with uterine rupture. Thus, an assessment of dangers of epidural analgesia in a trial-of-labor patient falls into three parts: (1) the incidence of uterine rupture, (2) the relative importance of the few signs and symptoms that may be abolished in the overall diagnosis of ruptured uterus (i.e., maternal tachycardia, uterine tenderness, and pain), and (3) the probability of severe bleeding.

The classic symptoms and signs of uterine rupture are well known.[140] Premonitory signs and symptoms are maternal restlessness, anxiety, tachycardia, and scar or lower uterine tenderness between contractions. Actual rupture is characterized by sudden, severe abdominal pain, pronounced fetal heart rate, decrease or cessation of uterine contractions, vaginal hemorrhage, hematuria if the bladder is involved, abdominal shape alteration, and possibly severe hypotension.

Before 1980, VBAC literature revealed few reports on the administration of epidural analgesia to patients undergoing trial of labor. There have been several reports since 1980 in the obstetric literature about the administration and outcome of regional anesthesia in patients undergoing trial of labor[141] (Table 8-8).

Whether use of epidural analgesia increases the incidence of cesarean section has been debated. Stovall et al reported the results of a 1-year prospective study of 272 VBAC patients with liberalized indications for trial of labor.[142] Oxytocin was used as needed, and epidural analgesia was used in patients who requested it. Patients requiring oxytocin augmentation of labor had more pain and therefore required an epidural block for analgesia during labor. Epidural analgesia was administered to 103 of 133 patients (77.4%) receiving oxytocin and only 50 of 139 patients (36%) who did not require oxytocin ($P < 0.001$). The incidence of cesarean section was 31% in patients receiving both an epidural and oxytocin, whereas it was 14% in the group with epidural and no oxytocin. Thus Stovall et al stated that the "negative effect" of epidural analgesia is correlated with the increased use of oxytocin. This study reaffirmed the findings of Flamm et al, who reported that oxytocin use decreased the vaginal delivery rate but epidural alone did not.[146]

A retrospective study[143] demonstrated that the use of oxytocin and epidural anesthesia is not contraindicated and in fact may enhance the success of VBAC shown in Table 8-9. The success rate of 94.2% in vaginal deliveries and the low rate of repeat cesarean section (5.8%) in patients with epidural anesthesia contraindicate the findings of Stovall.[142] Further, intrauterine pressure monitoring is more reliable for detecting impending uterine rupture than is pain during labor.

However, a recent randomized, controlled prospective study[144] demonstrated that epidural analgesia with an initial bolus of 0.25% bupivacaine followed by continuous infusion of 0.125% bupivacaine resulted in significant prolongation in the first and second stages of labor and a significant increase in frequency of cesarean delivery.[145] Further, Thorpe et al,[146] in a theoretic model depicting the dynamic effects of epidural on cesarean section rates over time, demonstrated that cesarean rate would increase several fold. Therefore, the use of low-dose bupivacaine infusion 0.625% becomes even more important to prevent the prolongation of the second stage of labor and the inci-

Table 8-9 VBAC and use of epidural anesthesia*†

Mode of delivery	With epidural anesthesia (n = 700)	Without epidural anesthesia (n = 172)	Total (n = 242)
Vaginal	66 (94.2%)	118 (68.6%)	184
Cesarean Section	4 (5.8%)	54 (31.4%)	58

*From Nguyen TV, Dinh RV, Suresh MS, et al: Vaginal birth after cesarean section at the University of Texas. *J Reprod Med* 1992; 37:10, 880.
†*p* < 0.00005.

dence of operative delivery, as well as to enhance the success of trial of labor in a patient undergoing VBAC.

Present evidence suggests that there is no need to withhold epidural analgesia from patients undergoing VBAC if certain conditions are fulfilled. These are (1) the scar is transverse in the lower segment, and (2) vaginal delivery is possible and safe.

Two precautions should be taken for care of VBAC patients laboring with an epidural block: (1) careful fetal heart rate and uterine monitoring, and (2) providing epidural analgesia with dilute local anesthetic concentrations. A sudden increase in baseline uterine tone or a sudden absence of uterine pressure, alone or coupled with evidence of acute fetal distress, mandates an immediate abdominal delivery. Higher concentrations (0.25% bupivacaine) may mask the pain of ruptured uterus.[149] The decision to use epidural analgesia in VBAC patients must take into consideration all the obstetric and anesthetic indications or contraindications.

Spontaneous hepatic rupture

Spontaneous rupture of the liver during pregnancy was first described in 1844 by Abercrombie.[148] Since then, reported cases have usually been associated with pregnancy-induced hypertension and have occurred in multiparous patients.[149,150] In the typical scenario, the patient, often labeled as preeclamptic, develops epigastric or right upper quadrant pain associated with nausea and vomiting. Right upper abdominal tenderness may be elicited on examination.[151] If the subcapsular hepatic hemorrhage extends beyond Glisson's capsule and intraperitoneal bleeding occurs, signs and symptoms of shock follow. Laboratory values may show evidence of a falling hematocrit, elevated liver enzymes and serum bilirubin, and a developing coagulopathy. The diagnosis is often made on clinical grounds; however, paracentesis, liver scan, ultrasonography, and computed tomography may be helpful for confirmation.[152] Also of note is the occasional finding of a right pleural effusion in patients with spontaneous liver rupture.[151] Liver bi-

opsy usually reveals fibrin thrombi extending up the hepatic arterioles to the periportal sinusoids, and periportal hemorrhagic necrosis.[153]

Expedient exploratory laparotomy is mandated for a patient in shock with evidence of intraperitoneal bleeding, because delay has been associated with increased mortality. Packing the liver and upper abdomen with abdominal lap-packs and providing adequate drainage of the abdomen is recommended in initial management.[152] The patient may be returned to the operating room at a later time to remove the packs once her condition has stabilized. Death is usually secondary to massive hemorrhage. In cases where bleeding is controlled by hepatic artery ligation or lobectomy, postoperative mortality is still high, secondary to hepatic failure and multisystem organ failure. In such cases, after arterial occlusion or partial liver resection, hepatic reserve is presumed to be insufficient to sustain life.[153]

Critical to the survival of patients who have had a spontaneous liver rupture is expedient decision making, usually involving the rapid decision to apply pressure to the bleeding points by packing the abdomen, to replace blood products, and to keep the patient warm before coagulopathy develops. In our experience it is better to return the patient to the operating room on numerous occasions to remove packs and repack the abdomen than it is to persist in fruitless efforts to contain the bleeding in a single protracted operation. With current ICU capabilities, the patient can be kept hemodynamically stable with blood and blood product replacement despite heavy blood loss as long as she is warm and her blood is clotting, but once the bleeding is complicated by coagulopathy the prognosis is frequently grave. Management in these patients is as described in the management of hemorrhagic shock.

CONCLUSION

Hemorrhage in the obstetric patient occurs unexpectedly and has potential for serious maternal and fetal morbidity and mortality. Various aspects of management of hemorrhagic shock have been reviewed.

Different aspects of antepartum hemorrhage, along with obstetric and anesthetic management guidelines, have also been reviewed. A well-equipped Labor and Delivery operative suite, along with expert obstetric, anesthesia, neonatal, and nursing teams, lends to the successful outcome for both mother and baby. Further, postoperative morbidity following obstetric hemorrhage is minimized by excellent critical care management.

REFERENCES

1. Koonin LM, Atrash AK, Lawson HW, et al: Maternal mortality surveillance, United States, 1979-1986. *MMWR CDC Surveill Summ* 1991; 40:1.
2. Rochat RW, Koonin LM, Atrash AK, et al: Maternal Mortality Collaborative: Maternal mortality in the United States. *Obstet Gynecol* 1988; 72:91.
3. Centers for Disease Control and Prevention: National Hospital Discharge Survey. *Healthy People* 2000:377.
4. Lund CJ, Donovan JC: Blood volume during pregnancy. *Am J Obstet Gynecol* 1967; 98:393.
5. Robson SC, Hunter S, Boys RJ, et al: Serial study of factors influencing changes in cardiac output during human pregnancy. *Am J Physiol* 1989; 256:H1060.
6. Ueland K, Hansen JM: Maternal cardiovascular hemodynamics. III. Labor and delivery under local and caudal anesthesia. *Am J Obstet Gynecol* 1989; 103:8.
7. Clark SL, Cotton DB, Lee W, et al: Central hemodynamic assessment of normal term pregnancy. *Am J Obstet Gynecol* 1989; 161:1439.
8. Assali NS, Brinkman CR III: Disorders of maternal circulatory and respiratory adjustments, in Assali NS (ed): *Pathophysiology of Gestational Disorders.* Vol I: *Maternal Disorders.* New York, Academic Press, 1972.
9. Kramer W, Saade G, Leibman B, et al: Maternal oxygen consumption and CO_2 production during the peripartum period in normal gestation. *Am J Obstet Gynecol* 1995; 172:319.
10. Pritchard JA, Baldwin RM, Dickey JC, et al: Blood volume changes in pregnancy and the puerperium. Red blood cell loss and changes in apparent blood volume during and following vaginal delivery, cesearean section, and cesarean section plus total hysterectomy. *Am J Obstet Gynecol* 1962; 84:1271.
11. Gonik B: Intensive care monitoring of the critically ill pregnant patient, in Creasky RK, Resnik P (eds): *Maternal-Fetal Medicine,* ed 2, Philadelphia, WB Saunders, 1989.
12. Baker RN: Hemorrhage in Obstetrics. *Obstet Gynecol Annu* 1977; 6:295.
13. Centers for Disease Control and Prevention. National Hospital Discharge Survey. *Healthy People* 2000:377.
14. Hibbard BM, Jeffcoate TNA: Abruptio placentae. *Obstet Gynecol* 1966; 27:155.
15. American College of Obstetricians and Gynecologists: Hemorrhagic shock. *ACOG Technical Bulletin: 82.* Washington, DC, 1984, p 1.
16. Millikan JS, Cain TL, Hansborough J: Rapid volume replacement of hypovolemic shock: A comparison of techniques and equipment. *J Trauma* 1984; 24:428.
17. Lowery BD, Cloutier CT, Carey LC: Electrolyte solutions in resuscitation in human hemorrhage shock. *Surg Gynecol Obstet* 1971; 133:273.
18. Modig J: Effectiveness of dextran 70 versus Ringer's acetate in traumatic shock and adult respiratory distress syndrome. *Crit Care Med* 1986; 17:454.
19. Hankeln K, Radel C, Beez M, et al: Comparison of hydroxyethyl starch and lactated Ringer's solution on hemodynamics and oxygen transport of critically ill patients with multisystem trauma and shock. *Arch Surg* 1983; 118:804.
20. Shatney CH, Deepika K, Militello PR, et al: Efficacy of hetastarch in the resuscitation of patients with multisystem trauma and shock. *Arch Surg* 1983; 118:804.
21. American College of Surgeons: Advanced trauma and life support course. Student manual: Shock. Chicago, *ACS* 1985, p 53.
22. Curran JW, Lawrence DN, Jaffe H, et al: Acquired immunodeficiency syndrome (AIDS) associated with transfusions. *N Engl J Med* 1984; 310:69.
23. Centers for Disease Control: Epidemiologic Notes and Reports: Human Immunodeficiency Virus Infection in Transfusion Recipients and Their Family Members. March 1987.
24. Consensus Conference Report: The impact of routine HLTV-III antibody testing of blood and plasma donors on public health. *JAMA* 1986; 256:1178.
25. Consensus Conference Report: Perioperative red blood cell transfusion. *JAMA* 1988; 260:2700.
26. Coveler LA, Werch JB, Todd CE: Rapid availability of blood for massive transfusion in a Trauma Center: A new approach using blood blocs. *Anesthesiology* 1991. vol 75, no 3A, Sept.
27. Stoelting RK: Anesthesia and co-existing disease, Stoelting RK, Dierdorf SF (eds): , ed 3. Edinburgh, Churchill Livingston, 1993.
28. Attar S, Boyd D, Layne E, et al: Alterations in coagulation and fibrinolytic mechanisms in acute trauma. *J Trauma* 1969; 9:939.
29. Green JR: Placental abnormalities: Placenta previa and abruptio placentae, in Creasy RK, Resnik ® (eds): *Maternal Fetal Medicine: Principles and Practice.* Philadelphia, WB Saunders, 1994, pp 592-612.
30. ACOG Technical Bulletin, no 78. July 1984.
31. NIH Consensus Conference: Fresh frozen plasma: Indications and risk. *JAMA* 1985; 253:551.
32. Chamberlain GVP, Philipp E, Howlett B, et al: *British Births,* 1970. London, Heinemann, 1978.
33. Pritchard JA: Genesis of severe abruption. *Am J Obstet Gynecol* 1970; 108:22.
34. Paintin DB: The epidemiology of antepartum haemorrhage: A study of all births in a community. *J Obstet Gynaecol Br Commonw* 1962; 69:614.
35. Hibbard BM, Hibbard ED: Aetiological factors in abruptio placentae. *Br Med J* 1962; 2:1439.
36. Knab DR: Abruptio placentae: An assessment of the time and method delivery. *Obstet Gynecol* 1978; 52:625.
37. Lunan CB: The management of abruptio placentae. *J Obstet Gynaecol British Commonw* 1973; 80:120.
38. Abdella TN, Sibai BM, Hays JM, et al: Relationship of hypertensive diseases to abruptio placentae. *Obstet Gynecol* 1984; 63:365.
39. Knuppel AR, Drukker JE: Bleeding in late pregnancy: Antepartum bleeding, in Hayashi RH, Castillo MS (eds): *High Risk Pregnancy: A Team Approach.* Philadelphia, WB Saunders, 1986.
40. Patterson MEL: The aetiology and outcome of abruptio placentae. *Acta Obstet Gynecol Scand* 1979; 58:31.
41. Fox H: *Pathology of the Placenta.* London, WB Saunders, 1978.
42. Nyberg DA, Cyr Dr, Mack LA, et al: Sonographic spectrum of placental abruption. *AJR* 1987; 148:161.
43. Gruenwald P, Levin H, Yousem H: Abruption and premature separation of the placenta. *Am J Obstet Gynecol* 1968; 102:604.

44. Harris BA: Marginal placental bleeding. *Am J Obstet Gynecol* 1952; 61:53.

45. Harris BA, Gore H, Flowers CE: Peripheral placental separation: A possible relationship to premature labor. *Obstet Gynecol* 1985; 66:774.

46. Spirt BA, Kagan EH, Rozanski RM: Abruptio placenta: Sonographic and pathologic correlation. *AJR* 1979; 133:877.

47. Hurd WW, Miodovnik M, Hertzberg V, et al: Selective management of abruptio placenta: A prospective study. *Obstet Gynecol* 1983; 61:467.

48. Jaffe MH, Schoen WC, Silver TM, et al: Sonography of abruptio placentae. *AJR* 1981; 137:1049.

49. McGahan JP, Phillips HE, Reid MH, et al: Sonographic spectrum of retroplacental hemorrhage. *Radiology* 1982; 142:481.

50. Page EW, King EB, Merril JA: Abruptio placentae: Dangers of delay in delivery. *Obstet Gynecol* 1954; 3:385.

51. Pritchard JA, Brekken AL: Clinical and laboratory studies on severe abruptio placentae. *Am J Obstet Gynecol* 1967; 97:681.

52. Green-Thompson RW: Antepartum haemorrhage. *Clin Obstet Gynaecol* 1982; 9:479.

53. Pritchard JA: Genesis of severe placenta abruption. *Am J Obstet Gynecol* 1970; 108:22.

54. Naeye RL, Harkness WL, Utts J: Abruptio placenta and perinatal death: A prospective study. *Am J Obstet Gynecol* 1977; 128:740.

55. Kettel LM, Branch DW, Scott JR: Occult placental abruption after maternal trauma. *Obstet Gynecol* 1988; 71:449.

56. Acker D, Sachs BP, Tracey KJ, et al: Abruptio placentae associated with cocaine use. *Am J Obstet Gynecol* 1983; 146:220.

57. Chasnoff IJ, Burns KA, Burns WJ: Cocaine use in pregnancy: Perinatal morbidity and mortality. *Neurotoxicol Teratol* 1987; 9:291.

58. Little BB, Snell LM, Palmore MK, et al: Cocaine use in pregnant women in a large public hospital. *Am J Perinatol* 1988; 5:206.

59. Schwartz RW: Pregnancy in physicians: Characteristics and complications. *Obstet Gynecol* 1985; 66:672.

60. Golditch IA, Boyce NE: Management of abruptio placenta. *J Am Med Assoc* 1970; 212:218.

61. De Valera E: Abruptio placenta. *Am J Obstet Gynecol* 1986; 100:599.

62. Sher G: Pathogenesis and management of uterine inertia complicating abruptio placentae with consumptive coagulopathy. *Am J Obstet Gynecol* 1977; 129:164.

63. Belfort MA, Moore PJ: The use of a cephalic perforator for delivery of the dead fetus in cases of severe abruptio placentae. *So Afr Med J* 1990; 77:80.

64. Clark SL, Phelan JP, Yeh SY, et al: Hypogastric artery ligation for obstetric hemorrhage. *Obstet Gynecol* 1985; 63:353.

65. Clark SL, Yeh SY, Phelan JP, et al: Emergency hysterectomy for the control of obstetric hemorrhage. *Obstet Gynecol* 1984; 64:376.

66. Montgomery L, Belfort M, Allon M, et al: Hypogastric artery ligation is an effective and safe alternative to hysterectomy in patients with severe postpartum hemorrhage. *Am J Obstet Gynecol* 1995; 172:291.

67. Schumaker B, Belfort MA, Kramer WB, et al: Adjunctive measures for control of hemorrhage in association with abdominal pregnancy. *J Mat Fet Med* (in press).

68. O'Leary J: Uterine artery ligation in the control of post cesarean hemorrhage. *J Reprod Med* 1995; 40:189.

69. Jansen RPS: Relative bradycardia: A sign of acute intraperitoneal bleeding. *Aust N Z J Obstet Gynaecol* 1978; 18:206.

70. Muldoon MJ: The use of central venous pressure monitoring in abruptio placentae. *J Obstet Gynaecol Commonw* 1969; 76:225.

71. Shubin H, Weil MH, Carlson RW: Bacterial shock. *Am Heart J* 1977; 94:112.

72. Czer LSC, Shoemaker WC: Optimal hematocrit value in critically ill postoperative patients. *Surg Gynecol Obstet* 1978; 147:363.

73. Oats JN, Vasey DP, Waldron BA: Effects of ketamine on the pregnant uterus. *Br J Anaesth* 1979; 51:1163.

74. Suresh MS, Solanki DR, Andrews JJ, et al: Comparison of Etomidate with thiopental for induction of anesthesia at cesarean section. *Anesthesiology* 1986; 65(3A)A400.

75. Andrews WW, Ramin SM, Maberry MC, et al: Effect of type of anesthesia on blood loss at elective repeat cesarean section. *Am J Perinatol* 1992; vol 9, no 3, 197.

76. Douglas RG, Buchman MI, MacDonald FA: Premature separation of the normally implanted placenta. *J Obstet Gynaecol Br Emp* 1955; 62:710.

77. Takagi S, Yoshida T, Togo Y, et al: The effects of intramyometrial injection of prostaglandin F2-alpha on severe postpartum hemorrhage. *Prostaglandins* 1976; 12:565.

78. Hayashi RH, Castillo MS, Noah ML: Management of severe postpartum hemorrhage with a prostaglandin F2-alpha analogue. *Obstet Gynecol* 1984; 63:806.

79. Hankins GDV, Berryman GK, Scott Jr RT, et al: Maternal arterial desaturation with 15-methyl prostaglandin F2-alpha for uterine atony. *Obstet Gynecol* 1988; 72:367.

80. Abdul Karim AW, Chevli AN: Antepartum hemorrhage and shock. *Clin Obstet Gynecol* 1976; 19:553.

81. Basu HK: Fibrinolysis and abruptio placentae. *J Obstet Gynaecol Br Commonw* 1969; 76:481.

82. Nelson SH, Suresh, MS: Lack of reactivity of uterine arteries from patients with obstetric hemorrhage. *Am J Obstet Gynecol* 1992; 166:1436.

83. Bick RL: Disseminated intravascular coagulation and related syndromes, in *Disorders of Hemostasis and Thrombosis,* New York, Thieme, 1985, pp 157-204.

84. Letsky EA: *Coagulation Problems During Pregnancy.* Edinburgh, Churchill Livingstone, 1985.

85. Collins JA: Recent developments in the area of massive transfusion. *World J Surg* 1987; 11:75.

86. Miller RD, Robbins TO, Toug MJ, et al: Coagulation defects associated with massive blood transfusions. *Ann Surg* 1971; 174:794.

87. Counts RB, Haisch C, Simon TL, et al: Hemostasis in massively transfused trauma patients. *Ann Surg* 1979; 190:91.

88. Reed RL, Heimback DM, Counts RB, et al: Prophylactic platelet administration during massive transfusion. *Ann Surg* 1986; 203:40.

89. NIH Consensus Conference: Fresh frozen plasma: Indications and risks. *JAMA* 1985; 253:551.

90. Stibbard BM, Jeffcoate TNA: Abruptio placentae. *Obstet Gynecol* 1966; 27:155.

91. Lunan CB: The management of abruptio placentae. *J Obstet Gynaecol Br Commonw* 1973; 80:120.

92. Mazze RI: Critical care of the patients with acute renal failure. *Anesthesiology* 1977; 47:138.

93. Belfort MA, Rokey R, Saade GR, et al: Rapid echocardiographic assessment of left and right heart hemodynamics in critically ill obstetric patients. *Am J Obstet Gynecol* 1994; 171:884.

94. Wilson RJ: Bleeding during late pregnancy, in Wilson RJ, Carrington ER, Ledger WJ (eds): *Obstetrics and Gynecology* St. Louis, Mosby, 1983.

95. Hibbard LT: Placenta previa, in Sciarra JJ (ed): *Gynecology and Obstetrics,* vol 2. New York. Harper & Row, 1981.

96. Wexler P, Gottersfeld KR: Second trimester placenta praevia: An apparently normal presentation. *Obstet Gynecol* 1977; 50:706.

97. Wexler P, Gottesfeld KR: Early diagnosis of placenta previa. *Obstet Gynecol* 1979; 54:231.

98. Clark SL, Koonings P, Phelan JP, et al: Placenta previa/accreta and prior Cesarean section. *Obstet Gynecol* 1985; 66:89.

99. Kelly JV, Iffy L: Placenta previa, in Iffy L, Kaminetsky HA (eds): *Principles and Practice of Obstetrics and Perinatology,* vol 2. New York, John Wiley & Sons, 1981.

100. Hibbard BM: Bleeding in late pregnancy, in Hibbard BM (ed) *Principles of Obstetrics.* London, Butterworth, 1988.

101. Crenshaw C, Jones DED, Parker RT: Placenta previa: A survey of twenty years experience with improved perinatal survival by expectant therapy and cesarean delivery. *Obstet Gynecol Surv* 1973; 28:461.

102. Silver R, Depp R, Sabbagha RE, et al: Placenta previa: Aggressive expectant management. *Am J Obstet Gynecol* 1984; 150:15.

103. Cotton DB, Read JA, Paul RH, et al: The conservative aggressive management of placenta praevia. *Am J Obstet Gynecol* 1980; 137:687.

104. Naeye RL: Placenta praevia: Predisposing factors and effects on the fetus and the surviving infants. *Obstet Gynecol* 1978; 52:521.

105. Newton ER, Barss V, Cetrulo CL: The epidemiology and clinical history of asymptomatic mid-trimester placenta praevia. *Am J Obstet Gynecol* 1984; 148:743.

106. Farine D, Peisner DB, Timor-Tritsch IE: Placenta previa—is the traditional diagnostic approach satisfactory? *J Clin Ultrasound* 1990; 18:328.

107. Konje JC, Ewings PD, Adewunmi OA, et al: The effect of threatened abortion on pregnancy outcome. *J Obstet Gynecol* 1992; 12:150.

108. Powell MC, Buckley J, Price H, et al: Magnetic resonance imaging and placenta previa. *Am J Obstet Gynecol* 1986; 154:565.

109. Macafee CHG: Placenta praevia: A study of 174 cases. *J Obstet Gynecol Br Emp* 1945; 52:313.

110. Johnson HW, Williamson JC, Greeley AV: The conservative management of some varieties of placenta praevia. *Am J Obstet Gynecol* 1945; 398:406.

111. Stallworthy J: Expectant management of placenta previa. *Am J Obstet Gynecol* 1951; 61:720.

112. Johnson HW: The conservative management of some varieties of placenta previa. *Am J Obstet Gynecol* 1945; 50:398.

113. Kramer W, Saade G, Goodrum L, Montgomery L, et al: Neonatal outcome after aggressive perinatal management of the very premature infant. *Am J Obstet Gynecol* 1995; 172:417.

114. Effect of corticosteroids for fetal maturation on perinatal outcomes. *NIH Consensus Statement* Feb 28-Mar 2, 1994; 12(2):1-24.

115. Brenner WE, Edelman DA, Hendricks CH: Characteristics of patients with placenta previa and results of "expectant management" *Am J Obstet Gynecol* 1978; 132:180.

116. Besinger RE, Niebyl JR: The safety and efficacy of tocolytic agents for the treatment of preterm labour. *Obstet Gynecol Surv* 1990; 45:415.

117. Sampson MB, Lastress O, Thomasi AM: Tocolysis with terbutaline sulphate in patients with placenta praevia complicated by premature labour. *J Reprod Med* 1984; 29:248.

118. Chestnut DH, Thompson CS, McLaughlin GL, et al: Does the intravenous infusion of ritodrine or magnesium sulfate alter the hemodynamic response to hemorrhage in gravid ewes? *Am J Obstet Gynecol* 1988; 159:1467.

119. Vincent RD, Chestnut DH, Sipes SL, et al: Does calcium chloride help restore maternal blood pressure and uterine blood flow during hemorrhagic hypotension in hypermagnesemic gravid ewes? *Anesth Analg* 1992; 74:670.

120. Hibbard LT: Placenta praevia. *Am J Obstet Gynecol* 1969; 104:172.

121. D'Angelo LJ, Irwin LF: Conservative management of placenta praevia: A cost benefit analysis. *Am J Obstet Gynecol* 1984; 149:320.

122. Kaunitz AM, Spence C, Danielson TS, et al: Perinatal and maternal mortality in a religious group avoiding obstetric care. *Am J Obstet Gynecol* 1984; 150:826.

123. Scott: Antepartum haemorrhage, in Whitfield CR (ed): *Dewhurst's Textbook of Obstetrics and Gynecology for Postgraduates,* ed 4, Oxford, Blackwell Scientific, 1986.

124. Myerscough PR: *Munro Kerr's Operative Obstetrics,* ed 10, London, Bailliere Tindall, 1982.

125. Aho AJ, Pulkkinen MO, Vaha-Eskeli K: Acute urinary bladder tamponade with hypovolemic shock due to placenta percreta with bladder invasion. Case report. *Scand J Urol Nephrol* 1985; 19:157.

126. Abboud TK, Gerard C, Go A, Zhu J: Anesthesia for placenta previa at Women's Hospital: 3 year survey. *SOAP Abstracts 25th Annual Meeting.* May 1993, p 19.

127. Sipes SL, Chestnut DH, Vincent RD, et al: Which vasopressor should be used to treat hypotension during magnesium sulfate infusion and epidural anesthesia? *Anesthesiology* 1992; 77:101.

128. Munson ES, Embro WJ: Enflurane, isoflurane, and halothane and isolated human uterine muscle. *Anesthesiology* 1977; 46:11.

129. Read JA, Cotton DB, Miller FC: Placenta accreta: Changing clinical aspects and outcome. *Obstet Gynecol* 1980; 56:31-4.

130. Cairo GM, Adler AD, Morris N: Placenta percreta presenting as intra-abdominal antepartum hemorrhage: Case report. *Br J Obstet Gynaecol* 1983; 90:491.

131. Sprung J, Cheng EY, Patel S: When to remove an epidural catheter in a parturient with disseminated intravascular coagulation. *Reg Anesth* 1992; 17:351.

132. Kamani AAS, Gambling DR, Christilaw J, et al: Anesthetic management of patients with placenta accreta. *Can J Anaesth* 1987; 34:6613.

133. Chestnut DH, Redick LF: Continuous epidural anesthesia for elective cesarean hysterectomy. *South Med J* 1985; 78:1168.

134. Chestnut DH, Dewan DM, Redick LF, et al: Anesthetic management for obstetric hysterectomy: A multiinstitutional study. *Anesthesiology* 1989; 70:607.

135. ACOG Committee Opinion: Committee on Obstetrics. Maternal and Fetal Medicine. *Anesthesia for Emergency Deliveries.* no 104, March 1992.

136. Golan A, Sandbank O, Rubin A: Rupture of the pregnant uterus. *Obstet Gynecol* 1980; 56:549.

137. Krishna Menon MK: Rupture of the uterus: A review of 164 cases. *J Obstet Gynaecol Br Commonw* 1962; 69:18.

138. O'Driscoll K: An obstetrician's view of pain. *Br J Anaesth* 1975; 47:1053.

139. Brundell M, Chakravarti S: Uterine rupture in labour. *Br Med J* 1975; 2:122.

140. McLean RA, Cochrane NE, Mattison ET: Maternal deaths due to rupture of uterus. *NY State J Med* 1979; 79:46.

141. Flamm BI: Vaginal birth after cesarean section: Controversies old and new. *Clin Obstet Gynecol* 1985; 28:735.

142. Stovall TG, Shaver DC, Solomon SK, et al: Trial of labor in previous cesarean section patients, excluding classical cesarean sections. *Obstet Gynecol* 1987; 70:713.

143. Nguyen Tu V, Dinh RV, Suresh MS, et al: Vaginal birth after cesarean section at the University of Texas. *J Reprod Med* 1992; 37(10):880.

144. Thorpe JA, Hu DH, Albin RM, et al: The effect of intrapartum epidural analgesia on nulliperous labor: A randomized, controlled, prospective trial. *Am J Obstet Gynecol* 1993; 169:851.

145. Chestnut DH, Vandewalker GE, Own CL, et al: The influence of continuous epidural bupivacaine analgesia on the second stage of labor and method of delivery in nulliparous women. *Anesthesiology* 1987; 66:774.

146. Thorpe JA, Hu DH, Albin RM, et al: Reply to Letters to Editor. *Am J Obstet Gynecol* 1994, 171(5):1401.

147. Rudick V, Niv D, Hetman-Peri M, et al: Epidural analgesia for planned vaginal delivery following previous cesarean section. *Obstet Gynecol* 1984; 64:621.

148. Abercrombie J: Case of hemorrhage of the liver. *London Med Gaz* 1844; 34:792.

149. Owen A, Kandalaft E: Spontaneous subcapsular hematoma and rupture of the liver during pregnancy. *Br J Obstet Gynecol* 1973; 80:852.

150. Jewett JF: Eclampsia and rupture of the liver. *N Engl J Med* 1977; 297:1009.

151. Mikotoff R, Weiss LS, Brandon LH, et al: Liver rupture complicating toxemia of pregnancy. *Arch Intern Med* 1967; 119:375.

152. Smith LG, Moise KJ, Dildy GA, et al: Spontaneous rupture of liver during pregnancy: Current therapy. *Obstet Gynecol,* 1991; vol 77, no 2, 171.

153. Aziz S, Merrell RC, Collins JA: Spontaneous hepatic hemorrhage during pregnancy. *Am J Surg* 1983; 146:680.

9 Postpartum Hemorrhage

W. Desmond Writer and Thomas F. Baskett

The third stage of labor lasts from the birth of the infant until delivery of the placenta, usually for only 5 to 10 minutes and rarely more than 30 minutes. While it is the shortest of the three stages, it carries the most risk to the mother.

In the United States, 10.9% of all direct maternal deaths between 1980 and 1985 resulted from hemorrhage, both antepartum and postpartum.[1] In Australia, for the triennium 1979 to 1981, postpartum hemorrhage accounted for 12.9% of all direct obstetric deaths.[2] Postpartum hemorrhage remains a clinical threat in the United Kingdom.[3] For the three years 1988 to 1990, direct maternal deaths from this cause doubled, compared with the previous triennium (1985 to 1987). Hemorrhage accounted for 15.5% of all direct maternal deaths, half of which were due to postpartum hemorrhage.[4] In Sweden, during the 1980s hemorrhage remained one of the main causes of direct maternal death, with a similar pattern in Europe.[4,5] In developing countries, where more than 98% of the world's maternal deaths occur, postpartum hemorrhage constitutes a leading cause of maternal mortality.[6]

A reduction in maternal mortality and morbidity due to postpartum hemorrhage can be achieved by careful prophylaxis, combined with anesthetic, nursing, and obstetric teamwork.

PHYSIOLOGIC MECHANISMS OF THE THIRD STAGE OF LABOR
Uterine contraction and retraction

After delivery of the infant the uterus continues to contract actively, causing its muscle fibers to shorten. This reduction in muscle fiber length is permanently sustained by retraction of uterine muscle, that property which maintains a permanent reduction in muscle fiber length after the active, energy-consuming contraction ceases.

Placental separation

The contraction and retraction of uterine muscle fibers after delivery considerably reduce the size of the placental implantation site. This causes the placenta to buckle and separate from the uterine wall. A secondary, much less important mechanism of placental separation involves the spiral arterioles, which continue to pump blood into the intervillous space while compression of the decidual veins by the uterine contraction prevents its egress. The resultant extravasation of blood, which dissects through the decidua spongiosa, facilitates placental separation.

Placental site hemostasis

As the placenta separates it leaves a very vascular site with torn blood vessels. The anatomic framework of the uterine muscle fibers, however, prevents hemorrhage from these vessels. Arranged in crisscross fashion, they form a latticework through which the blood vessels pass. As the fibers contract and retract, they compress the torn vessels. This muscular architecture constitutes the "physiologic sutures," or "living ligatures," of the uterus. Anything that interferes with this mechanism causes hemorrhage from the placental site.

CLINICAL MANAGEMENT OF THE THIRD STAGE OF LABOR

After delivery of the infant the cord is clamped and cut, and the appropriate cord blood samples are collected. The obstetrician then awaits the three signs of placental separation:

1. *The uterus rises and alters its shape from discoid to globular,* as the placenta separates and leaves the upper uterine segment.
2. *Bleeding* may occur with partial placental separation but may be absent because of containment of blood behind the membranes when complete separation has occurred.
3. *Cord lengthening* of 7 to 15 cm, the most reliable sign.

While awaiting these signs the obstetrician cups the uterine fundus with one hand but should not manipulate it because this may increase blood loss or stimulate a constriction ring, resulting in placental retention. When the clinical signs of separation occur, the obstetrician delivers the placenta by controlled cord traction.

PHARMACOLOGIC MANAGEMENT

Physicians who practice "traditional" management of the third stage await placental separation and delivery before administering an oxytocic drug. The socially and physiologically attractive view that immediate suckling after birth reduces blood loss and postpartum hemorrhage has not been supported by randomized controlled trial.[7]

Active management of the third stage, in contrast, entails giving an oxytocic agent with delivery of the anterior fetal shoulder. The data from randomized clinical trials demonstrate that active management shortens the third stage, reduces associated blood loss, and lessens the risk of postpartum hemorrhage by about 40%.[8,9] There seems little reason, therefore, not to embrace active management of the third stage as the evidence-based standard of care.[10] One argument advanced against it is the risk of placental retention, but the short $t_{1/2}$ of oxytocin (5 to 12 min), makes this unlikely, and clinical trials have not confirmed this risk. However, the longer-acting oxytocic drugs, ergometrine and prostaglandin analogues, can predispose the patient to retained placenta.[11-13]

Another potential risk of active management is asphyxia and trauma of an undiagnosed second twin, from oxytocin-induced uterine contraction. Although much less likely with the increased use of antenatal ultrasound, this can be overcome by delaying oxytocin administration until immediately after the infant has been delivered and the uterus palpated, to rule out a second fetus.

In our institution, we employ active management of the third stage of labor, administering oxytocin 5 IU intramuscularly (IM) or intravenously (IV), with delivery of the anterior shoulder.

PROPHYLAXIS OF POSTPARTUM HEMORRHAGE

Active management of the third stage reduces the risk of immediate bleeding, but in the 2 to 3 hours following delivery (sometimes called the fourth stage of labor), there remains a risk of uterine atony and hemorrhage. Although certain conditions (e.g., high parity, prolonged labor, prolonged intrapartum administration of oxytocin) increase the risk of uterine atony, hemorrhage sometimes occurs in women with no identifiable risk factors. Recent work demonstrates that many women have a protective endogenous oxytocin surge in late second- and third-stage labor. Those who fail to demonstrate this surge cannot be identified clinically, but they have an increased risk of hemorrhage and retained placenta.[14] Thus in all women after delivery we recommend the following routine:

1. Initial postpartum observation for 2 to 3 hours, *in the labor/delivery area.*
2. After the placenta has delivered, the uterine fundus should be firmly massaged and all clots expelled. The presence of clots in the uterus interferes with contraction and retraction, causing relaxation of the physiologic sutures, increased oozing from the placental site, more intrauterine clots, and thereby a vicious cycle.
3. Administration of an oxytocic drug for at least 2 hours postpartum. When the patient has an IV line, we add oxytocin, 20 to 30 IU, to 500 to 1000 mL crystalloid and infuse it to keep the uterus firmly contracted. If there is no IV line, ergometrine 200 μg or 15-methyl prostaglandin $F_{2\alpha}$ 250 μg can be given intramuscularly.
4. The uterine fundus must be checked and massaged every 15 minutes.
5. A full bladder must be emptied, since it may interfere with uterine contraction and retraction.

We make no apology for emphasizing the above routine. Most postpartum bleeding can be prevented or minimized by careful, consistent attention to the details of such a prevention protocol. This type of routine does not preclude the new parents from being with their newborn infant.

PHARMACOLOGY OF OXYTOCIC DRUGS

Oxytocic drugs used in the management of third stage labor fall into three categories:

1. Oxytocins
2. Ergot alkaloids
3. Prostaglandins

Although routine oxytocic drug use has become widespread, the preparation of choice differs between countries.[9,12] Oxytocin is widely used in North America, Syntometrine (a mixture of oxytocin, 5 IU, and ergometrine, 500 μg) is most popular in the United Kingdom, while ergometrine alone enjoys great popularity in Denmark. All oxytocic drugs significantly reduce the rate of postpartum hemorrhage, and their prophylactic administration diminishes the need for later oxytocic use. Oxytocic drugs differ in their physiologic and pharmacologic effects, especially those on the cardiovascular system.

Oxytocin

Naturally occurring oxytocin is a short-chain peptide secreted by the posterior pituitary (Fig. 9-1).[15,16] It derives from a larger precursor (prepro-oxyphysin) synthesized in the supraoptic and paraventricular hypothalamic nuclei. Endoplasmic reticulum degrades the precursor molecules to simpler peptides, which are then pack

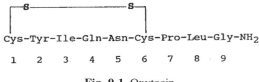

Fig. 9-1 Oxytocin.

aged into secretory granules in the Golgi apparatus and carried by axonal transport to the posterior pituitary. Sensory stimuli from cervix, vagina, and breast (nipple stimulation) promote oxytocin secretion from the posterior pituitary directly into the circulation.

All clinically used oxytocin preparations are now synthetic, and they lack the adverse effects of vasopressin, which frequently contaminated bioextracts.

Effects of oxytocin. Oxytocin acts mainly on the lactating breast to stimulate milk ejection and on the uterus, but it also has significant cardiovascular effects. In the uterus it stimulates the frequency and the force of uterine contractions.[17] The sensitivity of uterine musculature to oxytocin is enhanced in the presence of estrogen and is antagonized by progesterone. In late pregnancy, increased uterine sensitivity to oxytocin coincides with a pronounced increase in the number of myometrial (and endometrial) oxytocin receptors. By the end of pregnancy, receptor concentrations have increased 80-fold to 100-fold over those in the nonpregnant uterus.[18] The highest concentrations occur in early labor, 2 to 3 times higher than at term. This increase in receptors enhances oxytocin responsiveness by lowering the threshold for oxytocin-induced stimulation of contractions and by increasing the number of contractile units that respond, thus augmenting the force of contraction.[19]

Like all skeletal (striated) and smooth muscle, human myometrium requires the formation of actomyosin from the interaction of actin and myosin, in order to contract.[19] The process is complex and is regulated by calcium ions, the calcium-binding protein calmodulin, cAMP, and enzymes that effect phosphorylation and dephosphorylation of light-chain myosin (Fig. 9-2). All oxytocic agents act by mobilizing calcium.

The normal excitation of uterine muscle is tetanic, and an individual contraction results from a burst of rapid, repetitive action potentials. The force of the resulting contraction depends on the frequency of these potentials and the number of muscle filaments involved. Random asynchronous contractions maintain a baseline uterine tone, but for a significant contractile force to develop (in labor, for example), most muscle cells must contract simultaneously. In late pregnancy and labor, cellular contact zones ("gap junctions") appear between adjacent smooth muscle cells. In early labor, their

number further increases, and they permit rapid transmission of electrical or chemical signals between cells.[20] Calcium plays a major role in transmitting the excitatory signal from each muscle cell membrane to the contractile mechanism within the cell (excitation-contraction coupling).

Kawarabayashi et al[17] used isolated strips of term-pregnant myometrium to study the effects of oxytocin on its spontaneous electrical and contractile activity. Two types of action potential occur, plateau and spike, each of which causes spontaneous muscle contractions.[17] Oxytocin converts spike potentials to plateau potentials, thus promoting a sustained uterine contraction. In addition, oxytocin increases the frequency of spontaneous plateau potentials, in turn increasing the frequency of uterine contractions.

Oxytocin responsiveness diminishes in the absence of calcium, as well as after calcium antagonists (e.g., diltiazem). Oxytocin's effect on plateau potentials requires sufficient *extracellular* ionized calcium, and evidence suggests oxytocin may also evoke a uterine response in the absence of action potentials by releasing calcium from *intracellular* storage sites.[17,21] Elevated serum magnesium levels depress serum calcium by enhancing calcium excretion.[22] They may consequently reduce oxytocin responsiveness. High potassium concentrations induce a tonic uterine contraction, augmented by oxytocin.

Oxytocin has pronounced but transient relaxant effects on vascular smooth muscle; these effects increase with dosage. Weis and colleagues[23] measured these effects in healthy young women, who received oxytocin immediately following elective termination of pregnancy under general anesthesia with N_2O, O_2 and intermittent succinylcholine. Mean arterial pressure (MAP) decreased an average 30% in all subjects following an IV bolus of 0.1 IU/kg. Peak depression occurred after 40 seconds. Total peripheral resistance (TPR) declined approximately 50% from control. Heart rate (HR) increased an average of 30%, but this change lagged some 10 seconds behind the hypotension. Stroke volume (SV) and cardiac output (CO) increased, by 25% and 50% respectively, within 60 seconds (Fig. 9-3). Since these women were in early pregnancy, uterine contractility had less effect on their circulatory changes than would have occurred at term.

Thus, oxytocin's primary cardiovascular effect is to decrease TPR. Increased cardiac output, whether primary or secondary, offsets the hypotension from this decreased resistance and maintains regional blood flow. The hypotension does not represent myocardial depression.

The above results applied to bolus oxytocin. When given by continuous infusion, 10 IU/1000 mL at 60 drops/min, (approximately 35 mU/

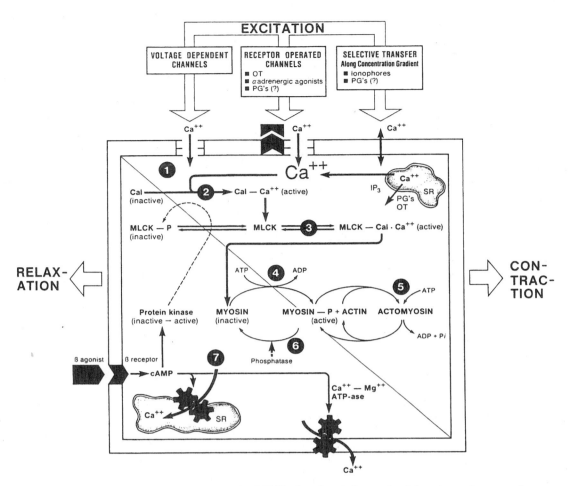

Fig. 9-2 The role of myosin light-chain (MLC) phosphorylation and calcium in uterine smooth muscle contraction. The diagonal separates the contracted from the relaxed state. The numbers indicate the sequence of events believed to occur following excitation: (1) intracellular calcium (Ca^{2+}) increases; (2) calmodulin binds to Ca^{2+} to form an active complex; (3) the calmodulin-Ca^{2+} complex interacts with myosin light-chain kinase (MLCK), forming an active complex; (4) this latter complex phosphorylates myosin, allowing subsequent activation of myosin ATPase by actin, with the formation of the actomysin complex (5); (6) when the Ca^{2+} level decreases, MLCK becomes inactivated, phosphatase dephosphorylates myosin, and muscle relaxation occurs. (7) Calcium enters the cell through voltage-dependent or receptor-operated channels. β-receptor activation leads to a reduction of intracellular Ca^{2+} via two possible mechanisms, both cAMP-dependent: *(a)* cAMP-dependent protein kinase is activated and phosphorylates MLCK rendering it inactive, and *(b)* Ca^{2+} is extruded from the cell by a membrane-associated cAMP-activated calcium ATPase. Calcium can also be taken up and released by sarcoplasmic vesicles through a Ca^{2+}-stimulated Mg-ATP-ase. Other organelles, especially mitochondria, can also take up and release calcium. (From Fuchs A-R, Fuchs F: Physiology of parturition, in Gabbe SG, Niebyl JR, Simpson JL, (eds): *Obstetrics: Normal and Problem Pregnancies,* ed 2, New York, Churchill Livingstone, 1991, p 155.)

minute), oxytocin produced no significant change in mean arterial pressure, and a slight but statistically insignificant increase in cardiac output. However, hypotension may result from bolus or infusion oxytocin administration in patients having concomitant regional anesthesia, especially in the presence of hypovolemia.[24]

Slater et al[25] described a possible anaphylactoid reaction to oxytocin, in which an atopic patient ex-

perienced severe pruritus, pronounced upper body urticaria, and systolic hypotension following IV oxytocin 5 IU and a dilute oxytocin infusion. However, skin tests failed to show significant hypersensitivity to oxytocin, and immunologic testing proved inconclusive. Certainly, hypotension and chest discomfort, together with pronounced facial flushing, not infrequently follow bolus oxytocin administration or a rapid infusion in awake moth-

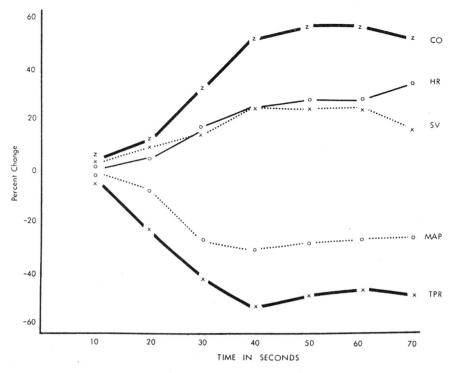

Fig. 9-3 Percent change in physiologic parameters with time and bolus oxytocin. *CO* = cardiac output; *HR* = heart rate; *SV* = stroke volume; *MAP* = mean arterial pressure; *TPR* = total peripheral resistance. (From Weis RF, Markello R, Mo B, et al: *Obstet Gynecol* 1975; 46:211–214. Used by permission.)

ers who are undergoing cesarean section.

When administered in high doses, oxytocin exhibits slight antidiuretic hormone–like activity, which can result in water intoxication if patients concomitantly receive excessive fluid volumes.[26] This effect has no significance with the doses employed in third-stage labor.

Dosage and elimination. Oxytocin acts effectively when administered by any parenteral route. In the management of placental delivery for third stage labor, we give oxytocin 5 to 7.5 IU prophylactically with delivery of the anterior fetal shoulder. The mother then receives an oxytocin infusion, for at least 2 hours postpartum, in a concentration of 40 to 60 IU/1000 mL crystalloid, at a rate of approximately 2 mL/kg/hr (80 to 120 mU/kg/hr). Since the $t_{1/2}$ ranges from 5 to 12 minutes, oxytocin infusions produce steady-state contractile effects after 30 to 60 min. Oxytocin's removal from plasma results from hepatic uptake and renal excretion. In pregnancy, the plasma concentration of oxytocinase increases approximately tenfold. This hormone derives from placenta but has little to do with the disappearance of oxytocin from plasma, although it may regulate local (uterine) oxytocin concentrations.[27]

Prostaglandin E_2 acts synergistically with oxytocin, and the simultaneous parenteral administration of both agents requires a substantial reduction in oxytocin dose.

Umbilical vein administration of oxytocin. A prolonged third stage may cause increased bleeding, or it may require manual removal of the placenta. In a number of recent studies, investigators evaluated administration of oxytocin into the umbilical cord vein of the in situ placenta in attempts to shorten the third stage. Golan et al[28] reported the effectiveness of oxytocin 10 IU injected in this manner, but the series lacked an appropriate control. In a randomized, double-blind, placebo-controlled study, Chestnut and Wilcox[29] found no significant difference between oxytocin 10 IU in 20 mL 0.9% NaCl and 20 mL of 0.9% NaCl alone, with respect to time to placental expulsion. Young et al[30] reported similar results in a comparable protocol, in which they injected oxytocin within 1 minute of cord clamping. However, when compared with IV oxytocin, a bolus of intraumbilical oxytocin 20 IU led to a shorter third stage than did an oxytocin infusion (20 IU/1000 ml Ringer's lactate, at 125 mL/hr) established immediately after placental delivery (4.1 vs. 9.4 minutes).[31]

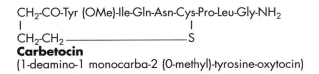

Carbetocin
(1-deamino-1 monocarba-2 (0-methyl)-tyrosine-oxytocin)

Fig. 9-4 Formula of carbetocin.

A recent metaanalysis of six randomized controlled trials suggested that umbilical vein administration of oxytocin is a promising treatment for retained placenta. However, the evidence is inconclusive, and we require further studies comparing different doses, volume and timing, before the practice can be adopted.[32]

Carbetocin

In 1992, Hunter et al[33] evaluated the effect of a long-acting synthetic oxytocin analogue, carbetocin (Fig. 9-4), which has a $t_{1/2}$ of 40 minutes, on uterine contraction in postpartum women. Forty women received IV carbetocin (8 to 30 μg) or IM carbetocin (10 to 70 μg) 24 to 48 hours postpartum. Intravenous injection produced a tetanic uterine contraction within 2 minutes, persisting approximately 6 minutes, followed by rhythmic contractions for an additional 60 ± 18 minutes. Intramuscular administration, similarly, caused uterine tetany within 2 minutes, which persisted 11 minutes, followed by rhythmic contractions for 119 ± 69 minutes. Approximately half the patients experienced flushing and warmth. Uterine cramping occurred in most women, and severe abdominal pain occurred in two women who received higher intravenous doses (50 to 100 μg). The investigators considered the prolonged effects of carbetocin advantageous when compared with oxytocin in third-stage labor.

Gambling et al[34] reported the preliminary results of a double-blind randomized phase III human study, which compared carbetocin with oxytocin for the prevention of uterine atony in women undergoing elective cesarean section. Group A subjects received oxytocin (5 U IV bolus immediately after delivery followed by an infusion of 20 U/1000 mL at 125 mL/hr for 8 hours), while group B women received a single IV bolus of carbetocin (100 μg) after delivery of the neonate. In the first 200 subjects analyzed, the investigators found no difference between carbetocin and oxytocin in intraoperative blood pressure, heart rate, presence of adverse reactions, and postoperative course. Dansereau et al[35] later reported the final results of this multicenter study, which included 696 enrolled subjects, with respect to the prevention of postcesarean uterine atony. The protocol allowed for women to receive additional oxytocin administration at any point in the study for inadequate uterine tone or persistent bleeding. The overall uterotonic intervention rate was 7.3%, but the odds of oxytocic treatment failure were 2.2 times higher in the oxytocic group (10% vs. 4.6%, $p < 0.05$). These studies confirmed carbetocin as a safe, more effective agent than oxytocin in preventing uterine atony at cesarean section. Currently, carbetocin awaits approval by the drug regulatory authorities in the United States and Canada. Further studies will be undertaken to investigate carbetocin's efficacy in the active management of third-stage labor after vaginal delivery. Of particular interest will be the question of whether its prophylactic use (intravenous or intramuscular) will increase the incidence of retained placenta. Carbetocin's effects appear to be intermediate between those of oxytocin and ergometrine. The latter drug, when given intravenously (0.5 mg) for the active management of third-stage labor, increases the need for manual removal of the placenta.[13] Oxytocin, in contrast, is effective because of its short half-life.

Ergot alkaloids

Ergot occurs naturally as the product of a fungus, *Claviceps purpurea,* which grows on rye and other cereal grains. The accidental ingestion of infected grains causes ergotism ("St Anthony's fire"), characterized by hallucinations, widespread vasospasm (which may progress to gangrene), and stimulation of uterine muscle, which may lead to abortion. The parent compound comprises several alkaloids, subdivided into two main groups: (1) amine alkaloids and their congeners and (2) amino-acid alkaloids.[15]

Of the amine alkaloids, only ergonovine (ergometrine) possesses any significant uterotonic effect. The amino-acid alkaloid ergotamine and its dihydro-derivative also have strong uterotonic effects. Ergometrine maleate is the pharmacologic preparation widely used for oxytocic effect, and the following discussion applies to this agent.

Effects of ergometrine

Following a small dose, uterine contractions increase in force, frequency, or both. With larger doses, contractions become still more forceful, resulting in a prolonged increase of uterine tone. This stimulant action appears to combine alpha-adrenergic, serotonergic, and other effects, and uterine sensitivity to ergometrine increases progressively throughout pregnancy. The potency of ergot alkaloids and their prolonged effects restrict ergometrine's use to the postpartum period for control of bleeding and the maintenance of uterine contraction.

The sensitivity of the gravid uterus normally ensures that a small dose produces a sustained response. Parenteral administration of 200 to 250 μg causes rhythmic uterine contractions within 2 to 3 minutes when given intramuscularly and 1 minute after IV injection. A tetanic contraction then persists for approximately 90 minutes, followed by a series of clonic contractions lasting an additional 90 minutes, or longer.[36] Ergometrine's plasma $t_{1/2}$ ranges between 0.5 and 2 hours, and its principal metabolism, by hydroxylation and demethylation, occurs in the liver.[15]

In the cardiovascular system, ergot alkaloids exert complex effects by interactions with tryptaminergic, dopaminergic, and alpha-adrenergic receptors. The resultant cardiovascular changes represent a mixture of agonist and antagonist actions at these receptor sites. Small doses of IV ergometrine (200 μg) produce weak peripheral vasoconstriction, demonstrable by forearm plethysmography.[37] The concomitant uterine contraction and peripheral vasoconstriction augment the central blood volume, causing increased mean arterial and central venous pressures. The pressor response may also be accompanied by reflex sinus bradycardia and nodal rhythm.[38] Johnstone[37] suggested that general anesthesia may obscure these effects, and postulated ergometrine as a cause of pulmonary edema following delivery. In normal parturients, the hypertensive response has little significance, but severe hypertension may occur in preeclamptic women or those with preexistent hypertension. Cerebral edema and eclamptic seizures have also accompanied hypertension due to an ergot preparation.[38,39] The combination of ergometrine and vasopressors administered to hypertensive mothers, even when separated by an interval of several hours, increases the risk of cerebrovascular accident.

Severe ergometrine-induced vasoconstriction may respond to IV chlorpromazine 15 to 25 mg (which will also combat the hypertension), IV nitroglycerin, or sodium nitroprusside.[36] Ergometrine can also induce coronary artery spasm and has been used as a provocative test.[40] Taylor and Cohen[41] ascribed one case of postpartum myocardial infarction to 200 μg IM. Should coronary spasm occur, prompt administration of nitroglycerin or calcium channel blockers may be advised.

In other body systems, ergometrine may also have profound effects. Crawford[42] described severe bronchospasm following administration of 250 μg IV. Bronchoconstriction may represent a tryptaminergic response, requiring treatment with chlorpromazine or the administration of general anesthesia and volatile agents. When given intravenously, ergometrine has a significant emetic effect and should not be given by this route to awake women having cesarean section.

Dosage and administration. Ergometrine may be administered intravenously or intramuscularly in a dose of 200 to 250 μg. The rare occurrences of nonfatal cardiac arrest, myocardial infarction, pulmonary edema, and intracerebral hemorrhage, which have all been attributed to ergometrine, suggest it should not be used *routinely.* When parturients fail to respond to oxytocin, ergometrine can be a most useful second-line drug, but it should not be given to hypertensive women or to those at increased cardiovascular risk. When given prophylactically for the active management of third-stage labor, ergometrine 0.5 mg IV significantly increases the need for manual removal of the placenta and the incidence of nausea, vomiting, after-pains, and hypertension. Its use for this purpose therefore appears undesirable.[13]

Prostaglandins

The prostaglandins PGE_2 and $PGF_{2\alpha}$ and the synthetic derivative 15-methyl $PGF_{2\alpha}$ have been used to achieve uterine contraction when other agents fail. Their administration produces strong contractions in the last two trimesters of pregnancy, and, as with oxytocin, the uterus demonstrates increased sensitivity as pregnancy proceeds. Prostaglandins occur in a wide variety of body tissues, including ovary and myometrium. Fetal membranes also contain prostaglandins as well as other degradation products of arachidonic acid. Prostaglandin concentrations in amniotic fluid, umbilical cord blood, and maternal blood, increase towards term and in labor.[15] In contrast to oxytocin, PGE_2 and $PGF_{2\alpha}$ receptors change little in the human myometrium during pregnancy and labor.

Prostaglandins, in vivo, originate close to their site of action, in the endometrial and myometrial cells. Each derives from the precursor arachidonic acid in a multistep process. Clear evidence exists of an in vivo interaction between prostaglandins and oxytocin, and a maximal response to oxytocin requires the presence of prostaglandins. Prostaglandin synthetase inhibitors diminish the sensitivity of the uterine oxytocin response.[21]

As with oxytocin, receptor binding of prostaglandins stimulates a second messenger mechanism and a chain of events that ultimately leads to muscle contraction (pharmacomechanical coupling). There is evidence that phosphoinositides constitute the second messenger and that receptor binding by the prostaglandins leads to their hydrolysis and subsequent Ca^{2+} release. The Ca^{2+} liberation promotes uterine contraction and accelerated synthesis of prostaglandins by a feedback loop.

Prostaglandins of the E and F series exert significant cardiovascular effects of concern to the anesthesiologist. Hughes and Hughes[43] closely followed the hemodynamic changes from PGE_2, after administration of serial doses by vaginal suppository (Fig. 9-5). Maternal systolic and diastolic blood pressures fell progressively from the first administration. While pulmonary artery pressures remained stable initially, they fell later. Pulmonary artery wedge pressure (PAWP) declined from 18

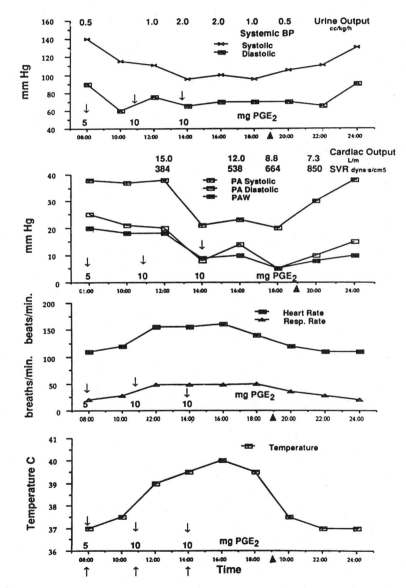

Fig. 9-5 Hemodynamic, respiratory, and temperature observations in a patient with preeclampsia before, during, and after administration of intravaginal PGE_2 suppositories. Delivery of the infant (▲) took place at 1930 hours. SVR = systemic vascular resistance; PA = pulmonary artery; PAW = pulmonary artery wedge; BP = blood pressure. (From Hughes WA, Hughes SC: *Anesthesiology* 1989; 70:713-716. Used by permission.)

mm Hg to 6–9 mm Hg. Maternal heart rate increased significantly from 105 beats/min to approximately 150 beats/min and declined steadily following the last prostaglandin dose. Maternal respiratory rate increased in a manner similar to the heart rate (Fig. 9-5). Finally, maternal temperature rose markedly until it peaked 2 hours after administration of the last prostaglandin dose.

Veber et al[44] described the paradoxical occurrence of severe hypertension following the IV administration of PGE_2. The patient received 0.5 mg PGE_2 by intramyometrial injection for the treatment of persistent uterine atony and postpartum hemorrhage, followed by a PGE_2 infusion (1 mg/500 mL). A few minutes later, her blood pressure increased from 100/70 mm Hg to 220/120 mm Hg, and the peripheral pulses in both arms became impalpable. After a decrease in infusion rate, blood pressure returned to normal, and peripheral bloodflow improved. The authors hypothesized this paradoxical response occurred because PGE_2 entered the systemic circulation, either because of a rapid infusion rate (with inadequate time for inactivation by the lung) or through a patent foramen ovale. In this manner, the central pressor effects of the prostaglandin (hypertension, tachycardia) would likely become apparent. Another possible explanation involved stimulation of renin release due to activation of the renin-angiotensin system by PGE_2.

Prostaglandin $F_{2\alpha}$, in contrast to PGE_2, has little effect on maternal heart rate, but it causes constriction of vascular and bronchial smooth muscle, an effect opposite to that of PGE_2. Pulmonary vascular resistance doubled in pregnant anesthetized women after the administration of $PGF_{2\alpha}$, but no change occurred with PGE_2.[45] In one woman who received an inadvertent intramyometrial overdose of $PGF_{2\alpha}$, we observed profound peripheral vasoconstriction and cyanotic extremities, although SaO_2 and arterial blood gases remained within normal limits. Douglas and associates[46] also reported the occurrence of severe hypertension and pulmonary edema in one parturient, following a massive overdose of intramyometrial $PGF_{2\alpha}$. In contrast to our patient, the woman's extremities were warm and appeared vasodilated. Douglas postulated a combination of increased pulmonary vascular resistance and decreased systemic resistance. Although $PGF_{2\alpha}$ normally causes vasoconstriction, with resultant hypertension, Douglas emphasized that hypotension may also occur.

In bronchial musculature, PGE_2 induces relaxation and antagonizes bronchoconstrictor substances. Prostaglandin $F_{2\alpha}$, in contrast, increases bronchial tone, especially in asthmatic patients.[47,48] These findings reemphasize the opposing effects prostaglandins have on various organ structures, as well as the possibility that paradoxical responses may occur.

Dosage and administration. Prostaglandins of the E and F series have no place in routine treatment of third stage labor. However, they frequently prove beneficial in the management of intractable postpartum hemorrhage and uterine atony. PGE_2 has been administered by vaginal suppository, IV infusion, and IM injection. $PGF_{2\alpha}$ has also been given intramuscularly and directly into the myometrium.

In 1976, Tagaki et al[49] described the first use of $PGF_{2\alpha}$ in atonic postpartum hemorrhage. In randomized trials, intramyometrial (IMM) injection proved superior to the IM or IV route. Over the past decade, the 15-methyl analogue of $PGF_{2\alpha}$ (Carboprost, Hemabate®) has become the prostaglandin of choice for atonic postpartum hemorrhage refractory to the standard oxytocic drugs (oxytocin and ergometrine). Its greater uterotonic effect, relative to the less desirable smooth-muscle stimulatory effects (vasoconstriction, bronchoconstriction, nausea and vomiting), confers definite advantages. Most authors agree the IV route should be avoided because of the greater chance of profound, undesirable smooth-muscle stimulation, although there are several individual cases where 15-methyl $PGF_{2\alpha}$ has been given intravenously without ill effect. Thus the choice of route lies between intramuscular and intramyometrial. Intramuscular injection is simple to administer, but the time to effect is reported to be 15 to 45 minutes.[50,51] In the patient with severe postpartum hemorrhage and/or shock and poor peripheral perfusion, this delay makes the intramuscular route inappropriate. Several studies[51-54] have reported IMM administration with rapid and effective onset of uterine contractions within 2 to 5 minutes. In four reports covering 75 cases in which the authors used the IMM route for atonic postpartum hemorrhage, the success rate was 70 of 75 cases (93%). Side effects were uncommon and mild. Blood pressure elevation occurred in 5% to 10%, but only one of the 75 cases required treatment. Approximately 10% had nonthreatening gastrointestinal complications in the form of nausea, vomiting, or diarrhea. Transient pyrexia (37.5 to 38.5° C) occurred in 2% to 5% of patients, for up to 24 hours. Oleen and Mariano[55] reported a one-year review of the use of 15-methyl $PGF_{2\alpha}$ in 12 obstetric units in the United States. They described 237 cases with a 95% success rate, when used in conjunction with other oxytocic drugs. Although they recommended the IM route, several women also received the drug by the IV and IMM routes, as well as by direct injection into the cervix. The overall success rate and mild nonthreatening side-effects were comparable to previous reports.

For intramyometrial injection we find it best to dilute the 1-mL ampule (250 μg) in 5 mL normal saline, and we inject this transabdominally through a 20-gauge spinal needle into two sites in the uterine fundus. We aspirate before injection to avoid intravascular placement. We expect some resistance during injection; this confirms that the needle tip is in the myometrium and not free within the uterine cavity. In the majority of cases a single dose proves successful. Occasionally, repeated injections become necessary, and up to eight doses (2 mg) can be given in cases of extreme need. The development of this $PGF_{2\alpha}$ analogue represents a major advance in providing a safe, effective choice in the management of uterine atony unresponsive to oxytocin and ergometrine. Although undiluted $PGF_{2\alpha}$ should not be injected intravenously, a dilute preparation (250 μg in 500 mL D5W), administered by infusion, effectively controlled postpartum hemorrhage in parturients unresponsive to other oxytocic drugs.[56] Currently, $PGF_{2\alpha}$ is unapproved for IV use, and further data are necessary.

Toxicity. The principal side effects of prostaglandins result from their stimulatory effects on smooth muscle throughout the body. Gastrointestinal effects predominate, followed by respiratory, cardiovascular, and neurologic manifestations. The transient pyrexia noted by Hughes and Hughes[43] probably represented a direct effect on hypothalamic thermoregulation. Prostaglandin-induced pyrexia occurs in approximately 12% of those who receive the 15-methyl analogue; it resolves after cessation of treatment.

Choice of oxytocic

Elbourne and co-workers,[12] having reviewed the evidence from 27 controlled trials of oxytocic drugs in third-stage labor, concluded the studies gave no support for continued use of ergot alkaloids alone. They found no evidence of greater effectiveness than other preparations, and noted the unwanted side effects described earlier. The authors considered the combination of oxytocin 5 IU and ergometrine 500 μg more effective in reducing the risk of postpartum hemorrhage than oxytocin alone. This combination may also ameliorate the individual vasodilator and vasoconstrictor properties of oxytocin and ergometrine, respectively.[10] However, one recent randomized controlled trial concluded there were few advantages, and several disadvantages (notably, hypertension and gastrointestinal side effects) for oxytocinergometrine, over oxytocin alone.[57] In North America, this combined preparation is unavailable,

perhaps because of concerns about ergometrine's adverse effects, and oxytocin remains the first-line choice.

Currently, evidence to support the routine administration of the more expensive $PGF_{2\alpha}$ analogue remains inadequate. It possesses no clear advantages over oxytocin, and it should be reserved for situations refractory to other oxytocic drugs.

Interactions of oxytocics with anesthetic agents

Inhalation anesthetics agents cause dose-related depression of uterine activity. In isolated pregnant and nonpregnant human myometrium, equipotent concentrations of enflurane, isoflurane, and halothane demonstrated this dose-dependent diminution of contractility.[58] At 1 MAC (minimum alveolar concentration) equivalent, halothane and all agents depressed uterine contractility by approximately 20%. Similarly, uterine responsiveness to oxytocic drugs during halothane or enflurane anesthesia relates to the dose of anesthetic. Concentrations exceeding 2 MAC block the uterine response to oxytocin. Lower concentrations, approximating 1.5 MAC, although relaxing the uterus, do not affect the oxytocin response.[59] Ketamine 2 mg/kg, administered to women undergoing second-trimester abortion increased intrauterine pressure comparably to ergometrine but caused no change in women having cesarean section at term.[60] In the immediate postpartum period, Marx and colleagues[61] failed to demonstrate increased uterine tone from ketamine, although uterine activity increased briefly.

While regional anesthesia may inhibit the reflex increase in oxytocin, which occurs with full cervical dilation in labor,[62] there is no evidence that regional or local anesthetic agents have any adverse effects on either postpartum uterine tone or oxytocin responsiveness.

OBSTETRIC CONSIDERATIONS IN POSTPARTUM HEMORRHAGE AND CLASSIFICATION OF POSTPARTUM HEMORRHAGE

Postpartum hemorrhage is classified as either (1) primary or (2) secondary.

PRIMARY POSTPARTUM HEMORRHAGE

Primary postpartum hemorrhage is defined as blood loss from the genital tract in excess of 500 mL within 24 hours of delivery. While the incidence is usually quoted as 2% to 5%, postpartum hemorrhage is often underreported, and the true incidence probably approximates 5% to 10%.[3] Clinical estimates of blood loss at delivery prove notoriously unreliable and often represent half the true deficit[63]; however, healthy parturients tolerate hemorrhage up to 1000 mL with relative impunity, and minimal changes occur in blood pressure and cardiac output.[64] Thus, in practical terms, clinical assessment, although it underestimates blood loss, usually indicates the level at which treatment should be initiated.

Causes of primary postpartum hemorrhage

1. *Uterine atony.*—Failure of uterine muscle to contract and retract adequately accounts for approximately 80% of all cases. Atony occurs more commonly in association with the following conditions:
   a. High parity
   b. Uterine overdistention (e.g., multiple pregnancy, polyhydramnios)
   c. Chorioamnionitis
   d. Placenta previa, due to partial or complete placental implantation in the lower uterine segment, which does not contract and retract as efficiently as the upper segment
   e. Prolonged labor
   f. Oxytocin-augmented labor
   g. Precipitate labor
   h. General anesthesia
   i. Uterine tocolytics
   j. Full bladder
2. *Mechanical factors preventing efficient contraction and retraction.*—These account for approximately 10% of cases.
   a. Retained placenta, or portions thereof
   b. Retained blood clots
   c. Uterine fibroids
   d. Uterine anomalies
3. *Genital tract lacerations.*—Episiotomy and lacerations of the uterus, cervix, vagina and perineum
4. Genital tract hematomas
5. Uterine inversion
6. Coagulation disorders (discussion beyond the scope of this chapter)

Obstetric management of primary postpartum hemorrhage. As most cases result from uterine atony, initial management should enlist and augment the physiologic mechanisms of hemostasis, by contracting the uterus. This can be achieved by:

1. Fundal massage
2. Intravenous oxytocin, 5 to 10 IU. After the initial bolus, an oxytocin infusion (oxytocin 30 IU in 500 mL crystalloid solution) should be initiated to keep the uterus firmly contracted.
3. Ergometrine, 200 to 250 µg, IM injection (IV only if necessary)

4. 15-methyl prostaglandin $F_{2\alpha}$, 250 µg IM, or directly into the myometrium

On occasion, the uterus responds to one oxytocic drug and not to another. (Oxytocin unresponsiveness not infrequently results from "down regulation" of oxytocin receptors, following a prolonged induction of labor). We usually follow the above regime, and start with oxytocin; if this fails, we give ergometrine as a second-line drug. If ergometrine fails, or contraindications to its use exist, 15-methyl prostaglandin $F_{2\alpha}$ becomes the oxytocic drug of choice.[50-54,65] Do not overlook the possibility of impaired Ca^{2+} activity (eg., in parturients receiving Mg SO_4). Oxytocin responsiveness requires Ca^{2+}, and calcium gluconate, 1 g IV, may prove beneficial in some situations.

Rarely, the uterus fails to respond to oxytocic drugs but contracts with *continuous fundal massage.* As a short-term measure, *bimanual uterine compression* may be employed (Fig. 9-6). The abdominal hand pulls the posterofundal aspect of the uterus forward, while the vaginal hand forms a fist in the anterior fornix and pushes the uterus up and out of the pelvis. This maneuver achieves a combination of uterine compression and massage.

Delivery of the placenta. If the placenta is not already delivered and oxytocic agents fail to stem the bleeding, placental delivery should be expedited (see section on Management of Retained Placenta).

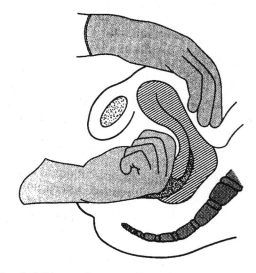

Fig. 9-6 Bimanual compression of the uterus. (From Baskett TF: *Essential Management of Obstetric Emergencies.* New York, John Wiley, & Sons, 1985, p 160. Used by permission.)

Genital tract lacerations. These must be identified and sutured (see section on Genital Tract Lacerations).

Uterine exploration. If bleeding continues despite a well-contracted uterus and the apparent exclusion of other causes, the uterus should be explored under anesthesia to rule out causes such as retained portions of placenta, uterine rupture, and incomplete uterine inversion. General anesthesia may be necessary to provide adequate uterine relaxation.

Surgical measures. When pharmacologic measures, uterine manipulation, and exploration fail to secure hemostasis, surgical measures such as uterine or hypogastric artery ligation, embolization, and postpartum hysterectomy may become necessary. Selective infusion of vasopressin into the pelvic vessels has successfully controlled postpartum bleeding and averted hysterectomy.[66]

ANESTHETIC CONSIDERATIONS IN POSTPARTUM HEMORRHAGE
Bleeding

We emphasized earlier that the expansion of maternal blood volume, by approximately 35%, which accompanies normal pregnancy, enables parturients to tolerate considerable bleeding with minimal physiologic change.[64] Immediately after delivery, maternal stroke volume, pulmonary blood volume, and central venous pressure (CVP) normally increase because of increased venous return as the uterus contracts and the effects of aortocaval compression disappear. In postpartum hemorrhage, however, uterine atony, if present, not only contributes to blood loss but also deprives the central circulation of the normal "autotransfusion" from the uterus. Robson[64] found that women who experienced postpartum hemorrhages ranging from 550 to 1900 mL normally maintained their blood pressure and cardiac output, although they had decreased stroke volume accompanied by tachycardia. They have diminished reserve to compensate for any additional blood loss, and they require immediate measures such as colloid and crystalloid replacement to avoid further deterioration. On occasion, the extent of postpartum blood loss proves unexpected, even alarming; mean arterial pressure and cardiac output may fall dramatically (Fig. 9-7). In all cases, the following immediate measures must be instituted, pending further assessment and management:

1. Establish two large-bore (14 to 16 gauge) IV lines
2. Infuse Ringer's lactate rapidly to correct the estimated immediate blood loss (1000 to 2000 mL)

3. Send immediately for 2 units ABO-Rh type-specific blood, and alert the blood bank to the possibility of the need for additional units.
4. Ensure the immediate availability of albumin, 5%, and if necessary, give 25 to 50 g (500 to 1000 mL) to help restore intravascular volume. (Alternative plasma expanders include hydroxyethyl starch and 25% albumin.)
5. Institute appropriate emergency measures to limit further bleeding, such as elevating the legs in the lithotomy position, administering additional/alternative oxytocic drugs, and giving inotropic agents such as dopamine 5 to 10 μg/kg/min.

After the above measures, insert a urinary catheter and establish a central venous line, if necessary, to monitor the effects of the blood loss and fluid replacement.

Use of blood and blood products in postpartum hemorrhage

Most obstetric units have adopted the "type and screen" procedure as an alternative to crossmatch for women having elective cesarean section; in the majority of centers the procedure is performed on all parturients.[67] Blood typing defines a woman's ABO and Rh status, while screening identifies almost all red cell alloantibodies in her serum.[67,68] Patients who have a positive antibody screen then require further study against an additional panel of reagent erythrocytes to identify the alloantibodies involved. In the presence of a negative type and screen, the serologic safety of ABO-Rh type-specific blood approximates 99.99%, and many blood banks have abandoned the crossmatch procedure in this situation.[67] The risk of receiving serologically incompatible blood, when a type-specific unit is given without a type and screen approximates 1:1000, a tenfold increase. In our unit, we formerly used the type and screen procedure in more than 90% of all parturients. If the patient had no antibodies, this enabled immediate availability of type-specific blood (5 to 10 minutes), in the event of unexpected bleeding. We now, unfortunately, use a "type and hold" procedure, which can delay the availability of blood in emergency situations.

Blood transfusion still constitutes a risk, and all patients have legitimate concerns about the safety of the blood supply. Hemolytic and nonhemolytic reactions occur in 3% to 5% percent of homologous transfusions.[69] The severity of these reactions varies from a clinically insignificant response to death. Hemolytic transfusion reaction remains the most common cause of acute transfusion death.[70] In 1980, 61% of deaths resulting from incompat-

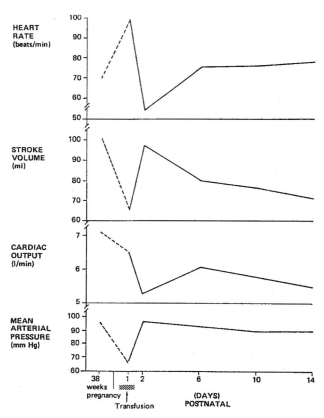

Fig. 9-7 Hemodynamic changes in a subject who experienced a massive primary postpartum hemorrhage (estimated blood loss 1900 mL) secondary to an atonic uterus. Exploration of the uterus was negative and the bleeding was eventually controlled with IV Syntocinon. She received 4 units of blood over the first 36 hours after delivery. The first postdelivery measurement was performed 12 hours after delivery. (From Robson SC, Boys RJ, Hunter S, et al: *Obstet Gynecol* 1989; 74:234-238. Used by permission.)

ible transfusion were due to clerical errors and administration of the wrong blood. While this no longer remains a major risk, nothing can replace scrupulous attention to detail, ensuring the recipient's blood is correctly labeled immediately at the point of origin.

The risk of transmissible disease depends on the donor population. Recent data suggested the following injection rates:[71]

· Hepatitis C <1/3000 units transfused
· Hepatitis B 1/200,000 units transfused
· HIV I 1/225,000 units transfused
· HTLV I or II 1/50,000 units transfused

Ninety percent of transfusion-related hepatitis results from hepatitis C, and 50% of these patients ultimately progress to chronic active hepatitis.

Other infections, which may be transmitted by transfusion, include syphilis, cytomegalovirus (CMV), Epstein-Barr virus, and parasites such as malaria and toxoplasmosis. Cytomegalovirus is carried in the neutrophils of asymptomatic donors, and up to 40% of Americans have experienced infection. Fetal transmission can produce serious sequelae, and CMV-negative blood should be given to immunocompromised patients and CMV-seronegative pregnant women, although only a small percentage of donors transmits the infection.[72]

The American Red Cross currently screens blood for syphilis, hepatitis B (HBsAg, and anti-HBc), HIV-1, anti-HTLV-I/II, anti-HIV-2, hepatitis C (anti-HCV), and alanine aminotransferase (as an indicator of chronic hepatitis).[72]

For the above reasons, anesthesiologists try to avoid blood transfusion in pregnant and postpartum women. In addition to the potential adverse effects for the recipient, transmission of some viruses and unidentified antigens may have hazardous effects in subsequent pregnancies. However, massive blood loss calls for vigorous resuscitation, including the use of colloids, red blood cells, and appropriate component therapy.

Uterine tone

As noted, uterine atony accounts for most cases of postpartum hemorrhage. Chorioamnionitis is the most common cause of failure to respond to first- and second-line oxytocic drugs (oxytocin, ergometrine) and to prostaglandin $F_{2\alpha}$.

In sufficient concentrations, all halogenated anesthetic agents cause uterine relaxation.[58,59] In women undergoing general anesthesia for cesarean section, this tocolytic effect may contribute to postpartum uterine atony, depending on the inspired concentration. Lamont et al[73] confirmed that isoflurane 0.5 MAC did not significantly affect uterine tone in women having general anesthesia for cesarean section. All subjects demonstrated reduced uterine tone immediately after delivery of the newborn and before placental delivery. However, the tone increased after placental delivery, and the investigators found no difference in immediate postpartum blood loss between mothers receiving $N_2O:O_2$ alone (70:30) and those having isoflurane to end-tidal concentrations of 0.6% to 0.7% (0.5 MAC). Progressive depression of uterine contractility does occur when volatile agent concentrations exceed 1 MAC.[58,59] In parturients who require general anesthesia for uterine exploration in primary postpartum hemorrhage, the anesthesiologist should not overlook the possibility that halogenated anesthetic agents may be the cause of persistent bleeding.

Other pharmacologic agents that predispose the patient to impaired uterine contractility include tocolytics such as isoxsuprine, ritodrine, and terbutaline; $MgSO_4$; nitrites, including sodium nitroprusside and nitroglycerin; dantrolene; and Ca^{2+} antagonists. One case report of postpartum atony and hemorrhage suggested dantrolene sodium as the possible cause.[74] Although no clear relationship could be established, the onset of atony coincided with the use of dantrolene, which, in isolated preparations of guinea-pig uterus, significantly decreases frequency and force of oxytocin-induced contractions.

The anesthesiologist should therefore discontinue all drugs that may interfere with uterine contraction, in order to achieve a desired oxytocic effect. Oxytocic agents should then be given as previously outlined, and if the uterus fails to respond, consideration should be given to such causes as chorioamnionitis and calcium deficiency.

In some clinical situations (e.g., retained placenta), increased uterine tone complicates the picture and may hinder easy removal of the placenta.

Traditionally, in these situations anesthesiologists induced rapid-sequence general anesthesia and increased the concentration of halogenated agents appropriately. Peng and colleagues[75] described a series of women in whom they achieved uterine relaxation and successful delivery of retained placenta by the use of IV nitroglycerin 500 μg with supplemental analgesia from IV fentanyl (50 to 100 μg) and/or mask nitrous oxide (40%). Ley and associates[76] also observed a reduction of intrauterine pressure from 38 to 23 mm Hg in one woman with a retained placenta who received such a dose. Other investigators recommend smaller doses of IV nitroglycerin in the management of retained placenta and other clinical situations, and they claim to achieve good to excellent uterine relaxation.[77,78]

Anesthetic techniques in postpartum hemorrhage: regional vs. general anesthesia

Because epidural and subarachnoid anesthesia cause peripheral vasodilation, they can exacerbate hypotension and shock in women with postpartum hemorrhage. For some years, an informal debate took place between leading obstetric anesthesiologists as to whether regional anesthesia should be initiated or extended in mothers with postpartum bleeding. This controversy resurfaced in discussions on the anesthetic management of patients with placenta accreta undergoing cesarean section. Kamani and colleagues[79] advocated general anesthesia for the procedure in women at risk of placenta accreta, while Chestnut et al[80] prospectively reviewed all elective and emergency obstetric hysterectomies over a 3-year period in five university hospitals and concluded epidural anesthesia was not contraindicated. Of 46 women who underwent hysterectomy, 12 received continuous epidural anesthesia and none required intraoperative induction of general anesthesia. The authors found no evidence that epidural anesthesia significantly affected blood loss, the volume of crystalloid replacement, or requirement for transfusion in the elective group. Arcario and others[81] reported significantly decreased intraoperative blood loss and need for fluid replacement in 180 women with placenta previa/accreta who underwent cesarean section or cesarean hysterectomy. While such results do not necessarily extrapolate to women with unexpected postpartum hemorrhage, they suggest that bleeding may not contraindicate regional anesthesia and that the technique may even decrease blood loss. Arcario[81] recommends avoiding regional anesthesia in patients with suspected placenta percreta because they undergo sudden, dramatic blood loss. In addition, in the face of rapid continuing blood loss, he acknowledges it may prove necessary to abandon regional anesthesia in favor of general anesthesia.

When bleeding is controlled and vital signs are stable, we consider the judicious institution of epidural or subarachnoid anesthesia acceptable, in women with primary postpartum hemorrhage. However, persistent bleeding, uncontrolled by pharmacologic agents and uterine massage and associated with signs of shock, contraindicates the establishment of regional anesthesia. In mothers with an epidural block in situ, augmentation of the block to provide uterine analgesia (T8–T10 level) is reasonable if vital signs are stable and resuscitation is in progress.

General anesthesia inevitably carries risks, notably the unexpected difficult intubation and pulmonary aspiration. The delayed gastric emptying, which results from narcotic analgesia in labor, further compounds this risk.[82] Therefore, the choice of technique becomes a matter of weighing the immediate and remote risks against the benefits. One advantage of general anesthesia is the tocolytic effect of volatile anesthetic agents, should it prove impossible to explore the uterus (e.g., in retained placenta). Since Peng and colleagues[75] described their achievement of good uterine relaxation and successful delivery of retained placenta by the use of IV nitroglycerin 500 μg with supplemental analgesia from IV fentanyl 50 to 100 μg, and/or nitrous oxide 40%, by mask, we have used a modification of their technique. We believe that nitrites (especially nitroglycerin) represent an important addition to the anesthesiologist's armamentarium. Most important, they invariably avoid the need for the administration of general anesthesia to reduce uterine tone.

General anesthesia. Women for whom the anesthesiologist considers general anesthesia desirable should receive 0.3 molar sodium citrate, 30 mL orally, immediately before induction of anesthesia, together with IV metoclopramide 10 mg, if the anesthesiologist's preference dictates. In some clinical situations (e.g., partially detached placenta), bleeding may persist until delivery of the placenta and the requirement for anesthesia becomes urgent. It may prove impracticable to obtain a comprehensive anesthetic history and salient functional enquiry, but preoperative assessment should not overlook the possibility of difficult intubation, or an adverse anesthetic reaction. Careful assessment of the maternal vital signs is mandatory.

With two IV lines in situ, immediate resuscitation should begin with crystalloid and colloid. When bleeding is heavy, we recommend that anesthesia not proceed until blood is immediately available to the operating room. We consider the following monitors and equipment necessary, either attached to the patient or in the operating room and able to be exclusively dedicated: ECG, automated blood pressure (BP) apparatus, pulse oximeter, end-tidal capnograph, nerve stimulator, temperature probe, and blood warmer. In addition, a precordial stethoscope may be applied. To facilitate the emergency resuscitation of bleeding parturients, our unit has a "blood cart" immediately available to the operating room. This contains all necessary equipment for rapid fluid/blood replacement.

Preoxygenation by the rapid 3 to 4 breath technique is normally effective, except in cases of significant hypovolemia and reduced cardiac output.[83] In this event, preoxygenation should be prolonged to allow for equilibration. If the mother delivered in the lithotomy position, we believe her legs should be placed flat before induction of anesthesia. This has a dual effect: (1) it enables re-evaluation of the mother's vital signs, since any "autotransfusion" from the legs may obscure significant hypovolemia, and (2) it avoids the increased intragastric pressure that accompanies the lithotomy position.

Anesthesia should be induced using a rapid sequence technique and an appropriate choice of induction agent. It may be necessary to attenuate the dose of thiopental (2 to 2.5 mg/kg) or to use a combination of thiopental/ketamine (thiopental 50 to 100 mg, plus ketamine 0.25 mg/kg) or ketamine 0.5 to 1 mg/kg alone.

After tracheal intubation, anesthesia may be continued with a "balanced" anesthetic technique: N_2O/O_2 (50:50), fentanyl (50 to 100 μg), and a volatile agent such as enflurane or isoflurane 0.5 to 1 MAC. When the airway is secure, the patient may be placed in the lithotomy position to permit uterine exploration. After evacuation of the atonic uterus, the patient who underwent general anesthesia may need increased oxytocic drug administration to achieve uterine contraction. She should be extubated awake in the left lateral position in the operating room, only when she is clearly able to maintain her airway. Uterine massage and additional oxytocic agents may be required in the recovery room.

Regional anesthesia. When women have an epidural catheter in situ, extension of the block, to secure anesthesia to T_8–T_{10}, provides excellent analgesia for uterine exploration. The procedure does not require profound abdominal relaxation, and sensory-blocking concentrations of local anesthetic (bupivacaine 0.25%; lidocaine 1%, with epinephrine) usually suffice. The block should be titrated, if time permits, and the maternal vital signs followed closely, with appropriate fluid replacement to avoid hypotension. (Although epinephrine promotes uterine relaxation by its beta-sympathomimetic effect, the small doses involved have little consequence. Epinephrine-containing local anesthetics cause a greater fall in peripheral resistance than do plain solutions, but they provide more satisfactory analgesia and their transient inotropic effects may prove beneficial.[84]) Epidural narcotic drugs (e.g., fentanyl 50 to 100 μg) enhance the quality of analgesia provided by these dilute solutions and enable uterine exploration without discomfort. Because of its hypotensive effect, I normally avoid 2-chloroprocaine, although it can be used to achieve a rapid block. Motor-blocking concentrations of other local anesthetics are unnecessary and should be avoided.

When inducing regional anesthesia de novo in mothers with no block in situ, a careful assessment of circulatory status is essential. Blood loss should be estimated; administration of crystalloid and/or colloid should be in progress and maternal vital signs stable. We consider it unwise to induce regional block unless these criteria can be satisfied. We generally perform the procedure with the patient in the left lateral position to minimize the effects of posture on the maternal blood pressure as the block becomes effective. Should it be necessary to perform it with the mother sitting (e.g., in obesity), careful attention must be paid to maternal blood pressure, and a minimal dose of local anesthetic should be injected before repositioning the patient supine. As before, an epidural block should be carefully titrated to secure a $T_8–T_{10}$ level; this may be supplemented with epidural narcotic drugs to enhance the quality of analgesia. When the patient has stable vital signs, subarachnoid block, in our view, represents an excellent alternative to epidural anesthesia. However, we consider it an unsuitable technique in the face of unstable blood pressure and continuing blood loss.

In the rare event that cesarean hysterectomy becomes necessary, the studies cited above suggest that continuation of regional anesthesia diminishes blood loss and morbidity. All anesthesiologists, however, recognize the occasional need to convert to general anesthesia in some situations (e.g., rapid and continuing blood loss).[81]

Retained placenta

The longer a placenta is retained, the greater the risk of postpartum hemorrhage. With active management of the third stage, placental delivery usually occurs within 5 to 10 minutes, and with traditional management, 10 to 15 minutes. If the mother has no active bleeding, we wait up to 30 minutes before undertaking manual removal of the placenta. The "30-minute rule" represents a balance between the need for anesthesia (with its attendant

risks) and the decreased likelihood of spontaneous placental delivery coupled with the increasing chance of primary postpartum hemorrhage. In practice it often takes an additional 20 to 30 minutes to prepare for safe anesthesia and manual removal. If the patient is stable and not bleeding, it is reasonable to proceed slowly because by waiting up to 60 minutes, the need for manual removal is halved.[85] In the case of active bleeding there should be no delay, and when epidural anesthesia is already in place, manual removal may be performed earlier. Using these guidelines, retained placenta occurs in approximately 2% of all deliveries.

Causes of retained placenta. Retention of a *separated placenta* may result from uterine atony or a uterine constriction ring.

Retention of *an adherent placenta* may be due to ordinary adherence or pathologic adherence. The latter signifies a deficient decidual reaction and occurs more frequently in patients with a history of previous uterine surgery (D & C, cesarean section, myomectomy), trauma, or infection. Depending on the extent of invasion, three degrees of pathologic adherence exist: *placenta accreta*—adherent to the myometrium; *placenta increta*—invades the myometrium; and *placenta percreta*—penetrates to the serosal layer of the uterus. Pathologic adherence occurs more commonly in placenta previa because of the limited decidual response over the lower uterine segment. The risk of *placenta previa accreta* significantly increases in patients with previous lower segment cesarean section scar(s).[86]

Management of retained placenta. If placental separation has occurred and its retention is due to uterine atony, the treatment of choice is to give an oxytocic drug and deliver the placenta by controlled cord traction when the uterus contracts. Active management of third-stage labor significantly decreases the likelihood of atonic separation.[8,9,10] Manual removal should be undertaken if hemorrhage, unresponsive to oxytocic drugs, occurs in association with a retained placenta. In patients in whom the retained placenta is accompanied by little bleeding, ordinary adherence or a constriction ring are common causes. In these cases the 30-minute rule applies, depending on the available facilities and anesthesia personnel. As discussed earlier, injection of oxytocin into the umbilical cord vein may cause separation and delivery of the placenta, in some cases.[28-32] No elevation of maternal plasma oxytocin levels results from this maneuver,[87] and it can prove useful in cases when anesthesia is inadvisable or unavailable. In very rare cases of placenta accreta, pathologic adherence involves the whole placenta. In such patients, the ap-

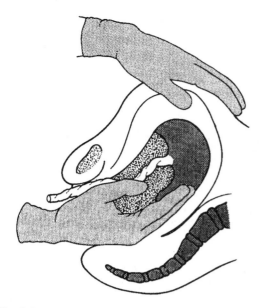

Fig. 9-8 Technique of manual removal of the placenta. From Baskett TF: *Essential Management of Obstetric Emergencies.* New York, John Wiley & Sons, 1985, p 160. Used by permission.)

propriate treatment is hysterectomy. More commonly, the areas of adherence involve only part of the placental site and, in these cases, "piecemeal" manual removal may prove feasible.

Technique of manual removal of the placenta (Fig. 9-8). One should place the right hand in the vagina and follow the umbilical cord up to the lower margin of the placenta. The fingers and thumb of this hand should be extended and kept together as one unit. The external (left) hand encircles the uterine fundus and pushes it firmly down onto the right hand. With a side-to-side motion of the right hand, create a plane of cleavage through the decidua spongiosa, separating the placenta from the uterine wall. Then grasp the placenta and slowly withdraw it from the uterus. It is important this be done slowly, because too rapid extraction of the placenta may invert the uterus if a small portion remains adherent to the uterine wall. Following removal of the placenta, reexplore the uterus with the right hand to ensure all placental fragments have been removed and the uterine wall is intact. At this point, any volatile anesthetic agent must be discontinued, and IV oxytocin must be initiated to achieve firm uterine contraction. The vagina and cervix should be checked for lacerations, which may have occurred during this manipulation.

Anesthetic considerations. Except in cases of partial placental detachment with brisk bleeding from open maternal venous sinuses, it may be necessary in some cases of retained placenta to secure

uterine relaxation. When general anesthesia is given, equipotent doses of halogenated agents produce comparable relaxation; the anesthesiologist's preference dictates the choice of drugs. Concentrations of 2.0 MAC or greater may temporarily be required to facilitate manual removal.

Since Peng[75] exploited the profound effect of nitrites on uterine relaxation by using nitroglycerin to avoid general anesthesia, the technique has gained in popularity. Although patients experienced blood losses between 400 and 900 mL (blood volume depletion estimated at 10% to 20%), these authors observed few side effects from nitroglycerin. Systolic and diastolic blood pressures fell by 8% and 5% respectively, which Peng et al.[75] described as "clinically unimportant." They observed no significant increase in heart rate. Uterine relaxation occurred 75 to 95 seconds following the administration of nitroglycerin. When necessary, patients had supplemental analgesia with IV fentanyl, 50 to 100 μg, or N$_2$O. Some had adequate relief from N$_2$O alone.

We now use a comparable technique to facilitate uterine relaxation in patients with a regional block in situ. However, we generally administer 100 to 250 μg in the first instance and we titrate additional nitroglycerin as necessary. Certainly, the use of nitroglycerin frequently circumvents the need for general anesthesia to provide uterine relaxation, and Peng[75] reported 100% success in his small series. Because regional anesthesia alone gives inadequate uterine relaxation, most patients need some additional tocolysis.

Following successful removal of the placenta, under general anesthesia all volatile agents or tocolytics must immediately be discontinued, and uterine contraction secured with an IV bolus of oxytocin 5 to 10 IU followed by an oxytocin infusion (40 to 60 IU/1000 mL).

For women without an epidural block in situ, we consider spinal anesthesia the technique of choice. If the placenta is trapped in the lower segment, or ordinarily adherent, excellent anesthesia can be achieved with as little as 40 to 50 mg hyperbaric (or isobaric) lidocaine, plus fentanyl, 25 μg. If the obstetrician suspects pathologic adherence, epidural anesthesia may be preferable because of the possibility of hysterectomy.

Placenta accreta

The incidence of placenta accreta has increased in recent years, pari passu with the increased cesarean section rate.[86] Although of low incidence in primigravid women and in those with no history of uterine surgery, there exists a strong association between placenta previa/accreta and the number of previous cesarean sections. After one cesarean section, a placenta previa in the current pregnancy carries a 24% risk of placenta accreta. After two or more cesarean sections, the risk exceeds 50%. In small focal accreta, treatment by uterine curettage may prove adequate, with uterine packing or suture of the uterine bed, as appropriate. However, more extensive adherence requires immediate hysterectomy, whether following vaginal delivery or cesarean section.[86]

Placenta accreta may present as primary postpartum hemorrhage in mothers having a trial of labor after previous cesarean section (VBAC), those with placenta previa in the current pregnancy (whether or not there is a uterine scar), and those in whom the placenta is adherent to the previous cesarean section scar. Bleeding from placenta accreta may be sudden and profound, and it depends on the extent to which the placenta invades the uterine wall and maternal venous sinuses.

In mothers having epidural anesthesia for cesarean section, bleeding from placenta accreta may cause dramatic hypotension, necessitating urgent volume replacement and supportive measures (e.g., phenylephrine infusion) to maintain vital signs and preserve consciousness. As noted previously, the question of whether or not to abandon the regional technique and proceed to general anesthesia in this emergency situation is controversial. In Chestnut's series, 21 of the 46 hysterectomies were emergency procedures, 50% of them for placenta previa and/or accreta.[80] Only 24% of emergency hysterectomies received regional anesthesia, which the anesthesiologists continued for the cesarean hysterectomy. In this small series, Chestnut could not compare regional and general anesthesia in the emergency group alone, although he demonstrated the safety of epidural anesthesia in *elective* situations. Emergency obstetric hysterectomy causes significantly greater blood loss, intraoperative hypotension, and fluid requirement. In Chestnut's study, mean intraoperative crystalloid requirement in women having emergency cesarean hysterectomies approximated 5400 mL as compared with 4100 mL in elective subjects.

Suboptimal operating conditions, maternal pain, nausea or vomiting, and a restless anxious patient usually mandate intraoperative induction of general anesthesia. We agree with Arcario[51] that failure to control blood loss invariably requires conversion to general anesthesia. However, when infused fluid volumes keep pace with blood loss, analgesia remains satisfactory, vital signs continue relatively stable, and the patient appears to tolerate the procedure well, regional anesthesia can be maintained. As the block wanes, it should be augmented cautiously with dilute concentrations of lo-

cal anesthetic, supplemented by epidural narcotic drugs as necessary.

When unexpected placenta accreta complicates vaginal delivery, the anesthesiologist must carefully appraise the patient's status. Persistent bleeding, inadequately controlled and accompanied by deterioration in vital signs, definitely contraindicates the initiation or augmentation of regional anesthesia.

Genital tract lacerations

Genital tract lacerations may bleed profusely. If the placenta has delivered and the uterus remains well contracted, laceration of the lower genital tract is the most common cause of continued hemorrhage. The common vulval sites include the *episiotomy,* and *perineal, periurethral,* or *periclitoral* lacerations. Their ready accessibility makes them suitable for suturing under either local anesthesia or the regional block established for delivery. Lower *vaginal* lacerations can similarly be identified and sutured. Lacerations higher up the vagina may require augmented epidural anesthesia or subarachnoid block to provide adequate exposure for suturing. Only rarely will general anesthesia be necessary. Following completion of the procedure, the obstetrician may wish to pack the vagina tightly and place an indwelling Foley catheter to avoid continual oozing and to prevent paravaginal hematoma formation. This applies particularly to spiral lacerations in the vaginal vault.

Small *cervical* lacerations occur commonly and usually do not bleed. Two pairs of ring forceps facilitate easy and painless cervical inspection. Lacerations most commonly involve the lateral aspect of the cervix. If less than 2 cm long and not bleeding, they do not require suture. Indeed, the cervix may be so friable that suturing provokes additional bleeding. Large or bleeding lacerations need suturing; ring forceps, placed on either side of the laceration for traction, will bring the laceration into view and facilitate placement of a continuous locking suture to achieve hemostasis. If bleeding continues despite the suturing, ring forceps can be applied for hemostasis and left in position for 1 to 2 hours if necessary.

Genital tract hematomas

Causes. Hematomas may arise from vessels damaged by the trauma and manipulation associated with forceps, breech or twin delivery, or paracervical/pudendal block. Inadequate repair of vaginal lacerations or episiotomy may, similarly, fail to secure underlying blood vessels. In some cases, the vessel causing the hematoma may rupture without laceration or disruption of the overlying vaginal skin. This may occur in normal spontaneous vaginal births, especially precipitate deliveries, or it may be associated with rapid distension and decompression of the vagina.

Clinical features. Vulval hematomas usually present as painful, tender swellings of the vulva, with pronounced dark blue discoloration of the overlying skin. Usually self-limiting, they occasionally extend into the tissues of the paravaginal space and ischiorectal fossa. Pain and swelling are dominant features.

Paravaginal hematomas are not visible externally, unless confluent with a vulval hematoma. They usually present within a few hours of delivery with excessive perineal pain, urinary retention, and rectal pressure. Signs of shock may be present because of the combination of blood loss and pain. Pelvic examination can prove extremely difficult because of the pain, but one can often feel a tense swelling encroaching on the vagina, on occasion obliterating the entire vaginal canal.

Broad ligament and retroperitoneal hematomas occur when a vessel ruptures and blood extravasates above the pelvic floor fascia. Blood may track between the leaves of the broad ligament, becoming palpable as a large mass on bimanual examination and pushing the uterus to one side. When a broad ligament hematoma occurs, rupture of the uterus should always be considered as a potential cause. Retroperitoneal hematomas may be very extensive and may track as far as the kidneys; they are also associated with profound hypovolemic shock.

Management. All cases require initial treatment with IV crystalloid and/or colloid, to treat or avert hypovolemic shock. Type-specific blood should be available in the event of persistent bleeding.

Vulval and *paravaginal hematomas* need incision and evacuation under regional block and occasionally under general anesthesia. Any bleeding points should be carefully secured, although commonly no bleeding site can be found. After evacuation of the hematoma, the vagina should be tightly packed with gauze and an indwelling Foley catheter then inserted. Both can be removed in 24 hours.

Broad ligament and *retroperitoneal hematomas* may be treated conservatively in the first instance, if the patient is not hypovolemic. If she remains stable, the hematoma may be self-limiting and thus may require no surgical intervention. Normally these will absorb in the coming weeks. If, however, the patient shows evidence of shock and the hematoma increases in size, the situation calls for more active treatment in the form of laparotomy, evacuation of clot, and ligation and suture of bleeding points. On occasion, the patient may need hys-

terectomy to achieve hemostasis. Rarely, internal iliac ligation or selective angiographic arterial embolization may be required. If facilities and personnel are available for this latter technique, it can be an adjunct to surgical management of paravaginal and retroperitoneal hematomas in which evacuation and packing fails to achieve complete hemostasis. On other occasions, it may take the place of surgery.[88]

Anesthetic considerations

Genital tract hematomas usually present some hours following delivery when the effects of any regional labor analgesia have waned and the epidural catheter has been removed. In the first edition of this book, we advocated general anesthesia as the technique of choice. We now consider spinal anesthesia to be the preferred technique, if the patient has stable vital signs and resuscitation is underway. (We also advise that a labor epidural block remain in situ postpartum if there is any suspicion of continuing postpartum hemorrhage. It may then be augmented to permit exploration and repair of any lacerations.) However, significant blood loss can occur following genital tract lacerations, and the sympathetic overactivity associated with intense pain may cause a spurious elevation of blood pressure, obscuring the signs of hypovolemia. Significant maternal hypotension and evidence of hypovolemia may only ensue following the induction of anesthesia and evacuation of the hematoma. The surgery can prove unexpectedly protracted because of the disorganized tissue planes and the friability that accompanies a slowly developing hematoma. In these cases, subarachnoid bupivacaine may be the local anesthetic of choice.

Acute uterine inversion

The incidence of this rare but potentially disastrous complication varies considerably, from 1:2,000 to 1:50,000 deliveries, depending on the standard of management of the third stage of labor.

Causes. While fundal insertion of the placenta appears to be an important prerequisite of uterine inversion, mismanagement of the third stage of labor, involving cord traction and/or fundal pressure on the relaxed uterus, is the cause in the vast majority of cases. Other, less common causes include a sudden rise in intraabdominal pressure (e.g., coughing and vomiting) when the uterus is relaxed, short umbilical cord, abnormal placentation (e.g., placenta accreta), and too rapid a withdrawal of the placenta during manual removal.

Clinical features. In *complete inversion* (Fig. 9-9), the uterus turns completely inside out and the uterine fundus passes through the cervix to lie in

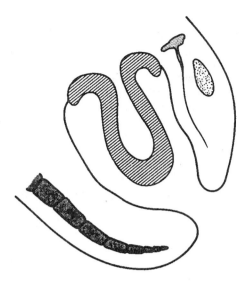

Fig. 9-9 Complete uterine inversion. (From Baskett TF: *Essential Management of Obstetric Emergencies.* New York, John Wiley & Sons, 1985, p 167. Used by permission.)

the vagina or even outside the introitus. Immediate and profound "neurogenic" shock, due to traction on the infundibulopelvic ligaments, round ligaments, and ovaries, accompanies the inversion. The patient becomes pale, hypotensive, and bradycardic. Hemorrhage and hypovolemic shock normally follow rapidly.

With *incomplete inversion,* the uterine fundus inverts but does not herniate through the cervix. Commonly these cases present with persistent postpartum hemorrhage, and the diagnosis becomes apparent during manual exploration of the uterus for bleeding. The uterine fundus may feel dimpled on abdominal palpation.

Management. In most cases, acute uterine inversion results from mismanagement of the third stage of labor, and should be considered preventable. The physician attempts to deliver the placenta by cord traction and/or fundal pressure ("fundus fiddling") before placental separation and firm uterine contraction occur. Routine active management of the third stage reduces the risk of acute uterine inversion. The earlier uterine contraction and placental separation, which result from prophylactic oxytocic administration, make premature cord traction less likely.

Although blood loss may not appear great, one should not assume the shock is entirely neurogenic. In a series of 28 cases of acute uterine inversion in our institution, all of which underwent replacement within 30 minutes, 54% of patients required blood transfusion.[89] Thus, IV crystalloid plus colloid must be rapidly infused as soon as the diag-

nosis becomes apparent, with at least 4 units of type-specific blood made available.

When any delay in uterine replacement occurs, constriction of the cervical ring leads to increased edema and uterine congestion, making attempted replacement more difficult as time passes. Thus an important principle of management is to replace the inversion as soon as possible. We recommend the following plan:

1. As soon as the inversion becomes diagnosed, one should try to replace the uterus *immediately.* This may be achieved without anesthesia, if accomplished before the cervical ring forms and the uterine fundus becomes congested. If the placenta remains attached, any attempt to remove it will increase the risk of hemorrhage and add to the delay. The uterine fundus should be cupped in the palm of the hand and pushed out of the pelvis toward the patient's umbilicus.

2. If this first single attempt at replacement without anesthesia is unsuccessful, one should not persist, because continued attempts will compound the patient's shock and will not succeed in replacing the uterus.

3. With the patient under general anesthesia, an attempt at manual replacement should then be repeated. It may be necessary to sustain upward pressure on the uterine fundus for several minutes to achieve replacement. Successful manual correction of the uterus usually results, if undertaken within 1 hour of the inversion.

4. If manual replacement fails, the hydraulic method of O'Sullivan should be tried.[90] The principle of this procedure is to distend the vaginal fornices with fluid, which pulls open the constricting cervical ring and facilitates replacement of the inversion. This may be achieved by placing tubing from a douche container into the posterior vaginal fornix with one hand and sealing the labia of the vulva around the forearm. The douche container is then elevated 1 to 2 meters, allowing the fluid to run into the fornices, so distending them and exerting traction on the constricting cervical ring. Before attempting this method, the obstetrician must repair all cervical and vaginal lacerations. O'Sullivan's method may be used when manual replacement of the uterus under general anesthesia fails, or when no anesthesiologist is available and immediate manual replacement is unsuccessful.

5. Recent reports suggested that tocolytic agents may successfully relax the cervical constric-

tion ring and allow manual replacement without recourse to general anesthesia.[91,92] The vasodilator effects of beta-sympathomimetic agents may worsen the hypotension; these should be used with caution. Magnesium sulphate 2 to 4 g given over 3 to 5 minutes, has less cardiovascular effect. The drug of choice to provide the short-term tocolysis required is intravenous nitroglycerin. Altabef et al[93] reported the successful replacement of an inverted uterus in one parturient, following two 50 μg doses of IV nitroglycerin.

6. If the above methods fail, laparotomy and surgical replacement becomes necessary. Huntington's technique employs tenacula to grasp the inverted uterine fundus in sequential fashion until the entire inversion has been corrected. On occasion the tightness of the constricting ring prevents this method, necessitating Haultain's procedure to incise the constricting ring posteriorly before the use of Huntington's routine.

7. Uterine inversion may occur at cesarean section.[94] On occasion, the epidural analgesia may not allow sufficiently adequate uterine relaxation to achieve replacement of the inverted uterus. It may then prove necessary to induce general anesthesia to achieve appropriate relaxation (although the tocolytic effect of intravenous nitroglycerin should first be assessed). In our own series, uterine inversion occurred on four occasions in 10,090 cesarean sections. In three instances, the patient had epidural anesthesia in place, and one required general anesthesia to permit replacement.[89]

8. In all cases, after replacement of the inversion, an oxytocin infusion should be continued for 12 hours to keep the uterus firmly contracted and to avoid recurrent inversion. Alternatively, 15-methyl prostaglandin $F_{2\alpha}$ may be used to reduce the risk of excessive oxytocin dosage and water intoxication.

Anesthetic considerations. Whether occurring at vaginal delivery or cesarean section, acute uterine inversion constitutes a true obstetric emergency.[94,95] In the absence of rapid diagnosis and prompt replacement, severe blood loss and shock develop. Profound and of rapid onset, classically the shock is described as "out of proportion to the observed blood loss." While the explanation for this may lie in intense vagal stimulation, generally the degree of blood loss is greater than appreciated and the shock appropriate. Watson et al[96] estimate average blood loss as 1800 mL; rapid treatment of the inversion will minimize this amount

and prevent further bleeding. Crystalloid and colloid should therefore be infused rapidly to correct any hypovolemia.

The inverted uterus can normally be readily reduced in those women who have an adequate epidural or subarachnoid block administered for delivery. Unfortunately, regional techniques do not provide the necessary uterine relaxation, and it may be necessary to provide tocolysis, (e.g., with IV terbutaline 250 μg, or nitroglycerin 100 to 200 μg). Sporadic reports of nitroglycerin's usage have appeared, but in view of the low incidence of uterine inversion, more experience is necessary before the technique can be confidently recommended. The time frame does not allow for establishment of a regional technique de novo. Moreover, general anesthesia, by enabling uterine relaxation, facilitates the uterine reduction (although it may take some 5 to 10 minutes to secure adequate tocolysis, by which time the inversion has usually been reduced[97]). Time is of the essence, and it will usually be necessary to administer general anesthesia with the woman in the lithotomy position, despite the increased regurgitation risk this entails. The anesthesiologist will also benefit from experienced help such as another anesthesiologist, nurse anesthetist, or experienced caseroom nurse, to assist with preparations for anesthesia, insert an additional IV line, and provide cricoid pressure for the rapid sequence induction. Immediately following successful uterine reduction, the patient should receive oxytocic drugs to enhance uterine tone.

Uterine inversion at cesarean section occurs with extreme rarity, although subclinical degrees of inversion are more common. Generally no serious sequelae, other than hypotension, occur, and the inversion may even be symptomless. Emmott and Bennett[94] described two such cases, one having general anesthesia and the other having epidural anesthesia. The latter patient remained remarkably comfortable throughout the inversion but became pale, sweaty, and distressed some 5 minutes later, without overt bleeding. Concurrently, blood pressure rapidly decreased and she had tachycardia (heart rate 130 beats/min) possibly a result of oxytocin. Alternatively, release of metabolic products into the general circulation following decompression of the uterine veins may have caused these changes.

Emmott and Bennett[94] suggest epidural anesthesia may minimize or prevent significant hypotension and discomfort during the period of inversion. They advocate uterine relaxation with terbutaline or ritodrine, or inhalation of amyl nitrite, should reduction not occur (IV nitroglycerin may, similarly, prove beneficial). If inversion occurs in women having general anesthesia, increasing the depth of anesthesia with a volatile agent will relax the uterus and facilitate reinversion, paradoxically preventing further hypotension.

Amniotic fluid embolism

This dramatic obstetric complication has an incidence between 1 in 8000 and 1 in 80,000, and an alleged mortality rate exceeding 80%. "Classic" precipitating factors include multiparity, a short "tumultuous" labor (sometimes oxytocin augmented), and intrauterine manipulations. Ten to 15% of cases present with postpartum bleeding, which progresses to disseminated intravascular coagulation in almost all who survive beyond 1 hour.[98]

Cardiorespiratory resuscitation dominates the immediate management, and, if unconscious, the patient requires tracheal intubation and ventilation, with inotropic support and external cardiac massage as appropriate.

The anesthetic considerations of postpartum hemorrhage apply. In addition, treatment of the bleeding calls for fresh blood, fresh frozen plasma, platelets, and cryoprecipitate to replace the depleted coagulation factors (see Chapter 24).

SECONDARY POSTPARTUM HEMORRHAGE

Abnormal bleeding, between 24 hours and 6 weeks postpartum, occurs in approximately 1% of pregnancies. Most cases present between 5 and 10 days postpartum.

Causes

1. Retained placental fragments
2. Chorioamnionitis (may accompany retained placental fragments)
3. Genital tract lacerations/hematoma
4. Submucous fibroid
5. Trophoblastic disease (although rare, an important complication to exclude)
6. Chronic uterine inversion

Management. Patients with heavy persistent bleeding, evidence of chorioamnionitis, or inadequate uterine retraction need immediate uterine exploration. There are two potential obstetric complications: (1) pathologic adherence of placental fragments to myometrium, causing focal placenta accreta, and (2) the increased risk of uterine rupture. These make dilation and curettage a potentially hazardous procedure.

From an anesthetic viewpoint, these patients demand careful preoperative assessment, as with all postpartum bleeding cases. Anemia, hypovolemia, and shock require fluid (rarely blood) replacement, according to the previous guidelines. Although several days may have elapsed since delivery, delayed gastric emptying should be assumed.

CONCLUSION

Because the postpartum period may be associated with multiple problems, continuous vigilance and good communication between obstetrician and anesthesiologist are essential for proper management.

REFERENCES

1. Rochat RW, Koonin LM, Atrash HK, et al: Maternal mortality in the United States: Report from the Maternal Mortality Collaborative. *Obstet Gynecol* 1988; 72:91.
2. Report on maternal deaths in Australia, 1979-81. Canberra, Australian Government Publishing Service, 1987.
3. Gilbert L, Porter W, Brown VA: Postpartum hemorrhage: A continuing problem. *Br J Obstet Gynaecol* 1987; 94:67.
4. Department of Health report on confidential enquiries into maternal deaths in the United Kingdom 1988-1990. London, HMSO, 1994, p 34.
5. Hogberg U, Innala E, Sandstrom A: Maternal mortality in Sweden, 1980-1988. *Obstet Gynecol* 1994; 84:240.
6. Harrison KA: Maternal mortality in developing countries. *Br J Obstet Gynaecol* 1989; 96:1.
7. Bullough CH, Msuku RS, Karonde L: Early suckling and postpartum haemorrhage: Controlled trial in deliveries by birth attendants. *Lancet* 1989; 2:522.
8. Prendiville WJ, Harding JE, Elbourne DR, et al: The Bristol third stage trial: Active versus physiological management of the third stage of labour. *Br Med J* 1988; 297:1295.
9. Prendiville W, Elbourne D, Chalmers I: The effects of routine oxytocic administration in the management of the third stage of labour: An overview of the evidence from controlled trials. *Br J Obstet Gynaecol* 1988; 95:3.
10. Prendiville W, Elbourne D: Care during the third stage of labour, in Chalmers I, Enkin M, Keirse MJN (eds): *Effective Care in Pregnancy and Childbirth.* Oxford, Oxford University Press, 1989, pp 1145.
11. Sorbe B: Active pharmacologic management of the third stage of labor: A comparison of oxytocin and ergometrine. *Obstet Gynecol* 1978; 52:694.
12. Elbourne D, Prendiville W, Chalmers I: Choice of oxytocic preparation for routine use in the management of the third stage of labor: An overview of the evidence from controlled clinical trials. *Br J Obstet Gynaecol* 1988; 95:17.
13. Begley CM: A comparison of 'active' and physiological management of the third stage of labour. *Midwifery* 1990; 6:3.
14. Thornton S, Davison JM, Baylis PH: Plasma oxytocin during the third stage of labor: Comparison of natural and active management. *Br Med J* 1988; 297:167.
15. Rall TW: Oxytocin, prostaglandins, ergot alkaloids, and other drugs; Tocolytic agents, in Gilman AG, Rall TW, Nies AS et al (eds): *The Pharmacological Basis of Therapeutics,* ed 8. New York, Pergamon Press, 1990:933.
16. Ganong WF: *Review of Medical Physiology,* ed 15. Norwalk, Conn, Appleton-Lange, 1991, pp 57.
17. Kawarabayashi T, Kishikawa T, Sugimori H: Effect of oxytocin on spontaneous electrical and mechanical activities in pregnant human myometrium. *Am J Obstet Gynecol* 1986; 155:671.
18. Fuchs A-R, Fuchs F, Husslein P, et al: Oxytocin receptors in the human uterus during pregnancy and parturition. *Am J Obstet Gynecol* 1984; 150:734.
19. Fuchs A-R, Fuchs F: Physiology of parturition, in Gabbe SG, Niebyl JR, Simpson JL (eds): *Obstetrics: Normal and Problem Pregnancies,* ed 2. New York, Churchill Livingstone, 1991, p 147.
20. Garfield RE, Hayashi RH: Appearance of gap junctions in the myometrium of women during labor. *Am J Obstet Gynecol* 1981; 140:254.

21. Carsten ME, Miller JD: A new look at uterine muscle contraction. *Am J Obstet Gynecol* 1987; 157:1303.
22. Bloss JD, Hankins GD, Hauth JC, et al: The effect of oxytocin infusion on the pharmacokinetics of intramuscular magnesium sulfate therapy. *Am J Obstet Gynecol* 1987; 157:156.
23. Weis FR, Markello R, Mo B, et al: Cardiovascular effects of oxytocin. *Obstet Gynecol* 1975; 46:211.
24. Stoelting RK: *Pharmacology and Physiology in Anesthetic Practice*, ed 2. Philadelphia, JB Lippincott, 1991: 415.
25. Slater RM, Bowles BJ, Pumphrey RS: Anaphylactoid reaction to oxytocin in pregnancy. *Anaesthesia* 1985; 40:655.
26. Saunders WG, Munsick RA: Antidiuretic activity of oxytocin in women postpartum. *Am J Obstet Gynecol* 1966; 95:5.
27. Amico JA, Seitchik J, Robinson AG: Studies of oxytocin in plasma of women during hypocontractile labor. *J Clin Endocrinol Metab* 1984; 58:274.
28. Golan A, Lidor AL, Wexler S, et al: A new method for the management of the retained placenta. *Am J Obstet Gynecol* 1983; 146:708.
29. Chestnut DH, Wilcox LL: Influence of umbilical vein administration of oxytocin on the third stage of labor: A randomized, double-blind, placebo-controlled study. *Am J Obstet Gynecol* 1987; 157:160.
30. Young SB, Martelly PD, Greb L, et al: The effect of intraumbilical oxytocin on the third stage of labor. *Obstet Gynecol* 1989; 71:736.
31. Reddy VV, Carey JC: Effect of umbilical vein oxytocin on puerperal blood loss and length of the third stage of labor. *Am J Obstet Gynecol* 1989; 160:206.
32. Carroli G: Management of retained placenta by umbilical vein injection. *Br J Obstet Gynecol* 1991; 98:348.
33. Hunter DJ, Schulz P, Wassenaar W: Effect of carbetocin, a long-acting oxytocin analog, on the postpartum uterus. *Clin Pharmacol Ther* 1992; 52:60.
34. Gambling DR, Dansereau J, Wassenaar W, et al: Double-blind randomized comparison of a single dose of carbetocin vs 8 hours oxytocin infusion after cesarean delivery: Safety data. *Anesth Analg* 1994; 78:S127.
35. Dansereau J, Gambling D, Joshi A, et al: Double-blind comparison of carbetocin vs oxytocin in preventing uterine atony post cesarean section. *Int J Gynecol Obstet* 1994;46 (Suppl 2):77.
36. Compendium of Pharmaceuticals and Specialties, ed. 29. Ottawa, Ontario, Canadian Pharmaceutical Association, 1994: 455.
37. Johnstone M: The cardiovascular effects of oxytocic drugs. *Br J Anaesth* 1972; 44:826.
38. Baillie TW: Influence of ergometrine on the initiation of the cardiac impulse. *J Obstet Gynaecol Br Commonw* 1969; 76:34.
39. Dua JA: Postpartum eclampsia associated with ergometrine maleate administration. *Br J Obstet Gynaecol* 1994; 101:72.
40. Fester A: Provocative testing for coronary arterial spasm with ergonovine maleate. *Am J Cardiol* 1980; 46:338.
41. Taylor GJ, Cohen B: Ergonovine-induced coronary artery spasm and myocardial infarction after normal delivery. *Obstet Gynecol* 1985; 66:821.
42. Crawford JS: Bronchospasm following ergometrine. *Anaesthesia* 1980; 35:397.
43. Hughes WA, Hughes SC: Hemodynamic effects of prostaglandin E$_2$. *Anesthesiology* 1989; 70:713.
44. Veber B, Gauthe M, Michel-Cherqui M, et al: Severe hypertension during postpartum haemorrhage after IV administration of prostaglandin E$_2$. *Br J Anaesth* 1992; 68:623.
45. Secher NJ, Thayssen P, Arnsbo P, et al: Effect of prostaglandin E$_2$ and F$_2$ alpha on the systemic and pulmonary circulation in pregnant anesthetized women. *Acta Obstet Gynecol* 1982; 61:213.
46. Douglas MJ, Farquharson DF, Ross PL, et al: Cardiovascular collapse following an overdose of prostaglandin F$_2$ alpha: A case report. *Can J Anaesth* 1989; 36:466.
47. Mathe A, Hedqvist P, Holmgren A, et al: Bronchial hyperreactivity to prostaglandin F$_2$ alpha and histamine in patients with asthma. *Br Med J* 1973; 1:193.
48. Fishburne JI, Brenner WE, Braaksma JT, et al: Bronchospasm complicating intravenous prostaglandin F$_2$ alpha for therapeutic abortion. *Obstet Gynecol* 1972; 39:892.
49. Tagaki S, Yoshida T, Togo Y, et al: The effect of intramyometrial injection of prostaglandin F$_2$ alpha on severe postpartum hemorrhage. *Prostaglandins* 1976; 12:565.
50. Toppozada M, El-Bossaty M, El-Rahman HA, El-Din AH: Control of intractable atonic postpartum hemorrhage by 15-methyl prostaglandin F$_2$ alpha. *Obstet Gynecol* 1981; 58:327.
51. Hayashi RH, Castillo MS, Noah ML: Management of severe postpartum hemorrhage with a prostaglandin F$_2$ alpha analogue. *Obstet Gynecol* 1984; 63:806.
52. Bruce SL, Paul RH, Van Dorsten JP: Control of postpartum uterine atony by intramyometrial prostaglandin. *Obstet Gynecol* 1982; 59:475.
53. Thiery M, Parewijck W: Local administration of 15-methyl PGF$_2$ alpha for management of hypotonic postpartum hemorrhage. *Z Geburtshilfe Perinatol* 1985; 189:179.
54. Bigrigg A, Chui D, Read MD: Use of intramyometrial 15-methyl prostaglandin F$_2$ alpha to control atonic postpartum haemorrhage following vaginal delivery and failure of conventional therapy. *Br J Obstet Gynecol* 1991; 98:734.
55. Oleen MA, Mariano JP: Controlling refractory atonic postpartum hemorrhage with Hemabate sterile solution. *Am J Obstet Gynecol* 1990; 162:205.
56. Granstrom L, Ekman G, Ulmsten U: Intravenous infusion of 15-methyl-prostaglandin F$_2$ alpha (Prostinfenem) in women with heavy postpartum hemorrhage. *Acta Obstet Gynecol Scand* 1989; 68:365.
57. McDonald SJ, Prendiville WJ, Blair E: Randomized controlled trial of oxytocin alone versus oxytocin and ergometrine in active management of third stage of labour. *Br Med J* 1993; 307:1167.
58. Munson ES, Embro WJ: Enflurane, isoflurane, and halothane and isolated human uterine muscle. *Anesthesiology* 1977; 46:11.
59. Marx GF, Kim YO, Lin CC, et al: Postpartum uterine pressures under halothane or enflurane anesthesia. *Obstet Gynecol* 1978; 51:695.
60. Oats JN, Vasey DP, Waldron BA: Effects of ketamine on the pregnant uterus. *Br J Anaesth* 1979; 51:1163.
61. Marx GF, Hwang HS, Chandra P: Postpartum uterine pressures with different doses of ketamine. *Anesthesiology* 1979; 50:163.
62. Goodfellow CF, Hull MG, Swaab DF, et al: Oxytocin deficiency at delivery with epidural analgesia. *Br J Obstet Gynaecol* 1983; 90:214.
63. Wallace G: Blood loss in obstetrics using a haemoglobin dilution technique. *J Obstet Gynaecol Br Commonw* 1967; 74:64.
64. Robson SC, Boys RJ, Hunter S, et al: Maternal hemodynamics after normal delivery and delivery complicated by postpartum hemorrhage. *Obstet Gynecol* 1989; 74:234.
65. Ananthasubramaniam L, Kuntal R, Sivaraman R, et al: Management of intractable postpartum hemorrhage secondary to uterine atony with intramuscular 15-methyl PGF2 alpha. *Acta Obstet Gynaecol Scand* 1988; 145(Suppl):17.
66. Herbert WN, Cefalo RC: Management of postpartum hemorrhage. *Clin Obstet Gynecol* 1984; 27:139.
67. Reisner LS: Type and screen for cesarean section: A prudent alternative. *Anesthesiology* 1983; 58:476.

68. Kelton JG, Perrault RA, Blajchman MA: Substitution of the "group-and-screen" for the full crossmatch in elective operations. *Can Anaesth Soc J* 1983; 30:641.

69. Gettinger A: Rational use of blood products and alternative fluids, in *39th Annual Refresher Course Lectures*. Chicago, American Society of Anesthesiologists, 1989, p 112.

70. Honig CL, Bove JR: Transfusion associated fatalities: A review of Bureau of Biologics report. *Transfusion* 1980; 20:653

71. Dodd RY: The risk of transfusion-transmitted infection. *N Engl J Med* 1992; 327:419.

72. Stehling LC: Blood transfusion/blood banking: the basics, in *45th Annual Refresher Course Lectures*. American Society of Anesthesiologists, 1994, p 264.

73. Lamont BJ, Pennant JH, Wallace DH, et al: Directly measured uterine tone and blood loss during anesthesia for cesarean section. *Anesth Analg* 1988; 67:S126.

74. Weingarten AE, Korsh JE, Neuman GG, et al: Postpartum uterine atony after intravenous dantrolene. *Anesth Analg* 1987; 66:269.

75. Peng AT, Gorman RS, Shulman SM, et al: Intravenous nitroglycerin for uterine relaxation in the postpartum patient with retained placenta. *Anesthesiology* 1989; 71:172.

76. Ley SJ, Scheller J, Jones BR, et al: Intrauterine pressure during administration of nitroglycerin for extraction of retained placenta. *Anesthesiol Rev* 1993; 20:95.

77. DeSimone CA, Norris MC, Leighton BL: Intravenous nitroglycerin aids manual extraction of a retained placenta, (letter). *Anesthesiology* 1990; 73:787.

78. Mayer DC, Weeks SK: Antepartum uterine relaxation with nitroglycerin at caesarean delivery. *Can J Anaesth* 1992; 39:166.

79. Kamani AS, Gambling DR, Christilaw J, et al: Anaesthetic management of patients with placenta accreta. *Can J Anaesth* 1987; 34:613.

80. Chestnut DH, Dewan DM, Redick LF, et al: Anesthetic management for obstetric hysterectomy: A multi-institutional study. *Anesthesiology* 1989; 70:607.

81. Arcario T, Greene M, Ostheimer GW, et al: Risks of placenta previa/accreta in patients with previous cesarean deliveries. *Anesthesiology* 1988; 69:A659.

82. O'Sullivan GM, Sutton AJ, Thompson SA, et al: Noninvasive measurement of gastric emptying in obstetric patients. *Anesth Analg* 1987; 66:505.

83. Norris MC, Dewan DM: Preoxygenation for cesarean section: A comparison of two techniques. *Anesthesiology* 1985; 62:827.

84. Scott DB, Littlewood DG, Drummond GB, et al: Modification of the circulatory effects of extradural block combined with general anaesthesia by the addition of adrenaline to lignocaine solutions. *Br J Anaesth* 1977; 49:917.

85. Selinger M, MacKenzie I, Dunlop P, et al: Intra-umbilical oxytocin in the management of retained placenta: A double blind placebo controlled study. *J Obstet Gynecol* 1986; 7:115.

86. Clark SL, Koonings PP, Phelan JP: Placenta previa/accreta and prior cesarean section. *Obstet Gynecol* 1985; 66:89.

87. Wilken-Jensen C, Strom V, Neilsen MD, et al: Removing a retained placenta by oxytocin: A controlled study. *Am J Obstet Gynecol* 1989; 161:155.

88. Chin HG, Scott DR, Resnik R, et al: Angiographic embolisation of intractable puerperal hematomas. *Am J Obstet Gynecol* 1989; 160:434.

89. Baskett TF: Unpublished data, 1989.

90. O'Sullivan GV: Acute inversion of the uterus. *Br Med J* 1945; 2:282.

91. Catanzarite V, Moffitt KD, Baker ML, et al: New approaches to the management of acute puerperal inversion. *Obstet Gynecol* 1986; 68:7S.

92. Grossman RA: Magnesium sulfate for uterine inversion. *J Reprod Med* 1981; 26:261.

93. Altabef KM, Spencer JT, Zinberg S: Intravenous nitroglycerin for uterine relaxation of an inverted uterus. *Am J Obstet Gynecol* 1992; 166:1237.

94. Emmott RS, Bennett A: Acute inversion of the uterus at caesarean section. *Anaesthesia* 1988; 43:118.

95. Harris BA: Acute puerperal inversion of the uterus. *Clin Obstet Gynecol* 1984; 27:134.

96. Watson P, Besch N, Bowles WA: Management of acute and subacute puerperal inversion of the uterus. *Obstet Gynecol* 1980; 55:12.

97. Plumer MH: Bleeding problems, in James FM, Wheeler AS, Dewan DM, (eds): *Obstetric Anesthesia: The Complicated Patient*, ed 2. Philadelphia, FA Davis, 1988, p 309.

98. Mainprize TC, Maltby JR: Amniotic fluid embolism: A report of four probable cases. *Can Anaesth Soc J* 1986; 33:382.

10 Neurologic and Muscular Diseases

Esther M. Yun, Bruce A. Meyer, Valerie M. Parisi, and Alan C. Santos

Anesthetic management of the pregnant patient with intercurrent neurologic or muscular disease is particularly challenging because the usual tenets of obstetric anesthesia may require modification. Fortunately, the occurrence of neuromuscular diseases during pregnancy is low, but with improved medical care one may expect a higher incidence of successful pregnancy among affected women.

Proper management of these patients should include early evaluation and consultation between the anesthesiologist, obstetrician, and neurologist. For example, neurologic disease may reduce the strength of intercostal and accessory muscles of respiration. Thus, careful assessment of pulmonary function and reserve before anesthesia is advisable.

Analgesia during labor and delivery may prove particularly beneficial for individuals with neuromuscular disease, notably in those with limited cardiorespiratory reserves. However, there has been a reluctance among anesthesiologists to use regional techniques in patients with chronic sensorimotor dysfunction based on a fear of litigation rather than sound medical contraindications. Although our knowledge is scarce and generally limited to case reports, it appears that chronic neurologic conditions are not exacerbated by regional anesthesia.[1,2] Nonetheless, it is important to engage in frank discussion with the parturient regarding the anticipated risks and benefits of the proposed anesthetic technique. Thus, it is crucial to document in the medical record the extent of neurologic deficit before undertaking anesthesia care.

BRAIN NEOPLASMS
Incidence and pathophysiology

Tumors occurring within the intracranial vault may be classified according to their potential for malignancy and mass effect, as well as the site of localization, which often results in focal neurologic deficits. The potential for malignancy is directly related to the tumor's histologic features. Expansion of an intracerebral tumor may be associated with a mass effect that, if sufficient, may obliterate the neighboring cortical sulci, compress the ipsilateral lateral ventricle, or shift the midline between the hemispheres. The potential for hernia-tion of the cingulate gyrus under the falx or herniation of the uncus (temporal lobe) into the tentorial notch is of greatest concern.[3] Such herniations are associated with profound, often life-threatening neurologic deficits due to compression of brain parenchyma and its blood supply, resulting in ischemia and infarction. In this respect, the location of the tumor is crucial. For instance, relatively little expansion in an area such as the cerebellum may cause enough of a mass effect to cause tonsillar herniation through the foramen magnum, resulting in fatal brain stem compression.

The most common primary intracranial tumors are those derived from cells (more accurately, from the progenitor cells) indigenous to the central nervous system (CNS). Such tumors generally fall under the category of gliomas, which for the most part are infiltrating neoplasms localized deep in the white matter of the brain parenchyma. Total resection is virtually impossible because of a lack of distinct tumor margins. The category of gliomas generally includes astrocytoma, glioblastoma multiforme, oligodendroglioma, ependymoma, and, in some classifications, medulloblastoma.[4] Astrocytoma may vary in malignant potential. Glioblastoma multiforme, the most aggressive of these tumors, is characterized by anaplasia (a high number of mitotic figures), hemorrhage, and necrosis. At the other end of the spectrum, less malignant astrocytomas have low-grade histology that often resembles proliferation of normal-appearing astrocytes.[5] An oligodendroglioma, as the name implies, has a cellular structure similar to oligodendrocytes. Like astrocytomas, these tumors usually occur deep within the white matter and have a tendency toward calcification and cyst formation. Histologic grade may vary; however, the benign type usually predominates.[6] Ependymomas, like other gliomas, are of neuroectodermal origin. They arise from the ependymal lining of the ventricular system and thus have characteristic features such as cilia or canal or rosette formation, depending on the degree of differentiation. Other relatively common intracranial tumors not classified under the broad category of gliomas include meningiomas, pituitary adenomas, and acoustic neuromas. Meningiomas are derived from the dura mater or arachnoid cells and are usually histologically benign. Unlike gliomas, these tumors have well-demarcated margins so that surgical resection is possible, if it becomes necessary because of localization or mass effect. For instance, a meningioma occurring in the cerebellopontine angle may require extirpation to alleviate progressive unilateral lower cranial nerve deficits, whereas a small meningioma occurring in the falx cerebri may be asymptomatic.

Pituitary adenomas are relatively common intracranial neoplasms. Clinical manifestations may be due to mass effect, causing progressive neurologic deficits and/or headache, or it may be related to increased hormonal production. Tumors extending into the suprasellar region may result in loss of bilateral temporal vision as a result of compression of the optic chiasm. Compression of the hypothalamus and adjacent temporal lobe may cause further neurologic deterioration.[4] Prolactin-secreting tumors are associated with amenorrhea, infertility, and galactorrhea; those producing growth hormone cause progressive acromegaly, and tumors secreting adrenocorticotropic hormone (ACTH) may be related to Cushing's syndrome. In some cases, pituitary function may be reduced. With the advent of magnetic resonance imaging (MRI), microadenomas of the pituitary measuring less than 1 cm in diameter are now detectable. Proton beam irradiation has been used to treat smaller tumors,[7] while surgical resection is usually necessary for the larger ones. In the case of prolactinomas, treatment with bromocriptine has been successful in reducing tumor mass.

Acoustic neuromas originate from the eighth cranial nerve. Bilateral acoustic neuromas may occur with neurofibromatosis. Neurologic deficits such as tinnitus, hearing loss, or dysequilibrium are referable to involvement of the nerve itself. Neighboring nerves may also be compressed, particularly in the cerebellopontine angle, resulting in ipsilateral facial weakness and numbness. Further growth may result in increased intracranial pressure (ICP) and/or obstructive hydrocephalus due to reduced cerebrospinal fluid (CSF) outflow.[8] In such cases, urgent surgical correction may be required.

Other intracranial tumors, such as craniopharyngioma, teratoma, chordoma, and pinealoma, occur less frequently and are beyond the scope of this chapter. However, intracranial metastases deserve special consideration because they represent a significant proportion of all tumors occurring in the CNS. The most common intracranial metastases are from lung, breast, and skin tumors.[3] Hematogenous spread of tumor cells gives rise to macroscopic tumors within the brain parenchyma; this is associated with significant edema and breakdown of the blood-brain barrier. Consequently, relatively small tumors can cause a significant mass effect. Metastases may also occur on the leptomeninges and dura; they are often associated with cranial nerve palsies, particularly if they occur at the base of the skull near the foramina through which the cranial nerves exit.[9]

Histologic diagnosis of intracranial tumors usually requires biopsy of either the intracranial mass or the suspected primary tumor, if metastatic origin is most likely. Appropriate therapy is based on the histologic tumor type. Gliomas may be debulked, though a surgical cure is not to be expected. Surgery is often followed by whole-brain irradiation. Adjuvant chemotherapy may also improve survival.[5,10] Benign tumors, causing neurologic deficit or a progressive mass effect, often necessitate surgery. Surgery for metastatic disease is considered if a single brain metastasis in an operable location is found. However, in most cases, radiation remains the mainstay of treatment for brain metastases. Dexamethasone is routinely administered to decrease vasogenic edema associated with both primary and metastatic malignant brain tumors.[11] However, improvement may not occur for up to 24 hours after its use.

Obstetric and anesthetic management

Obstetric management. An intracranial neoplasm occurring during gestation has serious implications for the management of pregnancy and of labor and delivery. The physiologic changes associated with pregnancy and the hemodynamic alterations occurring during labor are potentially hazardous to the mother with an intracranial neoplasm.

The incidence of brain neoplasms in pregnant women is no different than that of nonpregnant women. However, some tumors manifest greater potential for increased mass effect during pregnancy.[12-14] The exact cause is unknown, but it may be due to an increase in vascularity or to the direct effects of hormones on tumor growth or cell enlargement during pregnancy.

Maternal mortality related to intracranial neoplasms is 5% to 10%. The progression of symptoms is usually gradual. One exception may be pituitary adenomas, which can enlarge markedly during gestation because of hemorrhage into the tumor itself. Another is choriocarcinoma, since trophoblastic tissue proliferates in the arterial walls, also causing rupture and hemorrhage.[15]

Confounding rapid diagnosis of intracranial neoplasm during pregnancy is the fact that many of the associated symptoms such as vomiting, headaches and visual changes (which can also occur with preeclampsia) also occur during normal gestation. Furthermore, some preexisting tumors may only become symptomatic during the added stress of pregnancy or labor. If an intracranial neoplasm is diagnosed during pregnancy, the following should be considered: the malignant grade of the tumor, gestational age at the time of diagnosis, the impairment of neurologic function, the risks to mother and fetus of surgical versus medical management, and finally, the route of delivery.[16] Fortunately, the mother's condition usually improves in the postpartum period; however, in severe cases, neurosurgical intervention may be necessary during pregnancy.

Management of intracranial neoplasms during pregnancy should be guided by the same principles used in nonpregnant patients. Abortion has been considered by mothers with malignant neoplasms and uncontrollable seizures, markedly increasing intracranial pressure and/or visual failure. If the mother desires to keep the pregnancy, once fetal viability is reached delivery may be required if gestation itself exacerbates the disease or interferes with appropriate therapy.[17]

Pituitary tumors may require special attention during pregnancy, as the pituitary gland enlarges by up to 70% as a result of proliferation of prolactin-secreting cells. Management of a newly diagnosed pituitary tumor during pregnancy is based on the clinical condition of the patient, and consideration should be given to bromocriptine or steroid therapy.[18]

Occasionally, a parturient with a brain tumor and increased intracranial pressure (ICP) will present in labor or for elective cesarean section. Every effort should be made to reduce ICP during the peripartum period until surgical intervention becomes feasible. Steroids (dexamethasone) and diuretics are frequently used to reduce cerebral edema and increased ICP. The administration of osmotic diuretics such as mannitol may result in fetal hypovolemia because of a net flow of water from the fetus to the mother.[19] In women, administration of mannitol 200 g shortly before delivery alters volume and concentration of solutes in the fetus.[20] In light of this, furosemide may be a better choice. Hyperventilation, at least initially, is an effective method of quickly reducing cerebral edema. Unfortunately, it requires tracheal intubation and controlled ventilation. Vigorous hyperventilation leading to hypocapnia and alkalosis may result in reduced uteroplacental perfusion by decreasing venous return to the heart and, consequently, maternal cardiac output. Maternal hypocapnia and alkalosis can also produce fetal acidosis by umbilical and uterine vasoconstriction[21] as well as by the shifting of the oxyhemoglobin dissociation curve

to the left. Thus, when hyperventilation is necessary, fetal heart rate monitoring should be employed to detect untoward fetal effects.

Analgesia for labor and vaginal delivery. The anesthetic management of a parturient with an intracranial tumor requires an understanding of the physiologic changes occurring during pregnancy and the effects of various anesthetic agents on ICP.

ICP is normal during pregnancy and parturition.[22] However, as mentioned earlier, pregnant patients with a brain neoplasm may be more prone to develop cerebral edema as a result of increased blood volume, a decrease in colloid oncotic pressure, and sodium and water retention.[23]

A rapid change in ICP can be potentially lethal for patients with a CNS space-occupying lesion. For example, an increase in ICP may result in compression and ischemia of vital brain-stem cardiorespiratory centers while, on the other hand, a sudden decrease in extracranial pressure, such as may occur with inadvertent dural puncture and loss of CSF, may lead to tentorial herniation through the foramen magnum.[24,25]

Although most would agree that pain relief is important for parturients with intracranial hypertension, considerable controversy exists regarding the choice of analgesia to be used in patients with increased ICP. Subarachnoid block may not be appropriate because dural puncture and CSF leakage may, theoretically, enhance the risk of herniation. How significant this risk may be in practice, with the small-gauge pencilpoint needles used in obstetric anesthesia, is unknown and arguable. Proponents of epidural block argue that the technique offers superior pain relief as compared with other forms of analgesia. Indeed, peridural analgesia attenuates increases in ICP occurring in response to painful uterine contractions and, most notably, by abolishing involuntary skeletal muscle contractions and bearing-down efforts.[24,26,27]

On the other hand, concern exists regarding the potential for inadvertent dural puncture to occur with a large bore needle, which causes a sudden decrease in CSF pressure and possible tentorial herniation. Obviously the risk of dural puncture is reduced in the hands of an experienced operator. In this regard, the caudal approach may have significant advantages to lumbar placement since the dural sac ends at the second sacral vertebrae several centimeters above the sacral hiatus. Unfortunately, the caudal approach has a higher failure rate than the lumbar and requires greater volumes of drug for satisfactory analgesia.

Nonetheless, lumbar epidural analgesia has been used successfully and safely in several parturients with increased ICP.[23,28,29] Should the lumbar approach be chosen, the lateral recumbent position may be preferable to the sitting since the dural sac may be under less tension.[26] Rapid epidural administration of large volumes of drugs should also be avoided because this could potentially further increase ICP (Fig. 10-1).[29] It is the authors' preference to use a local anesthetic agent alone or in combination with a narcotic drug since, in our experience, the sole use of epidurally administered opioids may lead to incomplete analgesia and bearing-down efforts.

Other modes of analgesia, although not having the attendant risk of inadvertent dural puncture, may be even less desirable. Analgesia with systemically administered narcotics is incomplete and carries with it the risk of maternal sedation and hypercarbia, which in itself may increase ICP. Paracervical block provides good analgesia for the first stage of labor but carries with it an unacceptably high risk to the fetus and does not provide analgesia for the second stage of labor. Although not commonly used, bilateral lumbar sympathetic block (LSB) will provide adequate analgesia for the first stage of labor with minimal risk of dural puncture. However, labor may outlast the duration of blockade, requiring repeated administration. Intrapartum fetal and intraamniotic pressure monitoring are advisable because LSB may be associated with increased uterine activity.[30] A pudendal block is necessary for the second stage of labor. In general, assisted delivery is often required to avoid bearing-down efforts.

Anesthesia for cesarean section. There are little data to recommend an anesthetic technique with certainty. Based on general principles of management, for abdominal delivery, most anesthesiologists would choose general endotracheal anesthesia using a thiopental induction, hyperventilation, and control of blood pressure. Sodium nitroprusside or trimethaphan are frequently used to treat systemic hypertension, which often occurs during laryngoscopy and intubation. More recently, labetalol and esmolol have been used; however, high doses of the latter may lead to fetal acid-base derangements.[31] Severe hypocapnia, lower than 25 mm Hg, should be avoided, since it can cause uteroplacental insufficiency and is of no additional benefit in decreasing ICP. In addition, intravenous (IV) lidocaine and fentanyl may be given to blunt cardiovascular responses to intubation and to reduce the concentration of halogenated agents so as to avoid uterine atony. Most would use isoflurane for maintenance of anesthesia since it does not increase cerebral blood flow to the same extent as do other volatile agents.

Rapid-acting nondepolarizing muscle relaxants, particularly vecuronium, are suited for facilitation of tracheal intubation and maintenance of neuromuscular blockade. Use of succinylcholine is controversial in such a situation. In addition to routine monitoring, placement of an indwelling arterial catheter is strongly recommended for continuous monitoring of systemic blood pressure.

BENIGN INTRACRANIAL HYPERTENSION
Incidence and pathophysiology

Benign intracranial hypertension (BIH), also known as pseudotumor cerebri, is a chronic condition in which there is persistent elevation in ICP in the absence of an identifiable cause, such as intracranial mass, infection, or obstruction to CSF outflow. The etiology of the disease is unknown, but the disease has been attributed to hormonally induced changes in water and electrolyte balance,

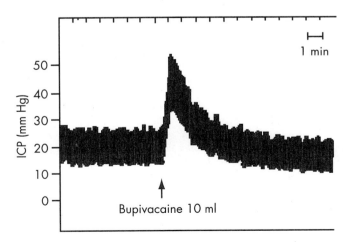

Fig. 10-1 Increase in ICP after epidural administration of bupivacaine 10 ml. (From Hilt H, Gramm HJ, Link J: *Br J Anaesth* 1986; 58:676.)

or to decreased CSF absorption.[32] Although it predominantly occurs in obese females after menarche,[33,34] the incidence in obstetric patients is approximately 19 per 100,000 patients. The incidence can be has high as 1 in 870 pregnancies at tertiary care hospitals.[35,36] The disease may manifest at any time during gestation, but it most commonly occurs in the first half of pregnancy.[37] Headache and/or visual disturbances are common, usually in conjunction with papilledema. Blindness can result in severe cases. The criteria for diagnosis include increased ICP with normal CSF composition in the absence of a space-occupying lesion and mental status deficit.

Obstetric and anesthetic management

Obstetric management. Benign intracranial hypertension is usually self-limiting, rarely life-threatening, and it does not adversely affect reproductive outcome.[35] Recurrence during subsequent pregnancies ranges from 10% to 30%.[37] Pregnancy itself may exacerbate the disease by causing water and electrolyte imbalances.[38] There does not appear to be an increased incidence of fetal wastage, congenital anomalies, or requirement for cesarean section among mothers having pseudotumor cerebri.

Therapy has generally consisted of analgesics and diuretics, most frequently a carbonic anhydrase inhibitor or furosemide. Use of diuretics during pregnancy carries the added risk of reducing intravascular volume, which results in uteroplacental insufficiency. Thus, maternal and fetal surveillance is suggested. Drainage of CSF with repeated lumbar punctures and occasional administration of steroids may be necessary.[38] In rare instances, continuous CSF drainage via placement of a lumbo-peritoneal shunt should be considered, particularly if the optic nerve is threatened by the disease. Despite these measures, if papilledema and visual field deficits persist, decompression of the optic nerve sheath may be required.[38]

Requirement for cesarean section should be based on the usual obstetric considerations. Although some authors recommend shortening the second stage of labor with operative vaginal delivery,[39] maternal and neonatal outcomes are generally excellent, and there is no data to specifically support this intervention.

Analgesia for labor and vaginal delivery. Epidural analgesia is preferred over systemic analgesics, since it avoids maternal sedation, respiratory depression, and hypercarbia. In addition, epidural analgesia reduces cardiovascular and ICP responses to pain associated with uterine contractions; epidural analgesia also abolishes the bearing-down reflex.[27,40] Avoiding further increases in ICP during labor is also important in preventing visual loss.

Continuous epidural analgesia has been successfully used for labor in parturients with benign intracranial hypertension.[41,42] However, as mentioned earlier, caution must be exercised to prevent further increases in ICP due to epidural injection of a large volume of solution (Fig. 10-1).[29] Unlike patients with intracranial hypertension due to neoplasm, the risk of cerebellar tonsillar herniation after dural puncture is not a major concern because increases in ICP are uniformly distributed.[37] In fact, lumbar puncture is used as a diagnostic as well as a therapeutic modality. However, two cases of cerebellar tonsillar herniation have been reported following diagnostic lumbar puncture in patients having BIH with focal neurologic deficits.[42] Thus, in patients with focal neurologic deficits suggestive of posterior fossa compression, the presence of low-lying cerebellar tonsils should be excluded radiologically, before lumbar puncture. In patients with a lumbar-peritoneal shunts, any analgesic technique is acceptable. However, if neuraxial analgesia is chosen, there may be a theoretical risk of puncturing the shunt.[43]

Anesthesia for cesarean section. Spinal or epidural block, in most instances, may be preferable to general anesthesia.[41,43] Spinal anesthesia (5% lidocaine 60 mg, with epinephrine 0.2 mg) has been used without untoward effects.[43] The hesitation among anesthesiologists to use neuraxial block secondary to the perceived risks of tonsillar herniation has already been discussed. Post–dural-puncture headache (PDPH) may occur in patients with BIH and may be difficult to differentiate from the primary disease.[44-46] Epidural blood patch has been used to treat PDPH in a patient with BIH who did not have papilledema.[45] Blood should be injected slowly, in small increments, thus avoiding sharp increases in ICP.

In patients with presumably normal ICP after lumbar-peritoneal shunt, general anesthesia would avoid the need for radiographic exposure of mother and fetus necessary to document shunt location before attempting regional anesthesia. Also, adequate sensory anesthesia following subarachnoid injection may be unpredictable because local anesthetic may run off into the peritoneum via the shunt.[43] If general anesthesia is chosen, a routine thiopentone-succinylcholine induction followed by cricoid pressure and endotracheal intubation has been used.[43] Anesthesia was maintained with 60% nitrous oxide and 0.5% to 1% isoflurane in oxygen, and atracurium was administered for muscle relaxation. In mothers who do not have a lumbar-peritoneal shunt but who require general anesthesia, hyperventilation and blood pressure control are recommended. Increasing the dose of thiopental and IV administration of lidocaine and/or fentanyl may blunt elevations in ICP during tracheal intubation.[47] Occasionally, it may be necessary to treat hemodynamic responses to intubation with nitroprusside, trimethaphan, or labetalol.

CEREBROVASCULAR DISEASES
Incidence and pathophysiology

Manifestations of cerebrovascular diseases, often sudden and catastrophic, are associated with hemorrhage or ischemic infarction. Spontaneous intracranial hemorrhage may occur in the subarachnoid space or it may be intraparenchymal. Subarachnoid hemorrhage (SAH) results primarily from rupture of a congenital aneurysm (CA) or arteriovenous malformation (AVM). In pregnant women, these occur with equal frequency, while in nonpregnant women, the former is more common.[48] Hemorrhage from either can occur at any time during pregnancy; however, the incidence of aneurysmal rupture appears to be progressively greater during the latter months of pregnancy, while the incidence of AVM rupture tends to increase during the second trimester and again during labor and delivery.[48,49]

A congenital aneurysm is usually located at the branch points of the major arteries forming the circle of Willis. Commonly, a rupture presents with sudden, severe headache, often described by the patient as the worst headache of her life. Many patients may recall an episode of severe headache a few days earlier, corresponding to a "sentinel bleed" before actual rupture. With extensive hemorrhage, ICP may increase and the patient may become obtunded. Focal neurologic deficits are related to parenchymal extension of subarachnoid blood or to herniation as a result of increased ICP. Should the patient survive the initial hemorrhage, the risk of rebleed from an aneurysm is highest during the ensuing week. In addition, there is a significant risk of ischemic stroke, beginning approximately 2 days after the initial hemorrhage and persisting for up to 10 days. The cause of ischemic stroke appears to be related to severe vasospasm provoked by the presence of blood in the subarachnoid space.[50] In contrast to aneurysms, arteriovenous malformations may be symptomatic for some time before the rupture. Seizures, focal neurologic deficits, and severe headache are common. Severe preeclampsia or eclampsia may, in some instances, be difficult to differentiate.

Nonhemorrhagic infarction results from ischemia of brain parenchyma supplied by an artery, usually as a result of thrombosis or embolism. Infarction occurs if collateral circulation to the ischemic area is not adequate. Morbidity from ischemic infarction is directly related to loss of neurologic function in the area of infarction. In the case of a large infarction, subsequent edema may cause a considerable mass effect and even herniation. Embolic infarction involves sudden occlusion of a vessel by a lodged embolus. Cardiomyopathy and atrial fibrillation are conditions that may predispose to thrombus formation. In the case of atrial fibrillation, conversion to sinus rhythm may cause a mural thrombus to dislodge. An embolic event is characterized by the sudden onset of neurologic deficit, which resolves, to some extent, over the ensuing 24 hours. Cerebral vein thrombosis or venous sinus thrombosis is uncommon in the general population, but it may be seen in patients with hypercoagulability and during the puerperium.[51,52] Hemorrhagic transformation of such an infarct is not uncommon and may also occur after infarction as a result of venous occlusion.

Overall, the risk factors for ischemic infarction are similar to those for atherosclerosis. Hypertension, hypercholesterolemia, and smoking are recognized risk factors. Systemic diseases associated with increased thrombotic risk or hyperviscosity also predispose to stroke. These include hematologic disorders with thrombocytosis, profound leukocytosis, severe anemia, and antithrombin III or protein C deficiencies.[53] Ischemic infarction is also a recognized complication of sickle cell anemia.

Vasculopathies such as fibromuscular dysplasia, systemic vasculitis, giant cell arteritis, and isolated vasculitis of the CNS can result in ischemic infarction. Collagen vascular diseases, including systemic lupus erythematosus, may be associated with ischemic infarction, particularly if lupus anticoagulant or anticardiolipin antibodies are present. Oral contraceptive use is associated with increased risk of ischemic infarction.[54] Other causes of drug-induced infarction include cocaine and excessive ethanol intake. A severe complicated migraine may also result in infarction due to prolonged vasospasm.

Cardiac risk factors for stroke in women of reproductive age generally include cardiomyopathies and paroxysmal atrial fibrillation. In the presence of a patent (or probe patent) foramen ovale, venous thrombosis may lead to paradoxical embolism.[55] Both rheumatic and nonrheumatic valvular heart disease are associated with embolic stroke. Bacterial endocarditis may also be a source of embolism. Mitral valve prolapse is associated with cerebral embolic events, particularly when redundant mitral valve leaflets are identified by echocardiogram.[56]

Diagnosis of patients with suspected arteriovenous malformation, aneurysms, or frank subarachnoid hemorrhage/infarction is made with computed tomographic (CT) scan (with and without contrast media). Magnetic resonance imaging (MRI) is often more sensitive in detecting small occlusive strokes and may be safely performed during pregnancy. In some cases, an arteriogram will be necessary to confirm physical or radiologic findings; this is not contraindicated during pregnancy. Maternal abdominal shielding should be performed. Lumbar puncture may also be required but should be performed cautiously if there is suspicion of increased intracranial pressure.

Obstetric and anesthetic management

Obstetric management. Pregnancy is associated with an increased risk of cerebral vascular accidents such as ischemic or hemorrhagic stroke or subarachnoid hemorrhage. For instance, the incidence of stroke during pregnancy ranges from 1 to 3,000 to 1 to 20,000; this is 13 times greater than the risk in nonpregnant age-matched women.[57,58] Risk factors for stroke during pregnancy are listed in Box 10-1. Whereas the majority of strokes in nonpregnant patients are related to atherosclerosis, arterial occlusion (usually of the middle cerebral artery) accounts for 60% to 80% of strokes occurring in pregnant women, most often in the second and third trimesters.[59] In contrast, stroke related to venous occlusion is more common during the first trimester.[59]

Prevention of stroke usually consists of control of hypertension, treatment of hypercholesterolemia, and change in lifestyle (moderate exercise and elimination of smoking and excessive alcohol intake). Anticoagulation is indicated in patients with a known risk for cardiogenic embolism.[60,61] Anticoagulation may also be of benefit in patients with circulating lupus anticoagulant, though long-term treatment with low-dose aspirin may also be effective.[54]

Subarachnoid hemorrhage occurs in 1 to 10,000 pregnancies with maternal mortality being as high as 80%.[62,63] In the general population, rupture of an intracranial aneurysm occurs more frequently than that of an arteriovenous malformation. During pregnancy, however, both vascular lesions result in cerebral hemorrhage with equal frequency.[63] Subarachnoid hemorrhage due to rupture of an arteriovenous malformation usually occurs during the second half of pregnancy or during labor. The risk of rebleed after rupture of an aneurysm is greater than following rupture of an arteriovenous malformation and is associated with high mortality. In pregnant women, the timing of the occurrence usually directs neurosurgical and obstetric management (Table 10-1). If rupture occurs prior to fetal viability, craniotomy and correction of the lesion may be carried out and pregnancy

---

BOX 10-1 RISK FACTORS AND CAUSES OF STROKE IN PREGNANCY

Hematologic Conditions
Hemoglobin SS, SC disease
Lupus anticoagulant
Polycythemia
Essential thrombocytosis
Deficiency of protein S or C
Deficiency of antithrombin III
Antiphospholipid antibodies
Systemic lupus erythematosus
Increase in Factor VIII
Paroxysmal nocturnal hemoglobinuria
Thrombotic thrombocytopenic purpura

Vasculopathy
Aneurysm
Arteriovenous malformation
Venous thrombosis
Atherosclerosis
Vasculitis
Syphilis
Systemic lupus erythmatosus
Tay-Sachs disease
Fibromuscular dysplasia
Arterial dissection (Moya-Moya disease)
Granulomatous angitis
Peripartum cardiomyopathy

Embolism
Peripartum cardiomyopathy
Nonbacterial thrombotic endocarditis
Fat or air embolism
Atrial fibrillation
Sick sinus syndrome
Infective endocarditis
Valvular heart disease
Mitral valve prolapse

Miscellaneous
Migraine
Alcohol intoxication
Drug abuse (Cocaine)
Metastatic choriocarcinoma
Eclampsia
Syphilis
Homocystinuria

---

allowed to continue. A normal spontaneous vaginal delivery at term will not be contraindicated. If rupture occurs nearer to term and the fetus is considered viable, a combined procedure of cesarean section followed by craniotomy may be appropriate.

Treatment of an unruptured arteriovenous malformation may involve a surgical approach, embo-

Table 10-1 Mode of delivery for patients with intracranial hemorrhage

Neurologic complication	Mode of delivery
Ruptured aneurysm	If clipped successfully, normal delivery
	If not clipped and rupture occurs in 3rd trimester, cesarean section at 38 weeks
	If not clipped and rupture occurs in 1st or 2nd trimester, vaginal delivery
Ruptured arteriovenous malformation	If excised before 35th week, normal delivery
	If not excised and pelvis is proved adequate, vaginal delivery without Valsalva maneuver
	If not excised and adequacy of pelvis is unproven, cesarean section at 38 weeks
Rupture of intraparenchymal vessel	Usually vaginal delivery without Valsalva maneuver

From Weibers DO: Subarachnoid hemorrhage in pregnancy, *Semin Neurol* 1988; 8:227.

lization, or proton beam irradiation.[64] Should hemorrhage occur due to a ruptured arteriovenous malformation, surgical resection and hematoma evacuation are to be considered to prevent further catastrophe related to a rebleed. Aneurysms found incidentally by angiography are usually considered for clipping if they are at least 1 cm in diameter. Medical management of patients after aneurysmal hemorrhage involves therapeutic measures, such as hyperventilation and osmotic diuretics, to decrease ICP. Careful attention must be directed to the prevention of hypertension, while relative hypotension must be avoided to ensure adequate cerebral perfusion during periods of vasospasm.

Concurrent delivery by cesarean section and repair of the aneurysm or arteriovenous malformation has been successfully accomplished.[65,66] Controlled intraoperative hypothermia and hypotension have been used. Fetal monitoring should be used during the procedure, since fetal bradycardia may occur in relation to hypothermia and hypotension.[67] After surgical correction, vaginal delivery appears to be safe. The use of regional anes-

thesia and a shortened second stage of labor with operative vaginal delivery may decrease the risk of secondary bleeding. Scheduled cesarean section is recommended for patients with a ruptured aneurysm or AVM that is unclipped.

Anesthesia for cesarean section. There are reports of good outcome following general endotracheal anesthesia administered for combined cesarean section and neurosurgical procedures.[65,66,68] The prevention of aspiration and fluctuations in systemic blood pressure in the mother, while at the same time avoiding undue fetal depression, constitutes a true anesthetic challenge.

Preoperative sedation may not be necessary because most patients may already be treated with agents such as phenobarbital or diazepam. Although the patient's anxiety should be allayed, undue sedation should be avoided because of the potential for hypercarbia and hypoxia to occur. Perioperative monitoring should include continuous blood pressure recording with the use of an indwelling arterial catheter. Prophylactic measures against aspiration pneumonitis should be taken. Cardiovascular responses to endotracheal intubation have been blunted with lidocaine (100 mg IV), propanolol (0.5 mg increments up to 3 mg), sodium nitroprusside (50 μg IV) and/or halothane by mask with continuous cricoid pressure.[65,68] Thiopental (150 to 350 mg) has been used for induction of anesthesia.[65,66,68] Succinylcholine may be used; however, it should be preceded by a defasciculating dose of a nondepolarizing muscle relaxant to minimize the risk of increasing ICP. Rapid-acting nondepolarizing muscle relaxants can also be used to facilitate intubation after using a priming dose.

Controlled induced hypotension may be useful at times. The fetus should be monitored (FHR) because hypotension may result in uteroplacental insufficiency. The choice of antihypertensive agent has been controversial. Concern has been expressed that the fetus might be particularly vulnerable to cyanide toxicity if nitroprusside is used because of a reduced concentration of thiosulphate, which is necessary for rhodanase detoxification of cyanide.[69] Indeed, in chronically instrumented pregnant ewes, high doses of nitroprusside resulted in fetal death.[69] However, in humans, relatively brief exposure to clinically accepted doses of the drug had no adverse effect on neonatal outcome or development.[70-73] Nitroglycerin has also been used, lower potential for toxicity being its main advantage.[74] However, it is slower acting, less potent and less unpredictable than nitroprusside.

Trimethaphan is a ganglionic blocking agent that may be slightly more effective in pregnant than in nonpregnant women. Potentiation of succinylcholine blockade may occur because trimethaphan inhibits plasma cholinesterase. Maternal mydriasis may affect interpretation of neurologic signs. Even when administered in large doses, trimethaphan is well tolerated by the fetus, except that it may result in meconium ileus.[63]

Monitoring of fetal heart rate may also be beneficial during cases in which hypothermia and hyperventilation will be used. A decrease in uterine blood flow related to an increase in uterine tone has been observed with profound maternal hypothermia (28° C).[75] However, moderate hypothermia, 28° to 32° C, has been used in several cases with good obstetric outcome.[76,77] Hyperventilation is often used during neurosurgical procedures to "slack the brain." However, severe hypocapnia <25 mm Hg can also have detrimental effects on the fetus by decreasing uterine blood flow.[78] Extreme hypocapnia may also increase the risk of cerebral vasospasm in the presence of subarachnoid hemorrhage.

After delivery of the infant, anesthesia may be modified as required for the neurosurgical procedure. In some patients a subarachnoid catheter may be placed for withdrawal of CSF during surgery, before induction of anesthesia. It would seem logical that, if possible, the catheter also be used for spinal anesthesia during the cesarean section.[68] This would decrease the risk of aspiration and fetal depression, as well as avoid hemodynamic changes associated with tracheal intubation under light anesthesia. There have been reports of neurologic deficits following the use of spinal catheters for continuous spinal anesthesia.[79] However, these reports pertained to the use of small-gauge catheters and not the larger-bore catheters used for drainage of CSF. Since most of the reported cases occurred with lidocaine, it would seem prudent to use bupivacaine as an alternative.[79]

Occasionally, one may be called on to provide anesthesia for cesarean section in a patient having an inoperable cerebrovascular lesion. Epidural anesthesia is preferred since it circumvents systolic hypertension resulting from intubation.[80] The level of sensory anesthesia should be extended slowly, allowing time for adequate hydration. Hypotension should be prevented since it may lead to vomiting that in turn can result in rupture of the intracranial lesion.[80] Administration of neuraxial opiates for postoperative analgesia is recommended to minimize pain and avoid hypertension. Management of a patient who already has the aneurysm or AVM corrected does not require any special treatment.

Analgesia for labor and vaginal delivery. Epidural analgesia is also preferred in patients undergoing labor and vaginal delivery who have had clipping or repair of an intracranial vascular lesion.

The second stage of labor might have to be shortened to minimize bearing-down efforts.

CORTICAL VEIN THROMBOSIS
Incidence and pathophysiology

Cortical vein thrombosis (CVT) is related to an obstruction of blood flow from the superior sagittal sinus and/or cortical veins. The resulting decrease in CSF absorption and increase in ICP may be manifested by headache, vomiting, seizures, and focal neurologic signs. Thrombosis may occur because of intracerebral blood flow stasis due to the fact that the longitudinal sinus and cerebral veins do not have valves. The pregnant patient, particularly the preeclamptic one, may be at increased risk because of injury of the endothelial lining of the cortical sinuses and veins during sudden changes in ICP accompanying uterine contractions and bearing-down efforts, and also because of hypercoagulability.[81-84]

The true incidence of the disease is difficult to estimate since it is often misdiagnosed or it goes undetected.[51,83] It most commonly occurs during the first postpartum month. A high index of suspicion must be maintained because the manifestations of the disease often mimic preeclampsia or even post–dural-puncture headache.[85] A diagnosis can usually be established by CT or MRI scans, or by angiography.[83,84]

Obstetric and anesthetic management

Obstetric management. Therapy should be directed at treating any underlying disorders such as infection, or at exchange transfusion for patients with sickle cell disease. Dehydration should be corrected, and early use of anticonvulsants may be beneficial.[83,84] Mortality is approximately 30% without treatment, but this can be reduced to 10% in patients who do not have active hemorrhage and receive aggressive care and anticoagulant therapy.[83,84] If the condition occurs antepartum, vaginal delivery with the avoidance of Valsalva maneuvers during the second stage has been recommended.[51]

Anesthetic considerations. Many patients with cortical vein thrombosis will require obstetric intervention because of its association with preeclampsia. In this setting, anesthetic management should avoid further jeopardy of an already compromised fetus and the critically ill mother.[82] The two overriding concerns for the anesthesiologist are the potential for raised ICP and coagulopathy. In emergency situations, or in the face of coagulopathy, general endotracheal anesthesia may be advisable. The technique for general anesthesia in patients with increased ICP has already been described, as have the concerns for the use of epidural anesthesia. With regional techniques, the potential for an asymmetric cerebral hematoma to cause brain-stem herniation should dural puncture occur is another consideration already discussed (see Brain Neoplasms). Also, significant untreated hypotension due to sympathetic block may reduce cerebral blood flow to areas that are compromised. Yet, considering the aforementioned, if labor and vaginal delivery are planned, carefully administered epidural block may be preferable to the use of systemic analgesics.

Postpartum headache in patients who have had regional anesthesia is often attributed to dural puncture. However, there have been several cases where CVT was misdiagnosed as PDPH and an epidural blood patch was performed, with subsequent neurologic deterioration.[83,84,86] It is a rare cause of peripartum headache, but it should be considered in the differential diagnosis of an atypical headache. Unlike PDPH, headache due to CVT is not positional, and it is usually accompanied by nausea, vomiting, and diaplasis.[84,87]

SEIZURE DISORDERS
Incidence and pathophysiology

A seizure may be defined as a repetitive synchronous electrical discharge in the cerebral cortex that may be local or general in its distribution. Thus, seizures can be classified as partial or generalized, depending on their localization. A partial seizure arises in a focal area of cerebral cortex and may or may not spread to involve adjacent areas. Partial seizures may be further subdivided into simple or complex subtypes based on the presence or absence of an alteration in consciousness. In contrast, a generalized seizure usually begins in both hemispheres simultaneously (Box 10-2). This distinction is often apparent by both electroencephalographic and clinical manifestations.[88]

Generalized seizures occurring during pregnancy and in the peripartum period may be related to gestation itself (e.g., eclampsia) or to preexisting conditions such as a cerebral vascular abnormality or neoplasm. Idiopathic epilepsy, usually characterized by the onset of grand mal seizures during childhood or early adult life, is possibly the most prevalent cause of convulsions during pregnancy.[89]

Maternal seizure disorders are perhaps the most common medical complications occurring during pregnancy.[90] The objective of therapy is to prevent recurrence in its most severe form, namely status epilepticus. On the other hand, the potential teratogenic effects of antiepileptic drugs must be considered. Whether chronic antiepileptic drug therapy reduces the risk of recurrent seizures is often debated.[91] Chronic use of anticonvulsant medi-

---

BOX 10-2   CLASSIFICATION OF SEIZURES

Generalized seizures

Convulsive
Tonic/clonic
Tonic only
Clonic only
Myoclonic
Atonic

Partial seizures

Simple
Motor only
Sensory only
Autonomic
Psychic (amnestic, cognitive, affective)

Complex
Impaired consciousness at onset
Impaired consciousness after onset

Partial, with evolution to generalized seizures
Simple
Complex

---

cation is unnecessary when seizures are provoked by factors that can be readily identified and corrected. Examples of this are seizures caused by physical injuries, vascular insults, and metabolic toxic disturbances.

The effect of pregnancy on epilepsy is unpredictable. In 35% to 45% of patients, the frequency of seizures may increase as a result of physiologic alterations in the mother, such as increased fluid retention or alkalosis related to vomiting or hyperventilation. The latter often leads to changes in the disposition of anticonvulsant drugs, resulting in subtherapeutic blood levels.[92,93] Sleep deprivation and stress can also contribute to recurrences. Fortunately, in only 10% of patients does pregnancy exacerbate the disease.[94,95] Maternal age, race, parity, or a history of recurrences during a prior pregnancy do not appear to correlate with gestational exacerbation of epilepsy. On the other hand, increasing seizure frequency prior to pregnancy, excessive weight gain, poor patient compliance with anticonvulsant therapy, anxiety, and insomnia do.[96]

Earlier studies concluded that epilepsy was associated with a higher incidence of obstetric complications such as preeclampsia, vaginal hemorrhage, premature rupture of amniotic membranes, and instrumental delivery,[97] although more recent data fail to confirm this observation.[98] Nonetheless, an increased frequency of stillbirth, microcephaly, and mental retardation has been observed in the offspring of epileptic mothers.[99,100] Furthermore, status epilepticus is associated with increased fetal and neonatal mortality, presumably because of acute hypoxia.

Obstetric and anesthetic management

Obstetric management. New onset of seizures occurring during the latter half of pregnancy or during the immediate postpartum period are most frequently due to eclampsia; however, other causes should be considered, including cerebrovascular disease, neoplasms and metabolic disorders. It is important to establish a diagnosis because the therapy and prognosis may differ considerably. Status epilepticus is unusual during pregnancy; in the nonepileptic patient, it may be indicative of eclampsia, encephalitis, meningitis, frontal lobe tumors, drug withdrawal, or other toxic metabolic conditions. Before the advent of effective anticonvulsants, status epilepticus during pregnancy was uniformly fatal to mother and fetus. Mortality is greater in pregnant women with the disease as compared with nonpregnant patients, and fetal loss approaches 50%.[101] Apnea and increased oxygen consumption during grand mal seizures can cause fetal hypoxia and acidemia. Noneclamptic status epilepticus does not improve with termination of pregnancy.[90] Therapy for status epilepticus in the pregnant patient is similar to that for the nonpregnant woman, but uterine displacement must be rigorously maintained. An airway should be immediately established and the seizure terminated with anticonvulsants. General anesthesia may be required in some cases to break the seizure. Fetal condition improves with maternal resuscitation, and emergency delivery is usually not indicated unless uncontrolled seizures are associated with eclampsia.[100] Due to vitamin K dependent clotting factor deficiencies, maternal and fetal hemorrhage may occur in up to 10% of pregnancies complicated by epilepsy.[100] Administration of vitamin K to the mother and neonate is an effective and preventative measure.[100]

Patients with epilepsy may be treated with a variety of medications selected according to their efficacy, cost, half-life, and side effects. Carbamazepine, phenytoin, trimethadione, valproic acid, and phenobarbital are equally effective for generalized seizures in nonpregnant patients. However, trimethadione has been associated with congenital malformations and should not be used during pregnancy. Likewise, valproic acid has been implicated in causing face-heart-limb malformations and lumbosacral meningomyelocele. During pregnancy, ethosuximide has become the drug of choice for

absence (petit mal) seizures, while clonazepam is preferred for the control of myoclonic and tonic seizures. Phenytoin has been associated with maternal side effects such as gingival hypertrophy, hirsutism, and coarsening of facial features, as well as with fetal hydantoin syndrome; it has thus been less commonly used during pregnancy.

The primary goal of obstetric management is to prevent or eliminate seizure activity. The following obstetric recommendations can be made: (1) A reevaluation of the advisability of chronic anticonvulsant therapy should occur before conception, (2) Patients should be informed about the teratogenic potential of antiepileptic medications, (3) Family history of congenital abnormalities should be evaluated, and (4) Folic acid and vitamin supplementation should be given. The lowest dosage and fewest anticonvulsants should be used to achieve optimal seizure control, and the plasma concentration should be measured on a monthly basis. The free unbound fraction of drug should be determined when highly protein bound medications such as phenytoin are used. Finally, in patients receiving phenytoin, parental vitamin K should be administered at the onset of labor.

Anesthetic considerations. The effects of chronic anticonvulsant therapy and the potential effects of anesthetic agents on the seizure threshold should be considered in selecting an anesthetic technique. In its most life-threatening form, status epilepticus, the disease may require rapid anesthetic intervention and intensive care.

Drug effects and interactions. The pharmacokinetics and dynamics of anticonvulsant drugs may be altered during pregnancy as a result of lower serum protein binding, unpredictable gastrointestinal absorption related to reduced gastric motility, and variable effects on volume of distribution, total clearance, and elimination half-life.[93,102-108] As a result, the effects of gestation on the pharmacokinetic profile of an individual drug are difficult to predict. Nonetheless, maternal serum concentrations of most anticonvulsant drugs decrease during pregnancy.[109,110] Determining the blood level of anticonvulsant remains the most reliable guide to dosage regimen, particularly during the second half of pregnancy or in the postpartum period.

Anticonvulsant drugs may directly increase the mother's sensitivity to the CNS-depressant effect of anesthetic agents, while induction or inhibition of hepatic microsomal enzymes may alter anesthetic drug requirement. For example, phenobarbital, being a potent enzyme-inducing agent, may increase the clearance of systemically administered drugs such as the narcotic analgesics. On the other hand, phenytoin use may lead to hepatitis, enzyme dysfunction, and prolongation of drug effect. Furthermore, the metabolic pathways of some anesthetic drugs may be altered by anticonvulsant therapy, which thus enhances their potential for renal or hepatic toxicity. For instance, phenobarbital has been shown in humans to enhance defluorination of methoxyflurane and halothane; this results in high fluoride levels and occasionally an antidiuretic hormone (ADH)–resistant diabetes insipidus.[111-113] In laboratory animals, pretreatment with phenobarbital enhances the incidence of fatal hepatitis after halothane exposure, particularly if combined with mild hypoxia.[114] Although enzyme induction has been shown to increase the hepatotoxicity of halogenated inhalation anesthetics in animal models, human data have been less convincing.[115]

Seizure threshold. Many agents used in anesthesia may provoke seizure activity, but not in the doses and concentrations usually administered during parturition.[116] Potent halogenated agents with a high number of fluoride ions are particularly prone to induce epileptiform EEG patterns.[117,118] Perhaps best described is the "spike and wave" pattern noted with enflurane, especially when administered at high doses (2.5 vol%) or in conjunction with hypocarbia (PCO_2 less than 25 mm Hg).[116-118] The data obtained in patients with seizure disorders have been inconclusive as to whether administration of enflurane in fact increases the frequency of convulsions.[116] With the use of the low concentrations appropriate in obstetric anesthesia, there is no evidence that enflurane is contraindicated in mothers with a history of epilepsy.[116,119,120]

Some narcotic analgesics such as fentanyl have been shown to be analeptic in laboratory animals and humans, although the doses employed far exceeded those used in obstetrics.[116,121,122] Aliphatic phenothiazines such as promethazine (Phenergan) may lower the seizure threshold and, at least in untreated epileptic patients, may cause generalized convulsions.[123]

Increased cortical seizure activity or frank convulsions have occurred following induction of general anesthesia with methohexital, ketamine, and etomidate.[124,125] Propofol is a new anesthetic agent currently being evaluated for obstetric use.[126] Isolated cases of propofol causing seizure-like activity in predisposed individuals have been reported.[127-129]

Although high doses and blood concentrations of local anesthetics result in seizures, it is reassuring that at the low blood concentrations that would be expected to occur during routine obstetric anesthesia, local anesthetics have been shown to be anticonvulsant.[129,130] Further, pregnancy itself does not reduce the seizure threshold for amide local anesthetics.[131,132]

Analgesia for labor and vaginal delivery. Analgesia during labor and delivery is particularly beneficial for the epileptic mother since it will prevent or reduce hyperventilation and anxiety. As already stated, respiratory alkalosis may exacerbate seizure disorders. Administration of systemic analgesics such as meperidine or butorphanol may be adequate. One should bear in mind that mothers treated with phenobarbital may be more sensitive to the CNS-depressant effects of opioids. On the other hand, chronic exposure to phenobarbital may result in increased narcotic requirement because of induced hepatic enzyme activity.

Regional techniques are safe and effective for labor analgesia. A retrospective review of 100 epileptic women undergoing vaginal delivery ($n = 74$) or cesarean section ($n = 13$) sought to evaluate the contribution of anesthetic technique to exacerbation of the disease.[133] Nineteen patients received general anesthesia, 48 spinal anesthesia, 21 peridural, and the remaining 12 pudendal block. No seizures were noted in patients receiving peridural anesthesia. In contrast, seizures did occur in 4 of 48 mothers given spinal anesthesia (1 of them was not taking anticonvulsant medications). One mother in the general anesthesia group, exposed to enflurane, had a seizure on the third day after postpartum tubal ligation. The small number of patients in this study does not allow firm conclusions to be drawn. However, the absence of seizures in mothers given peridural anesthesia is reassuring, reinforcing the general impression that this anesthetic technique should not be denied to the parturient with epilepsy. The seizures occurring after spinal anesthesia are more difficult to interpret. The authors suggested that an alteration in CSF dynamics due to subarachnoid block may exacerbate epilepsy. The more likely explanation for the difference in the incidence of convulsions between peridural and spinal anesthesia is that the blood levels of local anesthetic achieved after peridural (and pudendal) block may be anticonvulsant.[129,130] The contribution of surgery itself to the exacerbation of epilepsy was not studied.

Post–dural-puncture headache may occur in postpartum patients having seizure disorders. In nonepileptic patients, caffeine has been used to treat headache. However, caffeine also has CNS-stimulating effects, and it has been suggested that the drug be avoided in treating epileptic patients with PDPH.[134]

Anesthesia for cesarean section. The choice of anesthesia for cesarean section should be based on the usual considerations: maternal and fetal condition, the urgency of the procedure, the wishes of the patient, and skills of the anesthesiologist. In emergency situations, general anesthesia may be necessary. Thiopental remains an excellent induction agent to be followed by a mixture of nitrous oxide (50 vol%) in oxygen and 0.5 MAC of a potent inhalational agent for maintenance. Following delivery, the depth of anesthesia may be deepened by increasing the concentration of nitrous oxide and the IV administration of a narcotic drug and benzodiazepine. If nondepolarizing muscle relaxants are also given, neuromuscular function should be carefully monitored. Patients receiving chronic phenytoin therapy may be resistant to some nondepolarizing muscle relaxants.[135,136] The response to atracurium, however, is normal[137] (Fig. 10-2). In most situations regional anesthesia can be used, and it remains an excellent anesthetic technique for mothers with epilepsy.

Patients should also be closely observed in the recovery and postpartum period, since it has been reported that most seizures occur after delivery.[133] Anticonvulsant therapy should be continued throughout the fasting period, which may necessitate parenteral administration. Plasma drug levels of anticonvulsants should be checked at frequent intervals because postpartum drug requirements may be 50% less than what it was during pregnancy. Breastfeeding is not contraindicated.[137]

Newborn care. Initial evaluation of the neonate should include careful physical examination to document congenital anomalies, the risk of which is heightened in the offspring of epileptic women.[99,133] Anticonvulsants may be teratogenic; the most common malformations being midline facial clefts (21 per 1000) and congenital heart (43 per 1000). Phenytoin use during pregnancy can cause fetal hydantoin syndrome in approximately 10% of exposed fetuses.[138] Affected babies may have microcephaly, wide fontanelles, congenital heart malformation, skeletal abnormalities, hypertelorism, low-set ears, hyperplastic phalanges, digital thumb, dislocated hip, cleft palate or lip, and growth retardation, although not all need be present for the diagnosis to be made. The etiology is unclear; however, epoxide (a phenytoin metabolite) has recently been implicated.[138] Valproic acid, associated with an increased incidence of serious neural tube defects, should be avoided during pregnancy.

Neonatal administration of vitamin K (1 mg/kg) is particularly important for prevention of a bleeding diathesis related to reduced levels of coagulation factors as a result of maternal anticonvulsant medication. Infants whose mothers received anticonvulsant medications during pregnancy should have clotting studies performed 2 hours after the initial injection of vitamin K. In the nursery, the infant should also be carefully observed for signs and symptoms of drug withdrawal.

PARAPLEGIA/QUADRIPLEGIA

In women of childbearing age, spinal cord injury is usually a result of trauma caused by a motor vehicle accident, a fall down a flight of stairs (usually in an intoxicated state), diving into shallow water, a crush injury, or less commonly from a stab or gunshot wound. Neoplasms are rare causes of paraplegia in pregnant women, but infections such

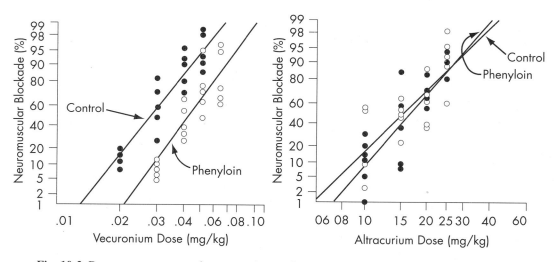

Fig. 10-2 Dose response curves for vecuronium and atracurium in patients taking chronic phenytoin therapy *(open circles)* and controls *(solid circles)*. (From Ornstein E, Matteo RS, Schwartz AE, et al: *Anesthesiology* 1987; 67:191.)

as HIV and tuberculosis may become more common. Injury to the spinal cord usually involves fracture or dislocation of the vertebrae, most frequently affected are the C1, C2, C4-C6, and T11, T12, L1, L2 vertebral levels.

Pathophysiology

The manifestations of spinal cord transection depend on the level of injury and duration of dysfunction.[139] In general, the initial phase (lasting less than 3 weeks) is characterized by flaccid paralysis, sensory anesthesia, and loss of reflex function below the level of the lesion. In the first 24 to 48 hours following a high cervical or thoracic transection there is also hemodynamic instability (spinal shock syndrome) associated with the loss of brain-stem regulatory mechanisms. The lack of cardioaccelerator innervation to the heart prevents a normal compensatory chronotropic response to fluctuations in blood volume or pressure. Pulmonary edema may also develop, presumably related to fluid overload.[140] Because of flaccid paralysis of intercostal muscles and inability to cough, respiratory complications are not infrequent. Poor respiratory reserve diminishes the paraplegic patient's ability to meet increased ventilatory demands from whatever cause, and during pregnancy, these difficulties are further compounded by upward displacement of the diaphragm (reduced functional residual capacity) and a greater dependence on "thoracic" breathing.[141]

A chronic state develops following a variable period of time, up to 3 weeks. It is characterized by continued paralysis, muscle spasticity, and disuse atrophy. These symptoms predispose the patient to the development of osteoporosis, rendering her more vulnerable to stress fractures. Other related problems such as decubitus ulcers are not infrequent. Paraplegic patients may also have impaired thermoregulation. As time progresses, renal involvement is probable because of chronic urinary tract infections and amyloidosis. Of particular concern during the chronic phase is the development of autonomic dysreflexia and the mass motor reflex.

Autonomic dysreflexia

Autonomic dysreflexia occurs most frequently with high spinal cord transection. It is estimated that up to 66% of parturients with a lesion above T6 will manifest the syndrome in response to distention of a hollow viscus such as uterus, bladder, or rectum.[142] Manifestations include malignant hypertension, bradycardia (rarely tachycardia), and diaphoresis, with cutaneous vasodilation above the level of injury and vasoconstriction below it[139] (Fig. 10-3). Severe headache and/or intracerebral hemorrhage may occur as a consequence of malignant hypertension, usually resulting in profound bradycardia.[142]

Although these may mimic preeclampsia, the incidence of preeclampsia is not increased by the presence of autonomic dysreflexia.[143] Elevations in blood pressure are a prominent feature of both diseases, but there are differences in the pattern of hypertension that may distinguish the two. Hypertension associated with autonomic hyperreflexia occurs rapidly with uterine contractions and dissipates during uterine diastole. In contrast, while additional increases in blood pressure may occur with uterine contractions in preeclamptic patients, hypertension is usually sustained and not periodic. In the postpartum period, hypertension associated with autonomic hyperreffexia resolves quickly with the loss of visceral stimulation, whereas with preeclampsia it does not resolve as readily or it may initially worsen.[142]

The effects of autonomic dysreflexia on maternal heart rate, however, are variable and determined by the height of cord lesion vis à vis the cardioaccelerator fibers. Unilateral pupillary dilation and nasal congestion may occur. The response to visceral stimulation in quadriplegic/paraplegic patients is further exaggerated by an enhanced sensitivity to catecholamines.[144,145] Fetal tachycardia may occur during autonomic dysreflexia; it is related to transplacental passage of maternal catecholamines.[146]

Mass motor reflex

The mass motor reflex is usually seen in conjunction with autonomic dysreflexia, but it may also occur independently.[147] Central input from an isolated muscle stretch receptor (spindle) normally causes contraction of a single muscle unit. In the absence of central inhibitory mechanisms, muscle contraction may extend to an entire muscle group, resulting in spasm. Unlike autonomic dysreflexia, the mass motor reflex occurs distal to the site of cord transection regardless of the level of injury.

Obstetric and anesthetic management

Obstetric anesthesia. After spinal cord injury, an initial period of amenorrhea, usually lasting for only a few months, may occur.[148] With improvements in medical care of quadriplegic/paraplegic patients, an increasing number are becoming pregnant.[149] Pregnancy rates and incidence of spontaneous abortions are not affected by spinal cord injury.[142,148] Nonetheless, during pregnancy special problems do occur in the quadriplegic/paraplegic patient that will require the close collaboration of the members of the perinatal care team.

Urinary tract infections (UTIs) are the most frequent complication related to pregnancy in these patients. Most authors recommend the administration of prophylactic antibiotics during pregnancy in spinal-cord–injured women, while others recommend against it.[150,151]

Decubitus ulcers pose significant problems particularly as the patient's weight increases during pregnancy and her ability to move is reduced. If decubiti develop, they may be a source of bacteremia and may cause a nutritional catabolic state. Further changes in hematocrit related hemodilution during pregnancy may predispose to decubiti. During labor and delivery, it is essential that appropriate skin care be taken using frequent changes in position and padding.[152]

Spasticity, particularly of the lower extremities, may prove problematic during labor and vaginal delivery. Continuous intrathecal infusion of baclofen (an antispasmodic agent) has been used in pregnant women to treat severe spasticity.[152] However, baclofen will not prevent autonomic dysreflexia.

It is controversial whether there is an increased risk of preterm labor and delivery occurring in spinal-cord–injured women.[150] However, because patients may not detect uterine activity, it has been suggested that cervical examinations begin at approximately 26 weeks' gestation. Furthermore, the patient herself may be educated to assess the occurrence of increased uterine activity by palpation and to recognize increased vaginal discharge as a potential sign of preterm labor. With technological developments, home uterine activity monitoring would seem to be an excellent modality for surveillance.[153] Labor and assisted vaginal delivery should be attainable in most cases. Cesarean section is reserved only for obstetric indications.

Analgesia for labor and vaginal delivery. Careful evaluation before anesthesia is mandatory. It should include documentation of sensory and motor deficits, as well as an assessment of renal and pulmonary reserve, if time permits. Prophylactic measures such as incentive spirometry and chest physical therapy may be required.

Spinal cord transection does not prevent labor, which is often painless, particularly if the level of injury is T10 or higher. Many paraplegic women are hospitalized before term to prevent delivery at home.[142,150,154,155] However, with the introduction of home uterine activity monitoring, more patients may remain at home until closer to term.[153] An assisted vaginal delivery is usually recommended.[150]

A major goal of management during parturition is the prevention of autonomic dysreflexia, or the mass motor reflex. Many agents have been used to treat autonomic dysreflexia, including nitroprusside, diazoxide, and hydralazine.[139]

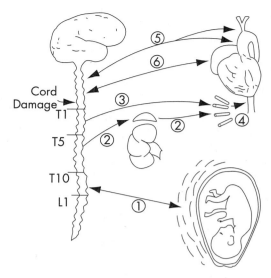

Fig. 10-3 Mechanism of cardiovascular changes in autonomic hyperreflexia. *1,* Afferent impulses from contracting uterus to spinal cord segments T10-L1. *2,* Efferent impulses from segments T5 to T9 to adrenal medulla causing discharge of catecholamines. *3,* Efferent impulses from sympathetic centers T1-L1 directly to vascular bed causing vasoconstriction. *4,* Increase in arterial blood pressure as a result of stimuli by 2 and 3. *5,* Afferent impulses from carotid sinus and aortic arch to cardiac centers in medulla oblongata. *6,* Efferent impulses through vagus nerve to heart causing bradycardia. (From Abouleish EI, Hanley ES, Palmer SM: *Anesth Analg* 1989; 68:523.)

Epidural or spinal anesthesia is particularly advantageous since it will prevent the reflex from occurring by interrupting noxious sensory input from the viscera, particularly the uterus[156,157] (Fig. 10-3). Epidural analgesia with intermittent injections of 0.25% to 0.5% bupivacaine has been used successfully for that purpose.[158,159] A single-injection subarachnoid block could be equally effective, but to overcome the unpredictability of anesthetic spread and limited duration of action, the use of a continuous subarachnoid catheter technique is preferable.

The dose of local anesthetic should be fractionated to prevent untoward systemic reactions or excessive rostral spread of anesthesia. Accidental intrathecal injection of local anesthetic may not be evident in these patients until respiratory embarrassment or total spinal anesthesia occurs. Transient hypotension can be prevented with adequate prehydration and uterine displacement. Ephedrine (5 to 10 mg IV) has been safely used in paraplegic patients to correct hypotension.[160] However, at least in theory, a potentially exaggerated response may occur.[144,145]

Varying success with the use of epidural opioids has been described.[161,162] Of potential benefit is the sparing of resting sympathetic tone that may already be impaired following cord transection.[160] One report pertains to a parturient with a bullet injury at T6.[161] Although uterine contractions were painless, they were accompanied by manifestations of autonomic dysreflexia. Epidural injection of preservative-free meperidine, 100 mg in 10 mL diluent, abolished all manifestations of dysreflexia. However, another group was not as successful with epidural injection of fentanyl alone.[162] During amniotomy, the patient sustained increases in blood pressure up to 225/135 mm Hg, accompanied by bradycardia. Fentanyl was discontinued, and an epidural injection of 0.25% bupivacaine (15 mL) terminated these untoward responses. This was followed by continuous epidural infusion of 0.125% bupivacaine (15 mL/hr), and no further cardiovascular instability was noted. The same authors suggested that a predominantly mu-receptor-selective narcotic, such as fentanyl, may not be effective in blocking nociceptive impulses that initiate autonomic dysreflexia. The success of meperidine may in part be due to its local anesthetic properties. Although not yet investigated, a predominantly kappa-agonist such as nalbuphine may be more effective than fentanyl.[162,163] Combinations of low concentrations of local anesthetic agents and narcotic drugs for epidural analgesia may prove most useful in preventing dysreflexia while preserving sympathetic tone.[164]

Epidural analgesia is also effective in preventing the mass motor reflex, but care must be taken in positioning or handling the patient in order to avoid undue stimulation.

Anesthesia for cesarean section. For abdominal delivery, regional anesthesia is a logical choice. If, however, general endotracheal anesthesia is deemed necessary, the use of depolarizing muscle relaxants is contraindicated over a period beginning 24 hours following cord injury, and extending for up to 1 year.[165,166] This is due to the risk of severe hyperkalemia and cardiac arrest, not preventable by pretreatment with nondepolarizing muscle relaxants. After that time period, hyperkalemia may occur, depending on the degree of muscle disuse and atrophy. Considering the alternatives available, it would seem prudent to avoid the use of succinylcholine altogether in paraplegic patients. General anesthesia with halothane has been used to suppress autonomic dysreflexia.[167] However, fairly deep levels of anesthesia were required, and in parturients this may lead to uterine atony and profuse bleeding. Arrhythmias have been reported in paraplegic patients receiving halo-

thane.[167] These may be related to the occurrence of hypercarbia during spontaneous ventilation, since arrhythmias were not a problem when ventilation was controlled.[160] Neonatal outcome is generally good in mothers with quadriplegia or paraplegia. In the postpartum period, thrombophlebitis has been reported and prophylactic therapy is recommended.[155] Special attention should be given to the prevention of pulmonary or urinary tract infections, anemia, and decubitus ulcers. As mentioned earlier, all three are related and quite common in patients with spinal injuries having impaired bladder or bowel function.

MULTIPLE SCLEROSIS
Incidence and pathophysiology

Multiple sclerosis (MS) is a chronic demyelinating disease that predominantly affects young adults. The disease afflicts females more frequently than males (3:2 ratio) and thus is not an uncommon neurologic disorder in women of childbearing age. The disease is characterized by the presence of plaques of inflammatory demyelination scattered throughout the white matter of the CNS, including the spinal cord. The cause is unclear, but it may be related to an immunologic response to viral infection.[168] Environmental, genetic, and geographic factors may also predispose individuals to the disease.[168] Symptoms include muscle weakness, ataxia, spasticity, diplopia, sphincter dysfunction, mental disturbance, and dysesthesia. In severe cases, paraplegia may also develop (Table 10-2).[169]

Diagnosis of MS may be difficult because symptoms are shared with other diseases such as systemic lupus erythematosus, sarcoidosis, Lyme disease, and neurosyphilis.[168,169] Multiple diagnostic criteria have been proposed to establish a clinical diagnosis of MS, since no one laboratory test can be considered diagnostic.[170] Common to all criteria is the presence of neurologic deficits, referable to white matter lesions, in more than one area of the CNS, and the occurrence of clinical deficits separated in time as well as in locale. Thus, MS is not a monophasic illness. The overall course of the disease may result in a gradual progression of deficits, but this is usually punctuated by periods of relapses and remissions, particularly in the early phases.

In addition to clinical manifestations, laboratory data also aid in establishing the diagnosis of MS. Cerebrospinal fluid abnormalities may include mononuclear pleocytosis, elevated immunoglobulin G, oligoclonal bands, and elevated myelin basic protein. Central conduction time of visual, auditory, and somatosensory evoked potentials may be prolonged because of demyelination.[171] Mag-

Table 10-2 Frequencies of signs and symptoms of multiple sclerosis from 157 autopsies

Symptoms	%	Signs	%
Muscle weakness	96	Spasticity and/or hyperreflexia	89
Ocular disturbance	85	Babinski sign	92
Urinary disturbance	82	Absent abdominal reflex	82
Gait ataxia	60	Dysmetria	79
Paresthesias	60	Nystagmus	71
Dysarthria	54	Impairment of vibratory sensation	61
Mental disturbance	47	Impairment of position sensation	52
Pain	19	Impairment of pain sensation	44
Vertigo	17	Facial weakness	42
Dysphagia	12	Impairment of touch sensation	29
Convulsions	6	Impairment of temperature sensation	17
Decreased hearing	6	Changes in state of consciousness	5
Tinnitus	5		

Adapted from Davis RK, Maslow A: *Obstet Gynecol Surv* 1992; 47:290.

netic resonance imaging is most useful in establishing the presence of white matter plaques.[172]

The most common neurologic deficits, such as gait difficulties, ataxia, and spastic paraparesis, are refereable to demyelination in the white matter of the spinal cord.[173] In addition, bladder control is often affected; this leads to increased urinary frequency and urgency as a result of detrusor-sphincter dyssynergia. With progression, bladder atony occur. This is best managed by intermittent catherization to avoid chronic high residual urinary volumes, which would increase the risk of urinary tract infections (UTIs). Subjective and objective sensory abnormalities may affect the limbs or trunk. Perineal and vaginal sensation may likewise be affected.

Demyelination of the brain stem may give rise to a number of symptoms. Diplopia is common as involvement extends to the medial longitudinal fasciculus. Other areas of demyelination in the brain stem and the neighboring cerebellum may result in dysequilibrium or true vertigo, truncal and appendicular ataxia, facial weakness and alteration in facial sensation, and disturbances of speech. Even a loss of the automaticity of breathing as a result of involvement of the medulla has been reported.[174]

Multiple sclerosis plaques in the subcortical white matter may be symptomatic, depending on their exact location. Often MRI scans reveal numerous subcortical and periventricular plaques that are clinically silent. However, contralateral motor and sensory symptoms may be observed when plaques involve the descending pyramidal tract or ascending thalamocortical radiations, respectively.

The optic nerve is another common site of involvement. It is the only cranial nerve affected because it is an extension of the CNS rather than a peripheral nerve. In many areas, optic neuritis may be the only initial manifestation of MS. Symptoms of optic neuritis include a sudden loss of central (central scotoma) and/or color vision.[175]

Exacerbations may be provoked by stress and a rise in core body temperature. Infection by itself, whether viral or bacterial, may be an exacerbating factor, even in the absence of fever. Thus, an evaluation for possible urinary tract infection should be among the first steps in the search for a cause of new clinical deterioration.

Medical therapy for specific neurologic dysfunction includes the use of baclofen or dantrolene in the treatment of painful flexor or extensor spasms of the lower extremities. Medications with anticholinergic effects, such as imipramine, are useful in treating urinary retention. Full urodynamic evaluation is helpful in assessing the extent of bladder dysfunction and its response to treatment.[176] The excessive fatigue experienced by some patients with MS may be alleviated by amantadine.[177]

Immunosuppressive therapy has also been used in an attempt to halt the progression of the disease.[178] Medications used for this purpose include ACTH and glucocorticoids, but these are generally reserved for patients experiencing severe exacerbations or rapid progressive clinical deterioration. The efficacy of immunosuppression in reversing the overall course of the illness has not been firmly established. Azathioprine and high-dose IV cyclophosphamide have also been used.[179] The use of nonpharmacologic immunosuppression by means of total lymphoid irradiation has also been reported.[180]

Prevention of urinary tract infections is important, particularly in patients with a history of recurrent urinary tract infections or an overdistended bladder.

Obstetric and anesthetic management

Obstetric management. Multiple sclerosis does not affect fertility or increase the incidence of spontaneous abortions. In general, MS does not adversely affect the course of pregnancy or obstetric outcome.[181,182] The potential for abnormal cardiovascular (autonomic dysreflexia) responses to occur during labor in a paraplegic patient has already been described and should also be considered in parturients with severe MS. Urinary tract infections are fairly common during pregnancy but may occur even more frequently with MS related to abnormal control of micturition. Antibiotic prophylaxis is recommended in patients having frequent and severe UTIs.

Magnesium sulfate or β-sympathomimetics may be used, if required, for the usual obstetric indications. Patients who have been treated with steroids should have replacement therapy during anticipated periods of stress such as labor. Cesarean section should be performed for obstetric indications only; however, operative or assisted vaginal delivery may be required because of maternal exhaustion during the second stage. There are no contraindications for MS patients to breastfeed, unless a treatment used during a postpartum relapse could potentially affect the baby via ingested breast milk.[182]

The frequency of MS relapses during pregnancy is similar to that in the nonpregnant population.[183,184] In one retrospective study, the risk of relapse decreased by 50% during pregnancy.[185] On the other hand, two prospective studies have demonstrated a significant (30% to 50%) increase in relapse rates during the first 3 months following delivery or elective termination of pregnancy.[185,186] The increased rate of relapse during these time periods has been attributed to maternal stress and fatigue.[182,187,188]

Surgery and anesthesia are generally well tolerated.[189] In severe cases, the extent of respiratory impairment should be evaluated if possible. Some peripartum factors, such as infection, stress, and hyperpyrexia, may exacerbate MS.[187,188,190,191]

Analgesia for labor and vaginal delivery. Most methods of analgesia may be beneficial in reducing stress. Epidural analgesia has been applied successfully[192,193] and may be particularly helpful in relieving abdominal and pelvic spasticity that may interfere with spontaneous delivery.[181] Nonetheless, controversy exists concerning the effects of epidural analgesia on the relapse rate in patients with MS. A retrospective review of 24 women with MS who were delivered vaginally under epidural (*n* = 9), local (*n* = 13), or general anesthesia (*n* = 2) detected no difference in the relapse rate among the three groups.[193] Although the number of patients was small, it is reassuring that the use of epidural blockade had no adverse effects on the course of the disease. Of interest is that the four women in the epidural group who experienced a relapse were given higher concentrations of bupivacaine 0.5% or lidocaine 2%. In contrast, no patient receiving a lower concentration of bupivacaine (0.25%) experienced exacerbation. The authors have suggested that relapses after prolonged epidural analgesia or after exposure to high local anesthetic dosage or concentrations are related to greater CSF levels of drug. Thus, only the lowest effective concentration and volume of local anesthetic should be given. The addition of a narcotic drug such as fentanyl or sufentanil make it possible to reduce the epidural local anesthetic requirement even further without affecting the quality of pain relief.[164,194] Experience with the use of neuroaxial opioids in patients with MS is limited, but no untoward short-term effects have been noted.[195,196]

Anesthesia for cesarean section. Bader et al also suggested that epidural anesthesia used for cesarean section in patients with MS does not aggravate the disease.[193] One of five patients studied had a relapse, although this may have been related to prolonged local anesthetic exposure because she received epidural analgesia for labor before the cesarean section.

More difficult to interpret are reports of relapses following subarachnoid block.[197,198] Spinal puncture itself does not affect the relapse rate,[199] but the potential effect of local anesthetic cannot be ruled out.[197,198] Drug concentrations in CSF have been estimated to be threefold to fourfold higher following subarachnoid block, compared with epidural administration.[200,201] It has been proposed that in individuals with MS, local anesthetic agents produce reversible inflammatory and degenerative neuronal changes.[202] Although some have suggested avoiding the use of 2-chloroprocaine in affected patients, there is no evidence indicating that the choice of local anesthetic affects the relapse rate.[193]

More important, the high sensory levels required for adequate analgesia during cesarean section may affect respiratory function by paralyzing the intercostal muscles.[203,204] For this reason, general anesthesia may be required in a small number of patients with MS who do not tolerate regional anesthesia.

General anesthesia itself does not exacerbate the course of MS.[193,198] As with other neurologic conditions, succinylcholine should be avoided in patients having severe musculoskeletal involvement because of the fear of possibly triggering massive potassium release from muscle tissue. However, in a state of remission, and with no other complications, succinylcholine may be used.[205] In all cases, particular attention must be directed to the prevention of pulmonary complications and the maintenance of normal body temperature. Pyrexia is of specific concern in MS patients for its damaging effects on neural tissue at sites of demyelination.[196]

MOTOR NEURON DISEASE
Incidence and pathophysiology

Motor neuron disease is a term applied to a group of related illnesses characterized by degeneration of motor neurons. As a rule, motor neuron disease is progressive, disabling, and ultimately fatal. Upper motor neurons with cell bodies in the cerebral cortex and axons extending into the brain stem or spinal cord, as well as the lower motor neurons of cranial nerve motor nuclei or anterior horn cells of the spinal cord, may be affected. Usually there is involvement of both as in amyotropic lateral sclerosis (ALS). But occasionally only the anterior horn cells of the spinal cord are affected, as in progressive muscular atrophy. Brain-stem motor involvement alone leads to progressive bulbar palsy. Upper motor neuron dysfunction is rarely present without degeneration of lower motor neurons, as with primary lateral sclerosis.

The combination of upper and lower motor neuron degeneration gives rise to paradoxical manifestations of progressive weakness and atrophy in the presence of preserved or even heightened deep tendon reflexes.

Patients may also be symptomatic as a result of brain-stem motor dysfunction. Progressive hoarseness and dysphagia are often present and may progress to total absence of phonation, drooling, and inability to swallow. Quadriplegia and progressive respiratory insufficiency may also ensue with spinal cord motor dysfunction. Placement of a feeding gastrostomy and/or artificial ventilation via endotracheal intubation or tracheostomy may be necessary.

Muscle cramps and spasms may respond to diphenhydramine. Emotional lability, often a feature of patients with progressive bulbar (brain stem) symptoms, may be ameliorated with low-dose amitryptiline or lithium. An indwelling urinary catheter may be required for optimal management of the bedridden patient. As the disease progresses, respiratory insufficiency and failure become manifest. A significant number of patients also have disorders of calcium homeostasis, which may result in resting tachycardia.[206] Severe forms of spinocerebellar degeneration have been associated with right ventricular hypertrophy, myocarditis, EEG changes, and even sudden death.[206]

Both poliomyelitis and amyotropic lateral sclerosis (ALS) are disorders that affect the anterior horn cells. Massive immunization programs have virtually eradicated poliomyelitis in the United States. ALS is relatively rare and usually has its onset in middle age.

Obstetric and anesthetic management

Obstetric management. Information regarding the effects of motor neuron disease on pregnancy is limited.[207,208] Generally speaking, pregnancy does not appear to be adversely affected by this group of disease.[207,209] Successful vaginal delivery has been reported, although the need for assisted delivery was noted.[207,210] In one series, pregnancy worsened motor and pulmonary dysfunction presumably related to mechanical effects of an enlarging uterus.[209] Bulbar involvement is common and, in conjunction with the physiologic changes of pregnancy, may further heighten the risk of aspiration. Successful pregnancy has also been reported with Werdnig-Hoffmann disease (spinal muscular atrophy), characterized by progressive anterior horn cell degeneration.[211] Unlike patients with spinal cord injury, pain pathways are intact but autonomic dysreflexia does not occur. Most have required cesarean section due to bony deformities of the pelvis.[211]

Anesthetic considerations. Data regarding anesthetic management of the pregnant patient with ALS are scant. However, two general concerns predominate. First, in mothers manifesting worsening bulbar dysfunction, the prevention of aspiration is of prime importance. The use of an H_2-antagonist and metoclopramide may be beneficial. Second, in more severely affected patients, pulmonary function and reserve may be very limited, to the point of requiring artificial ventilation. This should be taken into consideration when formulating an anesthetic plan.

Thiopental has been used for induction of general anesthesia.[190] Most anesthesiologists would agree that depolarizing muscle relaxants should be avoided and that there may be hypersensitivity to nondepolarizing muscle relaxants.[212] Anesthesia can be maintained with nitrous oxide and a potent inhalational agent. Higher concentrations of the latter may be useful in controlling spasticity, but in the parturient this may result in uterine atony and bleeding.

The effects of epidural or spinal anesthesia on the course of ALS are unknown. Nonetheless, in mildly affected laboring women, epidural analgesia may be preferable to systemic or inhalational analgesia in that it will provide better pain relief without depressing ventilation or airway reflexes. Epidural administration of local anesthetic in low concentrations combined with a narcotic drug may better preserve muscle function. Regardless of the choice of anesthesia, parturients with severe ALS should be carefully observed, particularly for respiratory compromise, in the postpartum period as well.

HEREDITARY MOTOR AND SENSORY NEUROPATHY
Pathophysiology

Charcot-Marie-Tooth (CMT) disease, the most common of these rare hereditary conditions, is characterized by distal muscular atrophy and sensory neuropathy of the lower extremities, extending in later life to the upper extremities.[213] The condition is attributed to slowly progressive degeneration of the peripheral nerves and roots. The disease is inherited as an autosomal dominant,[214] and two variants have been described. Type 1 is characterized by early onset (10 to 20 years of age) of foot drop, lower extremity muscle wasting (particularly of the peroneal and anterior tibialis muscles), decreased tendon reflexes and nerve conduction velocities, as well as sensory deficits in a "stocking-glove" distribution. Type II manifests itself in a similar manner but it begins in adulthood and has a slower course. In either type, foot deformities (high pedal arches) may be the only manifestation. Abnormalities in nerve conduction shown by studies performed on the patient and family members often aid in establishing a diagnosis.

Obstetric and anesthetic management

Obstetric management. Obstetric complications do not occur with greater frequency in patients with CMT disease. However, pregnancy may exacerbate the symptoms of CMT in up to half of patients with Type I disease, presumably because of endoneural edema,[214,215] whereas gestation has little effect on Type II CMT.[216]

Fortunately, recovery is usually complete following delivery, but exacerbation of the disease may be more severe with subsequent pregnancies. Although predominantly a disease of the extremities, it may involve intercostal muscles as well, and respiratory insufficiency has been reported to occur during pregnancy, particularly from the effects of an enlarging uterus.[215,216] Abnormalities of the cardiac conduction system may also be present. Creatine phosphokinase may be elevated, although there is no known association with malignant hyperthermia.[217]

Anesthetic considerations. Anesthetic management during labor and vaginal delivery should be based on the extent of the disease process. The use of regional anesthesia may be beneficial because it will reduce energy demands during labor. There

are only two case reports pertaining to obstetric anesthesia for patients with CMT disease.[216,218] Both parturients were given general endotracheal anesthesia for cesarean section because of poor respiratory reserve and severe progressive neurologic dysfunction. Unfortunately, the details of anesthetic management were described in only one of the cases.[216] Succinylcholine was avoided for fear of an exaggerated hyperkalemic response.[219] Scant evidence suggests that CMT disease does not alter the response to nondepolarizing muscle relaxants.[216,220] In severe cases, ventilatory support may have to be maintained in the postoperative period as well. In milder cases, regional anesthesia would be a suitable alternative to general anesthesia for cesarean section. Patients with longstanding neuropathies may have scoliosis, which may render regional techniques challenging.[218]

LANDRY-GUILLAIN-BARRÉ-STROHL SYNDROME
Incidence and pathophysiology

Landry-Guillain-Barré-Strohl (LGBS) syndrome (also known as acute idiopathic polyneuritis) is a disease of unknown cause. It is rare, occurring in 1 out of 250,000 women.[221] The syndrome is characterized by acute inflammatory polyradiculoneuropathy (inflammation of peripheral nerves and roots), and in two thirds of patients it is preceded by viral gastroenteritis, respiratory infection, vaccination, surgery, or malignancy.[222-225] It has been speculated that pregnancy may trigger the syndrome; however, this seems unlikely because the incidence of the disease is similar in pregnant and nonpregnant women.[226] Pathologic hallmarks include patchy demyelination of peripheral nerves and roots together with a variable inflammatory cell infiltrate.

Guillain-Barré syndrome usually presents with flaccid paralysis, which begins in the lower extremities and ascends to the upper extremities. This may be preceded by paresthesias and occasionally by painful dysesthesias of both extremities. Cranial nerves, with the exception of optic and auditory nerves, may also be involved.[225] Severe cases may require ventilatory support because the innervation of intercostal and accessory muscles of respiration and diaphragm may be affected. These manifestations typically progress to a maximum over 4 weeks, and recovery usually occurs within 6 months.[225] Abnormal nerve conduction, or in severe cases, complete block of motor conduction, may be present. There is typically an elevation of CSF protein concentration, but the cell count is normal. As with ALS, the increased risk of aspiration pneumonitis and respiratory failure is of greatest concern. In addition, there may be vasomotor instability resulting from chromatolysis of the cells belonging to the thoracolumbar autonomic nervous system.[227] Differential diagnoses include vitamin B_{12} deficiency, lead, arsenic or insecticide poisoning, and acute intermittent porphyria.

Obstetric and anesthetic management

Obstetric management. It has been suggested that pregnancy does not exacerbate the disease and that the offspring are unaffected.[228] However, there are three case reports that identified aspiration pneumonitis and/or respiratory failure as primary causes of mortality among women who contracted a severe form of the disease in the third trimester of pregnancy.[229-231] More recently, mortality in nonpregnant patients is estimated to be 3% to 4%, but it may be twice that during pregnancy.[232] Termination of pregnancy has little effect on the course of the disease.[232]

Treatment of LGBS syndrome is supportive, and nutritional status should be maintained. As with other neuromuscular diseases, respiratory compromise, measured by forced vital capacity and forced expiratory volume, provides a much more reliable assessment of respiratory function than do arterial blood gas measurements. The latter may often show little abnormality until the patient finally tires as a result of profound respiratory muscle weakness. Blood pressure lability due to autonomic dysfunction may also require intervention.

Plasmapheresis, when used early in the course of severe LGBS syndrome, may decrease the severity and length of illness. Steroids, however, are not as useful.

The prognosis is excellent, with 80% of pregnant patients having complete or near complete recovery. Neonatal outcome is also good, with a fetal survival rate of approximately 95%.[232] Vaginal delivery is preferable, although assisted delivery may be necessary during the second stage. Induction of labor should be performed only for obstetric indications. If mechanical ventilation is required, aortocaval compression and hyperventilation should be avoided to preserve placental perfusion.

Anesthetic considerations. Anesthetic considerations are similar to those for ALS. In mildly affected parturients, epidural analgesia appears to be suitable, and it would avoid the need for systemic analgesics. The notion that analgesia for all LGBS syndrome parturients be limited to psychoprophylaxis and local infiltration or pudendal block is no longer tenable.[233] Epidural anesthesia has been used in patients with LGBS syndrome without long-term effects.[1,234] No information was provided regarding the choice of drugs in one report[1]; bupivacaine was used in the other.[234]

Steiner et al attempted to implicate the use of epidural anesthesia in the development of LGBS in four patients.[235] However, the authors failed to exclude other, more likely triggering factors. On the other hand, Gautier reported a case in which a parturient developed LGBS syndrome 24 hours after delivery performed under epidural anesthesia. The authors suggested there was no relationship between conduction block and LGBS syndrome in light of the extremely short time interval between the administration of epidural anesthesia and the onset of LGBS.[236] Currently, there is no evidence that regional anesthesia should be withheld in patients with active LGBS syndrome or a history of the disease. In patients with impairment beyond T10, uterine contractions may be painless.[234]

Epidural anesthesia has been used for cesarean delivery in a patient with LGBS syndrome.[234] A reduced dose of local anesthetic may be required.[234] The patient did not require ventilatory support and recovered completely from LGBS syndrome within 3 to 4 months.

General endotracheal anesthesia is preferred for cesarean delivery in patients with bulbar dysfunction and respiratory insufficiency. Some have suggested that induction with ketamine may be preferable to a thiobarbiturate in view of vascular instability often observed in these patients.[190] The already described concerns regarding the administration of depolarizing and nondepolarizing muscle relaxants to individuals with advanced neuromuscular disease apply to LGBS syndrome patients as well. Indeed, there is one reported case of succinylcholine-induced hyperkalemia in a patient recovering from LGBS syndrome having an emergency cesarean section.[237]

FAMILIAL DYSAUTONOMIA
Incidence and pathophysiology

Familial dysautonomia (Riley-Day syndrome) is a rare, autosomal recessive, inherited disorder of the peripheral and autonomic nervous systems found largely in the Ashkenazi Jewish population.[238] The affected individuals have a reduced number of cells in the autonomic ganglia as well as fewer nerve fibers.[239] Catecholamine depletion may also occur.[240] Although prognosis is generally poor, substantial numbers of patients have been reaching adulthood as medical care has improved.[241] The effects of pregnancy on the course of the disease are unclear.[242]

The syndrome is associated with dysphagia, vomiting, intravascular volume depletion, pre–renal azotemia, extreme cardiovascular instability, pneumonia secondary to aspiration, localized sensory anesthesia, and impaired thermoregulation. Peripheral pain perception may be diminished, but visceral and peritoneal pain pathways remain intact. During periods of exacerbations (dysautonomic crisis) frequently triggered by stress, intractable vomiting, tachycardia, hypertension, flushing, and diaphoresis may occur.

Anesthetic considerations. Vomiting and aspiration pneumonitis are major concerns in these patients. Administration of H_2-antagonists and/or metoclopramide may prove beneficial. Pronounced cardiovascular instability may result from diminished autonomic function, baroreceptor insensitivity, decreased intravascular volume, and decreased norepinephrine synthesis.[243,244] The response to indirect-acting amines is unpredictable, whereas there is enhanced sensitivity to direct-acting agents.[245] Thus invasive monitoring of blood pressure may be useful. Careful IV hydration has been shown to reduce hemodynamic instability during anesthesia.[245] The extent of pulmonary impairment should be carefully assessed. Aspiration pneumonitis is common and can result in bronchiectasis.[246] The incidence of pulmonary complications is greatest during the postoperative period,[245] and many patients require postoperative ventilation.[245,247]

During parturition, despite areas of sensory anesthesia it is particularly important to provide adequate pain relief and to allay the patient's apprehension in order to prevent the occurrence of dysautonomic crisis. During dysautonomic crisis, high serum dopamine levels may occur[243]; diazepam has been used to treat dysautonomic crisis because it suppresses dopamine release.[245]

Administration of systemic analgesics to patients with familial dysautonomia is inadvisable in view of their predisposition to aspiration as well as their blunted compensatory responses to hypoxemia and hypercarbia.[246,248,249]

On the other hand, conventional spinal or epidural analgesia with the use of local anesthetics may cause hypotension due to uncorrected vascular volume, depletion of catecholamines, and deranged sympathetic tone.[240] In contrast, intrathecal and epidural injection of opioids such as morphine or fentanyl will provide adequate analgesia for the first stage of labor with less potential for blood pressure lability.[250,251] Since the duration of analgesia with neuroaxial opioids is limited, epidural or combined spinal-epidural technique will provide the ability to reinject without additional dural punctures. The potential for delayed respiratory depression reported with the use of morphine necessitates careful surveillance for up to 24 hours after drug administration. A pudendal or a true saddle block will be necessary for anesthesia during the second stage of labor and delivery.

For cesarean section, many anesthesiologists prefer general anesthesia in patients with familial dysautonomia. Thiopental has been used for induction, but only after intravascular volume replacement, which may also decrease the requirement for vasopressors.[245] The response to neuromuscular blockers is normal, and succinylcholine has been used without hyperkalemia or prolonged effect.[252] Patients with familial dysautonomia syndrome are exquisitely sensitive to the effects of anesthetic agents.[245] Nitrous oxide and 0.5 to 1.0 MAC of a potent inhalational agent may be used for maintenance. Fentanyl has been used for induction and as an adjuvant during surgical anesthesia in nonpregnant individuals.[247] In addition, many patients will benefit from controlled ventilation in the postoperative period.[245,247] Cesarean section under a field block using 1% lidocaine has also been reported.[238] However, uterine manipulation was noted to be painful. Local anesthetic toxicity is also of major concern and only a few obstetricians are trained in this technique.

NEUROECTODERMAL DISEASE
Pathophysiology

Neurofibromatosis and von Hippel-Lindau disease (VHLD) are known as the "phakomatoses." Tuberous sclerosis and Sturge-Weber disease are also included in this classification. Unfortunately, very little information is available. Several common features are present: skin or mucous membrane patches (phakes), undifferentiated embryonic cell tumors, localized hyperplastic structures, and congenital malformations.[253]

Neurofibromatosis

Neurofibromatosis (von Recklinghausen's disease) results from an overgrowth of the Schwann cells and fibroblasts of peripheral nerves originating from the neural crest. Since these are ubiquitous, there is the potential for involvement of numerous organs. Fortunately, the disease is most commonly limited to the skin, resulting in visible neurofibromas and café-au-lait spots. In rare cases, the condition is associated with a syndrome of multiple endocrine disorders, including hyperthyroidism and pheochromocytoma.[254-256] Pheochromocytoma should be suspected in patients manifesting neurofibromatosis and hypertension; it may be further aggravated by intimal fibrosis and renal artery stenosis.[257]

Obstetric and anesthetic management

Obstetric management. Pregnancy results in rapid growth of neurofibromas, occasionally leading to hemorrhage or sarcomatous degeneration.[255] Symptoms typically abate following delivery. The association between the disease and pregnancy-induced hypertension is unlikely in view of the already mentioned vascular changes noted in patients with neurofibromatosis.[255] Of greatest concern is the risk of developing intracranial hypertension as a result of rapid expansion of intracranial lesions. Steroids and diuretics may be useful, but surgical intervention is rarely required and ICP returns to normal in the postpartum period.

Anesthetic considerations. Systemic or regional analgesia is suitable for labor and vaginal delivery. Selection of a specific technique should be based on the disease process itself, as well as on the associated conditions. Careful attention to the size and location of neurofibromas is advisable. If they occur in the larynx or oropharynx, airway management may be difficult.[258] On the other hand, lesions along the spine may result in kyphoscoliosis and may cause technical difficulties in establishing epidural or spinal anesthesia. Cutaneous lesions at the site of needle puncture may create further difficulties.

The indication for cesarean section will, in most cases, influence anesthetic management. For instance, if the operation is necessitated by cephalopelvic disproportion due to pelvic neurofibromas, the choice of anesthesia is governed by the usual considerations for maternal and fetal welfare. On the other hand, as was discussed earlier, management may be more complex if abdominal delivery is indicated for more serious complications such as increased ICP.

In all patients, careful examination of the upper airway is recommended to rule out encroachment of the disease on the larynx. It has been shown that neurofibromatosis may result in an altered response to muscle relaxants, perhaps because of denervation sensitivity of the motor end-plate. There is increased or decreased sensitivity to succinylcholine, and increased sensitivity to nondepolarizing agents.[258-261] Regional anesthesia, if technically feasible, may circumvent some of the problems with general anesthesia. Complications due to associated pheochromocytoma may occur.[262]

von Hippel-Lindau disease

Pathophysiology. VHLD, also a neuroectodermal disorder, occurs in young women. It is inherited as an autosomal dominant with variable penetrance[263] and is manifested by angioblastic lesions, most often affecting the retina, but occasionally the cerebellum and spinal cord. The disease may be also associated with pheochromocytoma, cystic disease of the kidney or pancreas, or polycythemia related to hypernephroma.[263-265] Neurologic manifestations, which include dyses-

thesias and ataxia, are referable to the site(s) of lesion.

Anesthetic considerations. Limited information is available regarding the anesthetic management of VHLD. The possible presence of CNS hemangioblastomas, particularly involving the spinal cord, may create a potential risk during regional anesthesia. However, epidural anesthesia has been used in one patient with VHLD for cesarean delivery without untoward effects.[265] The risk of malignant hypertension with pheochromocytoma can be potentially life-threatening. A recent report described the anesthetic management for a combined cesarean section and pheochromocytoma resection in a patient with VHLD.[266] General anesthesia, with thiopental (4 mg/kg), lidocaine (1 mg/kg), and succinylcholine (1.5 mg/kg), was used to facilitate intubation, and N_2O (50%) and isoflurane (0.5%) were used for maintenance until delivery of the infant. Hemodynamic changes were managed with esmolol, labetalol, and nitroprusside as needed. After delivery, sufentanil, midazolam, and vecuronium were used as adjuvants to decrease the use of inhalational agents and the risk of uterine atony.

MUSCULAR DYSTROPHY
Pathophysiology

Muscular dystrophy is an inherited condition that may affect young adults. Variable muscle fiber size as well as increased amounts of fibrous connective tissue separating muscle fibers are pathologic hallmarks.[267] In severe cases, patients develop profound muscle weakness, particularly of proximal muscles, ultimately resulting in contractures and bone deformities. Muscle atrophy may also be present. Chronic aspiration and recurrent pneumonitis may occur as a result of bulbar muscle dysfunction. The myocardium may also be affected, leading to atrial tachyarrhythmias and cardiomyopathy. In advanced stages, involvement of intercostal and accessory muscles of respiration may reduce respiratory reserve and cause insufficiency, particularly during periods of stress such as labor.

Several types of muscular dystrophy have been described according to the age at onset and the grouping of affected muscles. Duchenne muscular dystrophy is the most common and perhaps the best described. It is rarely symptomatic in female patients since it is an X-linked recessive disorder and thus will not be discussed here. Fascioscapulohumeral (FSH) and limb-girdle (LG) dystrophies are the most common muscular dystrophies affecting women. Nemaline myopathy is a rare and slowly progressive muscular dystrophy.[268] These are hereditary disorders; FSH dystrophy and nemaline myopathy are transmitted as an autosomal dominant, whereas LG dystrophy may be inherited as either an autosomal dominant or recessive.

Facial weakness is a prominent feature of FSH dystrophy, but the extraocular muscles are generally spared. The patient's face may appear somewhat drawn and expressionless. Weakness of the orbicularis oris muscles results in difficulty in whistling or drinking through a straw. Wasting and atrophy of neck and shoulder muscles causes "winging" of the scapulae. Weakness in abduction of arms may actually be one of the first symptoms noted.[269] Other proximal upper extremity muscles, with the exception of the deltoid, may also be affected. Weakness of the wrist extensors, but not flexors, is often present, as is hip involvement, which often results in a compensatory lordosis. Bilateral foot drop may also be present. Fortunately, the progression of the disease is slow, and cardiac involvement has not been described.

Limb-girdle dystrophy is characterized by progressive weakness of the hip and shoulder musculature. It may appear early in the first to third decades or later in life. Unlike FSH dystrophy, deltoid weakness, as well as biceps atrophy, is often encountered. Neck weakness may also be seen.

Nemaline myopathy presents with diffuse muscular weakness of both smooth and skeletal muscles, decreased muscle mass, bony anomalies caused by hypotonia, and loss of deep tendon reflex.[270] Abnormal facies, characterized by prognathic mandible and high arched palate, restrictive lung disease, and rare cardiomyopathy may occur.

Anesthetic considerations. Muscular dystrophies are associated with a number of potential complications during anesthesia care such as pulmonary and cardiac dysfunction, hyperkalemia, malignant hyperthermia, sudden death, kyphoscoliosis, rhabdomyolysis, and renal failure.[271,272]

The goals of obstetric analgesia should be to limit cardiorespiratory demands imposed by labor and delivery and pain. If epidural analgesia is chosen, the level of block should be extended slowly, particularly in patients having cardiomyopathy and/or respiratory compromise. Pulmonary function tests may be useful in estimating respiratory reserve. Systemic analgesics provide less complete pain relief and may enhance the risk of aspiration and other respiratory complications.

Epidural anesthesia is generally suitable for cesarean section but may be technically challenging if severe kyphoscoliosis is present. If general anesthesia is preferred in view of obstetric complications or the severity of maternal disease, general precautions must be taken. In patients with nemaline myopathy particularly, the possibility of a difficult airway must be entertained. Indeed, a recent case report described difficulties with tracheal intubation in a parturient with nemaline myopathy undergoing an elective cesarean section.[268] An awake intubation may be necessary for these patients.

Succinylcholine should be avoided in patients with muscular dytrophies because its use may result in hyperkalemia, hyperthermia, and elevation of creatine phosphokinase. These mimic but do not always indicate the presence of malignant hyperthermia.[273] Although the association between muscular dystrophy and malignant hyperthermia is far from proved, all triggering agents, including potent inhalational agents, should be avoided.[273] The response to nondepolarizing muscle relaxants is usually normal,[274] but an unusually rapid recovery from atracurium was reported in one patient with FSH dystrophy.[269] Postoperative ventilatory support may be necessary. In addition, adequate pain relief may greatly improve postoperative pulmonary status.

MYOTONIC DYSTROPHY
Incidence and pathophysiology

Myotonic dystrophy is a relatively common neuromuscular disorder with a prevalence of 5 per 100,000 in the general population. It is inherited as an autosomal dominant with variable penetrance.[275,276] Myotonia is characterized by involuntary and sustained muscular contraction induced by various factors such as hypothermia, shivering, surgical or other mechanical stimulation, and various anesthetic agents.[276-278] Contraction is followed by a delay in relaxation. Furthermore, the disease may include gastrointestinal paresis and esophageal incompetence, abnormal insulin response to glucose load, cataract formation, frontal balding, and testicular atrophy.[275,276,279] Reduced pulmonary reserve, along with arrhythmias and cardiomyopathy, may also occur.[279-281]

Myotonia may often initially involve the muscles of hand grip and the face. A drawn face with prominent temporal and masseter muscle wasting and sagging of the lower part of the face aid in a clinical diagnosis. Nasal speech due to bulbar involvement is often apparent. Limb weakness is accompanied by myotonia, which may be perceived by the patient as cramping or may go unnoticed. Myotonia can often be elicited by having a patient grip an object and then attempt to release her grip quickly, at which point excessive myotonia prevents a quick release. Myotonia may also be triggered by percussion of distal muscles. Though myotonia may be bothersome, patients are usually more distressed and disabled by the associated progressive limb weakness.

Treatment is available for myotonic symptoms. Quinidine, procainamide, phenytoin, acetazolamide, and carbamazepine have all been used to treat myotonia,[267,282] but none of these treatments has been completely satisfactory. Cardiac muscle involvement commonly occurs and often becomes manifest in some degree of heart block or cardiomyopathy.

Obstetric and anesthesia management

Obstetric management. There are less then 30 cases of pregnancy reported in patients with myotonic dystrophy. There is controversy regarding the influence of the disease on fertility because gonadal atrophy may occur in males with the disease. Menstrual abnormalities and amenorrhea are also common, and pregnancy rates are low in severely affected women.[283] During pregnancy, muscle weakness and myotonia may be unchanged or may increase. Muscular function may deteriorate at any time, but most commonly in the third trimester. In some cases, the symptoms of the disease have been first diagnosed during pregnancy or in the postpartum period.[284] On the other hand, some patients experience significant improvement during pregnancy.[285] Factors that may worsen myotonia during pregnancy are en!argement of the uterus, progesterone effects on membrane potential, changes in potassium homeostasis, and decreased physical activity.[284]

High rates of fetal wastage, premature labor and delivery, and prolongation of the first, second, and third stages of labor have been commonly reported. Operative vaginal delivery is often required, and postpartum hemorrhage may occur.[285] Polyhydramnios is common[286] as well as fetal hydrops.[287] Abnormalities of fetal deglutition and unusual fetal movement patterns have also been reported.[288] Tocolytic agents may precipitate a dystrophic crisis.[289]

Obstetric management includes genetic counseling, prenatal diagnosis, careful ultrasound examination for findings consistent with the disease, and education and follow-up regarding premature labor. In the intrapartum period, careful attention to cardiorespiratory status and the need for oxytocin augmentation is necessary. Operative vaginal delivery or cesarean section should be reserved for the usual obstetric indications. There should be heightened vigilance in the postpartum period for hemorrhage.

Anesthetic considerations. A number of concerns arise in the anesthetic management of these patients. Weak intestinal mobility may delay gastric emptying, creating an even greater predisposition to aspiration than is generally associated with pregnancy. Administration of an H_2-receptor antagonist or metoclopramide may be particularly beneficial. As already mentioned, abnormal uterine contraction patterns and atony, resulting in postpartum hemorrhage, have been reported.[280,290] The CNS-depressant effects of anesthetics and analgesics appear to be increased in patients with myotonia.[275,279,291] Diminished respiratory reserve due to weakness of the diaphragm and the intercostal and accessory muscles may lead to further compromise.[275,280] Pulmonary function tests may be useful in gauging the extent of respiratory insufficiency.[275]

Epidural analgesia is preferred during labor, particularly if instrumental vaginal delivery is planned. Intrathecal administration of an opioid may be used, assuming adequate postpartum respiratory monitoring is available. Since shivering during conventional epidural anesthesia may precipitate myotonic crisis, it should be prevented by the addition of an epidural narcotic drug or by warming up the patient and the local anesthetic solution.[292,293] Intravenous fluids should also be warmed. Myotonia is caused by abnormal calcium metabolism[276]; thus, neither regional anesthesia nor general anesthesia with neuromuscular block will prevent it. However, local anesthetic directly infiltrated into the affected muscle may relieve myotonia.[294]

Both spinal and epidural anesthesia have been used for cesarean section.[276,280,281,295,296] Infiltration of uterine muscle with bupivacaine has been used to treat uterine atony unresponsive to oxytoxic drugs in a myotonic patient.[281]

If general anesthesia is necessary, care must be taken in the selection of drugs and doses administered because myotonics have increased sensitivity to the depressant effects of anesthetics.[275,276,280,297] An exaggerated response to propofol has been reported in patients with severe myotonic dystrophy,[279] whereas in those with mild disease the response is normal.[298] Succinylcholine should be avoided because fasciculations may induce muscle contractions.[299,300] Vecuronium (0.1 mg/kg) has been used for intubation during cesarean section.[280] The response to nondepolarizing muscle relaxants appears to be normal,[297] but an exaggerated response has also been reported to occur.[301,302] Therefore, short-acting nondepolarizing muscle relaxants may be preferable. Anticholinesterase agents may also trigger myotonia. On the other hand, incomplete reversal of neuromuscular blockade will merely lead to rapid respiratory insufficiency in these patients.[275,301] It is recommended to avoid halothane because it may be associated with greater postoperative shivering than other agents.[275,291] An acute myotonic crisis may be treated with quinidine (300 to 600 mg IV), large doses of steroids, or dantrolene.

Peripartum congestive heart failure (CHF), refractory to diuretics and vasodilators, occurred in a patient with myotonic dystrophy.[281] Because of cardiovascular decompensation, a cesarean section delivery was performed at 34 weeks gestation. Before delivery, the patient was treated with continuous arteriovenous hemofiltration (CAVH) to alleviate CHF, and the operation was successfully performed under epidural anesthesia.

Postoperative care for the myotonic dystrophy patient should include prevention of shivering and provision of adequate analgesia, and it should be noted that these patients may have a heightened sensitivity to CNS depressants.

Newborn care. Congenital newborn myotonia can be observed in the delivery room.[303] The affected infant may manifest hypotonia, respiratory difficulty, and, later on, feeding problems. Linkage analysis and polymerase chain reaction studies from both chorionic villous sampling and amniocyntesis may aid in early diagnosis.[304]

MYASTHENIA GRAVIS

Myasthenia gravis, an autoimmune disorder, is fully discussed in Chapter 19. Only a few important points will be stressed here.

Anesthetic considerations. Minimizing stress and pain is particularly important for the patient with myasthenia. Systemic or inhalational analgesia may be used, but pain relief is usually not as complete as with other techniques. An increased potential for respiratory compromise or aspiration in patients with myasthenia should be considered. Epidural analgesia is beneficial in that it affords the flexibility of allowing pain-free rest during the first stage of labor and adequate anesthesia for an assisted delivery.[305] Local anesthetic with differential blockade such as bupivacaine, with or without the addition of a narcotic drug, may better preserve muscle strength. The potential for systemic toxicity is heightened in patients who are receiving anticholinesterase drugs and who are given ester-type local anesthetics.[305] High blood levels of local anesthetic may also interfere with neuromuscular transmission. However, this is a theoretical concern, considering the doses used in obstetric anesthesia.[306] The administration of intrathecal opioids as previously described may also be used.

Regional anesthesia is an excellent technique for myasthenic parturients undergoing cesarean section. Occasionally, because of obstetric indications or, more commonly, because of bulbar dysfunction and/or poor respiratory insufficiency, general an-

esthesia may be preferable. Patients with myasthenia are particularly sensitive to the effects of muscle relaxants. Succinylcholine has been used; however, some have reported resistance to succinylcholine whereas others have described enhanced sensitivity.[301,306] If the drug is used in the face of anticholinesterase therapy, a reduced dose (50 mg) has been recommended.[307] Others, however, may prefer to use the full dose (1 mg/kg). Myasthenic patients are unusually sensitive to the effects of nonpolarizing muscle relaxants.[301] As little as a defasciculating dose of curare may abolish twitch response. Atracuricum (0.1 mg/kg) has been used for intubation.[308] Incremental doses (0.02 to 0.04 mg/kg) may be required for continued paralysis. Magnesium sulfate, which is often used in obstetrics, may exacerbate the symptoms of myasthenia.[309-311] In general, if the disease is well controlled, the patient can usually be extubated after reversal of neuromuscular blockade.[305] Even if general anesthesia is chosen, consideration should be given to the administration of intraspinal narcotics for postoperative pain relief. Attention must be directed to improving pulmonary function in the postoperative period.

Newborn care. Ten to fifteen percent of babies born to affected mothers will have transient neonatal myasthenia as a result of placental transfer of maternal antibodies.[312] Neonatal disease correlates poorly with the severity of maternal disease. Increased risk of arthrogryposis has been reported.[313] The syndrome may appear immediately in the delivery room or up to 4 days following birth, manifested by poor tone, weak reflexes, or frank respiratory insufficiency. It usually improves with an intramuscular injection of 0.5 to 1.0 mg edrophonium.[307]

ARNOLD-CHIARI MALFORMATION
Incidence and pathophysiology

In the 1890s, Chiari described four types of posterior fossa deformities associated with herniation of the cerebellum through the foramen magnum.[314-316] The features of the two more common types of Arnold-Chiari malformation (ACM), viz Type I and II, are summarized in Table 10-3. Type I is the more frequent of the two but is still an extremely rare disease in adults. Syringomyelia, cavitation of the spinal cord, occurs in 20% to 76% of patients with Type I ACM.[314,315,317-319] Type I malformation most probably occurs as a result of abnormal ICP gradients during embryologic development.[315,316,320]

The manifestations of Type I disease usually relates to cerebellar and cervical spinal cord involvement, namely, pain, particularly of the neck

Table 10-3 Pathology of Type 1 and Type II Arnold-Chiari malformation

Feature	Type I	Type II
Age group	Adult	Infant
Caudal displacement of cerebellar tonsils	Yes	Yes
Caudal displacement of inferior vermis and fourth ventricle	No	Yes
Caudal displacement of medulla oblongata	No	Yes
Dorsal kink of cervicomedullary junction	No	Yes
Course of upper cervical nerve roots	Normal	Usually cephalad
Spina bifida aperta	Usually absent	"Always" present
Hydrocephalus	May be present	"Always" present
Syringohydromyelia	May develop late	May develop early

Adapted from Carmel PW, Markesbury WR: *J Neurosurg* 1972; 37:544. Used by permission.

and occipital areas; weakness and numbness of the extremities; and paresthesias, ataxia and "clumsiness."[314-316,321,322] Reflexes may be increased or decreased and the gag reflex may be diminished. A definitive diagnosis is usually made with radiographs, CT or MRI scans, and myelography.[314-317] Posterior fossa decompression, by upper cervical laminectomy and occipital craniectomy, is the most widely accepted surgical procedure. Postoperative respiratory depression is a major concern, and relapses can occur.[316]

Syringomyelia

Syringomyelia is a fluid-filled cavity (syrinx) developing within the spinal cord. It is associated with Chiari I malformation and is assumed to be a slowly progressive degenerative disease of the spinal cord, leading to cavitations.[317,323] As with ACM, pain is usually the earliest manifestation followed by sensory and motor deficits, changes in reflexes, and spasticity.[324,325] Diagnosis is usually made on clinical manifestation, but it must be confirmed radiologically. Laminectomy may reduce the internal pressure of the cyst on the spinal cord, and CSF shunts may also be placed to prevent further expansion of the syrinx.[324]

Scoliosis, possibly resulting from paravertebral muscle weakness, has also been associated with Chiari I malformation and syringomyelia.[314,326,327] Some improvement of scoliosis may occur after posterior fossa decompression.[314]

Anesthetic management

Very little information is available regarding anesthetic management of patients with ACM and syringomyelia. Fear of herniation should not be of concern for those patients having had surgical decompression. There is no information available in untreated patients; however, because of the chronic nature of the disease, the risk of herniation is probably extremely low.

There is only one case report of a parturient with undiagnosed ACM Type I having epidural analgesia for labor and then spinal anesthesia for cesarean delivery.[328] Postoperatively, she was diagnosed as having a PDPH, which was not relieved by an epidural blood patch, and an MRI examination performed four days later revealed ACM Type I.

In general, careful positioning of the patient is required because pronounced flexion of the head may further compress the brain stem and provoke a respiratory arrest.[329] Vocal cord paralysis and stridor have also been observed with ACM, possibly a result of traction on the cranial nerves.[330]

The presence of associated syringomyelia also creates some concerns for regional anesthesia. It may be prudent to obtain an MRI study of the spinal cord to locate areas of cavitation before attempting regional anesthesia.[317,324] Scoliosis may also render regional techniques difficult to perform. Also of note is that general anesthesia has been used for emergency cesarean delivery in a patient with syringomyelia.[323]

CONCLUSION

Neurologic and muscular diseases are fortunately rare, but occasionally they will occur during pregnancy. Good communication among the members of the perinatal care team is essential to develop a plan of care. The extent of neurologic deficit should be well documented before any interventions. The patient should be included in these discussions and frank informed consent obtained.

REFERENCES

1. Crawford JS, James FM III, Nolte H, et al: Regional analgesia for patients with chronic neurological disease and similar conditions. *Anaesthesia* 1981; 36:827.
2. Crawford JS: Epidural analgesia for patients with chronic neurological disease. *Anesth Analg* 1983; 63:620.
3. Posner JB: Secondary neoplastic disease, in Asbury AK, McKhann GM, McDonald WI (eds): *Diseases of the Nervous System*. Philadelphia, WB Saunders, 1986, pp 1155-1168.
4. Adams RD, Victor M: *Principles of Neurology*. New York, McGraw-Hill, 1981, pp 440-474.

5. Shapiro WR, Shapiro JR: Primary brain tumors, in Asbury AK, McKhann GM, McDonald WI (eds): *Diseases of the Nervous System*. Philadelphia, WB Saunders, 1986, pp 1136-1154.

6. Smith MT, Ludwig CL, Godfrey AD, et al: Grading of oligodendrogliomas. *Cancer* 1983; 52:2107.

7. Kjellberg RN: A system of pituitary tumors: Bragg peak proton hypophysectomy, in Seydel HG (ed): *Tumors of the Nervous System*. New York, John Wiley & Sons, 1975, pp 145-174.

8. Harner SG, Laws ER: Clinical findings in patients with acoustic neuroma. *Mayo Clin Proc* 1983; 58:721.

9. Greenberg HS, Deck MDF, Vikram B, et al: Metastasis to the base of the skull: Clinical findings in 43 patients. *Neurology* 1981; 31:530.

10. Chang CH, Horton J, Schoenfeld D, et al: Comparison of postoperative radiotherapy and combined postoperative radiotherapy and chemotherapy in the multidisciplinary management of malignant gliomas. *Cancer* 1983; 52:997.

11. Steinberg ES, Santos AC: Surgical anesthesia during pregnancy, *Int Anaesthesiol Clin* 1990; 28:58.

12. Allen J, Eldrige R, Loerber T: Acoustic neuroma in the last months of pregnancy. *Am J Obstet Gynecol* 1974; 119:516.

13. Bickerstaff ER, Small JM, Guest IA: The relapsing course of certain meningiomas in relation to pregnancy and menstruation. *J Neurol Neurosurg Psychiatry* 1958; 21:189.

14. Enoksson P, Lundberg N, Sjosstedt S, et al: Influence of pregnancy on visual fields in suprasellar tumors. *Acta Neurol Scand* 1961; 36:525.

15. Donaldson JO: Neurologic emergencies in pregnancy. *Obstet Gynecol Clin North Am* 1991; 18(2):199.

16. Toakley G: Brain tumors and pregnancy. *Aust N Z J Surg* 1965; 35:148.

17. Simon RH: Brain tumors in pregnancy. *Semin Neurol* 1988; 8:214.

18. Magyar DM, Marshall JR: Pituitary tumors and pregnancy. *Am J Obstet Gynecol* 1978; 132:739.

19. Bruns PD, Linder RO, Drose VE, et al: The placental transfer of water from fetus to mother following the intravenous infusion of hypertonic mannitol to the maternal rabbit. *Am J Obstet Gynecol* 1963; 86:160.

20. Battaglia F, Prystowski H, Smission C, et al: Fetal blood studies. XIII. The effect of the administration of fluids intravenously to mothers upon the concentrations of water and electrolytes in plasma of human fetuses. *Pediatrics* 1960; 25:2.

21. Levinson G, Shnider SM, de Lorimier AA, et al: Effects of maternal hyperventilation on uterine blood flow and fetal oxygenation and acid-base status. *Anesthesiology* 1974; 40:340.

22. Marx GF, Orkin LR: Cerebrospinal fluid proteins and spinal anesthesia in obstetrics. *Anesthesiology* 1965; 26:340.

23. Finfer SR: Management of labour and delivery in patients with intracranial neoplasms. *Br J Anaesth* 1991; 67:784.

24. Marx GF, Scheinberg L, Romney SL: Anesthetic management of the parturient with intracranial tumor. *Obstet Gynecol* 1964; 24:122.

25. Abouleish E: Intracranial hypertension and caudal anaesthesia. *Br J Anaesth* 1987; 59:1478.

26. Marx GF, Zemaitis MT, Orkin LR: Cerebrospinal fluid pressures during labour and obstetrical anesthesia. *Anesthesiology* 1961; 22:349.

27. Marx GF, Oka Y, Orkin YR: Cerebrospinal fluid pressure during labor. *Am J Obstet Gynecol* 1962; 84:213.

28. Goroszenuik T, Howard RS, Wright JT: The management of labour using continuous lumbar epidural analgesia in a patient with a malignant cerebral tumor. *Anaesthesia* 1986; 41:1128.

29. Hilt H, Gramm HJ, Link J: Changes in intracranial pressure associated with extradural anaesthesia. *Br J Anaesth* 1986; 58:676.

30. Hunter CA Jr: Uterine motility studies during labor: Observations on bilateral sympathetic nerve block in the normal and abnormal first stage of labor. *Am J Obstet Gynecol* 1983; 85:861.

31. Eisenach JC, Castro MI: Maternally administered esmolol produces fetal β-adrenergic blockade and hypoxemia in sheep. *Anesthesiology* 1989; 71:718.

32. Johnston I: The definition of a reduced CSF absorption syndrome: A reappraisal of benign intracranial hypertension and related conditions. *Hypothesis* 1975; 1:1.

33. Thomas E: Recurrent benign intracranial hypertension associated with hemoglobin SC disease in pregnancy. *Obstet Gynecol* 1986; 67:7S.

34. Noronha A: Neurologic disorders during pregnancy and the puerperium. *Clin Perinatol* 1985; 12:695.

35. Peterson CM, Kelly JV: Pseudotumor cerebri in pregnancy. Case reports and review of the literature. *Obstet Gynecol Surv* 1985; 40:323.

36. Durcan FJ, Corbett JJ, Wall M: The incidence of pseudotumor cerebri. Population studies in Iowa and Louisiana. *Arch Neurol* 1988; 45:875.

37. Katz VL, Peterson R, Cefalo RC: Pseudotumor cerebri and pregnancy. *Am J Perinatol* 1989; 6:442.

38. Digre KB, Varner MW, Corbett JJ: Pseudotumor cerebri and pregnancy. *Neurology (Cleve)* 1984; 34:721.

39. Bullens C, De Vries W, Van Crevel H: Benign intracranial hypertension: A retrospective and follow-up study. *J Neurol Sci* 1979; 40:147.

40. Hopkins EL, Hendricks CH, Cibils LA: Cerebrospinal fluid pressure in labor. *Am J Obstet Gynecol* 1965; 93:907.

41. Polop R, Choed-Amphai E, Miller R: Epidural anesthesia for delivery complicated by benign intracranial hypertension. *Anesthesiology* 1979; 50:159.

42. Sullivan HC: Fatal tonsillar herniation in pseudotumor cerebri. *Neuro* 1991; 41:1142.

43. Abouleish E, Ali V, Tong RA: Benign intracranial hypertension and anesthesia for cesarean section. *Anesthesiology* 1985; 63:705.

44. Corbett J: The rational management of idiopathic intracranial hypertension. *Arch Neurol* 1989; 46:1049.

45. Lussos SA, Loeffler C: Epidural blood patch improves postdural puncture headache in a patient with benign intracranial hypertension. *Reg Anesth* 1993; 18:315.

46. Koppel BS, Kaunitz AM, Tuchman AJ: Pseudotumor cerebri following eclampsia. *Eur Neurol* 1990; 30:6.

47. Hamil JF, Bedford RF, Weaver DC et al: Lidocaine before endotracheal intubation: Intravenous or laryngotracheal? *Anesthesiology* 1981; 55:578.

48. Wiebers D: Subarachnoid hemorrhage in pregnancy. *Semin Neurol* 1988; 8:226.

49. Rish BL: Treatment of intracranial aneurysms associated with other entities. *South Med J* 1978; 71:553.

50. Heros RC, Zervas NT, Varsos V: Cerebral vasospasm after subarachnoid hemorrhage: An update. *Ann Neurol* 1983; 14:599.

51. Srinivasan K: Cerebral venous and arterial thrombosis in pregnancy and the puerperium: A study of 135 patients. *Angiology* 1983; 34:731.

52. Bousser MG, Chiras J, Bories J, et al: Cerebral venous thrombosis: A review of 38 cases. *Stroke* 1985; 16:199.

53. Adams HP, Butler MJ, Biller J, et al: Nonhemorrhagic cerebral infarction in young adults. *Arch Neurol* 1986; 43:793.

54. Tabachnik-Schor NF, Lipton SA: Association of lupus like anticoagulant and non-vasculitis cerebral infarction. *Arch Neurol* 1986; 43:851.

55. Lechat PH, Mas JL, Lascault G, et al: Prevalence of patent foramen ovale in patients with stroke. *N Engl J Med* 1988; 318:1148.

56. Nishimura RA, McGoon MD, Shub C, et al: Echocardiographically documented mitral-valve prolapse: Long-term follow-up of 237 patients. *N Engl J Med* 1985; 313:1305.

57. Wiebers DO, Whisnant JP: The incidence of stroke among pregnant women in Rochester, Minn, 1955 through 1979. *JAMA* 1985; 254:3055.

58. Rochat RW, Koonin LM, Atrash HK, et al: Maternal mortality in the United States: Report from the Maternal Mortality Collaborative. *Obstet Gynecol* 1988; 72:91.

59. Jennett WB, Cross NJ: Influence of pregnancy and oral contraception on the incidence of strokes in women of childbearing age. *Lancet* 1967; 1:1019.

60. Cerebral Embolism Study Group: Immediate anticoagulation of embolic stroke: A randomized trial. *Stroke* 1983; 14:668.

61. Cerebral Embolism Task Force: Cardiogenic brain embolism. *Arch Neurol* 1986; 43:71.

62. Reece EA, Chervenak FA, Coultrip L, et al: The perinatal management of pregnancy complicated by massive intracerebral hemorrhage. *Am J Perinatal* 1984; 1:266.

63. Minielly R, Yuzpe AA, Drake CG: Subarachnoid hemorrhage secondary to ruptured cerebral aneurysm in pregnancy. *Obstet Gynecol* 1979; 53:64.

64. Heros RC, Tu Y-K: Is surgical therapy needed for unruptured arteriovenous malformations? *Neurology* 1987; 37:279.

65. Lennon RL, Sundt TM, Gronert GA: Combined cesarean section and clipping of intracerebral aneurysm. *Anesthesiology* 1984; 60:240.

66. Whitburn RH, Laishley RS, Jewkes DA: Anaesthesia for simultaneous caesarean section and clipping of intracranial aneurysm. *Br J Anaesth* 1990; 64:642.

67. Van Buul BJA, Nijhuis JG, Slappendel R, et al: General anesthesia for surgical repair of intracranial aneurysm in pregnancy. Effects on fetal heart rate. *Am J Perinatology* 1993; 10:183.

68. Conklin KA, Herr G, Funy D: Anaesthesia for cesarean section and cerebral aneurysm clipping. *Can Anaesth Soc J* 1984; 31:451.

69. Naulty J, Cefalo RC, Lewis PE: Fetal toxicity of nitroprusside in the pregnant ewe. *Am J Obstet Gynecol* 1981; 139:708.

70. Newman B, Lam AM: Induced hypotension for clipping of cerebral aneurysm during pregnancy. *Anesth Analg* 1986; 65:675.

71. Donchin Y, Amirou B, Sahar A, et al: Sodium nitroprusside for aneurysm surgery in pregnancy. *Br J Anaesth* 1978; 50:849.

72. Rigg D, McDonogh A: Use of sodium nitroprusside for deliberate hypotension during pregnancy. *Br J Anaesth* 1981; 53:985.

73. Willoughby JS: Sodium nitroprusside pregnancy and multiple intracranial aneurysms. *Anaesth Intensive Care* 1984; 12:351.

74. Snyder SW, Wheeler AS, James FM III: The use of nitroglycerin to control severe hypertension of pregnancy during cesarean section. *Anesthesiology* 1979; 51:563.

75. Assali NS, Westra B: Effects of hypothermia on uterine circulation and on the fetus. *Pro Soc Exp Biol Med* 1962; 109:485.

76. Strange K, Halldin M: Hypothermia in pregnancy. *Anesthesiology* 1983; 58:460.

77. Boatman KK, Bradford VA: Excision of an internal carotid aneurysm during pregnancy employing hypothermia and vascular shunt. *Ann Surg* 1958; 148:271.

78. Motoyama EK, Rivard G, Acheson F, et al: Adverse effect of maternal hyperventilation on the fetus. *Lancet* 1966; 1:286.

79. Rigler ML, Drasner K: Distribution of catheter-injected local anesthesic in a model of the subarachnoid space. *Anesthesiology* 1991; 75:684.

80. Laidler JA, Jackson IJ, Redfern N: The management of caesarean section in a patient with an intracranial arteriovenous malformation. *Anaesthesia* 1989; 44:490.

81. Kendall D: Thrombosis of intracranial veins. *Brain* 1948; 71:391.

82. Heinz ER, Geeter D, Gabrielson ID: Cortical vein thrombosis in the dog with a review of aseptic intracranial venous thrombosis in man. *Acta Radiol Diagn* 1972; 13:105.

83. Younker D, Jones MM, Adenwala J, et al: Maternal cortical vein thrombosis and the obstetric anesthesiology. *Anesth Analg* 1986; 65:1007.

84. Gewirtz EC, Costin M, Marx G: Cortical vein thrombosis may mimic postdural puncture headache. *Reg Anesth* 1987; 12:188.

85. Mokri B, Jack CR, Petty GW: Pseudotumor syndrome associated with cerebral venous sinus occlusion and antiphospholipid antibodies. *Stroke* 1993; 24:469.

86. Hubbert CH: Dural puncture headache suspected, cortical vein thrombosis diagnosed. *Anesth Analg* 1987; 66:285.

87. Ravindran RS, Zandstra G, Viegas OJ: Postpartum headache following regional analgesia: A symptom of cerebral venous thrombosis. *Can J Anaesth* 1989; 36:705.

88. Porter RJ: Classification of epileptic seizures, in Laidlaw J, Richens A, Oxley J (eds): *A Textbook of Epilepsy,* ed 2. London, Churchill Livingstone, 1987.

89. Niedermeyer E: Abnormal EEG patterns (epileptic and paroxysmal), in Niedermeyer E, Lopes da Silva F (eds): *Electroencephalography: Basic Principles, Clinical Application and Related Fields,* ed 2. Baltimore, Urban and Schwarzenberg, 1987, pp 187-189.

90. Dalessio DJ: Current concepts seizure disorders and pregnancy. *N Engl J Med* 1985; 312:559.

91. So EL, Penry JK: Epilepsy in adults. *Ann Neurol* 1981; 9:3.

92. Allbert JR, Morrison JC: Neurologic diseases in pregnancy. *Obstet Gynecol Clin North Am* 1992; 19:765.

93. Jagoda A, Riggio S: Emergency department approach to managing seizures in pregnancy. *Ann Emerg Med* 1991; 20:80.

94. Knight AH, Rhind EG: Epilepsy and pregnancy: A study of 153 pregnancies in 59 patients. *Epilepsia* 1975; 16:99.

95. Montouris GD, Fenichel GM, McLain LW: The pregnant epileptic. *Arch Neurol* 1979; 36:601.

96. Suter C, Khingman WO: Seizure status and pregnancy. *Neurology* 1957; 7:105.

97. Bjerkedal T, Bahna SL: The course and outcome of pregnancy in women with epilepsy. *Acta Obstet Gynecol Scand* 1973; 52:245.

98. Hiilesmaa VK, Bardy A, Teramo K: Obstetric outcome in women with epilepsy. *Am J Obstet Gynecol* 1985; 152-499.

99. Nelson KB, Ellanberg JH: Maternal serizure disorder, outcome of pregnancy and neurologic abnormalities in the children. *Neurology* 1982; 32:1247.

100. Yerby S: Pregnancy and epilepsy. *Epilepsia* 1991; 32:S51.

101. Donaldson JO: *Neurology of Pregnancy,* ed 2. London, WB Saunders, 1989.

102. Dean M, Stock B, Patterson RJ, et al: Serum protein binding of drugs during and after pregnancy in humans. *Clin Pharmacol Ther* 1980; 28:257.

103. Simpson KH, Stakes AF, Miller M: Pregnancy delays paracetamol absorption and gastric emptying in patients undergoing surgery. *Br J Anaesth* 1988; 60:24.

104. Dam M, Christiansen J, Munck O, et al: Antiepileptic

drugs: Metabolism in pregnancy. *Clin Pharmacokinet* 1979; 4:53.

105. Lund CJ, Donovan JC: Blood volume during pregnancy. *Am J Obstet Gynecol* 1967; 98:393.

106. Santos AC, Pedersen H, Morishima HO, et al: Pharmacokinetics of lidocaine in nonpregnant and pregnant ewes. *Anesth Analg* 1988; 67:1154.

107. Ramsey R, Strauss R, Willmoore L: Status epilepticus in pregnancy: Effect of phenytoin malabsorption on seizure control. *Neurology* 1978; 28:85.

108. Yerby M: Problems and management of the pregnant woman with epilepsy. *Epilepsia* 1987; 28S:S29.

109. Hopkins A: Epilepsy and anticonvulsant drug. *Br Med J* 1987; 294:497.

110. Knott C, Williams C, Reynold F: Phenytoin kinetics during pregnancy and the puerperium. *Br J Obstet Gynaecol* 1986; 93:1030.

111. Van Dyke RA: Metabolism of volatile anesthetics. 3. Induction of microsomal dechlorinating and ether-cleaving enzymes. *J Pharmacol Exp Ther* 1966; 154:364.

112. Blake DA, Rozman RS, Cascorbi HF, et al: Biotransformation of fluroxene. 1. Metabolism in mice and dogs in vivo. *Biochem Pharmacol* 1967; 16:1237.

113. Van Dyke RA, Gandolfi AJ: Anaerobic release of fluoride from halothane: Relationship to the binding of halothane metabolites to hepatic cellular constituents. *Drug Metab Dispos* 1976; 4:40.

114. Gelman S, Rimerman V, Fowler KC, et al: The effect of halothane, isoflurane and blood loss on hepatotoxicity and hepatic oxygen availability in phenobarbital-pretreated hypoxic rats. *Anesth Analg* 1984; 63:965.

115. Green NM: Halothane anesthesia and hepatitis in a high risk population. *N Engl J Med* 1973; 289:304.

116. Modica PA, Tempelkoff R, White PF: Pro- and anticonvulsant effects of anesthetics (Part I). *Anesth Analg* 1990; 70:303.

117. Joas TA, Stevens WC, Eger EI II: Electroencephalographic seizure activity in dogs during anesthesia. *Br J Anaesth* 1971; 43:739.

118. Lebowitz MH, Blitt CD, Dillon JB: Enflurane-induced central nervous system excitation and its relation to carbon dioxide tension. *Anesth Analg* 1972; 51:355.

119. Wollman H, Smith AL, Neigh JL, et al: Cerebral blood flow and oxygen consumption in man during electroencephalographic seizure patterns associated with ethane anesthesia, in Brock M, Frieschi C, et al (eds): *Cerebral Blood Flow.* Berlin, Springer-Verlag, 1969, p 246.

120. Roizen MF: Anesthetic implications of concurrent diseases, in Miller RD (ed): *Anesthesia,* ed 2. New York, Churchill Livingstone, 1986, p 302.

121. Freman J, Ingvar DH: Effects of fentanyl on cerebral cortical blood flow and EEG in the cat. *Acta Anaesthesiol Scand* 1967; 11:381.

122. Carlson C, Smith DS, Keykhah MM, et al: The effects of high dose fentanyl on cerebral circulation and metabolism in rats. *Anesthesiology* 1982; 57:375.

123. Itil TM: Effects of psychotropic drugs in qualitatively and quantitatively analyzed human EEG, in Clark WG, del Guidice J (eds): *Principles of Psychopharmacology,* ed 2, New York, Academic Press, 1978, pp 261-277.

124. Evans DEN: Anesthesia and the epileptic patient: A review. *Anaesthesia* 1975; 30:34.

125. Hansen HC, Drenck NE: Generalized seizures after etomidate anaesthesia. *Anaesthesia* 1988; 43:805.

126. Dailland P, Cockshott ID, Lirzin JD, et al: Intravenous propofol during cesarean section: Placental transfer, concentration in breast milk and neonatal effects. A preliminary study. *Anesthesiology* 1989; 71:827.

127. Rampton AJ, Griffin RM, Durcan JJ, et al: Propofol and electroconvulsive therapy. *Lancet* 1988; 1:296.

128. Hodkinson BP, Frith RW, Mee EW: Propofol and the electroencephalogram. *Lancet* 1987; 2:1518.

129. Bohm E, Flodmark S, Petersen I: Effect of lidocaine (Xylocaine) on seizure and interseizure electroencephalograms in epileptics. *Arch Neurol Psychiatry* 1959; 81:550.

130. Merrel DA, Koch MAT: Epidural anaesthesia as an anticonvulsant in the management of hypertension and the eclamptic patients in labour. *S Afr Med J* 1980; 58:875.

131. Bucklin BA, Warner DS, Choi WW, et al: Pregnancy does not alter the threshold for lidocaine-induced seizures in the rat. *Anesth Analg* 1992; 74:57.

132. Santos AC, Arthur GR, Wlody D, et al: Comparative systemic toxicity of ropivacaine and bupivacaine in nonpregnant and pregnant ewes. *Anesthesiology* 1995; 82:734.

133. Aravapalli R, Abouleish E, Aldrete JA: Anesthetic implications in the parturient epileptic patient. *Anesth Analg* 1988; 67:S3.

134. Bolton VE, Leicht CH, Scanlon TS: Postpartum seizure after epidural blood patch and intravenous caffeine sodium benzoate. *Anesthesiology* 1989; 70:146.

135. Ornstein E, Matteo RS, Young WL, et al: Resistance to metocurine induced neuromuscular blockade in patients receiving phenytoin. *Anesthesiology* 1985; 63:294.

136. Ornstein E, Matteo RS, Schwartz AE, et al: The effect of phenytoin on the magnitude and duration of neuromuscular block following atracurium or vecuronium. *Anesthesiology* 1987; 67:191.

137. Commission on Genetics, Pregnancy and the Child, International League Against Epilepsy: Guidelines for the care of epileptic women of childbearing age. *Epilepsia* 1989; 30:34.

138. Buehler BA, Delimont D, Van Waes M, et al: Prenatal prediction of risk of the fetal hydantoin syndrome. *N Engl J Med* 1990; 322:1567.

139. Erickson RP: Autonomic hyperreflexia: Pathophysiology and medical management. *Arch Phys Med Rehabil* 1980; 61:431.

140. Quimby CW, Williams RN Jr, Greifenstein FE: Anesthetic problems of the acute quadriplegic patient. *Anesth Analg* 1973; 52:333.

141. Omatsu Y: Basal metabolism in pregnancy. *Kobe J Med Sci* 1957; 27:21.

142. McGregor JA, Meeurosen J: Autonomic hyperreflexia: A mortal danger for spinal cord-damaged women in labor. *Am J Obstet Gynecol* 1985; 151:330.

143. Young BK: Pregnancy in women with paraplegia. *Adv Neurol* 1994; 64:209.

144. DeBarge O, Christensen NJ, Corbett JL, et al: Plasma catecholamines in tetraplegics. *Paraplegia* 1974; 12:44.

145. Mathias CJ, Christensen NJ, Corbett JL, et al: Plasma catecholamines during paroxysmal neurogenic hypertension in quadriplegic man. *Circ Res* 1976; 39:204.

146. Young BK, Katz M, Klein S: Pregnancy after spinal cord injury: Altered maternal and fetal response to labor. *Obstet Gynecol* 1983; 62-59.

147. Stauffer ES: Long-term management of traumatic quadriplegia, in Pierce DS, Nicke VH (eds): *The Total Care of Spinal Cord Injuries.* Boston, Little, Brown & Co, 1977, p 81.

148. Comarr AE: Observation of menstruation and pregnancy among female spinal cord injury patients. *Paraplegia* 1966; 3:263.

149. Cross LL, Meythalar JM, Tuel SM, et al: Pregnancy, labor and delivery post spinal cord injury. *Paraplegia* 1992; 30:890.

150. Greenspoon JS, Paul RH: Paraplegia and quadriplegia:

Special considerations during pregnancy and labor and delivery. *Am J Obstet Gynecol* 1986; 155:738.

151. Ohry A, Peleg D, Goldman J, et al: Sexual function, pregnancy, and delivery in spinal cord injured women. *Gynecol Obstet Invest* 1988; 9:281.

152. Robertson D: Pregnancy and labor in the paraplegic. *Paraplegia* 1972; 10:209.

153. Verduyn WH: Spinal cord injured women, pregnancy, and delivery. *Paraplegia* 1986; 24:231.

154. Robertson DNS, Gultmann L: The paraplegic patients in pregnancy and labour. *Proc R Soc Med* 1963; 56:381.

155. Oppenhimer WM: Pregnancy in paraplegic patients: Two case reports. *Am J Obstet Gynecol* 1971; 110-784.

156. Katz VL, Thorp JM, Cefolo RC: Epidural analgesia and autonomic hyperreflexia: A case report. *Am J Obstet Gynecol* 1990; 162:471.

157. Ravindran RS, Cummins DF, Smith IE: Experience with the use of nitroprusside and subsequent epidural analgesia in a pregnant quadriplegic patient. *Anesth Analg* 1981; 60:61.

158. Stirt JA, Marco A, Conklin KA: Obstetric anesthesia for a quadriplegic patients with autonomic hyperreflexia. *Anesthesiology* 1979; 51:560.

159. Watson DW, Downey GO: Epidural anesthesia for labor and delivery of twins of a paraplegic mother. *Anesthesiology* 1980; 52:259.

160. Schonwald G, Fisk KJ, Perkash I: Cardiovascular complications during anesthesia in chronic spinal cord injured patients. *Anesthesiology* 1981; 55:550.

161. Baraka A: Epidural meperidine for control of autonomic hyperreflexia in a paraplegic parturient. *Anesthesiology* 1985; 62:688.

162. Abouleish EI, Hanley ES, Palmer SM: Can epidural fentanyl control autonomic hyperreflexia in a quadriplegic parturient? *Anesth Analg* 1989; 68:523.

163. Schmauss C, Yaksh TL: In vivo studies on spinal opiate receptor systems mediating antinociception. II. Pharmacological profiles suggesting a differential association of mu, delta and kappa receptors with visceral chemical and cutaneous stimuli in the rat. *J Pharmacol Ther* 1984; 228:1.

164. Cohen SE, Tan S, Albright GA, et al: Epidural fentanyl/bupivacaine mixtures for obstetric analgesia. *Anesthesiology* 1987; 67:403.

165. Stone WA, Beach TP, Hamilberg W: Succinylcholine: Danger in the spinal-cord-injured patient. *Anesthesiology* 1970; 32:168.

166. Tobey RE: Paraplegia, succinylcholine and cardiac arrest. *Anesthesiology* 1970; 32:359.

167. Alderson JD, Thomas DG: The use of halothane anesthesia to control autonomic hyperreflexia during transurethral surgery in spinal cord injury patients. *Paraplegia* 1975; 13:183.

168. Davis RK, Maslow A: Multiple sclerosis in pregnancy: A review. *Obstet Gynecol Survey* 1992; 47:290.

169. Cook SD, Troiano R, Bansil S, et al: Multiple sclerosis and pregnancy. *Adv Neuro* 1994; 64:83.

170. Izquierdo G, Hauw JJ, Lyon-Caen O, et al: Value of multiple sclerosis diagnostic criteria: 70 autopsy-confirmed cases. *Arch Neurol* 1985; 42:848.

171. McFarlin DE, McFarland HF: Multiple sclerosis. *N Engl J Med* 1982; 307:1183.

172. Stewart JM, Houser OW, Baker HL, et al: Magnetic resonance imaging and clinical relationships in multiple sclerosis. *Mayo Clin Proc* 1987; 62:174.

173. Hallpike JF: Clinical aspects of multiple sclerosis, in Hallpike JF, Adams CWM, Tourtellotte WW (eds): *Multiple Sclerosis*. Baltimore, Williams & Wilkins, 1983, p 129.

174. Boor JW, Johnson RJ, Canales L, et al: Reversible paralysis of automatic respiration in multiple sclerosis. *Arch Neurol* 1977; 34:686.

175. Matthews WB: Clinical aspects, in Matthews WB, Acheson ED, Batchelor JR, et al (eds): *McAlpine's Multiple Sclerosis*. New York, Churchill Livingstone, 1985, p 96.

176. Parsons CL: The bladder in multiple sclerosis, in Hallpike JF, Adams CWM, Tourtellotte WW (eds): *Multiple Sclerosis*. Baltimore, Williams & Wilkins, 1983, p 579.

177. Murray TJ: Amantadine therapy for fatigue in multiple sclerosis. *Can J Neurol Sci* 1985; 12:251.

178. Lisak RP: Overview of the rationale for immunomodulating therapies in multiple sclerosis. *Neurology* 1988; 38:5.

179. Hauser SI, Dawson DM, Lehrich JR, et al: Intensive immunosuppression in progressive multiple sclerosis: A randomized three-arm study of high-dose intravenous cyclophosphamide, plasma exchange and ACTH. *N Engl J Med* 1983; 308:173.

180. Devereux C, Toriano R, Zito G, et al: Effect of total lymphoid irradiation on functional status in chronic multiple sclerosis: Importance of lymphopenia early after treatment. *Neurology* 1988; 38:32.

181. McArthur JC, Young F: Multiple sclerosis in pregnancy, in Goldstein PJ (ed): *Neurological Disorders in Pregnancy*. Mt Kisco, NY, Futura Publishing, 1986, p 197.

182. Birk K, Smeltzer S, Rudick R: Pregnancy and multiple sclerosis. *Semin Neurol* 1988; 8:205.

183. Muller R: Studies on disseminated sclerosis with special reference to symptomatology, course and prognosis. *Acta Med Scand* 1949; 133:1.

184. McAlpine D, Compston N: Some aspects of the natural history of disseminated sclerosis. *Q J Med* 1952; 21:135.

185. Birk K, Ford C, Smeltzer S, et al: The clinical course of multiple sclerosis during pregnancy and the puerperium. *Arch Neurol* 1990; 47:738.

186. Roullet E, Verdier-Taillefer MH, Amarenco P, et al: Pregnancy and multiple sclerosis: A longitudinal study of 125 remittent patients. *Neurol Neurosurg Psychiatry* 1993; 56:1062.

187. Dalos NP, Rabins PV, Brooks BR, et al: Disease activity and emotional state in multiple sclerosis. *Ann Neurol* 1983; 13:573.

188. Muller R: Pregnancy in disseminated sclerosis. *Acta Psychiatr Neurol Scand* 1951; 26:397.

189. Ridley A, Schapira K: Influence of surgical procedures on the course of multiple sclerosis. *Neurology* 1961; 11:81.

190. Kadis LB: Neurological disorders, in Katz J, Benumof J, Kadis LB (eds): *Anesthesia and Uncommon Diseases,* ed 2. Philadelphia, WB Saunders, 1981.

191. Davis F: Pathophysiology of multiple sclerosis and related clinical implications. *Mod Treatment* 1970; 7:890.

192. Warren TM, Datta S, Ostheimer GW: Lumbar epidural anesthesia in a patient with multiple sclerosis. *Anesth Analg* 1982; 61:1022.

193. Bader AM, Hunt CO, Datta S, et al: Anesthesia for the obstetric patient with multiple sclerosis. *J Clin Anesth* 1988; 1:21.

194. Chestnut DH, Owen OL, Bates JN, et al: Continuous infusion epidural analgesia during labor: A randomized double-blind comparison of 0.0625% bupivacaine/0.0002% fentanyl versus 0.125% bupivacaine. *Anesthesiology* 1988; 68:754.

195. Leigh J, Fearnley SJ, Lupprian KG: Intrathecal diamorphine during laparotomy in a patient with advanced multiple sclerosis. *Anaesthesia* 1990; 43:640.

196. Berger JM, Outell R: Intrathecal morphine in conjunction

with a combined spinal and general anesthetic in a patient with multiple sclerosis. *Anesthesiology* 1987; 66:400.

197. Stenuit J, Marchand P: Les sequelles de rachi-anaesthesia. *Acta Neurol Belg* 1968; 68-626.

198. Bamford C, Sibley W, Laguna J: Anesthesia in multiple sclerosis. *Can J Neurol Sci* 1978; 5:41.

199. Schapiro K: Is lumbar puncture harmful in multiple sclerosis? *J Neurol Neurosurg Psychiatry* 1959; 22:138.

200. Cohen EN: Distribution of local anesthetic agents in the neuraxis of the dog. *Anesthesiology* 1968; 29:1002.

201. Bromage PR: Mechanism of action of extradural analgesia. *Br J Anaesth* 1975; 47:199.

202. Tui C, Preiss AL, Barchan I, et al: Local nervous tissue changes following spinal anesthesia in experimental animals. *J Pharmacol Exp Ther* 1944; 81:209.

203. Egbert LD, Tamersoy K, Deas TC: Pulmonary function during spinal anesthesia: The mechanism of cough depression. *Anesthesiology* 1961; 22:882.

204. Harrop-Griffiths AW, Ravalia A, Browne DA, et al: Regional anaesthesia and cough effectiveness. *Anaesthesia* 1991; 46:11.

205. Azar I: The response of patients with neuromuscular disorders to the muscle relaxants: A review. *Anesthesiology* 1984; 61:173.

206. Huxtable R: Cardiac pharmacology and cardiomyopathy in Friedrichs ataxia. *J Can Sci Neurol* 1978; 5:83.

207. Levine MC, Michaels RM: Pregnancy and amyotrophic lateral sclerosis. *Ann Neurol* 1977; 1:408.

208. Huston JW, Lingenfelder J, Mulder DW, et al: Pregnancy complicated by amyotrophic lateral sclerosis. *Am J Obstet Gynecol* 1956; 72:93.

209. Huston JW, Lingenfelder J, Mulder DW, et al: Pregnancy complicated by amyotrophic lateral sclerosis. *Am J Obstet Gynecol* 1956; 72:93.

210. Cohen BS, Felsenthal G: Peripheral nervous system disorders and pregnancy, in Goldstein PJ (ed): *Neurological Disorders of Pregnancy*. Mt Kisco, NY, Futura Publishing, 1986, p 167.

211. Carter GT, Bonekat HW, Milio L: Successful pregnancies in the presence of spinal muscular atrophy: Two case reports. *Arch Phys Med Rehabil* 1994; 75:229.

212. Rosenbaum KJ, Neigh JT, Strobel GE: Sensitivity to nondepolarizing muscle relaxants in amyotrophic lateral sclerosis: Report of two cases. *Anesthesiology* 1971; 35:358.

213. Harding AE, Thomas PK: The clinical features of hereditary motor and sensory neuropathy types I and II. *Brain* 1980; 103:259.

214. Rudnik-Schoneborn S, Rohrig D, Nicholson G, et al: Pregnancy and delivery in Charcot-Marie-Tooth disease type 1. *Neurology* 1993; 43:2011.

215. Pollock M, Nukada H, Kritchevsky M: Exacerbation of Charcot-Marie-Tooth disease in pregnancy. *Neurology* 1982; 32:1311.

216. Brian JE, Bayles GD, Quirk G, et al: Anesthetic management for cesarean section of a patient with Charcot-Marie-Tooth disease. *Anesthesiology* 1987; 66:410.

217. Richards WC: Anaesthesia and serum creatine phosphokinase levels in patients with Duchennes pseudohypertrophic muscular dystrophy. *Anaesth Intensive Care* 1972; 1:150.

218. Byrne DL, Chappatte OA, Spencer GT, et al: Pregnancy complicated by Charcot-Marie-Tooth disease, requiring intermittent ventilation. *Br J Obstet Gynaecol* 1992; 99:79.

219. Beach TP, Stone WA, Hamelberg W: Circulatory collapse following succinylcholine: Report of a patient with diffuse lower motor neuron disease. *Anesth Analg* 1971; 50:431.

220. Roelofse JA, Skipton EA: Anaesthesia for abdominal hysterectomy in Charcot-Marie-Tooth disease. *S Afr Med J* 1985; 67:605.

221. Hurwitz ES, Holman RC, Nelson DB, et al: National surveillance for Guillain-Barré syndrome: January 1978-March 1979. *Neurology* 1983; 33:150.

222. Hurley TJ, Brunson AD, Archer RL, et al: Landry-Guillain-Barré Strohl syndrome in pregnancy: Report of three cases treated with plasmapheresis. *Obstet Gynecol* 1991; 78:482.

223. Laufenberg HF, Sirus SR: Guillain-Barré syndrome in pregnancy. *Am Fam Physician* 1989; 39:147.

224. Nelson LH, McLean WT: Management of Landry-Guillain-Barré syndrome in pregnancy. *Obstet Gynecol* 1985; 65(3):25S.

225. Osler L, Sidell AD: The Guillain-Barré syndrome. The need for exact diagnostic criteria. *N Engl J Med* 1960; 262:964.

226. Raven H: The Landry-Guillain-Barré syndrome. *Acta Neurol Scand Suppl* 1967; 30:1.

227. Lichtenfeld P: Autonomic dysfunction in Guillain-Barré syndrome. *Am J Med* 1971; 50:72.

228. Graham JG: Neurological complications of pregnancy and anaesthesia. *Clin Obstet Gynecol* 1982; 9:333.

229. Elstein M, Legg NJ, Murphy M, et al: Guillain-Barré syndrome in pregnancy. *Anaesthesia* 1971; 26:216.

230. Rudolph JH, Norris RH, Garvey PH, et al: The Landry-Guillain-Barré syndrome in pregnancy: A review. *Obstet Gynecol* 1965; 26:265.

231. Sudo N, Weingold AB: Obstetric aspects of the Guillain-Barré syndrome. *Obstet Gynecol* 1975; 45:39.

232. Nelson LH, McLean WT: Management of Landry-Guillain-Barré syndrome in pregnancy. *Obstet Gynecol* 1985; 65:258.

233. Bravo RH, Katz M, Inturrisi M, et al: Obstetric management of Landry-Guillain-Barré syndrome. *Am J Obstet Gynecol* 1982; 142:714.

234. McGrady EM: Management of labour and delivery in a patient with Guillain-Barré syndrome. *Anaesthesia* 1987; 42:899.

235. Steiner I, Argon Z, Cahan C, et al: Guillain-Barré syndrome after epidural anesthesia: Direct nerve root damage may trigger disease. *Neurology* 1985; 35:1473.

236. Gautier PE, Pierre PA, Van Obbergh LJ, et al: Guillain-Barré syndrome after obstetrical epidural analgesia. *Reg Anaesth* 1989; 14:251.

237. Feldman JM: Cardiac arrest after succinylcholine administration in a pregnant patient recovered from Guillain-Barré syndrome. *Anesthesiology* 1990; 72:942.

238. Leiberman JR, Cohen A, Wiznitzer A, et al: Cesarean section by local anesthesia in patients with familial dysautonomia. *Am J Obstet Gynecol* 1991; 165:110.

239. Pearson J, Pytel B, Grover-Johnson N, et al: Quantitative studies of dorsal root ganglia and neuropathologic observation on spinal cords in familial dysautonomia. *Neurol Sci* 1978; 35:77.

240. Goodal G, Gillow SE, Atlon H: Decreased noradrenaline synthesis in familial dysautonomia. *J Clin Invest* 1971; 50:2734.

241. Axelrod FB, Abularrage JJ: Familial dysautonomia: A prospective study of survival. *J Pediatr* 1982; 101:234.

242. Porges RF, Axelrod FB, Richards M: Pregnancy in familial dysautonomia. *Am J Obstet Gynecol* 1978; 132:485.

243. Pearson J: Familial dysautonomia (a brief review). *J Auton Nerv Syst* 1979; 1:119.

244. Ziegler MG, Lake R, Kopin IJ: Deficient sympathetic nervous responses in familial dysautonomia. *N Engl J Med* 1976; 294:630.

245. Axelrod FB, Donenfeld RF, Danziger F, et al: Anesthesia in familial dysautonomia. *Anesthesiology* 1988; 68-631.

246. Axelrod FB, Nachtigal R, Dancis J: Familial dysautonomia: Diagnosis, pathogenesis and management, in Shulman I (ed): *Advances in Pediatrics*, Chicago, Year Book Publishers, 1974, pp 75-96.

247. Beilin B, Maayan C, Vatashsky E, et al: Fentanyl anesthesia in familial dysautonomia. *Anesth Analg* 1985; 64-72.

248. Edelman NH, Cherniack NS, Lahiri S: The effects of abnormal sympathetic nervous function upon ventilating response to hypoxia. *J Clin Invest* 1970; 41:1153.

249. Filler J, Smith AA, Stone S, et al: Respiratory control in familial dysautonomia. *J Pediatr* 1965; 66:509.

250. Baraka A, Noueihid R, Hajj S: Intrathecal injection of morphine for obstetric analgesia. *Anesthesiology* 1981; 54:136.

251. Abboud TK, Shnider SM, Dailey PA, et al: Intrathecal administration of hyperbaric morphine for the relief of pain in labour. *Br J Anaesth* 1985; 56:1351.

252. Meridy HW, Creighton RE: General anesthesia in eight patients with familial dysautonomia. *Can Anaesth Soc J* 1971; 18:563.

253. Pulst S: Prenatal diagnosis of the neurofibromatoses. *Clin Perinatol* 1990; 17:829.

254. Humble RM: Phaeochromocytoma neurofibromatosis and pregnancy. *Anaesthesia* 1967; 22:296.

255. Swapp GH, Main RA: Neurofibromatosis in pregnancy. *Br J Dermatol* 1973; 88:431.

256. Schimke RN, Hartmann WH, Prout TE, et al: Syndrome of bilateral pheochromocytoma, medullary thyroid carcinoma and multiple neuromas. *N Engl J Med* 1968; 279:1.

257. Bourke E, Gatenby PBB: Renal artery dysplasia with hypertension in neurofibromatosis. *Br Med J* 1971; 3:681.

258. Fisher MD: Anesthetic difficulties in neurofibromatosis. *Anaesthesia* 1975; 3:648.

259. Manser J: Abnormal responses in Von Recklinghausen's disease. *Br J Anaesth* 1970; 42:183.

260. Magbagbeola JAO: Abnormal responses with muscle relaxants in a patient with Von Recklinghausen's disease (multiple neurofibromatosis). *Br J Anaesth* 1970; 42:710.

261. Baraka A: Myasthenia response to muscle relaxants in Von Recklinghausen's disease. *Br J Anaesth* 1974; 46:701.

262. Strauss S, Pansky M, Lewinsohn G: Hemorrhagic pheochromocytoma in a pregnant patient with neurofibromatosis. *J Ultrasound Med* 1990; 9:165.

263. Cobb CA, Youmans JR: Sarcomas and neoplasms of blood, in Youmans JR (ed): *Neurological Surgery*, ed 3. Philadelphia, WB Saunders, 1990, pp 3153-3158.

264. Nibbelink DW, Peters BH, McCormick WF: On the association for pheochromocytoma and cerebellar hemangioblastoma. *Neurology* 1969; 19:455.

265. Matthews AJ, Halshaw J: Epidural anaesthesia in von Hippel-Lindau disease. *Anaesthesia* 1986; 41:853.

266. Joffe D, Robbins R, Benjamin A: Caesarean section and phaeochromocytoma resection in a patient with von Hippel-Lindau disease. *Can J Anaesth* 1993; 40:870.

267. Brooke MH: *A Clinician's View of Neuromuscular Diseases*, ed 2. Baltimore, Williams & Wilkins, 1986, p 158.

268. Stackhouse R, Chelmow D, Dattel BJ: Anesthetic complications in a pregnant patient with nemaline myopathy. *Anesth Analg* 1994; 79:1195.

269. Dresner DL, Ali HH: Anaesthetic management of a patient with facioscapulohumeral muscular dystrophy. *Br J Anaesth* 1989; 62:331.

270. Hudgson P, Gardner-Medwin D, Fulthorpe JJ, et al: Nemaline myopathy. *Neurology* 1967; 17:1125.

271. Brownell AKW, Paasuke RT, Elash A, et al: Malignant hyperthermia in Duchenne muscular dystrophy. *Anesthesiology* 1983; 58:180.

272. Sethna NF, Rockoff MA, Worthen HM, et al: Anesthesia-related complications in children with Duchenne muscular dystrophy. *Anesthesiology* 1988; 68:462.

273. Smith CL, Bush GH: Anaesthesia and progressive muscular dystrophy. *Br J Anaesth* 1985; 57:1113.

274. Cobham IG, Davis HS: Anesthesia for muscular dystrophy patients. *Anesth Analg* 1964; 43:22.

275. Aldridge LM: Anaesthetic problems in myotonic dystrophy. *Br J Anaesth* 1985; 57:1119.

276. Cope DK, Miller JN: Local and spinal anesthesia for cesarean section in a patient with myotonic dystrophy. *Anesth Analg* 1986; 65:687.

277. Castano J, Pares N: Anaesthesia for major abdominal surgery in a patient with myotonia dystrophica. *Br J Anaesth* 1987; 59:1629.

278. Fall LH, Young WW, Power JA, et al: Severe congestive heart failure and cardiomyopathy as a complication of myotonic dystrophy in pregnancy. *Obstet Gynecol* 1990; 76:481.

279. Speedy H: Exaggerated physiological responses to propofol in myotonic dystrophy. *Br J Anaesth* 1990; 64:110.

280. Blumgart CA, Hughes DG, Redfern N: Obstetric anesthesia in dystrophia myotonica. *Br J Anaesth* 1990; 64:26.

281. Dodds TM, Haney MF, Appleton FM: Management of peripartum congestive heart failure using continuous arteriovenous hemofiltration in a patient with myotonic dystrophy. *Anesthesiology* 1991; 75:907.

282. Munsat TL: Therapy of myotonia: A double-blind evaluation of diphenylhydantoin, procainamide and placebo. *Neurology* 1967; 17:359.

283. Hilliard GD, Harris RE, Gilstrap LC et al: Myotonic muscular dystrophy in pregnancy. *South J Med* 1991; 70:446.

284. Sarnat HB, O'Connor T, Byrne PA: Clinical effect of myotonic dystrophy on pregnancy and the neonate. *Am Neurol* 1976; 33:459.

285. Hopkins A, Wray S: The effect of pregnancy on dystrophia myotonia. *Neurology* 1967; 17:166.

286. Levine AB, Eddleman KA, Chitkara U, et al: Congenital myotonic dystrophy: An often unsuspected cause of severe polyhydramnios. *Prenatal Diagnosis* 1991; 11:111.

287. Afifi AM, Bhatia AR, Eyal F: Hydrops fetalis associated with congenital myotonic dystrophy. *Am J Obstet Gynecol* 1992; 166:929.

288. Hsu CD, Feng TI, Crawford TO, et al: Unusual fetal movement in congenital myotonic dystrophy. *Fetal Diagn Ther* 1993; 8:200.

289. Sholl JS, Hughey MJ, Hirschmann RA: Myotonic muscular dystrophy associated with ritodrine tocolysis. *Am J Obstet Gynecol* 1985; 151:83.

290. Webb D, Muir F, Faulkner J, et al: Myotonia dystrophica: Obstetric complications. *Am J Obstet Gynecol* 1978; 132:265.

291. Ravin M, Newmark Z, Saviello G: Myotonia dystrophia—An anesthetic hazard: Two case reports. *Anesth Analg* 1975; 54:216.

292. Matthews NC, Corser G: Epidural fentanyl for shaking in obstetrics. *Anaesthesia* 1988; 43:783.

293. Sevarino FB, Johnson MD, Lema MJ, et al: The effect of epidural sufentanil on shivering and body temperature in the parturient. *Anesth Analg* 1989; 68:530.

294. Shore RN, MacLachlan TB: Pregnancy with myotonic dystrophy: course, complications and management. *Obstet Gynecol* 1971; 38:448.

295. Hook R, Anderson EF, Noto P: Anesthetic management of a parturient with myotonia atrophica. *Anesthesiology* 1975; 43:689.

296. Harris MNE: Extradural anaesthesia and dystrophica myotonia. *Anaesthesia* 1984; 39:1032.

297. Mitchell MM, Ali HH, Savarese JJ: Myotonia and neuromuscular blocking agents. *Anesthesiology* 1978; 49:44.

298. Bouly A, Nathan N, Feiss P: Propofol in myotonic dystrophy. *Anaesthesia* 1991; 46:705.

299. Paterson IS: Generalized myotonia following suxamethonium: Case report. *Br J Anaesth* 1962; 34:340.

300. Thiel RE: The myotonic response to suxamethonium. *Br J Anaesth* 1967; 39:815.

301. Azar r I: The response of patients with neuromuscular disorders to muscle relaxants: A review. *Anesthesiology* 1984; 61:173.

302. Mudge BJ, Taylor RB, Vanderspek AFL: Perioperative hazards in myotonic dystrophy. *Anaesthesia* 1980; 35:492.

303. Vaniet TM: Dystrophia myotonic in childhood. *Br Med J* 1960; 2:1284.

304. Clark C, Kelly KF, Smith N, et al: Prenatal diagnosis for dystrophia myotonic using the polymerase chain reaction. *Prenat Diagn* 1991; 11:467.

305. Rolbin SH, Levinson G, Shnider SM, et al: Anesthetic consideration for myasthenia gravis and pregnancy. *Anesth Analg* 1978; 57:44.

306. Usubiaga JE, Wikinski JA, Morales RL, et al: Interaction of intravenously administered procaine, lidocaine and succinylcholine in anesthetized subject. *Anesth Analg* 1967; 46:39.

307. Hughes SC: Anesthesia for the pregnant patient with neuromuscular disease, in Shnider SM, Levinson G (eds): *Anesthesia for Obstetrics,* ed 2. Baltimore, Williams & Wilkins, 1987, pp 425-426.

308. Bell CF, Florence AM, Hunter JM, et al: Atracurium in the myasthenic patient. *Anaesthesia* 1984; 39-961.

309. Cohen BA, London RS, Goldstein PJ: Myasthenia gravis and preeclampsia. *Obstet Gynecol* (Suppl 1) 1976; 48:35S.

310. George WK, Haan CL: Calcium and magnesium in myasthenia gravis. *Lancet* 1962; 2:561.

311. Bashuk RG, Krendel DA: Myasthenia gravis presenting as weakness after magnesium administration. *Muscle Nerve* 1990; 13:708.

312. Plauche WC: Myasthenia gravis in pregnancy: An update. *Am J Obstet Gynecol* 1979; 135:691.

313. Plauche WC: Myasthenia gravis. *Clin Obstet Gynecol* 1983; 26:592.

314. Nohria V, Oakes WJ: Chiari I malformation: A review of 43 patients. *Pediatr Neurosurg* 1990-91; 16:222.

315. Payner TD, Prenger E, Berger TS, et al: Acquired Chiari malformations: incidence, diagnosis, and management. *Neurosurgery* 1994; 34:429.

316. Paul KS, Lye RH, Strang FA, et al: Arnold-Chiari malformation. *J Neurosurg* 1983; 58:183.

317. Olivero WC, Dink DH: Chiari I malformation with traumatic syringomyelia and spontaneous resolution: Case report and literature review. *Neurosurgery* 1992; 30:758.

318. Cahan LD, Bentson JR: Considerations in the diagnosis and treatment of syringomyelia and the Chiari malformation. *J Neurosurg* 1982; 57:24.

319. Isu T, Iwasaki Y, Akino M, et al: Hydrosyringomyelia associated with a Chiari I malformation in children and adolescents. *Neurosurgery* 1990; 26:591.

320. Gardner WJ: Hydrodynamic mechanism of syringomyelia: Its relationship to myelocele. *J Neurol Neurosurg Psychiatry* 1965; 28:247.

321. Dyste GN, Menezes AH, Vangilder JC: Symptomatic Chiari malformations: An analysis of presentation, management, and long-term outcome. *J Neurosurg* 1989; 71:159.

322. Menezes AH, Smoker WRK, Dyste GN: Syringomyelia, Chiari malformation and hydromyelia, in Youmans TR (ed): *Neurological Surgery,* ed 3, Philadelphia, WB Saunders, 1990, pp 1421-1459.

323. Roelofse JA, Shipton EA, Nell AC: Anaesthesia for caesarian section in a patient with syringomyelia. *S Afr Med J* 1984; 65:736.

324. Umbach I, Heilporn A: Review article: Post-spinal cord injury syringomyelia. *Paraplegia* 1991; 29:219.

325. Rossier AB, Foo D, Shillito J, et al: Posttraumatic cervical syringomyelia: incidence, clinical presentation, electrophysiological studies, syrinx protein and results of conservative and operative treatment. *Brain* 1985; 108:439.

326. Baker AS, Dove J: Progress scoliosis as the first presenting sign of syringomyelia. *J Bone Joint Surg* 1983; 65:472.

327. Bertren SL, Dravaric DM, Roberts JM: Scoliosis in syringomyelia. *Orthopaedics* 1989; 2:335.

328. Hullander RM, Bogard TD, Leivers D, et al: Chiari I malformation presenting as recurrent spinal headache. *Anesth Analg* 1992; 75:1025.

329. McComish PB, Bodley PO: Anesthesia for surgery of the posterior fossa. *Anesthesia for Neurological Surgery.* Chicago, Year Book Medical, 1971, pp 218-241.

330. Zalzal GH: Stridor and airway compromise. *Pediatr Clin North Am* 1989; 36:1389.

11 Respiratory Disease

Mark C. Norris and *Linda Chan*

RESPIRATORY CHANGES DURING PREGNANCY

Pregnancy induces significant anatomic and physiologic alterations in maternal respiratory function and gas exchange. Some of the changes that accompany normal pregnancy mimic pathologic states. Capillary engorgement of the respiratory mucosa can simulate inflammation by causing hyperemia and edema throughout the nasopharynx and tracheobronchial tree. These changes may be exacerbated by upper respiratory tract infection, fluid overload, or the edema associated with preeclampsia.[1] Vascular engorgement of the pulmonary circulation increases lung markings on chest roentgenograms and can resemble mild congestive heart failure.[1]

During pregnancy, up to 70% of normal women will perceive shortness of breath (dyspnea).[2-5] Fifteen percent notice this symptom in the first trimester and almost half report dyspnea before 19 weeks' gestation. By 31 weeks, 76% of women complain of dyspnea.[2] Cugell et al reported no correlation between changes in pulmonary function tests and the severity of dyspnea during pregnancy.[5]

Anatomic changes

Roentgenogram studies during pregnancy show a 4-cm elevation of the diaphragm and a 2.1-cm increase in the transverse diameter of the chest. The subcostal angle increases progressively from 68.5° in early pregnancy to 103.5° in late gestation. The increase in the subcostal angle occurs early, before significant uterine enlargement, and returns to normal within a few weeks after delivery.[6] Although the diaphragm is displaced upward during late gestation by the enlarging gravid uterus, its movement is not hindered. Indeed, diaphragmatic excursion with tidal breathing during pregnancy is greater than after delivery.[7]

Lung volumes

Progressive changes in lung volumes begin in the fifth month of pregnancy.[5,8,9] By term, reductions in both expiratory reserve volume (ERV) and residual volume (RV) decrease functional residual capacity (FRC) 18% to 25%.[5,10,11] These changes follow the upward displacement of the diaphragm by the enlarging uterus. Concurrently, to compensate for the smaller FRC, inspiratory capacity and inspiratory reserve volume increase. Investigators report slight increases or decreases in vital capacity (VC) and total lung capacity (TLC). However, the bulk of available data suggests that they remain unchanged. With a few exceptions, published reports of measurements of lung volumes in pregnancy agree with the aforementioned findings.[5-15] Figure 11-1 summarizes the changes in pulmonary volumes and capacities found in term pregnancy.

Airway function and pulmonary mechanics

Large airway (diameter > 2 mm) function, as measured by forced expiratory volume in one second (FEV_1), or the FEV_1 to forced vital capacity (FVC) ratio, does not change during pregnancy.[5,9,13-17] Lung compliance also remains unaltered.[10] However, total lung resistance (R_L) and small airway function do change. R_L decreases late in pregnancy. Approximately 80% of this decline results from changes in small airway resistance, presumably due to the bronchodilating effect of progesterone.[10,15]

Closing volume (CV), the lung volume below which small airways (diameter < 2 mm) in the dependent portion of the lung collapse, occurs well below the FRC in nonpregnant women.[18] ERV and FRC fall during normal pregnancy.[8,11,13,16-20] Late in gestation, airway closure occurs either close to or above FRC. As a result, atelectasis may occur during tidal breathing. The consequent ventilation/perfusion mismatching may impair arterial oxygenation.

Pulmonary diffusion capacity

Pulmonary diffusion capacity, as measured by carbon monoxide, appears unchanged[21,22] or elevated[23] during early pregnancy. By 24 to 27 weeks' gestation, the diffusing capacity decreases to a new equilibrium and remains depressed until term. Postpartum, diffusion capacity increases slightly over near term values.[23]

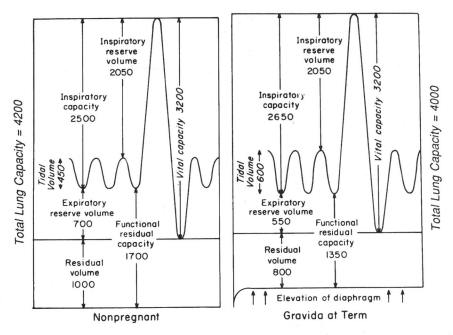

Fig. 11-1 Pulmonary volumes and capacities during pregnancy. (From Bonica JJ (ed): *Principles and Practice of Obstetric Analgesia and Anesthesia,* vol 1. Philadelphia, FA Davis, 1967, p 24.)

Pulmonary ventilation

Resting pulmonary ventilation increases,[4,5] peaking as early as the second or third month of gestation.[24,25] At term, minute ventilation rises 48% above nonpregnant rate. Oxygen consumption increases 21% and basal metabolic rate only 14% (Fig. 11-2).[4] Since respiratory rate remains constant during pregnancy, the increase in minute ventilation occurs because of a 40% increase in tidal volume[4,5] The plasma concentration of progesterone, a known respiratory stimulant,[26-28] rises significantly during gestation and may cause the hyperventilation of pregnancy.[4,5] Figure 11-3 summarizes the changes in pulmonary function occurring during pregnancy, before labor.

During labor, anxiety, pain and "controlled deep-breathing patterns" during uterine contractions can exaggerate the hyperventilation of pregnancy.[29-31] Some investigators report detrimental fetal effects from excessive maternal hyperventilation during labor.[32-34] Maternal hyperventilation-induced hypocarbia may decrease uterine blood flow as well as shift the O_2 dissociation curve to the left. It may also cause fetal hypoxemia and acidosis.[32,33] Pain relief lowers maternal oxygen consumption by reducing tidal volume and minute ventilation.[30,35,36]

Acid/base balance

The hyperventilation of pregnancy decreases the mean alveolar Pco_2 (P_Aco_2) and subsequently arterial Pco_2 ($Paco_2$) to 27 to 32 mm Hg.[24,25,37-40] Some investigators report a gradual decrease in $Paco_2$ beginning early in pregnancy.[37,38] Others found a low but constant level throughout gestation.[25,39] Painful labor incites a further fall in $Paco_2$,[41-43] and values as low as 17 mm Hg have been reported.[29] The mean $Paco_2$ during normal labor is 25 mm Hg.[30] When labor pain is abolished with regional analgesia, $Paco_2$ remains at its normal pregnancy baseline.[30,43]

The sensitivity of the respiratory center to CO_2 is greatly increased in pregnancy. Each 1 mm Hg rise in $Paco_2$ will increase minute ventilation 6 L/min instead of the 1.5 L/min rise seen in the nonpregnant state.[4]

The hyperventilation of pregnancy also induces a secondary increase in arterial Po_2. Maternal Pao_2 ranges between 106 and 108 mm Hg in the first trimester, and between 101 and 104 mm Hg in the last trimester.[25,39] Near term, maternal posture influences Pao_2, which may fall in the supine position.[44,45] The alveolar-arterial oxygen gradient (A-ao_2) is greater than 20 mm Hg in almost half of parturients in the supine position.[44] Underventilation secondary to airway closure above FRC probably causes this supine hypoxemia and widened A-ao_2 gradient.[44]

The pH of arterial blood reflects metabolic compensation for the maternal hyperventilation-induced respiratory alkalosis. Arterial pH generally ranges from 7.40 to 7.47.[24,25,38-40] The parturient

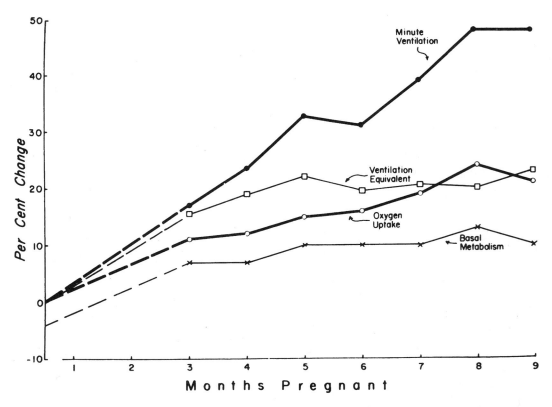

Fig. 11-2 Percent changes in minute ventilation, oxygen uptake, basal metabolism and the ventilatory equivalent for oxygen at monthly intervals throughout gestation. (From Prowse CM, Gaensler ES: *Anesthesiology* 1965; 26:384.)

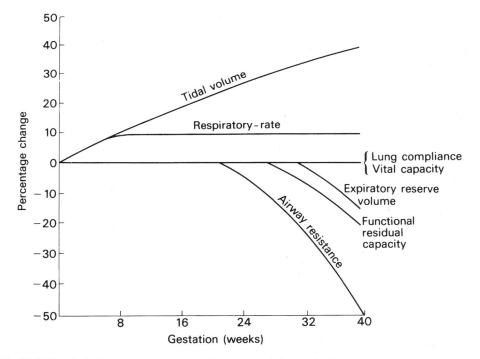

Fig 11-3 Trends in the percentage changes in aspects of the mechanics of ventilation during pregnancy, before the start of labor. (From Crawford JS (ed): *Principles and Practice of Obstetric Anesthesia,* ed 5. Oxford, Blackwell Scientific Publications, 1984, p 25.)

maintains this relatively normal arterial pH by increasing renal excretion of bicarbonate. The plasma bicarbonate falls to 21 to 18 mEq/L with a resultant base deficit of 3 to 4 mEq/L.[25,37-39] Progressive metabolic acidosis develops during labor in patients without adequate pain relief.[42,43,46-49] Alleviation of labor pain with effective epidural analgesia prevents this occurrence.[43]

Anesthetic implications of respiratory changes

Oxygenation. The respiratory changes that accompany pregnancy have important anesthetic implications. Two changes, the smaller FRC and the greater minute ventilation, significantly alter the rate and degree of nitrogen washout in parturients. These changes decrease the amount of nitrogen in the lungs and hasten its washout when the parturient breaths 100% oxygen. With a Magill breathing system, the time required to achieve 2% endtidal nitrogen concentration decreases progressively throughout pregnancy from 130 seconds in nonpregnant women to 104 seconds in the second trimester to 80 seconds in the third trimester (Fig. 11-4).[50] Using a circle breathing system, less time also is needed to achieve 5% end-tidal nitrogen.[51] End-tidal nitrogen falls to 5% after 110.8 ± 35.7 seconds in nonpregnant women but after only 54.5 ± 17.8 seconds in parturients past 18 weeks' gestation. These studies suggest that with either the Magill or circle breathing systems, parturients require only 2 minutes of 100% oxygen breathing to obtain adequate denitrogenation.[52] Although denitrogenation may be more that 95% complete after 2 to 3 minutes of oxygen breathing, a longer period of preoxygenation may still increase the body's oxygen stores and prolong the patient's tolerance for apnea.[53,54]

Lung oxygen stores and whole-body oxygen consumption are the main determinants of the rate at which hypoxemia develops during apnea. In parturients, a smaller FRC coupled with an increase in oxygen consumption markedly increases the risk of hypoxemia with maternal apnea. Critical hypoxemia can occur with alarming speed during induction of general anesthesia. Oxygen tension falls significantly more rapidly during apnea in parturients (139 ± 1 mm Hg/min) than in nonpregnant women (58 ± 8 mm Hg/min).[55] After 3 minutes denitrogenation, nonpregnant patients may tolerate over 10 minutes of apnea before oxygen saturation decreases below 90%.[56,57] Parturients desaturate much more rapidly. Baraka et al measured the time to 95% SaO_2 in pregnant and nonpregnant women.[58] Each group breathed 100% oxygen for 3 minutes. After induction and intubation, the endotracheal tube was left open to room air. In the pregnant women, oxygen saturation fell below 95% significantly faster than in the nonpregnant women (Fig. 11-5).

The decrease in FRC also facilitates the uptake of inhalation anesthetics. This effect, coupled with the 30% to 40% decrease in anesthetic requirement (MAC) that accompanies parturition,[59,60] places the parturient at risk for rapid and possibly unexpected induction of anesthesia.

Ventilation. Normally, the partial pressure of arterial CO_2 exceeds end tidal pco_2 by 3 to 5 mm Hg. This relationship changes significantly during pregnancy. Even early in gestation, the gradient between arterial and end tidal CO_2 narrows and $paco_2$ is only 0.5 mm Hg higher than end-tidal CO_2.[61] By the end of the first trimester the end-tidal CO_2 approximates $paco_2$. At term, the capnogram shows a steep phase III slope and end-tidal CO_2 can exceed mean alveolar (and arterial) pco_2 (Fig. 11-6).[62] Under general anesthesia, 50% of parturients have a higher end-tidal CO_2 than $paco_2$.[62] This trend reverses with delivery and $paco_2$ rises from 0.03 mm Hg to 0.78 mm Hg

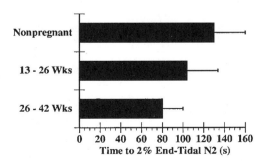

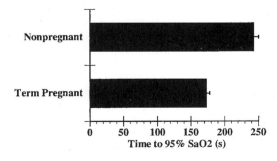

Fig. 11-4 Pregnancy speeds preoxygenation. Women breathed 100% oxygen via a tight fitting face mask. Time to 2% end-tidal nitrogen decreases progressively with increasing gestation. (Data from Byrne F, et al: *Anaesthesia* 1987; 148).

Fig. 11-5 Parturients are less tolerant of apnea than nonpregnant women. Subjects underwent rapid sequence induction and intubation after 3 minutes preoxygenation. Then the endotracheal tube was left open to room air until oxygen saturation fell to 95%. (Data from Baraka AS, et al: *Anesth Analg* 1992; 75:757).

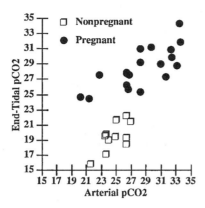

Fig. 11-6 Pregnancy narrows the gradient between arterial and end-tidal CO_2. (Data from Shankar KB, et al: *Anaesthesia* 1986; 41:698).

above end-tidal CO_2 by 25 minutes postpartum.[62] Still, up to 31% of women have higher end-tidal than arterial CO_2 during general anesthesia for postpartum tubal ligation.[63] Regression analysis suggests the relationship between arterial and end-tidal CO_2 returns to normal by eight days after delivery.[63]

Mechanical hyperventilation to a $paco_2$ of 22 mm Hg in anesthetized gravid ewes lowers fetal carotid po_2 by 8 mm Hg. Prolonged maternal hyperventilation may produce fetal asphyxia with severe hypoxemia and metabolic acidosis.[64] Maintaining maternal arterial or end-tidal CO_2 near 30 mm Hg will avoid the deleterious effects of mechanical hyperventilation on fetal oxygenation. Mechanical hyperventilation also can worsen fetal acid-base status by limiting maternal cardiac output and therefore placental blood flow.[65]

PREGNANCY AND PREEXISTING RESPIRATORY DISEASE

Even women with severe respiratory impairment adapt well to the demands of pregnancy. Unlike the healthy parturient, whose minute ventilation increases to a level well above that needed to satisfy her increased metabolic demands, the parturient with respiratory disease increases her minute ventilation only to match, not to exceed, her metabolic needs.[12] In the following sections of this chapter, we discuss the obstetric and anesthetic implications of a variety of respiratory diseases and problems that may occur concurrently with pregnancy.

Asthma

Incidence and classification. Asthma, the most common obstructive pulmonary disease seen in pregnancy, occurs in about 5% of adults in the United States[66] and complicates between 0.4 to

1.3% of pregnancies. [67-71] Hernandez et al reported a 0.15% to 0.2% incidence of status asthmaticus in his pregnant population.[69]

Asthma is a heterogeneous disease that can be broadly classified into two groups: allergic (extrinsic) and idiosyncratic (intrinsic). In allergic asthma serum levels of IgE increase; eosinophilia of the peripheral blood and bronchial secretions occurs. Skin reactions to intradermal injection of airborne antigens are positive and the bronchospastic response to inhalation allergens develops rapidly. These patients frequently have a personal or family history of atopic dermatitis and rhinitis. Patients with idiosyncratic asthma have a negative personal or family history of allergy, negative skin tests, normal serum IgE, and their symptoms cannot be classified on the basis of a defined immunologic mechanism. They develop bronchospasm following upper respiratory tract infection or from other undefined causes. Many patients will have features of each category and fall into a mixed group.[66]

Asthma represents a special type of airway inflammation causing smooth muscle spasm, microvascular leakage and bronchial hyperresponsiveness. These changes lead to intermittent coughing and wheezing. The chronic inflammatory changes of asthma are present even in cases of mild asthma. Bronchial biopsy specimens and lavage samples show epithelial shedding and multiple inflammatory cells including eosinophils and lymphocytes. Of these cells, the eosinophils are especially characteristic of asthma; they may release basic proteins that are especially toxic to airway epithelial cells. The intensity of bronchial hyperresponsiveness is related to the extent of airway inflammation and correlates with the severity of the disease and the need for treatment. Asthmatic patients typically exhibit a biphasic response to airway stimulation (Fig. 11-7). The immediate response, acute, stimulus-induced, bronchospasm, is relieved by β_2-agonists. A secondary, delayed response occurs 6 to 8 hours later and is characterized by edema formation and mucous secretion in addition to bronchospasm. This phase does not respond well to β_2-agonist therapy but does respond to corticosteroid or chromolyn treatment. Effective therapy of asthma must reduce airway inflammation as well as relieving acute bronchoconstriction.[72,73]

Obstetric management

Pregnancy and asthma. Uncontrolled asthma increases the risk of maternal and fetal death. The risks of growth retardation,[68,71,74-76] prematurity,[70,71,77,78] and preterm labor[79,80]; pregnancy induced-hypertension[81] also may rise. However, if maternal asthma is adequately controlled, maternal or perinatal outcome appear normal.[71,82] Poor control, while increasing fetal risk, does not always

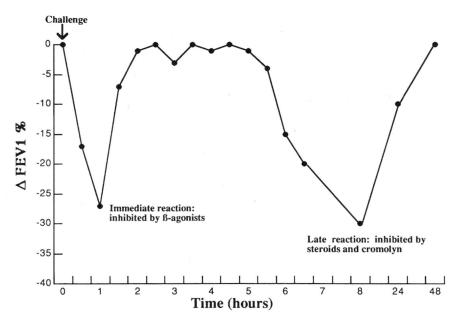

Fig. 11-7 Time course of bronchospasm following antigen challenge in asthmatic patients. The immediate, short-lived response is due to smooth muscle contraction and responds promptly to bronchodilators. The late response results from edema, inflammation, and mucous secretion as well as smooth muscle contraction. (Adapted from Pare PD, Gonzalez Montaner JS: Asthma, in Kelley WN (ed): *Textbook of Internal Medicine.* Philadelphia, JB Lippincott, 1989, pp 1873-1881).

yield a negative outcome. Good fetal outcome has followed even severe asthma-related respiratory failure.[82-84]

Pregnancy has no consistent effects on the course of asthma.[71] Gluck and Gluck summarized the effects of pregnancy on asthma in nine studies and found that symptoms improved in 36%, remained unchanged in 41%, and worsened in 23% of patients.[85] In a prospective study of 366 pregnancies in 330 women, Schatz and co-workers found that during pregnancy asthma improved in 28%, did not change in 33%, and worsened in 35% of cases.[86] Episodes of bronchospasm were significantly less frequent and less severe during the last month of pregnancy. Exacerbation of asthma occurred in 10% of women during labor and delivery. Half of these women required no treatment; some used inhaled bronchodilators. Only two of their patients required intravenous aminophylline. By 3 months after delivery, asthma reverted to its prepregnancy pattern in 73% of women. They also reported a significant concordance between the course of asthma between the first and subsequent pregnancies.

Deterioration of asthma during pregnancy may be more likely in women with severe disease.[71,75,76,85] These women may not experience the normally occurring decrease of IgE during gestation.[85] Other factors that may contribute to the deterioration of asthma during gestation include exposure to fetal antigens, decreased cell-mediated immunity, and an increased susceptibility to upper respiratory tract infection.[71,85,87] Factors that may improve the course of asthma during pregnancy include the progressive rise in the plasma cortisol,[88] a reduction of bronchomotor tone and airway resistance mediated by progesterone,[10,15,89,90] and an increase in serum cAMP inhibiting mast cell release of histamine.[85,91]

Prostaglandins may either improve or worsen the course of asthma in pregnancy. Serum concentrations of prostaglandin F_{2a} ($PGF_{2\alpha}$, a bronchoconstrictor) and prostaglandin E (PGE, a bronchodilator) both increase throughout gestation. Patients with asthma are more sensitive to the bronchoconstricting effects of $PGF_{2\alpha}$. PGE, normally a bronchodilator, can cause either bronchodilation or constriction in asthmatic subjects.[92] $PGF_{2\alpha}$ may aggravate asthma throughout pregnancy, and an increase in PGE at term may contribute to the alleviation of symptoms in the last trimester and during labor and delivery.[86,93] Exogenous $PGF_{2\alpha}$ may cause asthmatic symptoms[94] or status asthmaticus in susceptible parturients.[95,96] Consequently, one should avoid using $PGF_{2\alpha}$ to induce abortion in asthmatic women; one should use PGE, which may also cause bronchospasm in susceptible women, with caution.

Treatment of asthma during pregnancy. The medical management of asthma remains essentially unchanged by pregnancy[69-71] but now includes fetal surveillance and evaluation. Initial therapeutic goals include attempting to identify and reduce emotional stress and the exposure to known or suspected allergens and irritants. Identify specific inciting causes such as exercise, upper respiratory tract infection, the overuse of β- adrenergic antagonists, the use of aspirin or nonsteroidal antiinflammatory agents, or inadequate current therapy. Peak expiratory flow rate (PEFR) correlates with forced vital capacity (FEV_1) and normally does not change during pregnancy. PEFR can readily be measured with a portable peak flow meter. Daily measurement of PEFR can monitor therapy and provide early detection of acute asthmatic exacerbations. Each parturient with asthma should establish her own best baseline PEFR and the record PEFR every 12 hours throughout gestation. This daily record can then be evaluated at each prenatal visit. Should these daily PEFR measurements vary by more than 20%, changes in asthma therapy may be needed.[71] Optimal medical treatment may include the appropriate use of antibiotics, methylxanthines, chromones, β-adrenergic bronchodilators, supplemental oxygen, and corticosteroids. The choice of medications varies with the severity of asthma and the gestational age of the fetus. For a complete discussion of the management of asthma during pregnancy, one may study the National Institute of Health Report of the Working Group on Asthma and Pregnancy.[71]

Most asthma medications are considered safe during pregnancy.[71,78,97-101] The goals of pharmacotherapy in the asthmatic parturient are to maintain ventilation and oxygenation and prevent maternal death, respiratory failure, status asthmaticus, emergency room visits, disabling wheezing, and fetal hypoxemia or demise.[66,71] The obstetrician must closely monitor fetal well-being, especially after the second trimester, and during an acute asthma attack. External electronic fetal heart rate monitoring,[102] and ultrasound assessment of the fetal biophysical profile (presence of fetal movement, tone, breathing, and normal amniotic fluid volume),[103] provide important information about fetal status.[71]

Medical therapy of asthma varies from patient to patient depending largely on the frequency and severity of bronchospasm. Either a single drug or, more often, a combination of agents may be used. The five categories of drugs most commonly used in the treatment of asthma include methylxanthines, β-adrenergic agonists, glucocorticoids, chromones, and anticholinergics. While most asthma medications are safe for mother and fetus, some have potential adverse fetal and neonatal effects (Table 11-1).

The chromone cromolyn sodium inhibits degranulation of mast cells and the subsequent release of the chemical mediators of anaphylaxis. It may have additional similar effects on macrophages and eosinophils and also prevent neurally mediated bronchospasm. Cromolyn sodium effectively reduces the medication requirement and causes symptomatic improvement in approximately 75% of nonpregnant patients.[66,72] The drug both limits bronchial hyperresponsiveness to antigenic and other stimuli and prevents the late inflammatory response. Cromolyn is safe during pregnancy.[71,101,104]

Desensitization or immunotherapy with extracts of suspected allergens in 90 women throughout 121 pregnancies shows no increase in maternal or perinatal morbidity.[105] Anaphylaxis is a risk. While patients receiving treatments can be maintained at or slightly below their current dosages, immunotherapy should not be started during gestation.[71]

The anticholinergic atropine sulfate is a bronchodilator, but its use is limited by systemic side effects and slow onset (60 to 90 minutes).[66] Atropine has the theoretical risk of fetal tachycardia,

Table 11-1 Potential fetal and neonatal adverse effects of asthma drugs

Drug	Effect
Systemic corticosteroids	Impaired fetal growth
Theophylline	Fetal tachycardia (Maternal levels >20 μg/mL)
	Neonatal jitteriness, vomiting, tachycardia
	Neonatal levels >10 μg/mL, or maternal levels >12 μg/mL
Systemic $β_2$-agonists	Fetal tachycardia
	Neonatal tachycardia, hypoglycemia, tremor
Topical sympathomimetic decongestants	Fetal heart rate alterations attributed to uterine vasoconstriction
	Seen at high doses, perhaps only with overdose

Adapted from Report of the Working Group on Asthma and Pregnancy: Management of asthma during pregnancy, NIH Publication No 93-3279, 1993, p 14.

but little information exists concerning its chronic use during pregnancy. Ipratropium bromide, a quaternary derivative of atropine, is effective for treatment of acute exacerbations without atropine's side effects.[71] Animal studies and limited human experience suggest that anticholinergic medications are safe during pregnancy.[71]

Methyxanthines. Theophylline, a derivative of aminophylline, is the prototype methylxanthine used in the prophylaxis and treatment of asthma. This drug, an effective bronchodilator, works by an unknown mechanism. It increases cyclic AMP by preventing breakdown through inhibition of the enzyme phosphodiesterase. However, this effect, long thought to represent the primary action of theophylline, does not occur in vivo at therapeutically effective blood concentrations.[66,106] Other mechanisms by which theophylline may exert its bronchodilating effects include antagonism of the bronchoconstricting effects of adenosine.[66] The drug also has respiratory stimulating properties and augments the hypoxic ventilatory response. Other effects of theophylline include increasing the contractility of the diaphragm, improving right ventricular performance, and a mild diuretic action.[66] This drug, though commonly the first choice to treat asthma, has only weak bronchodilating effects. It does not reduce bronchial hyperresponsiveness; however it may have some antiinflammatory effects because it does inhibit the late bronchoconstriction reaction.[72]

Aminophylline is the only methylxanthine available for intravenous use, and it can be used readily in the treatment of an acute asthmatic attack. A loading dose of 6 mg/kg followed by 0.5mg/kg/hr maintenance infusion usually achieves therapeutic plasma concentrations of theophylline between 8 and 12 μg/mL.[66,71]

Theophylline is available in sustained-release formulations taken every 8 to 12 hours to a maximum dose of 900 mg per day.[107] The dose needed to achieve a therapeutic plasma concentration differs from patient to patient because individual metabolism of the drug varies widely. Theophylline is metabolized by the liver, and any changes in liver function will alter theophylline clearance.[66,107-109]

Pregnancy significantly alters the pharmacokinetics of theophylline. Renal excretion accounts for a significantly greater proportion of total theophylline elimination.[109,110] Clearance declines minimally during the first two trimesters of pregnancy but falls significantly in the third trimester.[108-110] Volume of distribution and elimination half life also increase significantly in the third trimester.[109,110] These changes can increase the risk of theophylline toxicity and may necessi-tate a reduction in drug dosage during the later part of gestation.[108] The most common symptoms of theophylline toxicity are nervousness, nausea, vomiting, anorexia, and headache. At plasma concentrations greater than 30 μg/mL, seizures and cardiac arrhythmias may occur.[66]

Theophylline readily crosses the placenta. Fetal tachycardia, neonatal jitteriness, and vomiting have been reported. However, adverse neonatal effects do not occur if maternal serum concentration does not exceed 12 μg/mL.[71] Approximately 1% or less of maternal theophylline is excreted in breast milk, a clinically insignificant amount for the newborn infant.[71]

Beta-adrenergic agonists. β-adrenergic agents dilate bronchial smooth muscle via interaction with the β_2-adrenergic receptor. The alpha and β_1-adrenergic receptors have no role in bronchial smooth muscle relaxation in humans; instead they produce many of the side effects of less β_2-selective agents. Clinically useful β-adrenergic agonists are catecholamines or derivatives of catecholamines that act directly on membrane receptors in smooth muscle. They activate adenylate cyclase, which converts adenosine triphosphate (ATP) to cyclic adenosine monophosphate (cAMP). Increased cAMP impedes the phosphorylation of myosin light-chain kinase and prevents its interaction with actin, blocking smooth muscle contraction.[111] β-adrenergic agonists also inhibit the chemical mediators of anaphylaxis, improve mucociliary transport, decrease the bronchoconstrictive effects of many airway irritants, and potentiate the bronchodilating effects corticosteroids.[111,112] However, these agents have no direct effects on the late inflammatory response.[72]

The major β-adrenergic agonists used for the treatment of asthma are metaproterenol, albuterol (salbutamol), salmeterol, terbutaline, fenoterol, isoetharine, and bitolterol mesylate. Epinephrine and isoproterenol, which are less β_2 selective, have considerable cardiac side effects.[66,111] The Collaborative Perinatal Project reported a slight increase in malformations in infants born to women who used epinephrine during pregnancy.[113] Current clinical experience does not support a teratogenic effect of epinephrine.[100,101] However, epinephrine significantly impairs uterine blood flow[114] and can cause transient fetal heart rate changes even in healthy fetuses.[115] While subcutaneous epinephrine may be used to treat severe acute exacerbations, it is not a first choice.[71]

β-agonists can be administered by aerosol, oral, subcutaneous, or intravenous routes. The onset varies with the specific drug and the route of administration. The inhaled catecholamines (epinephrine, isoproterenol, isoetharine) act within 1 to 3 minutes, peak in 5 to 15 minutes, and last 30 to 60 minutes. The inhaled catecholamine derivatives have a slower onset of bronchodilation (3 to 6 minutes), reach peak activity in 20 to 60 minutes, and remain effective for 4 to 6 hours. Salmeterol has a slightly slower onset, but it produces bronchodilation for up to 12 hours.[116] Subcutaneous epinephrine, terbutaline, fenoterol, or metaproterenol produce similar bronchodilation within a few minutes, peaking in 15 to 20 minutes. The therapeutic effects of epinephrine and fenoterol last 2 hours; metaproterenol and terbutaline last 3 to 4 hours. Orally, the drugs act within 30 minutes, peak after 1 to 2 hours, and last 3 to 6 hours. Parenterally administered β-adrenergic drugs have a rapid dose-related onset, but they vary in their duration.[111]

Inhaled β-adrenergic agonists are the primary drugs for the treatment of patients with an acute exacerbation of asthma.[117] Inhaled β-agonists are equally as effective as subcutaneous epinephrine in the treatment of acute asthma.[118,119] Intravenous β-adrenergic agonists offer no advantage over the inhalation route.[117,120] In acute asthma, combination therapy with theophylline increases the toxicity but not the efficacy of β-adrenergic agonist treatment.[117,120,121] However, adding corticosteroids to the treatment regimen is beneficial in severe exacerbations of asthma.[117,122,123]

Dosage of β-adrenergic agonists is limited by side effects: palpitations, tachycardia and tremor. Other side effects of β-agonists include restlessness, anxiety, weakness, sweating, headache, peripheral vasodilation, inhibition of uterine contractions, hyperglycemia and hypokalemia, and pulmonary edema.[111,124-126] Side effects are more common with parenteral administration when these agents are used in higher doses in the treatment of preterm labor.

Corticosteroids. Glucocorticoids are the most effective therapy available for patients with asthma.[127] These drugs have little or no direct bronchodilating actions; their beneficial effects derive mostly from their antiinflammatory functions, which reduce airway hyperreactivity.[66,127-129] Antiinflammatory effects include redistribution and reduction in the number of inflammatory cells in the circulation, blockade of bronchial hyperresponsiveness, reduction of microvascular leakage, and an inhibitory influence on the formation of leukotrienes and other metabolites of arachidonic acid. When adequate dosages are used for a sufficient time, steroids decrease mucus production and suppress the late-phase pulmonary reaction to inhaled allergen.[127] Synergism exists between corticosteroids and the β-adrenergic agonists. Corticosteroids reverse the tachyphylaxis of

β-adrenergic agonist by preventing internalization of β-adrenergic receptors and the uncoupling of those receptors from adenylate cyclase. In addition, steroid treatment restores the densities of β-adrenergic receptor, causes partial stimulation or enhancement of adenyl cyclase enzymes, and augments the bronchodilator effect of adrenergic agents. Steroids also may induce redistribution of pulmonary blood flow and improve ventilation-perfusion mismatching.[128,129] Because of their antiinflammatory actions, steroid inhalation may become first-line therapy for moderate to severe chronic asthma.[71,72,127]

The corticosteroids used in asthma are synthetic analogue of the adrenal cortical hormone hydrocortisone (cortisol), which bind to glucocorticoid receptors to produce their effects. Most of these compounds are modified to minimize binding to the mineralocorticoid receptors and the subsequent mineralocorticoid side effects. Systemically active steroid preparations may be administered via oral, topical, intramuscular or intravenous route. Oral inhalation treatment represents the most effective way to administer corticosteroids with the least risk of systemic side effects.[72] The onset of action usually requires 4 to 6 hours possibly because they act via steroid-mediated protein synthesis after transport to the cell nucleus.[128,129]

Corticosteroids, when used to treat asthma during pregnancy, do not increase the risk of congenital malformations.[71,74,78,97,98,100] Systemic corticosteroids may impair fetal growth and lower birth weight by 300 to 400 g.[71,80] Neonatal adrenal insufficiency did not occur in infants born to mothers receiving an average daily dose of 8.2 mg of prednisone during pregnancy.[78] Steroids are indicated in severe acute asthma when patients are refractory to standard bronchodilator therapy. Inhaled steroids are commonly used for maintenance therapy in patients with moderate to severe chronic asthma.[71,127] Early institution of steroid therapy in the emergency treatment of severe asthma averts respiratory failure, improving pulmonary function and clinical course, and thus reducing the need for hospitalization.[117,130,131]

When using corticosteroids in the management of acute asthma, one should begin with an intravenous loading dose of hydrocortisone 2.0 mg/kg followed by 2.0 mg/kg every 4 to 6 hours or a continuous intravenous infusion of 0.5 mg/kg/hr for 24 to 72 hours.[71] Oral prednisone, 40 to 60 mg per day, can be initiated when the patient is stabilized; this dose can be rapidly tapered over one week.[66,71] For chronic treatment, one should use the lowest possible dose or an alternate day regimen to avoid prolonged suppression of the pituitary-adrenal axis.[66,71,129] Prolonged use of oral corticosteroids may increase the risk of gestational diabetes, preeclampsia, and intrauterine growth retardation.[71,80,81] Mothers who are steroid-dependent will require supplementation with hydrocortisone during labor and delivery.[101]

Aerosolized corticosteroids are as effective as oral prednisone, and they can be used as an alternative to oral glucocorticoids in the treatment of asthma.[66,71,72,128] Commonly used inhaled steroid preparations, such as beclomethasone dipropionate, flunisolide, and triamcinolone acetonide, provide good symptomatic control in most patients with twice-daily dosing. These preparations present little risk of systemic side effects or adrenal suppression.[72] The dose required to achieve adequate symptomatic control varies considerably, with some patients requiring more than 500 µg/day. Women with unstable disease should take the drug four times daily. High-dose (>1.6 mg/day) inhaled corticosteroids may cause some adrenal suppression, and these patients might benefit from supplemental hydrocortisone during stressful periods.[73,127] The most common side effect of aerosol steroid therapy is oral candidiasis. Oral thrush can be controlled by rinsing the mouth or the use of a spacing device to decrease deposition of steroid in the upper airways. Other side effects include sore throat, cough, and rarely dysphonia.[66,123,128] Asthmatic patients who have post-inhalation coughing or wheezing from beclomethasone aerosol can usually tolerate triamcinolone aerosol.[132]

Anesthetic management. Because women with asthma have increased airway responses to chemical, pharmacologic, and physical stimuli, the perioperative period represents a time of considerable risk. Both vaginal and cesarean delivery present potential difficulties. During labor, pain, stress, and hyperventilation can combine to initiate or exacerbate an episode of bronchospasm. During cesarean delivery, both regional and general anesthesia can interact with a parturient's asthma. The anesthesiologist's goals when managing a woman with asthma include ensuring optimal preoperative pulmonary status, providing appropriate labor or cesarean delivery analgesia to facilitate a painless and stress-free childbirth, and preventing bronchospasm or aggressively treating any respiratory problems that may arise.

Preoperative assessment. When confronted with an asthmatic parturient, the anesthesiologist must perform as thorough a preoperative assessment as circumstances allow. Determine the presence and estimate the magnitude of any current respiratory impairment, assess the patient's current therapy, and plan an anesthetic tailored to both patient and clinical situation.[133] Preoperative assessment involves both history and physical examination. Important historical information includes the frequency and severity of attacks as well as medications necessary to achieve good control of symptoms. Some may report a history of asthma without an attack in many years and may require no medication. Others report more frequent symptoms requiring bronchodilator therapy. Of these more severely affected patients, one must differentiate between those in stable condition (without active disease) from those who have suffered recent deterioration and may have active wheezing.

Patients presenting with severe or active disease require closer questioning. Important additional information includes precipitating factors (cold air, exercise, stress, allergies, infection, abrupt withdrawal of corticosteroids, inadequate maintenance therapy), the cause and duration of the current attack, the resolution of previous attacks, and previous anesthetic experiences. One can identify the high-risk patient by noting an increased frequency of attacks, hospitalization with previous attacks, a long delay in seeking medical attention with this attack, a need for intensive care or intubation with previous attack, and current use of high-dose corticosteroids.[134]

The physical evaluation of the asthmatic patient attempts to assess the current degree of respiratory impairment. Wheezing, the common clinical finding of acute asthma, may be scattered and intermittent in mild attacks. With more severe impairment, one can hear wheezing throughout the lungs during both inspiration and expiration. It is also important to look for hyperinflation, hyperresonance, and accessory muscle use. As the attack worsens, the patient may become diaphoretic, refuse to lie supine, exhibit tachypnea and tachycardia, and develop an exaggerated, (>20 mm Hg) pulsus paradoxis.[117] (Pulsus paradoxis, typically < 5 mm Hg, represents the normal fall in systolic blood pressure that occurs with inspiration. The decrease in intrathoracic pressure accompanying inspiration augments venous return and right ventricular filling. This increased right ventricular volume displaces the interventricular septum into the left ventricle, limiting its filling and output. With airflow obstruction, greater negative intrathoracic pressures develop during inspiration, exacerbating these effects.) With very severe attacks, respiratory fatigue with decreased wheezing, hypoventilation, and ventilatory failure may occur.

Many patients with significant asthma regularly measure their peak expiratory flow rate (PEFR). This measurement correlates well with forced expiratory volume in one second (FEV_1), and can be used to asses both the severity of airflow obstruction and the response to therapy. Patients with an initial PEFR less than 100 L/min or less than 300

L/min after therapy are seriously ill and need intensive bronchodilator therapy.[134] Patients with no audible breath sounds, or with cyanosis, bradycardia exhaustion, confusion, or unconsciousness are near death.[135]

Women with mild disease require no further preoperative preparation. Parturients should continue their prophylactic medications throughout the peripartum period. Patients receiving long term oral corticosteroid treatment or on high-dose (>1600 μg/day, i.e., 32 puffs per day) inhaled corticosteroid medications may require supplementation with hydrocortisone 100 mg every 8 hours.[127,136] Infants of women with steroid-induced adrenal suppression may rarely suffer adrenal suppression themselves; they warrant careful observation but not prophylactic treatment.[137]

Parturients presenting with active wheezing should not undergo elective procedures. These patients must receive appropriate acute therapy and procedures delayed until they are in optimal respiratory condition. The woman who presents in active labor or in need of urgent or emergent cesarean delivery presents a significant anesthetic challenge and should begin receiving appropriate antiasthmatic treatment as soon as possible.

Analgesia for labor and delivery. Labor can prove emotionally and physically stressful. Both the pain and hyperventilation that accompany labor can incite bronchospasm. Adequate analgesia, by any technique, should alleviate maternal stress and limit the risk of bronchospasm. Systemic analgesics may provide adequate analgesia during the early phases of labor. However, be aware of the respiratory depressant properties of both opioid agonist and agonist-antagonist compounds. Women with active wheezing should not receive any potential respiratory depressants for fear of precipitating respiratory failure.

Lumbar epidural analgesia offers several advantages to the parturient with asthma. Effective epidural analgesia can block the increases in oxygen consumption and minute ventilation that occur with uterine contractions.[35,36] In one study, oxygen consumption and minute ventilation increased by 60% to 75% with uterine contractions in unmedicated labor.[138] After induction of epidural analgesia, these variables remained unchanged with uterine contractions (Fig. 11-8). In the second stage of labor, oxygen consumption and minute ventilation were 25% to 30% lower in women with adequate epidural analgesia (10 to 12 mL 3% 2-chloroprocaine) than in women having no analgesia or sedation only.[138]

Continuous epidural infusion techniques with dilute concentrations of local anesthetic agents and opioids can be especially useful in these patients.

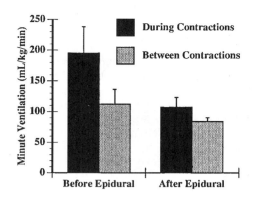

Fig. 11-8 Minute ventilation increases significantly during painful labor contractions (left columns). After successful induction of epidural analgesia, minute ventilation remains unchanged during contractions. (Data from Hägerdal M, et al: *Anesthesiology* 1983; 59:425).

When properly administered, these combinations can provide good, consistent analgesia with minimal maternal motor blockade and without the periodical return of pain that occurs with intermittent dosing techniques. Continuous infusion of 0.125% bupivacaine throughout the second stage of labor provides excellent maternal analgesia at the cost of a 50% increase in the incidence of forceps delivery.[139] Infusing 0.0625% bupivacaine combined with 0.0002% fentanyl also provides excellent second-stage analgesia and avoids the increased incidence of forceps deliveries.[140]

Epidural analgesia may prove especially useful in the care of the actively wheezing parturient. Younker et al reported a case in which induction of bupivacaine-fentanyl epidural analgesia appeared to enhance the therapeutic response to bronchodilators in a parturient in status asthmaticus. They recommend establishing epidural blockade before inducing labor in these women.[141]

Spinal blockade with local anesthetic drugs offers little to laboring women; however, subarachnoid injection of opioids (fentanyl, sufentanil or meperidine) can rapidly provide profound labor analgesia. When used as a part of a combined spinal-epidural technique, these drugs can prove useful in early labor[142] or in patients wishing to ambulate.[143] Because of the rapid onset of pain relief, others choose this technique for women in advanced labor.[144] Respiratory depression can follow intrathecal or epidural opioids.[145-149] These drugs should be used carefully in women with active wheezing.

Cesarean delivery. The choice of anesthesia for cesarean delivery depends on both fetal and maternal factors. The condition of the fetus and indication for cesarean delivery may determine anesthetic technique. The severity and current status of the mother's asthma as well as the interaction of anesthetic agents and techniques with her disease also must be considered.

Regional anesthesia. Spinal and epidural anesthesia can provide excellent operating conditions with good maternal comfort and neonatal outcome. However, both techniques have significant respiratory effects.

Regional anesthesia has little impact on inspiratory function or resting ventilation. Because the diaphragm is the principal muscle of inspiration, excessively high levels of sensory blockade, unlikely to occur in normal clinical circumstances, would be required to cause significant impairment of inspiration. In nonpregnant patients with mid to upper thoracic levels of sensory blockade, inspiratory capacity falls by 3% to 8% with epidural and spinal anesthesia.[150] Tidal volume, respiratory rate, and minute ventilation remain unchanged.[151,152] End-tidal CO_2 may fall slightly after spinal block (34.8 mm Hg to 31.6 mm Hg),[151] but remains unchanged after epidural local anesthetic.[152] Also, epidural blockade does not hinder the ventilatory response to hypoxemia.[152]

In contrast, expiratory function can be significantly altered by major conduction anesthesia. During quiet breathing, expiration is usually passive, but, with coughing, hyperventilation, or airway obstruction, active expiratory efforts are required. Spinal anesthesia can significantly impair abdominal muscle function and cough strength. In nonpregnant patients, even low spinal anesthesia (sensory blockade to S1) decreases cough strength by 34%; upper thoracic blockade decreases it by 94%.[153] In contrast, midthoracic levels of epidural blockade decrease cough strength by only 38%.[154] These differences occur not only because spinal anesthesia tends to produce more profound motor blockade than epidural anesthesia, but also because of differences in the level of motor block for a given level of sensory analgesia. With epidural blockade, motor weakness develops 4 to 5 segments below the sensory level. But with spinal anesthesia, motor block rises to within 2 to 3 dermatomes of the sensory level.[150] However, with the high levels of sensory blockade required for cesarean delivery, the differences between the two techniques diminish. In parturients, epidural sensory blockade to T8-T4 (mode T6) impairs peak expiratory flow rate by 11% after blockade is established and by 34% after delivery but before abdominal closure.[155] Spinal anesthesia to T3-C3 (mode T1) diminishes peak expiratory flow rate by a similar amount, (21%) (Fig. 11-9).[156,157] Thus despite some differences in their effects on motor function, spinal and epidural anesthesia do not ap-

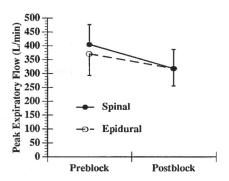

Fig. 11-9 Both spinal and epidural anesthesia impair cough effectiveness. Parturients received spinal or epidural anesthesia (level T3-4) for cesarean delivery. Peak expiratory flow rate fell significantly after either anesthetic. (Data from Harrop-Griffiths AW, et al: *Anaesthesia* 1991; 46:11.)

pear to differ greatly in their respiratory effects during cesarean delivery.

The literature contains little information about the respiratory effects of either regional technique in patients with asthma. Bronchial smooth muscle has little direct adrenergic innervation. However, airway smooth muscle contains many β_2 receptors that produce bronchodilation in response to circulating epinephrine.[158] Theoretically, high levels of regional block could decrease adrenal epinephrine output and allow unopposed vagal stimulation to incite bronchospasm. A very old series reported a 3.8% incidence of intraoperative respiratory complications in a mixed group of asthmatic patients receiving spinal anesthesia.[159] Shnider and Papper reported a 1.9% incidence of intraoperative wheezing in a group of patients receiving "regional anesthesia."[160]

There exist a few scattered case reports of significant bronchospasm in patients receiving spinal or epidural anesthesia.[161-163] In one case, an 18-year-old female patient with a history of asthma treated with theophylline and ephedrine received a spinal anesthetic for a therapeutic abortion. Fifteen minutes after induction, the sensory level had ascended to T5 and bilateral wheezes were noted. The patient responded promptly to treatment. The author suggested that diminished adrenal output of epinephrine resulting from lower thoracic sympathetic blockade contributed to the patient's bronchospasm.[161] Wang and Ong reported a case of bronchospasm during epidural anesthesia for cesarean delivery. Again, they attributed the event to a decrease in plasma epinephrine concentration.[162] Older literature contains sporadic reports of severe intraoperative bronchospasm and cardiac arrest in asthmatic patients receiving spinal anesthesia.[159]

Given the large number of patients with asthma who have received neuraxial anesthesia, this small number of case reports suggests coincidence, not causuality, as the etiology of perianesthetic bronchospasm associated with spinal or epidural block.

Both lumbar epidural and thoracic epidural blockade have been reported to relieve bronchospasm.[141,164] In patients with a history of bronchospasm, pulmonary sympathectomy induced by thoracic epidural block (C8–T6) did not change airway resistance.[165] The amount of inhaled acetylcholine needed to incite a 20% decrease in FEV_1 increased fourfold after epidural block (Fig. 11-10).[165] This protective effect may be due to systemically absorbed local anesthetic. A group of patients receiving intravenous bupivacaine also showed decreased sensitivity to inhaled acetylcholine.[165]

Clinically, either technique can be used successfully as long as good analgesia can be achieved and the patient is reassured about any sensations of chest heaviness or possible dyspnea. In acutely wheezing patients, epidural analgesia offers more control over the onset and extent of sensory blockade and seems preferable.

As with all anesthetized patients, appropriate monitoring is critical for safe perioperative care. In addition to blood pressure and ECG, women undergoing cesarean delivery with neuraxial block require pulse oximetry to monitor oxygenation. High thoracic levels of sensory blockade eliminate

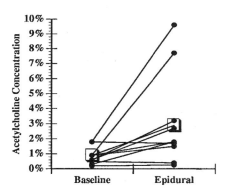

Fig. 11-10 Thoracic epidural anesthesia and bronchospasm. Patients with documented bronchial hyperreactivity had bronchospasm induced by breathing aerosolized acetylcholine (a potent bronchoconstrictor) before and after the induction of thoracic epidural anesthesia. Before sympathetic blockade, FEV_1 fell by 20% after inhalation of 0.9% acetylcholine. After epidural blockade (C4 to T6), FEV_1 fell by 20% only after inhalation of 2.9% acetylcholine. Intravenous bupivacaine infusion had a similar effect. (From Groeben H, et al: *Anesthesiology* 1994; 81:868).

spinal sympathetic outflow and abolish the normal cardiovascular response to hypoxemia.[166]

General anesthesia. Because of the risks of gastric acid regurgitation and aspiration, all parturients receiving a general anesthetic require a rapid sequence induction and endotracheal intubation. With her increased sensitivity to mechanical airway stimulation, this requirement presents a particular challenge in the woman with asthma. When planning and conducting a general anesthetic in these patients, one must be prepared to prevent and treat bronchospasm.

Bronchospasm can develop during general anesthesia even in patients without significant airway disease. In a survey of a large number of patients, bronchospasm occurred in 1.7 per 1000 anesthetics. Placing an endotracheal tube increased the incidence of intraoperative bronchospasm to 9.1 per 1000 anesthetics. The risk of airway constriction becomes even greater with the presence of significant obstructive pulmonary disease (21.9/1000) or active respiratory infection (41.1/1000).[167]

In patients without reactive airway disease, placing an endotracheal tube alone significantly influences pulmonary function and respiration. The tube itself presents a fixed, upper-airway obstruction, impeding peak inspiratory and expiratory air flow. This obstruction, when combined with inhalational anesthesia, alters respiratory function. Anesthesia impairs coordination between the chest wall and the abdomen, decreasing respiratory efficiency. Thus, while tidal volume and minute ventilation increase in response to expiratory resistance, end-tidal CO_2 also rises.[168] In addition, decreases in mid- and end-expiratory flow rates occur, suggesting endotracheal tube-induced constriction of smaller peripheral airways.[169] These effects are exaggerated in asthmatic patients, significantly increasing their risk of endotracheal tube-induced bronchospasm.[160] In addition to inciting reflex bronchospasm, this potent stimulus also may provoke the release of biochemical mediators of bronchospasm.[170]

Clinical strategies aimed at establishing an adequate depth of anesthesia and blocking reflex changes in airway caliber before attempting airway instrumentation can help diminish the risk of bronchospasm in the parturient with asthma.[133] Some of these approaches may include pretreatment with bronchodilators or anticholinergic medications, careful choice of induction drug and dosage, and use of adjuvant drugs during induction.

Preoperative administration of H_2 blocking drugs can raise maternal gastric pH and lower the risk of acid aspiration pneumonitis. In patients with asthma, unopposed H_2 receptor blockade increases the sensitivity to histamine-induced bronchoconstriction.[171,172] The concentrations needed to potentiate histamine effects are about the same with all H_2 receptor antagonists. Thus, airway constriction may be more likely with less potent drugs, which are given in higher concentrations.[173] The nonparticulate antacid 0.3 M sodium citrate also provides effective acid aspiration prophylaxis[174] and is probably a better choice in these women.

Anesthesiologists frequently administer anticholinergic agents, atropine or glycopyrrolate, before induction of general anesthesia. These drugs primarily limit the production of bothersome oral secretions. They also have significant bronchodilating effects, which may prove useful when anesthetizing an asthmatic parturient.[175]

Inhaled beta agonist or anticholinergic drugs are commonly used to treat bronchospasm. Kil et al studied the ability of these drugs to prevent endotracheal tube-induced increases in airway resistance.[176] Nonasthmatic patients inhaled placebo, ipratropium bromide 72 μg, or albuterol 360 μg one hour before surgery. The investigators then measured lung resistance after a fentanyl, thiopental, succinylcholine induction. Patients receiving ipratropium or albuterol had significantly lower lung resistance than those in the placebo group (Fig. 11-11). Three of 15 placebo-treated patients developed audible wheezing, while none of the 24 patients in the bronchodilator groups wheezed.

Choice of induction agent is important for the parturient with asthma. In dogs, thiopental neither causes nor prevents bronchospasm (Fig. 11-12).[160,177] However, in vitro thiopental (but not

methohexital) constricts tracheal muscle at concentrations similar to those seen clinically.[178] Experience with nonpregnant patients suggests that the endotracheal tube, not the induction agent, is more likely to incite bronchospasm.[160] If given in large enough doses, thiopental can provide adequate depth of anesthesia for intubation. However, large doses of thiopental (8mg/kg) also cause significant neonatal depression.[179] Thus thiopental, in the usual 3- to 4-mg/kg dose used in obstetric anesthesia, is not an appropriate induction agent for the parturient at significant risk for bronchospasm.

Ketamine may prove more useful in the management of patients with reactive airway disease. Case reports suggest that ketamine is a potent bronchodilator even in subanesthetic concentrations.[180-182] One must be careful using ketamine to treat severe bronchospasm; its sedative effects can contribute to respiratory depression in the patient in severe distress.[183] Early investigators noted increased pulmonary compliance and even relief of

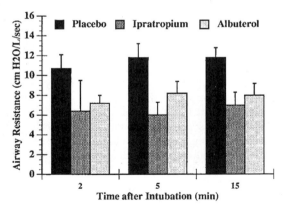

Fig. 11-11 Prophylactic bronchodilator treatment limits the increase in airway resistance that follows endotracheal intubation. Patients inhaled albuterol (360 μg) or ipratropium bromide (72 μg) one hour before surgery. Airway resistance, measured 2, 5, and 15 minutes after intubation, was significantly lower in the treated groups. Fewer patients in the treated groups developed wheezing after intubation. (From Kil H-K, et al: *Anesthesiology* 1994; 81:43).

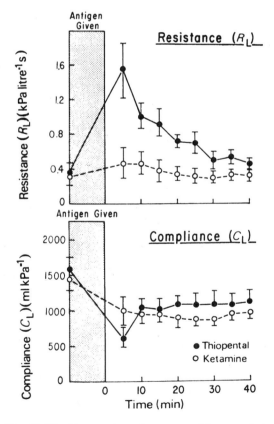

Fig. 11-12 Changes in pulmonary resistance and dynamic compliance in sensitized dogs anesthetized with ketamine or thiopental and then exposed to a 10-minute ascaris antigen challenge. (From Hirshman CA, Downes H, Farbood A, et al: *Br J Anaesth* 1979; 51:713-717.)

intraoperative wheezing after intravenous keta-mine.[184] Animal studies suggest that intravenous ketamine can prevent allergen-induced broncho-spasm (Fig. 11-12).[177] In vitro, ketamine relaxes tracheal smooth muscle and limits the response to various spasmogens.[185] Aerosolized ketamine appears to have neither protective nor therapeutic effects on histamine-induced bronchospasm.[186] Studies of ketamine's bronchodilating properties in anesthetized patients have yielded conflicting results. Corssen et al anecdotally reported relief of intraoperative bronchospasm with intravenous ke-tamine.[184] However, a more systematic study in nonpregnant adults could find no effect of keta-mine on aerosol-provoked increases in respiratory resistance (Fig. 11-13).[187]

Although ketamine may have some direct relax-ant effect on bronchial smooth muscle, its major effects are probably mediated by central catechol-amine release.[188,189] Preexisting sedation or gen-eral anesthesia, by depressing the central nervous system, inhibits ketamine's sympathomimetic properties[190] and probably accounts for the drug's inability to relieve intraoperative broncho-spasm.[187] Still, the preponderance of laboratory and clinical evidence suggests that ketamine is the agent of choice for rapid sequence induction in pa-tients with asthma.[133]

Seizure activity may complicate ketamine in-duction in patients receiving maintenance ami-nophylline therapy. Animal studies show that the combination of these two drugs lowers the thresh-old to electrically induced seizures by 10% to 20%.[191]

Propofol is rarely used for induction of parturi-ents. In vitro data, however, suggest that this drug may prove as potent as ketamine at inhibiting tra-

cheal smooth muscle contraction.[185] However, in dogs, both propofol and thiopental fail to protect against hypocapnia-induced bronchospasm.[192]

Some experts recommend using lidocaine to help prevent intubation-induced bronchospasm.[133] Intravenous local anesthetics are anecdotally re-ported to relieve bronchospasm after induction of anesthesia.[193] In animals, both intravenous and aerosolized lidocaine block reflex but not allergen-induced bronchoconstriction.[194,195] However, in patients with reactive airways, lidocaine aerosols often initially incite bronchospasm before having an occasional bronchodilator effect.[196] Lidocaine's protective effects occur at plasma concentrations of 1 to 4 μg/mL.[194,195] In gravid ewes, lidocaine at a plasma concentration of 40 μg/mL causes uter-ine hypertonus, uterine artery vasoconstriction, and fetal hypoxemia.[197] Smaller doses of lidocaine (1.5 mg/kg) appear to have no deleterious maternal or fetal effects (MC Norris, unpublished data).

After induction and intubation, one should main-tain anesthesia with 40% to 50% nitrous oxide in oxygen and a potent inhalation agent. In women with active wheezing, one should continue giving 100% oxygen. In addition to providing amnesia, potent inhalation agents may prove useful in treat-ing or preventing bronchospasm in these patients. Animal studies show that 1 to 1.5 MAC concen-trations of halothane, enflurane, isoflurane, and sevoflurane effectively treat or prevent antigen-induced and directly stimulated airway constric-tion.[198-201] Unfortunately, delivering 1 to 1.5 MAC end-tidal concentrations of potent agents during cesarean delivery may produce significant uterine relaxation and increase maternal blood loss. More recent studies have shown dose-related bronchodi-lation with potent agents.[200,202,203] In dogs, 0.6, 1.1, and 1.7 MAC halothane or isoflurane produce progressively greater degrees of airway dila-tion.[202,203] Halothane, however, is the more potent agent at lower concentrations (Fig. 11-14).[203,204]

The mechanism of the potent agents' effects on airway tone is complex. Halothane and enflurane decrease resting airway smooth muscle tone.[158,205] Halothane both increases airway caliber and de-creases pulmonary tissue resistance (pressure-volume hysteresis).[206] These drugs may exert their effects through blockade of vagal reflexes.[207] They reduce the amount of acetylcholine released from nerve terminals and the response of smooth muscle to direct muscarinic stimulation.[158,204] Other direct and indirect actions also have been re-ported.[158,192,204,208]

While halothane is the best choice for clinical use in parturients with asthma, it has some limita-tions. It sensitizes the myocardium to the arrhyth-mogenic effects of catecholamines.[173] Ventricular

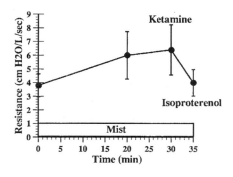

Fig. 11-13 Airway resistance in 20 healthy adults anes-thetized with thiopental, nitrous oxide, and meperidine and exposed to ultrasonic mist. Isoproterenol, 2 puffs de-livered by a metered dose inhaler, but not ketamine, 2 mg/kg IV, reversed the bronchoconstriction. (From Waltemath CA, Bergaman NA: *Anesthesiology* 1974; 41:473).

tachycardia and cardiac arrest have been reported in patients receiving both intravenous and oral aminophylline before receiving a halothane anesthetic.[209,210] Dogs given bolus doses or infusions of aminophylline, calculated to produce therapeutic levels of drug (10 to 20 µg/mL), immediately before induction of halothane anesthesia frequently develop ventricular arrhythmias[211] and exhibit enhanced epinephrine-induced arrhythmogenicity.[212] The sensitivity to epinephrine-induced arrhythmias appears diminished during chronic (6 weeks) aminophylline treatment.[212] Enflurane and isoflurane do not sensitize the myocardium to the effects of epinephrine and do not cause arrhythmias when combined with aminophylline.[213,214] Fortunately, fewer physicians are choosing chronic aminophylline therapy for their patients with asthma. In addition, aminophylline provides no additional bronchodilation during halothane anesthesia.[215]

Potent inhalation agents decrease uterine tone[216] and could increase blood loss at cesarean delivery. However, when used in low concentrations (<1 MAC), the uterus responds promptly to oxytocin and blood loss does not increase.[217,218]

Both theophylline[219] and the β-sympathomimetics[220,221] inhibit uterine activity. When combined with a potent inhalation agent, these agents can predispose to obstetric hemorrhage.[222] Should uterine hypotonus and excessive bleeding occur, one must stop any potent inhalation agent and β-sympathomimetic therapy if possible. One should enhance uterine contractility with additional oxytocin and uterine massage. Prostaglandin compounds should be avoided as they increase airway resistance[223] and can induce bronchospasm ($PGF_2\alpha$) in susceptible women.[95,224,225] (Patients with asthma are 8000 times

more sensitive to the bronchoconstricting actions of $PGF_2\alpha$ than normal controls.[226]) Ergotrates also may cause bronchoconstriction in some patients with asthma.[227]

After delivery, the anesthetic depth should be increased by additional nitrous oxide, if tolerated, and opioids. Both morphine and meperidine are associated with significant rises in plasma histamine concentrations while fentanyl and its cogeners are not.[228] Regardless of the opioid chosen, an adequate amount should be given to limit reflex responses to the endotracheal tube.

While succinylcholine has a long record of safety in asthmatic patients,[167] the nondepolarizing muscle relaxants present several potential problems. Curare releases histamine and increases airway resistance in normal patients. This effect is more pronounced in patients with significant pulmonary disease.[229] Pancuronium does not alter respiratory resistance[229] and has been used safely in patients with a history of bronchial asthma.[230] However, reports of bronchospasm associated with this relaxant have appeared.[231,232]

Presynaptic muscarinic receptors (M2) inhibit the release of acetylcholine. Blockade of these receptors by muscarinic antagonists (neuromuscular blocking drugs) removes this inhibition and could theoretically produce bronchospasm.[158] Gallamine is a potent M2 receptor antagonist. Animal studies suggest that pancuronium and atracurium enhance vagally mediated bronchoconstriction.[200] These drugs also may preferentially block inhibitory M2 receptors, augmenting the release of cholinergic neurotransmitter, and may induce bronchospasm in susceptible individuals. Vecuronium has no significant effect on pulmonary resistance.[200]

Intraoperatively, control ventilation can be used and normal and maintain arterial and end-tidal CO_2 should be maintained (27 to 32 mm Hg). In patients with bronchospasm, large, slowly delivered tidal volumes with a long expiratory phase can limit peak inspiratory pressures and prevent air trapping. In nonpregnant patients, high peak inspiratory pressures have proved more dangerous than hypercapnea. The current approach to these patients attempts to maintain normal oxygenation while minimizing hyperinflation and airway pressure,[135] using low tidal volumes (8 to 10 mL/kg, low rates (8 to 10/min) and high inspiratory flow rates (<70 L/min).[135,233] While hypercapnea usually results from this approach, as the patient responds to therapy, $Paco_2$ declines. In one series the mean time from intubation to $Paco_2$ < 45 mm Hg was 7.3 hours.[233] In severely ill patients, ventilation by an "educated hand" may prove more effective than a mechanical anesthesia ventilator.[234]

Cholinesterase inhibitors such as physostigmine,

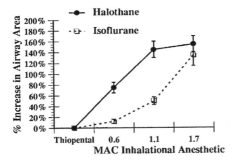

Fig. 11-14 Dose-response dilation of histamine-preconstricted airways to increasing concentrations of halothane and isoflurane. Halothane produced significantly more bronchodilation than isoflurane at 0.6 and 1.1 MAC. (From Brown RH, et al: *Anesthesiology* 1993; 78:1097).

neostigmine, and edrophonium can increase bronchial tone.[235] Fortunately, these actions are readily blocked by anticholinergic drugs. Reversal of neuromuscular blockade has little effect on bronchomotor tone. In healthy patients given neostigmine, 50 μg/kg and either atropine 20 μg/kg or glycopyrrolate 10 μg/kg, airway resistance decreases briefly in response to the anticholinergic drug and then increases slightly as a result of the neostigmine. This effect is mild and does not increase airway resistance to a level associated with bronchospasm.[236]

After reversal of neuromuscular blockade, extubation should be performed only after the parturient has awakened and regained her protective airway reflexes. Unfortunately, as with induction and intubation, the presence of an endotracheal tube in a lightly anesthetized patient can stimulate bronchospasm. Adequate doses of opioid analgesic (i.e., fentanyl 5 μg/kg after delivery) or lidocaine (1.5 mg/kg bolus) may prove useful in blunting the reflex responses to the endotracheal tube. In women with active wheezing, extubation should be delayed until the bronchospasm resolves and the patients respiratory status stabilizes.

Intraoperative bronchospasm. Intraoperative wheezing in an asthmatic patient is most likely due to bronchospasm. However, before instituting therapy, other causes should be considered. Possibilities include kinking or partial obstruction of the endotracheal tube, endobronchial intubation, pneumothorax, pulmonary edema, and aspiration of gastric contents and amniotic fluid embolus. In some important ways, therapy for intraoperative bronchospasm differs from the treatment of acute asthma in other settings. Aminophylline infusion has little place in the acute treatment of intraoperative bronchospasm. When administered in the presence of halothane, aminophylline can incite significant malignant ventricular arrhythmias.[209,210] In addition, halothane anesthesia inhibits the bronchodilating effects of intravenous aminophylline (Fig. 11-15).[215] These investigators suggest that halothane (1.5 MAC) blocks aminophylline-induced catecholamine release, preventing its therapeutic airway effects. It remains to be seen if other potent inhalation agents have similar effects. In contrast, the phosphodiesterase inhibitor amrinone does attenuate airway constriction during halothane anesthesia.[237] Aminophylline retains its efficacy during thiopental/fentanyl anesthesia.[215] In contrast, the β$_2$ selective sympathomimetic drug albuterol does provide additional protection against bronchospasm during halothane anesthesia (Fig. 11-16).[238]

Aerosolized selective β$_2$-adrenergic agonists are the treatments of choice for acute bronchos-

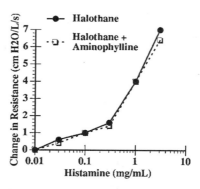

Fig. 11-15 Changes in pulmonary resistance in halothane anesthetized dogs (1.5 MAC) in response to aerosol histamine challenge the absence and presence of aminophylline. The addition of aminophylline does not add to the bronchodilation produced by halothane. (From Tobias JD, et al: *Anesthesiology* 1989; 71:5).

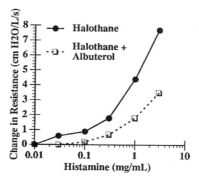

Fig. 11-16 Change in pulmonary resistance in response to aerosol histamine challenge in halothane anesthetized dogs (1.5 MAC) in the absence and presence of intravenous albuterol. Albuterol plus halothane produce significantly more bronchodilation than halothane alone. (From Tobias JD, Hirshman CA: *Anesthesiology* 1990; 72:105).

pasm.[239] Intraoperative β-adrenergic agents are most easily administered from a metered dose inhaler (MDI). A variety of methods have been suggested for connecting these devices to the anesthesia circuit.[240-244] Of these methods, both commercially available modified T-piece adapters or a simple device made from a tuberculin syringe and a T-piece adapter with a female Luer-lock side port can be readily available and are safe and easy to use. The ability of these adapters to deliver drug to the lung varies considerably.[245] The most efficient design incorporates an in-line spacer (Monaghan Aerochamber In-line Spacer; Monaghan, Littleton, Colo.) that helps minimize deposition of drug in the trachea. (Drug deposited in the trachea and oropharynx has no therapeutic effect. Absorption of this drug, however, does produce undesirable systemic effects like tachycardia and tremor.)[245]

When properly used by nonanesthetized patients, a MDI delivers 20% to 30% of each dose to the lungs. Several factors influence delivery efficiency when using MDIs in anesthetized patients and endotracheal tubes. Drug delivery increases with increasing tube size. Activating the MDI during continuous gas flow rather than before flow is initiated improves drug delivery.[246] Connecting a 19-gauge catheter to the tip of the MDI and inserting that catheter into the endotracheal tube before canister activation also may improve the efficiency of drug delivery.[247,248] In any case, one should titrate the drug to effect. Because of the lesser drug delivery compared with awake nonintubated patients, more puffs of drug will likely be needed.[246] One must carefully monitor the patient for both a therapeutic response and systemic side effects.

β-agonists also can be delivered by nebulizer.[249] Intravenous β-agonists are hazardous. There are few data to recommend their use over inhaled agents.[239]

The potent inhalation agents themselves have significant bronchial relaxing effects and have been used for prolonged periods (up to 7 days[250]) to treat refractory bronchospasm.[182,251-257] In most reported cases, patients respond to low concentrations of agent (<1 MAC). Respiratory resistance, hyperinflation and intrinsic positive end-expiratory pressure (PEEP) improve during treatment with potent agent.[256] If used in parturients, such a dose should not impair uterine responses to oxytocin or increase postpartum bleeding.[217] However, the combination of a potent agent and a β-sympathomimmetic can raise the risk of obstetric hemorrhage and should be used with care.[222]

Magnesium sulfate has some bronchodilator activity. Although not a first choice for the treatment of bronchospasm, it may prove useful in resistant patients.[258,259]

In summary, anesthetizing a parturient with significant bronchospastic disease can present a disconcerting challenge to the anesthesiologist. However, with careful attention to preoperative preparation and the choice of an anesthetic agent designed to avoid or minimize those factors that can incite bronchospasm, most anesthetics in these women should prove uneventful.

Cystic fibrosis

Obstetrical management

Incidence. Cystic fibrosis is the most frequent lethal genetic disorder in Caucasians. An autosomal recessive disorder with a gene frequency of 1 in 20, it affects approximately 1 in 2000 births.[260] In families with an affected living child, prenatal analysis of linked DNA probes with fetal DNA prepared from chorionic villus biopsy enables first-trimester diagnosis of cystic fibrosis.[261] The cystic fibrosis gene has been cloned and numerous mutations identified. Screening tests can now detect asymptomatic heterozygous carriers. The ability to detect the common mutations and the heterozygous carrier are major improvements in prenatal diagnosis, especially in families in which no DNA samples are available from an affected child.[262] However, the DNA-based blood or buccal cell test detects only 85% to 95% of cystic fibrosis cases; decision analysis suggests that routine prenatal cystic fibrosis-carrier screening may not be cost-effective.[263] Survival has lengthened due to improved medical care, and more women are reaching reproductive age. The median survival from the time of diagnosis is 22 years, and the median length of survival beyond the age of 18 years for affected women is 8 years.[264]

Pathophysiology. Cystic fibrosis primarily impairs exocrine gland function. Diseased glands secrete thick tenacious mucus, which readily obstructs their ducts. Sweat glands, mucous-secreting salivary glands, liver, pancreas, small intestine, respiratory tract, uterine cervix, and the male reproductive tract can be affected. Sweat contains elevated concentrations of sodium, potassium, and chloride. The clinical course of the disease varies with the severity of glandular dysfunction and the number of organ systems involved. Airway obstruction, bronchiolectasis, recurrent respiratory tract infections, peribronchial fibrosis, and emphysema are common. Airway obstruction by mucous plugs and parenchymal or peribronchial fibrosis from emphysema and infection produce combined obstructive and restrictive lung disease. Pulmonary disease and the progressive loss of pulmonary function accounts for greater than 95% of deaths. Other manifestations of cystic fibrosis include meconium ileus, malabsorption syndrome, failure to thrive, pancreatic insufficiency, recurrent pancreatitis, cholelithiasis, focal biliary cirrhosis, hepatic congestion secondary to cor pulmonale, portal hypertension, and male infertility.[260,265]

Abnormal ventilation in cystic fibrosis increases alveolar-arterial oxygen difference. This finding is the earliest manifestation of pulmonary dysfunction. Peripheral airway changes occur first, then obstruction of the large airways develops with a subsequent decrease in maximal mid-expiratory flow rates and FEV_1. RV and FRC rise as a result of air trapping and loss of elastic recoil. Even though VC is decreased, TLC remains normal or elevated.[260,266] With pulmonary insufficiency, even resting respiratory efforts increase oxygen consumption.[267] Respiratory infection, commonly with *Pseudomonas* and *Staphylococcus,* can produce rapid decompensation in patients with borderline pulmonary function.[267-269] Signs of impending respiratory failure include dyspnea, cyanosis, increased sputum production, hemoptysis and CO_2 retention.[260,264] Cystic fibrosis is a steadily progressive disease. Serial measurements of serial pulmonary function show variable deterioration with time. Pregnancy does not appear to alter this general trend.[266]

The prognosis of cystic fibrosis depends on the degree of pulmonary insufficiency.[260,267] Pregnancy outcome in these women correlates with the degree of respiratory compromise.[266] Poor prognostic factors include emphysema, atelectasis, bronchiectasis, VC less than 50% predicted, and cor pulmonale.[269-271] Indicators of the presence of cor pulmonale include right ventricular hypertrophy by electrocardiogram, Pao_2 less than 50 mm Hg (especially with $Pco_2 > 45$ mm Hg), VC less than 60% of predicted, clinical signs of congestive heart failure, and chest x-ray evidence of enlarged pulmonary artery or cardiac size.[260,267] The maternal mortality in pregnancy complicated by pulmonary hypertension and cor pulmonale is 31% to 53%, making this diagnosis an absolute contraindication to pregnancy.[272,273] Factors favoring long-term survival and good pregnancy outcome in cystic fibrosis include good clinical status (near-normal general activity, physical findings, nutritional status and chest x-ray findings), lack of pancreatic insufficiency and *S. aureus* alone in the lower respiratory tract flora.[264,266,269,274] Cohen et al reported the largest experience with cystic fibrosis in pregnancy. They found a direct relationship between pregnancy outcome and severity of maternal disease as determined by the presence or absence of pancreatic insufficiency, fat malabsorption, pulmonary hypertension and less than predicted VC. No congenital abnormalities occurred in the 129 pregnancies in this study. They advocated that women with poor clinical status avoid pregnancy.[274]

The treatment of cystic fibrosis in pregnancy is directed at maternal symptomatology and the specific organ systems involved. Use aerosolized β-adrenergic agonists and methylxanthine treatment as needed to relieve bronchospasm. Lung infections must be treated aggressively with appropriate antibiotics (avoiding tetracycline because of its adverse effects on the fetal bones and deciduous teeth). The inflammatory response to chronic infection speeds lung destruction in these patients. A recent study found that high-dose ibuprofen (200 mg twice daily) slowed the rate of pulmonary deterioration in patients with mild disease.[275] Unfortunately, nonsteroidal antiinflammatory drugs cross the placenta, and even short-term use can cause transient constriction of the ductus arteriosus.[276] Indomethacin exposure also increases the incidence of necrotizing enterocolitis, intracranial hemorrhage, and patent ductus arteriosus.[277] Pancreatic enzyme replacement should be continued in those women with pancreatic insufficiency. These patients must maintain caloric balance. In patients without diabetes, one should screen for gestational diabetes and treat as indicated with diabetic diet and insulin.[267,278] During labor and delivery, one must take care with fluid and electrolyte balance to avoid electrolyte depletion or congestive heart failure, especially in patients with cor pulmonale. Supplemental O_2 should be used as dictated by the maternal and fetal status.

Anesthetic management. When presented with a parturient with cystic fibrosis, one must consider how this disease will interact with the drugs and techniques chosen. As with the asthmatic patient, the preoperative assessment of a woman with cystic fibrosis centers on pulmonary function. One should review the most recently available pulmonary function tests. These patients often have moderate to severe pulmonary obstruction with decreased forced expiratory volumes and vital capacities.[279] One should inquire about a patient's current pulmonary status, general condition, and treatment regimen. On physical examination the patient's general status should be served; these women are frequently malnourished and dehydrated.[280] Because of their respiratory impairment, they may be unable to lie in the supine position, and they may be hypoxemic and have rales, wheezes, or rhonchi.[281]

The combination of dehydration and chronic disease may make intravenous access difficult. Some of these women will have permanent intravenous catheters, which may be used if needed.[282]

The literature contains little information concerning the anesthetic management of these women for obstetric procedures. Some basic principles apply, however. Maternal, and consequently fetal, oxygenation assume paramount importance during labor and delivery. Continuous monitoring of maternal oxygen saturation using pulse oximetry should prove useful in guiding the need for, and response to, supplemental oxygen therapy. Patients with acutely deteriorating respiratory function may benefit from invasive arterial and central monitoring.[282]

Painful labor increases maternal oxygen consumption and minute ventilation. Effective analgesia limits or prevents these respiratory demands. Systemic medication is of little use in relieving labor pain. In addition, patients with severe pulmonary disease may decompensate acutely when given respiratory depressant drugs such as opioid analgesics. Lumbar epidural analgesia will effectively relieve labor pain; it can be used safely in women with cystic fibrosis.[282] The height and density of blockade should be limited to minimize motor weakness and respiratory compromise. Some clinicians express concern about the stresses imposed by intravenous fluids and the possibility of hypotension.[281] Careful hydration and ephedrine therapy can limit these risks. For optimal pain control, one should initiate epidural analgesia early in labor. Maintaining analgesia with a continuous infusion of a dilute local anesthetic/opioid mixture will provide stable pain relief with minimal motor blockade and respiratory compromise. Continuing the infusion throughout the second stage will allow instrumental vaginal delivery and will minimize maternal work. Subarachnoid opioids also can provide effective pain relief for these patients.[281] However, they will not provide analgesia for the second stage of labor or delivery.

Should the obstetric situation indicate cesarean delivery, the anesthesiologist must choose between a regional and a general anesthetic technique. Regional anesthesia is often appropriate. However, women with severe respiratory impairment can have extreme difficulty lying in the supine position while awake and thus may not tolerate regional block. Should regional anesthesia be chosen, epidural blockade, by allowing careful, titrated dosing, may be the more appropriate technique.

Patients with cystic fibrosis commonly receive general anesthesia for other procedures.[283] Children with cystic fibrosis experience greater postoperative declines in pulmonary function after anesthesia and surgery when compared with healthy children (Fig. 11-17).[284] However, even repeated general anesthetics appear to have no long-term deleterious effects in these patients.

The pulmonary dysfunction caused by cystic fibrosis can directly precipitate several anesthetia problems. Pronounced V/Q mismatch can delay the uptake of inhalation anesthetics. These women have copious, viscous bronchial secretions. Wheezing may develop, possibly from bronchospasm, but more immediately threatening causes include endotracheal tube obstruction and pneumothorax. Profuse bronchial secretions, coughing, straining, and prolonged elimination of inhalation anesthetics complicate emergence. Before extubation, the patient must be thoroughly suctioned, fully awake, and well oxygenated.

To attempt to minimize postoperative respiratory impairment, these women should receive optimal analgesic therapy. In those receiving a regional anesthetic, spinal or epidural opioids should prove effective. After general anesthesia, one can use patient controlled intravenous analgesia.

In summary, parturients with cystic fibrosis may have extreme degrees of pulmonary impairment. However, with careful attention to the respiratory system and the choice of anesthetic technique best suited to an individual patient's needs, these women should traverse the peripartum period without undue difficulty.

Pulmonary infection

Pneumonia. Despite the advent of antibiotics, pneumonia remains the most common cause of infectious death in the United States.[285] Pneumonia complicates 0.04% to 0.08% of pregnancies.[286,287] In the preantibiotic era, pneumonia was frequent in pregnancy. Mortality most commonly occurred at term or immediately postpartum.[286-289] With the introduction of antibiotics, maternal mortality from pneumonia during pregnancy decreased from 20% to 3.5%.[288] In a population presenting early in the course of illness and with prompt institution of antibiotic treatment, no maternal deaths occurred.[287] Pneumonia in pregnancy is associated with cigarette smoking, cystic fibrosis, and acquired immunodeficiency syndrome (AIDS).[286,289] Other associated diseases include asthma, sickle cell disease, mitral valve diseases, alcoholism, nephrectomy, hepatitis A, and significant maternal anemia.[287] The perinatal mortality rate of pneumonia during pregnancy is between 40 to 115/1000 births.[286,287]

The advent of immunosuppressive drugs, the emergence of antibiotic-resistant forms of bacteria, and the increasing prevalence of AIDS and its associated opportunistic infections, have changed spectrum and treatment of pathognomic microbes.[286,290] Common pathogens causing pneumonia in pregnancy include *S. pneumoniae, H. influenzae, P. aeruginosa,* influenza A virus, *M. tuberculosis, E. coli, S. aureus,* and *P. carinii.* Direct treatment at the presumptive or culture-proven causative agent. Adequate fluid intake avoids dehydration. Antipyretic agents minimize the increased fetal oxygen consumption and consequent fetal hypoxemia in response to maternal hyperthermia.

Influenza, the best studied respiratory viral infection during pregnancy, places pregnant women at greater risk of death compared with the general population. Most maternal mortality occurs during the third trimester.[291,292] Maternal influenza infection confers no increased risk of serious fetal problems. Although controversial, the risk of congenital malformations and childhood cancers is probably not increased. While inactivated influenza vaccine is safe in pregnancy, gestation itself is not an indication for influenza immunization. The cri-

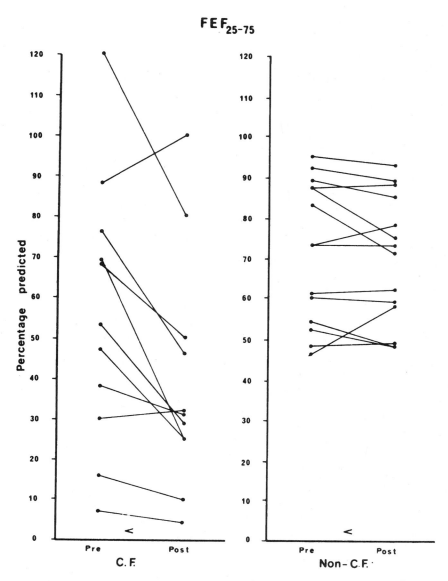

Fig. 11-17 FEF_{25-75} before and after anesthesia in children with and without cystic fibrosis. Data are expressed as percentage of predicted values based on the child's height. (From Richardson VF, Richardson CF, Mowat AP, et al: *Acta Paediatr Scand* 1984; 73:75-79.)

teria for influenza immunization in pregnancy are the same as for nonpregnant patients with chronic illness. Amantadine should be considered in the treatment of infected pregnant women at high risk of mortality because of heart disease, chronic anemia, diabetes, chronic pulmonary disease, chronic renal disease, or altered immune response.[292]

The other respiratory virus well studied during pregnancy is varicella (chicken pox). Even though varicella infection is common, its incidence in pregnancy is only 1 in 7500. Varicella infection in pregnancy carries a high risk of morbidity and

mortality for both mother and fetus. Maternal mortality from varicella pneumonia has been reported to be 41% as compared with 17% outside of pregnancy. The risks of abortion and prematurity are increased. Only one out of six pregnancies deliver without complications.[293,294] Even though experience with acyclovir antiviral therapy in pregnancy is limited, aggressive treatment may have a role in managing life-threatening disseminated varicella pneumonia.[294,295]

A variety of mycotic infections can complicate pregnancy, primarily in women who are immunosuppressed. Coccidioidomycosis, usually a benign pulmonary fungal infection, can occur in immunocompromised women.[296] The incidence in endemic areas is 1 in 500 to 1,000 pregnancies. Disseminated coccidiodomycosis can be fatal with mortality increasing to 91% in pregnancy (compared with 50% for nonpregnant women).[297] Experience with amphotericin B is limited in pregnancy, but case reports of its use for disseminated disease in all trimesters of pregnancy have noted no adverse fetal effects.[297,298]

Anesthetic management. When devising an anesthetic plan for a parturient with pneumonia, one should consider the risks of neuraxial infection. Patients with bacterial pneumonia may have bacteremia. Hematogenous spread of infection to the epidural or subarachnoid space can occur postpartum.[299] The presence of a foreign body (i.e., an epidural catheter) may increase this risk.[300] Lumbar puncture, commonly performed in confused patients with bacteremia, does not appear to significantly increase their risk of meningitis.[301] However, an animal study found a significantly increased risk of meningitis following dural puncture in chronically bacteremic *(E. coli)* rats.[302] No rats receiving appropriate antibiotic therapy before dural puncture, however, developed meningitis. If choosing regional anesthesia in a parturient with pneumonia, one should first initiate appropriate antibiotic therapy[303] and strongly consider a single injection technique to avoid the potential risk of an indwelling catheter. Patients should be observed carefully after delivery. Thorough investigations of any complaints of persistent back pain or leg weakness should be undertaken immediately. Epidural abscess may have a delayed presentation. Symptoms may develop gradually and not occur until a week or longer after delivery.[280,300,304]

Providing adequate labor analgesia for women with bacterial pneumonia can prove difficult. Narcotic analgesic agents and other respiratory depressants should be used with caution for fear of inducing further respiratory compromise. Paracervical and pudendal nerve block, when appropriate, may help. For cesarean delivery, general anesthesia can be used safely. Postoperatively, these women require optimal analgesia to minimize pain-induced respiratory compromise. Patient controlled analgesia should prove effective.

Tuberculosis. With the advent of effective drug therapy, mortality from tuberculosis has declined from 70 to 2.2 per 100,000 with the incidence of active disease falling by 30% from 1962 to 1972.[305] However, an active resurgence of tuberculosis currently exists among pregnant women. In New York City, the incidence of tuberculosis in pregnancy was 12.4 per 100,000 deliveries between 1985 and 1990 and has increased to 94.8 per 100,000 deliveries during 1991-1992.[306] This rising incidence of tuberculosis is accompanied by human immunodeficiency virus (HIV) infection and multidrug resistant strains of tuberculosis.[307,308] Neither pregnancy nor the peripartum period accelerate the progression of immunosuppression in HIV-infected women. However, HIV-infected patients are more susceptible to tuberculosis and have an increased risk of congenital transmission.[309]

Current pharmacotherapy of tuberculosis is complicated by the development of drug-resistant strains of mycobacterium. Initial isolates of *M. tuberculosis* should be tested for antimicrobial susceptibility. Several weeks may pass before the results are available. Initial treatment of active tuberculosis should follow the protocols from the Centers for Disease Control guidelines until drug susceptibility is demonstrated and drug resistance is excluded. A combination of isoniazid (INH), rifampin, pyrazinamide, and ethambutol or streptomycin are the drugs of choice for the treatment of tuberculosis in children and adults. Streptomycin should be avoided in pregnancy because of the risk for ototoxicity to the fetus.[310] Pyridoxine requirement increases in pregnancy, so pyridoxine supplement is recommended with INH treatment to decrease the risk of peripheral neuropathy.[311] The most important cause of treatment failure is poor compliance, which is associated with the emergence of drug resistance. Some experts suggest directly observed treatment of tuberculosis to increase patient compliance and to decrease treatment failure.[312]

All of the infants born to 1565 tuberculous mothers treated with combination chemotherapy were of average weight and none had congenital tuberculosis.[305] Congenital infection is uncommon but can occur *via* lymphohematogenous spread or fetal ingestion/aspiration of infected amniotic fluid.[122,313] Most infections develop postpartum from maternal contact. Untreated or inadequately treated congenital or neonatal tuberculosis carries a high mortality rate (45% to 50%); the prognosis is worse for premature infants. Treatment of congenital or neonatally acquired tuberculosis is similar to that for older children: chemotherapy with a four-drug combination of INH, rifampin, pyrazinamide, and either streptomycin or ethambutol for the first 2 months, followed by INH and rifampin for 4 to 10 months, depending on the of severity of the disease.[309]

Prompt diagnosis of tuberculosis during pregnancy with early treatment most effectively prevents congenital and neonatal disease.[122] The diagnosis of tuberculosis in pregnancy requires a high index of suspicion. Infection with *M. tuberculosis* may be identified with a positive purified protein derivative (PPD) tuberculin skin test (without a history of bacille Calmette-Guérin vaccination) and the definitive diagnosis confirmed by positive *M. tuberculosis* cultures and chest radiography.[310] Women with symptoms consistent with tuberculosis, those with recent contact with known infectious cases, patients who recently migrated from endemic areas, and patients with medical illness that predisposes them to tuberculosis should all be screened with PPD and diagnostic chest x-ray examination as indicated. Chest x-ray examination is not contraindicated in pregnancy when appropriate.[314] A negative PPD may not guarantee absence of disease in high-risk patients. In one study, 60% of parturients with tuberculosis had a negative PPD skin test; 55% of these women were HIV-seropositive. This finding emphasizes the importance of anergy in the interpretation of the PPD skin test result.[306] The decision to use preventive therapy in women with newly positive PPD but negative chest film and sputum culture during pregnancy should be made on an individual basis and depends on the patients estimated risk for progression to active disease. In general, preventive treatment with INH prophylaxis can be deferred until after delivery.[309]

Anesthetic management. The care of patients with adequately treated tuberculosis is dictated by the severity of their respiratory impairment, if any. Women with active tuberculosis can infect medical personnel and can contaminate anesthesia equipment. Disposable equipment must be used when possible, and one should place additional filters between the breathing circuit and anesthesia machine. Nondisposable equipment should be adequately disinfected with alcohol, phenol, or iodophor solutions or heat or gas sterilized before reuse. To avoid exposure and possible infection, health-care workers should wear face masks designed to filter 1 to 5 μm particles when taking care of patients with active disease.[315]

Sarcoidosis

Sarcoidosis is a chronic granulomatous disease of unknown etiology that affects virtually every organ system. Sarcoidosis produces a characteristic interstitial lung disease; 90% of patients have an abnormal chest x-ray result sometime during their course. Approximately 50% of patients develop permanent pulmonary abnormality; 10% to 20% will suffer progressive pulmonary fibrosis. Sarcoidosis is usually benign and self-limiting, characterized by frequent relapses alternating with periods of quiescence. Spontaneous recovery occurs in 50% of patients, while 15% to 20% have persistent disease. Death can occur in 10% of patients, most commonly as a result of cor pulmonale from pulmonary fibrosis. Hilar lymphadenopathy is common, as is involvement of the skin, eye, parotid gland, bone marrow, spleen, and liver. Sarcoidosis of the lung, eye, heart, and central nervous system confers the greatest risk of morbidity and mortality. The affected organs accumulate lymphocytes and mononuclear phagocytes, and they develop noncaseating granulomas that lead to architectural distortion and subsequent functional derangement.[316-319]

The prevalence of sarcoidosis in the United States is 10 to 40 in 100,000, with a ratio of black to white of 10-17:1. Most patients present between the ages of 20 and 40; both sexes are affected but females are slightly more susceptible than males.[316] Sarcoidosis is rare during pregnancy, accompanying between 0.023% and 0.047% of deliveries.[319-321] The true prevalence of severe pulmonary sarcoidosis in pregnancy is unknown.[311]

The diagnosis of sarcoidosis is imperfect and is made by a combination of clinical presentation and radiographic and histologic findings. The Kveim-Siltzbach skin test is limited by lack of standardization and availability. Chest x-ray findings of bilateral hilar adenopathy are characteristic but must be differentiated from other causes of lymphadenopathy. Angiotensin 1-converting enzyme is elevated in two thirds of patients, but this finding is both insensitive and nonspecific. The definitive diagnosis of sarcoidosis rests on the demonstration of noncaseating epithelioid granulomas from biopsy of involved organs, most often the lungs. However, other causes of granulomas such as infection and malignancy must be ruled out.[316,319]

Sarcoidosis does not affect fertility or the course of pregnancy. The disease usually improves or remains unchanged during gestation.[319,320,322-324] Two maternal deaths have been reported in pregnancy, one occurring in a women with coexisting preeclampsia.[318,322] Like other autoimmune diseases, the increase in circulating corticosteroids may help ameliorate sarcoidosis during pregnancy.[324] Exacerbation and relapse may occur in the puerperium, necessitating close follow-up during this period.[324-326] Transplacental transmission of sarcoidosis has not been reported.

Treatment of sarcoidosis is unchanged by pregnancy. Corticosteroid therapy can treat deteriorating pulmonary function, uveitis, and significant cardiac or neurologic abnormalities. However, steroids do not improve the permanent organ derangement of sarcoidosis.[316] Obstetrically, these women require no special treatment except lessening of the cardiovascular load in patients with significant cardiopulmonary involvement by shortening of the second stage of labor.[319] Sarcoidosis usually has little effect on anesthetic care. Rarely, patients may have granulomas of their vocal cords, increasing the risk of airway obstruction from postintubation swelling.[327]

Adult respiratory distress syndrome

Adult respiratory distress syndrome (ARDS), or noncardiogenic pulmonary edema, is a syndrome characterized by acute progressive respiratory failure with severe defects in oxygen transfer, diffuse pulmonary infiltrates, low static lung compliance, and normal cardiac filling pressures. A large number of disorders may lead to ARDS (Table 11-2), but the clinical presentation, respiratory pathophysiologic alterations, and specific treatment and management of the syndrome are similar regardless of the original inciting cause.[328-333] The prevalence of ARDS in pregnancy is unknown. The information available to date is limited to case reports.[334-338]

The mortality of ARDS is between 50% and 60%, an improvement over the virtually 100% mortality before the advent of mechanical ventilation with positive PEEP. Multiple organ system failure is common in ARDS and contributes to the extremely poor prognosis. Multiple organ system failure occurs in 93% of infected and 47% of noninfected patients. If drug overdose is the cause of ARDS, the mortality is low; if shock is the inciting cause, the mortality is high. ARDS persisting

Table 11-2 Conditions in pregnancy that may lead to adult respiratory distress syndrome

Infections	Hypovolemic shock
Pneumonia	Obstetrical hemorrhage
Aspiration	Massive blood transfu-
Bacterial	sion
Viral	Abruptio placentae
Fungal	DIC
Pyelonephritis	
Sepsis/Abscess	**Pancreatitis**
Chorioamnionitis	
Septic abortion	**Cancer**
	Pheochromocytoma
Preeclamp-	Carcinomatosis
sia/eclampsia	
	Embolus
Drugs	Amniotic fluid
Narcotics/barbiturates	Septic thrombi
β-adrenergic agonists	Trophoblasts
	(IUFD/GTD)
	Air/fat

*DIC = disseminated intravascular coagulation; IUFD = intrauterine fetal demise; GTD = gestational trophoblastic disease.

beyond 10 days is associated with significant interstitial fibrosis and emphysematous changes. However, some patients will recover without pulmonary sequelae.[329,331]

ARDS is a consequence of direct or indirect injury to the pulmonary capillary endothelium or to the alveolar epithelial lining. Direct causes include chemical injury from inhalation of noxious gases, focal pneumonia, or aspiration of gastric contents. Indirect damage is thought to be due to granulocyte aggregation and the secondary effects of the release of mediators of inflammation such as leukotrienes, thromboxanes, and prostaglandins. Alveolar-capillary membrane permeability increases in the presence of normal or low pulmonary microvascular hydrostatic pressures. Consequently, cellular elements and fluid extravasate into the lung interstitium and alveoli. The resulting edema decreases lung compliance and lung volume (decrease in FRC and increase in the dead space, D_V/D_T). The leakage of fluid and intravascular elements into the alveolar space causes alveolar collapse with ventilation-perfusion mismatch and diffusion impairment. This change widens the alveolar-arterial O_2 gradient. With progression of the disease, right-to-left shunting of blood away from collapsed alveoli worsens hypoxemia. At this time, the alveolar-arterial O_2 gradient is high and unresponsive to 100% oxygen administration. In this late stage of ARDS, endotracheal intubation, assisted mechanical ventilation with PEEP, and high inspired oxygen concentration (FIO_2) are all necessary. PEEP serves to decrease shunting and increase lung volume by opening collapsed alveoli.[328-333,337,339]

Therapy for ARDS is largely supportive, with the use of mechanical ventilation with PEEP to maintain oxygenation while treating any underlying disorder amenable to therapy. Optimal treatment includes early recognition of the disease process with prompt institution of aggressive therapy. Meticulous management of cardiac filling pressure is necessary to maintain an adequate cardiac output for organ perfusion while minimizing fluid extravasation through the leaky alveolar-capillary membranes. Cardiotonic, diuretic, bronchodilating, and sedative agents should be used as indicated. One should use the lowest possible combination of PEEP and FIO_2 to avoid barotrauma and pulmonary oxygen toxicity. If a drug is identified as the inciting cause of ARDS, it should be discontinued. Antibiotics are used only as needed for the treatment of primary infections. Evacuation of uterus is indicated in the presence of endometritis and chorioamnionitis to eliminate the source of sepsis. Immediate uterine evacuation is also necessary to eliminate the source of trophoblastic emboli in molar pregnancies and dead fetus syndromes associated with ARDS. Septic thrombophlebitis should be treated with antibiotic drugs as well as heparin. Coagulopathy should be treated with appropriate blood component replacement therapy.[329-331,333,339-345] During labor and delivery, epidural analgesia may be useful to decrease maternal oxygen consumption in severely ill parturients.[346]

REFERENCES

1. Mokriski BLK: Physiologic adaptation to pregnancy: The healthy parturient, in Norris MC: (ed) *Obstetric Anesthesia,* Philadelphia, JB Lippincott, 1993, pp 3-33.
2. Milne JA, Howie AD, Pack AI: Dyspnoea during normal pregnancy. *Br J Obstet Gynecol* 1978; 85:260.
3. Gilber R, Epifano L, Auchincloss JH: Dyspnea of pregnancy: a syndrome of altered respiratory control. *JAMA* 1962; 182:1073.
4. Prowse CM, Gaensler EA: Respiratory and acid-base changes during pregnancy. *Anesthesiology* 1965; 26:381.
5. Cugell DW, Frank NR, Gaensler EA, et al: Pulmonary function in pregnancy. I. Serial observations in normal women. *Am Rev Tuberc* 1953; 67:568.
6. Thomson KJ, Cohen ME: Studies on the circulation in pregnancy. II. Vital capacity observation in normal pregnant women. *Surg Gynecol Obstet* 1938; 66:591.
7. McGinty AP: Comparative effects of pregnancy and phrenic nerve interruption on the diaphragm and their relation to pulmonary tuberculosis. *Am J Obstet Gynecol* 1938; 35:237.
8. Craig DB, Toole MA: Airway closure in pregnancy. *Can Anaesth Soc J* 1975; 22:665.
9. Alaily AB, Carrol KB: Pulmonary ventilation in pregnancy. *Br J Obstet Gynaecol* 1978; 85:518.
10. Gee JBL, Packer BS, Millen JE, et al: Pulmonary mechanics during pregnancy. *J Clin Invest* 1967; 46:945.
11. Bevan DR, Holdcroft A, Loh L, et al: Closing volume and pregnancy. *Br Med J* 1974; 1:12.
12. Gazioglu K, Kaltreider NL, Rosen M, et al: Pulmonary function during pregnancy in normal women and in patients with cardiopulmonary disease. *Thorax* 1970; 25:445.
13. Baldwin GR, Moorthi DS, Whelton JA, et al: New lung function and pregnancy. *Am J Obstet Gynecol* 1877; 127:235.
14. Knuttgen HG, Emerson K Jr: Physiological response to pregnancy at rest and during excercise. *J Appl Physiol* 1974; 36:549.
15. Rubin A, Russo N, Goucher D: The effect of pregnancy upon pulmonary function in normal women. *Am J Obstet Gynecol* 1956; 72:963.
16. Milne JA, Mills RJ, Howie AD, et al: Large airways function during normal pregnancy. *Br J Obstet Gynaecol* 1977; 84:448.
17. Garrard GS, Littler WA, Redman CWG: Closing volume during normal pregnancy. *Thorax* 1978; 33:488.
18. Collins JV, Clark TJH, McHardy-Young S, et al: Closing volume in healthy non-smokers. *Br J Dis Chest* 1973; 67:19.
19. Holdcroft A, Bevan DR, O'Sullivan JC, et al: Airway closure and pregnancy. *Anaesthesia* 1977; 32:517.
20. Russell IF, Chambers WA: Closing volume in normal pregnancy. *Br J Anaesth* 1981; 53:1043.
21. Krumholz RA, Echt CR, Ross JC: Pulmonary diffusing capacity, capillary blood volumes, lung volumes and mechanics of ventilation in early and late pregnancy. *J Lab Clin Med* 1964; 63:648.
22. Bedell GN, Adams RW: Pulmonary diffusion capacity during rest and exercise: A study of normal persons and persons with atrial septal defect, pregnancy and pulmonary disease. *J Clin Invest* 1962; 41:1908.
23. Milne JA, Mills RJ, Coutts JRT, et al: The effect of human pregnancy on the pulmonary transfer factor for carbon monoxide as measured by the single-breath method. *Clin Sci Mol Med* 1977; 53:271.
24. Belchner JN, Cotter JR, Stenger VG, et al: Oxygen, carbon dioxide and hydrogen ion concentrations in arterial blood during pregnancy. *Am J Obstet Gynecol* 1968; 199:1.
25. Andersen GJ, James GB, Mathers NP, et al: The maternal oxygen tension and acid-base status during pregnancy. *J Obstet Gynaecol Br Commonw* 1969; 76:16.
26. Lyons HA, Antonio R: The sensitivity of the respiratory center in pregnancy and after the administration of progesterone. *Trans Assoc Am Physicians* 1959; 72:180.
27. Lyons HA, Huang CT: Therapeutic use of progesterone in alveolar hypoventilation associated with obesity. *Am J Med* 1968; 44:881.
28. Sutton FD Jr, Zwillich CW, Creagh CE, et al: Progesterone for outpatient treatment of Pickwickian syndrome. *Ann Intern Med* 1975; 83:476.
29. Miller FC, Petrie RH, Arce JJ, et al: Hyperventilation during labor. *Am J Obstet Gynecol* 1974; 120:489.
30. Fisher A, Prys-Roberts C: Maternal pulmonary gas exchange. *Anaesthesia* 1968; 23:350.
31. Crawford JS, Tunstall ME: Notes on respiratory performance during labour. *Br J Anaesth* 1968; 40:612.
32. Moya F, Morishima HO, Shnider SM, et al: Influence of maternal hyperventilation on the new born infant. *Am J Obstet Gynecol* 1965; 91:76.
33. Motoyama EK, Rivard D, Acheson F, et al: Adverse effect of maternal hyperventilation on the foetus. *Lancet* 1967; 1:286.
34. Coleman AJ: Absence of harmful effect of maternal hypocapnia in babies delivered at caesarean section. *Lancet* 1967; 1:813.
35. Marx GF, Macatagnay AS, Cohen AV, et al: Effects of pain relief on arterial blood gas values during labor. *New York State J Med* 1969; 69:819.
36. Sangoul F, Fox GS, Houle GL: Effect of regional analgesia on maternal oxygen consumption during the first stage of labor. *Am J Obstet Gynecol* 1975; 121:1080.
37. MacRae DJ, Palavradji D: Maternal acid-base changes in pregnancy. *J Obstet Gynaecol Br Emp* 1967; 74:11.
38. Lucius H, Gahlenbeck H, Kleine H-O, et al: Respiratory functions, buffer system, and electrolyte concentration of blood during human pregnancy. *Respir Physiol* 1970; 9:311.
39. Templeton A, Kelman GR: Maternal blood gases, (P_{AO_2}-Pa_{O_2}), physiological shunt and VD/VT in normal pregnancy. *Br J Anaesth* 1976; 48:1001.
40. Lim VS, Katz AI, Lindheimer MD: Acid-base regulation in pregnancy. *Am J Physiol* 1976; 231:1764.
41. Anderson GJ, Walker J: The effect of labour on the maternal blood-gas and acid-base status. *J Obstet Gynaecol Br Commonw* 1970; 77:289.
42. Fadl ET, Utting JE: Acid-base disturbance in obstetrics. *Royal Soc Med* 1970; 63:77.
43. Pearson JF, Davies P: Effect of continuous lumbar epidural analgesia on the acid-base status of maternal arterial blood during the first stage of labour. *J Obstet Gynecol Br Commonw* 1972; 80:218.
44. Awe RJ, Nicotra MB, Newsom TD, et al: Arterial oxy-

genation and alveolar-arterial gradients in term pregnancy. *Obstet Gynecol* 1979; 53:182.

45. Ang CK, Tan TH, Walters WAW: Postural influence on maternal capillary oxygen and carbon dioxide tension. *Br Med J* 1969; 4:201.

46. Cohen AV, Schulman H, Romney SL: Maternal acid-base metabolism in normal human parturition. *Am J Obstet Gynecol* 1970; 107:933.

47. Fadl ET, Utting JE: A study of maternal acid-base during labour. *Br J Anaesth* 1969; 41:327.

48. Low JA, Pancham SR, Worthington D, et al: Acid-base, lactate, and pyruvate characteristics of the normal obstetric patient and fetus during the intrapartum period. *Am J Obstet Gynecol* 1974; 120:862.

49. Jacobson L, Rooth G: Interpretative aspects of the acid-base composition and its variation in fetal scalp blood and maternal blood during labour. *J Obstet Gynaecol Br Commonw* 1971; 78:971.

50. Byrne F, Oruro-Dominah A, Kipling R: The effect of pregnancy on pulmonary nitrogen washout. *Anaesthesia* 1987; 42:148.

51. Norris MC, Kirkland MR, Torjman MC, et al: Denitrogenation in pregnancy. *Can J Anaesth* 1989; 36:523.

52. Russell GN, Smith CL, Snowdon SL, et al: Preoxygenation and the parturient patient. *Anaesthesia* 1987; 42:346.

53. Preoxygenation: Physiology and practice (editorial). *Lancet* 1992; 339:31.

54. Campbell IT, Beatty PCW: Monitoring preoxygenation. *Br J Anaesth* 1994; 72:3.

55. Archer GW, Marx GF: Arterial oxygen tension during apnoea in parturient women. *Br J Anaesth* 1974; 46:358.

56. Gambee AM, Hertzka RE, Fisher DM: Preoxygenation tecniques: Comparison of three minutes and four deep breaths. *Anesth Analg* 1987; 66:468.

57. Berthaud MC, Peacock JE, Reilly CS: Effectiveness of preoxygenation in morbidly obese patients. *Br J Anaesth* 1991; 67:464.

58. Baraka AS, Hanna MT, Jabbour SI, et al: Preoxygenation of pregnant and nonpregnant women in the head-up versus supine position. *Anesth Analg* 1992; 75:757.

59. Palahniuk RJ, Shnider SM, Eger EIII: Pregnancy decreases the requirements for inhaled anesthetic agents. *Anesthesiology* 1974; 41:82.

60. Gin T, Chan MTV: Decrease minimum alveolar concentration of isoflurane in pregnant humans. *Anesthesiology* 1994; 81:829.

61. Shankar KB, Moseley H, Ramasamy M, et al: Arterial to end-tidal carbon dioxide tension difference during anaesthesia in early pregnancy. *Can J Anaesth* 1989; 36:124.

62. Shankar KB, Moseley H, Kumar Y, et al: Arterial to end tidal carbon dioxide tension difference during caesarean section anaesthesia. *Anaesthesia* 1986; 41:698.

63. Shankar KB, Moseley H, Kumar Y, et al: Arterial to end-tidal carbon dioxide tension difference during anaesthesia for tubal ligation. *Anaesthesia* 1987; 42:482.

64. Motoyama EK, Rivard G, Acheson F, et al: Adverse effect of maternal hyperventilation on the foetus. *Lancet* 1966; 1:286.

65. Morishima HO, Moya F, Bossers AC, et al: Adverse effects of maternal hypocapnea on the newborn guinea pig. *Am J Obstet Gynecol* 1964; 88:524.

66. McFadden ER Jr: Asthma, in Isselbacher KJ, Braunwald E, Wilson JD, et al (eds): *Harrison's Principles of Internal Medicine,* ed 13. New York, McGraw-Hill, 1994, pp 1167-1172.

67. Clark SL: National Asthma Education Program Working Group on Asthma and Pregnancy National Institutes of Health, National Heart, Lung, and Blood Institute: Asthma and pregnancy. *Obstet Gynecol* 1993; 82:1036.

68. Gordon M, Niswander KR, Berendes H, et al: Fetal morbidity following potentially anoxigenic obstetric conditions. VII. Bronchial asthma. *Am J Obstet Gynecol* 1970; 106:421.

69. Hernandez E, Angell CS, Johnson WC: Asthma in pregnancy: Current concepts. *Obstet Gynecol* 1980; 55:739.

70. Schaefer G, Silverman F: Pregnancy complicated by asthma. *Am J Obstet Gynecol* 1961; 82:182.

71. Report of the Working Group on Asthma and Pregnancy: Management of asthma during pregnancy. NIH Publication No 93-3279. 14, 1993.

72. Barnes PJ: A new approach to the treatment of asthma. *N Engl J Med* 1989; 321:1517.

73. Pare PD, Gonzalez Montaner JS: Asthma, in Kelley WN (ed): *Textbook of Internal Medicine,* ed 2. Philadelphia, JB Lippincott, 1992, pp 1707-1717.

74. Fitzsimons RR, Greenberger PA, Patterson R: Outcome of pregnancy in women requiring corticosteroids for severe asthma. *J Allergy Clin Immunol* 1986; 78:349.

75. Derbes VJ, Sodeman WA: Reciprocal influences of bronchial asthma and pregnancy. *Am J Med* 1946; 1:367.

76. Williams DA: Asthma and pregnancy. *Allergy* 1967; 22:311.

77. Bahna SL, Bjerkedal T: The course and outcome of pregnancy in women with bronchial asthma. *Allergy* 1972; 27:397.

78. Schatz M, Patterson R, Zeitz S, et al: Corticosteroid therapy for the pregnant asthmatic patient. *JAMA* 1975; 233:804.

79. Doucette JT, Bracken MB: Possible role of asthma in the risk of preterm labor and delivery. *Epidemiology* 1993; 4:143.

80. Perlow JH, Montgomery D, Morgan MA, et al: Severity of asthma and perinatal outcome. *Am J Obstet Gynecol* 1992; 167:963.

81. Lehrer S, Stone J, Lapinski R, et al: Association between pregnancy-induced hypertension and asthma during pregnancy. *Am J Obstet Gynecol* 1993; 168:1463.

82. Schreier L, Cutler RM, Saigal V: Respiratory failure in asthma during the third trimester. *Am J Obstet Gynecol* 1989; 160:80.

83. Gilchrist DM, Fieldman JM, Werker D: Life-threatening status asthmaticus at 12.5 weeks gestation. Report of a normal pregnancy outcome. *Chest* 1991; 100:285.

84. Gruteke P, Askari A, Chatterjee TK, et al: Artifical ventilatory management in a severe, pregnant asthmatic: A case report. *Br J Clin Pract* 1992; 46:63.

85. Gluck JC, Gluck PA: The effects of pregnancy on asthma: A prospective study. *Ann Allergy* 1976; 37:164.

86. Schatz M, Harden K, Forsythe A, et al: The course of asthma during pregnancy, post partum, and with successive pregnancies: A prospective analysis. *J Allergy Clin Immunol* 1988; 81:509.

87. Jones E, Curzen P, Gaugas JM: Suppression activity of pregnancy plasma on mixed lymphocyte reaction. *J Obstet Gynecol* 1973; 80:603.

88. Nolten WE, Rueckert PA: Elevated free cortisol index in pregnancy: possible regulatory mechanisms. *Am J Obstet Gynecol* 1981; 139:492.

89. Raz S, Ziegler M, Caine M: The effect of progesterone on the adrenergic receptors of the urethra. *Br J Urol* 1973; 45:131.

90. Yannone ME, McCurdy JR, Goldfein A: Plasma progesterone levels in normal pregnancy, labor, and the puerperium. *Am J Obstet Gynecol* 1968; 101:1058.

91. Lichtenstein L, Margolis S: Histamine release in vitro: In-

hibition by catecholamines and methyxanthines. *Science* 1968; 161:902.

92. Mathe AA, Hedqvist P: Effect of prostaglandins F_2alpha and E_2 on airway conductance in healthy subjects and asthmatic patients. *Am Rev Respir Dis* 1975; 111:313.

93. Whalen JB, Clancey CJ, Farley DB, et al: Plasma prostaglandins in pregnancy. *Obstet Gynecol* 1978; 51:52.

94. Smith AP: The effects of intravenous infusion of graded doses of prostaglandins F_2alpha and E_2 on lung resistance in patients undergoing termination of pregnancy. *Clin Science* 1973; 44:17.

95. Fishburne JI Jr, Brenner WE, Braaksma JT, et al: Bronchospasm complicating intravenous prostaglandin F_2alpha for therapeutic abortion. *Obstet Gynecol* 1972; 39:892.

96. Hyman AL, Spannhake EW, Kadowitz QJ: Prostaglandins and the lung: State of the art. *Am Rev Respir Dis* 1978; 117:111.

97. Synder RD, Synder DL: Corticosteroids for asthma during pregnancy. *Ann Allergy* 1978; 41:340.

98. Greenberger PA, Patterson R: Beclomethasone diproprionate for severe asthma during pregnancy. *Ann Intern Med* 1983; 98:478

99. Schatz M, Zeiger RS, Harden KM, et al: The safety of inhaled β-agonist bronchodilators during pregnancy. *J Allergy Clin Immunol* 1988; 82:686.

100. Greenberger PA, Patterson R: Safety of therapy for allergic symptoms during pregnancy. *Ann Intern Med* 1978; 89:234.

101. Greenberger PA, Patterson R: The management of asthma during pregnancy and lactation. *Clin Rev Allergy* 1987; 5:317.

102. Freeman RK, Anderson G, Dorchester W: A prospective multiinstitutional study of antepartum fetal heart rate following MI. Contraction stress test versus nonstress test for primary surveillance. *Am J Obstet Gynecol* 1982; 143:771.

103. Manning FA, Morrison I, Lange IR, et al: Fetal assessment based on fetal biophysical profile scoring: Experience in 12,620 referred high-risk pregnancies. *Am J Obstet Gynecol* 1985; 151:343.

104. Wilson J: Use of sodium cromoglycate during pregnancy. *J Pharm Med* 1982; 8:45.

105. Metzger WJ, Turner E, Patterson R: The safety of immunotherapy during pregnancy. *J Allergy Clin Immunol* 1978; 61:268.

106. Bukowsky M, Nakatsu K, Hunt PW: Theophylline reassessed. *Ann Intern Med* 1984; 101:63.

107. Physician Desk Reference. Montvale, NJ, Medical Economics Data Production Co, 1995, pp 1271-1222.

108. Carter BL, Driscoll CE, Smith GD: Theophylline clearance during pregnancy. *Obstet Gynecol* 1986; 68:555.

109. Frederiksen MC, Ruo TI, Chow MJ, et al: Theophylline pharmacokinetics in pregnancy. *Clin Pharm Ther* 1986; 40:321.

110. Gardner MJ, Schatz M, Cousins L, et al: Longitudinal effects of pregnancy on the pharmacokinetics of theophylline. *Eur J Clin Pharm* 1987; 31:289.

111. Popa V: Beta-adrenergic drugs. *Clin Chest Med* 1986; 7:313.

112. Kalsner S: Mechanism of hydrocortisone potentiation of response to epinephrine and norepinephrine in rabbit aorta. *Circ Res* 1969; 24:383.

113. Heinonen OP, Slone D, Shapiro S: Birth defects and drugs in pregnancy. Littleton, Mass, Publishing Sciences Group, 1977.

114. Hood DD, Dewan DM, James FM III: Maternal and fetal effects of epinephrine in gravid ewes. *Anesthesiology* 1986; 64:610.

115. Leighton BL, Norris MC, Sosis M, et al: Limitations of epinephrine as a marker of intravascular injection in laboring women. *Anesthesiology* 1987; 66:688.

116. Brogden RN, Faulds D: Sameterol xinafoate: A review of its pharmacological properties and therapeutic potential in reversible obstructive airways disease. *Drugs* 1991; 42:895.

117. Fanta CH: Acute Asthma, in Weiss EB, Stein M (eds): *Bronchial Asthma. Mechanisms and Therapeutics,* ed 3. Boston, Little, Brown, 1993, pp 972-984.

118. Uden DL, Goetz DR, Kohen DP, et al: Comparison of nebulized terbutaline and subcutaneous epinephrine in the treatment of acute asthma. *Ann Emerg Med* 1985; 14:229.

119. Becker AB, Nelson NA, Simons FER: Inhaled salbutamol (albuterol) vs injected epinephrine in the treatment of acute asthma in children. *J Pediatr* 1983; 102:465.

120. Rossing TH, Fanta CH, Goldstein DH, et al: Emergency therapy in asthma: Comparison of the acute effects of parenteral and inhaled sympathomimetics and infused aminophylline. *Am Rev Respir Dis* 1980; 122:365.

121. Fanta CH, Rossing TH, McFadden ER Jr: Treatment of acute asthma: Is combination therapy with sympathomimetics and methylxanthines indicated? *Am J Med* 1986; 80:5.

122. Snider DE, Layde PM, Johnson MW, et al: Treatment of tuberculosis during pregnancy. *Am Rev Resp Dis* 1980; 122:65.

123. Williams MH Jr: Drugs five years after: Beclomethasone dipropionate. *Ann Intern Med* 1981; 95:464.

124. Caritis SN, Darby MJ, Chan L: Pharmacologic treatment of preterm labor. *Clin Obstet Gynecol* 1988; 31:635.

125. Benedetti TJ: Life-threatening complications of betamimetic therapy for preterm labor inhibition. *Clin Perinatol* 1986; 13:843.

126. Pisani RJ, Rosenow EC III: Pulmonary edema associated with tocolytic therapy. *Ann Intern Med* 1989; 110:714.

127. Barnes PJ: Inhaled glucocorticoids for asthma. *N Engl J Med* 1995; 332:868.

128. Morris HG: Mechanisms of action and therapeutic role of corticosteroids in asthma. *J Allergy Clin Immunol* 1985; 75:1.

129. Laurens RG Jr, Honig EG: Corticosteroids in the treatment of asthma. *South Med J* 1986; 79:1544.

130. Fanta CH, Rossing TH, McFadden ER Jr: Glucocorticoids in acute asthma: A critical controlled trial. *Am J Med* 1983; 74:845.

131. Littenberg B, Gluck EH: A controlled trial of methylprednisolone in the emergency treatment of acute asthma. *N Engl J Med* 1986; 314:150.

132. Shim CS, Williams MH Jr: Cough and wheezing from beclomethasone dipropionate aerosol are absent after triamcinolone acetonide. *Ann Intern Med* 1987; 106:700.

133. Kingston HGG, Hirshman CA: Perioperative management of the patient with asthma. *Anesth Analg* 1984; 63:844.

134. McDonald AJ: Asthma. *Emerg Med Clin North Am* 1989; 7:219.

135. Molfino NA, Slutsky AS: Near-fatal asthma. *Eur Respir J* 1994; 7:981.

136. Slinger PD: Perioperative respiratory assessment and management. *Can J Anaesth* 1992; 39:R115.

137. Schatz M: Asthma in pregnancy, in Dawson A, Simon RA (eds): *The Practical Management of Asthma,* New York, Grune & Stratton, 1984, pp 195.

138. Hagerdal M, Morgan CR, Sumner AE, et al: Minute ventilation and oxygen consumption during labor with epidural analgesia. *Anesthesiology* 1983; 59:425.

139. Chestnut DH, Vandewalker GE, Owen CL, et al: The influence of continuous epidural bupivacaine analgesia on the second stage of labor and method of delivery in nulliparous women. *Anesthesiology* 1987; 66:774.

140. Chestnut DH, Laszewski LJ, Pollack KL, et al: Continuous epidural infusion of 0.0625% bupivacaine-0.0002% fentanyl during the second stage of labor. *Anesthesiology* 1990; 72:613.

141. Younker D, Clark R, Tessem J, et al: Bupivacaine-fentanyl epidural analgesia for a parturient in status asthmaticus. *Can J Anaesth* 1987; 34:609.

142. Norris MC, Grieco WM, Borkowski M, et al: Complications of labor analgesia: Epidural versus combined spinal epidural techniques. *Anesth Analg* 1994; 79:529.

143. Collis RE, Baxandall ML, Srikantharajah ID, et al: Combined spinal epidural (CSE) analgesia: Technique, management and outcome of 300 mothers. *Int J Obstet Anesth* 1994; 3:75.

144. Abouleish A, Abouleish E, Camann W: Combined spinal-epidural analgesia in advanced labour. *Can J Anaesth* 1994; 41:575.

145. Palmer CM: Early depression following intrathecal fentanyl-morphine combination. *Anesthesiology* 1991; 6:1153.

146. Hays RL, Palmer CM: Respiratory depression after intrathecal sufentanil during labor. *Anesthesiology* 1994; 81:511.

147. Brockway MS, Noble DW, Sharwood-Smith GH, et al: Profound respiratory depression after extradural fentanyl. *Br J Anaesth* 1990; 14:971.

148. Negre I, Gueneron J-P, Ecoffey C, et al: Ventilatory response to carbon dioxide after intramuscular and epidural fentanyl. *Anesth Analg* 1987; 66:707.

149. Cohen SE, Labaille T, Benhamou D, et al: Respiratory effects of epidural sufentanil after cesarean section. *Anesth Analg* 1992; 74:677.

150. Freund FG, Bonica JJ, Ward RJ, et al: Ventilatory reserve and level of motor block during high spinal and epidural anesthesia. *Anesthesiology* 1967; 28:834.

151. Steinbrook RA, Concepcion M: Respiratory effects of spinal anesthesia: Resting ventilation and single-breath CO_2 response. *Anesth Analg* 1991; 72:182.

152. Saito Y, Sakura S, Kaneko M, et al: The effects of epidural anesthesia on ventilatory response to hypoxia. *J Clin Anesth* 1993; 5:46.

153. Egbert LD, Tamersy K, Deas TC: Pulmonary function during spinal anesthesia: The mechanism of cough depression. *Anesthesiology* 1961; 22:882.

154. Sharrock NE, Castellano P, Sanborn KV, et al: Correlation of cough strength and hemodynamics with recovery from sensory block during epidural anesthesia. *Reg Anesth* 1989; 14:S87.

155. Gamil M: Serial peak expiratory flow rates in mothers during caesarean section under extradural anaesthesia. *Br J Anaesth* 1989; 62:415.

156. Norris MC, Torjman M, Leighton BL, et al: Respiratory and motor function during bupivacaine spinal anesthesia for cesarean section. *Anesth Analg* 1990; 70:S283.

157. Harrop-Griffiths AW, Ravalia A, Browne DA, et al: Regional anaesthesia and cough effectiveness: A study in patients undergoing caesarean section. *Anaesthesia* 1991; 46:11.

158. Hirshman CA, Bergman NA: Factor influencing intrapulmonary airway calibre during anaesthesia. *Br J Anaesth* 1990; 65:30.

159. Converse JG, Smotrilla MM: Anesthesia and the asthmatic. *Anesth Analg* 1961; 40:336.

160. Shnider SM, Papper EM: Anesthesia for the asthmatic patient. *Anesthesiology* 1961; 22:886.

161. Mallampati SR: Bronchospasm during spinal anesthesia. *Anesth Analg* 1981; 60:838.

162. Wang CY, Ong GSY: Severe bronchospasm during epidural anaesthesia. *Anaesthesia* 1993; 48:514.

163. McGough EK, Cohen JA: Unexpected bronchospasm during spinal anesthesia. *J Clin Anesth* 1990; 2:35.

164. Bromage PR: Epidural Analgesia. *Epidural Analgesia.* Philadelphia, WB Saunders, 1978, p 638., pp 601-653.

165. Groeben H, Schwalen A, Irsfeld S, et al: High thoracic epidural anesthesia does not alter airway resistance and attenuates the response to an inhalational provocation test in patients with bronchial hyperreactivity. *Anesthesiology* 1994; 81:868.

166. Peters J, Kutkuhn B, Medert HA, et al: Sympathetic blockade by epidural anesthesia attenuates the cardiovascular response to severe hypoxemia. *Anesthesiology* 1990; 72:134.

167. Olsson GL: Bronchospasm during anaesthesia: A computer-aided incidence study of 136,929 patients. *Acta Anaesth Scand* 1987; 31:244.

168. Isono S, Nishino T, Sugimori K, et al: Respiratory effects of expiratory flow-resistive loading in conscious and anesthetized humans. *Anesth Analg* 1990; 70:594.

169. Gal TJ: Pulmonary mechanics in normal subjects following endotracheal intubation. *Anesthesiology* 1980; 52:27.

170. Hirshman CA: Airway reactivity in humans. *Anesthesiology* 1983; 58:170.

171. Nathan RA, Segall N, Glover GC, et al: The effects of H1 and H2 antihistamines on histamine inhalation challenges in asthmatic patients. *Am Rev Respir Dis* 1979; 120:1257.

172. Koga Y, Iwatsuki N, Hashimoto Y: Direct effects of H2-receptor antagonists on airway smooth muscle and on responses mediated by H1 and H2 receptors. *Anesthesiology* 1987; 66:181.

173. Hall KD, Norris FH Jr: Fluothane sensitization of the dog heart to action of epinephrine. *Anesthesiology* 1958; 19:631.

174. Dewan DM, Floyd HM, Thistlewood JM, et al: Sodium citrate pretreatment in elective cesarean section patients. *Anesth Analg* 1985; 64:34.

175. Gal TJ, Suratt PR: Atropine and glycopyrrolate effects on lung mechanics in normal man. *Anesth Analg* 1981; 60:85.

176. Kil H-K, Rooke GA, Ryan-Dukes MA, et al: Effect of prophylactic bronchodilator treatment on lung resistance after tracheal intubation. *Anesthesiology* 1994; 81:43.

177. Hirshman CA, Downes H, Farbood A, et al: Ketamine block of bronchospasm in experimental canine asthma. *Br J Anaesth* 1979; 51:713.

178. Curry C, Lenox WC, Spannhake EW, et al: Contractile responses of guinea pig trachea to oxybarbiturates and thiobarbiturates. *Anesthesiology* 1991; 75:679.

179. Kosaka Y, Takahashi T, Mark LC: Intravenous thiobarbiturate anesthesia for cesarean section. *Anesthesiology* 1969; 31:489.

180. Sarma VJ: Use of ketamine in acute severe asthma. *Acta Anaesthesiol Scand* 1992; 36:106.

181. Sarma VJ: Use of ketamine in acute severe asthma. *Acta Anaesthesiol Scand* 1992; 36:107.

182. Roy TM, Pruitt VL, Garner PA, et al: The potential role of anesthesia in status asthmaticus. *J Asthma* 1992; 29:73.

183. Smith JA, Santer LJ: Respiratory arrest following intramuscular ketamine injection in a 4-year-old child. *Ann Emerg Med* 1993; 22:613.

184. Corssen G, Gutierrez J, Reves JG, et al: Ketamine in the anesthetic management of asthmatic patients. *Anesth Analg* 1972; 51:588.

185. Pederson CM, Thirstrup S, Nielsen-Kudsk JE: Smooth muscle relaxant effects of propofol and ketamine in isolated guinea pig tracheal. *Eur J Pharmacol* 1993; 238:75.

186. Rock MJ, Reyes de la Rocha S, Lerner M, et al: Effect on airway resistance of ketamine by aerosol in guinea pigs. *Anesth Analg* 1989; 68:506.

187. Waltemath CL, Bergman NA: Effects of ketamine and halothane on increased respiratory resistance provoked by aerosols. *Anesthesiology* 1974; 41:473.

188. White PF, Way WL, Trevor AJ: Ketamine-Its pharmacology and therapeutic uses. *Anesthesiology* 1982; 56:119.

189. Stone DJ, Sarkar TK, Keltz H: Effect of adrenergic stimulation and inhibition on human airways. *J Appl Physiol* 1973; 34:624.

190. Kumar SM, Kothary SP, Zsigmond EK: Plasma free norepinephrine and epinephrine concentrations following diazepam-ketamine induction in patients undergoing cardiac surgery. *Acta Anaesthesiol Scand* 1978; 22:593.

191. Hirshman CA, Krieger W, Littlejohn G, et al: Ketamine-aminophylline-induced decrease in seizure threshold. *Anesthesiology* 1982; 56:464.

192. Nathan RA, Segall N, Schocket AL: A comparison of the actions of H1 and H2 antihistamines on histamine-induced bronchoconstriction and cutaneous wheal response in asthmatic patients. *J Allergy Clin Immunol* 1981; 67:171.

193. Brandus V, Joffe S, Benoit CV, et al: Bronchial spasm during general anaesthesia. *Can Anaesth Soc J* 1970; 17:269.

194. Downes H, Gerber N, Hirshman CA: I.V. lignocaine in reflex and allergic bronchoconstriction. *Br J Anaesth* 1980; 52:873.

195. Downes H, Hirshman CA: Lidocaine aerosols do not prevent allergic bronchoconstriction. *Anesth Analg* 1981; 60:28.

196. Weiss EB, Patwardhan AV: The response to lidocaine in bronchial asthma. *Chest* 1977; 72:429.

197. Greiss FC Jr, Still JG, Anderson SG: Effects of local anesthetic agents on the uterine vasculatures and myometrium. *Am J Obstet Gynecol* 1976; 124:889.

198. Hirshman CA, Bergman NA: Halothane and enflurane protect against bronchospasm in an asthma dog model. *Anesth Analg* 1978; 57:629.

199. Hirshman CA, Edelstein G, Peetz S, et al: Mechanism of action of inhalational anesthesia on airways. *Anesthesiology* 1982; 56:107.

200. Vettermann J, Beck KC, Lindahl SGE, et al: Actions of enflurane, isoflurane, vecuronium, atracurium and pancuronium on pulmonary resistance in dogs. *Anesthesiology* 1988; 69:688.

201. Mitsuhata H, Saitoh J, Shimizu R, et al: Sevoflurane and isoflurane protect against bronchospasm in dogs. *Anesthesiology* 1994; 81:1230.

202. Brown RH, Mitzner W, Zerhouni EA, et al: Direct in vivo visualization of bronchodilation induced by inhalational anesthesia using high-resolution computed tomography. *Anesthesiology* 1993; 78:295.

203. Brown RH, Zerhouni EA, Hirshman CA: Comparison of low concentrations of halothane and isoflurane as bronchodilators. *Anesthesiology* 1993; 78:1097.

204. Yamamoto K, Morimoto N, Warner DO, et al: Factors influencing the direct actions of volatile anesthetics on airway smooth muscle. *Anesthesiology* 1993; 78:1102.

205. Kochi T, Hagiya M, Mizuguchi T: Effects of enflurane on contractile response of canine trachealis muscle. *Anesth Analg* 1989; 69:60.

206. Warner DO, Vettermann J, Brusasco V, et al: Pulmonary resistance during halothane anesthsia is no determined only by airway caliber. *Anesthesiology* 1989; 79:453.

207. Shah MV, Hirshman CA: Mode of action of halothane on histamine-induced airway constriction in dogs with reactive airways. *Anesthesiology* 1986; 65:170.

208. Lindeman KS, Baker SG, Hirshman CA: Interaction between halothane and the nonadrenergic, noncholinergic inhibitory system in procine trachealis muscle. *Anesthesiology* 1994; 81:641.

209. Roizen MF, Stevens WC: Multiform ventricular tachycardia due to the interaction of aminophylline and halothane. *Anesth Analg* 1978; 57:738.

210. Richards W, Thompson J, Lewis G, et al: Cardiac arrest associated with halothane anesthesia in a patient receiving theophylline. *Ann Allergy* 1988; 61:83.

211. Stirt JA, Berger JM, Roe SD, et al: Halothane-induced cardiac arrhythmias following administration of aminophylline in experimental animals. *Anesth Analg* 1981; 60:517.

212. Prokocimer PG, Nicholls E, Gaba DM, et al: Epinephrine arrhythmogenicity is ehanced by acute, but not chronic, aminophylline administration during halothane anesthesia in dogs. *Anesthesiology* 1986; 65:13.

213. Stirt JA, Berger JM, Roe SD, et al: Safety of enflurane following administration of aminophylline in experimental animals. *Anesth Analg* 1981; 60:871.

214. Stirt JA, Berger JM, Sullivan SF: Lack of arrhythmogenicity of isoflurane following administration of aminophylline in dogs. *Anesth Analg* 1983; 62:568.

215. Tobias JD, Kubos KL, Hirshman CA: Aminophylline does not attenuate histamine-induced airway constriction during halothane anesthesia. *Anesthesiology* 1989; 71:723.

216. Munson ES, Embro WJ: Enflurane, isoflurane and halothane and isolated human myometrium. *Anesthesiology* 1977; 46:11.

217. Wallace DH, Cosentino SL, Shearer VE, et al: The effect of isoflurane 1% or low-dose and regional anesthesia on uterine tone at cesarean section. *Anesthesiology* 1989; 71:A874.

218. Moir DD: Anaesthesia for caesarean section: An evaluation of a method using low concentrations of halothane and 50 percent of oxygen. *Br J Anaesth* 1970; 42:136.

219. Lipshitz J: Uterine and cardiovascular effects of aminophylline. *Am J Obstet Gynecol* 1978; 131:716.

220. Andersson KE, Bengtsson LP, Gustafson I: The relaxing effect of terbutaline on the human uterus during term labor. *Am J Obstet Gynecol* 1975; 121:602.

221. Lipshitz J, Baillie P: The effects of fenoterol hydrobromide (partusisten) aerosol on uterine activity and the cardiovascular system. *Br J Obstet Gyneacol* 1976; 83:864.

222. Vinall PS, Jenkins DM: Salbutamol and haemorrhage at spontaneous abortion. *Lancet* 1977; 1:1355.

223. Smith AP: The effects of intravenous infusion of graded doses of prostaglandins F_2alpha and E_2 on lung resistance in patients undergoing termination of pregnancy. *Clin Sci* 1973; 44:17.

224. O'Leary AM: Severe bronchospasm and hypotension after 15-methyl prostaglandin $F_{2\alpha}$ in atonic post partum haemorrhage. *Int J Obstet Anesth* 1994; 3:42.

225. Kreisman H, Van de Wiel W, Mitchell CA: Respiratory function during prostaglandin-induced labor. *Am Rev Resp Dis* 1975; 111:564.

226. Mathé AA, Hedqvist P, Holmgren A, et al: Bronchial hyperreactivity to prostaglandin $F_{2\alpha}$ and histamine in patients with asthma. *Br Med J* 1973; 1:193.

227. Louie S, Krzanowski JJ Jr, Bukantz SC, et al: Effects of ergometrine on airway smooth muscle contractile responses. *Clin Allergy* 1985; 15:173.

228. Flacke JW, Flacke WE, Bloor BC, et al: Histamine release by four narcotics: A double-blind study in humans. *Anesth Analg* 1987; 66:723.

229. Crago RR, Bryan AC, Laws AK, et al: Respiratory flow resistance after curare and pancuronium, measured by forced oscillations. *Can Anaesth Soc J* 1972; 19:607.

230. Nana A, Cardan E, Leitersdorfer T: Pancuronium bromide: Its use in asthmatics and patients with liver disease. *Anaesthesia* 1972; 27:154.

231. Heath ML: Bronchospasm in an asthmatic patient following pancuronium. *Anaesthesia* 1973; 28:437.

232. Clark RM: Reaction to pancuronium? *Br J Anaesth* 1973; 45:997.

233. Bellomo R, McLaughlin P, Tai E, et al: Asthma requiring mechanical ventilation: A low morbidity approach. *Chest* 1994; 105:891.

234. Silverman MS, Bishop MJ: Manual vs mechanical ventilation in a model of bronchospasm: Does the "educated hand" exist? *Anesthesiology* 1989; 71:A441.

235. Miller MM, Fish JE, Patterson R: Methacholine and physostigmine airway reactivity in asthmatic and non-asthmatic subjects. *J Allergy Clin Immunol* 1977; 60:116.

236. Hammond J, Wright D, Sale J: Pattern of change of bronchomotor tone following reversal of neuromuscular blockade. Comparison between atropine and glycopyrrolate. *Br J Anaesth* 1983; 55:955.

237. Lenox WC, Hirshman CA: Amrinone attenuates airway constriction during halothane anesthesia. *Anesthesiology* 1993; 79:789.

238. Tobias JD, Hirshman CA: Attenuation of histamine-induced airway constriction by albuterol during halothane anesthesia. *Anesthesiology* 1990; 72:105.

239. Kelley HW, Murphy S: Beta-adrenergic agonists for acute, severe asthma. *Ann Pharmacother* 1992; 26:81.

240. Duckett JE, Zebrowski M: A simple device for delivering bronchodilators into the anesthesia circuit. *Anesthesiology* 1985; 62:699.

241. Diamond MJ: Delivering bronchodilators into the anesthesia circuit. *Anesthesiology* 1986; 64:531.

242. Bush GL: Aerosol delivery devices for the anesthesia circuit. *Anesthesiology* 1986; 65:240.

243. Gold MI, Marcial E: An anesthetic adaptor for all metered dose inhalers. *Anesthesiology* 1988; 68:964.

244. Koska AJ III, Bjoraker DG: An anesthetic adapter for all metered dose inhalers that is readily available to all. *Anesth Analg* 1989; 69:266.

245. Bishop MJ, Larson RP, Buschman DL: Metered dose inhaler aerosol characteristics are affected by the endotracheal tube actuator/adapter used. *Anesthesiology* 1990; 73:1263.

246. Crogan SJ, Bishop MJ: Delivery efficiency of metered dose aerosols given via endotracheal tubes. *Anesthesiology* 1989; 70:1008.

247. Taylor RH, Lerman J: High-efficiency delivery of salbutamol with a metered-dose inhaler in narrow tracheal tubes and catheters. *Anesthesiology* 1991; 74:360.

248. Peterfreund RA, Niven RW, Kacmarek RM: Syringe-actuated metered dose inhalers: A quantitative laboratory evaluation of albuterol delivery through nozzle extensions. *Anesth Analg* 1994; 78:554.

249. Vichitvejpaisal P, Oranee S-X, Suthiporn U: The use of nebulized salbutamol in patients with bronchospasm during anaesthsia: A clinical trial. *J Med Assoc Thai* 1991; 74:397.

250. Andrews WM, Ramin SM, Maberry MC, et al: Effect of type of anesthesia on blood at elective repeat cesarean section. *Am J Perinatol* 1992; 9:197.

251. Schwartz SH: Treatment of status asthmaticus with halothane. *JAMA* 1984; 251:2688.

252. Bayliff CD, Koch JP, Faclier G: The use of halothane in the treatment of status asthmaticus. *Drug Intell Clin Pharm* 1985; 19:307.

253. Rosseel P, Lauwers LF, Baute L: Halothane treatment in life-threatening asthma. *Intensive Care Med* 1985; 11:241.

254. Bierman MI, Brown M, Muren O, et al: Prolonged isoflurane anesthesia in status asthmaticus. *Crit Care Med* 1986; 14:832.

255. Parnass SM, Feld JM, Chamberlin WH, et al: Status asthmaticus treated with isoflurane and enflurane. *Anesth Analg* 1987; 66:193.

256. Maltais F, Sovilj M, Goldberg P, et al: Respiratory mechanics in status asthmaticus. Effects of inhaled anesthesia. *Chest* 1994; 106:1401.

257. Otte RW, Fireman P: Isoflurane anesthesia for the treatment of refractory status asthmaticus. *Ann Allergy* 1991; 66:305.

258. McLean RM: Magnesium and its therapeutic uses: A review. *Am J Med* 1994; 96:63.

259. Skobeloff EM, Kim D, Spivey WH: Magnesium sulfate for the treatment of bronchospasm complicating acute bronchitis in a four-months'-pregnant woman. *Ann Emerg Med* 1993; 22:1365.

260. Wood RE, Boat TF, Doershuk CF: Cystic fibrosis. *Am Rev Respir Dis* 1976; 113:833.

261. Dry PJ, Wake S, Robertson CF, et al: Analysis of DNA probes for the prenatal diagnosis of cystic fibrosis. *Med J Aust* 1989; 151:131.

262. Lemna WK, Feldman GL, Kerem BS, et al: Mutation analysis for heterozygote detection and the prenatal diagnosis of cystic fibrosis. *N Engl J Med* 1990; 322:291.

263. Lieu TA, Watson SE, Washington AE: The cost-effectiveness of prenatal carrier screening for cystic fibrosis. *Obstet Gynecol* 1994; 84:903.

264. Huang NN, Schidlow DV, Szatrowski TH, et al: Clinical features, survival rate, and prognostic factors in young adults with cystic fibrosis. *Am J Med* 1987; 82:871.

265. Di Sant'Agnese PA, Davis PB: Cystic fibrosis in adults: 75 cases and a review of 232 cases in the literature. *Am J Med* 1979; 66:121.

266. Corkey CWB, Newth CJL, Corey M, et al: Pregnancy in cystic fibrosis: A better prognosis in patients with pancreatic function? *Am J Obstet Gynecol* 1981; 140:737.

267. Valenzuela GJ, Comunale FL, Davidson BH, et al: Clinical management of patient with cystic fibrosis and pulmonary insufficiency. *Am J Obstet Gynecol* 1988; 159:1181.

268. Novy MJ, Tyler JM, Shwachman H, et al: Cystic fibrosis and pregnancy. *Obstet Gynecol* 1967; 30:530.

269. Palmer J, Dillon-Baker C, Tecklin JS, et al: Pregnancy in patients with cystic fibrosis. *Ann Intern Med* 1983; 99:596.

270. Larsen JW: Cystic fibrosis and pregnancy. *Obstet Gynecol* 1972; 39:880.

271. Taussig LM, Kattwinkel J, Friedewald WT, et al: A new prognostic score and clinical evaluation system for cystic fibrosis. *J Pediatr* 1973; 82:380.

272. McCaffrey RM, Dunn LJ: Primary pulmonary hypertension and pregnancy. *Obstet Gynecol Surv* 1964; 19:567.

273. Morgan Jones A: Eisenmenger syndrome in pregnancy. *Br Med J* 1965; 1:1627.

274. Cohen LF, Di Sant'Agnese PA, Friedlander J: Cystic fibrosis and pregnancy: A national survey. *Lancet* 1980; 2:842.

275. Konstan MW, Byard PJ, Hoppel CL, et al: Effect of high-dose ibuprofen in patients with cystic fibrosis. *N Engl J Med* 1995; 332:848.

276. Moise KJ Jr, Huhta JC, Sharif DS, et al: Indomethacin in the treatment of premature labor. *N Engl J Med* 1988; 319:327.

277. Norton ME, Merrill J, Cooper BAB, et al: Neonatal complications after the administration of indomethacin for preterm labor. *N Engl J Med* 1993; 329:1602.

278. Grand RJ, Talamo RC, Di Sant'Agnese PA, et al: Pregnancy in cystic fibrosis of the pancreas. *JAMA* 1966; 195:993.

279. Lamberty JM, Rubin BK: The management of anaesthesia for patients with cystic fibrosis. *Anaesthesia* 1985; 40:448.

280. Dawson P, Rosenfeld JV, Murphy MA, et al: Epidural abscess associated with postoperative epidural analgesia. *Anaesth Intens Care* 1991; 19:569.

281. Hyde NH, Harrison DM: Intrathecal morphine in a parturient with cystic fibrosis. *Anesth Analg* 1986; 65:1357.

282. Howell PR, Kent N, Douglas MJ: Anaesthesia for the parturient with cystic fibrosis. *Int J Obstet Anesth* 1993; 2:152.

283. Olsen MM, Gauderer MWL, Girz MK, et al: Surgery in patients with cystic fibrosis. *J Pediatr Surg* 1987; 22:613.

284. Richardson VF, Robertson CF, Mowat AP, et al: Deterioration in lung function after general anaesthesia in patients with cystic fibrosis. *Acta Paediatr Scand* 1984; 73:75.

285. Fick RB, Reynolds HY: Changing spectrum of pneumonia: News media creation or clinical reality? *Am J Med* 1983; 74:1.

286. Madinger NE, Greenspoon JS, Ellrodt AG: Pneumonia during pregnancy: Has modern technology improved maternal and fetal outcome? *Am J Obstet Gynecol* 1989; 161:657.

287. Benedetti TJ, Valle R, Ledger WJ: Antepartum pneumonia in pregnancy. *Am J Obstet Gynecol* 1982; 144:413.

288. Oxorn H: The changing aspects of pneumonia complicating pregnancy. *Am J Obstet Gynecol* 1955; 70:1057.

289. Hopwood HG: Pneumonia in pregnancy. *Obstet Gynecol* 1965; 25:875.

290. Minkoff H, de Regt RH, Landesman S, et al: *Pneumocystis carinii* pneumonia associated with adult immunodeficiency syndrome in pregnancy: A report of three maternal deaths. *Obstet Gynecol* 1986; 67:284.

291. Greenberg MW: Maternal mortality in the epidemic of Asian influenza. *Am J Obstet Gynecol* 1958; 76:897.

292. Kort BA, Cefalo RC, Baker VV: Fatal influenza a pneumonia in pregnancy. *Am J Perinatol* 1986; 3:179.

293. Landsberger EJ, Hager WD, Grossman JHIII: Successful management of varicella pneumonia complicating pregnancy: A report of three cases. *J Reprod Med* 1986; 31:311.

294. Harris RE, Rhoades FR: Varicella pneumonia complicating pregnancy: Report of a case and review of the literature. *Obstet Gynecol* 1965; 25:734.

295. Grover L, Kane J, Kravitz J, et al: Systemic acyclovir in pregnancy: A case report. *Obstet Gynecol* 1985; 65:284.

296. Purtilo DT: Opportunistic mycotic infections in pregnancy women. *Am J Obstet Gynecol* 1975; 122:607.

297. Harris RE: Coccidioidomycosis complicating pregnancy. *Obstet Gynecol* 1966; 28:401.

298. Ellinoy BR: Amphotericin B usage in pregnancy complicated by cryptococcosis. *Am J Obstet Gynecol* 1973; 115:285.

299. Ready LB, Helfer D: Bacterial meningitis after epidural anesthesia. *Anesthesiology* 1989; 71:989.

300. Strong WE: Epidural abscess associated with epidural catheterization: A rare event? Report of two cases with markedly delayed presentation. *Anesthesiology* 1991; 74:943.

301. Eng RHK, Seligman SJ: Lumbar puncture-induced meningitis. *JAMA* 1981; 245:1456.

302. Carp H, Bailey S: The association between meningitis and dural puncture in bacteremic rats. *Anesthesiology* 1992; 76:739.

303. Chestnut DH: Spinal anesthesia in the febrile patient. *Anesthesiology* 1992; 76:667.

304. Ngan Kee WD, Jones MR, Thomas P, et al: Extradural abscess complicating extradural anaesthesia for caesarean section. *Br J Anaesth* 1992; 69:647.

305. Schaefer G, Zervoudakis IA, Fuchs FF, et al: Pregnancy and pulmonary tuberculosis. *Obstet Gynecol* 1975; 46:706.

306. Margono F, Mroueh J, Garely A, et al: Resurgence of active tuberculosis among pregnant women. *Obstet Gynecol* 1994; 83:911.

307. Hamburg M: The challenge of controlling tuberculosis in New York City. *NY State J Med* 1992; 92:291.

308. Frieden TR, Sterling T, Pabllo-Mendez A, et al: The emergence of drug-resistant tuberculosis in New York City. *N Engl J Med* 1993; 328:521.

309. Cantwell MF, Shehab ZM, Costello AM, et al: Brief report: Congenital tuberculosis. *N Engl J Med* 1994; 330:1051.

310. Centers for Disease Control: Guidelines for preventing the transmission of mycobacterium tuberculosis in health-care facilities. *MMWR* 1994; 43:59.

311. Jacob RF, Abernathy RS: Management of tuberculosis in pregnancy and the newborn. *Clin Perinatol* 1988; 15:305.

312. Iseman MD, Cohn DL, Sbarbaro JA: Directly observed treatment of tuberculosis: We can't afford not to try it. *N Engl J Med* 1993; 328:576.

313. Ramos AD, Hibbard LT, Craig JR: Congenital tuberculosis. *Obstet Gynecol* 1974; 43:61.

314. Swartz HM, Reichling BA: Hazards of radiation exposure for pregnant women. *JAMA* 1979; 239:1907.

315. Centers for disease control: Guidlines for prevention of TB transmission in hospitals. Atlanta, U.S. Department of Health and Human Services, Public Health Service, HHS Publication No (CDC) 1982; 82-8371.

316. Crystal RG: Sarcoidosis, in Isselbacher KJ, Braunwald E, Wilson JD, et al (eds): *Harrison's Principles of Internal Medicine,* vol 13. New York, McGraw-Hill, 1994, pp 1679-1684.

317. Fanbury BL (ed): Sarcoidosis and other granulomatous diseases of the lung. New York, Marcel Dekker, 1983.

318. Given FT Jr, Di Benedetto RL: Sarcoidosis and pregnancy: Report of 5 cases and 1 maternal death. *Obstet Gynecol* 1963; 22:355.

319. O'Leary JA: Ten-year study of sarcoidosis and pregnancy. *Am J Obstet Gynecol* 1962; 84:462.

320. Reisfield DR: Boeck's sarcoid and pregnancy. *Am J Obstet Gynecol* 1958; 75:795.

321. Gallagher JP, Douglass LH: Sarcoidosis and pregnancy. *Obstet Gynecol* 1953; 2:590.

322. Dines DE, Banner EA: Sarcoidosis during pregnancy: Improvement in pulmonary function. *JAMA* 1967; 200:726.

323. Fried KG: Sarcoidosis and pregnancy. *Acta Med Scand* 1964; 176(425S):218.

324. Mayock RL, Sullivan RD, Greening RR, et al: Sarcoidosis and pregnancy. *JAMA* 1957; 164:158.

325. Wilson-Holt N: Post partum presentation of hypercalcaemic sarcoidosis. *Postgrad Med J* 1985; 61:627.

326. Eggelmeijer F, Dijkmans BAC: Sarcoidosis post partum: a description of four cases. *Br J Rheum* 1989; 28:270.

327. Wills MH, Harris MM: An unusual airway complication with sarcoidosis. *Anesthesiology* 1987; 66:554.

328. Hanley ME, Bone RC: Acute respiratory failure: Pathophysiology, causes, and clinical manifestations. *Postgrad Med J* 1986; 79:166.

329. Ingram RH Jr: Adult respiratory distress syndrome, in Isselbacher KJ, Braunwald E, Wilson JD, et al (eds): *Harrison's Principles of Internal Medicine,* vol 13. New York, McGraw-Hill, 1994, pp 1240-1243.

330. Hyers TM, Fowler AA: Adult respiratory distress syndrome: Causes, morbidity and mortality. *Fed Proc* 1986; 45:25.

331. Bell RC, Coalson JJ, Smith JD, et al: Multiple organ sys-

tem failure and infection in the adult respiratory distress syndrome. *Ann Intern Med* 1983; 99:293.

332. Elliott CG, Zimmerman GA, Orme JF, et al: Case report: Granulocyte aggregation in adult respiratory distress syndrome (ARDS): Serial histologic and physiologic observations. *Am J Med Sci* 1985; 289:70.

333. Andersen HF, Lynch JP, Johnson TRB: Adult respiratory distress syndrome in obstetrics and gynecology. *Obstet Gynecol* 1980; 55:291.

334. Feldman JM: Adult respiratory distress syndrome in a pregnant patient with a pheochromocytoma. *J Surg Oncol* 1985; 29:5.

335. Stratta P, Canavese C, Colla L, et al: Adult respiratory distress syndrome following administration of nitroprusside in postpartum acute renal failure (letter). *Clin Nephrol* 1989; 31:117.

336. Kaufman BS, Kaminsky SJ, Rackow EC, et al: Adult respiratory distress syndrome following orogenital sex during pregnancy. *Crit Care Med* 1987; 15:703.

337. Raphael JH, Bexton MDR: Combined high frequency ventilation in the management of respiratory failure in late pregnancy. *Anaesthesia* 1993; 48:596.

338. Hanley ME, Bone RC: Acute respiratory failure. Pathophysiology, causes and clinical manifestations. *Post Grad Med* 1986; 79:166.

339. Sosin D, Krasnow J, Moawad A, et al: Successful spontaneous vaginal delivery during mechanical ventilatory support for the adult respiratory distress syndrome. *Obstet Gynecol* 1986; 68:19S.

340. Pruett K, Faro S: Pyelonephritis associated with respiratory distress. *Obstet Gynecol* 1987; 69:444.

341. Wilkins I, Mezrow G, Lynch L, et al: Amnionitis and life-threatening respiratory distress after percutaneous umbilical blood sampling. *Am J Obstet Gynecol* 1989; 160:427.

342. Elkington KW, Greb LC: Adult respiratory distress syndrome as a complication of acute pyelonephritis during pregnancy: Case report and discussion. *Obstet Gynecol* 1986; 67:18S.

343. Orr JW, Austin JM, Hatch KD, et al: Acute pulmonary edema associated with molar pregnancies: A high-risk factor for development of persistent trophoblastic disease. *Am J Obstet Gynecol* 1980; 136:412.

344. Russi EW, Spaetling L, Gmur L, et al: High permeability pulmonary edema (ARDS) during tocolytic therapy: A case report. *J Perinatol Med* 1988; 16:45.

345. MacLennan FM, Thomson MAR, Rankin R, et al: Fatal pulmonary oedema associated with the use of ritodrine in pregnancy. *Br J Obstet Gynaecol* 1985; 92:703.

346. Ackerman WE,III, Molnar JM, Juneja MM: Beneficial effect of epidural anesthesia on oxygen consumption in a parturient with adult respiratory distress syndrome. *South Med J* 1993; 86:361.

12 Cardiac Disease

Mark D. Johnson and *Daniel H. Saltzman*

Advances in medical technology have allowed increasing numbers of patients with congenital heart disease to survive to childbearing age. Hence pregnant patients may present with any type of cardiac disease. Pathophysiologic changes of the disease process will be stressed by the physiologic changes of pregnancy. Labor and delivery further compound these stresses. In addition, these patients are subject to all of the diseases and obstetric emergencies associated with pregnancy (e.g., gestational diabetes, preeclampsia, placenta previa, abruptio placentae, acute fetal distress, amniotic fluid embolism, uterine atony).

Difficult decisions regarding maternal-fetal triage or life and death priorities must be addressed early. These questions must be discussed with the patient, her spouse, and the entire management team. In some situations where, for instance, the mother would be unlikely to survive a "crash induction," the fetus may have to be a secondary consideration even in the event of acute fetal distress. On the other hand, if the mother's condition is absolutely terminal, the fetus may take priority.

In this chapter we first address a few important issues that are relevant for all parturients with cardiac disease. Following this, obstetric and anesthetic management are discussed in detail related to some special situations. Finally, the management of valvular problems is concisely reviewed.

TEAM APPROACH

Effective management of pregnant patients with severe cardiac disease requires a coordinated team approach, and important points regarding this are summarized in Boxes 12-1 and 12-2. Communication between the obstetrician, cardiologist, perinatologist, nursing staff, anesthesiologist, and patient is essential. Decisions about therapeutic abortion, when to deliver, route of delivery, anesthetic management, and maternal-fetal priorities need to be made early. Logistical problems regarding nursing and staff availability, operating room time, intensive care unit (ICU) space, travel, or in-house management should also be considered.[1]

Pregnant patients with heart disease can develop all of the problems associated with pregnancy.

Contingency plans for obstetric emergencies should be formulated early.

CARDIAC DISEASE

The frequency of cardiac disease in pregnancy has remained relatively constant over the past 15 years.[2] The prevalence of heart disease during pregnancy ranges from 0.4% to 4.1%.[3] However, the relative proportion of rheumatic heart disease appears to have recently decreased and congenital heart disease increased. This change is attributable to both a decline in the frequency of rheumatic carditis as well as improved surgical correction of congenital heart lesions, thus creating a new category of patients who are now reaching childbearing age. Table 12-1 describes the New York Heart Association (NYHA) functional classification of cardiac disease.

Counseling of women with cardiac disease is best performed prior to conception. This will allow for a thorough evaluation that includes discussing needed invasive procedures such as cardiac catheterization with fluoroscopy that are better performed during the nonpregnant state to avoid potential fetal risks. In addition, patients with surgically correctable lesions should undergo repair before pregnancy to improve both maternal and fetal prognosis. Table 12-2 describes maternal mortality risks with various cardiac lesions. It must be remembered that some of these mortality figures were obtained over long periods of time prior to modern cardiac, obstetric, and anesthetic care. Therefore with modern care, outcome may be better in selected groups.[4]

PHYSIOLOGIC CHANGES OF PREGNANCY AND THE STRESS OF LABOR

The cardiovascular (Table 12-3) and pulmonary changes associated with pregnancy include an increase in circulatory blood volume, the "physiologic anemia of pregnancy," an increase in cardiac output accomplished by increases in both heart rate and stroke volume and an overall increase in cardiac work,[5] a decrease in functional residual capacity (FRC), and increased oxygen

BOX 12-1 IMPORTANT POINTS TO CONSIDER IN MANAGING PARTURIENTS WITH CARDIAC DISEASE

1. Pregnant patients can have any type of cardiac disease.
2. The physiologic changes of pregnancy.
3. The stress of labor and delivery.
4. Two patients: mother and fetus.
5. Preventing cardiovascular complications is more effective than treating problems after they occur. Thus, aggressive monitoring and tight control of cardiovascular parameters are warranted.
6. Adequate sedation, analgesia, and anesthesia are essential to minimize endogenous catecholamine secretion and cardiovascular stress.
7. Regional anesthesia (carefully titrated continuous epidural or continuous spinal), when not contraindicated by coagulopathy, infection, or neurologic deficit, is advantageous.
8. Postoperative ICU monitoring.
9. Postoperative analgesia: epidural or spinal narcotics, patient-controlled analgesia.
10. Multidisciplinary team approach: communicate.

BOX 12-2 MANAGEMENT ISSUES: CARDIAC DISEASE IN PREGNANCY

1. Maternal condition: stabilize, optimize.
2. Fetal condition: maturity, distress.
3. Maternal/fetal medical priorities.
4. When should the fetus be delivered?
5. Route of fetal delivery (vaginal vs. cesarean).
6. Extent of invasive monitoring.
7. Anesthetic management: regional vs. general.
8. Contingency plans for obstetric emergencies.

Table 12-1 New York Heart Association functional classification*

Class I	Asymptomatic
Class II	Symptomatic with exertion
Class III	Symptomatic with normal activities
Class IV	Symptomatic at rest

*Maternal mortality ranges from 0.4% among patients in class I or II to 6.9% in Class III or IV.[2]

Table 12-2 Maternal mortality risk associated with pregnancy*

Group I (mortality <1%)	Group II (mortality 5%-15%)	Group III (mortality 25%-50%)
Atrial septal defect†	Mitral stenosis with atrial fibrillation	Pulmonary hypertension
Ventricular septal defect†	Artificial valve	Coarctation of aorta, complicated
Patent ductus arteriosus†	Mitral stenosis, NYHA Classes III and IV	Marfan's syndrome with aortic involvement
Pulmonic/tricuspid disease	Aortic stenosis	
Corrected tetralogy of Fallot	Coarctation of aorta, uncomplicated	
Porcine valve	Uncorrected tetralogy of Fallot	
Mitral stenosis, NYHA classes I and II	Previous myocardial infarction	
	Marfan's syndrome with normal aorta	

*From Clark SL, Phelan JP, Cotton DB (eds): *Critical Care Obstetrics*. Oradell, NJ, Medical Economics Books, 1987, p 63. Used by permission.
†Uncomplicated.

consumption with associated increased minute ventilation, increased respiratory rate, and decreased $Paco_2$ and buffering capacity. **Aortocaval compression can have a significant effect on venous return as early as the *20th* week of gestation.**

The peak periods of cardiovascular stress (increased cardiac output) occur at 28 to 32 weeks' gestation, in labor and delivery, and in the postpartum period for about 12 to 24 hours (Fig. 12-1). In addition to the peak periods of increased cardiac output, the enlarging uteroplacental unit can increase the risk of venous stasis and limit ambulation in the final weeks of pregnancy.

Labor imparts significant additional cardiovascular stress (Table 12-4). In the first stage of labor, significant increases in heart rate, cardiac output, and systemic and central pressures occur with each contraction. Pain and temporary autotransfusion from the uterus (200 to 400 ml) that occur with each contraction are both causative factors. Patients usually hyperventilate during contractions, which can lower maternal $Paco_2$ and reduce placental perfusion. Epidural anesthesia can sig-

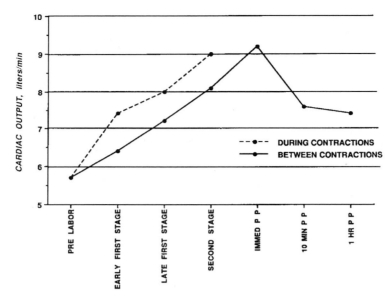

Fig. 12-1 Changes in cardiac output during and in between uterine contractions. *PP* = postpartum.

Table 12-3 Cardiovascular changes nonpregnant compared with 40 weeks' gestation*

Variable	Direction of change	Average change
Blood volume	↑	+35%
Plasma volume	↑	+45%
Red blood cell volume	↑	+20%
Cardiac output	↑	+40%
Stroke volume	↑	+30%
Heart rate	↑	+15%
Femoral venous pressure	↑	+15 mm Hg
Total peripheral resistance	↓	−15%
Mean arterial blood pressure	↓	−15 mm Hg
Systolic blood pressure	↓	−0 to 15 mm Hg
Diastolic blood pressure	↓	−10 to 20 mm Hg
Central venous pressure	No change	

*From Cheek TG, Gutsche BB: Maternal physiologic alterations during pregnancy, in Shnider SM, Levinson GL (eds): *Anesthesia for Obstetrics*. Baltimore, Williams & Wilkins, 1987, p 6. Used by permission.

nificantly blunt these cardiovascular changes and minimize hyperventilation[6]; it can also stabilize maternal heart rate and transcutaneous P_{O_2} (Fig. 12-2).

Pushing during the second stage of labor involves considerable physical work and should be avoided by using outlet forceps in the patient with cardiac disease. Even if the patient's epidural analgesic is completely adequate and she perceives absolutely nothing, some cardiovascular instability will occur at delivery.

Table 12-4 Cardiac output: labor and delivery

Labor stage	Cardiac output increase (%)*
Early first	15
Late first	30
Second	45
5 minutes postpartum	65
1 hour postpartum	30–50

*Additional 15% increase during contractions.

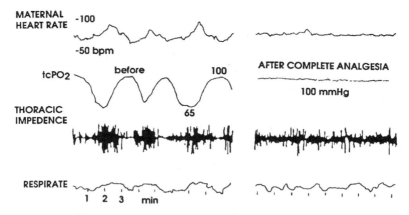

Fig. 12-2 Maternal hyperventilation during painful uterine contractions resulting in hypoventilation between contractions with a corresponding fall in transcutaneous oxygen tension (transcutaneous Po_2) to 65 to 70 mm Hg. After effective epidural analgesia to Po_2 is maintained at a stable 100 mm Hg. (From Huch R, Huch A, Lubbers DW: *Transcutaneous Po₂*, New York, Thieme-Stratton, 1981, p 139. Used by permission.)

In addition, blood loss may be expected to be about 500 ml for an uncomplicated vaginal delivery, and 1000 to 1500 ml if a cesarean delivery is undertaken. The acute changes in blood volume, the reduction of aortocaval compression with the evacuation of the uterus, the loss of the placental shunt, and rapid hormonal shift often result in postdelivery tachycardia. The cardiac output continues to increase for many hours postdelivery.

Oxytocin (Pitocin) can produce sudden hypotension and should not be administered as a rapid bolus in the postpartum cardiac patient.

INVASIVE MONITORING: WHAT ARE THE NORMAL VALUES AT TERM?

Until recently, no measured data were available regarding normal central pressures and cardiac output in healthy women at term gestation. Only pregnant patients sick enough to require invasive central monitoring for diagnostic purposes underwent radial arterial and pulmonary artery catheter placement. Thus "normal values" at term were extrapolated from animal studies and from nonpregnant women.

Capeless and Clapp,[7] using m-mode echocardiography, reported that cardiac output increased 1 L/min by the 8th week of gestation, primarily by increasing stroke volume, which accounts for more than 50% of the total change in cardiac output in pregnancy (Figs. 12-3 and 12-4). Significant changes in the maternal cardiovascular system occur prior to the third trimester of pregnancy (Table 12-5). They also observed that systemic vascular resistance had fallen significantly to 70% of pre-conceptual values by 8 weeks' gestation. These physiologic changes that occur during the embryonic period are important when taking care of pregnant patients having operative procedures performed during the first trimester.

Clark et al[8] recently studied ten healthy primiparous volunteers between 36 and 38 weeks' gestation. Each patient then served as her own nonpregnant control between 11 and 13 weeks postpartum. All patients were measured in the left lateral recumbent position. Tables 12-6 to 12-8 present the mean hemodynamic profiles for these patients. The authors documented a 43% increase in cardiac output, 17% increase in pulse, 21% decline in systemic vascular resistance, 34% decline in pulmonary vascular resistance, 14% decline in colloid oncotic pressure, and a 28% decline in colloid oncotic pressure minus pulmonary capillary wedge pressure.[8] Clark et al also used invasive techniques to measure cardiac output and compared them with other methods.[9] The values are shown in Tables 12-7 and 12-8. There was no significant change between nonpregnant and third-trimester values with respect to mean arterial pressure, central venous pressure, pulmonary capillary wedge pressure, and left ventricular stroke work index.

Absence of an increase in pulmonary capillary wedge pressure or central venous pressure in pregnant patients in the face of marked increases in intravascular volume reflects the decrease in systemic vascular resistance and pulmonary vascular resistance associated with pregnancy that allow systemic and pulmonary vasculature to accommodate higher volumes at normal vascular pressures.

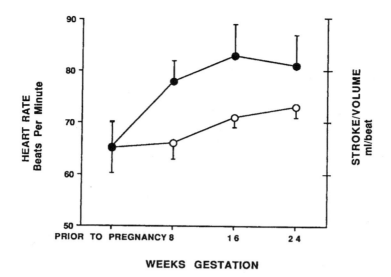

Fig. 12-3 Stroke volume *(closed circles)* and heart rate *(open circles)* components of cardiac output during four study periods. (From Capeless EL, Clapp JF: *Am J Obstet Gynecol* 1989; 161:1449. Used by permission.)

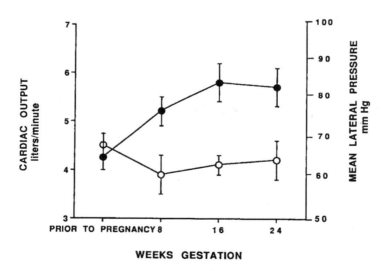

Fig. 12-4 Cardiac output *(closed circles)* and mean arterial pressure *(open circles)* components of SVR during four study periods. (From Capeless EL, Clapp JF: *Am J Obstet Gynecol* 1989; 161:1449. Used by permission.)

MONITORING
Electrocardiogram

All cardiac patients should have a standard 12-lead electrocardiogram (ECG) and rhythm strip run with the patient in the left uterine displacement position to establish a base line. A five-lead monitor with diagnostic mode should be used during any procedure. The ability to monitor two leads simultaneously (leads II and V5) is helpful.

Blood pressure

Blood pressure (BP) should be measured with a standard sphygmomanometer and cuff in *both* arms and used to calibrate any Doppler type automated BP device or arterial line. The morbidity associated with a carefully placed 20-gauge radial arterial line (in a patient with a normal Allen's test) is extremely small—if appropriate nursing protocols are followed. An arterial line is indicated in

Table 12-5 Cardiovascular measurements*†

	Before pregnancy	**8 weeks' gestation**	**16 weeks' gestation**	**24 weeks' gestation**	**Significance**	**P value**
Heart rate (beats/ min)	65 ± 3	68 ± 4	72 ± 3	73 ± 3	Before pregnancy vs. 16	<0.05
					Before pregnancy vs. 24	<0.05
End-diastolic volume (ml)	109 ± 9	122 ± 9	125 ± 8	126 ± 8	Before pregnancy vs. 8	<0.05
					Before pregnancy vs. 16	<0.01
					Before pregnancy vs. 24	<0.001
Stroke volume (ml)	65 ± 5	79 ± 5	83 ± 6	81 ± 5	Before pregnancy vs. 8	<0.02
					Before pregnancy vs. 16	<0.001
					Before pregnancy vs. 24	<0.001
Ejection fraction (%)	61 ± 2	64 ± 4	66 ± 2	64 ± 2	All time periods	NS
Cardiac output (L/ min)	4.2 ± 0.4	5.2 ± 0.3	5.9 ± 0.4	5.7 ± 0.3	Before pregnancy vs. 8	<0.01
					Before pregnancy vs. 16	<0.01
					Before pregnancy vs. 24	<0.001
Mean arterial pressure (mm Hg)	69 ± 3	62 ± 4	69 ± 2	67 ± 4	Before pregnancy vs. 16	<0.05
Systemic vascular resistance (dynes·sec·cm^{-3})	1,376 ± 143	969 ± 76	926 ± 68	930 ± 82	Before pregnancy vs. 8	<0.05
					Before pregnancy vs. 16	<0.01
					Before pregnancy vs. 24	<0.01

*From Capeless EL, Clapp JF: *Am J Obstet Gynecol* 1989; 161:1449. Used by permission.
†Data presented are mean ± SEM. NS = not significant.

Table 12-6 Central hemodynamic changes*

	Nonpregnant	**Pregnant**
Cardiac output (L/min)	4.3 ± 0.9	6.2 ± 1.0
Heart rate (beats/min)	71 ± 10.0	83 ± 10.0
Systemic vascular resistance (dyne·cm·sec^{-5})	1,530 ± 520	1,210 ± 266
Pulmonary vascular resistance (dyne·cm·sec^{-5})	119 ± 47.0	78 ± 22
Colloid oncotic pressure (mm Hg)	20.8 ± 1.0	18.0 ± 1.5
Colloid oncotic pressure–pulmonary capillary wedge pressure (mm Hg)	14.5 ± 2.5	10.5 ± 2.7
Mean arterial pressure (mm Hg)	86.4 ± 7.5	90.3 ± 5.8
Pulmonary capillary wedge pressure (mm Hg)	6.3 ± 2.1	7.5 ± 1.8
Central venous pressure (mm Hg)	3.7 ± 2.6	3.6 ± 2.5
Left ventricular stroke work index (g·m·m^{-2})	41 ± 8	48 ± 6

*From Clark SL, Cotton DB, Lee W, et al: *Am J Obstet Gynecol* 1989; 161:1439. Used by permission.

Table 12-7 Comparison: hemodynamic method of cardiac output determination*

Mean difference from Fick determination

Thermodilution	Pulsed Doppler	Cont. Wave Doppler	Elec. Imped.
20%	15%	36%	27%

*From Clark SL, Cotton DB, Lee W: Central hemodynamic assessment of normal pregnancy (abst). *Am J Obstet Gynecol* 1989; 161:1439.

Table 12-8 Position effects on cardiac output via Fick principle in normal pregnant patients at 36 to 38 weeks' gestation*

L. Lat	R. Lat	Supine	Knee-Chest	Sitting	Standing
6.6 ± 1.4	6.8 ± 1.3	6.0 ± 1.4†	6.9 ± 2.1	6.2 ± 2.0	5.4 ± 2.0†

*From Clark SL, Cotton DB, Lee W: Central hemodynamic assessment of normal pregnancy (abst). *Am J Obstet Gynecol* 1989; 161:1439.
†$P < 0.05$.

all moderate-to-severe valve lesions, congenital heart disease, pump failure syndrome, Marfan's syndrome, and ischemic coronary disease. It is much easier to place an arterial line electively than to do so during an acute decompensation episode. An arterial line is more accurate than most automated Doppler systems; it also gives a continuous reading, it is less traumatic to the patient (than a cuff inflating every few minutes), and it allows arterial blood gases to be drawn as needed. Some automated Doppler BP systems read an artificially low diastolic BP in preeclamptic patients.

Noninvasive capillary oximetry (finger pulse oximetry)

Capillary oximetry is a very useful tool because it gives an indication of respiratory function at the end-organ vessels. It is sensitive and noninvasive. Continuous capillary oximetry is vital in cases of congenital heart disease involving intercardiac shunts. Any treatment which increases the capillary oxygen saturation (O_2Sat) (positioning, blood pressure change, ventilatory change or drug) is potentially good, whereas any event that lowers the capillary O_2Sat is a potential sign of worsening of the shunt picture, the V/Q matching, and/or the cardiac output.

Temperature monitoring

Maintenance of normothermia minimizes both oxygen consumption and changes in vascular resistance and arrhythmias. Tympanic membrane laser temperature probes (intermittent) give an accurate core temperature and are more accurate than skin probes. The core temperature can also be continuously read from an in-dwelling pulmonary arterial (PA) catheter.

Central monitoring

The risks and benefits must be weighed whenever invasive monitoring is considered. Supplemental oxygen, BP, ECG and O_2Sat monitoring should be used, with adequate analgesia, sedation, and local anesthesia given prior to line placement. Left uterine displacement must be maintained. The patient should be maintained in the Trendelenberg position for the shortest possible duration during central line placement.

A central venous pressure (CVP) catheter, carefully placed in the superior vena cava (SVC), above the right atrium, is appropriate and indicated for all cardiac patients. In addition to CVP monitoring, it provides access to the central circulation for drug administration. By changing it to a cordus over a wire, it provides for pacer or PA-line placement, in an emergency. Potential complica-

tions include hemorrhage, infection, nerve injury, pneumothorax, and air embolism.

A PA catheter allows the measurement of filling pressures (RA/CVP, PA directly, and LA indirectly via the wedge pressure). It allows for calculation of cardiac output by thermodilution using the Fick principle. With the cardiac output and pressure values, the systemic vascular resistance (SVR) and pulmonary vascular resistance (PVR) can be calculated.

Monitoring CVP and PA wave forms will reveal tricuspid and mitral regurgitation, respectively (new onset is often indicative of ischemic papillary muscle dysfunction). Blood samples can be obtained from the PA catheter to directly measure O_2Sat. This can be used to follow changes in shunt associated with atrial septal defect (ASD), ventricular septal defect (VSD), or anomalous anatomy. Finally, using specialized PA catheters, continuous mixed venous O_2Sat can be followed via fiberoptic bundles. PA catheters equipped with multiple electrodes or channels for pacer wires can be used to temporarily pace patients.

Forrester, Diamond, and Swan reported that in the setting of acute myocardial infarction (MI), the CVP often does not accurately reflect the left ventricular (LV) filling pressure, whereas the PA wedge pressure does.[9a] Kaplan reported that subendocardial ischemia can often be detected earlier using the PA wedge pressure.[9b] Specifically, in evaluating the PA wedge, an A-wave of greater than 15 torr or a V-wave greater than 20 torr as compared to a 1-mm ST depression in lead II or V5 may be an earlier indicator of ischemia.

Indications for a PA catheter vs. CVP catheter

The use of a PA catheter is warranted in patients with an ejection fraction less than 0.4, a left ventricular end-diastolic pressure (LVEDP) greater than 18 torr, or cardiac index (cardiac output/body surface area [CO/BSA]) less than 2.0). Clinical indications include pregnant patients: s/p M.I., significant coronary artery disease (CAD), congestive heart failure (CHF), pulmonary edema, LV dysfunction (wall motion abnormalities via echocardiogram), peripartum cardiomyopathy, sepsis, pulmonary embolus (including amniotic fluid embolus), moderate-to-severe preeclampsia, shock, major aortic surgery, moderate-to-severe regurgitant valvular disease, pulmonary hypertension, and any situation where major rapid volume shifts may occur or where pulmonary vascular resistance or systemic vascular resistance must be tightly controlled.

Patients with tight aortic stenosis in the absence of other lesions can generally be managed *without* a PA catheter. These patients tolerate reduction in SVR or cardiac output (e.g., onset of arrhythmia) poorly. A CVP catheter will provide sufficient information about the volume status. An arterial line is absolutely essential. Blood pressure (SVR) should be maintained with Neo-Synephrine, IV volume support, and avoidance of aortocaval compression. The placement of a PA catheter can precipitate arrhythmias and its use should be carefully weighed against this risk.

The use of a PA catheter in patients with Eisenmenger's syndrome is generally not indicated. In this case, the risks of precipitating an arrhythmia, the risk of the PA catheter passing through a defect between the right and left circulation (ASD, VSD, etc.), and trauma and infection outweigh the value of any data the PA catheter might provide. Cardiac output data determined by thermodilution will be inaccurate due to the shunt. The status of the shunt and the effect of therapy on the shunt can be followed with the capillary oxygen saturation (the finger pulse oximeter).

There is a small risk of precipitating a Right Bundle Branch Block with "floating" a PA catheter. This must be considered in patients with pre-existing Left Bundle Branch Block; that is, complete atrioventricular (AV) block could occur.

Risks associated with placement of a PA catheter include venous or arterial hemorrhage and hematoma, arrhythmia, pneumothorax, infection, valve trauma, myocardial trauma, pulmonary artery rupture, pulmonary vasculature ischemia, air embolism, micro shock, cerebral ischemia, and neurovascular trauma. In experienced hands the risks are small and can be further reduced with careful attention to sterile technique. PA catheters should be continuously monitored and never allowed to remain in the "wedged" position. An occlusive dressing around the cordus sight (tegaderm) will minimize the possibility of air being drawn into the central circulation along the side of the cordus by a pressure gradient.

Vascular access via the right internal jugular vein has several advantages. It presents a relatively straight approach to the superior vena cava and is associated with less risk of pneumothorax, compared with the subclavian approach. The external jugular vein may be used if it is present; it offers the advantage of minimal risk (cutaneous hematoma as opposed to carotid puncture with the internal jugular approach). However, the likelihood of getting a cordus and central line/PA line to pass into the central circulation via the external jugular approach is less than when the internal jugular approach is used. No matter what approach is chosen, the patient should receive face mask oxygen and sedation during the placement. The BP, ECG, finger pulse O_2Sat, and fetal heart rate should be monitored and aortocaval compression avoided.

A properly placed PA catheter can act as a nidus for clot formation. This may be enhanced by the pregnant patient's so-called "hypercoaguable state." Heparin-coated PA catheters may reduce this risk. The indwelling PA catheter's position through actively moving valves in the beating heart can traumatize valve and myocardium.

During a long labor, when data from the PA catheter are needed only intermittently, the use of a sterile cellophane sleeve over the PA catheter (outside the patient) can allow the PA catheter to be advanced (floated forward with the balloon up), a reading taken, and the catheter withdrawn (balloon down) out of heart into the SVC and can be kept sterile. The proximal junction of the sleeve over the PA catheter should be covered with antibiotic ointment and sealed with a tegaderm. Caution should be taken to prevent saline from the CVP port to fill the sleeve.

Conceptually, the cardiovascular system can be analyzed in terms of its different components: pump, pipes, and circulating fluid (volume and pressure). The system is actually two separate two-stage pumps (the right heart and the left heart) in continuous series. It has two separate circuits, the pulmonary circuit (low pressure) and the systemic circuit (high pressure), both of which carry the entire cardiac output.

Pump. Actually this is two 2-stage pumps set up in series and electrically controlled to work in tandem. The coordinated pumping action is controlled by an electrical system with complex feedback and fine tuning circuits. The heart can work efficiently over a range of heart rate by varying stroke volume and contractility. As volume (preload) increases, the heart is stretched and the contractile force increases within the physiologic range. Oxygen is the rate-limiting factor in myocardial (fuel) substrate utilization. The major issues involved in pump function are rate, rhythm, preload, and the myocardial oxygen supply–demand relationship.

Pipes. The vascular system includes the arterial tree (with both resistance and capacitance components), the capillary bed, and the venous tree (with both resistance and capacitance components).

Circulating fluid. This is a relatively noncompressible slurry of cells and fluid, with properties of viscosity and both laminar and non–laminar flow characteristics.

The fluid–mechanical relationship between these components can be illustrated using an analogy to Ohm's law:

$$E = IR$$

where, in electric circuit theory, E is voltage, I is current, and R is resistance. Thus:

Voltage = Current × Resistance

Translated into fluid–mechanics theory:

Pressure = Flow × Resistance

In the body, for the systemic circuit:

Blood Pressure = Cardiac Output × Systemic Vascular Resistance

In the pulmonary circuit:

Pulmonary Pressure = Cardiac Output × Pulmonary Vascular Resistance

Thus:

$$SVR = \frac{\text{Drop in pressure across the systemic circuit}}{CO}$$
$$= \frac{MAP - CVP}{CO}$$
$$PVR = \frac{\text{Drop in pressure across the pulmonary circuit}}{CO}$$
$$= \frac{PA - wedge}{CO}$$

MAP (mean arterial pressure) can be measured with an arterial line. The CVP, PA, and wedge pressures can be measured directly with the PA catheter. The cardiac output (CO) can be calculated using the Fick equation with thermodilution. With these values, the SVR and PVR can be calculated.

Clinical management

1. Avoid aortocaval compression—hip roll.
2. Check SAT (finger pulse oximeter)—oxygen as needed.
3. Check ECG.
   a. *Rate* (60-100) R_X: Increase with atropine, glycopyrolate, ephedrine, pacer
   Decrease with beta blockers
   b. *Rhythm* R_X: Preserve normal sinus rhythm (NSR), antiarrhythmic agents as required
   c. *ST changes* (ischemia)
   R_X: Optimize myocardial oxygen supply/demand

4. Obtain filling pressures:
   Mean arterial pressure → A-line
   CVP, PA, PA wedge → PA line
5. Obtain cardiac output → PA line thermodilution
6. Calculate:

$$SVR = \frac{\overline{MAP} - CVP}{CO} \times 80$$
Normal pregnancy (NL P_G) = 600 to 900 dyne/sec/cm^5
$$PVR = \frac{\overline{PA} - wedge}{CO} \times 80$$
NL P_G = 60 to 80 dyne/sec/cm^5

7. Correct volume, pressure/resistance. See Figure 12-5.
8. Evaluate cardiac function. See Figure 12-6.

Cardiac arrhythmias

The approach to arrhythmias occurring during pregnancy is, in general, similar to that for nonpregnant patients. It is important to carefully evaluate the pregnant patient for evidence of any underlying organic heart disease or any predisposing factors, and to determine the risk of mortality or major morbidity as a consequence of the arrhythmia. The decision regarding the necessity of antiarrhythmic therapy will ultimately be made after weighing the benefit of therapy against the risk of adverse effects to both the mother and the fetus.

During pregnancy, palpitations and benign arrhythmias are frequent. The incidence of paroxysmal atrial tachycardia is higher during pregnancy,[10] but the arrhythmia is usually well tolerated. Labor and delivery exert cardiovascular stress in "normal" patients. Upshaw[11] examined 13 pregnant women without cardiac disease and noted that all had arrhythmias when continuously monitored during labor, most of them asymptomatic. Atrial and ventricular premature contractions as well as sinus tachycardia and asymptomatic supraventricular tachycardia were reported in his series.

The use of antiarrhythmic drug therapy in pregnancy must also take into consideration fetal safety, particularly in regard to organogenesis and the potential for malformations. In 1979, the Food and Drug Administration (FDA) established five drug categories (A, B, C, D, X) with regard to potential adverse pregnancy and fetal effects.[12] Category A and B are believed to be relatively safe for use during pregnancy. Category C drugs are those in which there is little or no information available regarding their safety during pregnancy. Category D medications are those in which there may be some risk to the fetus, but the benefits may outweigh the risk. Category X drugs are thought

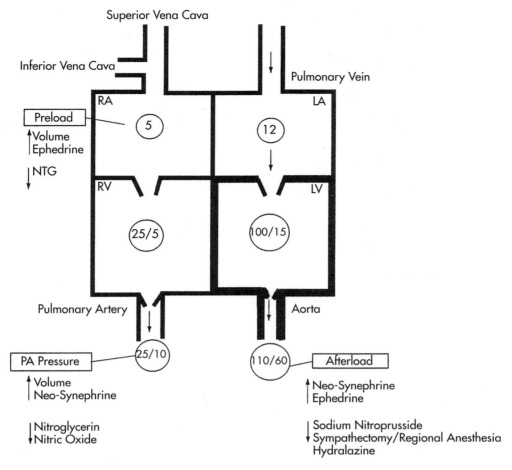

Fig. 12-5 Diagram of correct volume pressure/resistance.

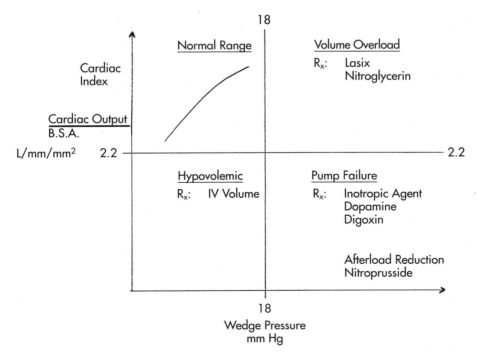

Fig. 12-6 Diagram illustrating cardiac function.

to be associated with fetal malformations and are thus contraindicated during pregnancy. Table 12-9 lists antiarrhythmic agents and their FDA categories.

Maternal cardioversion has been reported on several occasions (Table 12-10) and appears safe for the fetus.[13-20] The use of antiarrhythmic therapy in pregnancy has been reviewed by Rotmensch et al.[21] Detailed descriptions of the drugs are included in Table 12-11. Digoxin and quinidine can be used for the usual indications and, in therapeutic doses, have not been shown to be harmful to the fetus. Procainamide is also considered safe during pregnancy. Chronic therapy with procainamide is a frequent cause of drug-induced lupus syndrome. Prolonged treatment stimulates antinuclear antibodies in 50% to 70% of patients, with systemic lupus syndrome occurring in 20% to 30% of these.[22] In most cases, complete remission follows discontinuation of therapy.

Disopyramide, a drug useful in the treatment and prophylaxis of ventricular tachyarrhythmias, has been associated with preterm labor.[23] The mechanism of this apparent myometrial effect is not known, however. Since data supporting disopyramide use in pregnancy is lacking, it cannot be recommended as a first-line antiarrhythmic drug during pregnancy.

Beta-blocker therapy is appropriate in some tachyarrhythmias. In a critical review, Rubin[24] concluded that beta-blocker therapy with inderal is not associated with adverse fetal outcome. The incidence of intrauterine growth retardation (IUGR) is probably more a function of the disease for which beta-blockers are prescribed (i.e., maternal hypertension) than a complication of beta-blocker therapy itself. Labetalol, a relatively nonselective alpha, beta-1 blocker, preserves placental perfusion. It is a useful agent in preeclampsia. Esmolol, a short-acting selective beta-1 blocker, is rapidly titratable because of its short half-life. However, it is not as advantageous to placental perfusion and its rapid placental transfer can affect the fetal heart rate.

Amiodarone, a new Class III antiarrhythmic agent with noncompetitive alpha- and beta-adrenergic inhibition effects, has a very long half-life. Its use in pregnancy can result in hypotension that is difficult to treat.

There are limited U.S. data on verapamil, a calcium-channel blocking agent, for use as an antiarrhythmic agent during pregnancy, but European data indicate a lack of teratogenic effects or poor pregnancy outcome.[25] Pregnant patients treated with calcium channel blockers (such as Nifedapine) to control hypertension may be at increased risk for uterine atony and postpartum hemorrhage.

Phenytoin, a common anticonvulsant, has unique antiarrhythmic properties. It is used in the

Table 12-9 Antiarrhythmic agents*

Drug	FDA category
Amiodarone	C
Bretylium tosylate	C
Digoxin	C
Disopyramide	C
Encainide	B
Flecainide	C
Lidocaine	B
Mexiletine	C
Procainamide	C
Propranolol	C
Quinidine	C
Tocainide	C
Verapamil	C

*From Meller J, Goldman ME: Arrhythmias in pregnancy, in Elkayam U, Gleicher N (eds): *Principles of Medical Therapy in Pregnancy.* New York, Alan R Liss, 1982, p 114. Used by permission.

Table 12-10 Electrical cardioversion in pregnancy: published reports*

Arrhythmias	Trimester	DC shock (W/sec)	Outcome	Authors
Supraventricular tachycardia	1, 2, 3	100 (7 episodes)	Three normal deliveries	Schroeder et al[14]
Supraventricular tachycardia	2	?	Arrhythmia sustained until delivery	Robards et al[15]
Atrial fibrillation	2	100	Normal delivery	Vogel et al[16]
Atrial fibrillation	3	300	Cesarean section for fetal distress	Grand et al[17]
Atrial flutter	1	100	Normal delivery	Sussman et al[18]
Atrial flutter	1	100	Normal delivery	Meitus[19]
Ventricular fibrillation	2	300	Normal fetal ECG	Curry et al[20]

*From Briggs GG, Freeman RK, Yaffe SJ: *Drugs in Pregnancy and Lactation.* Baltimore, Williams & Wilkins, 1983, p xxi. Used by permission.

Table 12-11 Guide to the use of antiarrhythmic drugs in pregnancy*†

Drug	Route of administration	Clinical application	Therapeutic concentration	Placental transfer UV/MV ratio	Secreted in breast milk	Use in pregnancy	Comment
Lidocaine	Parenteral	"Choice" in ventricular tachyarrhythmias digitalis toxicity	2-4 µg/ml	0.5-0.7	Yes	Safe	Toxic doses and fetal acidosis may cause CNS and cardiovascular depression in the neonate
Quinidine	Oral	Paroxysmal atrial tachyarrhythmias‡	2-5 µg/ml	~1.0	Yes	Relatively safe	Excessive doses may lead to premature labor, very occasionally neonatal thrombocytopenia
Procainamide	Oral, parenteral	Termination and prophylaxis in atrial tachyarrhythmias	4-8 µg/ml (+NAPA 8-16 µg/ml)	?	?	Relatively safe	High incidence of maternal antinuclear antibodies and lupus-like syndrome with chronic use
Phenytoin	Oral, parenteral	Digitalis toxicity, refractory ventricular tachyarrhythmias	10-18 µg/ml	0.8-1.0	Yes, at low concentration	Not recommended for chronic use§	High risk of malformations ("fetal hydantoin syndrome"); bleeding disorder
Disopyramide	Oral, parenteral	Atrial and ventricular tachyarrhythmias	3-7 µg/ml	~0.4	Yes	Probably safe#	One report documents uterine contractions in association with the drug
Verapamil	Oral, parenteral	Paroxysmal supraventricular tachycardia; rate control in chronic atrial fibrillation	15-30 ng/ml¶	~0.4	?	Probably safe#	Rapid IV injection may occasionally cause maternal hypotension and fetal distress
Digoxin	Oral, parenteral	Paroxysmal supraventricular tachyarrhythmias; rate control in chronic atrial fibrillation	1-2 µg/ml¶	~1.0	Yes, at equal to maternal serum concentration	Safe	Adjust dosage when quinidine is given concomitantly
Propranolol	Oral, parenteral	Termination and prophylaxis in atrial and ventricular tachyarrhythmias; rate control in chronic fibrillation	75-100 ng/ml¶	~1.0	Yes	Relatively safe	Chronic administration may be associated with IUGR, premature labor, neonatal hypoglycemia, bradycardia, and respiratory depression

*From Rotmensch HH, Elkayam U, Frishman W: *Am J Cardiol* 1971; *27*:445. Used by permission.
†*UV/MV* = umbilical venous/maternal venous concentration; *NAPA* = N-acetylprocainamide; *IV* = intravenously; *ECG* = electrocardiogram.
‡Prior digitalization recommended.
§Probably safe as acute therapy of digitalis-induced arrhythmia.
#These drugs have not been studied extensively enough in pregnant patients to establish absolute safety, but no serious adverse effects to the fetus have been reported.
¶Large interindividual variation.

treatment of primary digitalis-induced tachya-rrhythmias.[26,27] It is known to be teratogenic in some animals and there is ample evidence implicating it in human malformations.[25] Therefore, considering its significant obstetric toxicity, its use should be restricted to the acute management of digitalis-induced arrhythmias unresponsive to alternate therapy.

Lidocaine is considered safe for use in pregnancy and is the agent of choice in the emergency management of ventricular arrhythmias. It should be noted that newborns exposed to lidocaine via maternal epidural administration were shown to manifest subtle transient neonatal depression and neurobehavioral changes[28]; however, this was refuted by subsequent observers.[29,30]

FETAL CARDIAC ARRYTHMIAS

Fetal cardiac arrythmias may be associated with fetal heart failure leading to nonimmune fetal hydrops and fetal death. The treatment of fetal arrythmias involves giving the mother potent antiarrythmic medications that cross the placenta and thus treat the fetus in utero. Sustained tachyarrythmias, most of which are supraventricular tachycardia (SVT), are clinically the most important for the fetus. The most common agents given to the mother to treat a fetus with SVT are digoxin or adenosine.

Mothers receiving digoxin should be monitored for evidence of digoxin toxicity. Possible maternal side effects of adenosine include dyspnea, flushing, and chest pain. These medications can interact with the anesthetic techniques or drugs used for this purpose.

VASOACTIVE MEDICATIONS AND UTEROPLACENTAL PERFUSION

Ephedrine is the agent of choice for hypotension associated with regional anesthesia in the pregnant patient (in conjunction with intravenous volume loading).[31-36] Butterworth et al,[37] in a dog model using cardiopulmonary bypass and an indwelling spinal catheter, demonstrated that high spinal anesthesia reduced arterial resistance and dilated venous capacitance beds, in addition to reducing heart rate, by blocking cardiac sympathetics and leaving the parasympathetic system unopposed. Subsequent ephedrine, given intravenously, increased arterial resistance (increased blood pressure) and constricted venous capacitance vessels (autotransfusion) in addition to its inotropic and chronotropic effect. Thus, ephedrine acts on the cardiovascular system in a manner almost exactly reciprocal to the effects of sympathectomy associated with high spinal or epidural anesthesia. In a subsequent study,[38] the cardiovascular effects of dopamine were shown to be very

similar to those of ephedrine. On the other hand, phenylephrine only increased the arterial resistance, with little effect on the venous capacitance beds (and has no significant inotropic or chronotropic effect).

Ralston et al[39] evaluated the effect of several vasoactive agents on placental perfusion in a chronically instrumented pregnant sheep model. The vasoactive agents were given intravenously until the maternal blood pressure was elevated 25%; the ephedrine was found to maintain the best placental perfusion. It is important to remember that autoregulation does not occur in the placental vessels. Thus, placental perfusion is almost completely dependent on the maternal systemic pressure.[39] Placental vessels usually maintain maximal dilation. The effect of systemically administered alpha-agonists (phenylephrine) on placental vessels is partial constriction. The normal placenta has considerable vascular reserve. However, in a compromised placenta, systemic alpha-agonists may exert a significant detrimental effect.

Clinically, vasopressors are not routinely given to normotensive patients, i.e., pregnant patients usually do not receive vasopressors with the intent of raising the blood pressure to supernormal levels. Rather, hypotension associated with sympathectomy caused by spinal or epidural anesthetics is treated with the goal of restoring the maternal blood pressure to its normal baseline. In this clinical situation the beneficial effects of alpha-agonists on placental perfusion (increasing the maternal blood pressure to normal) generally outweigh any detrimental effect caused by constriction of placental vessels. Studies in this context, as reported by Ramanathan and Grant[40] and Moran et al,[41] phenylephrine is an effective and safe agent to treat maternal hypotension associated with regional anesthesia (Fig. 12-7).

Ephedrine is the agent of choice to treat hypotension in normal pregnant patients. However, in some types of cardiac disease where tachycardia and arrhythmias are poorly tolerated or in ischemic situations in which an increase in heart rate and contractility may compromise the myocardial oxygen supply/demand ratio, ephedrine may not be the agent of choice. Phenylephrine can be an appropriate and lifesaving agent in the pregnant patient when carefully titrated to maintain baseline blood pressure and systemic vascular resistance (i.e., in maternal myocardial infarction, aortic stenosis, idiopathic hypertrophic subaortic stenosis (IHSS), and Eisenmenger's syndrome).

During labor fetal effects of any of these agents can be followed with continuous fetal heart rate monitoring and intermittent fetal scalp capillary blood pH sampling.

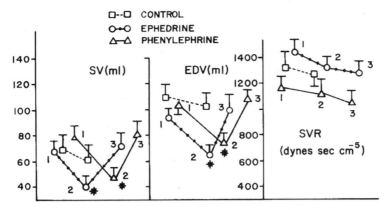

Fig. 12-7 Stroke volume (SV), end diastolic volume (EDV), and systemic vascular resistance (SVR) before anesthesia (1), during hypotension (2), and after therapy with ephedrine or phenylephrine (3). An asterisk (*) significantly different from *1* and *3* ($P < 0.01$). Measurements in the control group were obtained before anesthesia and T6 sensory level. (From Ramanathan S, Grant GJ: *Acta Anaesth Scand* 1988; 32:559. Used by permission.)

CARDIOVERSION, DEFIBRILLATION, AND CARDIAC PACING

Synchronous and asynchronous cardioversion, defibrillation, overdrive, and direct pacing can be accomplished in the pregnant patient. As the cardiopulmonary reserve is reduced in pregnancy, these techniques should be rapidly applied when indicated. The axis of the heart is shifted up and rotated dorsally by the gravid uterus. Optimal cutaneous electrode placement is anterior-posterior over the heart, both to maximize current concentration in the maternal myocardium and to reduce stray current from affecting the fetus.

In patients at risk for supraventricular tachycardia (SVT), heart block, ventricular-tachycardia or V-fibrillation, adhesive large-surface–area anterior/posterior cutaneous electrodes should be prophylactically applied, and the defibrillator or external pacer should be kept ready. During cardioversion, micro shock (via indwelling central lines) or macro shock (stray current conduction via internal or external fetal monitors, ECG lines, etc.) must be avoided.

In high-risk patients, a central line (which can be rapidly changed over a wire), a cordus introducer sheath (for floating a temporary pacer), or a pacing PA catheter can be placed prior to delivery.

Cardiac pacing may be required temporarily during general anesthesia in the intubated pregnant patient. The use of an esophageal electrode requires much lower current levels and has less likelihood than external pacing electrodes of precipitating an arrhythmia in the fetus.

Pregnant cardiac patients are prone to arrhythmia problems, coronary ischemia/MI, valvular lesions, and pump failure (cardiomyopathy, etc.).

In addition to the status of the pregnancy and the routine medical history and physical examination, these patients must receive a standard cardiac workup (keeping the pregnancy in mind). Care must be taken to limit fetal exposure to radiation and teratogenic drugs. Appropriate shielding should be used. After 20 weeks' gestation, pregnant patients may experience hypotension secondary to aortocaval compression if they lie flat on an examining or radiology table. Therefore, left lateral uterine displacement should be maintained.

The workup should include a physical examination with special attention to cardiac auscultation, airway assessment and classification, examination of the spine (for regional access), an ECG and rhythm strip, a cardiac echocardiography, and, where indicated, cardiac catheterization or MRI. The ECG should be reviewed for rate, rhythm, axis, hypertrophy, and ischemia. A room air saturation should be obtained by finger pulse oximeter. The echocardiography should be reviewed for ejection fraction, wall motion, valve area, and regurgitant fraction. Where indicated, cardiac catheterization should be used to determine shunt, cardiac output, and chamber saturation values.

A team approach should be developed early in the pregnancy between the patient and her family, the obstetrician, anesthesiologist, cardiologist, and nursing service. The intensive care unit and cardiothoracic surgical team should be included as indicated. Contingency plans for cardiac and obstetric emergencies should be worked out and discussed in advance. Educating the patient and keeping her advised of all possible plans will reduce anxiety associated with the fear of the unknown, especially during emergent procedures.

Vagal bradycardia

Glycophyrolate is a vagolytic agent. It is a highly charged quaternary ammonium salt that does not cross the placenta. It is a very useful agent to manage maternal bradycardia or nausea and vomiting caused by increased vagal tone. In the event of a bradycardic crisis, atropine has a faster onset. Atropine does cross the placenta and will increase fetal heart rate. Ephedrine is also useful to increase maternal heart rate. It also crosses the placenta and will increase fetal heart rate.

Inotropic agents

The management of cardiac failure with inotropic agents is appropriate with drugs including digitalis, dopamine, nonepinephrine, or epinephrine.

Jelsema et al reported on the use of amrinone, a phosphodiesterase inhibitor, to treat heart failure in pregnancy as an alternative agent.[41a] Fishburne et al reported that amrinone did not significantly alter uterine blood flow in the gravid baboon[41b] (see Table 12-12).

Patients with cardiac disease may be stressed beyond their myocardial reserve as cardiac output increases to meet the physiologic demands of pregnancy. Such increases in cardiac output occur at 32 to 34 weeks' gestation, with labor, and with spontaneous vaginal or operative delivery, and it may continue for many hours postpartum. Infection, fever, anxiety, toxemia, hypovolemia, and acute blood loss can compound this increased demand.

By definition, pregnant patients are relatively young, and in the normal population the incidence of ischemic heart disease is very low. Normal pregnant patients have significant myocardial reserve.

This cannot be assumed for any type of pregnant cardiac patient. Anything that increases the work of the heart increases the myocardial oxygen demand, such as the increased cardiac output with delivery, the immediate postpartum period, or an increased metabolic rate related to pain, infection, or anxiety. Decreases in myocardial oxygen supply (hypotension, hypovolemia, anemia, decreased oxygen saturation, reduced myocardial filling time, coronary spasm, or occlusion) can result in myocardial ischemic injury. Morbidity occurring in the postpartum period may be due to an event at that time, or it may be secondary to an unrecognized ischemic event that occurred during labor or delivery. Careful monitoring and tight control of cardiovascular parameters before, during, and after delivery can reduce the incidence of ischemic events.

TIGHT CONTROL VS. MINIMALISM

When managing a pregnant patient with severe cardiac disease the concept of minimal intervention to reduce alteration of maternal or fetal homeostasis appears initially appealing. In normal healthy pregnant patients, pregnancy is a "natural physiologic state" and minimal intervention is a commendable goal. However, pregnant patients with severe cardiac disease are cardiac patients and pregnancy only exacerbates their problems. Invasive monitoring and tight hemodynamic management during anesthesia in cardiac patients with ischemic heart disease has been shown to reduce mortality.[42-44] A pregnant patient must be managed as any other cardiac patient (except that the fetus must be kept in mind). Generally it is much easier to prevent problems by maintaining tight control

Table 12-12 Sympathomimetic amines

Drug	Usual IV dosage	Adrenergic Effect		Arrhythmogenic potential
		α	β	
Epinephrine (Adrenalin)	0.5-1.0 mg 1-200 μg per min	+ ++	++ +++	+++ +++
Norepinephrine (Levophed)	2-80 μg per min	+++	++	++
Dopamine (Intropin)	1-2 μg/kg per min 2-10 μg/kg per min 10-30 μg/kg per min	+ ++ +++	+* ++* ++	+ ++ +++
Dobutamine (Dobutrex)	2-30 μg/kg per min	+	+++	++
Isoproterenol (Isuprel)	2-10 μg/min	0	+++	+++
Amrinone† (Inocor)	2-15 μg/kg per min	0	0*	++

*Increases renal and splanchnic blood flow.
†Phosphodiesterase inhibitor.

of cardiovascular parameters with continuous monitoring and prophylactic intervention than to treat a cardiovascular problem after it occurs. The anesthetic and obstetric management of the pregnant patient with severe heart disease is no place for the faint of heart (no pun intended) or the inexperienced. Tight control of every cardiovascular and pulmonary parameter, in combination with optimal analgesia and anesthesia throughout the peripartum and postpartum periods, is essential to maximize survival of both mother and fetus.

ADEQUATE SEDATION AND ANALGESIA

Healthy pregnant patients have considerable cardiovascular reserve. To avoid fetal exposure to medication, sedation is not routinely given prior to delivery. In pregnant patients with severe cardiac disease, narcotic and sedative medication should be considered prior to any invasive monitoring, anesthetic, or surgical procedure to minimize the cardiovascular stress response. Good communication and rapport between the care team and the patient will significantly reduce anxiety.

PREVENTION OF BACTERIAL ENDOCARDITIS

When routine surgical antibiotic prophylaxis is used in normal healthy pregnant patients it is usually given after fetal delivery (if the procedure is obstetric). For a pregnant patient with valvular heart disease, prosthetic heart valves, congenital heart disease, IHSS, and mitral valve prolapse, complicated by mitral insufficiency, antibiotic prophylaxis should be administered prior to any anesthetic, surgical, or invasive monitoring procedure. The current recommendations are indicated in Table 12-13.[1]

Shivering

Shivering, a common occurrence in labor, can increase oxygen consumption 100% to 150%. This may become critical in a patient with minimal cardiopulmonary or uteroplacental reserve. The cause of this phenomenon involves a number of factors, including: cool intravenous (IV) fluids, anxiety, sweating and evaporation, changes in hormonal levels, small quantities of fetal blood and/or amniotic fluid getting into the maternal systemic circulation, and drug and anesthetia effects.

Spinal or epidural anesthesia can contribute to this phenomenon in four ways. First, the IV volume load will reduce body temperature if it is cooler than body temperature. Second, the sympathectomy associated with a spinal or epidural anesthetic agent will cause dilation of peripheral vessels, bringing warm core temperature blood to the body surface. This can result in net heat loss if the patient is not well covered or if the room is cool. Third, the blocking of afferent pain and temperature signals carried by the spinolthalmic tracts to the brain may induce shivering. Finally, detectable blood levels of local anesthetic agents (lidocaine apparently more than bupivacaine) may induce shivering.

Modalities that may be useful to minimize shivering include warming (to body temperature) IV fluids and local anesthetics; warming mattresses forced hot air blanket systems head and extremity covers; and radiant warmers and warmed/humidified gases if general anesthesia is used. Spinal and epidural narcotics may be helpful (especially fentanyl, sufentanyl, and meperidine). The use of sedative medication such as diphenhydramine, diazepam, or midazolam may be considered.

Air embolism at delivery

Any situation in which the operative site is higher than the heart can produce a negative venous gradient that can draw ambient air into an open vein, resulting in air embolism. This can occur when the uterus is retracted up out of the abdomen for posterior repair during cesarean-section, especially if the patient is in the Trendelenberg position. A number of studies have reported that the incidence of small air emboli (detectable with a Doppler placed over the pulmonary artery at a resolution level of

Table 12-13 Genitourinary or gastrointestinal procedures*

Ampicillin, gentamicin	50 mg/kg (maximum dose 2.0 g) and 2 mg/kg (maximum dose 80 mg), respectively, IV 30 min before procedure and repeat 8 hr after initial dose
Penicillin-allergic patients:	
Vancomycin, gentamicin	20 mg/kg (maximum dose 1.0 g) and 2 mg/kg (maximum dose 80 mg), respectively, IV 1 hr before procedure
Alternative low-risk patient regimen:	
Amoxicillin	50 mg/kg (maximum dose 3.0 g) orally 1 hour before procedure, then 25 mg/kg 6 hr after initial dose

*From Dajani AS, Bisno AL, Chung KJ, et al: Prevention of bacterial endocarditis: Recommendations by the American Heart Association. *JAMA* 1990; 264:2912-2922.

air bubbles of 0.2 ml or greater) is not uncommon. Large volumes of air can result in pulmonary artery obstruction and V/Q mismatch with resultant drops in oxygen saturation. If the patient is intubated, decreased end-tidal carbon dioxide and increased end-tidal nitrogen may be seen. Only rarely do small emboli result in ischemia or chest pain in normal patients. In cardiac patients, especially with shunts or valve lesions (e.g., interconnection of right-left circulation), these small emboli can have more serious consequences. In cardiac patients, the risks of retracting the uterus out of the abdomen for repair and concurrent Trendelenberg position should be a concern. A high level of suspicion and vigilance must be maintained for evidence of air emboli in this position. In addition, in cardiac patients every precaution should be taken to minimize IV air emboli (including taking air out of IV bags and use of bubble traps). It is worth noting that 5% to 8% of patients have a patent foramen ovale.

Superventricular tachycardia

It is not uncommon for normal patients to develop a sinus or superventricular tachycardia at or immediately after delivery (vaginal or operative, with or without anesthesia). This may be related to increased catecholamic levels, changing circulating blood volume (with associated hypotension), loss of placental shunt, or fetal blood emboli, amniotic fluid emboli, or air emboli.

Postpartum management includes evaluating and treating the patient for pain, anxiety, hypovolemia, hypotension or hypothermia, checking the oxygen saturation, and considering infectious causes. An ECG and rhythm strip should be obtained to rule out ischemic changes, to screen for undiagnosed pre-excitation syndromes and to review P-wave morphology. Widerhorn et al reported an increased incidence of superventricular arrhythmias in pregnancy in patients with Wolff-Parkinson-White syndrome (WPW).[44a] The heart sounds should be auscultated to rule out undiagnosed valve lesions (especially mitral valve prolapse) or shunts. Iatrogenic tachycardia secondary to patient sensitivity to administered ephedrine should be considered. This is usually of short duration consistent with the half-life of ephedrine. When vagal maneuvers such as carotid massage, volume expansion, or controlled elevation of blood pressure with carefully titrated Neo-Synephrine are ineffective, antiarrhythmic agents should be considered if the heart rate is limiting the cardiac filling time.

Repeated serial doses of calcium channel blockers are often not effective in treating postpartum SVT, but these patients usually respond to beta-blockers. When not contraindicated (asthma, reduced ejection fraction, etc.), postpartum esmolol is initially the drug of choice because it can be titrated, it rapidly dissipates, and it is beta-2 selective.

Peripartum patients with cardiac disease may tolerate SVT poorly. If antiarrythmic agents are ineffective or contraindicated, and the patient's cardiopulmonary status is deteriorating (decreased oxygen saturation with supplemental oxygen, hypotension, or evidence or ischemia/angina), rapid synchronized cardioversion should be considered.

HEART SURGERY AND CARDIOPULMONARY BYPASS

Surgical management of acutely decompensated valvular or congenital heart disease may be the best or the only effective treatment (when medical therapy has been maximized) even in the pregnant patient. Over the last 25 years an increasing number of successful open heart procedures have been reported during pregnancy, including over 100 cases in which cardiopulmonary bypass has been used. The first reports of the use of extracorporeal bypass in pregnancy appeared in 1965.[45] Hawthorne carried out the first valve replacement in pregnancy in 1967.[46] In 1969, Zitnik reported a series of 20 cases using cardiopulmonary bypass during pregnancy with 1 maternal loss and a 33% fetal mortality.[47]

In 1983, Becker reviewed 68 open heart procedures with 1 maternal death and an 80% fetal survival rate.[48] Definitive cardiac surgery is remarkably safe and effective during pregnancy and the rate of fetal survival is very respectable, especially considering the 100% fetal mortality rate with either maternal demise or therapeutic abortion to reduce the stress of pregnancy and maternal cardiac decompensation.[49,50] Evidence of subsequent developmental anomalies has, thus far, been minimal. Necessary cardiac surgery should not be withheld because of pregnancy.

The optimal timing of cardiac surgery during pregnancy is during the second trimester prior to the 30th week of gestation (Box 12-3). This avoids fetal drug exposure and surgical stress during fetal organogenesis (which occurs in the first trimester) and the increased cardiovascular demands of the growing fetus after 32 weeks' gestation. The risk of spontaneous labor unresponsive to tocolysis is also increased as the mother approaches term.

Anesthetic considerations include avoiding uterine aortocaval compression both prior to, during, and after cardiopulmonary bypass, and prevention of gastric aspiration. High-dose narcotic induction and anesthetic technique are optimal. Narcotics (fentanyl and morphine), neuromuscular blocking

BOX 12-3   SURGICAL CONSIDERATIONS
DURING PREGNANCY

If at all possible, cardiac surgery should be done before the third trimester.

Necessary corrective cardiac surgery should not be
withheld on the basis of pregnancy, since maternal
mortality is comparable to that in the nonpregnant
state and surgery is often curative.

When the fetus is viable, intraoperative fetal heart and
uterine monitoring helps determine the effect of procedures on the fetus and detect premature labor in a
patient under sedation.

agents (succinylcholine, pancuronium), and volatile agents (halothane, enflurane, and isoflurane)
have a long safety record for use during pregnancy.
It is probably prudent to avoid benzodiazepines at
least during the first trimester because of possible
teratogenic effects. Scopalamine can be used for
amnesia, and diphenhydramine is a useful sedative
in conjunction with narcotic agents. As placental
perfusion is pressure-dependent, careful maintenance of maternal blood pressure is paramount.
Hypotension should be aggressively treated with
intravenous volume loading, ephedrine, and/or
phenylephrine, depending on the underlying cardiac lesion.

During cardiopulmonary bypass, high normal
range mean perfusion pressure should be maintained (preferably greater than 60 mmHg). The fetus tolerates nonpulsatile flow of cardiopulmonary
bypass surprisingly well. (Fetal umbilical artery
blood flow is normally only 11 ml/100 g fetal
weight with a normal oxygen saturation of 52% to
65%.) On bypass, maintenance of maternal Pa_{O_2}
in the 200 to 300 mmHg range is probably optimal. Maternal blood volume and hematocrit should
be maintained with intravenous crystalloid and
blood replacement. Mild hypothermia (32° C or
greater) is well tolerated by the fetus. At lower core
temperatures the risk of fetal arrhythmias and fetal cardiac arrest becomes significant.

When possible, fetal heart rate monitoring and
maternal tocodynametry should be used intraoperatively and postoperatively. During cardiopulmonary bypass the fetal heart variability is minimal
and the baseline heart rate is reduced. This is probably secondary to fetal exposure to high-dose narcotics as well as hypothermia and nonpulsatile
blood flow. After rewarming, the fetal heart rate
increases and often a compensatory fetal tachycardia is transiently seen.[51] The fetal heart rate vari-

ability then returns to normal. These patients need
to be monitored for the onset of premature labor
for several days postoperatively. If labor begins,
tocolytic therapy should be instituted with magnesium sulfate or beta-agonists such as terbutaline or
ritodrine (depending on the cardiovascular status
and type of cardiac disease).

The risks associated with heparin anticoagulation and the use of protamine are comparable to
their use in nonpregnant patients undergoing cardiopulmonary bypass. Warfarin is teratogenic and
should be avoided. The development of porcine
prosthetic valves that do not require postoperative
anticoagulation has improved maternal and fetal
prognosis.[52,53]

ANTICOAGULANTS

Anticoagulant use during pregnancy is indicated
for the treatment and prophylaxis of thromboembolic disease as well as for the prevention and
treatment of systemic embolism, which can be associated with valvular heart disease. Heparin does
not cross the placenta and therefore should not directly affect the fetus, whereas oral anticoagulants
such as warfarin do cross the placenta and have
the potential to adversely affect the fetus. The literature with respect to this topic is difficult at times
to interpret because patients receiving anticoagulants have coexisting conditions that are independently associated with adverse fetal outcomes.
Ginsberg and Hirsh[54] analyzed the literature taking the confounding factors into consideration. In
their analysis, when the frequencies of fetal and
neonatal deaths in those pregnancies without co-
morbid conditions are calculated, the rates were
2.5% in the heparin-treated patients, 16.8% in the
oral anticoagulant patients, and 11.5% when both
anticoagulants were used. The 2.5% fetal neonatal
death rate in the heparin-treated patients is similar
to the death rate in the normal population. They
concluded that the reported high rate of adverse fetal outcome associated with heparin therapy can be
explained by the frequent presence of co-morbid
conditions and the higher rate of uncomplicated
prematurity. They further concluded that heparin
therapy does not cause adverse fetal outcome
whereas warfarin therapy does. Warfarin has been
shown to cause warfarin embryopathy and central
nervous system abnormalities, consisting of nasal
hypoplasia and/or stippled epiphyses after in utero
exposure to oral anticoagulants during the first trimester. In their literature review this occurred in
45 of 970 pregnancies associated with oral anticoagulant therapy.

Iturbe-Alessio et al[55] reported on anticoagulant
therapy in 72 pregnancies associated with valvular
heart disease and reviewed the rate of congenital

malformations following maternal warfarin therapy. Warfarin embryopathy was reported in 10 of 35 (28.6%) of infants exposed to warfarin between the 6th and 12th weeks of gestation. No case of warfarin embryopathy occurred in the 19 patients in whom heparin was substituted for warfarin between the 6th and 12th weeks of gestation. Therefore, once pregnancy is recognized in these patients they should be switched to therapeutic heparin. Maternal complications can occur in any patient on such therapy. Anticoagulant-induced bleeding has clearly been reported and therefore patients should be followed carefully for this complication. In addition, heparin has been associated with osteoporosis in patients receiving long-term subcutaneous heparin (i.e., longer than 6 months) for ischemic heart disease. Since pregnant patients can be receiving heparin for longer than 6 months, one should beware of this complication. A report by Zimran[56] suggests that the bone abnormalities seen pathologically may be reversible after discontinuation of heparin therapy. Clearly, all oral anticoagulant therapy should be avoided in the weeks before delivery to avoid potential fetal bleeding caused by the trauma of delivery in the anticoagulated fetus.

REGIONAL VS. GENERAL ANESTHESIA

Regional anesthesia, meaning carefully titrated continuous epidural or continuous spinal anesthesia, when not contraindicated by anticoagulation, coagulopathy, infection, or anatomic defects, provides a number of advantages (for both mother and fetus) over general anesthesia in the pregnant cardiac patient. The pregnant patient with cardiac disease often has reduced cardiovascular reserve that will be further taxed by the physiologic changes of pregnancy as the gestation proceeds. Minimizing sudden changes in cardiovascular and pulmonary parameters and reducing or preventing the stress response are important considerations in the management of these patients.

Endotracheal intubation, although a stimulating and stressful procedure, is mandatory when general anesthesia is used for pregnant patients. When continuous epidural anesthesia is compared with a standard obstetric (rapid sequence induction) general anesthetic using thiopental and succinylcholine for cesarean section, the acute effect of intubation on systemic and central pressures versus the stability afforded by epidural anesthesia can be appreciated. The standard obstetric general anesthetic rapid sequence induction does little to blunt the stress response. In fact the anesthetic is kept intentionally "light" to minimize fetal drug exposure. This is completely inadequate for the cardiac patient. The cardiovascular response to intubation can be blunted with prior administration of la-

betalol or esmolol, but many cardiac patients with reduced left ventricular function will tolerate this poorly. If a general anesthetic is required, a modified high-dose narcotic technique is preferable because it will provide considerably more cardiovascular stability. High-dose narcotic induction is slower than a standard rapid sequence induction, which slightly increases the risk of gastric aspiration, but this can be minimized by pretreatment with sodium bicitrate (30 ml by mouth) and metoclopramide (10 mg intravenously 30 minutes before induction) and maintenance of cricoid pressure.

When a high-dose narcotic induction is used, the fetus will be exposed to some level of narcotic, and depending on induction to delivery time, it may be narcotized. This is only a minor problem if the pediatric team is prepared, since the newborn can certainly be ventilated and naloxone can be administered to reverse any narcotic depression. The mother will require positive pressure ventilation. This affects the thoracic pressure and, in some cardiac patients, especially those with congenital heart disease, it can significantly alter V/Q matching, venous return, cardiac output, shunt size, and even shunt direction. Maternal postoperative ventilation will be required and careful attention to the timing and technique of extubation is needed to minimize "bucking on the tube," which can have profound cardiovascular effects. Finally, even a high-dose narcotic technique does not completely block the stress response. As with any general anesthetic, it does not block afferent noxious stimuli but instead reduces the perception and response to them in the central nervous system.

Continuous epidural and continuous spinal anesthesia block afferent nerve transmission and thus minimize the release of endogenous catecholamines, antidiuretic hormone (ADH), and other neuroendocrine transmitters associated with the stress response.[57] Hypotension associated with the abrupt sympathectomy caused by single-shot spinal techniques relatively contraindicates this approach in severe cardiac disease. Conversely, carefully titrated continuous epidural or continuous spinal anesthesia used with appropriate monitoring, adequate intravenous volume loading, and judicious vasopressor therapy can safely provide excellent anesthesia and maintain a stable cardiovascular state. Continuous regional anesthesia is not contraindicated and may be the anesthetic of choice in pregnant patients with tight aortic stenosis,[58] IHSS,[59] mitral stenosis,[60] Eisenmenger's syndrome,[61] and recent myocardial infarction.[62]

The advantages of continuous conduction anesthesia include an awake patient who can cooperate and report the onset of more symptoms, avoidance of intubation and the effects of positive pressure ventilation on thoracic pressures, good cardiovascular stability with minimal endogenous stress response, T4 or higher sensory levels, blocking of the sympathetic outflow to the heart and hence reduction in heart rate and possibly coronary artery spasm, and finally, reduction of afterload that in turn can increase cardiac output and reduce cardiac work. Postoperative pain management can be achieved successfully with epidural or spinal narcotics with minimal fetal drug exposure. There is some evidence that lumbar epidural anesthesia may even improve ventricular function in patients with angina.[63]

Continuous catheter techniques also allow a degree of flexibility. Low segmental conduction anesthesia can be induced for labor and if the clinical picture changes, the level can be brought up for cesarean delivery. Finally, in cardiac patients who have ventricular arrhythmias, or who have recently sustained a myocardial infarction, continuous epidural infusion with lidocaine can result in therapeutic lidocaine blood concentration for prophylaxis or treatment of these arrhythmias.[64] At the conclusion of surgery, the local anesthetic block

and sympathectomy may be permitted to wear off while analgesia is maintained with epidural or spinal narcotics. The resolution of the sympathectomy and concomitant autotransfusion must be expected and allowed for in the management plan.

CARDIOPULMONARY RESUSCITATION

Cardiopulmonary resuscitation (CPR) in the pregnant patient is complicated by the physiologic changes of pregnancy. The pregnant patient's expanded blood volume, physiologic anemia, decreased FRC, and increased oxygen consumption significantly reduce her cardiopulmonary reserve. After 20 weeks' gestation, aortocaval compression becomes a significant factor and lateral uterine displacement must be maintained or uterine compression of the aorta and especially the vena cava will reduce venous return and make chest compression futile. The increased risk of aspiration of gastric contents warrants immediate intubation with a cuffed endotracheal tube.[65] Songster and Clark[66] outlined the protocol for the treatment of lethal dysrhythmias in parturients; this is presented in Table 12-14).

Table 12-14 Protocols for lethal dysrhythmias*

Ventricular fibrillation
1. Defibrillate at 200-300 J. Repeat if ineffective.
2. Intubate and ventilate with oxygen. Give epinephrine, 0.5-1.0 mg IV. Repeat every 5 min. Give sodium bicarbonate, 1 mEq/kg (75-100 mg). Repeat with half the dose every 10 min as needed.
3. Defibrillate at 360 J; repeat.
4. Give bretylium, 10 mg/kg IV (750-1000 mg).
5. Defibrillate at 360 J; repeat.
6. After the maximum dose of bretylium, or as an alternative, one may give lidocaine hydrochloride or procainamide hydrochloride as an adjunct to defibrillation.
7. Give 1 mg/kg of lidocaine as an initial bolus, followed after 10 min by 0.5 mg/kg. This may be repeated until a total dose of 225 mg is reached, followed by maintenance infusion at 2 to 4 mg/min.
8. Give 100 mg of procainamide over 5 min, repeated every 5 min. Stop bolus dosage on noting hypotension, suppression of dysrhythmia, a 50% increase in width of the QRS complex, or on reaching a total dose of 1 g. Maintenance is 1-4 mg/min.

Asystole
1. Intubate and ventilate with oxygen. Give epinephrine, 0.5-1.0 mg IV. Repeat every 5 min. Give sodium bicarbonate, 1 mEq/kg (75-100 mg). Repeat with half the dose every 10 min as needed.
2. Give atropine, 1.0 mg IV.
3. Give calcium chloride 10% solution, 5 ml IV. Repeat every 10 min.
4. Give isoproterenol infusion 2-20 μg/min.
5. Arrange for pacemaker placement.

Electromechanical dissociation
1. Intubate and ventilate with oxygen. Give epinephrine, 0.5-1.0 mg IV. Repeat every 5 min. Give sodium bicarbonate, 1 mEq/kg (75-100 mEq). Repeat half the dose every 10 min as needed.
2. Give calcium chloride 10% solution, 5 ml, IV. Repeat every 10 min.
3. Give isoproterenol infusion, 2-20 μg/min.
4. Consider hypovolemia, tension pneumothorax, and cardiac tamponade as possible causes, and treat appropriately.

*From Songster GS, Clark SL: *Contemp Obstet Gynecol* Nov 1985. Used by permission.

Both elective cardioversion and emergency defibrillation have been successfully carried out in pregnant patients. The risk of electrical induction of fetal arrhythmias can be minimized by careful electrode placement. The left breast should be pushed out of the way and a wide posterior back electrode used if available.[20,67,68]

In addition to an electrocardiogram (ECG) monitor to assess rhythm, a securely placed finger pulse oximeter (or alternatively an ear oximeter probe clipped to the nose so that the inner aspect of the clip is in the nostril and the outer is on the lateral aspect of the nose) will give an indication of the effectiveness of chest compressions. Transabdominal fetal heart monitoring should be used to assess the fetus.

If a pregnant patient near term in a hospital setting does not initially respond to CPR, emergency cesarean delivery of the fetus should be considered for both fetal and maternal indications.[69,70] Patients with artificial heart valves are at increased risk of cardiac trauma secondary to closed chest cardiac massage. Open chest cardiac massage, which is much more effective at maintaining cardiac output, should be considered whenever it appears that the resuscitation is going to be prolonged. Whenever a pregnant patient with severe cardiac disease is electively taken to the operating room, communication with the perfusionist and the cardiothoracic surgical team is advisable, since timely institution of cardiopulmonary bypass (either femoral artery/femoral vein or via sternotomy) may be lifesaving as a last resort.

Pregnant patients are more susceptible to local anesthetic neurotoxicity and cardiotoxicity. Bupivacaine is 10 to 15 times more cardiotoxic than lidocaine, but it is commonly used in pregnant patients both because it is largely protein bound in the maternal blood and because of its long duration and differential sensory motor block at low concentrations.[71] A massive intravascular amide local anesthetic overdose resulting in maternal asystole essentially anesthetizes both the heart's electrical conduction system and the myocardial cell contractile apparatus. Bupivacaine has a strong affinity for myocardial tissue and will exert its effect for many hours.

If this situation is confirmed by failure of closed chest in CPR to restore cardiac function, then immediate cesarean delivery of the fetus is warranted (its heart will also soon be exposed to significant local anesthetic levels). The mother should be intubated, ventilated, and converted to open-chest CPR to maintain adequate circulatory perfusion until cardiopulmonary bypass can be instituted. The institution of open chest CPR and then cardiopulmonary bypass to treat local anesthetic cardiotoxicity, though drastic, has been successfully used.[72]

GENERAL OBSTETRIC MANAGEMENT

In this section we will discuss the general management of parturients with cardiac disease. More specific recommendations will be described with the different pathophysiologic conditions. Pregnancy obviously imposes an extra burden to the already deranged cardiovascular system. In a mild disease state the residual reserve capacity will be able to take care of the pregnancy without deleterious effect. However, in parturients with severe cardiac problems specifically associated with severe cardiac symptoms in the nonpregnant state, the residual cardiac function reserve may be nonexistent. In such a situation, the cardiologist and the obstetrician should discuss and critically investigate the cardiac problems and the cardiac reserve function to ultimately make a rational choice with input from the patient regarding the termination or continuation of the pregnancy.

Once the pregnancy is allowed to continue, careful medical management is the hallmark of successful outcome. The patient should see her cardiologist and obstetrician as frequently as necessary. Patients with severe cardiac problems or with a history of decompensation should be seen weekly and special consideration must be given between 28 to 36 weeks' gestation. Radiographic studies should be avoided, if at all possible. However, if necessary, they can be done after the third month with proper shielding. Cardiac catheterization may be necessary in an unusual circumstance and should only be carried out if the data are extremely important in making vital decisions.

Physical activity and emotional problems should be addressed by the obstetrician. Physical exertion should be limited if there is associated dyspnea, palpitation, or fatigue. Emotional problems may also ameliorate cardiac conditions. Hence, the patient should be counseled if necessary in this regard.

Attention to the patient's diet has become an important issue, and a nutritionally adequate diet with supplemental vitamins and iron should be maintained. This will minimize anemia, which if present will increase myocardial work. Excessive weight gain, either due to overeating or excessive salt intake, may be detrimental to patients with severe cardiac disease. If the patients are on diuretic therapy, potassium supplementation may be necessary. Prevention of infection is also an important issue, and close supervision by the obstetric team is necessary. Finally, vigilant attention for any signs of congestive heart failure is crucial in the weekly visit. History of gradual weakness, and increasing exertional dyspnea together with the presence of auscultatory basal rales, may be a confirmatory diagnosis. Selective cardiac patients should be admitted to the hospital a few weeks before delivery for closer monitoring.

Vaginal delivery vs. cesarean section

McGarry and Pearson[73] compared the duration of labor in 256 patients with "cardiac disease" with 23,510 patients without "cardiac disease" during the period of 1965 to 1969. They reported no difference in the length of labor between these two groups and the majority of patients delivered within 12 hours. Even considering the inherent physical effort associated with labor and vaginal delivery, the majority of obstetricians believe that there is less morbidity and mortality associated with vaginal delivery than with cesarean delivery. However, most agree that assistance of delivery during the second stage of labor is indicated to avoid the bearing-down effort. With the rapid improvements in invasive monitoring and anesthetic techniques, the perioperative mortality of cesarean section has been reduced significantly. The ultimate choice of route of delivery must be individualized and, if necessary, abdominal delivery can always be considered if the patient situation changes. Following delivery, judicious use of oxytocin is important to reduce postpartum hemorrhage. Methergine should be avoided if possible because of the possibility of increased cardiovascular stress secondary to acute hypertension. Close supervision of these patients in the postpartum period for 48 to 96 hours is mandatory.

PERIPARTUM CARDIOMYOPATHY

Peripartum cardiomyopathy is an uncommon and poorly understood phenomenon involving unexpected cardiovascular decompensation in the peripartum period. Idiopathic myocardial failure associated with the puerperium was first described in the 19th century. Peripartum cardiomyopathy was described as a separate disease entity in the 1950s.[74-77] It is defined as the onset of primary heart failure of indeterminate cause in a patient with no previous evidence of heart disease, occurring during the last month of pregnancy or during the first 6 postpartum months.[74]

The incidence of peripartum cardiomyopathy has been reported as 1 in 3000 to 1 in 15,000, representing less than 1% of all cardiovascular disease occurring during pregnancy. It occurs most commonly in the second postpartum month.[74] These patients usually present with evidence of left ventricular failure, including paroxysmal nocturnal dyspnea, dyspnea on exertion, edema, gallop rhythms, and distended neck veins. Since many of these signs and symptoms can occur during normal pregnancy, early diagnosis is often difficult. Emboli to cerebral and systemic circulation occur in up to 25% of these cases.[78-80] Cardiomegaly is a hallmark of the disease. The laboratory workup is usually nondiagnostic. Electrocardiography may show low voltage, T-wave inversion, conduction defects, and evidence of left ventricular hypertrophy. Echocardiography may demonstrate dilated, hypokinetic ventricular function.[81]

The diagnosis is initially one of exclusion after other causes of congestive heart failure are ruled out. Invasive monitoring is warranted and usually reveals high wedge pressure and low cardiac output.[80] Endomyocardial biopsy usually shows degenerative changes. Intracellular and extracellular deposition of fibrous material and often mural thrombi are seen with light microscopy. Postmortem findings generally include biventricular hypertrophy with grossly enlarged hearts, pale myocardium with endocardial thickening, mural thrombi, and normal heart valves and coronary arteries.[82]

Factors that correlate with a diagnosis of peripartum cardiomyopathy include maternal age greater than 30 years, multiparity, multiple gestations, toxemia, obesity, and breastfeeding. Peripartum cardiomyopathy has been reported more often in tropical and subtropical zones. Nutritional factors have been questioned but not demonstrated.[76]

Cardiomyopathy can be classified by pathophysiology as restrictive hypertrophic or congestive. The congestive cardiomyopathies include familial, alcoholic, neuromuscular disease, and peripartum cardiomyopathy. Etiologic classification of cardiomyopathies include nutritional (Beri-Beri), metabolic (thyroid dysfunction, anemia), toxic (chemical-alcohol, sulfonamides, carbon tetrachloride, or bacterial [diphtheria toxin]), infectious (viral, rickettsial, protozoal, bacterial), ischemic coronary artery disease, syphilis, polyarteritis, giant cell arteritis), infiltrative (sarcoidosis, amyloidosis, hemachromatosis), collagen vascular (lupus), neuromuscular (muscular dystrophy, Friedreich's ataxia, polymyositis), and traumatic (mechanical, electrical, radiation).[83] The etiology is unknown and the phenomenon may be a multifactorial disorder, requiring interaction of genetic, autoimmune, nutritional, endocrine, and/or metabolic factors.

An overall mortality rate of 30% to 60% has been reported, with 10% to 20% occurring during the initial hospitalization. The recurrence rate in subsequent pregnancies of patients that survive peripartum cardiomyopathy has been estimated at 50% to 80% with a mortality rate of 60%.[75] However, patients who have undergone heart transplantation after severe peripartum cardiomyopathy have been reported to successfully deliver in subsequent pregnancies and survive without evidence of recurrent disease.[84] Prognosis appears to be linked to the duration of cardiomegaly. The patients in whom cardiomegaly does not resolve within 6 months have a very poor prognosis.[75]

The management of peripartum cardiomyopathy initially centers on improving the low output congestive heart failure. Invasive monitoring (following the wedge pressure and cardiac output) is warranted in the acute phase until the cardiac output is stabilized and adequate. These patients should be maintained in an upright position with uterine displacement. Supplemental oxygen and occasionally intubation and ventilation with positive end-expiratory pressure are required. Inotropic support initially with dopamine or dobutamine and subsequent digitalization is often necessary. Afterload reduction and diuretic therapy may be helpful. In severe cases amrinone may be useful.

Expeditious delivery of the fetus (cesarean section or vaginal delivery with outlet forceps to minimize pushing) may be necessary both to protect the fetus and to limit further cardiovascular stress imposed by pregnancy. Anticoagulant therapy with intravenous heparin during pregnancy and long-term anticoagulant treatment with warfarin after fetal delivery are necessary because of the high risk of stasis related to embolization.

In patients with severe left ventricular failure, intraaortic balloon counter pulsation may be required. Extreme cases of peripartum cardiomyopathy have required subsequent heart transplantation. The longterm management of chronic peripartum cardiomyopathy includes prophylactic anticoagulation, digitalization, sodium restriction, rest (with adequate ambulation to minimize venous stasis), possible avoidance of oral contraceptives, and avoidance of further pregnancy until the cardiomegaly resolves completely. Intensive nursing support is essential in the management of these patients.[85]

Both regional and general anesthetic techniques have been reported in peripartum cardiomyopathy patients.[86] Prior to delivery, anticoagulation must be withheld and the coagulation status normalized. Carefully titrated regional anesthetic techniques (continuous epidural or continuous spinal) offer a number of advantages. Regional techniques reduce afterload with minimal effect on contractility, thus improving cardiac output and reducing myocardial work. The titration of local anesthetic and volume loading/vasoactive medication should be based on wedge pressure. By blocking afferent noxious stimuli, the release of stress-related hormones (catecholamines, ADH, etc.) is reduced. Regional anesthesia may minimize the incidence of venous sta-

sis emboli. Spinal and epidural narcotic agents are also useful for postoperative analgesia before the reimplementation of anticoagulant therapy. When general anesthesia is used, the myocardial depressive effects of volatile agents and thiopental and ketamine are of concern. "Cardiac induction" with high-dose fentanyl is preferred. These patients require prolonged postoperative monitoring in an ICU.

IDIOPATHIC HYPERTROPHIC SUBAORTIC STENOSIS

Idiopathic hypertrophic subaortic stenosis was first described in the 1960s as an obstructive cardiomyopathy with a variety of clinical presentations.[87] Hypertrophic changes in ventricular muscle may reduce ventricular outflow, producing a cardiovascular picture resembling aortic stenosis. Obstructive changes may also obstruct ventricular inflow in a manner similar to mitral stenosis or distort the mitral valve, resulting in coexisting mitral regurgitation. These patients may complain of episodic palpitations and chest pain and may avoid cardiac stimulants such as caffeine.

The history of this disorder is not as yet fully defined. The pathophysiology of IHSS can best be understood by considering the pressure gradient across the ventricular outlet (aortic valve). Anything that increases this gradient will further stress the cardiovascular system. Increases in contractility will compound the obstructive effect of the hypertrophied muscle, thus increasing the obstruction. Decreases in left ventricular end diastolic volume (LVEDV) (preload) or acute reduction of systemic vascular resistance (SVR) will worsen the obstructive effect. Tachycardia will also reduce cardiac output by reducing the effective ventricular filling and ejection time.

Pregnancy and its associated physiologic changes may affect this disorder in conflicting ways. Initially, the expanded intravascular volume may have a beneficial effect by increasing the LVEDV. However, as the gestation progresses, the increase in cardiac output of the SVR may have a negative effect. The expanded uterus will cause aortocaval compression in certain body positions and this will reduce venous return and have a detrimental effect.[88]

Beta-blocking agents are useful in managing IHSS. The reduction of contractility improves the obstruction, and lower heart rates allow for greater ventricular filling and ejection times. Thus, IHSS patients are usually chronically managed with beta-blockers. Sympathomimetic agents including digoxin, epinephrine, ephedrine, and calcium chloride should be avoided because they will increase the occlusive effect. Diuretics should also be used with great caution.

The management of IHSS patients for labor and delivery will depend on the clinical severity of their symptoms and on coexisting problems. Antibiotic prophylaxis to prevent endocarditis should be given. The volume status of these patients must be carefully followed. Arterial monitoring and central pressure monitoring is useful in severe cases. Adequate uterine displacement should be maintained. Sufficient intravenous volume loading with warmed (37° C) crystalloid is essential. Beta-blockade should be maintained by continuing the patient's usual medications. Intravenous esmolol infusion can be titrated to prevent tachycardia. Continuous epidural anesthesia should be instituted early and maintained with local anesthetic/narcotic infusion. Blood pressure should be aggressively managed with intravenous volume expansion and phenylephrine titration. Supplemental oxygen by face mask should be administered. Continuous ECG and finger pulse oximetry monitors should be used.

In all but the most severe cases, labor and vaginal delivery are not contraindicated, but excessively long or stressful trials of labor should be avoided. If cesarean delivery is required for obstetric reasons, regional anesthesia is *not* contraindicated.[89] However, "single shot" and rapid inductions are to be avoided.[90,91] Slowly titrated continuous epidural or continuous spinal anesthesia with aggressive blood pressure support, carefully managed with continuous invasive monitoring, can provide a stable cardiovascular state. If a general anesthetic induction is used, additional beta-blockade (preferably with a rapidly titratable agent such as esmolol) is necessary prior to the stress of intubation. (Maternal beta-blockade exposes the fetus to beta-blockade and thus fetal heart rate monitoring is less reliable to detect fetal stress. If fetal status is questioned, fetal scalp pH analysis should be considered.) Intraoperative blood loss should be continuously measured and replaced.

Finally, IHSS patients should be monitored in an ICU for 24 hours postoperatively. Resolution of sympathectomy associated with continuous epidural or continuous spinal anesthesia should not present problems because it will result in an increased SVR and autovolume transfusion. Adequate postoperative analgesia should be maintained with epidural or spinal narcotics or patient-controlled analgesia (PCA) if available.

MITRAL VALVE PROLAPSE

Mitral valve prolapse is the most common congenital heart lesion. It is defined as the pathologic protrusion of the mitral leaflet into the left atrium during systole. It is present in approximately 6% of the general population and may be present in 12% to 17% of women of childbearing age.[92] Mi-

tral valve prolapse has been classified as primary (idiopathic), which is commonly associated with characteristic changes in body habitus, blood pressure, and evidence of labile hemodynamics, or as secondary, which is when the prolapse is associated with connective tissue disease or cardiac disease that reduces the size of the left ventricle. Marfan's syndrome has been most commonly associated with mitral valve prolapse. The classification system is listed in Box 12-4.

Mitral valve prolapse associated with nonspecific symptoms, ECG abnormalities, and dysrhythmias was termed *mitral valve prolapse syndrome* in the 1960s.[93] These symptoms include fatigue, dizziness, chest pain, palpitation, and dyspnea. Savage et al[92] examined the general population with mitral valve prolapse and reported no increase in symptoms of atypical or anginal chest pain, dysp-

---

BOX 12-4   ETIOLOGY OF MITRAL VALVE PROLAPSE SYNDROME*

Primary (idiopathic)
Familial
Nonfamilial

Secondary
Definite or probable cause
   Marfan's syndrome
   Floppy valve syndrome
   Rheumatic endocarditis
   Occlusive coronary artery disease
   Congestive cardiomyopathy
   IHSS
   Myocarditis
   Mitral valve surgery
   Trauma
   Left atrial myxoma
   Polyarteritis nodosa
   Left ventricular aneurysm
   Ehlers-Danlos syndrome
   Relapsing polychondritis
   Lupus erythematosus
   Muscular dystrophy
   Wolff-Parkinson-White syndrome
   Osteogenesis imperfecta
   Pseudoxanthoma elasticum

Probable association
Congenital heart disease (atrial septal defect, patent ductus arteriosus, Ebstein's anomaly, corrected transposition of great vessels)
Athlete's heart
Turner's syndrome
Noonan's syndrome
Congenital prolonged Q-T syndrome

---

*From Degani S, Abinader EG, Scharf M: *Obstet Gynecol Surv* 1989; 44:642. Used by permission.

nea, or syncope. Therefore, close evaluation of all pregnant patients with these complaints is necessary, and symptoms should not be ascribed automatically to mitral valve prolapse syndrome.

Mitral valve prolapse syndrome has a generally benign course. The prognosis depends on whether it is primary or secondary to another cardiac problem. The course is infrequently complicated by progression of mitral insufficiency, ruptured chorda tendinae, transient ischemic attacks, infective endocarditis, and sudden death from dysrhythmia.[94] The risk of sudden death in mitral valve prolapse patients who do not have mitral regurgitation does not seem to be appreciable over the background risk. However, the 2% to 4% of patients with severe mitral regurgitation comprise a group that may have a 50- to 100-fold greater rate of sudden death, with an annual mortality rate in this subset of 94 to 188 per 100,000.[95,96]

The recommendations of the Committee on Rheumatic Fever and Infective Endocarditis of the American Heart Association suggest antibiotic prophylaxis only for patients with mitral valve prolapse complicated by mitral insufficiency. Vaginal hysterectomy is the only gynecologic procedure specifically listed in which antibiotic prophylaxis is recommended. Uncomplicated vaginal delivery is stated to rarely if ever precipitate endocarditis.[96]

Routine prophylaxis is also thought unnecessary in cesarean section, uterine dilation and curettage, and therapeutic abortions when these procedures do not involve patients in whom infection is suspected.[97,98] Antibiotic prophylaxis is considered appropriate in the presence of regurgitant murmur or if there are indications of an infection.

Pregnancy in patients with mitral valve prolapse usually follows an uneventful course. Rayburn and Fontana[99] noted pregnancy outcome did not significantly differ in the group with mitral valve prolapse versus a control group of pregnancies uncomplicated by cardiac disease. The incidence of spontaneous abortion, preterm delivery, low birth weight, neonatal mortality, cesarean section, and antenatal hospitalization was not significantly increased in pregnancies associated with mitral valve prolapse. In a separate study, Tang et al[100] observed a similar result. Shapiro et al[101] speculated that labor and delivery might be less complicated and quicker in patients with mitral valve prolapse because of an increased laxity of joints and connective tissue that can be associated with this population. However, no statistical difference in the rate of cervical dilation during the first stage of labor, rate of cesarean sections, oxytocin augmentation, birth weights, or Apgar scores were noted.

Beta-adrenergic blocking agents are useful in the management of both atrial and ventricular premature beats, supraventricular and ventricular tachycardia, and other arrhythmias associated with mitral valve prolapse. Older reports of studies using beta-blockers during pregnancy were met with concern, since propranolol was linked to IUGR and neonatal depression. However, it is difficult to separate the effects of the disease, such as maternal hypertension, from the treatment (i.e., beta-blockers during pregnancy). Recent reports of well-controlled prospective studies have provided reassuring data regarding the use of beta-adrenergic blockers during pregnancy.[96] Thus, the use of these drugs to control chest pain, palpitation, or arrhythmias during pregnancy complicated by mitral valve prolapse should certainly be considered when clinically warranted.

Anesthetic considerations

Mitral valve prolapse is the most common cardiac lesion seen in pregnancy, with an estimated incidence of 0.5% to 17%. In the young adult age group it is more commonly seen in women. Its spectrum of presentation ranges from clinically insignificant and unrecognized to significant debilitation due to chest pain, dysrhythmia, and mitral regurgitation.

History may include episodes of dyspnea on exertion, palpitations, chest pain, dizziness, and fainting. Auscultation usually reveals a systolic murmur (mitral regurgitation) and a middle to late systolic click murmur caused by abrupt decelerations of the prolapsed leaflet.[102] Electrocardiographic evidence is seen in up to 70% of these patients and may include dysrhythmias, ST segment changes, T-wave inversion, and QT interval prolongation.[103,104] Mitral valve prolapse may be associated with other cardiovascular lesions including IHSS, Marfan's syndrome, atrial septal defect, coronary artery disease, and periarteritis nodosa. Conditions that cause or are associated with mitral valve prolapse are listed in Box 12-5.

The pathophysiology of mitral valve prolapse involves congenitally oversized, redundant valve leaflets, especially the posterior leaflet, and increased length of the chorda tendinae. This allows the leaflets to prolapse with resultant regurgitation during systole.[105] Chest pain and arrhythmias may be related to associated coronary artery spasm or compression of the circumflex artery by the posterior leaflet.[106] Decreases in LVEDV can exaggerate the prolapse and worsen associated symptoms.

The workup of a pregnant patient with the diagnosis of mitral valve prolapse should include a thorough history and physical examination, ECG, chest x-ray examination, echocardiography, and

---

BOX 12-5   CONDITIONS CAUSING OR ASSOCIATED WITH MITRAL VALVE PROLAPSE

Primary mitral valve prolapse
Marfan's syndrome
Floppy valve syndrome
Rheumatic endocarditis
Coronary artery disease
Congestive and hypertrophic cardiomyopathy
Myocarditis
Trauma
Left atrial myxoma
Polyarteritis nodosa
Systemic lupus erythematosus
Left ventricular aneurysm
Ehlers-Danlos syndrome
Pseudoxanthoma elasticum
Pulmonary emphysema
Relapsing polychondritis
Muscular dystrophy
Wolff-Parkinson-White syndrome
Inherited disorders of metabolism (Hunter-Hurler syndrome, Sanfilippo's syndrome, Fabry's disease, Sandhoff's disease)

Osteogenesis imperfecta
Straight back syndrome
Thoracic skeletal abnormalities
Neuroectomesodermal histocysplasia
Hyperthyroidism
Willebrand's syndrome
Platelet abnormalities
Migraine
Hypomagnesemia
Anxiety neurosis, neurocirculatory asthenia, autonomic dysfunction
Congenital heart disease (atrial septal defect, ventricular septal defect, patent ductus arteriosus, aortopulmonary window, complete absence of left pericardium, membranous subaortic stenosis, supravalvular aortic stenosis, Ebstein's anomaly, corrected transposition of great vessels, infundibular pulmonary stenosis, Uhl's anomaly)
Congenital prolonged QT syndrome
Athlete's heart

---

cardiology consult to identify any coexistent problems. Medical management of dysrhythmias and chest pain should be optimized and may include beta-blocker or calcium-channel blocker therapy.

Anesthetic management goals include avoiding decreases in LVEDV, minimizing increases in cardiac output and heart rate, providing adequate analgesia and anesthesia, and preventing and treating arrhythmias. The psychological changes of pregnancy and the stress of labor and delivery complicate the management. The effects of maternal antiarrhythmic drugs on fetal heart rate monitoring should be noted. Maternal monitoring should include a baseline 12-lead ECG, followed by continuous ECG rhythm monitoring. Maternal antiarrhythmic drugs should be continued. Antibiotic prophylaxis for bacterial endocarditis should be given prior to anesthetic or delivery. Careful attention to volume status is necessary. Aortocaval compression can exaggerate mitral valve prolapse symptoms by reducing venous return. Intravenous volume preloading with warmed (37° C) crystalloid solution is useful to maintain preload LVEDV and minimize shivering. Acute decreases in the SVR should be avoided, since this would also reduce LVEDV and increase mitral valve prolapse. Thus, if regional conduction anesthesia is required, a carefully titrated continuous epidural or spinal catheter should be used. Agents that acutely raise heart rate or cardiac output should be avoided or used with caution (epinephrine, ephedrine, ketamine, atropine, pancuronium). Hypotension should be aggressively managed with intravenous volume expansion, and phenylephrine is the pressor of choice. Adequate analgesia and/or anesthesia will minimize pain and reduce endogenous catecholamines, thereby reducing arrhythmogenicity and mitral valve prolapse. Supplemental oxygen by nasal prongs or face mask is advisable.[107]

Vaginal delivery can be managed with continuous epidural analgesia/anesthesia. Adjunctive epidural fentanyl is especially useful since it tends to improve the block, reduce local anesthetic requirements, and reduce maternal shivering and discomfort. Cesarean delivery can be managed with continuous epidural or continuous spinal anesthesia, although care must be taken to support the blood pressure and maintain the SVR. Usually, a carefully titrated regional anesthetic will provide more cardiovascular stability than a standard obstetric rapid sequence general anesthetic. Initial induction of a standard obstetric general anesthetic using thiopental will first result in hypotension, followed by significant cardiovascular stimulation on intubation.

The standard obstetric rapid sequence induction of general anesthesia consists of a very light anesthetic, at least until the fetus is delivered. This will predispose the patient to cardiovascular instability and increase the likelihood of arrhythmias. The

Table 12-15 Effects of volatile anesthetic agents on cardiovascular parameters (starting from baseline in normal awake patient)*

	Halothane	Enflurane	Isoflurane
Heart rate	↓	—	↑
SVR	↓	↓	↓ ↓
Contractility	↓ ↓	↓	↓
Most common arrhythmia	PVCs/PACs	Nodal rhythm	SVT

*PVC = premature ventricular contraction; PAC = premature atrial contraction; SVT = supraventricular tachycardia.

ideal choice of volatile anesthetic agent (until the fetus is delivered) is probably halothane (Table 12-15) since it tends to slow the heart rate, reduce contractility, and maintain SVR. Enflurane would be the second choice and isoflurane the least useful. If the patient has clinically severe mitral valve prolapse symptoms, the use of a high-dose narcotic induction is warranted. Ventilation should be maintained with a relatively slow inspiratory flow rate setting to minimize the efforts of positive pressure ventilation on intrathoracic pressure.

WOLFFE-PARKINSON-WHITE SYNDROME

An inherited anomaly of the atrial conduction system, Wolffe-Parkinson-White (WPS) syndrome is a condition in which patients have aberrant conduction pathways that can bypass the normal SA-node to AV-node conduction path. These patients are prone to SVT associated with retrograde or antegrade conduction. The ECG is characterized by a short PR interval and a delta R-wave slope. It is not clear whether the hormonal and cardiovascular changes of pregnancy increase conduction phenomenon in these patients. While a rapid ventricular rate may be controlled by digitalization, the effect of calcium-channel blockers or beta-blockers is unpredictable and may increase aberrant conduction. Adenosine should be considered. If the patient becomes unstable (hypotensive, reduced oxygen saturation), immediate synchronized cardioversion is indicated. Note that aortacaval compression must be avoided.

Agents which should be avoided include ephedrine, epinephrine-containing solutions, and meperidine. If blood pressure support is required, volume expansion and Neo-Synephrine should be used. Carefully titrated epidural analgesia is the most controllable. Ajunctive epidural fentanyl is helpful to augment analgesia. If general anesthesia is required, it has been reported that fentanyl or sufentanil and lorazepam has no effect on conduction, and ethrane is the agent of choice to increase refractoriness and suppress SVT.[41c] Droperidol also suppresses conduction in aberrant pathways.

MARFAN'S SYNDROME

In addition to the concerns regarding possible difficult intubation, airway management, and restrictive pulmonary status, the cardiovascular considerations are paramount in pregnancy. Patients with Marfan's syndrome are at risk for acute and catastrophic dissection of their abdominal and especially thoracic aorta because of cystic medial necrosis.[108] Pregnancy may significantly increase this risk as a result of sustained increases in cardiac output, hormonal changes with associated effects on connective tissue, and the stress and pain of labor and delivery.[109-111] The key to managing these patients is tight blood pressure control and minimization of vascular shear stress (dp/dt). Acute changes in contractility and sudden increases in blood pressure increase shear stress. These patients are managed during their pregnancy with beta-blockers and/or calcium-channel blocker therapy. These drugs should be continued at the time of delivery. An indwelling arterial line with continuous blood pressure monitoring is necessary. A central venous pressure catheter is useful to administer vasoactive medications. Additional beta-blockade with esmolol or labetalol should be instituted before delivery. Volume status should be optimized. Continuous epidural or continuous spinal anesthesia should be the anesthetic of choice, and carefully titrated blood pressure should be supported with intravascular volume expansion and slow, careful phenylephrine titration. Ephedrine, epinephrine, calcium chloride, dopamine, dobutamine, or digoxin should be avoided as should Methergine to prevent increases in contractility. Tachycardia should be aggressively treated. It is essential that the anesthesiologist be continually present to monitor changes in blood pressure and to titrate vasoactive medications. This is also true in the immediate postoperative period since the cardiac output continues to increase in the postpartum period. Blood loss should be replaced continuously since it is lost with appropriate crystalloid or blood products. Pain and anxiety must be prevented even if significant sedation is required. The Valsalva maneuver is to be avoided; thus outlet forceps or cesarean section should be used for delivery.

PRIMARY PULMONARY HYPERTENSION

The diagnosis of primary pulmonary hypertension in pregnancy is ominous. The maternal mortality rate is greater than 50% and will correlate with the severity of the hypertension. As the changes in the pulmonary vasculature progress, the vessels become less and less able to react, and the pulmonary vascular resistance (PVR) increases and becomes relatively fixed. Pregnancy in these patients is relatively contraindicated and therapeutic abortion should be considered.[112,113]

The stress of pregnancy further exacerbates the effects of increased pulmonary vascular resistance. As the cardiac output requirements increase, cyanosis may increase and the right heart's workload is increased. These patients should be followed during pregnancy with serial blood gas analysis and finger pulse oximetry. As soon as the fetus has mature lungs, delivery should be considered. Maternal dexamethasone treatment should be given early to mature the fetal lungs.

Pulmonary artery catheter monitoring is necessary at delivery or operation to follow changes in the PVR. Oxygen is the best pulmonary vascular vasodilator and should be administered prior to, during, and after delivery with the use of high-flow rebreathing mask systems to achieve an F_{IO_2} of at least 40%. Intravenous nitroglycerin may be useful to reduce PVR because of its reduction of preload and direct pulmonary vasoactive effects. Isoproterenol or dobutamine may be of some benefit in treating failure in end-stage disease.[114]

Adequate perioperative analgesia and anesthesia are imperative and continuous epidural or continuous spinal technique with local anesthetics in combination with narcotics is useful to blunt the stress of labor.[115-117] Expeditious delivery with outlet forceps or cesarean section is warranted.

Nitric oxide is an exciting new experimental agent that can be added to the breathing mixture (5 to 20 parts per million) to treat pulmonary hypertension when other treatments have not been adequate. To date, there have been reports of little effect on placental perfusion.

TERMINATION OF PREGNANCY

Despite recent significant advances in monitoring technology, cardiovascular pharmacology, obstetric and perinatal medicine, critical care science, and anesthetic techniques, some cardiovascular entities are still essentially incompatible with maternal survival if a pregnancy is carried to term. Maternal mortality is almost certain if a mother with end-stage *primary* pulmonary hypertension carries

a gestation to term. In such a situation, absolute prevention of pregnancy and/or its termination is warranted to save the mother's life. Even if not interrupted, fetal morbidity and mortality is very high.

Women with uncorrected severe mitral stenosis, Eisenmenger's complex, and Marfan's syndrome also have high mortality rates and should conceive only after careful and thorough counseling about their relative risk of mortality and of the possibility of becoming a postdelivery cardiac cripple.[118-120] Nevertheless, reports of patients with mitral stenosis, Eisenmenger's syndrome, and Marfan's syndrome who have successfully carried a gestation to term are now appearing in the literature.

The anesthetic management of termination of pregnancy will, of course, depend on the stage of gestation and the patient's cardiovascular status. It is often tempting to manage first-trimester therapeutic abortions with sedation and local anesthesia (paracervical block). However, patients with cardiac disease severe enough to require therapeutic abortion have the potential for sudden cardiovascular decompensation that can be triggered by pain, anxiety, blood loss, and sympathetic or vagal reflexes. Carefully titrated regional anesthesia (spinal or epidural) to a level of T9-10 with epidural or spinal fentanyl is optimal. Adequate sedation is both appropriate and medically indicated. While these procedures are usually of short duration, attention to adequate monitoring, volume status, antibiotic prophylaxis, bubble traps, patient temperature, and postoperative monitoring is still essential. The postoperative management team should be vigilant for signs of bleeding and alteration in coagulation status.

PREGNANCY AFTER MATERNAL HEART TRANSPLANTATION

Cardiac transplantation has become an accepted mode of therapy for many types of end-stage heart disease, both congenital and acquired. Five-year survival rates now exceed 65% and the use of new immunosuppressive regimens have significantly improved the quality of life.[121-124] A number of patients have been reported to have successfully carried a pregnancy to term and delivered normal healthy infants after orthotopic heart transplantation. Both vaginal delivery and cesarean section have been reported.[125-127]

Patients who have received organ transplants must be maintained on immunosuppressive therapy to prevent organ rejection.[128] This usually includes cyclosporine, prednisone, and antibiotics, and must be continued throughout the pregnancy. Strict attention to sterile technique is especially important. Prophylactic antibiotics and prophylactic "stress doses" of steroids are indicated before anesthetics and surgical procedures. Cyclosporine concentrations may change abruptly after delivery because of acute changes in maternal circulatory blood volume and volume of distribution and should be followed with serial blood levels.[123]

Despite exposure to immunosuppressive drugs, fetal effects appear to be minimal. Many successful deliveries of apparently normal infants have been reported in immunosuppressed mothers who have undergone renal,[129] hepatic,[130] and bone marrow[131] transplantation.

Periodic transvenous right atrial myocardial tissue biopsy is performed in cardiac transplant patients to follow evidence of allograft rejection. When carried out in pregnant patients (as early as 20 weeks' gestation), attention should be maintained to provide supplemental oxygen and avoid aortocaval compression during the procedure. This includes uterine displacement and the use of a lead shield, not a lead apron, applied directly to the mother's abdomen for fetal protection, if fluoroscopy is used.

In the absence of allograft rejection, the transplanted heart usually maintains excellent ventricular function. However, the transplanted heart is completely devoid of direct autonomic innervation. The baseline heart rate is usually slightly increased in cardiac transplant patients since the predominant underlying vagal tone present in most healthy young adults is not expressed through direct innervation. Interestingly, cardiac transplant recipients can increase and regulate their cardiac output in response to exercise (although the response time is slower), probably through the Starling mechanism, by regulating their preload and afterload. As ventricular function and thus cardiac output are significantly dependent on the Starling mechanism, the maintenance of adequate preload (intravascular volume loading) is especially important.

Only direct-acting vasoactive agents will affect the heart rate (atropine will not increase the heart rate, isoproterenol will, etc.). Unlike normal patients, sympathectomy associated with high spinal or epidural anesthesia will not cause bradycardia by blocking the cardiac sympathetics since these fibers have already been surgically ablated.

Cardiac transplant patients may be more sensitive to beta-mimetics (epinephrine being the most clinically significant) because of receptor up regulation. Camann et al.[127] reported the onset of tachycardia possibly associated with epinephrine 1:200,000 used in 2% lidocaine given for epidural anesthesia. The resulting tachycardia was profound and was managed with intravenous esmolol.

In the absence of allograft rejection, the patient has a relatively "good heart" and a fairly young and hopefully otherwise healthy body. These patients should be able to handle the stress of labor and delivery.

The mode of delivery, either vaginal or abdominal, should be decided on obstetric grounds. Noninvasive monitoring, including automated blood pressure cuff, ECG, finger pulse oximetry, and fetal heart rate monitoring, is usually adequate. Invasive monitoring (central venous pressure, pulmonary artery, A-line) poses a risk of infection and arrhythmias that must be weighed against the volume of the data to be gained.

The avoidance of endogenous catecholamines associated with pain is important. The induction of continuous epidural analgesia early in labor is optimal. This also allows the level to be brought up rapidly in the event of an obstetric emergency, thus avoiding the need for a general anesthetic. Blood pressure should be maintained with intravenous volume loading, ephedrine, or phenylephrine. Continuous epidural or continuous spinal techniques allow careful titration and greater control of cardiovascular parameters. Epidural or spinal narcotics are advantageous.

If general anesthesia is used, thiopental may have an exaggerated depressant effect on the cardiac output. Ketamine may cause excessive tachycardia in these patients because of changes in beta-receptor sensitivity. A high-dose fentanyl technique will produce the most stable induction (although the onset time will be longer).

MYOCARDIAL INFARCTION

Myocardial infarction is a rare complication of pregnancy. It was first described by Katz in 1922.[132] Subsequently, over 80 cases have been reported and the relative incidence has been estimated at 1 in 10,000 deliveries.[133-137] Most of these myocardial infarctions occurred in the third trimester. Maternal age may play a significant role since more than half of the women were 35 years of age or older. While many of the earlier cases occurred in women with other significant underlying disease (toxemia, diabetes, familial hyperlipidemia, etc.), cases in which obvious underlying disease is not present are appearing more frequently in the recent literature (Box 12-6).

The incidence of myocardial infarction in pregnancy appears to be increasing. This may correlate with the increased mean maternal age of many women who postpone beginning their families until after completing their education and establishing their careers. The unfortunate increase of smoking among young women, stress in the workplace, and the exponential increase in the maternal use of cocaine may all be contributing factors.[138]

BOX 12-6   MYOCARDIAL INFARCTION IN PREGNANCY

Etiology
  Atherosclerosis
  Diabetes
  Hyperlipidemia
  Smoking
  Hypertension
Thrombus
Spasm
Congenital defect
Preeclampsia
Arrhythmia
Substance abuse
Embolism
Stress
  Supply/demand
  Catecholamines

The etiology of myocardial infarction in pregnancy is probably multifactorial (Box 12-6). Of the cases presently published in the literature, angiography or autopsy studies demonstrated significant coronary atherosclerosis in about 40% of the patients, coronary aneurysms or obstruction in about 10%, evidence of coronary thrombosis in 30% to 40%, and normal coronary arteries in 10% of the cases. Thus, in addition to coronary artery disease, thrombus formation and coronary spasm probably contribute to the cause. Alterations in the levels of many coagulation factors, hepatic function, volume of distribution, and an increased tendency toward venous stasis result in a relatively procoagulant state during pregnancy. This is balanced by an increase in fibrinolytic activity. Older patients may statistically have a greater amount of atherosclerotic coronary damage that could act as a template and catalyst for thrombus formation. Smoking, in addition to its effect on atherosclerosis, enhances platelet aggregation and may increase the risk of thrombus formation. An ischemic placenta may release renin,[139] and Sasse et al postulated that this might result in coronary spasm.[140] Finally, cocaine has significant vasoactive effects, and in addition to its affect on endogenous catecholamine levels, it may precipitate coronary spasm.[141-147]

The overall mortality rate for patients who sustain myocardial infarction during pregnancy is about 30%. The risk of death increases as the time of initial infarct approaches term. The highest mortality seems to occur at the time of the initial infarct, and at delivery if it occurs soon thereafter. Myocardial infarction that occurs in the postpartum period in patients with severe preeclampsia has a particularly dismal survival rate. Fetal survival appears to be strongly linked to maternal survival. No data are available on fetal morbidity.[148]

The initial stabilization of the pregnant patient who has sustained myocardial infarction must be aggressive since she is at risk for sudden death and should include immediate evaluation and support of her vital signs and CPR if required (see previous section on CPR). High-flow oxygen should be instituted, left lateral uterine displacement should be maintained, and an intravenous line established. The patient should be immediately transported to an intensive care unit (ICU). Sublingual nitroglycerin and parenteral morphine should be given in addition to a lidocaine bolus and prophylactic lidocaine infusion. Electrocardiographic monitoring should be established and an arterial catheter placed. Intravenous nitroglycerin should be started and titrated against symptoms of angina and ECG evidence of ischemia. Nitroglycerin therapy should not be discontinued if or when maternal hypotension develops. Instead, maternal mean blood pressure should be maintained in a normal range with intravenous phenylephrine infusion. Severe tachyarrhythmias should be controlled with beta-blocker therapy (preferably a beta-selective agent). Finger pulse oximetry is useful (especially in sedated nonintubated patients) and will serve as an indicator of respiratory depression, V/Q mismatch, and unexpected maternal shunt. Fetal heart monitoring should be used to observe fetal well-being. A pulmonary artery catheter should be placed to guide fluid and vasopressor therapy. If the patient has sustained myocardial injury, higher than normal wedge pressures may be required to maintain adequate cardiac output by pushing the ventricular function to a higher level on the Starling curve. A sudden rise in wedge pressure or wave-form evidence of tricuspid or mitral regurgitation may be early indications of new ischemia.

Significant items in the history and physical examination include obesity, smoking, familial and personal hyperlipidemia or heart disease, hypertension, toxemia, evidence of arrhythmia, venous stasis, congenital heart defects, obstetric history, drug allergies, and drug use/abuse. A toxicology screen (cocaine) should be obtained.

The diagnostic workup should include serial 12-lead ECG, serial cardiac isoenzyme determination, coagulation profile, electrolyte profile, hematocrit, routine liver enzymes, BUN, creatinine, glucose, urinalysis, and baseline arterial blood gases. Two-dimensional echocardiography should be obtained to evaluate left ventricular and valve function and ejection fraction. If there is evidence of ongoing or progressive ischemia or infarction, immediate cardiac catheterization should be considered (with lead shielding of the abdomen that does not compress the abdomen). If a discrete coronary circulation defect is visualized, intracoronary lytic therapy or percutaneous transluminal coronary angioplasty (PTCA) may be effective to prevent further progression of myocardial damage. A case of successful PTCA in a pregnant patient with ongoing infarction has been reported.[148] Operative revascularization (coronary artery bypass grafting using cardiopulmonary bypass) has been reported in the pregnant patient.[149,150] Patients in acute left ventricular failure can be managed with digitalization (and rarely furosemide). If this therapy is not adequate, dopamine, dobutamine, or norepinephrine may be required despite their effects on placental perfusion. Tachycardia should be avoided. In the patient with severe myocardial dysfunction (congestive heart failure with low ejection fraction, not responsive to dopamine or norepinephrine) stabilization with an intraaortic balloon pump is a consideration. However, the coagulation-related risks of emboli are very high.

Prophylactic "low-dose" subcutaneous heparin should be started to reduce the risk of deep vein thrombosis associated with venous stasis and bedrest. If there is evidence of significant ventricular dyskinesis, hypokinesis, or ventricular aneurysm, intravenous heparin and maintenance of a partial thromboplastin time (PTT) at twice normal levels should be used to minimize the risk of mural thrombosis and emboli.[151-153] Heparin does not cross the placenta. Prior to delivery, the heparin will need to be stopped (usually 6 hours before surgery) and the PTT allowed to return to normal. Protamine or fresh frozen plasma can be used to normalize the PTT in the emergency situation.

Intravenous systemic thrombolytic therapy with streptokinase and urokinase are now often used to treat acutely evolving myocardial infarction in nonpregnant patients.[154] In the acute setting, thrombolytic therapy has been shown to reduce mortality rates and limit infarct size.[155,156] When used in pregnant patients, streptokinase and urokinase have been associated with significant maternal bleeding, premature labor, and dysfunctional uterine contractions.[157] Thus, systemic thrombolytic therapy is not routinely used in pregnancy. The direct application of a thrombolytic agent to a coronary thrombus at coronary angiography has not yet been reported in pregnant patients. Dipyridamole has not been associated with any maternal/fetal problems. Theoretically, aspirin could result in maternal or fetal hemorrhage and fetal premature closure of the ductus arteriosus in utero. Aspirin is generally avoided in pregnancy. However, aspirin therapy in severe preeclampsia may be beneficial and it

may prove useful in pregnant myocardial infarction patients in the future.[158,159]

The management of the pregnant patient who has sustained an acute myocardial infarction requires a coordinated team approach with careful intradisciplinary communication. The patient needs to be maintained in a critical care setting during her initial stabilization, during her delivery, and for several days in the postpartum period. Invasive monitoring and tight control of all cardiovascular parameters are essential. Rao et al. demonstrated that invasive monitoring and intensive management based on the monitoring data significantly improve the outcome and reduce the mortality in acute myocardial infarction patients who undergo anesthesia and surgery.[160] The first 3 months after a myocardial infarction carry the greatest mortality rate.[161] Pregnant myocardial infarction patients will almost assuredly undergo anesthesia for a procedure (delivery) within this high-risk 3-month period. They will also most likely undergo an abdominal procedure (cesarean delivery) that correlates with an increased risk of mortality.[162] While they are recuperating at bedrest their risk of stasis increases and the stress on their cardiovascular system caused by the demands of pregnancy also heightens.

Many clinicians have had some experience with pregnant patients with various cardiac valve lesions. While challenging, these patients generally have good myocardial function and cardiovascular reserve. Carefully managed with attention to their particular anomalies, they usually do remarkably well. It is a mistake to think of the pregnant patient who has suffered an acute myocardial infarction as being in the same situation as the patients with valve lesions. The myocardial infarction patient has sustained an injury to the myocardium. The pump is damaged and will function less efficiently. The cardiovascular reserve is usually limited or nonexistent and may be overwhelmed by the ever-increasing demands of pregnancy. Finally, the myocardial oxygen supply/demand relationship is tenuous. These patients are at great risk. The key to successful management of the pregnant patient who has suffered an acute myocardial infarction is attention to detail, tight control over all cardiovascular parameters using invasive monitoring, and *optimizing the myocardial oxygen supply/demand relationship* (Fig. 12-8).[163]

The major determinant of myocardial oxygen demand is heart rate. Other factors include contractility, myocardial wall tension (preload/afterload consideration) and the patient's metabolic state (temperature, shivering). Increased heart rate should be managed with adequate analgesia, appropriate volume management (titrated against the wedge pressure) and with the use of beta-

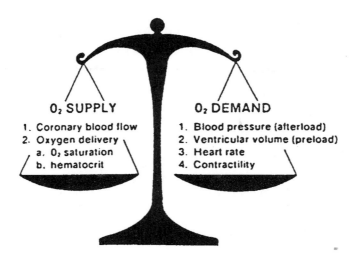

Fig. 12-8 Myocardial oxygen supply and demand balance. (From Reich DL, Brooks JL, Kaplan JA: Uncommon cardiac diseases, in Katz J, Benumof JF, Dadis LB (eds): *Anesthesia and Uncommon Diseases,* Philadelphia, WB Saunders, 1990, p 347. Used by permission.)

blocking agents. (The normal heart rate of a pregnant woman is increased 10 to 20 beats/min at term.)

The myocardial oxygen supply (Box 12-7) will depend on the oxygen content of the blood (affected by hemoglobin, inspired Fio_2, V/Q matching, 2,3-diphosphoglycerate [2,3-DPG] level, and temperature). The coronary perfusion pressure (CPP) (mostly during diastole) can be approximately equal to the mean diastolic blood pressure of the aortic root minus the left ventricular-end diastolic pressure. Other related factors include the coronary luminal diameter at any atherosclerotic blockage or coronary anomaly and the phenomenon of spasm. Coronary perfusion pressure can be increased by reducing the LVEDP (with nitroglycerin, which also improves endocardial perfusion and reduces coronary spasm). The mean arterial pressure should be maintained at normal baseline levels with phenylephrine when nitroglycerin is being used to optimize the CPP.

It is worth noting that not only does maternal hyperventilation (a ubiquitous response to labor) have a possible detrimental effect on placental perfusion, it also may reduce coronary perfusion.[164,165] Pregnant patients at term normally have a resting Pco_2 of about 32 mm Hg. When hyperventilation is superimposed, the Pco_2 can be significantly reduced. Epidural analgesia can reduce or eliminate this response.[6] (Avoiding labor altogether is another option.) Factors affecting suitable management are described in Box 12-8.

The timing of the delivery will require a risk/benefit analysis based on maternal cardiovascular stability and fetal lung maturity. If possible, it is

---

BOX 12-7   DETERMINANTS OF MYOCARDIAL OXYGEN SUPPLY

Oxygen content = Hemoglobin (g%) $\times$ Sao_2 $\times$ 1.34

Hemoglobin
Fio_2
V/Q
pH
Temperature
2,3-DPG

CPP $\approx$ MDP $-$ LVEDP
Rheology

BOX 12-8   FACTORS AFFECTING MANAGEMENT

Maternal status
  Arrhythmias
  Ejection fraction
  Wall motion abnormalities
  Valvular regurgitation
  Congestive heart failure
  Anticoagulation
  Time since infarct

Fetal status
  Development status
  Physiologic status
  Labor

desirable to maintain the fetus in utero until its lungs are determined to be mature (e.g., L/S ratio, saturated phosphatidylcholine). This process may already be accelerated because of maternal stress, and dexamethasone therapy can be considered. It is probably prudent to deliver the fetus as soon as it is mature to limit the continued stress of pregnancy on the mother. In the event of uncontrollable maternal decompensation, immediate fetal delivery is warranted regardless of fetal maturity since maternal considerations take precedence. Also, if the mother is not doing well, the fetus will be doing worse. Teleologically, the blood supply to the uteroplacental unit is maximum and autoregulation is absent in this circulation.

In most cases, vaginal delivery is suboptimal and should be avoided. The stress of labor and delivery is considerable. Cardiology consultants often quote the slightly increased morbidity and mortality associated with cesarean section vs. vaginal delivery taken from huge demographic pregnancy studies. This, of course, is not applicable to these patients since the patients in those series who underwent cesarean delivery generally had more complications than those who underwent vaginal delivery. Also these data do not look at patients who suffered a myocardial infarction. Hankins, in his review of 68 cases of myocardial infarction in pregnancy, noted a slightly increased, but not statistically significant, survival rate in patients who underwent vaginal delivery.[166] This series includes patients from 1925 to 1985. The patients are from different eras and areas, and different medical standards, surgical techniques, and anesthetic techniques were used. The majority did not undergo any type of invasive monitoring. Thus, while interesting historically, this review has little clinical relevance today. (The relative considerations to vaginal vs. cesarean delivery are listed in Table 12-16.)

It is preferable to plan the cesarean delivery electively to avoid the risks of labor and/or emergency scenarios and to allow for adequate personnel availability. Continuous epidural anesthesia with phenylephrine when necessary, and adequate intravenous volume loading and vasopressors carefully titrated against blood pressure and wedge pressure provide the optimal combination of cardiovascular system control. The awake patient may also provide additional warning of myocardial ischemia by reporting angina. An epidural block brought to the T3 dermatome interrupts cardiac sympathetics, thus slowing the heart rate and possibly preventing sympathetically mediated coronary spasm.[167,168] Epidural narcotics improve the quality of the anesthetic and can be used postoperatively to manage postoperative analgesia. If technical problems make epidural anesthesia inadequate, continuous spinal anesthesia, carefully titrated to effect, is the next best option. If regional anesthesia is contraindicated (coagulopathy, infection), a standard high-dose narcotic cardiac induction is required. Under no circumstances should a standard thiopentone/succinylcholine rapid sequence general anesthetic induction be used even for fetal distress.

If the patient is allowed to deliver vaginally, she should be brought in the operating room on high-flow oxygen mask and be adequately sedated and properly monitored, and she should undergo epidural induction in the same fashion as a patient for cesarean section. A high analgetic level should be maintained to keep the heart rate slow, ensure analgesia, and provide for immediate cesarean delivery in the event of fetal distress or maternal decompensation. The patient should not be allowed to push and outlet forceps should be applied.

Postoperatively, the patient should be carefully monitored in the ICU for several days. Adequate

Table 12-16 Advantages and disadvantages of vaginal delivery and elective cesarean section in parturients with myocardial infarction

	Vaginal delivery	Cesarean section
Advantages	Avoids surgical stress Minimal blood loss Early ambulation Hemodynamic stability	Avoids prolonged unpredictable labor Hemodynamic control Able to time delivery
Disadvantages	Prolonged labor; stressful labor can be unpredictable	Surgical stress Increased metabolic demands Hemorrhage Postoperative infection Postoperative pulmonary complications

analgesia should be assured (epidural or spinal narcotics or PCA).

EISENMENGER'S SYNDROME

Eisenmenger's syndrome is a complex combination of cardiovascular pathophysiology that includes (1) clinical cyanosis; (2) a communication between the right and left circulatory systems (atrial septal defect, ventricular septal defect, or aortopulmonary anomaly) that allows bidirectional shunting; and (3) pulmonary hypertension at systemic pressure levels that is relatively fixed, secondary to elevated pulmonary vascular resistance. The "Eisenmenger complex" was originally described in 1897 by Victor Eisenmenger in an article on congenital defects of the ventricular system.[169] Wood redefined the complex more precisely in 1958 as "pulmonary hypertension at systemic level, due to high pulmonary vascular resistance, with reversed or bidirectional shunt through a large ventricular septal defect."[170] Eisenmenger's syndrome may occur as the pathophysiologic end result of several congenital heart defects if untreated or incompletely treated (atrial septal defect, ventricular septal defect, patent ductus arteriosus, tetrology of Fallot, etc.). It develops as a result of chronic right heart volume overload that eventually results in hypertrophic changes in the pulmonary vasculature. The right heart volume overload is initially caused by left-to-right shunt. Eventually, as the pulmonary vascular resistance increases and the right-sided pressures increase, some bidirectional, right-to-left shunting begins. In the developmental stages, before the pulmonary vascular resistance becomes fixed, surgical correction (closure of the anomalous defect) may be feasible.[171,172]

The mortality rate associated with an Eisenmenger's syndrome patient carrying a pregnancy to term is very high. The physiologic changes of pregnancy, including the increased cardiac output, increased heart rate, increased blood volume, reduced FRC, altered V/Q matching, increased coagulability, increased oxygen consumption, pain and stress of labor, acute blood loss, and loss of the placental shunt at delivery, all combine to place an extremely high demand on a patient with no cardiac reserve. Jones[173] reported a 27% mortality rate and Gleicher et al[174] reported a 30% mortality rate when pregnancy was carried to term in these patients. Mortality associated with pregnancy in Eisenmenger's syndrome patients peaks at delivery and during the first postpartum week.[173,174] The mortality rate associated with therapeutic abortion in Gleicher's series was about 7%.[174]

Eisenmenger's syndrome develops slowly as a result of chronic right-sided overload. Patients compensate physiologically and function adequately at lower oxygen saturation levels that would never be acutely tolerated by a normal person. In the absence of pregnancy, a significantly high incidence of mortality occurs in the third to fourth decade.

Management of the pregnant patient with Eisenmenger's syndrome is very challenging. These patients should be counseled regarding maternal and fetal mortality and be offered the option of therapeutic abortion. At the Brigham and Women's Hospital, from 1986 to 1989, we have managed seven Eisenmenger's syndrome patients who underwent therapeutic abortion at 13 to 18 weeks' gestation without fatality. The anesthetic was managed as follows. Patients were premedicated with 30 ml of oral sodium bicitrate and 10 mg intravenous metoclopramide. Prophylactic ampicillin, 2 g, and gentamycin, 80 mg, were given intravenously. Mask oxygen was administered with high-flow rebreathing masks. Monitoring included finger pulse oximetry, 5-lead ECG, and automated blood pressure measurements. The first three patients were also followed with radial arterial catheters. No central monitoring was used. The patients were sedated with intravenous morphine and diazepam or midazolam. Intravenous volume loading was accomplished with warmed Ringer's lactate using a bubble trap and filter for a total of 1200 to 1400 ml over 20 minutes. Continuous epidural anesthesia was induced with the patient in the sitting position and a loss of resistance to saline technique (to minimize possible air bubble emboli). Incremental doses of 2% lidocaine without epinephrine were carefully titrated until an anesthetic block to T10 was obtained. Blood pressure was maintained with intravenous phenylephrine. Fentanyl, 50 μg in 10 ml of normal saline, was then given via the epidural catheter. Care was taken to keep the patients warm to minimize shivering. Blood loss was promptly replaced with 25% albumin. All of these patients had an unremarkable intraoperative and postoperative course.

Finger pulse oximetry is a very useful monitoring technique in Eisenmenger's syndrome.[175] It is an ideal indicator of changes in shunt fraction and direction. An arterial line allows continuous blood pressure monitoring and is very helpful in shortening the therapeutic response time to treat acute hypotension.

Central monitoring is more controversial.[176] A central venous pressure catheter is helpful in following preload. Care must be taken to avoid air emboli and to maintain strict sterile technique.

(The anatomic defect can permit direct right-to-left circulation passage of air or bacteria, bypassing the filtering effect of the lungs. These patients have an increased incidence of central nervous system infection.) Some authors advocate the use of pulmonary artery catheters. However, the pulmonary artery catheter may inadvertently traverse the anomalous defect (especially if the catheter is placed without fluoroscopy). Its placement may also cause arrhythmias, emboli to left circulation, infarction, transseptal or transdefect passage of the catheter, or pulmonary artery rupture/infarct. On the other hand, the information to be gained from the pulmonary artery line is limited. In the patient with fixed pulmonary resistance the pulmonary artery pressure is known to be at systemic levels. Hypertrophic changes in the pulmonary circulation make wedge pressures unreliable. Fick thermodilution cardiac output determinations will be spurious because of the shunt from the anatomic defect. Thus, in most cases, the data to be obtained from pulmonary artery monitoring are not worthy of the risks associated with this technique.[177]

The highest incidence of sudden death occurs in pregnant patients during the peripartum and early postpartum period. The causes include embolism, arrhythmia, right heart overload, myocardial infarction, and acute drops in SVR. Emboli (air clot or tissue) can bypass the lungs and affect the cerebral or coronary circulation. Acute arrhythmias in Eisenmenger's syndrome patients are particularly dangerous as these patients have little or no cardiac reserve and need the atrial kick and regular rhythm to keep up with the increased workload. Increased right heart pressures and volume can be caused by pain-induced endogenous catecholamines and the stress of pushing. This can overload the right heart and cause it to fail. Increased pulmonary pressures may precipitate pulmonary edema and worsen V/Q matching. As the right-sided pressure increases, the right-to-left shunt through the anatomic defect can increase, bypassing the lungs and reducing systemic saturation. A sudden drop in SVR can also reduce left-sided pressures and increase the right-to-left shunt.[178]

Chronic pulmonary vascular hyperplasia makes vasoactive agents (including isoproterenol and prostacyclin) relatively ineffective in reducing pulmonary vascular resistance. These agents may be considered in the event that any component of the increased pulmonary vascular resistance is believed to still be reactive in early stages of the disease. Oxygen is the most effective pulmonary circulation vasodilator.

If the patient intends to carry her pregnancy to term, continuous management with communication between all members of the care team will be required. The patient should be monitored with serial finger pulse oximetry and arterial blood gases. Reduction in saturation from the early pregnancy baseline is indicative of decompensation. Avoidance of upper respiratory tract infections and/or their prompt treatment is essential. Bedrest with regular periods of ambulation may be required as the gestation continues. Anticoagulation with heparin (initially subcutaneous "minidose" eventually upgraded to continuous intravenous heparin drip near term) should be considered to minimize the risk of a stasis venous emboli. Care to avoid positions that promote aortocaval compression should be stressed. Supplemental oxygen should be considered. As soon as the fetus is deemed viable and fetal lung maturity is diagnostically demonstrated, an elective delivery should be considered to avoid the continually increasing cardiovascular stress associated with gestation. A cesarean delivery is prudent to avoid the stress associated with labor. If for any reason labor is induced, adequate sedation/analgesia/anesthesia and continuous monitoring in an ICU is essential (monitoring has already been discussed in detail). Outlet forceps should be considered to minimize the effects of maternal pushing.

The effects of positive pressure ventilation on venous return, V/Q matching, pulmonary pressures, and shunt through the anatomic defect are particularly worrisome in Eisenmenger's syndrome patients. If general anesthesia is required, a slowly induced high-dose narcotic technique is essential. Volatile agents must be used with caution because of their effects on contractility, SVR, and possible arrhythmogenecity. Precautions must be taken to avoid gastric aspiration (since a slowly titrated high-dose narcotic induction is not a rapid sequence induction). Precautions should include routine pretreatment with cimetidine, metoclopramide, and sodium bicitrate. Cricoid pressure should be used after neuromuscular blockade is established until the endotracheal tube position is verified and its cuff inflated.

If not contraindicated, a carefully titrated continuous epidural anesthetic is probably the technique of choice.[61] Heparin must be stopped and coagulation status determined to be normal (prothrombin time, partial thromboplastin time, platelet count). Regional anesthesia may reduce the risk of postoperative venous stasis emboli. Regional anesthesia does pose the risk of reducing the SVR. However, when slowly and carefully titrated against blood pressure (arterial line) and oxygen saturation (finger pulse oximetry), with judicious intravenous volume loading and intravenous phenylephrine drip, the level can be adequately raised with minimal blood pressure fluctuations. The adjunctive use of epidural morphine/fentanyl (or spinal morphine/fentanyl) minimizes intraoperative peritoneal symptoms and allows adequate anesthesia for cesarean delivery at lower local anesthetic dermatome block levels, thus reducing the sympathectomy. Intrathecal or epidural narcotics alone are not adequate, even for labor analgesia.[179]

Lidocaine 2% without epinephrine for epidural block is probably the best choice. Epinephrine given epidurally, even in 1:200,000 concentrations, can be absorbed and can cause tachycardia in some patients. This would be poorly tolerated in the Eisenmenger's syndrome patient. The addition of fentanyl (50 mcg) with lidocaine will improve the quality of the block. Bupivacaine is 10 to 15 times more cardiotoxic than lidocaine, and chloroprocaine's extremely fast action, short duration, and antagonism of amides and epidural narcotics make them less attractive. Prior to placement of monitoring lines or epidural catheter, prophylactic cardiac antibiotics should be administered. Adequate sedation should also be used to avoid maternal anxiety–induced endogenous catecholamine release. If epidural anesthesia is technically difficult and not clinically adequate, a *continuous* catheter spinal technique should be considered. Adequate anesthesia must be absolutely demonstrated before surgery begins. Intraoperative blood loss should be aggressively replaced.

Pregnant patients with Eisenmenger's syndrome are susceptible to all of the usual obstetric emergencies (abruptio placentae, placenta previa, toxemia, amniotic fluid embolism, gestational diabetes, and acute fetal distress). Decisions about maternal/fetal priorities and contingency plans should be made early in pregnancy with thorough communication between the patient and members of the care team. A "crash induction" is never indicated in these patients even if fetal demise is imminent. (If the patient is allowed to labor, maintenance of an epidural level of analgesia adequate for rapid cesarean delivery in the case of acute fetal distress is an option.)

Postoperatively, Eisenmenger's syndrome patients should be followed in an ICU for several days (significant mortality occurs during this period). The resolution of the sympathectomy associated with regional anesthetic techniques should be carefully controlled. Sudden increases in sympathetic tone, catecholamine levels associated with pain, and circulatory blood volume that occur after delivery can precipitate right-sided volume overload, pulmonary edema, and right heart failure. If general anesthesia is used, avoidance of "bucking on the endotracheal tube" is important prior to extubation since this can acutely increase thoracic pressures. Adequate analgesia is mandatory postoperatively to minimize endogenous catecholamines and to allow early ambulation. Epidural or spinal narcotics are very useful for postoperative pain management. If this option is not technically possible, continuous PCA should be used.

VALVULAR DISEASE

Cardiovascular valve disease can be congenital or acquired. The incidence of acquired rheumatic valve disease has been steadily decreasing in the developed countries because of antibiotic therapy, but rheumatic heart disease is still common in many third world countries. Most pregnant patients with valvular disease are otherwise basically healthy and have good ventricular function. While the incidence of clinically significant atherosclerotic coronary disease is low in this patient population, alterations in the myocardial oxygen supply/demand relationship can precipitate myocardial ischemia in some patients with valve disease. The increased blood volume and cardiac output associated with pregnancy can overload stenotic valve lesions (Fig. 12-9) and may increase the regurgitant fraction in mitral or aortic insufficiency.[180]

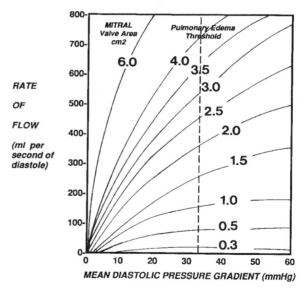

Fig. 12-9 Relationship between mean diastolic gradient pressure across the mitral valve and rate of flow across the mitral valve per second of diastole, as predicted by the Gorlin formula. (From Wallace AG: Pathophysiology of cardiovascular disease, in Smith LH Jr, Their SO (eds): *Pathophysiology: The Biological Principles of Disease. The International Textbook of Medicine,* vol 1, Philadelphia, WB Saunders, 1981, p 1192. Used by permission.)

Pregnant patients with clinically significant valvular heart disease need cardiac consultation early in their pregnancy to evaluate the extent of their disease and reserve and to establish baseline function. Noninvasive echocardiography can document valve area (Table 12-17), regurgitant fraction, and ventricular function. A baseline 12-lead ECG should be obtained to document evidence of ischemia, left ventricular hypertrophy, or arrhythmias. Arrhythmias should be treated and anticoagulation is indicated for atrial fibrillation (see section on anticoagulants). Antibiotic prophylaxis is indicated prior to any surgical procedure and prior to delivery. In the case of rapidly decompensating aortic or mitral disease (Box 12-9), open heart surgery with cardiopulmonary bypass should not be withheld. While it is prudent for the prospective mother to have her cardiac function evaluated and if necessary undergo valve replacement prior to pregnancy, this is often not possible. If open heart surgery is required during pregnancy, the optimal time to undertake it is during the second trimester (see section on Heart Surgery and Cardiopulmonary Bypass).

In the presence of good left ventricular function, the cardiovascular management of patients with valve disease involves mostly plumbing considerations, i.e., pharmacologic control of volumes and pressures (preload, afterload), pipe

resistance (SVR, pulmonary vascular resistance, etc.) and pump rate (heart rate). Invasive monitoring is essential and the effects of vasoactive medications on placental perfusion must be considered.

Low, carefully titrated continuous epidural (or in some cases continuous spinal) analgesia, with appropriate monitoring, is optimal for labor and vaginal delivery for any of the valve lesions. In patients with tight aortic stenosis, coronary perfusion is critically dependent on blood pressure (maintenance of SVR). Carefully titrated continuous epidural analgesia can be used safely even in patients with tight aortic stenosis provided that the patient is *continuously* monitored with an arterial line and blood pressure (SVR) is continuously maintained with intravenous volume replacement and phenylephrine drip. The block can be kept at a low level and augmented with epidural narcotics. Epidural anesthesia can be used safely for cesarean delivery, but the patient must be constantly monitored

Table 12-17 Valve area calculation

Gorlin formula
$$\text{Valve area (cm}^2) = \frac{\text{Flow (ml/sec)}}{K \times \text{Pressure gradient (mm Hg)}}$$

Mitral valve area

$$\text{Flow} = \frac{\text{Cardiac output}}{K \times \text{Diastolic filling time}}$$

$K = 31$

Pressure gradient = Left atrial pressure
                    − Left ventricular end-diastolic pressure

Normal mitral valve area = 4–6 cm^2

Critical mitral valve area:
  <2.5 cm^2 = symptoms
  <1.0 cm^2 = severe

- -

Aortic valve area

$$\text{Flow} = \frac{\text{Cardiac output}}{K \times \text{Systolic ejection period}}$$

$K = 44.5$

Pressure gradient = Left ventricular systolic
                    pressure − Aortic systolic pressure

Normal aortic valve area = 2.6–3.5 cm^2

Critical aortic valve area = 0.75 cm^2

BOX 12-9 PATHOPHYSIOLOGY OF VALVULAR DISEASE

Aortic stenosis

Etiology: Rheumatic fever, congenital

Pathophysiology: Smaller aortic valve orifice → left ventricular hypertrophy and ultimately ischemia → fixed stroke volume and ultimately left ventricular failure with reduced left ventricular output and pulmonary transudation

Mitral stenosis

Etiology: Rheumatic fever

Pathophysiology: Smaller mitral valve orifice → decreases left ventricular filling and output → increases left atrial and pulmonary capillary wedge pressure → pulmonary hypertension and ultimately right ventricular failure

Aortic insufficiency

Etiology: Rheumatic fever, trauma

Pathophysiology: Incompetent aortic valve → regurgitation of blood to left ventricle → left ventricular stress and dilation → ultimately decreased left ventricular contractile force → left ventricular output → pulmonary hypertension → ultimately right ventricular failure

Mitral insufficiency

Etiology: Rheumatic fever, trauma

Pathophysiology: Incompetent mitral valve → systolic regurgitation of blood to left atrium → dilation of left ventricular function → left ventricular failure with reduced left ventricular output → pulmonary hypertension and ultimately right ventricular failure

by an anesthesiologist at the bedside until the block and sympathectomy has completely resolved.

The basic considerations of cardiovascular management for the common valve lesions are reviewed in Table 12-18.

STENOTIC LESIONS
Aortic stenosis

Ideally, severe aortic stenosis should be treated with a valve replacement *before* the pregnancy or during pregnancy in the second trimester. Aortic stenosis in a pregnant patient may be congenital or secondary to rheumatic fever. (While the incidence of rheumatic fever–induced lesions declined in the 1970s and 1980s in the U.S. population as a result of extensive use of antibiotics, it is still seen in third world countries. There has been a resurgence in the United States, associated with immigration.

The incidence of symptomatic aortic stenosis in the pregnant patient is rare because it usually takes 30 to 40 years for the effects of rheumatic fever to result in critical stenosis and significant left ventricular hypertrophy (LVH). Patients may present with angina, dyspnea, on exertion or syncope. These symptoms may correlate with decreased survival. Sudden death may occur if an arrhythmia or hypotension develops.

The normal valve area in an adult is approximately 2.6 to 3.5 cm^2. The critical aortic valve area is 0.75 cm^2 or a 75% reduction in area, and increased left ventricular systolic pressure becomes significant. Hemodynamically significant aortic stenosis correlates with a pressure gradient across the aortic valve of 50 mm Hg or greater. As increased pressure is needed to eject the stroke volume through a stenotic valve, concentric hypertrophy of the left ventricle develops. This results in a precarious myocardial oxygen supply/demand balance. Decreased left ventricular compliance develops and the stroke volume becomes relatively fixed. The limiting factor to forward flow (cardiac output) becomes the valve area. Reduction in afterload (SVR) does not result in significant increases in forward flow but may seriously reduce coronary filling during diastole. The atrial kick becomes an increasingly important factor in left ventricular filling.

Pregnant patients who have reached 32 to 34 weeks' gestation with no cardiac symptoms and no ECG evidence of ischemia will probably tolerate labor and delivery. Aortocaval compression can be lethal. Two large IV access lines are recommended. Supplementary oxygen is a prudent measure during labor. Monitoring should include an A-line, backup blood pressure cuff, finger pulse oximeter,

FHM, and CVP. A PA-line is usually avoided because of the risk of precipitating an arrhythmia (assuming the aortic stenosis is an isolated valve lesion).

Every effort should be made to keep the patient warm, maintain an adequate preload, keep the heart rate normal, and maintain sinus rhythm. A Neo-Synephrine drip should be immediately available and titrated to maintain the patient's baseline blood pressure. A constantly monitored arterial line is mandatory. Subacute bacterial endocarditis (SBE) prophylaxis is appropriate.

A continuous epidural analgesia, very carefully, slowly titrated to T10 is effective for labor. Epidural fentanyl is quite helpful to maximize the block while minimizing local anesthetic requirements. The blood pressure should be maintained with IV Neo-Synephrine and IV volume (one can consider 5% plasminate and 25% salt-poor albumin). If there is any question of fetal problems, the level should be *slowly* raised to T6 (to facilitate surgical delivery if required). Bradycardia must be treated with glycopyrolate (small doses of atropine or ephedrine may be used, but extreme care should be observed to avoid tachycardia or arrhythmias). If the patient is anxious, sedation with diazepam and diphenhydramine is prudent to reduce the likelihood of tachyarrhythmias. Epinephrine in local anesthetic solution should be used cautiously. If an operative delivery is required, a crash induction is *contraindicated*. If practical, the indwelling continuous epidural should be slowly, carefully raised. It is essential to ensure a "solid block." Pain may induce arrhythmias. If a general anesthetic is required, after an additional dose of sodium citrate and metoclopramide a slow high-dose narcotic induction should be conducted, keeping in mind the risk of gastric aspiration. Meperidine and pancuronium should probably be avoided to minimize the risk of tachycardia. Volatile anesthetic agents may reduce contractility, induce hypotension, or cause an arrhythmia or tachycardia and should be used with caution.

Postoperative monitoring in the ICU setting is essential until the patient stabilizes (at least 24 hours). Postoperative pain management with epidural *narcotic drugs* (no local anesthesia) is ideal.

Mitral stenosis

Mitral stenosis is the most common cardiac valvular lesion seen in pregnancy. It is most often caused by fusion of the mitral valve leaflets secondary to rheumatic fever. The normal mitral valve area in an adult is 4 to 6 cm^2. A valve area of less than 2.5 cm^2 usually correlates with symptoms, and a valve area less than 1.0 cm^2 is severe. Dilated left atria develops (often evidenced by a "mitral P

Table 12-18 Clinical management of valvular disease

	Aortic stenosis	Mitral stenosis	Aortic insufficiency	Mitral regurgitation
History	Syncope Angina Dyspnea on exertion Sx decreased survival compared with other lesions Sudden death Increased incidence CAD	Prolonged Hx with CHF and low output syndrome Cardiac cachexia	Long asymptomatic period Multiple etiologies Sx may be worse at rest than with exercise Acute vs chronic	Long asymptomatic Multiple causes Acute vs chronic Ischemic?
Pathophysiology	Concentric hypertrophy Decreased LV compliance Pressure work	LV diastolic defect Increased LAP Increased PAP Pulmonary HTN, TR, RV failure Associated LV dysfunction	Eccentric hypertrophy Cor bovinum LV volume overload Increased LV compliance	Eccentric hypertrophy LV volume overload Increased LV compliance if ischemic LV dysfunction exists
Maternal Oxygen Balance	Precarious Rx decrease BP aggressively with α-agonist	Generally okay LV "protected" unless associated LV dysfunction exists	Low O_2 costs (compared with AS)	CAD? Rapid decreased wall tension = O_2 cost (even lower than AI)
Rate	Keep normal (70-80)	Slow Is digitalization adequate? Need adequate filling time Avoid tachycardia	Slight increase keeps heart small (diminishes O_2 requirements) (80-100)	Normal to slightly increased (80-100)
Rhythm	Sinus Atrial kick provides 40% filling in severe AS	Usually AF Consider monitoring MAP Consider digitalization	Not usually a problem	Often AF Consider digitalization

238

(CVP) (Wedge) Preload	Keep full LVEDP is much greater than LAP or PAW Avoid venodilation Increase or maintain	Maintain Usually on diuretics PAW follows LVEDP except with severe tachycardia CVP reveals RV function	Keep full (patients usually are) Maintain	Reduce slightly Will improve cardiac output
(SVR) Afterload	Maintain Avoid decrease of SVR at all costs Maintain BP with IV volume, phenylephrine	Decreased RV afterload beneficial Consider dobutamine rather than dopamine	Vasodilator Rx may help to decrease regurgitant fraction	Reduce (will improve cardiac output)
Contractility	Maintain Usually LVH Avoid depression (avoid volatile anesthetics)	Maintain Usually okay unless RV failure exists	Maintain Usually good Inotrope may decrease heart size	Maintain
Anesthetic Approach	Regional anesthesia (carefully titrated continuous technique can be used with constant attention to BP and SVR) Phenylephrine drip and good IV access necessary A-line monitoring required If general anesthesia is used, high-dose narcotic is required	Regional or general anesthesia with A-line and PA monitoring	Regional anesthesia is technique of choice Continuous epidural Continuous spinal	Regional anesthesia is technique of choice Continuous epidural Continuous spinal

AF = atrial fibrillation; AI = aortic insufficiency; AS = aortic stenosis; CAD = coronary artery disease; CHF = congestive heart failure; CVP = central venous pressure; HTN = hypertension; Hx = history; IV = intravenous; LAP = left atrial pressure; LV = left ventricle; LVEDP = left ventricular end-diastolic pressure; LVH = left ventricular hypertrophy; MAP = mean arterial pressure; PA = pulmonary artery; PAP = pulmonary artery pressure; PAW = pulmonary artery wedge pressure; RV = right ventricle; Rx = therapy; Sx = symptoms; TR = tricuspid regurgitation.

wave" on the ECG), and the pulmonary system becomes congested. In cases in which the stenosis has been gradual, the pulmonary lymphatic system hypertrophies and helps to minimize pulmonary edema. In severe cases, pulmonary hypertension and right heart failure can develop. These patients develop a low-output state and congestive heart failure. As the left atria dilates, the patient may develop atrial thrombi and is at risk for systemic emboli. Therefore, many of these patients are anticoagulated. This is necessary if the patient has developed atrial fibrillation. Digitalization is appropriate if the cardiac output is inadequate or if atrial fibrillation develops.

The left ventricular oxygen supply/demand balance is usually "protected," but the right heart is at risk of failure. The heart rate should be kept slow (adequate digitalization and good analgesia and sedation) to maximize LV filling time. Care should be observed to maintain normothermic and minimize shivering. Many of these patients have been treated chronically with diuretics. While care should be used to avoid volume overload, adequate filling pressures must be maintained. Except with severe mitral stenosis and rapid tachycardia, the wedge pressure is useful to demonstrate trends. The CVP is a rough gauge of the RV function.

Monitoring should consist of an arterial line, a finger pulse oximeter, an ECG, a fetal heart rate monitor (FHR), and a PA line. One should note that the pulmonary artery system will be disturbed and that obtaining a wedge pressure may be challenging. The cardiac output is still reliable. If an inotropic agent is needed, dobutamine is a good choice. Nitroglycerin is useful to manage pulmonary hypertension and right-sided volume overload. Nitric oxide may be a useful agent (5 to 20 parts per million), but data on its use in this setting is still lacking. SBE prophylaxis is appropriate.

If the patient is not anticoagulated, a slowly titrated continuous epidural analgesia is appropriate for labor. Epidural fentanyl is useful to improve analgesia, reduce the likelihood of shivering, and reduce local anesthetic requirements. If operative delivery is required, an epidural block should be used via slow titration, if it is not contraindicated by coagulation status. Drop in blood pressure should be treated with 25% albumin (small volume, significant osmotic effect), ephedrine, or Neo-Synephrine.

Ideally, this lesion should be treated before the patient becomes pregnant or during the pregnancy in the second trimester with valve replacement. Percutaneous catheter balloon valvuloplasty (venous transseptal approach) may be considered in some patients.

Hypoxia and acidosis will increase pulmonary vasoconstriction and thus supplemental oxygen is prudent throughout labor and in the postoperative period.

Maternal "pushing" in labor should be minimized or avoided.

REGURGITANT VALVE LESIONS
Aortic insufficiency

Aortic insufficiency may be acute or chronic. Acute aortic insufficiency is usually associated with trauma or a dissecting aortic aneurysm (Marfan's syndrome) and it must be treated with cardiac bypass and valvular surgery. Patients with a chronic aortic insufficiency usually develop cardiac complication after the childbearing age.

Long-standing aortic insufficiency increases the work of the heart because of the regurgitant fraction. It gradually results in eccentric hypertrophy and increased left ventricle compliance as a result of left ventricular overload. Compensatory mechanisms to maintain cardiac output include increased heart rate and contractility.

Monitoring should include an arterial line, a finger pulse oximeter, an FHR monitor, and a PA catheter. The thermodilution calculation of the cardiac output (done in the right heart) will reflect the net cardiac output for the heart as it is arrested in series with the left heart. SBE prophylaxis is appropriate. The volume status (preload) should be maintained. Slight increases in heart rate reduce left ventricular distention and oxygen requirements. After load reduction, sodium nitroprusside, hydralazine, or regional analgesia or anesthesia may help to reduce the regurgitant fraction and improve cardiac output.

Continuous regional analgesia is the anesthetic technique of choice for labor and delivery, whereas regional anesthesia can be used for cesarean section. Hypotension should be treated with volume replacement and ephedrine. The SVR should be slightly reduced. General anesthesia can be induced with high-dose narcotic drugs or, in less severe cases, with rapid sequence induction with etomidate.

Mitral insufficiency

Acute mitral insufficiency (MI) is often secondary to papillary muscle dysfunction associated with acute MI (see MI in pregnancy). It can also be secondary to ruptured chordea tendinea associated with infarctive endocarditis. Chronic MI is rarely an isolated lesion but usually is associated with mitral stenosis.

Mitral insufficiency results in volume overload of the left ventricle (but low pressure as a result of the venting effect of the incompetent valve into the more pliable left atria). Left atrial enlargement and eventual overload and congestion of the pulmonary circuit can occur. A regurgitant fraction of greater than 0.6 is considered severe. SBE prophylaxis is appropriate. Monitoring should include an A-line, a finger pulse oximeter, an ECG, an FHM, and a PA-line. V-waves may be seen on the PA trace with mitral stenosis. Reducing SVR will improve forward flow. A slightly increased heart rate is advantageous. Digitalization should be considered if atrial fibrillation results. (One should note the concomitant risk of thromboemboli and anticoagulation issues.) Continuous regional anesthesia, carefully titrated, is advantageous. General anesthesia may be considered in an aortic insufficiency.

Tricuspid regurgitation

Seen with tricuspid stenosis secondary to rheumatic fever, tricuspid regurgitation is most commonly a functional anomaly due to dilation of the right ventricle, secondary to pulmonary hypertension. Because of the capacitance of the vena cava and the compliance of the right atria, the CVP elevation is usually slight.

Management involves treatment of the underlying pulmonary hypertension. SBE prophylaxis is appropriate. One should note that in patients with patent foramen ovale right-to-left shunting is possible, especially in the setting of right heart failure and left ventricular afterload reduction.

REFERENCES

1. *Med Lett* 26(562), January 6, 1984.
2. McFaul PB, Dornan JC, Lamki H, et al: Pregnancy complicated by maternal heart disease: A review of 519 women. *Br J Obstet Gynaecol* 1988; 95:861.
3. Sullivan JM, Ramanathan KB: Management of medical problems in pregnancy: Severe cardiac disease. *N Engl J Med* 1985; 313:304.
4. Clark SL, Phelan JP, Cotton DB (eds): *Critical Care Obstetrics.* Oradell, NJ, Medical Economics Books, 1987, p 63.
5. Cheek TG, Gutsche BB: Maternal physiologic alterations during pregnancy, in Shnider SM, Levinson GL (eds): *Anesthesia for Obstetrics.* Baltimore, Williams & Wilkins, 1987, p 6.
6. Huch R, Huch A, Lubbers DW: *Transcutaneous Po_2.* New York, Thieme-Stratton, 1981, p 139.
7. Capeless EL, Clapp JF: Cardiovascular changes in early phase of pregnancy. *Am J Obstet Gynecol* 1989; 161:1449.
8. Clark SL, Cotton DB, Lee W, et al: Central hemodynamic assessment of normal term pregnancy. *Am J Obstet Gynecol* 1989; 161:1439.
9. Clark SL, Cotton DB, Lee W: Central hemodynamic assessment of normal pregnancy (abst). *Am J Obstet Gynecol* 1989; 161:1439.
9a. Forrester JS, Diamond G, McHugh TJ, et al: Filling pressure in the right and left sides of the heart in acute myocardial infarction: A reappraisal of central-venous-pressure monitoring. *N Engl J Med* 1971; 285:190.
9b. Kaplan JA, Wells PH: Early diagnosis of myocardial ischemia using the pulmonary arterial catheter. *Anesth Analg* 1981; 60:789.
10. Meller J, Goldman ME: Arrhythmias in pregnancy, in Elkayam U, Gleicher N (eds): *Principles of Medical Therapy in Pregnancy.* New York, Alan R Liss, 1982, p 114.
11. Upshaw CB: A study of maternal electrocardiograms recorded during labor and delivery. *Am J Obstet Gynecol* 1970; 107:17.
12. Briggs GG, Freeman RK, Yaffe SJ: *Drugs in Pregnancy and Lactation.* Baltimore, Williams & Wilkins, 1983, p xxi.
13. Ueland K, McAnulty JH, Ueland FR, et al: Special considerations in the use of cardiovascular drugs during pregnancy. *Clin Obstet Gynecol* 1981; 24:809.
14. Schroeder JS, Harrison DC: Repeated cardioversion during pregnancy: Treatment of refractory paroxysmal atrial tachycardia during three successive pregnancies. *Am J Cardiol* 1971; 27:445.
15. Robards GJ, Saunders PM: Refractory supraventricular tachycardia complicating pregnancy. *Med J Aust* 1973; 2:278.
16. Vogel JHK, Pryor R, Blount SG: Direct current defibrillation during pregnancy. *JAMA* 1965; 193:970.
17. Grand A, Bernard J: Cardioversion et grosesse: Consequences foetalies. *Nouv Presse Med* 1973; 2:2327.
18. Sussman HI, Duque D, Lesser ME: Atrial flutter with 1 : 1 conduction: Report of a case in a pregnant woman successfully treated with DC countershock. *Dis Chest* 1966; 49:99.
19. Meitus ML: Fetal electrocardiography and cardioversion with direct current countershock. *Dis Chest* 1965; 48:324.
20. Curry JJ, Quintana FJ: Myocardial infarction with ventricular fibrillation during pregnancy treated by direct current defibrillation with fetal survival. *Chest* 1970; 58:82.
21. Rotmensch HH, Elkayam U, Frishman W: Antiarrhythmic therapy during pregnancy. *Am J Cardiol* 1971; 27:445.
22. Condmi JJ, Blumgren SE, Vaughn JH: The procainamide induces lupus syndrome. *Bull Rheum Dis* 1970; 20:604.
23. Leonard RF, Braun TE, Levy AM: Initiation of uterine contractions by disopyramide during pregnancy. *N Engl J Med* 1978; 299:84.
24. Rubin PC: Beta blockers in pregnancy. *N Engl J Med* 1978; 305:1323.
25. Dicke JM: Cardiovascular drugs in pregnancy, in Elkayam U, Gleicher N (eds): *Principles of Medical Therapy in Pregnancy.* New York, Alan R Liss, 1982, p 646.
26. Conn RD: Diphenylhydantoin sodium in cardiac arrhythmias. *N Engl J Med* 1965; 272:277.
27. Atkinson AJ, Davison R: Diphenylhydantoin as an antiarrhythmic drug. *Ann Rev Med* 1974; 25:99.
28. Scanlon JW, Brown WV, Weiss JB, et al: Neurobehavioral responses of newborn infants after maternal epidural anesthesia. *Anesthesiology* 1974; 40:121.
29. Kileff ME, James FM, Dewan DM, et al: Neonatal neurobehavioral responses after epidural anesthesia for cesarean section using lidocaine and bupivacaine. *Anesth Analg* 1984; 63:413.
30. Abboud TK, Khoo SS, Miller F, et al: Maternal and neonatal responses after epidural anesthesia with bupivacaine, 2-chloroprocaine, or lidocaine. *Anesth Analg* 1982; 61:638.
31. Brizgys RV, Dailey PA, Shnider SM, et al: The incidence and neonatal effects of maternal hypotension during epidural anesthesia for cesarean section. *Anesthesiology* 1987; 67:782.
32. Hollmen AL, Jouppila R, Jouppila P: Regional anesthesia and uterine blood flow. *Ann Chir Gynaecol* 1984; 73:149.
33. Hollmen AL, Jouppila R, Albright GA, et al: Intervillous

blood flow during cesarean section with prophylactic ephedrine and epidural anaesthesia. *Acta Anaesthesiol Scand* 1984; 28:396.

34. Shnider SM, DeLorimier AA, Holl JW, et al: Vasopressors in obstetrics: Correlation of fetal acidosis with ephedrine during spinal hypotension. *Am J Obstet Gynecol* 1968; 102:911.

35. Wright RG, Shnider SM, Levinson G, et al: The effect of maternal administration of ephedrine on fetal heart rate and variability. *Obstet Gynecol* 1981; 57:734.

36. Levinson G, Shnider SM: Vasopressors in obstetrics. *Clin Anesth* 1974; 10:77.

37. Butterworth JF, Piccione W, Bernizbeitia LD, et al: Augmentation of venous return by adrenergic agonists during spinal anesthesia. *Anesth Analg* 1986; 65:612.

38. Butterworth JF, Austin JC, Johnson MD, et al: Effect of total spinal anesthesia on arterial and venous responses to dopamine and dobutamine. *Anesth Analg* 1987; 66:209.

39. Ralston DH, Shnider SM, deLorimier AA: Effects of equipotent ephedrine, metaraminol, mephentermine and methoxamine on uterine blood flow in the pregnant ewe. *Anesthesiology* 1974; 40:345.

40. Ramanathan S, Grant GJ: Vasopressor therapy for hypotension due to epidural anesthesia for cesarean section. *Acta Anaesthesiol Scand* 1988; 32:559.

41. Moran DH, Perillo M, Bader AM, et al: Phenylephrine in treating maternal hypotension secondary to spinal anesthesia. *Anesthesiology* 1989; 71:A857.

41a. Jelsema RD, Bhaha RK, Gangsly S: Use of intravenous amrinone, in the short-term management of refractory heart failure in pregnancy. *Obstet Gynecol* 1991; 78:935.

41b. Fishburne JL Jr, Dormer KJ, Payne GG et al: Effects of amrinone and dopamine on uterine blood flow and vascular responses in the gravid baboon, *Am J Obstet Gynecol* 1988; 158:829.

41c. Sharpe MD, Dolkowski WB, Murkin JM: The electrophysiologic effects of volatile anesthetics and sufentanil on the nodal atrioventricular conduction system and accessory pathway in WPW syndrome, *Anesthesiology* 1994; 80:63.

42. Topkins MJ, Artusio JF: Myocardial infarction and surgery. *Anesth Analg* 1964; 23:716.

43. Steen PA, Tinker JH, Tarhan S: Myocardial reinfarction after anesthesia and surgery. *JAMA* 1978; 16:2566.

44. Rao TLK, El-Etr A: Anticoagulation following placement of epidural and subarachnoid catheters. *Anesthesiology* 1981; 55:618.

44a. Widerhorn J, Widerhorn AL, Rahimtoola SH, et al: WPW syndrome during pregnancy: Increased incidence of supraventricular arrhythmias. *Am Heart J* 1992; 123:796.

45. Ueland K: Cardiac surgery and pregnancy. *Am J Obstet Gynecol* 1965; 92:148.

46. Hawthorne J, Buckley M, Grover J, et al: Valve replacement during pregnancy. *Ann Intern Med* 1967; 67:1032.

47. Zitnik R, Brandenburg R, Sheldon R, et al: Pregnancy and open heart surgery. *Circulation* 1969; 39:257.

48. Becker RM: Intracardiac surgery in pregnant women. *Ann Thorac Surg* 1983; 36:453.

49. Meffert WG, Stansel HC: Open heart surgery during pregnancy. *Am J Obstet Gynecol* 1968; 102:1116.

50. Levy DL, Warriner RA, Burgess GE: Fetal response to cardiopulmonary bypass. *Obstet Gynecol* 1980; 56:112.

51. Katz J, Hook R, Barash P: Fetal heart rate monitoring in pregnant patients undergoing surgery. *Am J Obstet Gynecol* 1976; 125:267.

52. Tenebaum J: Pregnancy can be safe after cardiac surgery. *Contemp Obstet Gynecol* April 1985; 137.

53. Eilen B, Kaiser IH, Becker RM, et al: Aortic valve replacement in the third trimester of pregnancy: Case report and review of the literature. *Obstet Gynecol* 1981; 57:119.

54. Ginsberg JS, Hirsh J: Use of anticoagulants during pregnancy. *Chest* 1989; 95:156S.

55. Iturbe-Allessio I, Fonseca MDC, Mutchinik O, et al: Risks of anticoagulant therapy in pregnant women with artificial heart valves. *N Engl J Med* 1986; 315:1390.

56. Zimran A, Shilo S, Fisher D, et al: Histomorphometric evaluation of reversible heparin-induced osteoporosis in pregnancy. *Arch Intern Med* 1986; 164:386.

57. Yeager MP: Regional anesthesia for the patient with heart disease. Pro: Regional anesthesia is preferable to general anesthesia for the patient with heart disease. *J Cardiothorac Anesth* 1989; 3:793.

58. Easterling TR, Chadwick HS, Otto CM, et al: Aortic stenosis in pregnancy. *Obstet Gynecol* 1988; 72:113.

59. Boccio RV, Chung IH, Harrison DM: Anesthetic management of cesarean section in a patient with idiopathic hypertrophic subaortic stenosis. *Anesthesiology* 1986; 65:663.

60. Hemming GT, Whalley DG, O'Connor PJ, et al: Invasive monitoring and anesthetic management of a parturient with mitral stenosis. *Can J Anaesth* 1987; 34:182.

61. Spinnato JA, Kraynack BJ, Cooper MW: Eisenmenger's syndrome in pregnancy: Epidural anesthesia for elective cesarean section. *N Engl J Med* 1981; 804:1215.

62. Stokes IM, Evans J, Stone M: Myocardial infarction and cardiac arrest in the second trimester followed by assisted vaginal delivery under epidural analgesia at 38 weeks' gestation, case report. *Br J Obstet Gynaecol* 1984; 91:197.

63. Baron JF, Coriat P, Mundler O, et al: Left ventricular global and regional function during lumbar epidural anesthesia in patients with and without angina pectoris: Influence of volume loading. *Anesthesiology* 1987; 66:621.

64. Juneja MM, Ackerman WE, Kaczorowski DM, et al: Continuous epidural lidocaine infusion in the parturient with paroxysmal ventricular tachycardia. *Anesthesiology* 1989; 71:305.

65. Rees GAD, Willis BA: Resuscitation in late pregnancy. *Anaesthesia* 1988; 43:347.

66. Songster GS, Clark SL: Cardiac arrest. *Contemp Obstet Gynecol* Nov 1985; 141.

67. National Conference on Cardiopulmonary Resuscitation and Emergency Cardiac Care: Standards and guidelines for cardiopulmonary resuscitation (CPR) and emergency cardiac care (ECC). *JAMA* 1980; 244:453.

68. McIntyre KM, Lewis AJ: *Textbook of Advanced Cardiac Life Support.* Dallas, American Heart Association, 1983.

69. DePace NL, Betesh JS, Kotler MH: Postmortem cesarean section with recovery of both mother and offspring. *JAMA* 1982; 248:971.

70. Selden BS, Burke TJ: Complete maternal and fetal recovery after prolonged cardiac arrest. *Ann Emerg Med* 1988; 17:346.

71. Moller R, Covino BG: Cardiac electrophysiologic effects of lidocaine and bupivacaine. *Anesth Analg* 1988; 67:107.

72. Long WB, Rosenblum S, Grady IP: Successful resuscitation of bupivacaine-induced cardiac arrest using cardiopulmonary bypass. *Anesth Analg* 1989; 69:403.

73. McGarry J, Pearson JF: Time of onset and duration of labour in women with cardiac disease. *Lancet* 1973; 1:483.

74. Demakis JG, Rahimtoola SH: Peripartum cardiomyopathy. *Circulation* 1971; 44:964.

75. Demakis JG, Rahimtoola SH, Sutton GC, et al: Natural course of peripartum cardiomyopathy. *Circulation* 1971; 44:1053.

76. Homans DC: Current concepts: Peripartum cardiomyopathy. *N Engl J Med* 1985; 312:1432.

77. Veille JC: Peripartum cardiomyopathies: A review. *Am J Obstet Gynecol* 1984; 148:805.

78. Julian DG, Szekely P: Peripartum cardiomyopathy. *Prog Cardiovasc Dis* 1985; 27:223.

79. Hodgman MT, Pessin MS, Homans DC, et al: Cerebral embolism as the manifestation of peripartum cardiomyopathy. *Neurology* 1982; 32:668.

80. Walsh JJ, Burch GE, Black WC, et al: Idiopathic myocardiopathy of the puerperium (post partal heart disease). *Circulation* 1965; 32:19.

81. Silverman RI, Ribner IIS: Peripartal cardiomyopathy, cardiac problems in pregnancy, in Elkayam U, Gleicher N (eds): *Diagnosis and Management of Maternal and Fetal Disease.* New York, Alan R Liss, 1982, p 95.

82. Sakakibura S, Sekiguchi M, Konno S, et al: Idiopathic post partum cardiomyopathy: Report of a case with special reference to its ultrastructural changes in the myocardium as studied by endomyocardial biopsy. *Am Heart J* 1970; 80:395.

83. Glick G, Braunwald E: The cardiomyopathies and myocarditides, in Isenbacher KJ, Adams RD, Braunwald E, et al (eds): *Harrison's Principles of Internal Medicine.* New York, McGraw-Hill, 1980, p 1141.

84. Camann W, Goldman G, Johnson M, et al: Cesarean delivery of a patient with a transplanted heart. *Anesthesiology* 1989; 71:618.

85. Sirignoano R: Peripartum cardiomyopathy. *J Cardiovasc Nurs* 1987; 2:24.

86. Malinow AM, Butterworth JF, Johnson MD, et al: Peripartum cardiomyopathy presenting at cesarean delivery. *Anesthesiology* 1985; 63:545.

87. Turner GM, Oakley CM, Dixon HG: Management of pregnancy complicated by hypertrophic obstructive cardiomyopathy. *Br Med J* 1968; 4:281.

88. Kolibash AJ, Ruiz DE, Lewis RP: Idiopathic hypertrophic subaortic stenosis in pregnancy. *Ann Intern Med* 1975; 82:791.

89. Boccio RV, Chung IH, Harrison DM: Anesthetic management of cesarean section in a patient with idiopathic hypertrophic subaortic stenosis. *Anesthesiology* 1986; 65:663.

90. Loubser P, Suh K, Cohen S: Adverse effects of spinal anesthesia in a patient with idiopathic hypertrophic subaortic stenosis. *Anesthesiology* 1984; 60:228.

91. Baraka A, Jabbour S, Itani I: Severe bradycardia following epidural anesthesia in a patient with idiopathic hypertrophic subaortic stenosis. *Anesth Analg* 1987; 66:1337.

92. Savage DD, Garrison RJ, Devereux RD, et al: Mitral valve prolapse in the general population. I. Epidemiologic features: The Framingham Study. *Am Heart J* 1983; 106:571.

93. Degani S, Abinader EG, Scharf M: Mitral valve prolapse and pregnancy: A review. *Obstet Gynecol Surv* 1989; 44:642.

94. Kligfield P, Levy D, Devereux RB, et al: Arrhythmias and sudden death in mitral valve prolapse. *Am Heart J* 1987; 113:1316.

95. Devereux RB: Inheritance of mitral valve prolapse: Effect of age and sex on gene expression. *Ann Intern Med* 1982; 97:826.

96. Cowles T, Gonik B: Mitral valve prolapse in pregnancy. *Semin Perinatol* 1990; 14:34.

97. Shulman ST, Amren DP, Bisno AL, et al: Prevention of bacterial endocarditis: A statement for health professionals by the committee on rheumatic fever and infective endocarditis of the council on cardiovascular disease in the young. *Circulation* 1984; 70:1123A.

98. Kaye D: Prophylaxis for infective endocarditis: An update. *Ann Intern Med* 1986; 104:419.

99. Rayburn WF, Fontana ME: Mitral valve prolapse and pregnancy. *Am J Obstet Gynecol* 1981; 141:9.

100. Tang LCH, Chan WYW, Wong VCW, et al: Pregnancy in patients with mitral valve prolapse. *Br J Gynaecol Obstet* 1985; 23:217.

101. Shapiro EP, Trimble EL, Robinson JC, et al: Safety of labor and delivery in women with mitral valve prolapse. *Am J Cardiol* 1985; 56:806.

102. Cheitlin MD, Byrd RC: The click-murmur syndrome: A clinical problem in diagnosis and treatment. *JAMA* 1981; 245:1357.

103. Jeresaty RM: Mitral valve prolapse-click syndrome. *Prog Cardiovasc Dis* 1973; 15:623.

104. Gooch AS, Vicencio F, Maranhao V, et al: Arrhythmias and left ventricular asynergy in the prolapsing mitral leaflet syndrome. *Am J Cardiol* 1972; 29:611.

105. Barlow JB, Pocock WA: The problem of non-ejection systolic clicks and associated mitral systolic murmurs: Emphasis on the billowing mitral leaflet syndrome. *Am Heart J* 1975; 90:636.

106. Buda AJ, Levene JL, Myers MG, et al: Coronary artery spasm and mitral valve prolapse. *Am Heart J* 1978; 95:457.

107. Thiagarajah S, Frost EAM: Anaesthetic considerations in patients with mitral valve prolapse. *Anaesthesia* 1983; 38:560.

108. Dalen JE, Alpert JS, Cohn LH, et al: Dissection of the thoracic aorta. *Am J Cardiol* 1974; 34:803.

109. Pyritz RE: Maternal and fetal complications of pregnancy in Marfan's syndrome. *Am J Med* 1981; 71:784.

110. Ferguson JE, Ueland K, Stinson EB, et al: Marfan's syndrome: Acute aortic dissection during labor, resulting in fetal distress and cesarean section, followed by successful surgical repair. *Am J Obstet Gynecol* 1983; 147:759.

111. Ehas B, Berkowitz RL: The Marfan syndrome and pregnancy. *Obstet Gynecol* 1976; 47:358.

112. Slomka F, Salmeron S, Zetlaoui P, et al: Primary pulmonary hypertension and pregnancy: Anesthetic management for delivery. *Anesthesiology* 1988; 69:959.

113. Weir EK: Diagnosis and management of primary pulmonary hypertension, in Wier EK, Reeves JT (eds): *Pulmonary Hypertension.* New York, Futura, 1984, p 142.

114. Simonneau G, Herve P, Baudouin C, et al: Short and long term effects of vasodilators in primary pulmonary hypertension: Predictive value of prostacyclin acute infusion. *J Crit Care* 1986; 1:117.

115. Sorenson BM, Korshin JD, Fernandes A, et al: The use of epidural analgesia for delivery in a patient with pulmonary hypertension. *Acta Anaesthesiol Scand* 1982; 26:180.

116. Robinson DE, Leicht CH: Epidural analgesia with low-dose bupivacaine and fentanyl for labor and delivery in a parturient with severe pulmonary hypertension. *Anesthesiology* 1988; 68:285.

117. Abboud TK, Nouhihed R, Daniel J: Intrathecal morphine for relief of labor pain in a parturient with severe pulmonary hypertension. *Anesthesiology* 1983; 59:477.

118. Nora JJ, Nora AH: *Genetics and Counseling in Cardiovascular Disease.* Springfield, Ill, Charles C Thomas, 1978, p 155.

119. German JL, Ehlers KA, Engle MA: Familial congenital heart disease. II. Chromosomal studies. *Circulation* 1966; 34:517.

120. Ehlers KA, Engle MA: Familial congenital heart disease: Genetic and environmental factors. *Circulation* 1966; 34:503.

121. Painvin GA, Reece IJ, Cooley DA, et al: Cardiopulmonary allotransplantation, a collective review: Experimental process and current clinical status. *Tex Heart Inst* 1983; 10:372.

122. Cabrol C, Gandjbackhch I, Pavie A, et al: Heart transplantation at Lapitie Hospital, Paris 1968-1984. *Heart Transplant* 1984; 4:27.

123. Shumway NE: Recent advances in cardiac transplantation. *Transplant Proc* 1983; 15:1223.

124. McGregor CGA, Jamieson SW, Oyer PE, et al: Heart transplantation at Stanford University. *J Heart Transplant* 1984; 4:31.

125. Lowenstein B, Vain N, Perrone S, et al: Successful pregnancy and vaginal delivery after heart transplantation. *Am J Obstet Gynecol* 1988; 158:589.

126. Key T, Resnik R, Dittrich C, et al: Successful pregnancy after cardiac transplant. 1989; 160:367.

127. Camann W, Goldman G, Johnson MD, et al: Cesarean delivery in a patient with transplanted heart. *Anesthesiology* 1989; 71:136.

128. Kossoy LR, Herbert CM, Wentz AC: Management of heart transplant recipients: Guidelines for the obstetrician-gynecologist. *Am J Obstet Gynecol* 1988; 159:490.

129. Lou RJ, Scott JR: Pregnancy following renal transplantation. *Clin Obstet Gynecol* 1985; 28:339.

130. Newton ER, Turskoy N, Kaplan M, et al: Pregnancy and liver transplantation. *Obstet Gynecol* 1988; 71:499.

131. Deeg HJ, Kennedy MS, Sanders JE, et al: Successful pregnancy after marrow transplantation for severe aplastic anemia and immunosuppression with cyclosporine. *JAMA* 1983; 250:647.

132. Katz H: About the sudden natural death in pregnancy: During delivery and the puerperium. Arch Gynaekol 1922; 115:283.

133. Hankins GDV, Wendall GD, Leveno KJ, et al: Myocardial infarction during pregnancy: A review. *Obstet Gynecol* 1985; 65:139.

134. Trouton TG, Sidhu H, Adgey AJ: Myocardial infarction in pregnancy. *Int J Cardiol* 1988; 18:35.

135. Lamb MA: Myocardial infarction during pregnancy: A team approach. *Heart Lung* 1987; 16:658.

136. Sperry KL: Myocardial infarction in pregnancy. *J Forensic Sci* 1987; 32:1464.

137. Laughlin MP, From RP, Choi W: Recent myocardial infarction in a parturient. *Anesthesiol Rev* 1986; 8:43.

138. Hands ME, Johnson MD, Saltzman DH, et al: The cardiac, obstetric and anesthetic management of pregnancy complicated by acute myocardial infarction. *J Clin Anesth*, in press.

139. Skinner SL, Lumbers ER, Semonds EM: Renin concentration in human fetal and maternal tissues. *Am J Obstet Gynecol* 1968; 101:529.

140. Sasse L, Wagner R, Murray FE: Transmural myocardial infarction during pregnancy. *Am J Cardiol* 1975; 35:448.

141. Ludmer PL, Selwyn AP, Shook TL, et al: Paradoxical vasoconstriction by acetylcholine in atherosclerotic coronary arteries. *N Engl J Med* 1986; 315:1046.

142. Coleman D, Ross TF, Naughton JL: Myocardial ischemia and infarction related to recreational cocaine use. *West J Med* 1982; 13:444.

143. Kossawsky WA, Lyori AF: Cocaine and acute myocardial infarction: A probable connection. *Chest* 1984; 85:729.

144. Schachne JS, Roberts BH, Thompson PD: Coronary-artery spasm and myocardial infarction associated with cocaine use. *N Engl J Med* 1984; 310:2665.

145. Howard RE, Hueter DC, Davis GJ: Acute myocardial infarction following cocaine abuse in a young woman with normal coronary arteries. *JAMA* 1985; 254:95.

146. Pasternack PF, Colvin SB, Bauman FG: Cocaine-induced angina pectoris and acute myocardial infarction in patients younger than 40 years. *Am J Cardiol* 1985; 55:847.

147. Cregler LL, Mark H: Relation of acute myocardial infarction to cocaine abuse. *Am J Cardiol* 1985; 56:794.

148. Cowan NC, DeBelder MA, Rothman MT: Coronary, angioplasty in pregnancy. *Br Heart J* 1988; 59:588.

149. Majdan JF, Walinsky P, Cowchock S, et al: Coronary artery bypass surgery during pregnancy. *Am J Cardiol* 1983; 52:1145.

150. Bernal JM, Miralles PJ: Cardiac surgery with cardiopulmonary bypass during pregnancy. *Obstet Gynaecol Surg* 1986; 41:1.

151. Veterans Administration Hospital: Anticoagulants in acute myocardial infarction: Results of a cooperative trial. *JAMA* 1973; 225:724.

152. Davis M, Ireland M: Effect of early anticoagulation on the frequency of left ventricular thrombi after anterior wall acute myocardial infarction. *Am J Cardiol* 1986; 57:1244.

153. Hall JG, Pauli RM, Wilson KM: Maternal and fetal sequelae of anticoagulation during pregnancy. *Am J Med* 1980; 68:122.

154. The I.S.A.M Study Group: A prospective trial of intraveous streptokinase in acute myocardial infarction (I.S.A.M.). *N Engl J Med* 1986; 314:1465.

155. Anderson JL, Marshall HW, Bray BE, et al: A randomised trial of intracoronary streptokinase in the treatment of acute myocardial infarction. *N Engl J Med* 1983; 308:1312.

156. Kennedy JW, Ritchie JL, Davis KB, et al: Western Washington randomized trial of intracoronary streptokinase in acute myocardial infarction. *N Engl J Med* 1983; 309:1477.

157. Pfeifer GW: The use of thrombolytic therapy in obstetrics and gynaecology. *Aust Ann Med (Suppl)* 1970; 19:1928.

158. Corby DG: Aspirin in pregnancy: Maternal and fetal effects. *Pediatrics* 1978; 62:930.

159. Stuart MJ, Gross SJ, Elrad H, et al: Effects of acetylsalicylic-acid ingestion on maternal and neonatal hemostasis. *N Engl J Med* 1982; 307:909.

160. Rao TK, Jacobs KH, El-Etr AA: Reinfarction following anesthesia in patients with myocardial infarction. *Anesthesiology* 1983; 59:499.

161. Topkins JH, Artusio JF: Myocardial infarction and surgery, a five year study. *Anesth Analg* 1964; 23:716.

162. Tarhan S, Moffitt EA, Taylor WF, et al: Myocardial infarction after general anesthesia. *JAMA* 1972; 220:1451.

163. Reich DL, Brooks JL, Kaplan JA: Uncommon cardiac diseases, in Katz J, Benumof JL, Dadis LB (eds): *Anesthesia and Uncommon Diseases*. Philadelphia, WB Saunders Co, 1990, p 347.

164. Rowe G, Castillo C, Crampton C: Effects of hyperventilation on systemic coronary hemodynamics. *Am Heart J* 1962; 63:67.

165. Rowe G: Responses of the coronary circulation to physiologic changes and pharmacologic agents. *Anesthesiology* 1974; 41:182.

166. Hankins GDV, Wendall GD, Leveno KJ, et al: Myocardial infarction during pregnancy: A review. *Obstet Gynecol* 1985; 65:135.

167. Curletta JD, DeLeon OA: Epidural anesthesia in patients with coronary artery disease (letter). *Anesthesiology* 1990; 72:214.

168. Peters J, Kutkuhn B, Medert HA, et al: Sympathetic blockade by epidural anesthesia attenuates the cardiovascular response to severe hypoxemia. *Anesthesiology* 1990; 72:134.

169. Eisenmenger VZ: *Clin Med* 1897; 32:1.

170. Wood P: The Eisenmenger syndrome or pulmonary hypertension with reversed control shunt. *Br Med J* 1958; 2:701.

171. Young D, Mark W: Fate of the patient with Eisenmenger's syndrome. *Am J Cardiol* 1971; 28:658.

172. Young D, Mark W: Fate of the patient with Eisenmenger syndrome. *Am J Med* 1971; 28:679.

173. Jones AM: Eisenmenger syndrome in pregnancy. *Br Med J* 1965; 1:1627.

174. Gleicher R, Midwall J, Hochberger D, et al: Eisenmenger's syndrome and pregnancy. *Obstet Gynecol Surv* 1979; 34:721.

175. Garber SZ, Choi HJ, Tremper KK, et al: Use of a pulse oximeter in the anesthetic management of a pregnant patient with Eisenmenger's syndrome. *Anesthesiol Rev* 1988; 15:59.

176. Devitt JW, Noble WH, Byrick RJ: A Swan-Ganz catheter related complication in a patient with Eisenmenger's syndrome. *Anesthesiology* 1982; 57:335.

177. Robinson S: Pulmonary artery catheters in Eisenmenger's syndrome: Many risks, few benefits. *Anesthesiology* 1983; 58:588.

178. Midwall J, Jaffin H, Herman MV, et al: Shunt flow and pulmonary hemodynamics during labor and delivery in the Eisenmenger syndrome. *Am J Cardiol* 1978; 42:299.

179. Abboud TK, Raya J: Intrathecal morphine for relief of labor pain in a parturient with severe pulmonary hypertension. *Anesthesiology* 1983; 59:477.

180. Wallace AG: Pathophysiology of cardiovascular disease, in Smith LH Jr, Thier SO (eds): *Pathophysiology: The Biological Principles of Disease. The International Textbook of Medicine.* Philadelphia, WB Saunders, 1981, p 1192, vol 1.

13 Renal Disease

Michael N. Skaredoff and *Richard E. Besinger*

Diseases of the kidney during pregnancy put both the mother and fetus at risk. Normal physiologic alterations observed during pregnancy can exacerbate preexisting renal disease and may also contribute to many disease states unique to pregnancy. A sound knowledge of the physiologic changes that occur during pregnancy is necessary for the proper management of renal disease in parturients. This knowledge also allows the physician to avoid the various pitfalls involved in the detection and diagnosis of renal disease during the pregnant state. These clinical maxims must be tempered by the fact that our scientific and clinical understanding of renal physiology and pathophysiology during pregnancy is still developing.

The first section of this chapter will provide a basic understanding of physiologic alterations observed in the kidney during pregnancy. The remainder of the chapter will be devoted to the diagnosis and clinical management of chronic and acute pathophysiologic processes in the pregnant patient. The diagnostic tests and appropriate interventions necessary for the proper obstetric and anesthetic management of these special patients will be outlined. As usual with medical disorders during pregnancy, the ultimate treatment goal is to stabilize the compromised maternal physiologic state in order to provide an adequate environment for the developing fetus and optimize the maternal-fetal conditions for a safe delivery.

NORMAL PHYSIOLOGIC ALTERATIONS DURING PREGNANCY

The issue of changes of renal function and their contribution to disease in pregnancy is beyond the scope of this chapter but they have been presented in detail in the proceedings of the First International Symposium on Renal Function and Disease in Pregnancy held in Chicago in September 1986.[1] Table 13-1 summarizes these changes.

Anatomic alterations

The length of the human kidney, as estimated in intravenous pyelograms (IVPs) during pregnancy, increases by approximately 1 cm.[2] It appears that 70% of this increase in size has occurred by the third trimester.[3] It is thought that this increase in kidney weight and length is attributable to incremental increases in renal interstitial[3] and vascular volumes.[4]

The most striking anatomic alteration during pregnancy is dilation of the urinary collecting system. These physiologic changes can be observed as early as the first trimester[5]; by the third trimester 97% of pregnant women showed evidence of urostasis or hydronephrosis.[6] While most of the observed dilation of the urinary collecting system resolves within 48 hours after delivery, some dilation may persist for up to 4 months after delivery.[5] The observed dilation is usually worse on the right side, presumably due to the dextrorotation of the gravid uterus. The exact etiology of "physiologic hydroureter" of pregnancy is uncertain but has been ascribed to both humoral and mechanical factors.[7] It has been postulated that elevated levels of progesterone, gonadotropins, and prostaglandin E_1 (PGE_1) produce a decrease in smooth muscle tone and contractility in the gravid ureter. It is also suggested that ureteral compression by the iliac artery at the pelvic brim and by the enlarged uterine veins in the pelvis contribute to ureteral dilation during pregnancy. The incidence of vesicoureteric reflux is also higher in parturients and this, in combination with urostasis, contributes to the higher incidence of pyelonephritis in pregnant women with asymptomatic bacteriuria.[8] Bladder capacity initially increases in early gestation due to mechanical and hormonal influences, but then diminishes as rapid fetal growth occurs in the third trimester.[7]

The clinical significance of physiologic hydroureter during pregnancy lies mainly in its impact on a variety of tests of renal function during pregnancy. Severe ureterodilation can give the erroneous impression of obstructive uropathy, which can be difficult to diagnose in the gravid patient. Though technically difficult to perform, single-shot IVP and retrograde pyelography may be considered to rule out true obstruction in the symptomatic pregnant patient. It is unclear whether Foley catheter drainage of the gravid bladder in the patient with suspected obstruction is helpful. Timed urine collections to evaluate renal function are potentially inaccurate because of the large volumes of urine that may remain in the gravid urinary collecting system. This can be minimized by having the patient avoid lying in the supine position for 30 minutes before the beginning and end of the collection period. Because of persistent ureteral dilation during the postpartum period, elective radiologic examination of the urinary tract should be deferred until at least 16 weeks' postpartum.

Renal hemodynamics

Renal blood flow (RBF), as measured by p-aminohippurate clearance, increases markedly during pregnancy with a midpregnancy peak of 60% to 80% over nonpregnant values, followed by a significant fall in the third trimester that appears unrelated to the effect of posture.[9,10] Upright or supine positions in late pregnancy can significantly alter RBF, prompting the recommendation that pregnant women with preeclampsia or underlying renal disease maintain a modified bedrest schedule in a left lateral position.

Glomerular filtration rate (GFR), as measured by inulin or creatinine clearance, appears to parallel the rise in RBF by increasing by 25% to 50% throughout pregnancy.[10] Therefore, creatinine clearances during normal pregnancy typically range from 150 cc/min to 200 cc/min (Fig. 13-1). This increase in GFR is observed as early as 8 weeks' gestation with a plateau occurring during the second trimester. The increase in RBF seems

Table 13-1 Normal changes in the renal system during pregnancy*†

Item	Change	Comment
Kidney size	Length increases 1 cm by x-ray	Postpartum size reduction is normal
Dilation	Resembles hydronephrosis	Not to be confused with obstructive uropathy
	More prominent on *right side*	
Increased renal hemodynamics	GFR and RBF increase by about 25%-40%	Serum creatinine, BUN *decrease;* albumin, amino acids, glucose *increase*
Renal H$_2$O handling	Osmoregulation altered	Serum osmolality about 10 mOsm *less*
		Serum Na about 5 mEq/L *less*
Change in acid base status	Renal bicarbonate threshold decreases	Serum bicarbonate is 4-5 mEq/L *less*

*Adapted from Barron WM, Lindheimer MD: Renal function and volume homeostasis during pregnancy, in Gleicher N (ed): *Principles of Medical Therapy in Pregnancy.* New York, Plenum Press, 1985, p 779.
†GFR = glomerular filtration rate; RBF = renal blood flow; BUN = blood urea nitrogen.

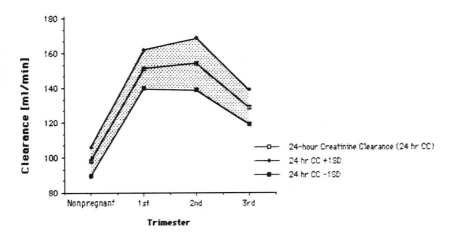

Fig. 13-1 Graph demonstrating significant increases in renal plasma flow as demonstrated by 24-hour creatinine clearance during normal human pregnancy. (Data from Davison J: Renal disease, in de Swiet M (ed): *Medical Disorders in Obstetric Practice.* Oxford, Blackwell Scientific Publications, 1989, p 309.)

to be out of proportion to the observed increase in GFR.[10] There does not appear to be a significant decrease in GFR in the third trimester, though accurate calculation of GFR is highly dependent on positional changes, sample sizes, and appropriate body surface corrections in late pregnancy.[9] Despite these theoretical limitations, the clinical use of 24-hour urine collections remains the mainstay of diagnosis for preexisting or new-onset alterations in GFR. This significant increase in GFR during pregnancy produces lower serum values for creatinine and blood urea nitrogen (BUN), in addition to providing an explanation for enhanced urinary excretion of protein, amino acids, and water-soluble vitamins.[9] It appears that glomerulotubular balance is usually maintained during pregnancy because of increased tubular resorption.

The physiologic mechanisms for the observed increase in RBF and GFR are undefined in humans, but animal studies suggest a variety of potential explanations for this dramatic change in renal hemodynamics during pregnancy.[11,12] Increased RBF and GFR with progressing gestation is probably mediated by equal vasodilation of preglomerular and postglomerular resistance vessels with equal distribution of these effects to all nephron units.[11] Altered sensitivity to prostanoids and renin-angiotensin control mechanisms of vascular reactivity have been implicated in this physiologic alteration.[12,13] Decreased sensitivity to angiotensin, vasopressin, and epinephrine during normal pregnancy has been clearly documented, as well as the observation that pregnancies destined to develop preeclampsia fail to demonstrate this decreased response to pressors.[13] This appears to be a progesterone-mediated event that has been linked to local production of vasodilatory prostanoids, down-regulation of pressor receptors, and postreceptor alterations in response.[12,13] Circulating renin levels are increased during pregnancy with myometrium and chorion contributing to substrate production, but the majority of elevation in renin levels is probably attributable to increased vasodilatory prostanoid production (PGE, PGI_2) in the pregnant kidney.[14] Circulating renin levels are very sensitive to postural and dietary alterations in pregnancy, and they form the physiologic basis for the rollover test to evaluate for impending preeclampsia.[15] The contribution of volume expansion to the observed increase in RBF and GFR will be discussed in the following section.

Volume homeostasis

The mean weight gain during pregnancy approximates 12 kg for primigravidas, with multigravidas gaining about 1 kg less.[16,17] Approximately 60% of the weight gain during pregnancy is attributable to water retention.[17] No data exist to suggest the upper limits of acceptable weight gain, but 20 kg is frequently quoted. Preliminary clinical data exist to suggest that women with smaller increments in plasma volume in pregnancy are associated with lower birth weight and poor pregnancy outcome. Weight gains outside the normal limits for pregnancy have obvious consequences for fetal growth, uteroplacental blood flow, and the development of pregnancy-induced hypertension. Obviously a basic understanding of volume homeostasis during pregnancy is necessary to identify pathologic alterations in water and salt metabolism in the high-risk pregnancy.

Utilizing deuterium oxide as a tracer, investigators have estimated that total body water increases by 7 to 8 L during pregnancy.[17,18] The largest increase in body water during pregnancy is attributable to a 20% to 25% expansion in plasma volume.[17] Plasma volumes begin to increase as early as 5 weeks, accelerate in the second trimester, peak near 32 weeks, and remain elevated until term. It is estimated that only 1300 mL of extracellular fluid is present in the interstitial space during normal pregnancy, though it can be as high as 5 to 7 L in pathologic pregnancies.[18] The maximum increase in interstitial fluid occurs after the 32nd week of gestation. This increase in maternal plasma volume and interstitial space constitute a physiologic "hypervolemia" that is sensed as normal by the sodium and water metabolic control mechanisms of the pregnant woman.

Despite the fact that total body sodium increases by 1000 mEq during pregnancy, with 60% of this increased sodium remaining in the maternal compartment,[19] the serum plasma osmolarity decreases by 8 to 10 mOsm/kg below nonpregnant values.[20] The osmotic threshold for both vasopressin release and onset of thirst appears to decrease by 10 mOsm/kg and represents the resetting of the osmostat during pregnancy.[21] The metabolic clearance of vasopressin increases dramatically in the third trimester.[21] The loop of Henle is the major site of water and sodium reabsorption, and the concentrating ability of the gravid kidney appears intact despite a tendency for hypotonic urine production during pregnancy. Water excretion also appears to be impaired in later gestation and may represent a postural-induced phenomenon.[20] Therefore, the clinical use of random urine specific gravity measurements to assess maternal volume status may be erroneous in the supine patient or patients with existing renal disease.

With the increase in GFR during pregnancy, the daily filtered sodium load is increased by 30% to 50% to as much as 35,000 mEq.[22] In addition to reabsorption of this increased sodium load, the

BOX 13-1 FACTORS INCREASING SODIUM FILTRATION

Renal plasma flow
Glomerular filtration
Prostaglandin
Progesterone
Arginine vasopressin
Melanocyte stimulating hormone

gravid kidney is able to reabsorb an additional 2 to 5 mEq of sodium for fetal and maternal stores.[22] The ability of the gravid kidney to reabsorb this increased load represents the largest renal adjustment during pregnancy. Sodium reabsorption appears to be promoted by aldosterone, deoxycorticosterone, estrogens, renin-angiotensin, and postural effects, while sodium excretion is promoted by the competitive inhibition of aldosterone by progesterone, vasopressin, natriuretic hormones, and vasodilating prostaglandins[22] (see Box 13-1). Despite this level of knowledge of sodium metabolism during pregnancy, its contribution to the hypertensive diseases of pregnancy remains unknown. In addition, there are no existing clinical data to support the use of diuretic therapy in the treatment of pregnancy-induced hypertension or excessive weight gain. In the attempt to minimize fluid retention and stabilize blood pressure, use of hypotonic saline solutions is preferable when caring for the high-risk pregnant patient with preexisting renal compromise.

The initiating events for these significant physiologic alterations in volume homeostasis are still obscure, but two conflicting hypotheses exist at the present time.[23] An overfill maternal state can be theorized where a hormonally induced primary renal sodium and water retention produces secondary increases in GFR, RBF, and cardiac output. Alternatively, a primary enlargement of the maternal vascular compartment may occur in response to vasodilatory prostaglandins and placental arteriovenous shunting effects, thus presumably producing secondary renal and sodium retention. Regardless of the initiating scenario, the recognition of a physiologic "hypervolemic" state during pregnancy is essential in the clinical management of the high-risk pregnancy.

Tubular function

Clinically detectable glucosuria is more common in the gravid patient.[9,23] Glucose excretion increases soon after conception and may exceed nonpregnant levels by a factor of 10, with approximately 5% of the filtered glucose being excreted during normal pregnancy.[10] It appears that the maximum tubular reabsorption remains unchanged throughout gestation, resulting in an increased glucose excretion secondary to a progressively increasing GFR.[9] Therefore, the presence of glucosuria in pregnancy is not diagnostic for diabetes, though new onset of glucosuria in early gestation may warrant further evaluation.

Net reabsorption of urea in the kidney is a passive event and is directly related to the rate of urine flow. Conflicting data exist regarding urea excretion during pregnancy,[9,23] but it is agreed that plasma BUN levels are significantly decreased in normal pregnancy.[10] Serum levels of BUN and creatinine at the upper limits of normal may be associated with impending renal compromise (Fig. 13-2).

Plasma uric acid levels decrease by 25% over nonpregnant values.[24] This alteration is seen as early as 8 weeks, and a progressive increase in serum levels is noted in the third trimester. This initial alteration is probably due to increased fractional excretion of and a decrease in net tubal reabsorption of uric acid. Elevated random serum uric acid is a popular, though potentially erroneous, laboratory determination to evaluate progressive renal compromise in pregnancy-induced hypertension (Fig. 13-2).

Paradoxically, potassium excretion is decreased despite elevated aldosterone levels and alkaline urine.[20,23] The result is the retention of 350 mEq of potassium, which probably reflects the effect of progesterone on aldosterone response. In general, routine potassium supplement of 10 to 20 mEq in the fasting patient is all that is required during pregnancy.

Bicarbonate reabsorption and hydrogen ion excretion during pregnancy appears to be intact.[25] Plasma bicarbonate levels decrease by an average of 4 mEq/L in response to the physiologic pregnancy-induced respiratory alkalosis. This renal compensation maintains the average pregnant serum pH at 7.44 with a corresponding average P_{CO_2} value of 31 mm Hg. This renal effect and accelerated maternal metabolic rate predispose the parturient to acute metabolic acidosis in the face of an acute insult. In addition, maternal blood gas determinations must be interpreted in view of this compensated respiratory alkalotic state.

Aminoaciduria occurs during pregnancy and is reflected by lower serum values. This effect is probably related to cortisone influences on tubal reabsorption mechanisms.[20] More important, normal tubular protein reabsorption is unable to handle the increased filtered protein load.[23] This results in a physiologic gestational proteinuria of 150 to 300 mg during normal pregnancy. Any 24-

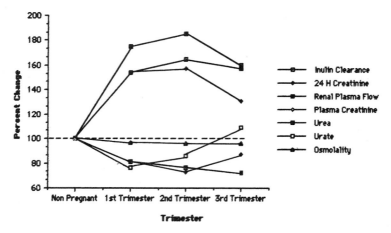

Fig. 13-2 Graph manifesting percent change of various renal parameters during normal human pregnancy. (Data from Davison J: Renal disease, in de Swiet M (ed): *Medical Disorders in Obstetric Practice*. Oxford, Blackwell Scientific Publications, 1989, p 309.)

hour proteinuria greater than 300 mg should be considered pathologic and indicative of preexisting or progressive renal damage.

Postpartum physiologic changes

Anatomic alterations in the urinary collecting system may persist up to 4 months postpartum, but the majority of patients will have normal collecting systems by 6 weeks as previously discussed.[7] Bladder hypotonia in the immediate postpartum period is common, with bladder volumes normalizing by 6 weeks.[7]

Glomerular filtration increases immediately postdelivery and begins decreasing by the sixth postpartum day.[4,10] This commonly results in a diuresis of 2 to 3 L within the first 72 hours, which resembles a postobstructive diuresis. Over the next 8 weeks GFR returns to normal, while for unknown reasons RBF remains depressed below nonpregnant values for up to 24 weeks.[10]

Tubular function normalizes rapidly with a significant improvement in proteinuria and glucosuria in the immediate postpartum period.[23] Normalization of renal acid base regulation requires a longer interval.[20]

CHRONIC RENAL DISEASE AND PREGNANCY
Prepregnancy counseling

Because of the different obstetric conditions as well as varying degrees of chronic renal insufficiency, the impact of pregnancy on a particular patient should be considered by the state of renal function prior to conception. The consideration of pregnancy in the face of chronic renal disease must be balanced between maternal and fetal prognosis (Fig. 13-3). Based on the type and severity of ma-

ternal renal disease, the potential for a good fetal outcome may directly conflict with the long-term prognosis for the mother. Such a balance can be ascertained by evaluating:

1. Type of preexisting chronic renal disease
2. General health status
3. Presence or absence of hypertension
4. Current renal function
5. Prepregnancy drug therapy

The influence of preexisting renal disease on pregnancy varies greatly according to the etiology and type of the renal disease[26] (Table 13-2). Most women with diabetic nephropathy demonstrate normal increases in GFR with progressive gestation, and pregnancy does not appear to accelerate renal deterioration.[27,28] Patients with adult polycystic kidney disease likewise do well during pregnancy in the absence of preexisting hypertension.[29] Similarly, individuals with chronic urolithiasis,[30] previous pyelonephritis,[26] permanent urinary diversion,[31] solitary kidney, and pelvic kidneys[32] do well despite an increase in infectious risks during pregnancy.

On the other hand, women with preexisting collagen vascular diseases such as lupus erythematosus and systemic sclerosis may be at significant risk during pregnancy. In general, relapse of lupus nephritis during pregnancy is rare if maternal disease has been in remission for 6 months prior to conception.[33,34] Severe flares of lupus nephritis can occur in the postpartum period, prompting the recommendation to increase steroid coverage in patients at risk during this critical period.[34] Onset of renal involvement during pregnancy from scleroderma can lead to rapid deterioration.[35] The significant risk of new-onset hypertension with im-

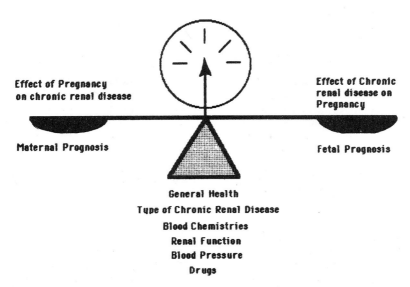

Fig. 13-3 Pregnancy and renal disease—a dynamic balance regarding maternal and fetal safety and successful outcome must be reached.

Table 13-2 Specific renal diseases and their interaction with pregnancy*

Disease	Effects/comments
Systemic lupus erythematosus	Good prognosis if in remission
	Need to increase steroids postpartum
Scleroderma	If onset during pregnancy, then rapid downhill course
Periarteritis nodosa	Poor fetal prognosis
	Maternal death rate increased
Chronic glomerulonephritis	If no hypertension, little effect
Reflux nephropathy	Increased chance of sudden hypertension/deterioration of renal function
Pyelonephritis	Exacerbation with bacteriuria
Diabetic nephropathy	Increased chance of infection, edema, pre-eclampsia
Polycystic disease	Minimal renal impairment or hypertension
Permanent urinary diversion	Urinary tract infection common
	Renal function may decline during pregnancy
	Cesarean section may be necessary for abnormal presentation
Postnephrectomy solitary and pelvic kidneys	Minimal interference with pelvic labor/delivery
Urolithiasis	Increased infections

*Adapted from Davison J: Renal disease, in de Swiet M (ed): *Medical Disorders in Obstetric Practice*. Oxford, Blackwell Scientific Publications, 1989, p 330.

munoglobulin A (IgA) nephropathy during pregnancy may deter a high-risk mother from considering pregnancy. A similar concern in individuals with reflux nephropathy during pregnancy has been voiced.[36] Perhaps one of the most controversial areas is the effect of pregnancy on primary glomerular disease.[37] The concern rests on the argument that increasing GFR during pregnancy is maladaptive and in the long run will produce further renal compromise. While the clinical outcome data are reassuring in most cases,[38] it appears that the severity of preexisting renal compromise will ultimately determine the risk for these patients.[37] It has been suggested that certain types of primary glomerular disease, including membranoproliferative glomerulonephritis and focal glomerular sclerosis, appear to be more sensitive to pregnancy effects.[37] Nephrotic syndrome due to a variety of causes carries little maternal risk if renal function is normal and hypertension is absent.

It is now recognized that the presence of preexisting chronic hypertension and/or onset of hypertension during pregnancy is an important determinant of perinatal morbidity and mortality.[39] This is due to increased rates of intrauterine growth retardation (IUGR) and preterm deliveries for uncontrollable hypertension or superimposed preeclampsia.[38-40] The presence of hypertension prior to conception increases the risk of IUGR fivefold and doubles the prematurity rate.[38,39] Even more important for maternal considerations is the presence of uncontrolled hypertension during pregnancy of patients with moderate or severe renal insufficiency because it can cause progression to end-stage renal disease.[38,40-42] While control of hypertension during pregnancy is paramount to a good outcome, the inability to accurately predict which patient will exhibit uncontrollable hypertension mandates thorough risk counseling of the hypertensive renal patient.

Functional renal status is an important indicator of maternal and fetal prognosis during pregnancy.[39,40] However, in patients with renal disease, pathology may be both clinically and biochemically silent. An individual can lose up to 50% of her functional nephrons before exhibiting alterations in creatinine clearance. After this point, a further small decrease in functioning nephrons will cause dramatic increases in serum creatinine values. Therefore, evaluation of renal function is best based on timed creatinine clearances rather than on random plasma concentrations. Use of such renal function tests can be helpful for prepregnancy counseling as well as for structuring a prenatal care plan for these high-risk patients.

Women with chronic renal disease but normal or mildly decreased prepregnancy renal function (serum creatinine < 1.5 mg/dL or creatinine clearance >100 cc/min) usually have a successful obstetric outcome and pregnancy does not adversely affect the course of their disease.[39] Most patients show incremental increases in GFR, and increased proteinuria is observed in up to 50% of these gestations.[43] The prevalence and severity of hypertension, renal function abnormalities, and proteinuria are considerably lower between pregnancies and during long-term follow-up.[39] This group of patients can usually contemplate pregnancy with little risk.

The prognosis is more guarded when renal function is moderately impaired (serum creatinine between 1.5 and 2.5 mg/dL or a creatinine clearance between 50 and 100 cc/min).[39] Those individuals with a 50% loss of renal function still have a 90% chance of a good obstetric outcome, but approximately 25% of these patients will exhibit long-term renal deterioration.[39,41,43] A significant number of

these patients also exhibit accelerated hypertension during pregnancy.[39,41] While these clinical data are encouraging from the obstetric standpoint, contemplation of pregnancy places the mother at significant long-term risk of end-stage renal disease.

Most women with severe renal insufficiency (serum creatinine >2.5 mg/dL or creatinine clearance <50 cc/min) are anovulatory and hence incapable of conception. However, occasional pregnancies do occur and are associated with dismal maternal and fetal outcomes.[39] Approximately 50% of the pregnancies will have poor obstetric outcomes and 50% of the pregnant patients will exhibit end-stage renal disease within 1 year.[44] Needless to say, these individuals should be actively discouraged from attempting pregnancy.

Prenatal care

Once the patient with renal problems has decided to become pregnant, it is clear that good antenatal care is a major factor in reducing maternal and perinatal morbidity.[43] The goals of such prenatal care should be directed toward:

1. Recognition and control of hypertension.
2. Recognition of deteriorating renal function.
3. Maintenance of maternal and fetal nutrition in the severely proteinuric patient.
4. Early detection and treatment of asymptomatic bacteriuria.
5. Assessment of fetal growth patterns and well-being.

Early recognition and prompt treatment of these abnormalities in the renal patient will minimize their impact on the course of pregnancy. Prenatal care plans for these high-risk patients must provide surveillance for deteriorating renal function, urogenital infections, and altered fetal development. Such prenatal care must be individualized to the patient's type of disease, preexisting renal compromise, and different potential complications of pregnancy.

Baseline evaluations of the pregnant patient with renal disease should be directed toward detecting altered renal function, degree of preexisting hypertension, presence of anemia, evidence of abnormal chemistries, and compromised end-organ function. Timed urine collection, complete blood counts, and routine serum chemistries are usually helpful in this task. Hypertensive patients should be evaluated for preexisting retinopathy and cardiomyopathy. These baseline studies will also serve for comparison later in the gestation if potential complications should arise.

Clinic visits every 2 weeks in early pregnancy are in order and home blood pressure monitoring should be instituted in patients with preexisting hypertension. Prenatal visits should document weight, blood pressure, and proteinuria, in addition to evaluating fetal development. Initial urine cultures should be performed with aggressive treatment and follow-up of asymptomatic bacteriuria when identified. Baseline sonographic studies of the fetus should be performed prior to 20 weeks to establish dates and evaluate the fetus at risk for drug-induced anomalies. The presence of hypertension, severe proteinuria, or clinical evidence of altered fetal growth warrants the initiation of serial sonography to evaluate interval fetal growth.

Pregnancies at risk for uteroplacental insufficiency should start weekly antepartum surveillance at 32 weeks. The presence of uncontrolled hypertension warrants aggressive therapy, including hospitalization. Modified bed rest is usually recommended in the hypertensive patient, based on the belief that it is conducive to improved blood pressure control and improved fetal growth. A high index of suspicion for superimposed pregnancy-induced hypertension is warranted in the previously well-controlled hypertensive pregnancy that is exhibiting worsening hypertension, disproportionate proteinuria, and deteriorating renal function. The astute clinician must vigilantly look for the early signs of superimposed pregnancy-induced hypertension in the patient chronically receiving antihypertensive agents since these medications can theoretically mask the initial labile blood pressures associated with this disease. Evidence of impending pregnancy-induced hypertension warrants hospitalization if the pregnancy is preterm, and further time can be bought for the fetus with conservative management.

While progressive increases in proteinuria should be expected as the pregnancy progresses, new-onset or disproportionate proteinuria during the prenatal period mandates further evaluation. Serial timed urine collections are indicated in patients with significant preexisting renal compromise. Severe proteinuria with or without renal compromise places the patient at risk for nephrotic syndrome. In general, a high-protein diet contributes to the progression of glomerular disease, prompting the recommendation of low-protein diets for the chronic renal patient.[45] However, the risk of further renal compromise for the pregnant patient with nephrotic syndrome must be balanced with the fetal need for protein substrate for normal development. Therefore, a high-protein diet is usually recommended for these specific patients in the presence of massive proteinuria.

The case of the pregnant patient presenting with flank pain should always raise a high index of suspicion for occult pyelonephritis. Urolithiasis must also be a diagnostic consideration in these patients, particularly in the presence of microscopic hematuria.

Clinical or sonographic evidence of severe alterations in fetal growth or deteriorating placental function mandates hospitalization for closer monitoring and evaluation of fetal well-being. Therapy is directed toward improving uteroplacental blood flow and is accomplished by left-sided bedrest and control of hypertension. It should be understood that overaggressive control of maternal blood pressure is not without its toll on uteroplacental blood flow; generally it is best to keep diastolic pressures above 90 mm Hg in pregnant patients with chronic hypertension to maintain an adequate pressure-head in the uteroplacental circulation. Based on the degree of fetal growth retardation, daily fetal biophysical surveillance may be indicated. Abnormal biophysical testing of the compromised fetus should be treated with immediate delivery.

New-onset renal disease during pregnancy offers a diagnostic challenge to the clinician. Interpretation of available clinical data must include consideration of the physiologic alterations of pregnancy. Use of radiographic and nuclear medicine methods of urologic evaluation is best limited during pregnancy but should be considered if the information is deemed valuable to further management of the pregnancy. While pregnancy has been considered a relative contraindication to renal biopsy in the past, more recent clinical experience suggests a complication rate similar to that of nonpregnant individuals.[46] Gross hematuria remains the major complication; it occurs in 1% to 5% of patients. Routine tests to exclude an underlying bleeding diathesis and abstinence from drugs that interfere with clotting should precede any renal biopsy. If the clinical information derived from a renal biopsy can have a significant impact on the further management of the pregnancy, then the risks are usually deemed acceptable.

Issues regarding delivery

Most perinatologists approach the issue of timing of delivery in the high-risk pregnancy in terms of risk-benefit analysis. Any decision to deliver a premature fetus for maternal indications must be balanced with the age-adjusted survival and morbidity statistics for a fetus at that gestational age. In the modern era, neonatal survival begins at 25 weeks and approaches 100% at 32 weeks in most institutions. Still, a significant degree of neonatal morbidity exists for the preterm fetus even after 32 weeks' gestation because of intraventricular hemorrhage and chronic lung disease. It should be obvious that a fetus with abnormal biophysical testing indicative of uncompromised hypoxia mandates immediate delivery in any potentially survivable fetus. Most obstetricians agree that documented fetal lung maturation and/or attainment of the 37th week of gestation should serve as delivery end-points in the compromised high-risk pregnancy.

However, any decision in the conservative management of a pregnancy with deteriorating renal status or progressive superimposed pregnancy-induced hypertension must be balanced against the maternal risks.

Progressive renal failure can theoretically be treated with hemodialysis or peritoneal dialysis in an attempt to temporize the maternal status until a term delivery is possible.[47] A significant number of successful pregnancies are being reported in patients requiring chronic dialysis. However, the majority of cases associated with deteriorating renal function during late pregnancy warrant delivery for the preservation of maternal renal function. The presence of uncontrollable hypertension, severe deterioration in GFR, or the onset of severe pregnancy-induced hypertension usually dictates delivery of the pregnancy for maternal indications. In the absence of these complications, conservative management of the pregnancy to buy time for further fetal maturation is usually successful but not without maternal risks. Decisions regarding the route of delivery are usually based on obstetric considerations only.

Intrapartum management. Once the parturient is admitted for delivery, special attention must be paid to the current renal function and blood pressure status of the patient. Baseline evaluation of electrolytes, complete blood count, and degree of proteinuria should be assessed. A reassuring state of fetal well-being must be documented, and continuous electronic fetal heart rate monitoring during the labor is the usual rule.

During labor the patient should be monitored for worsening hypertension or the onset of superimposed pregnancy-induced hypertension, since this is a common occurrence during the rigors of labor. Fluid administration should be restricted to maintenance levels to prevent fluid overload in the pregnant patient with borderline renal function. If the patient is unable to take her current antihypertensive medication orally during labor, an intravenous equivalent must be administered to prevent hypertension. As discussed previously, these powerful medications must be titrated to prevent significant alterations in uteroplacental blood flow caused by overaggressive therapy. For this reason, maternal diastolic blood pressures should be kept *above* 90 mm Hg in the patient with chronic hypertension.

Continuous epidural anesthesia provides significant benefits for the hypertensive patient during labor, including pain control, renal vasodilation effects, and improved uteroplacental blood flow.[48]

Drugs for the acute management of severe hypertension during labor are listed in Table 13-3. Intravenous hydralazine is the most widely used drug for rapid control of blood pressure during pregnancy and its main advantage is the extensive experience with its use. It is a potent vasodilator with greater activity on arteries than on veins, it has a short duration of effect, and it is reportedly a vasodilator of uteroplacental circulation.[49] Nevertheless, hydralazine produces significant maternal symptomatology including reflex tachycardia, headache, tremor, flushing, nausea, and vomiting. Hydralazine may be given initially as 10 mg intravenously, followed by 5 to 10 mg at 20- to 30-minute intervals, with the realization that the full drug effect will not be apparent for 30 to 45 min-

Table 13-3 Drugs for acute intrapartum management of severe hypertension

Drug	Dosage	Comments
Hydralazine (Apresoline)	2.5-20 mg	Effects begin in 15 min; last 3-4 hr
Labetalol (Normodyne)	20-40 mg over 2 min	α- and β-blocker
		Bronchospasm less likely than with other β-blockers
Diazoxide (Hyperstat)	1-3 mg/kg as a rapid injection	Effects begin in 1-2 min; last 6-7 hr
		Dose unable to be titrated
Nifedipine (Procardia)	10-20 mg PO	Resultant vasodilation may result in reflex tachycardia
Nitroprusside (Nipride)	1-8 μg/kg/min	Cyanide toxicity possible
Trimethaphan (Arfonad)	10-200 μg/kg/min	Does NOT cross placenta
		Resultant reflex tachycardia may require a β-blocker

utes. Alternatively, a continuous infusion may be administered after the initial bolus dose.

Recently, the supplier of hydralazine has unilaterally discontinued the drug's availability in the United States, based on purely economic reasons. Several obstetric societies have an application to the FDA to designate hydralazine as an orphan drug. Its uniform dosing, ease of administration, and long-standing obstetric experience make it a first-line agent in the treatment of preeclampsia. Many hospitals, having recently depleted their stores of hydralazine, have been forced to utilize other antihypertensive agents for patients with severe hypertension. (Fortunately this agent is available at the present time.—*Editor*.)

Labetalol, also of use in the acute management of hypertension, has become the preferred drug of choice among obstetricians when hydralazine is not available. Labetalol has the advantage of providing both alpha and beta effects, which theoretically preserve uteroplacental blood flow during therapy. Labetalol can be administered intravenously in a bolus dose or as a continuous infusion. Initial doses of 10 to 20 mg can be given over a 2-minute period, and repeat dosing at 10-minute intervals can be given up to a total of 300 mg. The maximum physiologic effect of labetalol usually occurs within 5 minutes of each injection. A continuous infusion of 1 to 5 mg per minute can be safely used during pregnancy to control a severely hypertensive patient. Obstetricians are beginning to feel more comfortable with labetalol as a potential replacement for hydralazine.

Diazoxide is a potent vasodilator, but its tendency toward excessive hypotension and its dramatic ability to produce fetal bradycardia due to altered uteroplacental blood flow limits its clinical use.[50] Diazoxide also produces a significant antinaturetic effect on the renal tubules, producing significant sodium and water retention.[51] Similar concerns for uteroplacental blood flow can be voiced regarding the acute use of nifedipine in this clinical situation. In patients failing to respond to these therapies, intravenous nitroprusside may be considered in view of its rapid onset and offset of action. However, its potent effect on uteroplacental circulation and the potential for fetal cyanide poisoning must be balanced with the maternal risk of uncontrolled severe hypertension.[52]

CHARACTERISTICS, DIAGNOSIS, AND OBSTETRIC MANAGEMENT OF CHRONIC RENAL FAILURE

Chronic renal failure is defined by a progressive and irreversible loss of functioning nephrons. The consequences of this loss of nephron function are anemia, fluid and electrolyte imbalances, and an inability to excrete certain drugs.[53]

Anemia

The primary cause of anemia in the overwhelming majority of chronic renal failure patients is a decrease in erythropoietin.[54,55] As is obvious, the body must compensate for a hemoglobin value that may reach levels as low as 4.5 g/dL. At first the cardiac output increases and there is an increasing shift of the oxyhemoglobin dissociation curve to the right.[56]

When the hemoglobin value falls below 9 g/dL, blood viscosity as well as systemic vascular resistance (SVR) decreases and the cardiac output increases primarily from an increased stroke volume. By and large, the pulse rate remains normal.

Oxygen transport is further improved by shifting the dissociation curve to the right. This is accomplished in two ways. At first, there is an increase in 2,3-diphosphoglycerate (2,3-DPG) that increases in response to the fall in hemoglobin concentration. In addition, renal failure patients have a moderate acidosis that further moves the curve to the right. However, acidemia has a tendency to decrease 2,3-DPG production and paradoxically, a uremic patient with erythropoetin-deficiency anemia has *less* 2,3-DPG than an otherwise normal anemic patient.[56]

Often the question arises as to what level the hemoglobin or hematocrit must be in order for a surgical operation to be safely executed. There is no known "safe level" above which elective surgery may be done. Each case must be judged in its clinical context. Factors considered are age of the parturient, level of sympathetic nervous system activity, and presence of coronary artery disease. The last factor deserves special mention because at present there is a national trend for professional women to put off having children until their late 30s or even early 40s, at which time the presence of coronary artery disease may be of more than academic interest.

Transfusion of packed cells is sometimes indicated. However, it should be borne in mind that 2,3-DPG levels in stored blood are low, although levels increase during the first 24 hours after transfusion. Another hazard to keep in mind is the possibility of a fluid overload leading to congestive heart failure, owing to the impaired ability to excrete fluid. As with all blood products, the risks of transmission of communicable diseases such as hepatitis (type B and type non-A, non-B) [57] and acquired immunodeficiency syndrome (AIDS) as well as more seldom encountered varieties must be weighed against the possible benefits.

Fluid imbalance

In anuric patients fluid elimination depends totally on dialysis, apart from insensible losses, which average approximately 500 cc per 24 hours. It is extremely rare for pregnancy to occur in this state, so the typical parturient with renal disease falls in the state between anuria and normality.

If the fluid balance is severe enough or persists for a long time, several consequences may occur:

1. The parturient may develop hypertension—entirely unrelated to the preeclamptic disease process—that may be severe enough to cause an encephalopathy with associated seizure, making the differential diagnosis of this process with eclampsia necessary (indeed, both processes may be present!).
2. Occasionally severe hypertension may push the parturient into congestive heart failure, necessitating multiple drug therapy. Peripheral edema and pulmonary edema may be present. Adequate dialysis will reverse the problems of edema, including pericardial effusions. In addition, the need for extensive antihypertensive therapy may be substantially lessened.
3. It is important, however, to be aware that 5% to 10% of patients have renin-dependent hypertension that does *not* respond to hemodialysis or ultrafiltration.

Electrolyte disturbances

The electrochemical derangements in the renal failure patient are many and varied. These patients may present with acidemia, *hypo*natremia, *hyper*chloremia, *hypo*calcemia, *hyper*phosphatemia, and *hyper*magnesemia as well as *hyper*kalemia.[58]

Hypermagnesemia is primarily a disease of medication. It usually occurs only in those patients taking magnesium-containing antacids or cathartics. Manifestation of hypermagnesemia is primarily muscle weakness; this is because of the competition of magnesium ion with calcium-binding release sites at the neuromuscular junction. The antidote is a slow infusion of calcium chloride, with concurrent indicated ventilatory support. It is recommended that the parturient take as little of these substances as is medically necessary.

Hyperkalemia, on the other hand, is a product of deranged or absent renal function and may occur in inadequately treated end-stage renal disease.

Manifestations may be absent, but when they do occur, they can be amplified by concomitant hyponatremia, hypocalcemia, or acidosis. Neuromuscular signs of hyperkalemia include weakness, paresthesia, areflexia, and muscular or respiratory paralysis. Cardiac manifestations are frequent when the serum potassium level is greater than 8 mEq/L. Manifestations include bradycardia, hypotension, ventricular fibrillation, and cardiac arrest. The electrocardiogram (ECG) demonstrates, in sequence, tall peaked T waves, depressed ST segments, a decreased amplitude of the R wave, a prolonged PR interval, diminished to absent P waves and ultimately, widening of the QRS complexes with prolongation of the QT interval, resulting in a sine-wave pattern.

Treatment of hyperkalemia may be affected by measures that antagonize the effects of potassium, force cellular entry of potassium, or actually remove potassium from the body. Therapeutic measures should depend on the degree of hyperkalemia and the severity of the manifestations.

Calcium immediately antagonizes the cardiac toxicity of hyperkalemia particularly if hypocalcemia is also present. Calcium gluconate, 5 to 10 mL of a 10% solution, may be injected intravenously over a 2-minute period. (If the patient is also receiving digitalis, administration of this drug is sufficiently dangerous that it should be given with *extreme* caution.[53])

Respiratory or a metabolic alkalosis causes rapid movement of potassium into the cells. *Sodium bicarbonate,* 45 mEq intravenously, may be given over a 5-minute period, and this may be repeated after 10 to 15 minutes if ECG abnormalities persist. However, large quantities of bicarbonate may be contraindicated owing to concurrent fluid overload and congestive heart failure.

Glucose-insulin solutions may also reduce the serum potassium level by causing potassium to return to the intracellular compartment. Usually 1 unit of regular insulin is given for each 2 g of glucose infused (200-300 mL 20% glucose containing 20-30 units of insulin may be given intravenously over a 30-60 minute period). If concern for fluid overload is paramount, then a 50% glucose plus insulin solution may be slowly given intravenously.[59,60]

Cation exchange resins reduce the serum potassium level more slowly but have the advantage of actually removing potassium from the body. Sodium cycle resins are preferable to hydrogen cycle carboxylic resins, which induce acidosis. This is doubly important in the parturient, in which the normal pH of pregnancy is already raised. These agents may be given rectally or orally. Rectal administration involves 50 g of polystyrene sulfonate (Kayexalate) and 50 g of sorbitol added to 200 mL water to make a retention enema. Oral administration is 20 to 50 g Kayexalate suspended in 15 mL sorbitol.[61]

Dialysis is indicated when conservative methods fail.

The question of appropriate blood potassium levels often arises. There is no scientific basis for the often quoted figure of 5.5 mEq/L. This level can be and is often safely exceeded provided there are no ECG changes of hyperkalemia and care is taken to avoid further increases in serum levels due to internal shifts.

Uremia

Uremia involves all organ systems. Of interest to the anesthesiologist is the immunologic system, which is impaired in this condition. Sepsis is the leading cause of death in these patients. Thus, it is of paramount importance to utilize ultra-aseptic techniques in placing any catheter, whether it be for urine (Foley), hemodynamic monitoring, epidural analgesia, spinal anesthesia, or even for a straightforward intravenous infusion. Obviously, multiple attempts will increase the chance of infection in these compromised patients. All sites should be thoroughly cleaned and the site should be prepared using an antiseptic such as Povidone or Betadine. The operator should be gowned and gloved.[62]

Coagulation abnormalities are also of great concern since birthing, whether via the vaginal or the operative route, involves a substantial amount of blood loss. In addition, modern obstetric anesthesia practice encourages the use of regional anesthetic techniques. Uremic patients may have problems related to platelet dysfunction,[63] which can be reversed with adequate dialysis. In any event, at the present time only a few institutions will perform a mandatory Ivy bleeding time to evaluate this portion of the coagulation system. Normality varies from institution to institution but falls within a range of roughly 3 to 7 minutes. The prothrombin time and partial thromboplastin time are not usually affected by renal disease; however, complete coagulation parameters should be checked before the administration of regional anesthesia.

Uremia affects multiple systems and multiple sites. The nervous system is no exception. These patients experience peripheral neuropathies, and it is most prudent to get a thorough history. Although there is little in the literature to point to a cause and effect relationship, it is medicolegally more prudent to forego regional anesthesia techniques in such patients unless there are compelling obstetric or anesthetic indications for it.[58]

Autonomic neuropathies are also found. In these patients, in contrast, regional techniques may be indicated.

The central nervous system can also be affected, in which case there may be central depression or central irritability, or altered consciousness, resulting in inappropriate behavior. In these circumstances, it may be wise to avoid regional anesthesia. In the emergent obstetric circumstance, general anesthesia may be indicated. At the same time, one must take into consideration that general anesthesia is fraught with its own risks and cautions. Since the blood-brain barrier is altered, there is an increased sensitivity to central nervous system–depressant drugs.

The gastrointestinal system is especially important to consider in the parturient with renal failure. Gastric emptying time is delayed in pregnancy and this phenomenon is also present in the non-pregnant individual with renal failure. In the parturient with renal failure, this effect is enhanced. It is important to notice that while many uremic side effects are alleviated or eliminated by dialysis, this therapy does *not* correct slow gastric emptying. Administration of metoclopramide (Reglan), 10 mg intravenously, preoperatively is recommended.[64]

Hyperdynamic circulation associated with chronic renal failure can increase the clearance of local anesthetic, thus shortening the duration of the local anesthetic blockade.

ANESTHETIC MANAGEMENT

The following detailed discussion of anesthetic management for patients with chronic renal failure will also be a guide for parturients with other renal problems.

General anesthetic considerations

Adequate preoperative preparation is mandatory. If the parturient is receiving dialysis therapy, it is highly encouraged to have the dialysis instituted before the induction of labor or cesarean section. After dialysis is completed, a complete battery of laboratory tests should be drawn to provide the anesthesia and obstetric teams with a set of baseline values.

Monitoring. As with any other obstetric patient, the parturient with renal failure should have the same standard of monitoring that is available in the main operating suite. This would include precordial stethoscope, blood pressure cuff, pulse oximeter, end-tidal carbon dioxide monitor, and ECG, the last of which is mandatory to detect changes related to hyperkalemia or hypokalemia. Standard of care during labor mandates the use of electronic fetal monitoring, and there is no known reason not to have this device applied during labor. Ideally, fetal monitoring should be continued not only in the labor room but also during transport to the operating theater where the delivery or cesarean section is to be performed.

In addition, *central venous access* may be desirable not only for more precise fluid management but also because peripheral venous access may be difficult or impossible to obtain or because all available sites are being used as dialysis sites. An *arterial line* may also be useful, especially in the more unstable parturient (i.e., the one who was unable, for a variety of reasons, to benefit from dialysis before surgery).

Positioning. Positioning is critical, especially in those parturients with arteriovenous fistulas. These should be carefully protected. Left uterine displacement should also be mandatory.

Ventilation. Ventilation parameters are especially important for these patients. Parturients in renal failure have a significant anemia (due to suppressed erythropoetin), and maneuvers that are of little importance in a normal patient become quite significant. Hyperventilation is to be avoided (i.e., causing the $Paco_2$ to fall below 30 mm Hg) as the hemoglobin curve is shifted to the left, hindering oxygen unloading. By the same token, hypoventilation is likewise discouraged because it may increase acidosis and it will increase the level of hyperkalemia.

Anesthetic drugs

Renal failure patients can and do have abnormal reactions to anesthetic drugs; this is in addition to the differences in general sensitivity to anesthetic drugs that such parturients exhibit. Uremic patients have abnormal protein binding, and highly protein-bound drugs such as thiopental[65] may cause prolonged or exaggerated effects.

Finally, drugs dependent on renal excretion should be used with extreme caution. Gallamine (Flaxedil), an older nondepolarizing muscle relaxant,[66] is almost exclusively excreted via the kidneys. Cases have been reported in which the only treatment for reversing the blockade was by dialysis. Muscle relaxants such as vecuronium (Norcuron[67]) and pancuronium (Pavulon)[66] have substantially prolonged rates of excretion in the patient with renal failure.

By the same token, mivacurium (Mivacron)[68,69,70] and rocuronium (Zemuron)[71-74] have been found to have prolonged effects in renal failure patients due to decreased clearance via the kidney.

Anesthetic management of the emergent parturient (for fetal distress) is modified (in the presence of hyperkalemia) in that the use of succinylcholine is relatively contraindicated because this drug will transiently increase serum potassium levels by at least 1 mEq/L. In the patients in whom ECG changes may already have appeared, the addition of another milliequivalent may have dangerous consequences. In addition, pseudocholinesterase levels may be significantly decreased and recovery from succinylcholine may be significantly prolonged. Hence, the nondepolarizing muscle relaxants vecuronium (Norcuron) or atracurium (Tracrium) are recommended neuromuscular blockers. Narcotic drugs such as fentanyl (only 10% of an injected dose of fentanyl appears in urine)[67] are conjugated in the liver and they are less affected. Currently used inhalation anesthetics (halothane and isoflurane) are little involved with the kidney and so may be used without difficulty.[75,76] Some patients receiving enflurane[77] for more than 9.5 hours at one sitting have peak serum inorganic fluoride levels in the 30 to 40 μmol/L range[78] and thus this agent should be avoided. The new fluorinated ether desflurane (I-653) has also been examined for evidence of fluoride ion. In phenobarbital-pretreated or ethanol-pretreated rats given I-653, the increase in serum inorganic fluoride and in urinary excretion of organic or inorganic fluoride is quite small, several-fold smaller than that found with isoflurane.[79-81]

Regional anesthesia may very well be the anesthetic technique of choice in many instances. In abdominal surgery, the use of regional anesthesia results in significantly decreased blood loss,[82] but this modality has its major complications as well. Hypotension, total spinal blockade, and local anesthetic toxicity are just a few. Absolute or relative contraindications to regional anesthetic procedures include hypovolemia, hemorrhage, coagulation abnormalities, bacteremia, septicemia neuropathy, or patient refusal.

Spinal (subdural, subarachnoid) anesthesia is a very satisfactory technique for surgery of the lower abdomen because it is simple and it has a high success rate. The greatest danger is hypotension secondary to sympathetic blockade, but adequate intravenous hydration with an electrolyte solution and vasopressor therapy (ephedrine) will prevent serious falls in blood pressure. A postspinal headache is not a serious complication, though it can at times be quite unpleasant. It usually subsides spontaneously within 3 days. In those few patients whose headache persists, a caffeine infusion or an epidural blood patch may be considered. Contraindications to spinal anesthesia include severe hypertension, hypotension, hypovolemia, and hemorrhage in addition to those described above.

Epidural blockade offers advantages over spinal anesthesia. The onset of anesthesia is slower than with spinal block and thus the development of profound hypotension is less precipitous and more easily prevented or treated. To include the placement of an epidural catheter in the technique offers additional flexibility. The local anesthetic agent can now be injected in small increments at selected intervals, and a desired level of anesthetic blockade can be more slowly and safely obtained and maintained regardless of the duration of surgery. Leaving the epidural catheter in place after completion of surgery allows subsequent injection of narcotic drug to provide postoperative pain relief for several days. Regional anesthesia should be contraindicated in the presence of coagulopathy or bacteremia and septicemia.

Patients should be monitored carefully during recovery for rebound hypertension, which may be catastrophic and may require prompt vasodilator therapy.

RENAL TRANSPLANT PARTURIENT
Obstetric and anesthetic management

The parturient with a transplanted kidney deserves special mention. Renal transplantation usually improves reproductive performance and allows end-stage renal patients to successfully carry a pregnancy to term.[44,83] While these transplant patients appear to have an increase in first-trimester miscarriage rates up to 40%, approximately 90% of continuing pregnancies will produce viable offspring.[44] It does not appear that pregnancy alters the graft rejection rate significantly.[84] The best predictor of good perinatal outcome in these high-risk patients is the presence of normal renal function prior to conception and the resolution of preexisting hypertension with transplantation.[85] Despite the apparent favorable outlook for these patients, approximately 30% of mothers will develop pregnancy-induced hypertension, 20% of these pregnancies will exhibit IUGR, and in 45% of pregnancies the fetus will be delivered prematurely for a variety of indications.[44]

Since a large percentage of renal allograft recipients demonstrate secondary hyperparathyroidism, transient neonatal hypocalcemia is a theoretical and described risk in these pregnancies.[86] Prospects for a vaginal delivery are dependent on the location of the pelvic kidney, but cesarean section is usually required only for obstetric indications. Despite these risks, the available data on subsequent infant development, though limited, are encouraging.[44]

Many of these women have had chronic medical conditions leading to renal failure (such as diabetes mellitus), and the key to management of these women is to be mindful of their underlying condition. A successfully transplanted kidney functions as well as the original, and a transplant patient's fluid and electrolyte balance is every bit as fine-tuned as that of a healthy person. For documentation purposes, an electrolyte and clotting profile is drawn along with a complete blood count. In contrast to the dialysis patient, there is no need for anticoagulation. Regional anesthesia may be used at will.

Since there is generally a history of decreased resistance to infection and since the patient may be maintained on low-dose immunosuppressant drugs (cyclosporine dose adjusted to blood levels in the range of 500 to 700 ng/mL in whole blood as measured by radioimmunoassay), careful sterile technique is observed throughout the procedure and antibiotics are given to the parturient after birth of the baby. Obviously these immunosuppressed patients are at risk for urinary tract infection and therefore should have cultures done regularly and be given urosuppressive medications.[83] In addition, renal transplant patients are at significant risk for primary and recurrent infections by cytomegalovirus, which carries a significant risk for the fetus.[87] The potential fetal risks from the various immunosuppressive agents used in these patients will be discussed in the next section.

Some former recipients may also be receiving chronic steroid therapy. For these parturients, steroid coverage typically would be 100 mg hydrocortisone intravenously as well as 100 mg intramuscularly just before surgery. The intramuscular injection may be repeated until the patient can resume her oral dose of the steroid drug (usually 5 mg prednisone daily).[88]

CHRONIC DRUG THERAPY IMPLICATIONS

Many renal patients considering pregnancy are receiving a variety of medications that can theoretically affect the fetus. Some of these common medications are listed in Table 13-4. The most common class of chronic medications used in renal patients are the antihypertensive agents. While there is long-standing experience with most antihypertensive medications in the nonpregnant patient, in the gravid patient the effects of such chronic therapy on fetal development, uteroplacental blood flow, and postdelivery development is based on only a limited experience.

The most widespread clinical experience in pregnancy has been with methyldopa. It is the preferred antihypertensive medication for use during pregnancy. It is usually well tolerated by the mother, not believed to be teratogenic, and follow-up of exposed infants for up to 7 years after birth have shown no significant abnormalities.[89] Doses of up to 3 to 4 g per day may be required for appropriate blood pressure control during pregnancy.[90]

There is widespread experience in the use of beta-blockers in women with mild to moderate hypertension during pregnancy.[91] Early reports of their use described adverse fetal effects such as bradycardia, hypotension, hypoglycemia, and fetal distress.[49] It is also theoretically possible that beta-blockade may mask fetal heart rate evidence of fe-

Table 13-4 Antihypertensive agents used in pregnancy

Drug	FDA class*	Comments
Methyldopa	C	Safety during pregnancy is well documented
		Initial lethargy and drowsiness
Propranolol	C	Rare incidence of neonatal hypoglycemia and bradycardia
		Possible masking of fetal distress; possible bronchospasm, insomnia, dizziness, depression, and hyperglycemia in mother; possible association with IUGR
Labetalol	C	Tremulousness, flushing, headache
		Theoretical advantage of beneficial alpha blockage on uteroplacental blood flow
Furosemide	C	Possible masking of superimposed pregnancy-induced hypertension
Thiazides	D	Neonatal thrombocytopenia
Clonidine	C	Limited clinical experience
Nifedipine	C	Limited clinical experience
		Significant risk of maternal hypotension
		Animal studies suggest significant alterations in uteroplacental blood flow and fetal cardiovascular responses
Captopril	C	Possible teratogenic effects in animals

*A = controlled studies in pregnant humans fail to demonstrate a risk to the fetus and the possibility of fetal harm is remote. B = animal studies do not demonstrate a fetal risk but controlled studies in pregnant humans are lacking. In addition, animal studies may show an adverse effect but controlled studies in humans fail to confirm it. C = studies in animals have revealed an adverse effect and there are no controlled studies in humans available. Drugs should be given only if the potential benefit justifies the risk to the fetus. D = there is positive evidence of human fetal risk, but the benefits from use in pregnant humans may be acceptable in a high-risk clinical setting. X = studies in either animals or humans demonstrate serious fetal abnormalities or other risks that clearly outweigh any possible benefit in the pregnant human.

tal distress.[90] This class of drugs is not thought to be associated with teratologic events, but the clinical experience is still forthcoming. However, with further clinical experience, it appears that beta-blockers rarely produce these effects in the neonate and that the effects of uncontrolled hypertension during pregnancy far outweigh the risk of their use.[90,91] Dosages of beta-blockers vary according to the drug and are the same as for nonpregnant individuals.[90]

The use of beta-blockers during pregnancy has been associated with the development of IUGR. While the beta-blockage of the uteroplacental vasculature has been implicated, several randomized trials with methyldopa reveal similar birth weights, suggesting that the underlying hypertensive effects are more important determinants of altered fetal growth.[91,92]

Because of the theoretical advantages of simultaneous alpha- and beta-blockade, the use of labetalol during pregnancy might alleviate these concerns. While the clinical experience with labetalol is still growing, it is believed to be safe and effective in the control of chronic hypertension during pregnancy. Initial dosages are started at 100 mg three to four times daily and can be increased to 1200 mg daily.[90] In a small randomized trial, labetalol produced better blood pressure control and larger birth weights when compared with methyl-

dopa,[92] but these results were not confirmed in a larger randomized trial.[93] In addition, teratogenic data are still minimal at this time; therefore, these agents should be reserved for methyldopa failures or severe hypertensives requiring multiple agents.

Chronic diuretic therapy is generally thought to be contraindicated for blood pressure control during pregnancy because of theoretical risk of vascular depletion and sodium wasting during pregnancy.[90] Diuretic use clearly does not prevent the onset of pregnancy-induced hypertension and may in fact mask some of the early clinical signs of preeclampsia.[94,95] While intermittent or chronic use of furosemide for other indications during late pregnancy may be safe, teratogenic experience in the first trimester is minimal.[52] Conversely, use of the thiazide diuretics during late pregnancy has been clearly associated with neonatal thrombocytopenia[52] and thus should be avoided during pregnancy.

While angiotensin-converting enzyme inhibitors have a theoretical advantage for the control of renovascular-induced hypertension, they should not be used during pregnancy because of undefined teratogenic risks in animal studies.[96] Similarly, chronic use of calcium-channel blockers during pregnancy is controversial despite their clinical use in Europe as a tocolytic agent.[97] However, chronic use of calcium-channel blockers for blood pressure control is probably contraindicated because of ani-

Table 13-5 Immunosuppressive agents used in pregnancy

Drug	FDA class*	Comment
Prednisone	B	Considered safe in pregnancy
		Maternal risks include glucose intolerance, peptic ulcer disease, osteoporosis, and delayed wound healing
		Fetal risks considered minimal, but possible immunosuppression
Cyclosporine	D	Limited experience in pregnancy
		Potentially nephrotoxic and hepatotoxic
Azathioprine	D	Maternal risks of infection and/or neoplasia
		Increased teratogenicity and fetal loss in animals
		Lymphopenia, transient chromosomal aberrations, and undefined fertility risks for exposed human fetuses

*For a key to FDA drug classification during pregnancy, see Table 13-4.

mal model reports of significant alterations in uteroplacental blood flow that resulted in fetal demise.[98] Clonidine, though probably safe in pregnancy, is not recommended for use in parturients because of the lack of clinical experience.[52]

Renal transplant patients may be receiving a variety of immunosuppressive agents that can be theoretically detrimental to the fetus (Table 13-5). Prednisone, commonly used in these patients to decrease cell-mediated responses to the allograft, has the disadvantages of increased risk of infection, malignancy, and poor healing. Additional maternal side effects include glucose intolerance, peptic ulcer disease, and osteoporosis. Prednisone and prednisolone cross the placenta to only a limited extent and are thought to present little teratologic risk to the developing fetus.[99] Immunosuppression of the fetus does not appear to be a significant clinical concern.[100] Judicious use of prednisone is clearly justified in all patients requiring immunosuppressive therapy during pregnancy.

On the other hand, azathioprine is a potent immunosuppressive purine analogue that readily crosses the placenta into the fetal compartment.[101] The evidence of increased congenital anomalies and fetal wastage in animals, the presence of chromosomal aberrations and lymphopenia in exposed human neonates, and the concern for future fetal fertility are all issues associated with azathioprine use in pregnancy.[102] While human teratologic data remain sketchy, it is clear that these other concerns can be limited by adjusting azathioprine dosages in the third trimester to maintain maternal leukocyte counts within normal limits.[103]

Little is known about the maternal and fetal effects of cyclosporine administration during pregnancy.[104] While it is documented that the drug crosses the placenta into the fetal compartment,[105] it is also clear that although human data are lacking, cyclosporines are a unique class of immuno-

suppressant agents without apparent myelotoxicity, teratogenicity, or mutagenicity in most animal species.[106] Cyclosporine has long-term nephrotoxic effects,[107] and its possible effects during pregnancy on renal hemodynamics and sodium regulation remain undefined.

Despite the possible risks with these immunosuppressant agents, it is usually prudent to continue these medications during pregnancy to prevent allograft rejection. It seems that the fetal and maternal risks from these immunosuppressive agents are acceptable when considering the overall long-term health of the transplant parturient.

A variety of antibiotics are considered safe for the treatment of infections of the urinary tract during pregnancy.[108] Two classes of antibiotics for the treatment of urinary tract infections are suitable in the patient with chronic renal disease. Widespread experience has shown that broad-spectrum penicillins and the cephalosporins are safe in pregnancy. Similarly, a trimethoprim-sulfonamide combination or nitrofurantoin appears to be well suited for use during pregnancy. The aminoglycosides can be given cautiously in cases of microbial resistance or severe infection, with frequent monitoring of serum levels to avoid nephrotoxicity. Conversion to oral therapy may be considered for use during the 48 to 72 hours after pyrexia has resolved and for as long as 10 to 14 days. A variety of urosuppressive antibiotics are summarized in Table 13-6.

Most of these patients do not pose any anesthetic problems because of their normal kidney function. For labor and delivery, an epidural analgesia may be an ideal choice. For cesarean section, if the patients are receiving hypotensive drugs, regional anesthesia should be used carefully and epidural anesthesia might be an ideal choice. General anesthesia may be necessary in urgent situations. A meticulous aseptic technique is mandatory in such cases. (Detailed anesthetic management is

Table 13-6 Antibiotic agents commonly used in pregnancy

Drug	FDA class*	Comment
Penicillins	B	Safety well established in pregnancy
Cephalosporins	B	Probably safe for use in pregnancy
		5%-10% cross-reactivity in penicillin-sensitive patients
Nitrofurantoin	B	Probably safe in pregnancy
		Possible neonatal thrombocytopenia
		Contraindicated in G6PD deficiency†
Gentamicin	C	No reported teratogenic effects
		Possible fetal ototoxicity
		8th cranial nerve toxicity with kanamycin and streptomycin
Tetracycline	D	Adverse effects on fetal teeth and bones
		Potential for maternal liver toxicity
Trimethoprim/sulfonamide	C/B	Probably safe in pregnancy
		Theoretical contribution to hyperbilirubinemia in neonates if given in late pregnancy
Mandelic acid	C	Limited experience in humans

*For a key to FDA drug classification during pregnancy, see Table 13-4.
†G6PD = glucose-6-phosphate dehydrogenase.

discussed in the section on Characteristics, Diagnosis, and Obstetric Management of Chronic Renal Failure, p. 255.)

ACUTE RENAL FAILURE DURING PREGNANCY
Obstetric and anesthetic management

Acute renal failure during pregnancy is a medical emergency that requires prompt and precise treatment. Acute renal failure in civilian surgical patients in 1989 had a 50% mortality rate. Although this is an improvement over the 90% mortality found in soldiers wounded in World War II, it is not very much better than the 53% mortality experienced by American soldiers in Korea when dialysis was available. Indeed, in Vietnam, the mortality approached 77%. What has been found is that early, aggressive intervention may limit mortality.[109]

Acute tubular necrosis. The causes of acute renal failure are many and varied. They may include trauma (primarily crush injuries such as those resulting from automobile accidents), extensive surgery, or obstetric complications such as disseminated intravascular coagulopathy or amniotic fluid embolism. In addition, a parturient may become ill with a disease process that necessitates a nephrotoxic agent. Finally, it has been recorded that those parturients who have had a cardiac arrest from accidental intravenous injection of a long-acting anesthetic agent such as bupivacaine or etidocaine may have renal failure as a sequela.

Renal failure in trauma and obstetric accidents is often accompanied by considerable extrarenal injury, and patient survival is often dictated by the amount of extrarenal injury sustained. The ultimate course of acute tubular necrosis may range from a case demonstrating mild and short-lasting tubular damage with a quick recovery to one involving extensive damage and a protracted course (Table 13-7).

The functional hallmarks include renal vasoconstriction in which renal blood flow may be reduced to 50% of normal. Cellular damage is due to local ischemia. Glomerular filtration rate is reduced to essentially zero and there is evidence of tubular damage.

Pathogenesis. The initiation phase of perioperative acute renal failure often occurs during the period when the anesthesiologist is directly responsible for the patient's welfare and when vigorous intervention is likely to be effective. Renal hypoperfusion is secondary to hemodynamic factors. The most common causes in the surgical and obstetric population are external and/or internal fluid loss or, more seldom, sepsis. Nephrotoxins may be a cause, but they are rarely involved. What essentially occurs is tubular dysfunction with or without tubular obstruction that then results in decreased GFR and RBF.

Pathological studies of renal tissue in patients with acute renal failure have yielded equivocal results. It is probable that the real damage is in the medullary cells. Medullary cells perform a large amount of the metabolic work in the form of sodium chloride transport. Medullary blood flow is normally low, and under normal conditions the rate of oxygen delivery may be very close to the oxy-

Table 13-7 Causes of renal failure in obstetrics*

Pathophysiologic derangement	Obstetric complication
Hypovolemia/hypotension	Abortion
	Hemorrhage secondary to placenta previa
	Hyperemesis gravidarum
	Adrenocortical failure
	Postpartum hemorrhage due to soft-tissue trauma
Hypovolemia/hypotension/coagulopathy	Pregnancy-induced hypertension
	Hemorrhage secondary to placental abruption
	Blood transfusion reactions
	Amniotic fluid embolism
	Drug reactions
	Acute fatty liver
	Hemolytic uremic syndrome
Hypovolemia/hypotension/coagulopathy/infection	Chorioamnionitis
	Pyelonephritis
	Septic abortion
	Puerperal sepsis
Urinary tract obstruction	Surgically induced damage to ureters
	Pelvic hematoma
	Broad ligament hematoma

*Adapted from Davison J: Renal disease, in de Swiet M (ed): *Medical Disorders in Obstetric Practice.* Oxford, Blackwell Scientific Publications, 1989, p 373.

gen demands of the transporting epithelial cells. In the presence of medullary ischemia, cellular anoxia may occur, initiating the events associated with acute renal failure. Cell death is due to accumulation of cellular calcium.[110]

Pathogenesis of toxin-induced acute tubular necrosis is different from that of ischemic acute tubular necrosis. Histologic studies suggest that toxins such as heavy metals and aminoglycoside antibiotics produce damage mostly in the proximal tubule.

CLINICAL SYNDROMES OF ACUTE RENAL FAILURE

Acute renal failure may be classified as either *prerenal* or *intrinsic* renal failure (*postrenal* failure will be addressed in a later section).

Prerenal failure generally involves the principle of renal hypoperfusion with concomitant or resultant impaired renal function. It may reflect the normal renal response to sense volume depletion. Reflex changes promoting salt (primarily sodium) and water conservation are set in motion, and as a result patients with renal hypoperfusion are *oliguric* and therapy generally involves volume correction.

Ischemia

Intrinsic intrarenal failure is primarily due to ischemic tubular damage, which in turn is due to a combination of vasoconstriction *and* ischemia.

Ischemia can be the *sole* inciting event or it may be the end result of a series of bodily insults. Ischemia may be originally due to prolonged prerenal failure. It is increasingly due to extensive trauma and burns. Extensive surgical procedures, with concomitant complications such as hemorrhagic hypotension, may also contribute to renal ischemia. Finally, sepsis and septic shock with the release of various toxins may also contribute to the cause. With such a great range of inciting events, there is a great range of severity.

Diagnosis

It is of obvious importance to identify whether the problem is prerenal, intrinsic renal, or postrenal failure because therapy for each broad category is unique.

One should begin with the patient's thorough history and physical examination. History should include questions regarding exposure to nephrotoxic agents, history of muscle damage (to rule in or out myoglobin as a factor), cardiac disease, or hepatic disease.

The physical examination should address the state of hydration and should discover whether there is a state of volume depletion. One should note any acute weight loss and consider carefully signs of hypovolemia: reduced blood pressure, resting tachycardia, and orthostatic hypotension. In addition, signs and symptoms of cardiac insufficiency or failure should be sought. This is of great importance since acute renal failure in a well-hydrated patient without cardiac or hepatic disease strongly suggests *intrarenal* failure.

Beyond a thorough history and physical examination, diagnosis of this condition often depends on inspection of the urinary sediment (Table 13-8). Inspection of the urinary sediment may be of critical importance in distinguishing between prerenal and intrarenal failure. By and large, prerenal failure syndromes reveal little urinary sediment with few formed elements. In contrast, intrarenal failure reveals active urinary sediment with "muddy" pigmented casts, epithelial cells, and epithelial cell casts.

Urinary electrolytes may also be diagnostic. In prerenal failure the kidneys are attempting to conserve volume and the urine sodium is low while the osmolarity is high. In intrarenal failure the tubular epithelium itself is disrupted and filtered sodium is unable to be resorbed completely; urinary sodium is elevated while osmolarity is reduced to isotonicity.[111]

Using the fractional sodium excretion criterion, one may further refine the diagnosis. The technique involves measuring the sodium and creatinine concentrations in a spot urine sample and relating them to the simultaneous serum values for sodium and creatinine. The ratio of urine-to-plasma sodium concentration is divided by the ratio of urine-to-plasma creatinine concentration, and the result is multiplied by 100[111]:

$$\text{Fractional sodium excretion} = 100 \times \frac{Na_{urine}/Na_{plasma}}{Cr_{urine}/C_{plasma}}$$

In prerenal failure the fractional excretion is less than 1%; in intrarenal failure the fractional excretion ranges from 1% to 3%.

This ratio is valid in *both* oliguric and nonoliguric renal failure. Fractional chloride excretion might be superior to the fractional excretion of sodium, but this awaits further evaluation.[112]

Nephrotoxic renal failure

Nephrotoxic renal failure (i.e., nonischemic failure) is generally of slower onset and longer duration, and less likely to be oliguric. The kidney is susceptible to a variety of nephrotoxins, both endogenous and exogenous. The endogenous toxins include myoglobin and hemoglobin, which primarily originate from crush injuries; uric acid from tumor lysis; oxalic acid from primary and acquired hyperoxaluria; and myeloma proteins from multiple myeloma. The exogenous nephrotoxins cover a wide range of substances. Of interest to the anesthesiologist is the anesthetic agent methoxyflurane, which was known to release fluoride ion, the causative agent in nonoliguric renal failure.[67,77] Although methoxyflurane is essentially unobtainable for human anesthetic practice, this agent is still widely used in small-animal veterinary practices. While modern veterinary anesthesia technique, like human technique, employs scavenger systems and modern agents such as isoflurane, there are enough older practices that have not been updated.

Myoglobin-induced renal failure. Myoglobin-induced renal failure is generally due to muscle damage released myoglobin into the circulation. Myoglobin may be released via a vascular occlusion of an extremity or from protracted ischemia from pressure immobilization. An example would be a patient comatose from a drug overdose with resultant rhabdomyolysis. Bacterial and viral infections may also cause myoglobinemias.

Although myoglobin is toxic to renal epithelial cells, a degree of vasoconstriction and/or ischemia must be present for acute renal failure to develop. Usually these patients have a substantial tissue injury (overwhelming sepsis or trauma). The clinical picture is thus one of intravascular volume depletion with concomitant hemoconcentration that has already been implicated in renal injury. It is now quite probable that oliguria will also occur.

Table 13-8 Urinary findings in renal hypoperfusion and acute tubular necrosis

Parameter	Renal hypoperfusion	Acute tubular necrosis
Urinary sediment	Normal, few hyaline and granular casts	Renal epithelial cells and epithelial cell casts, granular muddy pigmented cell casts
Urine specific gravity	>1.020	<1.015
Urine osmolality (mOsm/kg)	>450	<400
Urine sodium (mEq/L)	<20	>20
Urine:plasma creatinine concentration ratio	>40	<20
Fractional sodium excretion (FE_{Na}), %	<1	>1

Criteria for diagnosis include occult blood in the urine but no red blood cells in the urinary sediment. The BUN/creatinine ratio is less than 10. Laboratory serum investigations show an increase in the enzymes alanine transaminase, aspartate transaminase, and creatinine phosphokinase. In addition there is a marked increase in uric acid. Patients with myoglobin-induced renal failure have hyperkalemia and hyperphosphatemia as well as an occasional *decrease* in serum calcium.

The clinical course is dependent on a clinical triad: a nephropathy due to myoglobin toxicity, a myopathy-related muscle damage, and a peripheral neuropathy secondary to entrapment in anatomic compartments compressed by swelling and edema of damaged muscle tissue. There is a profound oliguria and a significant catabolism related to the degree of muscle injury. Hemodialysis, rather than peritoneal dialysis, is the therapy of choice for patients needing dialysis therapy, and daily treatments may be necessary. The prognosis is generally good provided adequate support is maintained.

Drug-induced renal failure. Drug-induced renal failure is usually associated with the aminoglycoside group of antibiotic agents.[106] The primary offenders are kanamycin, gentamycin, and tobramycin. Gentamycin is of special interest to the obstetrician since it is commonly used in treating gram-negative pelvic infections. Somewhat less offensive are amikacin and netilmicin. Volume depletion (more common to obstetric patients) is a major risk factor. Each drug is associated with decreased renal function. There is poor correlation between peak and trough levels and the development of acute renal failure. In fact renal failure may develop and worsen after the antibiotic therapy is terminated because of the continued effects of drug accumulated in renal tissue.

A second group of drugs commonly associated with renal failure are the nonsteroidal antiinflammatory drugs. The mechanism of interference with renal function is that these drugs inhibit the enzyme cyclooxygenase.[114] The importance of this enzyme is that it is involved with a critical step in the synthesis of prostaglandins. In the renal system, prostaglandins regulate renal blood flow. In the absence or suppression of this enzyme with resultant prostaglandin suppression, extreme renal vasoconstriction may occur.

Interstitial nephritis. Interstitial nephritis may occur secondary to allergic drug reactions such as methicillin nephritis.[115,116] The drugs that are known to cause these problems are the penicillins and cephalosporins as well as the sulfonamides, rifampin, and the nonsteroidal antiinflammatory drugs. Diagnosis is by examination of the renal sediment. Typically the urinary sediment contains white blood cells, including eosinophils, and red blood cells. Proteinuria is mild. Bacterial infections with resultant sepsis may lead to ischemic renal damage. Disseminated intravascular coagulopathy may supervene, leading to acute cortical necrosis. In this case the prognosis is far graver. More commonly, bacterial infection leads to acute glomerular disease.

Glomerulonephritis. Glomerulonephritis is a process that takes place via immune mechanisms. The classic example is poststreptococcal glomerulonephritis, but the process may be triggered by either gram-positive or gram-negative bacteria; virus or yeast are rare vectors. Acute renal failure is caused by fulminant glomerulonephritis. The diagnosis is again via the urine where 3 to 4+ protein can be observed, along with sediment that shows red blood cells and red cell casts. Serologic studies showing a depressed serum complement and elevated antibody titers to one or more streptococcal antigens will confirm the diagnosis.

There are a number of other causes for acute renal failure; these are listed in Table 13-2. Most of these are related to arterial occlusive disease.

Postrenal failure

Postrenal failure is usually a mechanical problem secondary to acute urinary tract obstruction. There is a history of urinary tract disease and there is an abrupt cessation of urine output. The physical examination usually reveals a suprapubic bladder and/or flank fullness. The causes may be linked to the disease process or they may be iatrogenic (cut ureter(s) during hysterectomy, especially cesarean hysterectomy). Radiographic examinations are excellent for diagnosis of acute urinary obstruction and are often all that is necessary for diagnosis of postrenal failure. Renal ultrasound is becoming the investigation of choice because it is completely noninvasive and it has a high degree of sensitivity as well as a high degree of specificity. A negative result essentially allows one to concentrate on prerenal and intrarenal causes.

MANAGEMENT AND THERAPEUTIC AGENTS FOR ACUTE RENAL FAILURE

The mainstay of therapy is to limit the magnitude and duration of renal ischemic insults that initiate acute renal failure. All efforts to improve perfusion, including volume expansion, pulmonary artery catheterization, inotropic support (i.e., dopamine), and vasodilation should be employed. Solute excretion should be promoted.

By the same token, one should consider diagnostic data with caution. The most useful parameter is urine volume. The resuscitation of patients with significant perioperative oliguria should be aggressive enough to restore urine flow and systemic perfusion, or it should be continued until oliguria persists despite a pulmonary artery pressure of 18 mm Hg or more following the administration of dopamine and diuretics.

The second most useful parameter is hemodynamic measurements. This is useful in situations in which empirical volume expansion does *not* restore urine flow.

Finally, few far-reaching decisions can be made from formulas or spot blood determinations.

There are a variety of therapeutic maneuvers, all of which are useful in their appropriate context. For prerenal failure, volume repletion and renal perfusion are the critical concepts for the prevention of acute renal failure. For intrinsic renal failure, removing the cause as quickly as possible is paramount. For example, in ischemic-caused acute tubular necrosis, stabilization of cardiac function and general surgical management is needed, whereas in nephrotoxic-induced acute renal failure, the toxin must be removed. Azotemia may progress despite timely removal. When a known nephrotoxin (e.g., amphotericin B) is given, side effects may be blunted with a high-salt diet and intravenous saline infusions.

Diuretic agents are the first line of therapy, despite lack of good evidence regarding efficacy.

Mannitol,[116-118] an osmotic diuretic, has been shown to protect against experimental renal failure and is used extensively in acute renal failure in humans. In the pregnant renal failure patient, this otherwise extremely useful therapy is to be used with extreme caution since the fetus can be significantly dehydrated.[119]

Mannitol, in conjunction with sodium bicarbonate, is effective in myoglobinuric acute renal failure. Bicarbonate minimizes toxicity of myoglobin on the tubule by alkalinizing the tubular fluid. While the bicarbonate is not especially harmful to the fetus, mannitol is still being employed and the caveats for mannitol alone still apply.[120]

Furosemide (Lasix) acts in several ways. It is a renal vasodilator[121] that interferes with sodium transport within the loop of Henle. Since shutting down sodium transport will reduce cellular oxygen consumption, furosemide may preserve tubular integrity by reducing demand. Use of this drug in the clinical setting has produced equivocal results.[122] It is indeed ototoxic and it is recommended to be used with caution up to 500 mg.

Dopamine (Intropin) is an intermediary product of catecholamine metabolism. Among its unique actions is that it stimulates specific dopaminergic receptors, causing renovascular dilation. This particular effect is limited to doses ranging from 0.5 to 1.0 μg/kg/min. At higher doses vasoconstriction

begins to take place. Dopamine's efficacy in acute tubular necrosis is yet unknown.

Calcium-channel blockers appear to reduce the level of vasoconstriction. The mechanism appears to be one of retardation of intracellular calcium buildup.[123] Pretreatment with this drug may be effective when administration of drugs with nephrotoxin activity seems likely. Such drugs would include cisplatin, cyclosporine, and radio contrast agents.

There are some issues regarding drug therapy that should be addressed. Adjustment of drug doses is mandatory, especially if excretion is either wholly or preferentially via the kidneys. Magnesium and potassium loads must be minimized. Drugs that are wholly excreted by the kidney such as gallamine (Flaxedil) should be avoided whenever possible. It should be noted here that *no form of pharmacologic therapy is routinely effective.* Finally, the role of nutrition remains controversial. It is still recommended to be careful about nitrogen-containing foods, since a protein load is difficult to excrete and may cause clouding of memory or even frank coma.

Citrate infusions and *prostacyclin* are anticoagulants that have promise for the nonpregnant patient, but they are *contraindicated* for the parturient.

Management of acute renal failure

Dialysis. Most renal failure patients are well controlled by acute and chronic dialysis; however, there are several iatrogenic complications that must be addressed. The *indications for dialysis* are volume overload, refractory acidosis, and hyperkalemia and excessive nitrogen compounds. Aggressive dialysis may result in hypovolemia and electrolyte depletion. Inadequate dialysis can result in fluid overload and electrolyte excess. *Dialysis should be left to a skilled nephrologist.* The key issues are timing of institution of dialysis, frequency, and methods of anticoagulation. Chronic acidosis is well-tolerated in the *nonpregnant* patient. However, the numbers of parturients undergoing dialysis are rather sparse, and the changes successfully endured by a pregnant patient and the fetus are less known. The primary recommendation might be that the fetus is likely to be less tolerant of electrolyte changes and while dialysis must be continued, close monitoring of the parturient's fluid and electrolyte status is mandatory.

Prophylactic dialysis has gained favor in some circles.[124] Some studies indicated that there is reduced mortality/morbidity if dialysis is started early. Hemodialysis is the modality of choice. Peritoneal dialysis can be used in certain circumstances.

The use of *anticoagulants* requires experienced management. Heparin either intravenously or subcutaneously is the mainstay as it does *not* cross the placenta.

Diagnosis and management of acute oliguria

Oliguria is defined as a urine volume of less than 0.5 mL/kg/hr in an acutely stressed patient.[125] It has been found that the most common cause of oliguria and subsequent acute renal failure is prolonged renal hypoperfusion. Obviously it is far more efficacious to prevent acute renal failure than it is to treat it.[109,126] It is important to bear in mind that both the duration (the longer the interval permitted between the insult and the commencement of therapy, the greater the chance of acute renal failure) *and* the magnitude are critical in determining the severity of acute renal failure.

Diagnostic tests in acute oliguria. It is difficult to differentiate prerenal from intrarenal oliguria. (Postrenal oliguria can be ruled in or out in a very straightforward manner, with various radiologic and physical techniques.) Consequently, therapy of patients with acute oliguria must usually be undertaken in the absence of information that can accurately predict whether the patient will or will not develop acute renal failure.

With oliguria due to prerenal causes, urine osmolality is usually higher (>500 mOsm), the urine sodium is usually higher (>40 mEq/L) and the renal failure index is less than 1%. It is also important to remember that use of these indices is limited in the acute situation. Giving diuretics increases urinary sodium and decreases urine osmolality. It is best to take a sample *before* diuretics are given to minimize potential confusion.

For oliguria secondary to intrarenal causes, the osmolarity is usually less than 350 mOsm, the urine sodium is less than 20 mEq/L, and the renal failure index is greater than 2%.[127]

If the above tests are equivocal, Swan-Ganz catheterization can be instituted. The primary question to be answered is: Can volume be given without inducing pulmonary edema? If the pulmonary artery occlusion pressure (PAOP) is less than 18 mm Hg, then volume expansion is usually well tolerated; if PAOP lies between 18 and 25 mm Hg, then one ought to proceed with caution; a PAOP of greater than 25 mm Hg indicates that volume expansion will be of little benefit. Other modalities, such as dopamine or other inotropic-derived support, should be considered. (Fig. 13-4).

Postrenal oliguria is generally secondary to some obstructive process. The tests are quite simple, ranging from checking the urinary catheter to various radiologic tests (IVP) to rule out problems of ureteral patency or integrity.

Management and therapeutic interventions. If possible, the magnitude and duration of renal ischemic insults that initiate acute renal failure should be limited. All efforts to improve perfusion, including volume expansion, pulmonary artery catheterization, inotropic support (dopamine), and vasodilation should be employed. Second, solute excretion should also be addressed.[128]

Diagnostic data should be considered with caution. The most consistent monitoring parameter is urine volume. The resuscitation of patients with significant perioperative oliguria should be aggressive enough to restore urine flow and systemic perfusion, or it should be continued until oligura persists despite a pulmonary pressure of 18 to 25 mm Hg or more following the administration of dopamine and diuretics. Hemodynamic measurements (cardiac index, PAOP) is useful in situations in which empirical volume expansion *does not* restore urine flow.

In acute oliguria, the goal of therapy is to increase urine production since the morbidity/mortality from nonoliguric renal failure is significantly less than from oliguric or anuric renal failure.

Mannitol is one of the mainstays of traditional renal failure therapy since it can limit renal damage produced by a fixed ischemic insult. Production of a solute diuresis is superior to volume expansion. Again, it should be borne in mind that mannitol should be preferentially used after delivery since, as mentioned earlier, this drug crosses the placenta and is known to cause fetal dehydration.

Furosemide (Lasix)[129,130] decreases experimental renal failure in animals with a fixed ischemic insult. Large doses can convert oliguric acute renal failure to nonoliguric acute renal failure.[131,132] Nonoliguric renal failure permits easier management of fluid and electrolyte balance. Even though azotemia still develops, nonoliguric renal failure may be associated with decreased morbidity and mortality.[122,133]

Timing is important. The majority of the animal models involve the administration of furosemide *before* the initiation phase or immediately after conclusion of an ischemic or nephrotoxic insult; those studies clearly show that furosemide limits renal damage. In contrast, the majority of *clinical studies* consist of the administration of furosemide to oliguric patients in whom a rise in serum creatinine has already been documented, i.e., during the maintenance phase. In that setting the results are far less impressive.

Adding low-dose *dopamine (Intropin)* (0.5-1 µg/kg/min) to high-dose furosemide may convert oliguric to nonoliguric renal failure.[134] In addition, dopamine limits renal damage produced by fixed

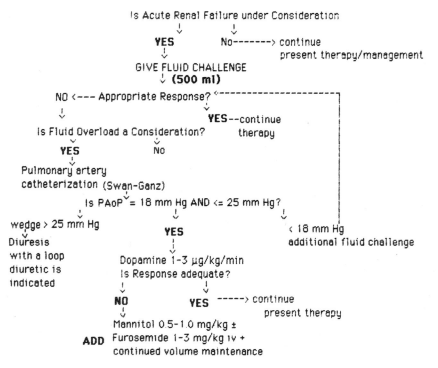

Fig. 13-4 The algorithm for oliguria presupposes that the primary reason for oliguria is *prerenal;* good medical practice requires that diagnostic tests be done in the appropriate intervals to differentiate between prerenal, intrarenal, and postrenal disease. (Adapted from Prough D: The assessment and management of acute oliguria, in American Society of Anesthesiologists, 35th Annual Refresher Course Lectures and Clinical Update Program, Lecture no. 241, New Orleans, 1984.)

renal insults. The mechanism is the renal vascular dilation caused by stimulation of dopaminergic receptors in the kidney.

Anesthetic management in parturients with this problem should revolve around the treatments that have been mentioned. Regional anesthesia (epidural) may be used if the clotting parameters are normal; in the presence of abnormal clotting values and severe bacteremia or septicemia, general anesthesia may be mandatory. (Detailed anesthetic management is discussed in the section on Characteristics, Diagnosis, and Obstetric Management of Chronic Renal Failure.)

REFERENCES

1. Lindheimer MD, Baylis C (eds): Symposium on renal function and disease in pregnancy. *Am J Kidney Dis* 1987; 9:243.
2. Bailey RR, Rolleston GL: Kidney length and ureteric dilatation in the puerperium. *J Obstet Gynaecol Br Commonw* 1971; 78:55.
3. Cietak KA, Newton JR: Serial quantitative nephrosonography in pregnancy. *Br J Radiol* 1985; 58:405.
4. Dunlop W, Davison JM: Renal hemodynamics and tubular function in human pregnancy. *Clin Obstet Gynecol* 1987; 1:769.
5. Fried AM: Hydronephrosis of pregnancy: Ultrasonographic study and classification of asymptomatic women. *Am J Obstet Gynecol* 1979; 135:1066.
6. Cietak KA, Newton JR: Serial qualitative nephrosonography in pregnancy. *Br J Radiol* 1985; 58:399.
7. Freidman AJ: The urinary tract in pregnancy. *Am UroGynecol Soc Rep* 1987; 7:1.
8. MacDonald P, Alexander D, Catz C, et al: Summary of a workshop on maternal genitourinary infections and the outcome of pregnancy. *J Infect Dis* 1983; 147:596.
9. Davison JM: Overview: Kidney function in pregnant women. *Am J Kidney Dis* 1987; 9:248.
10. Davison JM, Dunlop W: Renal hemodynamics and tubular function in normal human pregnancy. *Kidney Int* 1980; 18:152.
11. Baylis C: The determinants of renal hemodynamics in pregnancy. *Am J Kidney Dis* 1987; 9:260.
12. Conrad KP: Possible mechanisms for changes in renal hemodynamics during pregnancy: Studies from animal models. *Am J Kidney Dis* 1987; 9:253.
13. Gant NF, Whalley PJ, Everett RB, et al: Control of vascular reactivity in pregnancy. *Am J Kidney Dis* 1987; 9:303.
14. Bay WH, Ferris TF: Factors controlling plasma renin and aldosterone during pregnancy. *Hypertension* 1979; 1:410.
15. Gant NF, Chand S, Worley RJ, et al: A clinical test useful in predicting the development of acute hypertension in pregnancy. *Am J Obstet Gynecol* 1974; 120:1.
16. Thomson AM, Billewicz T: Clinical significance of weight trends during pregnancy. *Br Med J* 1957; 1:243.

17. Hytten FE: Weight gain in pregnancy, in Hytten FE, Chamberlain G (eds): *Clinical Physiology in Obstetrics.* Oxford, Blackwell Scientific Publications, 1981, pp 193-233.

18. Chesley LC: *Hypertension in Pregnancy.* East Norwalk, Conn, Appleton-Century-Crofts, 1978, pp 190-228.

19. Davison JM, Vallotton MB, Lindheimer MD: Plasma osmolality and urinary concentration and dilution during and after pregnancy. *Br J Obstet Gynaecol* 1981; 88:472.

20. Weinberger MH, Kramer NJ, Petersen P, et al: Sequential changes in renin-angiotensin-aldosterone systems in normal and abnormal pregnancies, in Lindheimer MD, Katz AI, Zuspan FP (eds): *Hypertension in Pregnancy.* New York, John Wiley & Sons, 1976, pp 263-268.

21. Lindheimer MD, Barron WM, Durr J, et al: Water homeostasis and vasopressin release during rodent and human gestation. *Am J Kidney Dis* 1987; 9:270.

22. Gallery EDM, Brown MA: Control of sodium excretion in human pregnancy. *Am J Kidney Dis* 1987; 9:290.

23. Schrier RW, Durr JA: Pregnancy: An overfill or underfill state. *Am J Kidney Dis* 1987; 9:284.

24. Dunlop W, Davison JM: The effect of normal pregnancy upon renal handling of uric acid. *Br J Obstet Gynaecol* 1977; 84:13.

25. Lim VS, Katz AI, Lindheimer MD: Acid-base regulation in pregnancy. *Am J Physiol* 1976; 231:1764.

26. Lindheimer MD, Katz AI: Gestation in women with kidney disease: Prognosis and management. *Clin Obstet Gynecol* 1987; 1:921.

27. Kitzmiller JL, Brown ER, Phillippe M, et al: Diabetic nephropathy and perinatal outcome. *Am J Obstet Gynecol* 1981; 141:741.

28. Reece EA, Coustan DR, Hayslett JP, et al: Diabetic nephropathy: Pregnancy performance and fetomaternal outcome. *Am J Obstet Gynecol* 1988; 159:56.

29. Milutinovic J, Fialkow PJ, Agodoa LY: Fertility and pregnancy complications in women with autosomal dominant polycystic kidney disease. *Obstet Gynecol* 1983; 61:566.

30. Miller DR, Kakkis J: Prognosis, management and outcome of obstructive renal disease in pregnancy. *J Reprod Med* 1982; 27:199.

31. Barret RJ, Peters WA: Pregnancy following urinary diversion. *Obstet Gynecol* 1983; 62:556.

32. Klein EA: Urologic problems during pregnancy. *Obstet Gynecol Surv* 1983; 39:605.

33. Hayslett JP, Lynn RI: Effect of pregnancy upon lupus nephropathy. *Kidney Int* 1980; 18:207.

34. Bobrie G, Liote F, Houillier P, et al: Pregnancy in lupus nephritis and related disorders. *Am J Kidney Dis* 1987; 9:339.

35. Mor-Josef S, Navot D, Rabinowitz R, et al: Collagen disease in pregnancy. *Obstet Gynecol Surv* 1984; 39:67.

36. Jungers P, Joillers P, and Forget D: Reflux nephropathy and pregnancy. *Clin Obstet Gynecol* 1987; 1:955.

37. Katz AI, Lindheimer MD: Does pregnancy aggravate primary glomerular disease? *Am J Kidney Dis* 1985; 6:261.

38. Surian M, Imbasciati E, Cosci P, et al: Glomerular disease and pregnancy: A study of 123 pregnancies in patients with primary and secondary glomerular disease. *Nephron* 1984; 36:101.

39. Davison JM, Katz AI, Lindheimer MD: Kidney disease and pregnancy: Obstetrics outcome and long-term renal prognosis. *Clin Perinatol* 1985; 12:497.

40. Jungers P, Forget D, Houillier P, et al: Chronic renal disease and pregnancy. *Arch Nephrol* 1986; 15:103.

41. Bear RA: Pregnancy in patients with renal disease: A study of 44 cases. *Obstet Gynecol* 1976; 48:13.

42. Hou S: Pregnancy in women with chronic renal disease. *N Engl J Med* 1985; 312:836.

43. Katz AI, Davison JM, Hayslett JP, et al: Pregnancy in women with renal disease. *Kidney Int* 1980; 18:192.

44. Katz AI, Lindheimer MD: Effects of pregnancy upon the natural course of kidney disease. *Semin Nephrol* 1984; 4:252.

45. Brenner BM, Meyers TW, Hostetter TH: Dietary protein intake and the progressive nature of kidney disease. *N Engl J Med* 1982; 307:652.

46. Packham D, Fairley KF: Renal biopsy: Indications and complications in pregnancy. *Br J Obstet Gynaecol* 1987; 94:935.

47. Hous S: Peritoneal and hemodialysis in pregnancy. *Clin Obstet Gynecol* 1987; 1:1009.

48. Jouppila P, Jouppila R, Hollmen A, et al: Lumbar epidural analgesia to improve intervillous blood flow during labor in severe preeclampsia. *Obstet Gynecol* 1982; 59:158.

49. Rubin PC: Beta-blockers in pregnancy. *N Engl J Med* 1981; 305:1323.

50. Neuman J, Weiss B, Rabello Y, et al: Diazoxide for acute control of severe hypertension complicating pregnancy: A pilot study. *Obstet Gynecol* 1979; 53(suppl):50S.

51. Koch-Weser J: Diazoxide. *N Engl J Med* 1976; 294:1271.

52. Berkowitz RL: Anti-hypertensive drugs in the pregnant patient. *Obstet Gynecol Surv* 1980; 35:191.

53. Bastron RD: Anesthetic considerations for patients with endstage renal disease, in Barash PG (ed): *Refresher Course in Anesthesiology.* Philadelphia, JB Lippincott, 1985, p 1.

54. Fisher JW, Moriyama Y, Rege AB, et al: The role of inhibitors of heme synthesis and bone marrow erythroid colony forming cells in the mechanism of anemia of renal insufficiency. *Proc Dial Transplant Forum* 1974; 4:141.

55. Eschbach JW, Funk D, Adamson J, et al: Erythropoiesis in patients with renal failure undergoing chronic hemodialysis. *N Engl J Med* 1967; 276:653.

56. Lichtman MA, Murphy MS, Byer BJ, et al: Hemoglobin affinity for oxygen in chronic renal disease: Effect of hemodialysis. *Blood* 1974; 43:417.

57. LaMont JT: The liver, in Vandam LD (ed): *To Make the Patient Ready for Surgery.* Reading, Mass, Addison-Wesley, 1984, p 53.

58. Reese GN, Appel SH: Neurological complications of renal failure. *Semin Nephrol* 1981; 1:137.

59. Skeie B, Askanazi J, Khambatta H: Nutrition, fluid, and electrolytes, in Barash PG, Cullen BF, Stoelting RK (eds): *Clinical Anesthesia.* Philadelphia, JB Lippincott, 1989, pp 744.

60. Mecca RS: Postanesthesia recovery, in Barash PG, Cullen BF, Stoelting RK (eds): *Clinical Anesthesia.* Philadelphia, JB Lippincott, 1989, pp 245-246.

61. Rosenfeld MG (ed): *Manual of Medical Therapeutics,* ed 25. Boston, Little, Brown & Co, 1986, pp 48-51.

62. Skaredoff MN, Poppers PJ: Anesthesia for vascular access, in Waltzer WC, Rapaport FT (eds): *Angioaccess.* New York, Grune & Stratton, 1984, pp 51-52.

63. Horowitz HI: Uremic toxins and platelet function. *Arch Intern Med* 1970; 126:823.

64. Zelnick EB, Goyal RK: Gastrointestinal manifestations of chronic renal failure. *Semin Nephrol* 1981; 1:124.

65. Hilgenberg JC: Renal disease, in Stoelting RK, Dierdorf SF (eds): *Anesthesia and Coexisting Disease.* New York, Churchill Livingstone, 1983, p 394.

66. Buzello W, Agoston S: Kinetics of intercompartmental disposition and excretion of tubocurarine, gallamine, alcuronium and pancuronium in patients with normal and impaired renal function. *Anaesthesist* 1978; 27:319.

67. Maddern PJ: Anaesthesia for the patient with impaired renal function. *Anaesth Intensive Care* 1983; 11:321.

68. Mangar D, Kirchoff GT, Rose PI, et al: Prolonged neuromuscular block after mivicurium in a patient with end-stage renal disease. *Anesth Analg* 1993; 76(4):866.

69. Phillips BJ, Hunter JM: Use of mivacurium chloride by constant infusion in the anephric patient. *Br J Anaesth* 1992; 68:492.

70. Cook DR, Freeman JA, Lai AA, et al: Pharmacokinetics of mivacurium in normal patients and in those with hepatic or renal failure. *Br J Anaesth* 1992; 69:580.

71. Szenohradszky J, Caldwell JE, Sharma ML, et al: Interaction of rocuronium (ORG 9426) and phenytoin in a patient undergoing cadaver renal transplantation: A possible pharmacokinetic mechanism. *Anesthesiology* 1994; 80:1167.

72. Szenohradszky J, Fisher DM, Segredo V, et al: Pharmacokinetics of rocuronium bromide (ORG 9426) in patients with normal renal function or patients undergoing cadaver renal transplantation. *Anesthesiology* 1992; 77:899.

73. Cooper RA, Maddineni VR, Mirakuhr RK, et al: Time course of neuromuscular effects and pharmacokinetics of rocuronium bromide (ORG 9426) during isoflurane anesthesia in patients with and without renal failure. *Br J Anaesth* 1992; 71:222.

74. Khuenl-Brady KS, Pomaroli A, Pühringer F, et al: The use of rocuronium bromide (ORG 9426) in patients with chronic renal failure. *Anaesthesia* 1993; 48:873.

75. Boucher BA, Witt WO, Foster TS: The postoperative adverse effects of inhalational anesthetics. *Heart Lung* 1986; 15:63.

76. Crowhurst JA, Rosen M: General anaesthesia for caesarean section in severe preeclampsia: Comparison of the renal and hepatic effects of enflurane and halothane. *Br J Anaesth* 1984; 56:587.

77. Mazze RI, Trudell JR, Cousins MJ: Methoxyflurane metabolism and renal dysfunction: Clinical correlation in man. *Anesthesiology* 1971; 35:247.

78. Mazze RI, Calverly RK, Smith NT: Inorganic fluoride nephrotoxicity: Prolonged enflurane and halothane anesthesia in volunteers. *Anesthesiology* 1977; 46:265.

79. Gelman S, Fowler KC, Smith LR: Regional blood flow during isoflurane and halothane anesthesia. *Anesth Analg* 1984; 63:557.

80. Koblin DD, Eger EI II, Johnson BH, et al: I-653 resists degradation in rats. *Anesth Analg* 1988; 67:534.

81. Eger EI II: Inhaled anesthetics: A look into the future. Presented at IARS 63rd Congress, 1989 Review Course Lectures pp 91-93.

82. Davis FM, Laurenson VG: Spinal anaesthesia or general anaesthesia for emergency surgery in elderly patients. *Anaesth Intensive Care* 1981; 9:352.

83. Davison JM: Renal transplantation and pregnancy. *Am J Kidney Dis* 1987; 9:374.

84. Whetam JCG, Cardella C, Harding M: Effect of pregnancy on graft function and graft survival in renal cadaver transplant patients. *Am J Obstet Gynecol* 1983; 145:193.

85. Davison JM, Lindheimer MD: Pregnancy in women with renal allografts. *Semin Nephrol* 1984; 4:240.

86. Schoenike SL, Kaldenbaugh HH, Kaplan AM, et al: Transient hypoparathyroidism in an infant of a mother with a renal transplant. *Am J Dis Child* 1978; 132:530.

87. Chatterjee SN, Fiala M, Weiner J, et al: Primary cytomegalovirus and opportunist infections: Incidence in renal transplant recipients. *JAMA* 1980; 240:2446.

88. Shaw BW, Wood RP: Immunosuppressive therapy in organ transplantation, in Gelman S (ed): *Anesthesia and Organ Transplantation.* Philadelphia, WB Saunders, 1987, pp 38-39.

89. Cockburn J, Moar VA, Ounsted M, et al: Final report of study on hypertension during pregnancy: The effects of specific growth and development of the children. *Lancet* 1982; 1:647.

90. Naden RP, Redman CWG: Antihypertensive drugs in pregnancy. *Clin Perinatol* 1985; 12:521.

91. Gallery EDM, Saunders DM, Hunyor SN, et al: Randomized comparison of methyldopa and oxprenolol for treatment of hypertension in pregnancy. *Br Med J* 1979; 1:1591.

92. Lamming GD, Broughton-Pipkin F, Symonds EM: Comparison of the alpha and beta blocking drug labetalol and methyldopa in the treatment of moderate and severe pregnancy-induced hypertension. *Clin Exp Hypertens* 1980; 2:865.

93. Redman CWG: *The Investigation of Labetalol in the Management of Hypertension in Pregnancy.* Princeton, NJ, Excerpta Medica, 1982; pp 101-110.

94. Flowers CE, Grizzle JE, Easterling WE, et al: Chlorothiazide as a prophylaxis against toxemia of pregnancy: A double blind study. *Am J Obstet Gynecol* 1962; 84:919.

95. Weseley AC, Douglas GW: Continuous use of chlorothiazide for the prevention of toxemia in pregnancy. *Obstet Gynecol* 1962; 19:355.

96. Pipkin FB, Turner SR, Symonds EM: Possible risk with captopril in pregnancy: Some animal data. *Lancet* 1980; 1:1256.

97. Ulmsten U: Treatment of normotensive and hypertensive patients with preterm labor using oral nifedipine, a calcium antagonist. *Arch Gynecol* 1984; 236:69.

98. Ducsay CA, Thompson JS, Wu At, et al: Effects of calcium entry blockers (nicardipine) tocolysis in rhesus macaques: Fetal plasma concentrations and cardiorespiratory changes. *Am J Obstet Gynecol* 1987; 157:1482.

99. Lau RJ, Scott JR: Pregnancy following renal transplantation. *Clin Obstet Gynecol* 1985; 28:339.

100. Korsch BM, Klein JD, Negrete VF, et al: Physical and psychological follow-up of offspring of renal allograft recipients. *Pediatrics* 1980; 65:275.

101. Sarrikoski S, Seppala M: Immunosuppression during pregnancy: Transmission of azathioprine and its metabolites from mother to fetus. *Am J Obstet Gynecol* 1973; 115:1100.

102. Weil R, Barfield N, Shroter GPJ, et al: Children of mothers with kidney transplant. *Transplant Proc* 1985; 17:1569.

103. Davison JM, Dellagrammatikas, Parkin JM: Maternal azathioprine therapy and depressed hemopoiesis in the babies of renal allograft recipients. *Br J Obstet Gynaecol* 1985; 92:233.

104. Ross WB, Richard T, Williams GL, et al: Cyclosporine and pregnancy. *Transplantation* 1988; 45:1142.

105. Venkataramanan R, Koneru B, Wang CC, et al: Cyclosporine and its metabolites in mother and baby. *Transplantation* 1988; 46:468.

106. Ryffel B, Donatsch P, Madorin M, et al: Toxicologic evaluation of cyclosporin-A. *Arch Toxicol* 1983; 53:107.

107. Kaskel FJ, Devarajan P, Arbiet LA, et al: Cyclosporine nephrotoxicity: Sodium excretion, autoregulation and angiotensin II. *Am J Physiol* 1987; 252:F733.

108. Chapman ST: Prescribing in pregnancy: Bacterial infections in pregnancy. *Clin Obstet Gynecol* 1986; 13:397.

109. Tilney NL, Lazarus JM: Acute renal failure in surgical patients. *Surg Clin North Am* 1983; 63:357.

110. Humes HD: Role of calcium in pathogenesis of acute renal failure. *Am J Physiol* 1986; 250:F579.

111. Miller TJ, Anderson RJ, Linas SL, et al: Urinary diagnostic indices in acute renal failure. *Ann Intern Med* 1978; 89:47.

112. Anderson RJ, Gabow PA, Gross PA: Urinary chloride concentration in acute renal failure. *Miner Electrolyte Metab* 1984; 10:92.

113. Humes HD: Aminoglycoside nephrotoxicity. *Kidney Int* 1988; 33:900.
114. Clive DM, Stoff JS: Renal syndromes associated with non steroidal antiinflammatory drugs. *N Engl J Med* 1984; 310:563.
115. Linton AL, Clark WQF, Driedger AA, et al: Acute interstitial nephritis due to drugs: Review of the literature with a report of nine cases. *Ann Intern Med* 1980; 93:735.
116. Appel GB, Kunis CL: Acute tubulointerstitial nephritis, in Brenner BM, Stein JH (eds): *Contemporary Issues in Nephrology.* Vol 4: *Tubulo-Interstitial Nephropathies.* New York, Churchill Livingstone, 1983, pp 151-185.
117. Warren S, Blantz R: Mannitol. *Arch Intern Med* 1981; 141:493.
118. Battaglia F, Prkystowsky H, Smisson C, et al: Fetal blood studies. XIII. The effect of administration of fluids intravenously to mothers upon the concentrations of water and electrolytes in plasma of human fetuses. *Pediatrics* 1960; 25:2.
119. Bruns PD, Linder RO, Drose VE, et al: The placental transfer of water from fetus to mother following the intravenous infusion of hypertonic mannitol to the maternal rabbit. *Am J Obstet Gynecol* 1963; 86:160.
120. Eneas JF, Schoenfeld PY, Humphreys MH: The effect of mannitol-bicarbonate infusion on the clinical course of myoglobinuria. *Arch Intern Med* 1979; 139:801.
121. Fink M: Are diuretics useful in the treatment of prevention of acute renal failure? *South Med J* 1982; 75:329.
122. Anderson RJ, Linas SL, Berns AS, et al: Nonoliguric acute renal failure. *N Engl J Med* 1977; 296:1134.
123. Schrier RW, Arnold PE, Van Putten J: Cellular calcium in ischemic acute renal failure: Role of calcium entry blockers. *Kidney Int* 1987; 32:313.
124. Conger JD: The use of prophylactic dialysis in acute renal failure. *Contemp Dial* 1980; 1:36.
125. Gregory IC: Anaesthesia and the kidney, in Churchill-Davidson HC (ed): *A Practice of Anaesthesia.* Philadelphia, WB Saunders, 1978, pp 1242.
126. Schrier RW: Acute renal failure. *Kidney Int* 1979; 15:205.
127. Goldstein MB: Acute renal failure. *Med Clin North Am* 1983; 67:1325.
128. Rosenthal MH: Heart-lung-kidneys: Management interrelationships. American Society of Anesthesiologists, 34th Annual Refresher Course Lectures and Clinical Update Program, Atlanta, 1983, p 106.
129. Hanley MJ, Davidson K: Prior mannitol and furosemide infusion in a model of ischemic acute renal failure. *Am J Physiol* 1981; 241:F556.
130. de Torrente A, Miller PD, Cronin RE, et al: Effects of furosemide and acetylcholine in norepinephrine-induced acute renal failure. *Am J Physiol* 1978; 235:F131.
131. Brown CB, Ogg CS, Cameron JS: High dose furosemide in acute renal failure: A controlled trial. *Clin Nephrol* 1981; 15:90.
132. Kleinknecht D, Ganeval D, Gonzalez-Duque LA, et al: Furosemide in acute oliguric renal failure. *Nephron* 1976; 17:51.
133. Shin B, Mackenzie CF, McAslan C, et al: Postoperative renal failure in trauma patients. *Anesthesiology* 1979; 51:218.
134. Linder A: Synergism of dopamine and furosemide in diuretic-resistant, oliguric acute renal failure. *Nephron* 1983; 33:121.

14 Endocrine Disorders

Donald H. Wallace and *Larry C. Gilstrap III*

The obstetric anesthesiologist is alerted to the potential for complications when the obstetrician requests consultation for a pregnant woman with an endocrine disorder. Clinical features of the individual pregnancy and endocrine disorder often point to the pathophysiologic alterations that signal end-organ dysfunction. Hormone levels that are excessively high or low perioperatively may be hazardous, and even when replacement or other therapy achieves normal levels, abnormal responses to anesthesia and surgery do occur. Replacement therapy with synthetic hormone is guided by both measurement of blood levels and clinical response. A clinical record of body weight and cardiorespiratory parameters normal for the stage of pregnancy, absence of glucosuria, and history free of medication suggest absence of significant endocrine dysfunction. Advances in knowledge allow continual examination of the safety of current practices for both mother and fetus in the presence of endocrine disorder.

Endocrine cells synthesize hormones that are polypeptides, proteins, iodinated thyronines, catecholamines, and melatonin from amino acids, and steroid hormones derived from cholesterol (Table 14-1). During transport in the blood (Fig. 14-1), there is binding of hormones to plasma proteins, especially of the steroid group and "other" group. There is dynamic equilibrium between the circulating concentrations of free and bound hormone:

$$\frac{[\text{Free hormone}]\,[\text{protein}]}{[\text{Bound hormone}]} = K$$

where K is the dissociation constant. Circulation of stored hormone limits the effects of inactivating systems in the blood and ensures the availability of free hormone at the target cell receptor. Free hormone binds to the target cell and serves as the "first messenger" or "key" of a "lock" of membrane receptor protein with specific sites for hormone binding.

Feedback mechanisms (Fig. 14-2) allow rapid fine tuning so that release of hormone is matched to target tissue requirements. Direct negative (metabolite) feedback regulates insulin and blood glucose levels, and a change in these levels affects the rate of secretion of insulin. Hypothalamus-pituitary-target organs systems are tightly coordinated so that hormonal signals from the hypothalamus stimulate or inhibit secretion of distinct anterior pituitary cells, responsible for secretion of a specific hormone.[1] In contrast to the secretion of most anterior pituitary hormones by stimulating hormones, prolactin secretion is tonically inhibited by dopamine. From the central nervous system (CNS) hypothalamus indirect or long-loop negative feedback controls release of adenohypophyseal hormones that stimulate the secretion of thyroid hormones, adrenocortical hormones, and gonadal hormones (GHs). There is direct negative feedback controlling the release of adenohypophyseal hormone. Short-loop negative feedback controls release of adenohypophyseal hormones, with the hypothalamus producing, releasing and inhibiting hormones. Gonadal hormones and other adenohypophyseal hormones have short-loop negative feedback control of secretion of controlling hypothalamic hormones. Positive feedback mechanisms exist between female sex hormones and 17β-estradiol and progesterone, and gonadotropins follicle-stimulating hormone (FSH) and luteinizing hormone (LH). Intracellular feedback loops operate within endocrine cells such as the inhibition of thyroid hormone synthesis by iodide.

A hormone-receptor interaction may result in direct membrane effects, intracellular effects involving "second messenger" systems, and nuclear actions. Since the discovery that formation of cyclic adenosine monophosphate (cAMP) was the intermediate step between epinephrine-hepatic cell membrane receptor interaction and glycogenolysis in the liver,[2] other hormones have been shown to involve cAMP in one or more of their actions (Table 14-1). cAMP is formed from ATP by adenylate cyclase, which is membrane-bound. Coupling of a hormone receptor to an enzyme allows the hormonal signal to be greatly amplified. The three components of hormone-sensitive adenylate cyclate systems identified include the peptide hormone receptor, the coupling unit G, and

Table 14-1 Hormones synthesized by endocrine cells*†

Hormone	Structure	Principle site of synthesis	Target tissue with "2nd messenger" cAMP
GnRH	Polypeptide	Hypothalamus	Adenohypophysis
TRH	Polypeptide	Hypothalamus	Adenohypophysis
Somatostatin	Polypeptide	Hypothalamus	
FSH	Protein	Adenohypophysis	
LH	Protein	Adenohypophysis	Ovary, testis
GH	Protein	Adenohypophysis	
Prolactin	Protein	Adenohypophysis	
TSH	Protein	Adenohypophysis	Thyroid
ACTH	Polypeptide	Adenohypophysis	
ADH	Polypeptide	Neurohypophysis	Kidney
Oxytocin	Polypeptide	Neurohypophysis	
T_3	Other	Thyroid	
T_4	Other	Thyroid	
CT	Polypeptide	Thyroid	
PTH	Polypeptide	Parathyroids	Kidney, bone
$1,25\text{-}(OH)_2D_3$	Steroid	Kidneys	
Epinephrine	Other	Adrenal medulla	Liver, adipose tissue
Norepinephrine	Other	Adrenal medulla	
Aldosterone	Steroid	Adrenal cortex	
Cortisol	Steroid	Adrenal cortex	
17 β-Estradiol	Steroid	Gonads, placenta	
Progesterone	Steroid	Gonads, placenta	
Testosterone	Steroid	Gonads	
Insulin	Polypeptide	Pancreatic islets	
Glucagon	Polypeptide	Pancreatic islets	Liver, adipose tissue
Melatonin	Other	Pineal	
Gastrin	Polypeptide	Stomach	
PGs	Other	Various	

*Adapted from Laycock J, Wise P: *Essential Endocrinology,* ed 2. New York, Oxford Medical Publications, 1983.
†cAMP = cyclic adenosine monophosphate; GnRH = gonadotropin-releasing hormone; TRH = thyrotropin-releasing hormone; FSH = follicle-stimulating hormone; LH = luteinizing hormone; GH = gonadal hormone; TSH = thyroid-stimulating hormone; ACTH = adrenocorticotropic hormone; ADH = antidiuretic hormone; T_3 = triiodothyroinine; T_4 = thyroxine; CT = cortical hormone; PTH = parathyroid hormone; $1,25(OH)_2D_3$ = dihydroxycholecalciferol; PG = prostaglandin.

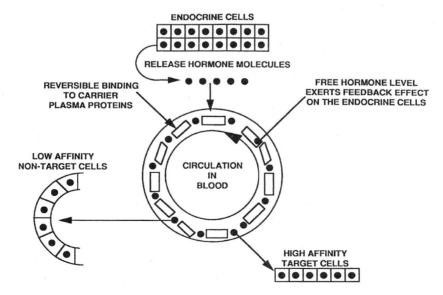

Fig. 14-1 Endocrine cells during transport in the blood. (Adapted from Laycock J, Wise P: *Essential Endocrinology,* ed 2. New York, Oxford Medical Publications, 1983.)

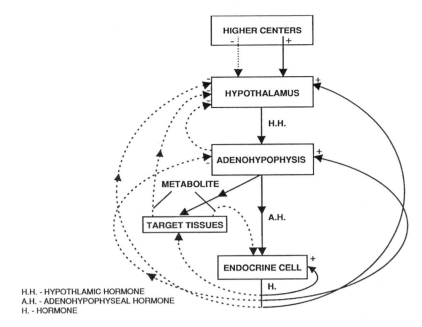

Fig. 14-2 Negative and positive feedback control of hormone synthesis/release. (Adapted from Laycock J, Wise P: *Essential Endocrinology*, ed 2. New York, Oxford Medical Publications, 1983.)

catalytic cyclase[3] (C). The hormone receptor does not act directly with the catalytic cyclase; it interacts with the coupling unit,[4] and G is activated only when GTP is bound, forming active hormone-receptor-G protein-GTP complex which then binds to catalytic cyclase to activate this enzymatic formation of cAMP. G is inactive when GDP is bound, and formation of hormone-receptor-G increases removal of inhibitory GDP and facilitates (preferential) binding of GTP. GTP hydrolysis to GDP, which results in a conformational change of G unable to bind to C, reverses the activation of adenylate cyclase. Steroid hormones penetrate the cell membrane, and there are specific cytoplasmic receptors that are protein molecules. The steroid-receptor complexes so formed appear able to influence protein synthesis at the nuclear level. Cortisol and estrogens also stimulate protein synthesis at the nuclear level. Cortisol and estrogens stimulate protein synthesis mainly at the transcription stage, and other hormones act at nuclear level at the translation stage.

Transport of hormones to a specific target DNA segment is possibly illustrated by progesterone-receptor complexes. The progesterone receptor is a dimeric molecule comprised of two subunits, A and B. After entering the cell nucleus, subunit B of the dimer binds to a specific nonhistone protein on the DNA. Dissociation of the subunits allows subunit A to attach to a sequence of DNA located near to the specific nonhistone protein. The binding of subunit A may initiate binding of RNA polymerase to the DNA segment, and it is possible that this is necessary for synthesis of mRNA molecules, the first stage in synthesis of new protein on the cytoplasmic free ribosomes for intracellular proteins, and on the rough endoplasmic reticulum for secretory proteins.

Endocrine function of the placenta includes striking increase in formation of steroid hormones. Of the steroids (estrogens and progesterone) produced in the placenta, 90% enter maternal blood and 10% enter fetal blood. Placental production of hormones also includes human placental lactogen (HPL), human chrorionic gonadotropin (HCG), chorionic adrenocorticotropics (ACTH), human chorionic thyrotropin (HCT), and hypothalamic-like releasing and inhibiting hormones (thyrotropin-releasing hormone [TRH], gonadotropin-releasing hormone [GnRH], luteinizing hormone releasing hormone [LHRH], corticotropin-releasing factor [CRF], and somatostatin). Plasma levels of renin, angiotensinogen, and angiotensin II are greatly elevated.

Variations in the circulating levels of hormone have been focused on as the primary factor determining both the concentration of hormone in body fluids and the formation of the hormone receptor complex causing biological activity. The receptor is also subject to extensive regulation, like the control of hormone synthesis, secretion, and transport. The importance of the receptor in the formation of active hormone receptor complex is shown when decrease in a specific receptor results in a deficiency state, despite the presence of normal or supranormal concentrations of hormones in those patients. Also, increases in receptor concentrations in the presence of normal circulating levels of hormone may result in an endocrine excess state.

It is not uncommon for clinicians to encounter a pregnant woman with an endocrine disorder. In women of childbearing years the most common endocrinopathy is diabetes mellitus. Glucose homeostasis involves balance between glucose production by the liver and peripheral uptake/utilization by peripheral tissue, especially muscle. From the beta cell regulator of the system, insulin release is adjusted so that this balance of glucose supply and peripheral uptake achieves euglycemia. However, plasma concentrations of insulin are frequently supranormal if impaired glucose tolerance exists, suggesting resistance to the action of insulin is responsible for the impaired glucose tolerance. Apparent insensitivity to insulin is associated in part with the obesity that often accompanies noninsulin-dependent diabetes mellitus (NIDDM).[5] Manifestations of the insulin-resistance syndrome also include hypertension, dyslipidemia, and coronary, cerebral, and peripheral artery disease.[6] The pathogenesis of NIDDM remains unclear[7]; glucose production increases, clearance of glucose from the circulation falls, and insulin release after meals is slowed.[8] Currently, associations are being sought between hyperglycemia, hypertension, and insulin resistance, which are characteristic of NIDDM, and polymorphisms in candidate genes. Insulin receptor expression may be down-regulated in skeletal muscle and adipocytes, leading to insulin resistance in severe obesity.[9] Interestingly, pharmacologic correction of insulin resistance has been achieved in the obese[10]; this also induced a small but significant reduction in blood pressure.

Resistance to thyroid hormone[11] is linked to abnormalities in the T_3-receptor-B gene.[12] The degree of hypothyroidism correlates with the magnitude of elevation of the serum cholesterol, with decreased clearance of cholesterol caused by decrease in LDL receptors. In hypothyroid patients the elevation of serum LDL cholesterol concentration and response to thyroxine treatment are strongly correlated with the genotype of the LDL-receptor gene.[13] Basic mechanisms regulated or influenced by T_3 include cardiac function, lipid me-

tabolism, pituitary hormone secretion, and neural development. In pregnant women fetal and maternal thyroid physiologies differ, but these interact by means of the placenta and amniotic fluid, [14] with resulting modulation including transfer to the fetus of iodine and small but important amounts of thyroid hormone. Currently, the role of thyroid hormones in fetal growth and development remains unclear. With greater understanding of the disease process, it is anticipated that therapy for Graves' disease will allow modulation of the disease, more so than current therapies, which effectively reduce synthesis and secretion of thyroid hormones. Although current therapies depend on remission of Graves' disease, advances in knowledge of hyperthyroidism are expected following the recent cloning of the TSH receptor.[15] Better knowledge of interactions between these receptors or other thyroid antigens and the immune system is needed.[16] There has long been recognition of the integration of homeostatic mechanisms by the nervous and endocrine systems, with recent information about neuroendocrine interaction with the immune system to adapt to infection, inflammation, and tissue injury. Findings that link immune and neuroendocrine function provide explanations for the response of the pituitary and adrenal glands to infection and inflammation, as well as for the alterations in pituitary-thyroid and pituitary-gonadal function that occur in patients with nonendrocine disease.[17] Cytokines secreted locally in most endocrine tissues exert paracrine regulatory effects in response to circulating toxins and cytokines; circulating cytokines have inhibiting actions on the hypothalamus, pituitary, and target glands reducing pituitary-thyroid and pituitary-gonadal function. In addition, adrenal disease and diseases of the pituitary present endocrine disorders of a significant challenge to the anesthesiologist and obstetrician caring for these women.

In summary, etiologies of endocrine disorders (Fig. 14-3) include biosynthesis disorder, target-cell receptor defects, and failure of feedback control. Altered inactivation may follow increased enzyme induction of the P-450 microsomal system by drugs and chemicals administered to treat a disorder, leading to unwanted side effects. Autoimmune disease and antibodies to thyroid cell components cause excessive thyroid hormone production in Graves' disease, and decreased hormone production in autoimmune thyroiditis and adrenalitis. Ectopic hormone syndromes associated with excessive production of hormones by tumors include antidiuretic hormone (ADH) and oatcell bronchial carcinoma, ectopic thyrotropin, and frequently choriocarcinoma and occasionally bron-

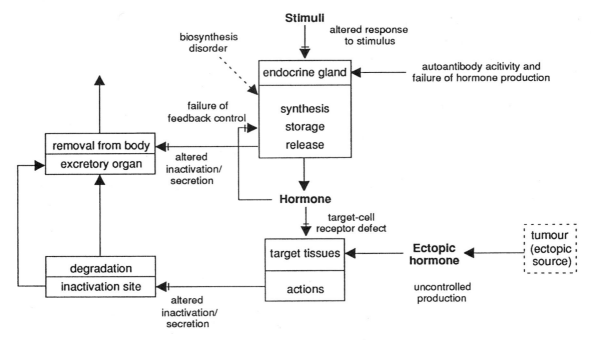

Fig. 14-3 Etiologies of endocrine disorders. (Adapted from Laycock J, Wise P: *Essential Endocrinology*, ed 2. New York, Oxford Medical Publications, 1983.)

chogenic carcinoma. Benign endocrine tumors affecting multiple organs have recently been classified into two major groups, multiple endocrine adenomatosis (MEA) types 1 and 2. In addition, there are autoimmune polyendocrine deficiency states.

DIABETES MELLITUS

It is now well accepted that pregnancy exerts certain diabetogenic effects. For example, there is increased insulin resistance during pregnancy that is probably related to HPL and to estrogen and progesterone. Human placental lactogen has both a lipolytic and carbohydrate sparing effect. There is also a paradoxical tendency to fasting hypoglycemia and ketonuria during pregnancy.

Since the advent of insulin in the early 1920s, there has been a significant improvement in perinatal and maternal morbidity and mortality in pregnancies complicated by diabetes. Before this time, infertility was the rule and maternal and fetal mortality were high.[18]

Incidence

The exact incidence of diabetes complicating pregnancy is not known, especially if one considers gestational diabetes or diabetes appearing or diagnosed for the first time during pregnancy. Although some recommend routine screening for all pregnant women for gestational diabetes,[19] others recommend screening only for certain at-risk women.[20] If only patients with risk factors (see Box 14-1)

BOX 14-1   RECOMMENDATIONS FOR SCREENING PREGNANT WOMEN FOR GESTATIONAL DIABETES[4]

All women*
Only women at risk
　Previous unexplained stillbirth
　Family history of diabetes
　Previous macrosomic infant
　Previous unexplained malformed infant
　Women 30 years of age and older
　Presence of glucosuria or hypertension

---

*No unanimity of opinion. See text.

are screened for gestational diabetes, it is estimated that 50% or more of patients will be missed.[21] Currently there is no unanimity of opinion regarding universal versus selective screening. The American College of Obstetricians and Gynecologists has recently suggested that selective screening for gestational diabetes may be appropriate in some clinical settings such as teen clinics, while universal screening may be more appropriate for populations with a high risk for gestational diabetes.[20] In certain populations, such as native Americans, the prevalence of diabetes is so high that screening is not necessary and these women should simply have a diagnostic test as discussed below.[20]

It is estimated that diabetes complicates[18] 2% to

Table 14-2 Classification of diabetes complicating pregnancy*

Class	Age onset (yr)	Duration (yr)	Vascular disease	Therapy
	Progestational diabetes			
A	Any	Any	None	A-1, diet only
B	Over 20	Less than 10	None	Insulin
C	10 to 19 or	10 to 19	None	Insulin
D	Before 10 or	More than 20	Benign retinopathy	Insulin
F	Any	Any	Nephropathy	Insulin
R	Any	Any	Proliferative retinopathy	Insulin
H	Any	Any	Heart disease	Insulin

Class	Fasting plasma glucose		Postprandial plasma glucose
	Gestational diabetes		
A-1	Less than 105 mg/dL	and	Less than 120 mg/dL
A-2	More than 105 mg/dL	and/or	More than 120 mg/dL

*From American College of Obstetricians and Gynecologists: *ACOG Technical Bulletin*, no. 92, May 1986. Used by permission.

3% of all pregnancies and that 90% of all cases of diabetes during pregnancy are gestational.[20] The incidence for pregestational or insulin-dependent diabetes mellitus (IDDM) in pregnancy[19] is less than 1% (0.1% to 0.5%).

Classification. Diabetes is generally classified as either insulin-dependent (Type 1) or as non–insulin-dependent (Type 2). In gestational diabetes, diabetes is first diagnosed during pregnancy. Although there is less than unanimity of opinion regarding the clinical utility of the Priscilla White classification system,[20] it is still commonly used (shown in Table 14-2). Pregnancy outcome is related to age of onset and duration of diabetes as well as the presence or absence of the vascular diseases outlined. Patients with preexisting vascular diseases are especially at risk for development of pregnancy-induced hypertension or preeclampsia. It would also appear that the degree of metabolic or glucose control is also related to neonatal morbidity and mortality.[20]

Diagnosis. Since the diabetogenic effects of pregnancy are generally maximized in the second half of pregnancy, screening is begun at 24 to 28 weeks' gestation.[20,21] Women with a history of gestational diabetes may actually benefit from earlier screening; such women should be retested at 24 to 28 weeks if the initial screen is negative or normal.[20] Initial screening should be performed with a 50-g oral glucose load followed by a plasma glucose determination 1 hour later.[20,21] Values in excess of 140 mg/dL are considered abnormal and are an indication for a 3-hour glucose tolerance test (GTT).[20-23] The normal values for the 3-hour GTT are summarized in Table 14-3.[20,21,24] The diagnosis of diabetes is based on two abnormal values.

Table 14-3 Three-hour oral glucose tolerance test[4,5,6]

	Whole blood (mg%)	Plasma (mg%)
Fasting	90	105
1 hr	165	190
2 hr	145	165
3 hr	125	145

Class A diabetes is based on two abnormal values with a normal fasting blood sugar. Gestational diabetes with fasting hyperglycemia is generally designated as A-2 diabetes (Table 14-2).

Adverse effects. The major adverse effect of gestational diabetes with fasting euglycemia is macrosomia (birth weight >4500 g) with the attendant risk of shoulder dystocia and need for operative delivery.[20] However, the perinatal mortality in this group of patients approaches that of the general population.

Insulin-dependent diabetes, on the other hand, may be associated with significant perinatal morbidity and mortality as well as maternal morbidity. Mothers with IDDM have a threefold to fourfold increased risk of pregnancy-induced hypertension. During the first half of pregnancy, these patients are more likely to experience hypoglycemia (secondary to hyperemesis), while in the latter half of pregnancy they are more prone to ketoacidosis. They are also at increased risk of developing urinary tract infections. These mothers are also much more likely to delivery prematurely and to be delivered by cesarean section. In a review of the literature from 1965 to 1985 of pregnancy compli-

Table 14-4 Maternal complications according to diabetic classification†

| Complication* | Classification | | |
	Gestational (%)	B, C (%)	D, F, R (%)
Pregnancy-induced hypertension	10	8	16
Ketoacidosis	0	8	7
Pyelonephritis	4	2	5
Hydramnios	5	18	19
Preterm labor	0	8	8
Cesarean section	20	42	58

†Adapted from Cousins L: Pregnancy complications among diabetic women: Review 1965-1985. *Obstet Gynecol Surv* 1987; 42(3):140.
*All complications significantly different ($p < 0.05$) except for pyelonephritis ($p = $ NS).

cations among diabetic women, Cousins found that the risk of pregnancy-induced hypertension was significantly increased in classes D, F, and R diabetic patients over nondiabetic patients (Table 14-4).[25]

The adverse effects of IDDM on the fetus and newborn are summarized as follows:[20]

· Fetal death
· Congenital malformation
· Macrosomia
· Hypoglycemia
· Respiratory distress syndrome
· Hypocalcemia
· Hyperbilirubinemia
· Polycythemia

Of all the various complications, congenital malformations are associated with the highest frequency of both morbidity and mortality. Pregnant women with IDDM have a twofold to threefold increased risk over the general population of having a baby with a congenital malformation. Common malformations include neural tube defects (anencephaly and spina bifida), cardiac defects, skeletal defects (caudal regression syndrome), renal anomalies, and gastrointestinal anomalies. There have been published reports that poor diabetic control preconceptually and during the first trimester may be related to the increase in the malformation rate seen in infants of mothers with IDDM and that tight control to achieve euglycemia may decrease the risk.[20,26,27,28] Unfortunately, recent evidence does not support these findings.[29]

Patients with gestational diabetes and fasting euglycemia can be managed by diet alone consisting of 30 to 35 kcal/kg of ideal body weight. Approximately 50% of the calories should be from carbohydrates, 30% from fat, and 20% from protein.[19,20]

All pregnant women with IDDM should have multisystem evaluation at the start of pregnancy to include ophthalmologic evaluation, renal function tests, electrocardiogram, and a complete physical examination.

It is now generally accepted that diabetic control should be kept as close to euglycemic as possible, with fasting glucose levels between 50 to 105 mg/dL.[3] This is best accomplished through insulin and diet as outlined above. Oral hypoglycemic agents should not be utilized during pregnancy because they may cause fetal hyperinsulinemia and profound protracted neonatal hypoglycemia.[20] Generally, patients can be followed as outpatients every 1 to 2 weeks with hospitalization reserved for poor control or complications such as acute pyelonephritis. The condition of the fetus can be monitored periodically with serial ultrasound and either the nonstress test and/or the contraction stress test. Patients with an abnormality seen with any of these tests should be hospitalized for further evaluation and possible delivery, depending on gestational age.

Obstetric and anesthetic management. The timing of delivery is based on many factors, including gestational age, fetal lung maturity, and fetal status as determined by various tests of fetal well-being. Pregnant patients with gestational diabetes not requiring insulin can generally be allowed to go into spontaneous labor. The cesarean section rate is not much greater in these patients than in the general population. Sedation with small intravenous boluses of Demerol and Phenergan is frequently ordered by the obstetrician to supplement nonpharmacologic methods of pain control during early active labor.[30,31] When satisfactory pain relief is achieved by these methods, local infiltration and pudendal nerve blocks are utilized as needed for delivery.

Epidural analgesia has proved to be the "Cadil-

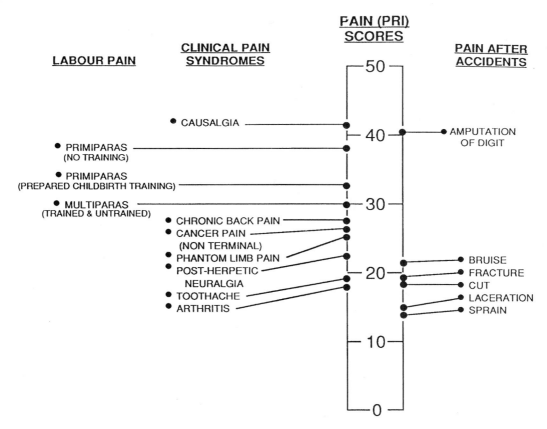

Fig. 14-4 Comparisons of severity of pain from various conditions. (From Melzack R: *Pain* 1984; 19:325.)

lac" of methods to control severe pain that nullipara or multipara parturients may experience during labor (Fig. 14-4). Severe pain during labor such as that from surgical stimulation causes afferent transmission of nociceptive information and stimulation of the hypothalamic-hypophyseal endocrine system. Unrelieved severe pain results in a maternal stress response accompanied by increased circulating levels of catecholamines that are counterregulatory and that oppose insulin activity and affect glucose homeostasis.[32] Regional anesthesia has been shown to advantageously decrease circulating levels of catecholamines,[33,34] and there is reduced potential for vasoconstriction of uteroplacental vessels causing critical reductions in uteroplacental blood flows in parturients with chronic uteroplacental insufficiency. Current practices of epidural anesthesia initiate a limited segmental block with incremental boluses of dilute local anesthetic solutions. Each 3-ml epidural bolus of 0.25% bupivacaine serves as a test dose, and gradual extension of the segmental block, which

includes sacral segments, occurs. Guidelines for epidural doses of selected agents (Table 14-5)[35] and for maintenance of a more selective block with continuous epidural infusions of dilute bupivacaine/fentanyl solutions[36] are useful in high-risk populations. In the diabetic population it is also essential to maintain euglycemia, to avoid aortocaval compression by adequate uterine tilt, and to measure brachial cuff pressures (NIBPs) frequently at the bedside. In addition, it is important to avoid the use of glucose-containing crystalloid solutions during acute hydration[37,38]; it is known too that if greater than 6g/70kg/hr of dextrose-containing solutions are administered, then neonatal hypoglycemia may result.[39,40] Even small boluses of intravenous fluids to minimize hypotension should be dextrose-free,[39] and ephedrine should be used prophylactically to avoid maternal hypotension.[38,41] Although there is potential for maternal hypotension during regional anesthesia, several evaluations of maternal, fetal, and neonatal effects support the choice of regional tech-

Table 14-5 Continuous epidural analgesia for labor and vaginal delivery

Local anesthetic	First dose* by height			Supplementary dose by height			Onset (min)	Duration (min)	Interval between doses (min)
	<5 ft 0 in	5 ft 0 in–5 ft 6 in	5 ft 6 in–6 ft 0 in (+)	<5 ft 0 in	5 ft 0 in–5 ft 6 in	5 ft 6 in–6 ft 0 in (+)			
Bupivacaine 0.25%	6	9	10-15	3	6	9	5-12	90-150	120
0.5%									
0.125% CIE† (range, 8-15 mL/hr)									
2-Chloroprocaine 2.0%	6	9	10-15	3	6	9	5-10	40-60	45-60
Lidocaine 1.5%	6	9	10-15	3	6	9	5-10	60-75	≈60

*Includes 3 mL local anesthetic test dose.
†CIE = continuous infusion epidural.

niques in this population.[38,41,42] Epinephrine-containing test doses[43] present limitations, including reliability in interpretation of the test in the pregnant population.[44,45] Although intravenous epinephrine was demonstrated to cause dose-related but transient decreases in uterine blood flow in pregnant laboratory animals,[46,47] there are concerns[45-47] for the parturient that epinephrine-containing local anesthetic solutions can cause reduction in uteroplacental blood flows[48] that increases the risk of uteroplacental insufficiency.

Combined spinal-epidural technique has been reported in nondiabetic parturients[49] requesting regional analgesia, who may not have time to achieve adequate epidural analgesia before delivery. Also, perineal pain may be rapidly and completely relieved by low-dose intrathecal plain 0.25% bupivacaine (5 mg). The epidural catheter is of value if analgesia must be prolonged, or to extend the block for operative delivery, or treat inadequate intrathecal block. Although hypotension occurred in 2 of 30 parturients, it responded to fluids and ephedrine[49]; it is recommended that the anesthesiologist closely monitor the parturient at the bedside for at least 30 minutes if this method is used. Other recent reports confirm selective analgesia of rapid onset may be accomplished by intrathecal injection of opioids,[50-53] the duration of analgesia being about 2 hours. Currently, reports are lacking on the use of these combined spinal-epidural methods for labor analgesia in the diabetic population. Further maternal hypotension observed with intrathecal sufentanil was comparable to that with intrathecal bupivacaine.[50] An important recommendation is that the anesthesiologist remain at the bedside for at least 30 minutes with monitoring of blood pressure and respiratory rate after intrathecal injection of opioid.

KETOACIDOSIS

Ketoacidosis is especially hazardous from both an obstetric and anesthetic standpoint. Although this complication is relatively uncommon in modern obstetrics, previously undiagnosed diabetic women may actually present for the first time with ketoacidosis during pregnancy. Ketoacidosis may result in both maternal and fetal mortality. Fetal loss may be as high as 50%.

It is of paramount importance to correct this serious metabolic derangement before the initiation of anesthesia and subsequent delivery. Treatment consists of correction of both dehydration (which is often pronounced) and hyperglycemia, as well as monitoring fetal status. Identification and correction of underlying causes such as infection or beta-agonist therapy is also important. One proto-

---

BOX 14-2 MANAGEMENT PROTOCOL FOR KETOACIDOSIS IN PREGNANCY

I. Hydration
   A. 1000 mL of 0.9% saline over 1 hr, 1000 mL over next 2 to 3 hrs
   B. Adjust rate according to urine output
   C. Change to D_5NS when glucose falls to less than 250 mg/dL
II. Correction of hyperglycemia
   A. Insulin 0.1 U/kg IV push
   B. Insulin 5 to 10 U/h infusion
   C. Reduce insulin to 1 to 2 U/h when glucose is <150 mg/dL
III. Correction of electrolyte and acidosis
   A. KCl 20 to 40 mEq/L to IV fluids when urine output adequate
   B. Sodium bicarbonate 44 mEq in IV fluids for arterial pH < 7.10
IV. Identify and correct underlying causes

Adapted from Clark SL, Cotton DB, Hankins GDV, et al: Diabetic ketoacidosis in pregnancy. In *Handbook of Critical Care Obstetrics.* Blackwell Scientific Publications, Oxford, 1994, pp 163-173.

BOX 14-3 PROTOCOL FOR CESAREAN DELIVERY IN THE DIABETIC WOMAN*

1. First surgical case in morning
2. Hold morning insulin
3. Two intravenous lines
   A. Balanced electrolyte solution (for hydration)
   B. Glucose-containing solution (125–150 mL/hr)
4. Preoperative antacids
5. Blood glucose and electrolytes before surgery
6. Regular insulin (5–10 U) intravenously as needed for significant hyperglycemia (i.e., blood sugar ≥200 mg/dL)

---

*Modified from Gilstrap LC, Hankins GDV: The high risk patient, in Phelan JP, Clark SL (eds): *Cesarean Delivery.* New York, Elsevier, 1988, p 161.

---

col for the management of diabetic ketoacidosis in pregnancy is summarized in Box 14-2.

PROTOCOL FOR CESAREAN DELIVERY IN THE DIABETIC WOMAN

For cesarean section, either regional anesthesia or general anesthesia is acceptable. The cesarean section rate, significantly increased for the patient with IDDM, ranges from approximately 50% to 80%.[55] The surgery should be scheduled as the first case in the morning. The usual morning insulin should be withheld (Box 14-3) and the patient should be managed with a sliding scale following delivery (Table 14-6). All gravidas receive antacid prophylaxis with nonparticulate antacid,[56-58] uterine tilt if in the supine position, and 100% oxygen via clear face mask for preoxygenation.[59]

Since hypotension is common during regional anesthesia, a preload with 1 to 2 L of crystalloid and the prophylactic use of ephedrine is needed to minimize this problem. Continuous epidural anesthesia established by incremental epidural boluses (3 to 5 mL) of 2-chloroprocaine (3%), lidocaine (2%), or bupivacaine (0.5%) gradually raises the cephalad spread of segmental block to a T_4 level. We prefer the ice test initially to detect as early as possible the loss of temperature discrimination secondary to sympathetic blockade. The onset of hypotension is immediately observed when blood pressure is measured noninvasively each minute, and it is our practice to continually display the systolic and diastolic pressures. It is also common practice in our institution to combine spinal and epidural methods of regional anesthesia. When monitoring systolic and diastolic pressure each minute by Dynamap, we have found no significant difference in the incidence of hypotension with epidural or combined spinal-epidural methods.[60]

In the combined single interspace technique,[61] lumbar puncture is performed with a long 25-gauge needle through a 17-gauge Tuohy needle previously placed in the epidural space by loss-of-resistance method. After injection of hyperbaric bupivacaine (12 mg, or 10.5 mg plus fentanyl 15 μg), the 25-gauge needle is withdrawn and the epidural catheter is secured in place. In the two-interspace technique, the epidural catheter is placed and the intrathecal injection is made separately through the adjacent midlumbar interspace. This combined method offers the advantages of rapid onset of surgical analgesia; minimum maternal blood levels and risk of serious local anesthetic toxicity; and reduced placental transfer of local anesthetic to the fetus. Supplementary epidural boluses of local anesthetic or opioid intraoperatively are available should surgery require an extended operative time. If intrathecal fentanyl (15 μg) is not administered, epidural fentanyl (50 to 100 μg) is given to increase intraoperative comfort and the duration of postoperative analgesia. If epidural morphine (Duramorph, 3.5 mg) is administered for long-duration pain control, we monitor vital signs in the extended care unit for at least 12 hours because of the risk of delayed onset of respiratory depression.

The steps for general anesthesia are summarized in Box 14-4. Monitoring inspired and end-tidal concentrations of physiologic and anesthetic gases by in-line medical mass spectrometer allows the obstetric anesthesiologist to control ventilation so

Table 14-6 Suggested sliding scale for postcesarean insulin injection in the diabetic mother*

Serum glucose†	Regular insulin (units)‡
150	0
150–200	2
200–250	4
250–300	6
300–350	8
>350	Consider insulin infusion pump

*From Gilstrap LC, Hankins GDV: The high risk patient, in Phelan JP, Clark SL (eds): *Cesarean Delivery.* New York, Elsevier, 1988, p 160. Used by permission.
†Checked every 4 hours.
‡Given subcutaneously.

BOX 14-4   STEPS FOR GENERAL ENDOTRACHEAL ANESTHESIA

Intravenous catheter, 18- or 16-gauge
Pressure bag to acutely infuse crystalloid
Administer antacid prophylaxis 15 to 60 min preinduction

Preinduction

Uterine displacement and preoxygenation (100%) via clear face mask
Blood pressure, pulse oximeter, and ECG monitors attached and checked
Screen placed to allow access for tracheal intubation
Abdomen prepared and draped
Cricoid cartilage identified
Assistant applies cricoid pressure before patient loses consciousness

Induction

Rapid sequence induction
Thiopental and succinylcholine
Cricoesophageal compression until tracheal intubation confirmed with inflated cuff seal

Inspired gas mixture

50% N_2O : 50% O_2
Enflurane 0.5%–1.0%, halothane 0.5%, or isoflurane 0.75% until delivery

Monitoring

Inspired and end-tidal concentrations of O_2, CO_2, N_2, and anesthetic gases (SARA, or equivalent systems)

Additional agents

Fentanyl or morphine after delivery
Decompress stomach with large-bore suction catheter
Maintain patient's relaxation
Monitor relaxation and limit dosage with the peripheral nerve stimulator
Extubate when awake

that oxygenation remains optimal and hypercarbia is avoided.[59] Good neonatal outcome is also associated with properly administered general anesthesia, which is essential when immediate delivery is indicated.

Diabetic patients have a greater incidence of delayed gastric emptying,[62] significant features of autonomic dysfunction including orthostatic hypotension, pulse rate variability, and sweat response. The diabetic stiff-joint syndrome[63] may be associated with difficulty in tracheal intubation by direct laryngoscopy. Failure to intubate the trachea following rapid sequence induction is an emergency managed by commencement of failure of intubation protocol[64] with the goal of restoring maternal oxygenation (Box 14-5 and Fig 14-5). Following restoration of maternal oxygenation and recovery of the mother, a period of intrauterine resuscitation allows the anesthesiologist and obstetrician to plan further management. A fiberoptic oral tracheal intubation with the patient awake and sedated may then be performed. The risk of serious epistaxis in the obstetric patient mandates careful preparation of the nasal airways if fiberoptic or blind nasal intubation is to be attempted. In addition to difficult intubation associated with stiff-joint syndrome in diabetic patients, the overall incidence of failed tracheal intubation in the obstetric population exceeds the incidence of difficult intubation in the general surgical population (approximately 1:500[66] vs. 1:2000[67]). The life-threatening "can't intubate, can't ventilate" situation is rare in the general surgical population (1:10,000 Benumof).[68] Further, 6 out of 8 anesthesia-related maternal deaths were due to difficult or failed tracheal intubation, as in the 1985-1987 Report on Confidential Enquiries into Maternal Deaths in England and Wales.[69] The

LMA as well as TTJV and the OTC have been recommended by the American Society of Anesthesiologists as nonsurgical techniques if an anesthetized patient cannot be intubated or mask-ventilated. The triple airways technique to clear the airways and restore ventilation and oxygenation requires the help of a third person to ventilate with 100% oxygen while others hold the face mask and apply jaw thrust to elevate the jaw and chin.[64] It has been recently suggested the LMA may be useful in failed obstetric intubation, with the note that hasty surgical attempt at tracheostomy or cricothyroidotomy has proved dangerous and time-consuming. Indeed, 3 of 10 anesthesia-related deaths in the 1982-1984 RCE[70] were associated with failed tracheostomy. An algorithm has been proposed,[71] and the LMA[71] has been reviewed for obstetric anesthesia and neonatal resuscitation, including its use as an airway intubator by fiberoptic and other methods. There is controversy concerning the need to release cricoid pressure during insertion of the LMA in some patients, and there has been report of difficulty during attempts to intubate the trachea through the LMA. A decision to perform spinal or epidural anesthesia is an often appropriate alternative. (See Chapter 20 for further information regarding diabetic parturients.)

THYROID DISEASE

The thyroid gland undergoes significant changes during pregnancy. Because of the increased vascularity and hyperplasia, the thyroid gland is readily palpable during pregnancy. There is also an increase in serum triiodothyronine (T_3) and thyroxine (T_4) levels as measured by radioimmunoassay (Table 14-7). Concomitant with the increase, the serum levels of thyroid-binding globulin (TBG) also increase, the net result being that the amount of actual free hormone is not significantly increased above that in the nonpregnant woman.[72]

Hypothyroidism

Incidence. Hypothyroidism is an uncommon complication of pregnancy because most women thus affected also suffer from infertility secondary to chronic anovulation. As of 1988, there had been

---

BOX 14-5   FAILED INTUBATION PROTOCOL

1. Help!
2. Maintain cricoesophageal compression
3. Left lateral position
4. Head-down tilt
5. Bag and mask with 100% oxygen
6. Improve airway if necessary by:
   A. Triple airway maneuver
   B. Release cricoid pressure
7. Airway?
   A. If clear, inhalational anesthesia; continue cricoesophageal compression
   B. If partially obstructed, LMA; continue 100% oxygen/assist ventilation/allow to recover
   C. If completely obstructed, transcricothyroid or transtracheal ventilation with 100% oxygen

Table 14-7 Changes in thyroid function during pregnancy*

Total T_4	Increased
Total T_3	Increased
Free T_4	Unchanged
Free T_3	Unchanged
TSH	Unchanged
TBG	Increased

T_4 = thyroxine; T_3 = triiodothyronine; TSH = thyroid-stimulating hormone; TBG = thyroid-binding globulin.

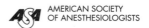

AMERICAN SOCIETY OF ANESTHESIOLOGISTS

DIFFICULT AIRWAY ALGORITHM

1. Assess the likelihood and clinical impact of basic management problems:

    A. Difficult intubation
    B. Difficult ventilation
    C. Difficulty with patient cooperation or consent

2. Consider the relative merits and feasibility of basic management choices:

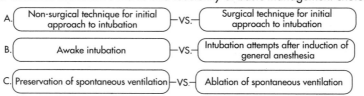

A. Non-surgical technique for initial approach to intubation —vs.— Surgical technique for initial approach to intubation

B. Awake intubation —vs.— Intubation attempts after induction of general anesthesia

C. Preservation of spontaneous ventilation —vs.— Ablation of spontaneous ventilation

3. Develop primary and alternative strategies:

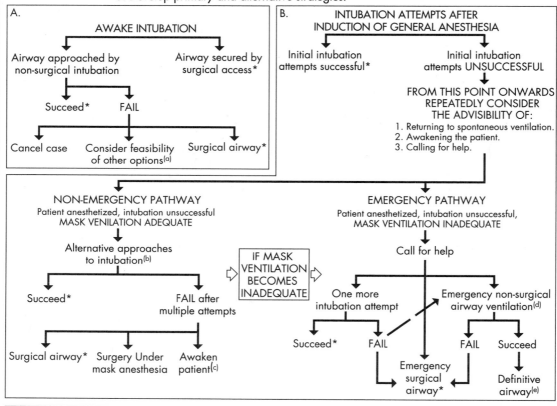

A. AWAKE INTUBATION

- Airway approached by non-surgical intubation
- Airway secured by surgical access*

Succeed* / FAIL

- Cancel case
- Consider feasibility of other options(a)
- Surgical airway*

B. INTUBATION ATTEMPTS AFTER INDUCTION OF GENERAL ANESTHESIA

- Initial intubation attempts successful*
- Initial intubation attempts UNSUCCESSFUL

FROM THIS POINT ONWARDS REPEATEDLY CONSIDER THE ADVISIBILITY OF:
1. Returning to spontaneous ventilation.
2. Awakening the patient.
3. Calling for help.

NON-EMERGENCY PATHWAY
Patient anesthetized, intubation unsuccessful
MASK VENILATION ADEQUATE

Alternative approaches to intubation(b)

Succeed* / FAIL after multiple attempts

- Surgical airway*
- Surgery Under mask anesthesia
- Awaken patient(c)

IF MASK VENTILATION BECOMES INADEQUATE

EMERGENCY PATHWAY
Patient anesthetized, intubation unsuccessful,
MASK VENTILATION INADEQUATE

Call for help

- One more intubation attempt
- Emergency non-surgical airway ventilation(d)

Succeed* / FAIL

FAIL / Succeed

Emergency surgical airway*

Definitive airway(e)

• CONFIRM INTUBATION WITH EXHALED CO_2

(a) Other options include (but are not limited to): surgery under mask anesthesia, surgery under local anesthesia infiltration or regional nerve blockade, or intubation attempts after induction of general anesthesia.

(b) Alternative appoaches to difficult intubation include (but are not limited to): use of different laryngoscope blades, awake intubation, blind oral or nasal intubation, fiberoptic intubation, intubating stylet or tube changer, light wand, retrograde intubation, and surgical airway access.

(c) See awake intubation.

(d) Options for emergency non-surgical airway ventilation include (but are not limited to): transtracheal jet ventilation, laryngeal mask ventilation, or esophageal-tracheal combitube ventilation.

(e) Options for establishing a definitive airway include (but are not limited to): returning to awake state with spontaneous ventilation, tracheotomy, or endotracheal intubation.

Fig 14-5 Difficult airway algorithm. (Courtesy American Society of Anesthesiologists.)

less than 100 cases of untreated hypothyroidism completing pregnancy reported.[73]

Etiology. Recently Davis and colleagues reported their findings in 16 pregnancies in 14 overtly hypothyroid women and 12 pregnancies in women with subclinical hypothyroidism.[73] The three most common etiologies of hypothyroidism in these 26 women were subtotal thyroidectomy (38%), treatment with radioiodine (27%), and primary hypothyroidism (27%).

Diagnosis. The diagnosis of hypothyroidism can be difficult to make during pregnancy since many normal pregnant women experience fatigue and tiredness and even hair loss. In the series reported by Davis et al,[73] the most common signs and symptoms included delayed deep tendon reflexes (69%), fatigue (44%), hair loss (44%), dry skin (38%), and brawny edema (19%).

The diagnosis of hypothyroidism can be confirmed by demonstrating a low T_4 uptake and a high thyroid-stimulating hormone (TSH) level. In the series by Davis et al,[73] the mean T_4 was 2.8 μg/dL (normal usually 8 to 16 μg/dL in pregnancy) and the mean TSH was 88 mIU/mL (normal <10 mIU/dL).

Effects on pregnancy. Women with hypothyroidism who do conceive have a higher frequency of spontaneous abortions and early pregnancy losses. In addition, as pointed out by Davis et al,[73] women with both overt and subclinical hypothyroidism may have an increased risk of preeclampsia, placental abruption, anemia, cardiac dysfunction, and postpartum hemorrhage. These authors also reported an increased risk in the frequency of low birth weight in infants, as well as increased perinatal morbidity and mortality.

Treatment. The treatment of hypothyroidism during pregnancy is essentially the same as for the nonpregnant patient (i.e., thyroid replacement). Synthroid, 0.1 mg per day, is generally satisfactory. Very little, if any, of this drug crosses the placenta and there are no known adverse fetal effects.

Obstetric and anesthetic management. In the otherwise uncomplicated pregnant patient, replacement therapy with Synthroid is monitored during the antepartum management. During labor it should be remembered that psychological support is to be maximized and that the hypothyroid parturient is at serious risk of respiratory depression with opioids. The stress of labor, similar to surgical stress, may unmask decreased adrenal cortex function if delivery cannot be delayed. Other serious end-organ effects include cardiomegaly, cardiomyopathy, conduction abnormalities with reductions in heart rate and stroke volume, and anemia. In addition to the typical myxedematous changes (puffy periorbital tissue, large tongue, and rough doughlike skin), pericardial effusion, pleural effusion, ascites, and peripheral edema may be present. When adequate replacement therapy has been accomplished, either regional or general anesthesia is satisfactory for operative delivery. If surgery cannot be delayed in the hypothyroid parturient, induction of anesthesia occurs with baroreceptor responses impaired and decrease of intravascular volume. At still greater risk is the patient with severe angina and severe hypothyroidism.

Emergency cesarean delivery under general anesthesia is conducted with careful attention to cardiorespiratory parameters. In-line mass spectrometry or equivalent monitoring at the bedside offers assurance that the hypothyroid patient is free of hypoxia and hypercarbia. Respiratory control mechanisms and the physiologic responses to hypoxia and hypercarbia are abnormal in the hypothyroid population, and we avoid these increased risks by using this noninvasive method of monitoring. When replacement therapy is considered adequate, rapid sequence induction with minimal doses of thiopentone or ketamine and succinylcholine is acceptable. In some hypothyroid patients nitrous oxide alone may result in unconsciousness. Minimal doses of opioids and benzodiazepines, as well as avoidance of volatile agents, are measures recommended for maintenance. Strict control of low doses of muscle relaxants by nerve stimulator monitoring is desirable because of the reduced skeletal muscle activity that characterizes hypothyroidism. Balanced electrolyte solutions should be infused because there is reduced free water clearance; central venous pressure (CVP) and other invasive monitoring may be indicated in the presence of hypovolemia and abnormal baroreceptor reflexes. Placental abruption and preeclampsia are additional serious risks in this population.

The onset of hypothyroidism is often insidious, whereas prior thyroid surgery or medical treatment warns of this possibility. Reduced β-adrenergic receptor populations, with a change to α-receptor from β-receptor function, is associated with reduced circulating levels of thyroid hormones.[74] Overall, anesthetic management focuses on critical myocardial and hemodynamic effects of depressant drugs during hypothyroidism, altered metabolism and inactivation of drugs, primary adrenal insufficiency, electrolyte and free water clearance abnormalities, hypoglycemia, delayed gastric emptying, and skeletal/respiratory muscle dysfunction. An altered conscious state and impaired ventilatory response to hypoxemia and coma are potentially life-threatening.

Hyperthyroidism

Incidence. Unlike hypothyroidism, hyperthyroidism is not an uncommon complication of pregnancy. It has been estimated to complicate 0.2%

of all pregnancies, and it may result in significant maternal and neonatal morbidity.[75] In a recent series reported by Davis et al, there were 60 cases of overt thyrotoxicosis in nearly 120,000 pregnant women for an incidence of 1 in 2000.[76]

Etiology. The most common etiology of thyrotoxicosis in pregnant women is Graves' disease.[75] Graves' disease appears to be an autoimmune disorder with the production of antibodies such as thyroid-stimulating antibodies and long-acting thyroid stimulator in some patients.[77] Other less common causes include hydatiformole, thyroiditis, and a toxic adenoma. It has been reported that women with Graves' disease frequently undergo remission during pregnancy and are at risk of exacerbation during the postpartum period.[75,78]

Diagnosis. The common signs and symptoms of hyperthyroidism are:

· Heat intolerance
· Nervousness
· Irritability and emotional lability
· Tachycardia
· Tremors
· Hyperreflexia
· Exophthalmos
· Goiter or enlarged thyroid
· Bruit

Some of these symptoms, such as fatigue and heat intolerance, may occur in normal pregnant women. Laboratory findings of hyperthyroidism include an elevated total T_3 and T_4 above the normal pregnancy elevations. The free thyroxine index, which corrects the T_4 for the elevated TBG seen in pregnancy, is also elevated. The T_3 resin uptake, which is normally low in pregnancy secondary to increased TGB, is normal or elevated in patients with hyperthyroidism. As expected, the TSH will be low.

Pathophysiology. As pointed out in a study by Davis et al,[76] pregnancy complications are directly related to the degree of metabolic control. In this series, there was an increased incidence of premature labor (22%) and stillbirths (10%). If premature labor does develop, β-adrenergic receptor agonists are contraindicated since they may precipitate thyroid storm.[79]

Maternal heart failure may also occur in uncontrolled thyrotoxicosis; it did occur in 12% of the patients in the study reported by Davis et al.[76]

An exaggerated hypermetabolic state of thyrotoxicosis, thyroid storm, fortunately rarely occurs during pregnancy and when it does occur, it is usually in the poorly controlled patient. Clinical signs and symptoms include high fever, tachycardia, agitation, and severe dehydration.[75] Thyroid storm, a serious life-threatening complication with up to 25% mortality, must be recognized and treated promptly.[75] It may be precipitated by a variety of factors such as infection, labor, or surgery such as cesarean section. The following is a summary of the treatment of thyroid storm[75,76,80]:

1. Intravenous hydration
2. Propylthiouracil: 1 g orally or through nasogastric tube, then 300 mg every 6 hours
3. Potassium iodide: 1 g orally or sodium iodine 0.5 : 1 g IV every 8 hours
4. Cooling blanket
5. Propranolol: 40 to 80 mg orally or 0.15 mg/kg intravenously
6. Acetaminophen 325 mg rectally every 3 hours
7. Hydrocortisone 100 mg IV every 8 hours
8. Treatment of infection or other precipitating cause
9. Electrocardiographic (ECG) monitoring
10. Transfer to intensive care unit

Neonatal thyrotoxicosis occurs in approximately 1% of newborns of mothers with Graves' disease[75]; it is caused by transplacental passage of thyroid-stimulating antibodies. It is generally transient in nature, lasting 1 to 3 months.

Treatment. The treatment of thyrotoxicosis in the nonpregnant patient includes radioactive iodine, surgery, or an antithyroid drug; however, radioactive iodine is contraindicated in pregnancy. Although surgery is a satisfactory choice during pregnancy, the most common therapy involves medical treatment with one of the thiomide drugs such as propylthiouracil (PTU) or methimazole. Both of these drugs cross the placenta and may cause hypothyroidism or goiter in the fetus if given in large enough doses over a long enough time. The most commonly used drug is PTU. Aplasia cutis has been reported in the newborns of mothers treated with methimazole; thus it is not recommended for use during pregnancy.[75] The usual starting dose of PTU is 100 to 150 mg every 8 hours (400 to 600 mg daily), after which the patient should be continued on the lowest possible dose to maintain a euthyroid or slightly hyperthyroid state.[75] Side effects of the thiomides include agranulocytosis, maternal hypothyroidism, or goiter formation, or hypothyroidism in the fetus.[75]

In the report by Davis et al,[76] doses larger than 600 mg per day were required in approximately one third of the patients, yet only 1 infant of 60 was hypothyroid. Those infants who do develop hypothyroidism or goiter generally respond satisfactorily to medical management without significant sequelae.

Obstetric and anesthetic management. Pregnant women with well-controlled hyperthyroidism generally tolerate labor without significant complications. Excessive anxiety and inadequate pain control during labor may activate the sympathetic nervous system, and early and judicious sedation is indicated. Pain during active labor can become severe (Fig. 14-4), and epidural analgesia should be initiated once active labor is established. The associated blockage of the sympathetic nervous system is advantageous; conduction blockade of the B fibers is restricted initially by limited segmental block, which extends gradually following 3 mL epidural boluses of bupivacaine 0.25%. Continuous epidural infusion of a dilute solution of bupivacaine (0.1% with fentanyl 2 µg/ml) maintains analgesia while minimizing motor blockade. There is potential for exaggerated circulatory responses to sympathomimetics. Acute hydration with 0.5 to 1.0 L of Ringer's lactate solution is recommended in an attempt to avoid hypotension. Should a vasopressor be required, 20 to 40 µg boluses of phenylephrine should be the pressor of choice, because adverse fetal effects have not been observed with these doses.[82] Excessive circulating thyroid hormones are associated with an increase in β-adrenergic receptors.[74] Epinephrine should not be added to local anesthetic solutions because of the risk of exaggerated circulatory responses in the thyrotoxic population.

Labor and/or delivery may rarely evoke thyroid storm in the poorly controlled or uncontrolled hyperthyroid patient (the management of such patients is explained in the section, Hyperthyroidism–Effects on Pregnancy). Propranolol reduces the peripheral effects of thyroid hormones on the cardiovascular system, and PTU reduces the synthesis of thyroid hormones, including those that follow administration of iodide. Steps to lower body temperature include infusion of cold crystalloid solutions, which also corrects dehydration. Rapid sequence induction with thiopentone and succinylcholine and balanced endotracheal anesthesia (see Box 14-4) avoids drugs such as ketamine[83] that stimulate the sympathetic nervous system. If there is exophthalmos, special care to protect the eyes is essential. Altered or accelerated drug metabolism is also possible in the hyperthyroid state. The advantages of isoflurane are that it is stable, it reduces adverse sympathetic nervous system responses, and it does not sensitize the myocardium to catecholamines. If the hyperthyroid patient has become euthyroid at the time of surgery, liver function tests have not been altered postoperatively by halothane or enflurane, which are more extensively metabolized.[84] Caution is indicated in use of these agents in the presence of skeletal muscle weakness, a frequent feature of hyperthyroidism. The peripheral nerve stimulator allows continual monitoring

to prevent overdosage and facilitate reversal with glycopyrrolate and neostigmine without excessive changes in the heart rate.

The anesthesiologist should evaluate the effectiveness of predelivery therapy planned to render the parturient euthyroid. Sudden exacerbations of the cardiovascular system abnormalities may reduce cardiac reserve and may increase the potential for arrhythmias. Other organ system compromise includes dehydration secondary to diarrhea, hypercalcemia, anemia, and thrombocytopenia. Propylthiouracil prevents incorporation of iodide into the tyrosine molecules of thyroglobulin. Propylthiouracil blocks deiodination of T_4 by the liver, and steroids also block the deiodination of T_4 to more potent T_3. In addition, there is a greater incidence of myasthenia gravis, which reinforces the cautious dosage and monitoring of neuromuscular blocking agents previously recommended. Significant enlargement of the thyroid gland can be associated with obstruction of the trachea or a bronchus. Emergency management of thyroid storm (see section on Hyperthyroidism–Effects on Pregnancy) includes vigorous hydration, selection and use of antithyroid agents, iodides, glucocorticoids, and β-adrenergic blocking agents. However, propranolol is contraindicated in the presence of congestive cardiac failure, bronchial asthma, and chronic obstructive pulmonary disease.

Excessive anxiety and activation of the sympathetic nervous system remain management issues in the awake hyperthyroid parturient, even with successful regional analgesia and sympathetic nervous system blockade. Sedation with increasing dosage of midazolam leads to loss of recall of delivery, greater risk of respiratory depression, and hazard of gastric acid aspiration, as well as increased transplacental transfer to the fetus.

Thyroid nodules

The presence of a solitary thyroid nodule during pregnancy presents a diagnostic dilemma because radionucleotide scanning is contraindicated during pregnancy. Because of this, fine-needle aspiration is recommended to rule out malignancy,[79] reported to occur in almost half of the women with solitary nodules.[85] If carcinoma is found, then surgery is indicated. Medullary thyroid carcinoma is usually associated with secretion of large amounts of calcitonin, and in combination with pheochromocytoma as an autosomal dominant disorder classified as multiple endocrine neoplasia (MEN), type 2.

Multiple endocrine neoplasia/adenomatosis

Two major groups (type 1 and type 2) have been identified, and the mode of inheritance of these syndromes appears to be autosomal dominant. Currently, no related histocompatibility types have been identified, and when one endocrine adenoma is identified the question of other adenomatosis type I (Wermer's syndrome) includes parathyroid adenoma or hyperplasia, pancreatic β-cell islet adenoma, pituitary adenoma, carcinoid syndrome, and adrenal cortical adenoma (Cushing's syndrome or hyperaldosteronism). Multiple endocrine adenomatosis type 2 (Sipple's syndrome) includes parathyroid adenoma or hyperplasia, pheochromocytoma, C cell tumors (medullary thyroid cell carcinoma, thymus, parathyroid), and associated multiple cutaneous and mucosal neuromas, neurofibromas, and ganglioneuromas.

Hyperparathyroidism

The literature includes about 100 cases of hyperparathyroidism complicating pregnancy,[79] and parathyroid storm characterized by hypercalcemia and convulsions has been reported among four cases described by Whalley.[86] Hyperemesis, weakness, renal calculi, pancreatitis, and psychiatric disorders are clinical features of hyperparathyroidism. Parathyroid adenoma and carcinoma and ectopic sites such as carcinoma of the lung, breast, and kidney secrete excessive parathyroid hormone (PTH), resulting in hypercalcemia. Hypertension and an electrocardiogram with short QT and prolonged PR intervals, the need for careful positioning because of osteoporosis, and risk of pathologic fractures are concerns when anesthesia is planned. Cautious use of neuromuscular blocking agents monitored by a peripheral nerve stimulator is essential. Emergency treatment of hypercalcemia is considered if plasma levels exceed 7.5 mEq/L; mithramycin (25 μg/kg over 4 hours) will reduce plasma levels in 12 to 36 hours. Because of polyuria and polydipsia, most patients are dehydrated, and 1 to 2 L of normal saline is given initially to replace lost volume, after which diuresis with furosemide and continued saline is given initially to replace lost volume, and measurement of serum electrolytes and magnesium levels are indicated. Neonatal tetany has led at times to a search identifying maternal parathyroid adenoma.[79]

ADRENAL GLAND DISEASE

Diseases of the adrenal gland are relatively uncommon during pregnancy. However, Addison's disease or adrenal insufficiency, Cushing's syndrome or excess glucocorticoid production, and pheochromocytomas or catecholamine-producing tumors have all been reported in pregnancy.

Addison's disease

Incidence. The exact incidence of Addison's disease is unknown, but it is sufficient to say that the disease is uncommon.

Etiology. Primary adrenal failure is known as Addison's disease. Adrenal insufficiency may also occur secondary to pituitary failure, adrenal destruction, and surgical removal. In the not too distant past, adrenal tuberculosis was not an uncommon cause of adrenal insufficiency.[87]

Pathophysiology and diagnosis. The signs, symptoms, and laboratory findings of adrenal insufficiency may point to a deficiency in both cortisol and aldosterone. The related findings in the former include hyperpigmentation, weakness, fatigue, nausea, hypotension, and hypoglycemia, while findings attributable to the latter include hyponatremia, hyperkalemia, and volume depletion.[88] Nausea, vomiting, weakness, fatigue, and hyperpigmentation are also common symptoms of normal pregnancy, which makes the diagnosis of Addison's disease difficult to determine during pregnancy.

Since plasma cortisol is increased in normal pregnancy (along with cortisol-binding globulin), the diagnosis of Addison's disease is based primarily on symptomatology and response to ACTH stimulation.[88] Patients with Addison's disease fail to show the expected rise in cortisol following ACTH administration.

Effects on pregnancy. With proper steroid replacement, the majority of women should have an essentially uncomplicated pregnancy with minimal risk.[88] However, one must also be alert to the possibility of acute adrenal insufficiency, which is a life-threatening condition. Although adrenal crisis is more common in the previously undiagnosed patient with Addison's disease, it can also appear during times of stress such as labor and delivery, infection, and surgery.

The overall prognosis for the fetus and newborn is good, although some have reported an increased risk of intrauterine growth retardation.[88,89]

Treatment. Treatment of pregnant women with Addison's disease is basically the same as for the nonpregnant patient (i.e., replacement of glucocorticoids and mineralocorticoids, if necessary). Prednisone, 7.5 mg orally each day, is generally satisfactory for routine glucocorticoid requirements; fluorohydrocortisone, 0.1 mg per day, provides adequate mineralocorticoid coverage (Box 14-6).[88]

The dose of glucocorticoid should be increased during periods of stress such as labor and delivery, as outlined in Box 14-6.

Obstetric and anesthetic management. Most women with adrenal insufficiency tolerate labor well with the addition of parenteral corticosteroids as outlined in Box 14-6. Current practices for epidural analgesia (Table 14-5) during labor and for operative delivery are appropriate. General anesthesia, as summarized in Box 14-4, is recommended, with certain modifications.

If unexplained intraoperative hypotension should occur, confirmation of adequate infusion of hydrocortisone (Box 14-6) is essential. However, evidence that primary adrenal insufficiency is a major determinant is lacking.[90] If emergency surgery is necessary, infusion of hydrocortisone and intravenous fluid administration controlled by invasive hemodynamic monitoring is indicated. Doses of anesthetic agents should be administered in small increments because drug-induced myocardial depression is a major hazard. Perioperatively, glucose levels and electrolyte plasma levels must be measured frequently. Skeletal muscle weakness is a clinical feature warning of the need for small initial doses of neuromuscular blocking agents and maintenance of neuromuscular blockade carefully controlled by peripheral nerve stimulator monitoring.

Adrenocortical insufficiency, whatever its etiology, is associated with the potential for hypotension and circulatory collapse. Autoimmune diseases causing primary hypoadrenalism and hypothyroidism, enzyme defect in synthesis of cortisol, and secondary adrenal insufficiency following surgery or irradiation for pituitary or hypothalamic tumor share the hazard of glucocorticoid deficiency. Chronic oral doses of steroids are the most common adrenal suppressor. Chronic adrenal insufficiency features hyperpigmentation, hyponatremia, hypovolemia, and hyperkalemia. Supplemental steroids should be administered and fluid balance and electrolyte values normalized. A small effect on wound healing is a risk of this supplementation.

BOX 14-6 GLUCOCORTICOID AND MINERALOCORTICOID REPLACEMENT IN PREGNANT WOMEN WITH ADRENAL INSUFFICIENCY

Routine replacement[50]

Prednisone, 7.5/day (or equivalent), orally
Fluorohydrocortisone, 0.1 mg/day, orally

Labor, delivery, surgery, stress[50]

Hydrocortisone, 100 mg intravenously every 8 hrs for labor and delivery and stress
Hydrocortisone, 100 mg perioperatively for cesarean section and other surgery

Adrenal crisis

Hydration
Maintain blood pressure
Hydrocortisone, 100 mg intravenously every 8 hrs (or equivalent)

Cushing's syndrome

Incidence. Cushing's syndrome complicating pregnancy is extremely rare; as of 1986 there had been only 33 cases reported.[91-93] This is probably related to the fact that many of these women are infertile secondary to anovulation.[94]

Etiology. Cushing's syndrome may be caused by adrenal hyperplasia, an adrenal adenoma, or adrenal carcinoma. In a literature review in 1986, Koerten et al reported 41 pregnancies in 33 women with Cushing's syndrome.[91] Of these 33 women, an adrenal adenoma was present in 15 (45%), adrenal hyperplasia in 12 (36%), and carcinoma in 6 (19%).

Diagnosis. Signs and symptoms of Cushing's syndrome include weakness, muscle atrophy, edema, increased weight gain, hypertension, abdominal striae, and easy bruising.[91] These patients may also have abnormal glucose tolerance.

As previously mentioned, pregnant women have elevated cortisol levels, but much of this is bound. Women with Cushing's syndrome do not show the normal diurnal variation in cortisol levels and will fail to demonstrate suppression of baseline urinary 17-hydroxycorticoid levels following dexamethasone suppression. Ultrasonography or computed tomography may be helpful in ruling out an adenoma.

Effects on pregnancy. Cushing's syndrome is associated with significant morbidity in both mother and fetus. Of the 41 pregnancies reviewed by Koerten et al, 17 (41%) were associated with preterm births, 7 (17%) with spontaneous abortions, and 4 (10%) with stillbirths. Only one third of the pregnancies resulted in term births. Of the 15 women with adrenal adenomas, 44% developed pulmonary edema and 100% developed hypertension.[91] Complications were less common in women with hyperplasia.

Treatment. Once the diagnosis of Cushing's syndrome is confirmed, prompt treatment is of paramount importance. In the series reviewed by Koerten et al,[91] 7 women underwent either unilateral or bilateral adrenalectomy during pregnancy (12 to 20 weeks' gestation) and 1 received pituitary irradiation (24 weeks' gestation). Of these 8 pregnancies, there were 5 term births, 2 premature births, and 1 spontaneous abortion. Thus, surgery would appear to result in the most favorable outcome with regard to pregnancy.

Medical therapy for Cushing's syndrome during pregnancy has also been reported. Gormley et al reported on the successful management of a pregnant woman with Cushing's syndrome treated with metyrapone.[93] Kasperlik-Zaluska et al[94] reported the successful treatment of a woman with Cushing's syndrome through two separate pregnancies with the drug cyproheptadine, an antiserotonin.

Successful use of this agent has also been described by Montgomery and Welbourne.[95]

Obstetric and anesthetic management. Severe hypertension is the most significant maternal complication encountered during labor and delivery. Control of hypertension and recognition of the clinical features of glucocorticoid excess are essential when planning analgesia and anesthesia. Evaluation of cardiovascular function and plasma glucose, electrolytes, and acid base parameters precedes regional analgesia or general anesthesia. Central obesity, muscle wasting, osteoporosis and potential for vertebral body collapse, and thinning and bruising of skin are features that present technical problems if regional analgesia is planned. During labor skillful use of fine-gauge needles and assistance of midlumbar sagittal ultrasound scanning are advantageous for patient comfort, as is choice of needle length.[96] Hematologic abnormalities including thrombocytopenia may preclude use of regional methods.

Polyuria and diabetes mellitus are frequent; management for diabetes disorder has already been discussed. Psychiatric disturbance may preclude use of regional methods. Severe- or malignant-phase hypertension may be associated with cardiac failure and may need invasive monitoring. Depending on the severity, regional anesthesia may be avoided. Increased vascular response to pressors is potentially hazardous. Aortocaval compression may lead to hypotension and add to fetal risks of acidemia. Intrathecal preservative-free morphine for labor analgesia and long-duration pain control is possibly advantageous in this complex disorder. Many of these women will require operative delivery. Fluid retention and hypokalemic alkalosis are important features; hypokalemia must be corrected. Other complications of iatrogenic glucocorticoid excess include cataracts, glaucoma, aseptic necrosis of bone, and pancreatitis. Continuous CVP and radial arterial blood pressure monitoring and correction of electrolyte abnormalities are essential in the presence of serious dysfunctions. Additional risks include increased potential for bleeding and hypovolemia. Hydralazine administered following admission to the labor and delivery unit may require supplementation during preoxygenation for general anesthesia if time permits, systolic and diastolic blood pressures should be reduced to the range of 140–150/90–100. Intravenous lidocaine, 100 mg, in addition to hydralazine can blunt the pressor response to laryngoscopy and tracheal intubation. Alternatively, in our practice severe hypertension is controlled with 50 μg boluses of nitroglycerin (dose range 50 to 200 μg), followed by rapid sequence induction (see Box 14-

4). Intravenous opioids after cord clamping are given for pain control intraoperatively. This will control, however not eliminate, release of corticol secondary to surgical stimulation.

Pheochromocytoma

Incidence. Like other diseases of the adrenal gland, pheochromocytomas are rare during pregnancy. In 1971 Schenker and Chavers[97] reviewed 112 pregnancies in 89 patients with a pheochromocytoma. More recently Schenker and Granat reviewed an additional 50 patients for a total of 162 pregnancies.[97,98]

Diagnosis. The clinical signs and symptoms of 139 pregnant women with a pheochromocytoma is summarized in Table 14-8.[98] Almost all (95%) patients with a pheochromocytoma will have one or more of the following symptoms: headache, palpitations, and excessive perspiration.[98] Many normal pregnant women will also complain of one or more of these symptoms.

Various biochemical tests have been employed to detect excessive catecholamine secretion associated with pheochromocytoma. Measurements of either urinary catecholamines (or their metabolites) or serum catecholamines have been used. There is no unanimity of opinion regarding the single best test, but measurement of plasma catecholamines appears to have the highest sensitivity while measurement of urinary vanillylmandelic acid has the lowest.[99] Various provocative tests with phentolamine or histamine are generally not recommended for use during pregnancy.[99] Bravo and Gifford[99] have recently reported on their experience with the clonidine suppression test, which suppresses catecholamines in patients with essential hypertension but not with pheochromocytoma. However, there is little or no published information regarding this test during pregnancy, and clonidine may cause significant hypotension, a potentially serious side effect during pregnancy.

The localization of pheochromocytoma can be

Table 14-8 Signs and symptoms in pregnant women with a pheochromocytoma*

Symptom	Approx. percentage
Hypertension	80-85
Headache	65-70
Palpitation	35-40
Sweating	30-35
Blurred vision	18-20
Anxiety	15

*Adapted from Schenker JG, Granat M: *Aust N Z J Obstet Gynaecol* 1982; 22:1-10.

made with a reasonable degree of accuracy (96%) with a computed tomographic scan and occasionally with ultrasound.[99] Selective arteriography is difficult to perform during pregnancy, and it should be used only when the other techniques fail to demonstrate the site(s) of the tumor.

Effects on pregnancy. Pheochromocytomas complicating pregnancy carry significant risks for both mother and fetus. In the 139 cases reviewed by Schenker and Granat,[98] there were 56 (40%) maternal deaths. Of these 56 deaths, 14 occurred during the antepartum period, 1 intrapartum, and 36 within 3 days of delivery. The most common causes of death were cardiovascular accidents, cardiac arrest, and arrhythmias.

Of the 162 pregnancies reported by Schenker and Granat, only 47% of the fetuses survived.[98] Twelve percent of the pregnancies aborted, 23% resulted in intrauterine deaths, and 17% resulted in intrapartum or postpartum deaths.

Treatment. The cure for pheochromocytoma is surgery with removal of the tumor. However, for the pregnant patient at or near term when the diagnosis is made, medical management with phenoxybenzamine may prove advantageous until the patient can be delivered.[98] It would appear that cesarean section is associated with a maternal mortality rate lower than with vaginal delivery, and it is possible that the tumor may be resected at the time of cesarean delivery.[98] It may be necessary to use intravenous nitroprusside to control blood pressure in these patients. The sodium nitroprusside solution is prepared by adding 50 mg of sodium nitroprusside solution to 500 mL of 5% dextrose solution. An infusion pump administers the precise dose to control the blood pressure (average adult dose 3 μg/kg/min, maximum dose not to exceed 800 μg/min).[100] Infusion can be terminated immediately when the adrenal vein is clamped. Recovery from infusion is typically observed in 1 to 2 minutes, avoiding rapid fall in blood pressure as the tumor is removed.

Obstetric and anesthetic management. Of all the pregnant patients with endocrine disorders, those with pheochromocytoma present the greatest challenge to both obstetrician and anesthesiologist. If a cesarean section is planned for a patient with a known pheochromocytoma, therapy with phenoxybenzamine precedes scheduling elective cesarean delivery. Beta-adrenergic blocking agents should not be used for arrhythmias or blood pressure control until α-adrenergic blockade has been achieved with phenoxybenzamine.[98] Paradoxical hypertension can occur if propranolol is given before α-adrenergic blockade with phenoxybenzamine. After α-blockade is established, control of

heart rate, arrhythmias, and blood pressure with β-adrenergic blocking agents is indicated. Minimal dosage of propranolol is recommended in the presence of cardiomyopathy where β-adrenergic blockade has the potential to increase left ventricular dysfunction. Cardiomyopathy and myocardial infarction may result from sustained excess of circulating catecholamines. Cardiovascular causes of death include myocardial infarction, cardiac failure, or intracerebral hemorrhage, which also results in hyperglycemia.

Duration of therapy after initiation of α-adrenergic blockade with phenoxybenzamine to prevent vasoconstriction with catecholamines is usually 10 to 14 days. When α-blockade is adequate, blood pressure should not exceed 160–170/90; tilt test should result in orthostatic hypotension of not less than 80/55 mm Hg.[102] Decreases in hematocrit also indicate increased intravascular volume from pretreatment volume following α_1- and α_2-receptor blockade. Electrocardiographic monitoring should be free of ST-T changes, and premature ventricular contractions should be infrequent.

Continuous radial arterial blood pressure monitoring is essential, and arterial blood gases, hematocrit, plasma electrolytes, and blood glucose concentrations should be continually evaluated. A central venous catheter, or Cordis sheath and pulmonary artery catheter, is essential to monitor intravascular volume. A pulmonary artery catheter is indicated when there is history of cardiac failure; in the presence of left ventricular dysfunction it is important to monitor left side filling pressures, which may not be predictable from central venous or right atrial pressures. Hemodynamic monitoring also allows an attempt to achieve optimal myocardial oxygen balance and permits continual evaluation of the effects of vasodilators, vasopressors, ionotropic agents, and filling pressures.

Sedation is important to reduce maternal anxiety in the presence of a pheochromocytoma.[103] Oral diazepam the night before surgery and again 2 hours before induction is recommended to reduce anxiety and activation of the sympathetic nervous system. Preparation for induction of general anesthesia includes all normal noninvasive monitoring (see Box 14-4) and monitored intravenous sedation with fentanyl and small doses of midazolam. Cannulation of the radial artery and placement of a second large peripheral intravenous cannula (14- or 16-gauge) under local anesthesia allows for rapid infusion of warmed crystalloid or colloid solution. To prevent or limit a significant increase in blood pressure and heart rate at induction, alfentanil (20 to 30 μg/kg) or fentanyl (2 to 3 μg/kg), and lidocaine (1 to 2 mg/kg) is recommended to reduce the incidence of ventricular arrhythmias immediately before injection of thiopentone sodium (2 to 4 mg/kg). Tracheal intubation and controlled ventilation with nitrous oxide/oxygen and isoflurane or enflurane is acceptable for maintenance of anesthesia. Monitoring by in-line mass spectrometer, optimal oxygenation, normocarbia, and adequate depth of surgical anesthesia are confirmed. A peripheral nerve stimulator monitors neuromuscular blockade throughout the procedure, and if succinylcholine (1.5 mg/kg) has been injected to facilitate tracheal intubation, neuromuscular blockade is maintained with vecuronium or atracurium.

A comparative study of four methods of anesthesia in the nonpregnant population[103] included combined regional anesthesia and balanced endotracheal anesthesia with nitrous oxide/oxygen. All methods of general anesthesia and the combined method were satisfactory, and all resections of pheochromocytoma were elective after α-adrenergic blockade was evaluated to be optimal and β-adrenergic-blockade was added to control arrhythmias and tachycardia. Intraoperative hypertension was controlled with sodium nitroprusside and increased depth of anesthesia. Hypotension was corrected by fluid boluses, decreased anesthetic concentration, and phenylephrine. Propranolol was used in 0.1- to 0.5-mg intravenous boluses to treat arrhythmias. All 24 patients in the study population survived without major organ sequelae.[103]

Parenteral magnesium has been shown to reduce systematic vascular resistance and slightly reduce mean arterial pressure in severe preeclampsia.[104] Magnesium sulfate infusion at rates of 2.0 to 2.5 g/min during general anesthesia and resection of pheochromocytoma in a nonpregnant woman has successfully inhibited catecholamine drive during surgery.[105] Magnesium sulfate has been shown to inhibit release of catecholamines from adrenal medulla[106,107] and peripheral adrenergic nerve terminals;[108] to directly block catecholamine receptors; and to have direct dilator effect on vascular walls.[109]

Although there is blockade of the sympathetic nervous system with regional analgesia, postsynaptic α-adrenergic receptors can still respond to the direct effects of sudden increase in the circulating levels of catecholamines. Other considerations include reduced sympathetic nervous system activity during onset of hypotension associated with ligation of the veins of the tumor, and the possibility of inadequate anesthesia if high abdominal exploration is necessary. Surgery should not be performed with the patient in the supine position,

and selection of combined regional and general anesthesia may be beneficial. Although cesarean section and resection of pheochromocytoma has been reported, these procedures have been performed separately at this medical center.[110]

DISEASES OF THE PITUITARY GLAND
Microadenomas

Incidence. Pregnancy in women with microadenomas was once rare. However, with the development of bromocriptine for the treatment of pituitary adenomas and hyperprolactinemia, pregnancy is much more common.

Etiology. The majority of pituitary tumors encountered during pregnancy are microadenomas and are associated with hyperprolactinemia.

Diagnosis. Pregnant women with microadenomas have few symptoms. Prior to treatment and pregnancy, most of these women presented with amenorrhea, galactorrhea, and infertility.

The main laboratory finding in women with microadenomas is elevated prolactin or hyperprolactinemia, which is a test that is relatively easy to obtain. The diagnosis can be confirmed by a computed tomographic scan, which is rarely necessary during pregnancy.

Effects on pregnancy. The majority of pregnant women with microadenomas are asymptomatic. In one the largest series reported (over 200 women), less than 2% of the patients developed symptoms during pregnancy.[111] A small number of patients demonstrated enlargement or growth of the tumor during pregnancy, but they were asymptomatic. Development of symptoms is much more common for macroadenomas, occurring in approximately 15% of such women.[112]

Treatment. The majority of pregnant women with pituitary adenomas require no specific therapy during pregnancy. Routine visual fields and measurement of prolactin are not necessary in the asymptomatic patient, and computed tomographic scanning is indicated only for the presence of significant symptoms.[112] If symptomatic enlargement occurs, these patients can be treated with bromocriptine.

Obstetric and anesthetic management. The majority of these patients require no unusual care during labor. Operative delivery is reserved for obstetric indications, and either regional or general anesthesia may be used.

Diabetes insipidus

This is a very rare condition complicating pregnancy following surgical removal or tumor destruction of the pituitary gland and hypothalamo-hypophyseal system. There is complete or partial deficiency of ADH secretion. Treatment consists primarily of vasopressin replacement with synthetic analogue vasopressin, L-deamino-8-D-arginine vasopressin, or desmopressin, which has a longer duration of action, freedom from allergic reaction, and reduced vasopressor activity. Labor may be complicated by dysfunctional contractions and there may be an increase in operative deliveries.[113] Either regional or general anesthesia may be used in these patients.

Inadequate release of ADH is also associated with head injury, and like the reversible trauma of the posterior pituitary that may occur during pituitary surgery, it is transient and lasts about 24 hours. Normally the stimulus of a 20 mOsm increase in plasma osmolarity activates the osmoreceptors in the hypothalamus, and release of ADH follows. Diagnosis of central diabetes insipidus requires the kidney to respond to exogenous ADH.[100] Diminished response to the test of 5 U (0.25 mL) of aqueous vasopressin injected subcutaneously with measurement of urine osmolarity 1 hour later indicates nephrogenic diabetes insipidus.[100] Postoperative diuresis and osmotic diuresis that accompanies hyperglycemia and glucosuria must be excluded when the diagnosis of diabetes insipidus is considered. The goal of accurate daily monitoring is to prevent dehydration and avoid water intoxication.

Variables helpful in evaluation of the maintenance of normal water balance are body weight, fluid intake and output, serum sodium concentration, plasma, osmolarity, and renal function. When the patient is alert, has a urine output less than 5 L/day, and is permitted oral fluids, drinking is encouraged in the presence of partial diabetes insipidus. If no fluids are permitted, intravenous 5% dextrose and water is administered to replace urine volume plus insensible losses. Intranasal desmopressin, 0.1 or 2.0 mL once or twice daily, or parenteral vasopressin, 5 U in 1 L of 5% dextrose and water at 1 mL/min, is recommended.[100]

The syndrome of inappropriate ADH secretion (SIADH) may occur secondary to various pathophysiologies such as cerebral tumor or accident; trauma; pulmonary disease, including bronchogenic carcinoma and other tumors; endocrinopathies such as hypoadrenalism and hypothyroidism; and hepatic cirrhosis. The syndrome is clinically recognized when urinary sodium is elevated and there is a decreased plasma level that reflects the expansion of intravascular volume. Neurologic symptoms may occur when plasma sodium levels are less than 125 mEq/L, and management of free water loss necessary to elevate serum sodium from 110 to 125 mEq/L should avoid elevating serum sodium at greater than 1 to 2 mEq/L/hr in the urgent management of symptomatic SIADH.[113]

CONCLUSION

Basic understanding of the pathophysiologic processes of endocrine abnormalities is absolutely necessary to take care of the parturients with endocrine disorders. Early anesthetic evaluation is mandatory.

REFERENCES

1. Vance ML: Hypopituitarism. *N Eng J Med* 1994; 330:1651.
2. Sutherland EW, Rall TW: The relation of adenosine 3',5' phosphate and phosphorylase to the actions of catecholamines and other hormones. *Pharmacol Rev* 1960; 12:265.
3. Ross EM, Gilman A: Biochemical properties of hormone-sensitive adenylate cyclase (review). *Annu Rev Biochem* 1980; 49:533.
4. Rodbell M: The role of hormone receptors and GTP-regulatory proteins in membrane transduction. *Nature* 1980; 284 (5751):17.
5. Keen H: Insulin resistance and the prevention of diabetes mellitus. *N Eng J Med* 1994; 331:1226.
6. Reaven GM: Role of insulin resistance in human disease. *Diabetes* 1988; 37:1595.
7. Leahy JL, Boyd AE: Diabetes genes in non-insulin-dependent-diabetes mellitus. *N Eng J Med* 1993; 328:56.
8. Defronzo RA, Bonadonna RC, Ferrannini E: Pathogenesis of NIDDM: A balanced overview. *Diabetes Care* 1992; 15:318.
9. Garg A: in Datta S (ed): *Common Problems in Obstetric Anesthesia*. St. Louis, Mosby, 1994, p 94.
10. Nolan JJ, et al: Improvement in glucose tolerance and insulin resistance in obese subjects treated with troglitazone. *N Eng J Med* 1994; 331:1118.
11. Brent GA: The molecular basis of thyroid hormone action. *N Eng J Med* 1994, 331:847.
12. Refetoff S, Weiss RE, Usala SJ: The syndromes of resistance to thyroid hormone.
13. Wiseman SA, Powell JT, Humphries SE, et al: The magnitude of the hypercholesterolemia of hypothyroidism is associated with variation in the low density lipoprotein receptor gene. *J Clin Endocrinol Metab* 1993; 77:108.
14. Burrow GN, Fisher DA, Reed Larsen P: Maternal and fetal thyroid function. *N Eng J Med* 1994; 331:1072.
15. Libert F, Lefort A, Gerard C, et al: Cloning, sequencing, and expression of the human TSH receptor.
16. Franklyn JA: The management of hyperthyroidism. *N Eng J Med* 1994; 330:1731.
17. Reichlin S: Neuroendocrine-immune interactions. *N Eng J Med* 1993; 329:1246.
18. Leveno KJ, Whalley PJ: Dilemmas in the management of pregnancy complicated by diabetes. *Med Clin North Am* 1982; 66:1325.
19. Gabbe SG: Management of diabetes mellitus in pregnancy. *Am J Obstet Gynecol* 1985; 153:824.
20. American College of Obstetricians and Gynecologists: Diabetes and pregnancy. *ACOG Technical Bulletin,* no 200, Dec 1994.
21. Landon MB, Gabbe SG: Diabetes and pregnancy. *Med Clin North Am* 1988; 72:1493.
22. American Diabetes Association: Summary of recommendations of the Second International Workshop Conference

on Gestational Diabetes Mellitus. *Diabetes* 1985; 34(suppl 2):123.

23. O'Sullivan JB, Mahan CM: Criteria for the oral glucose tolerance test in pregnancy. *Diabetes* 1964; 13:278.

24. American College of Obstetricians and Gynecologists: Diabetes and pregnancy. *ACOG Technical Bulletin*, no 92, May 1986.

25. Cousins L: Pregnancy complications among diabetic women: Review 1965-1985. *Obstet Gynecol Surv* 1987; 42(3):140.

26. Mills JL: Malformations in infants of diabetic mothers. *Teratology* 1982; 25:385.

27. Cousins L: Congenital anomalies among infants of diabetic mothers: Etiology, prevention, prenatal diagnosis. *Am J Obstet Gynecol* 1983; 147:333.

28. Miller LS, Hare JW, Cloherty JP, et al: Elevated maternal hemoglobin A_{1c} in early pregnancy and major congenital anomalies in infants of diabetic mothers. *N Eng J Med* 1981; 304:1331.

29. Mills JL, Knobb RH, Simpson JL, et al: Lack of relation of increased malformation rates in infants of diabetic mothers to glycemic control during organogenesis. *N Eng J Med* 1988; 318:671.

30. Read GD: Childbirth without fear. *NY Harper* 1944, p 192.

31. Lamaze F: *Painless Childbirth: Psychoprophylactic Method.* Chicago, Henry Regenery, 1970.

32. Cohen P: Signal integration at the level of protein kinases, protein phosphates and their substrates. *Trends Biochem Sci* 1992; 17:408.

33. Shnider SM, Abboud TK, Artral R, et al: Maternal endogenous catecholamines decrease during labor after lumbar epidural anesthesia. *Am J Obstet Gynecol* 1983; 147:13.

34. Abboud TK, Artal R, Hendriksen EH, et al: Effects of spinal anesthesia on maternal circulating catecholamines. *Am J Obstet Gynecol* 1982; 142:252.

35. Wallace DH: Epidural anesthesia for vaginal delivery, in Datta S, Ostheimer GW (eds): *Common Problems in Obstetric Anesthesia.* Chicago, Year Book Medical Publishers, 1987, pp 140.

36. Chestnut DH, Owen CL, Bates JN, et al: Continuous infusion epidural analgesia during labor: A randomized double-blind comparison of 0.0625% bupivacaine/0.002% fentanyl versus 0.125% bupivacaine. *Anesthesiology* 1988; 68:754.

37. Datta S, Brown WU Jr: Acid-base status in diabetic mothers and their infants following general or spinal anesthesia for cesarean section. *Anesthesiology* 1977; 47:272.

38. Datta S, Brown WU Jr, Ostheimer GW, et al: Epidural anesthesia for cesarean section in diabetic parturients: Maternal and neonatal acid base status and bupivacaine concentration. *Anesth Analg* 1981; 60:574.

39. Kenepp NB, Shelley WC, Kumar S: Effects on newborn of hydration with glucose in patients undergoing cesarean section with regional anesthesia. *Lancet* 1980; 1:645.

40. Kenepp NB, Kumar S, Shelley WC, et al: Fetal and neonatal hazards of maternal hydration with 5% dextrose solutions prior to cesarean section. *Lancet* 1982; 1:1150.

41. Datta S, Kitzmiller JL, Naulty JS, et al: Acid-base status of diabetic mothers and their infants following spinal anesthesia for cesarean section. *Anesth Analg* 1982; 61:662.

42. Ramanathan S, Khoo P, Avismendy J: Perioperative maternal and neonatal acid base status and glucose metabolism in patients with insulin-dependent diabetes mellitus. *Anesth Analg* 1991; 73:105.

43. Moore DC, Batra MS: The components of an effective test dose prior to epidural block. *Anesthesiology* 1981; 55:693.

44. Cartwright PD, McCarroll SM, Antzaka C: Maternal heart rate changes with a plain epidural test dose. *Anesthesiology* 1986; 65:226.

45. Leighton BL, Norris MC, Sos KM, et al: Limitations of epinephrine as a marker of intravascular injection in laboring women. *Anesthesiology* 1987; 66:688.

46. Hood DD, Owen DM, Jones FM: Maternal and fetal effects of epinephrine in gravid ewes. *Anesthesiology* 1986; 64:610.

47. Chestnut DH, Owen CL, Brown CK, et al: Does labor affect the variability of maternal heart rate during induction of epidural anesthesia? *Anesthesiology* 1988; 68:622.

48. Marx GF, Elstein ID, Schuss M, et al: Effects of epidural block with lignocaine and lignocaine-adrenaline on umbilical artery velocity waveform ratios. *Br J Obstet Gynecol* 1990; 97:517.

49. Stacey RGW, Watts SS, Kadim MY, et al: Single space combined spinal-extradural technique for analgesia in labour. *Br J Anaesth* 1993; 71:499.

50. D'Angelo RD, Anderion MT, Philip J, et al: Intrathecal sufentanil compared to epidural lignocaine for labor analgesia. *Anesthesiology* 1994; 19(4):243.

51. Camann WR, Denney RA, Holby ED, et al: A comparison of intrathecal, epidural, and intravenous sufentanil for labor analgesia. *Anesthesiology* 1992; 77:884.

52. Camann WR, Mintzer BH, Denney RA, et al: Intrathecal sufentanil for labor analgesia: Effects of added epinephrine. *Anesthesiology* 1993; 73:870.

53. Arkoosh VA, Sharkey SJ, Norris MC, et al: Subarachnoid labor analgesia fentanyl and morphine versus sufentanil and morphine. *Reg Anesth* 1994; 19(4):243.

54. Clark SL, Cotton DB, Hankins GDV, et al: Diabetic ketoacidosis in pregnancy, in *Handbook of Critical Care Obstetrics.* Blackwell Scientific Publications, Oxford, 1994, p 163.

55. Gilstrap LC, Hankins GDV: The high-risk patient, in Phelan JP, Clark SL (eds): *Cesarean Delivery.* New York, Elsevier, 1988, p 155.

56. Gibbs CP, Tanner TC: Effectiveness of bicitra as a preoperative antacid. *Anesthesiology* 1984; 61:973.

57. Sullivan GM, Bullingham RE: Assessment of gastric activity and antacids effect in pregnant women by a noninvasive radiotelemetry technique. *Br J Anaesth* 1984; 91:973.

58. Crawford JS, Potter SR: Magnesium trisilicate mixture BP: Its physical characteristics and effectiveness as a prophylactic. *Anesthesiology* 1984; 39:535.

59. Bogod DG, Rosen M, Rees GAD: Maximum FiO_2 during caesarean section. *Br J Anaesth* 1988; 61:255.

60. Shearer VE, Wallace DH, Ramin S: Adverse neonatal effects of prophylactic ephedrine during regional anesthesia for cesarean delivery (abstr no B-7). 21st Annual Meeting of the Society for Obstetric Anesthesia and Perinatology, Seattle, May 1989.

61. Wallace DH, Cosentino SL, Shearer VE, et al: The effect of isoflurane 1% or low-dose and regional anesthesia on uterine tone at cesarean section. *Anesthesiology* 1989; 71:A874.

62. Thomas DJ: Diabetic gastroparesis. *Anaesth* 1984; 39:1143.

63. Salzarulo HH, Taylor LA: Diabetic stiff joint syndrome as a cause of difficult endotracheal intubation. *Anesthesiology* 1986; 64:366.

64. Tunstall ME: Failed intubation drill. *Anesthesiology* 1976; 31:850.

65. Practice guidelines for management of the difficult airway: A report by the American Society of Anesthesiologists Task Force on Management of the Difficult Airway. *Anesthesiology* 1993; 78:597.

66. Davies JM, Weeks S, Crome LA, et al: Difficult intubation in the parturient. *Can J Anaesth* 1989; 36:668.
67. Samsoon GLT, Young B Jr: Difficult tracheal intubation: A retrospective study. *Anaesth* 1987; 42:487.
68. Benumof JL, Scheller MS: The importance of transtracheal jet ventilation in the management of the difficult airway. *Anesthesiology* 1989; 71:769.
69. Dept. Of Health, and others: Report on Confidential Enquiries into Maternal Deaths in the United Kingdom 1985-1987. London, HMSO, 1991.
70. Dept. Of Health, and others: Report on Confidential Enquiries into Maternal Deaths in the United Kingdom 1982-1984. London, HMSO, 1987.
71. Brimacomb J, Berry A: The laryngeal mask airway for obstetric anesthesia and neonatal resuscitation. *Int J Obstet Anesth* 1994; 3:211.
72. Osathanondh R, Tulchinsky D, Chupra IJ: Total and free thyroxine and triiodothyronine in normal and complicated pregnancies. *J Clin Endocrinol Metab* 1976; 42:98.
73. Davis LE, Leveno KJ, Cunningham FG: Hypothyroidism complicating pregnancy. *Obstet Gynecol* 1988; 72:108.
74. Maze M: Clinical implications of membrane receptor function in anesthesia. *Anesthesiology* 1981; 55:160.
75. Burrow GN: The management of thyrotoxicosis in pregnancy. *N Eng J Med* 1985; 313:562.
76. Davis LE, Lucas MJ, Hankins GDV, et al: Thyrotoxicosis complicating pregnancy. *Am J Obstet Gynecol* 1989; 160:63.
77. Hollingsworth DR: Graves' disease. *Clin Obstet Gynecol* 1983; 26:615.
78. Amino N, Tanizawa O, Mori H, et al: Aggravation of thyrotoxicosis in early pregnancy and after delivery in Graves' disease. *J Clin Endocrinol Metab* 1982; 55:108.
79. Cunningham FG, MacDonald PC, Gant NF: Medical and surgical illnesses complicating pregnancy in Williams Obstetrics, ed 18. Norwalk, Conn, Appleton & Lange, 1989, p 824.
80. Clark SL, Cotton DB, Hankins GDV, et al: Thyroid storm in pregnancy, in *Handbook of Critical Care*. Blackwell Scientific Publications, Oxford 1994, p 153.
81. Matsuura N, Fujieda K, Iida Y, et al: TSH receptor antibodies in mothers with Graves' disease and outcome in their offspring. *Lancet* 1988; 1:14.
82. Moran DH, Perillo M, Laporta RF, et al: Phenylephrine in the prevention of hypotension following spinal anesthesia for cesarean delivery. *J Clin Anesth* 1991; 3:301.
83. Kaplan JA, Cooperman LH: Alarming reactions to ketamine in patients taking thyroid medication: Treatment with propranolol. *Anesthesiology* 1971; 35:229.
84. Seino H, Doho S, Aiyoshi Y, et al: Postoperative hepatic dysfunction after halothane or enflurane anesthesia in patients with hyperthyroidism. *Anesthesiology* 1986; 64:122.
85. Rosen IB, Walfish PG: Pregnancy as a predisposing factor in thyroid neoplasia. *Arch Surg* 1986; 121:1287.
86. Whalley PJ: Hyperparathyroidism and pregnancy. *Am J Obstet Gynecol* 1963; 86:517.
87. Brent F: Addison's disease and pregnancy. *Am J Surg* 1950; 79:645.
88. O'Shaughnessy RW, Hackett KJ: Maternal Addison's disease and fetal growth retardation. *J Reprod Med* 1984; 29:752.
89. Osler M: Addison's disease and pregnancy. *Acta Endocrinol* 1962; 41:67.
90. Knudson L, Christiansen LA, Lorentzen JE: Hypotension during and after operation in glucocorticoid-treated patients. *Br J Anaesth* 1981; 53:295.
91. Koerten JM, Morales WJ, Washington SR, et al: Cushing's syndrome in pregnancy: A case report and literature review. *Am J Obstet Gynecol* 1986; 154:626.
92. Grimes EM, Gayez JA, Miller GL: Cushing's syndrome during pregnancy. *Obstet Gynecol* 1973; 42:550.
93. Gormley MJJ, Hadden DR, Kennedy TL, et al: Cushing's syndrome in pregnancy: Treatment with metyrapone. *Clin Endocrinol* 1982; 16:283.
94. Kasperlik-Zaluska A, Migdalska B, Hartwig W, et al: Two pregnancies in a woman with Cushing's syndrome treated with cyproheptadine. *Br J Obstet Gynaecol* 1980; 87:1171.
95. Montgomery DAD, Welbourne RB: Cushing's syndrome: 20 years after adrenalectomy. *Br J Surg* 1978; 65:221.
96. Wallace DH, Currie JM, Santos R: Indirect sonographic guidance for epidural anesthesia in obese pregnant patients. *Reg Anesth* 1992; 17:233.
97. Schenker JG, Chavers I: Pheochromocytoma and pregnancy. *Obstet Gynecol Surv* 1971; 26:739.
98. Schenker JG, Granat M: Pheochromocytoma and pregnancy: An updated appraisal. *Aust N Z J Obstet Gynaecol* 1982; 22:1.
99. Bravo EL, Gifford RW. Pheochromocytoma: Diagnosis, localization and management. *N Engl J Med* 1984: 311:1298.
100. Smith RJ, Dluhy RG, Williams GH: Endocrinology, in Vandam LD (ed): *To Make the Patient Ready for Anesthesia: Medical Care of the Surgical Patient*, ed 2. Menlo Park, Calif, Addison-Wesley, 1984, p 145.
101. Litt L, Roizen MF: Endocrine and renal function, in Brown DL (ed): *Risk and Outcome in Anesthesia*. Philadelphia, JB Lippincott, 1988, p 120.
102. Egbert LD, Battit BE, Turndorf H: The value of the preoperative visit by an anesthetist. *JAMA* 1963; 185:553.
103. Roizen MF, Horrigan M, Koike EI, et al: A prospective randomized trial of four anesthetic techniques for resection of pheochromocytoma. *Anesthesiology* 1982; 57:A43.
104. Cotton DB, Gonik B, Dorman KF: Cardiovascular alterations in severe pregnancy-induced hypertension: Acute effects of magnesium sulfate. *Am J Obstet Gynecol* 1984; 148:152.
105. James MFM: The use of magnesium sulfate in the anesthetic management of pheochromocytoma. *Anesthesiology* 1985; 62:188.
106. Douglas WW, Rubin RP: The mechanism of catecholamine release from the adrenal medulla and the role of calcium in stimulus-secretion coupling. *J Physiol* 1963; 167:288.
107. Lishajko F: Releasing effect of calcium and phosphate on catecholamines, ATP and protein from chromaffin granules. *Acta Physiol Scand* 1970; 79:575.
108. Kirpekar SM, Misu Y: Release of noradrenaline by splenic nerve stimulation and its dependence on calcium. *J Physiol* 1967; 188:219.
109. Altura BM, Altura BT: Magnesium ions and contraction of vascular smooth muscle in relationship to some vascular diseases. *Fed Proc* 1981; 40:2674.
110. Stoneham J, Wakefield C: Phaeochromocytoma in pregnancy. *Anaesth* 1983; 38:654.
111. Moltich ME: Pregnancy and the hyperprolactinemic woman. *N Engl J Med* 1985; 312:1364.
112. Hime ML, Richardson JA: Diabetes insipidus and pregnancy: Case report, incidence and review of literature. *Obstet Gynecol Surv* 1978; 3:375.
113. Narins RG, Lazarus MJ: Renal system, in Vandam LD (ed): *To Make the Patient Ready for Anesthesia: Medical Care of the Surgical Patient*, ed 2. Menlo Park, Calif, Addison-Wesley, 1984, p 81.

15 Trauma and Orthopedic Problems

David Anthony Rocke and *Jack Moodley*

TRAUMA

Trauma is a leading cause of death in young women, accounting for some 20% of nonobstetric causes of maternal death.[1] The major anatomic and physiologic changes of pregnancy may influence evaluation of the injured pregnant patient by altering both the signs and symptoms of injury and the results of the laboratory tests.[2] Pregnancy may also affect both the pattern and severity of injury. Although the attending physicians must remember that they have two patients, treatment priorities are the same as for the nonpregnant patient and are directed initially at maternal stabilization. Nevertheless, monitoring and evaluation techniques should encompass both mother and fetus. Several reviews have addressed problems encountered with the pregnant trauma victim.[3-9]

Anatomic and physiologic changes

Genitourinary. During the first trimester the thick-walled uterus remains an intrapelvic organ. After 12 weeks the uterus begins to rise out of the pelvis and encroach on the peritoneal cavity, restricting the intestines to the upper abdomen. During the second trimester the small fetus remains mobile and cushioned by the amniotic fluid. By the third trimester the uterus is large and thin-walled, and after 36 weeks the fetal head is usually fixed in the pelvic brim. Following trauma the amniotic fluid itself could be a source of embolism or a cause of disseminated intravascular coagulation.

The bladder, attached to the lower segment of the uterus and to the cervix, becomes more susceptible to injury as the uterus enlarges. Ureteral dilation is common from as early as 6 weeks, and this must be kept in mind when evaluating excretory pyelograms. The placenta reaches maximal size at 36 to 38 weeks and is devoid of elastic tissue predisposing to shear forces between the placenta and uterus and leading to an increased likelihood of abruptio placentae. The placental vasculature itself, while maximally vasodilated, is extremely sensitive to catecholamines. Direct trauma to the uterus may result in the release of high concentrations of placental thromboplastin and/or plasminogen activator from the myometrium. The anatomic changes in the uterus, while protecting other intraabdominal organs, increase the likelihood of uterine penetration or rupture, abruptio placentae, and premature rupture of the membranes.

Gastrointestinal tract. The enlarging uterus displaces the peritoneum from sites of trauma, leading to a diminished response to peritoneal irritation. The usual signs of guarding, rebound, and rigidity are often diminished and sometimes absent, thus delaying diagnosis. Rearrangement of the abdominal viscera may also result in atypical pain referral. As mentioned earlier, the enlarging uterus compresses bowel into the upper abdomen and while acting in a protective capacity in blunt trauma may result in injury to multiple loops of small bowel following penetrating injury.

Although pregnancy per se has recently been shown not to significantly delay gastric emptying,[10] all pregnant patients who have suffered trauma should still be regarded as having a full stomach. The use of narcotic drugs for pain relief significantly reduces gastric emptying, which will be also delayed if the patient goes into labor. Airway protection and aspiration prophylaxis are the same as for the traumatized nonpregnant patient; these include the use of antacids such as 30 ml 0.3 *M* sodium citrate and the placement of a nasogastric tube as appropriate.

Diaphragm. The enlarged uterus also causes the diaphragm to be elevated some 4 cm, and the anterior-posterior diameter of the chest is increased. These changes will be seen on chest radiograph, which will also demonstrate cephalization of the pulmonary vasculature, widening of the mediastinum, and apparent but not actual cardiac enlargement.

Cardiac. The hemodynamic changes of pregnancy are well known. These include a 30% to 50% increase in cardiac output from the 10th week. The cardiac output is highly dependent on maternal position as term approaches, and vena caval compression when the patient is in the supine position can result in a 30% to 40% reduction. Heart

296

rate increases by 15 to 20 beats per minute and must be considered in interpreting the tachycardiac response to hypovolemia. Blood pressure at term is near-normal, whereas the second trimester is usually accompanied by a small 5- to 15-mm decrease in systolic and diastolic blood pressure. The resting central venous pressure is usually unchanged by pregnancy, and the response to volume is the same as in the nonpregnant state. However, lower extremity venous hypertension is common in late pregnancy. Electrocardiographic changes include a 15-degree left axis shift and flattened or inverted T waves in leads III and AVF, as well as in the precordial leads. Ectopic beats may also be a normal phenomenon.

Blood and plasma. At 34 weeks' gestation, plasma volume increases by 40% to 50% and is accompanied by an 18% to 30% increase in red cell volume, resulting in a hematocrit of 32% to 34% and a hemoglobin of 10.5 to 11 g/dl. Patients who have taken iron supplementation have a slightly higher hemoglobin and hematocrit. Overall, blood volume increases by some 48% and allows the mother to lose a significant amount of blood at delivery without adverse hemodynamic effects. In the pregnant trauma patient the usual hemodynamic responses to blood loss do not occur until the patient loses between 1500 and 2000 ml of blood. Because pregnant patients lose relatively fewer red cells during hemorrhage, their oxygen-carrying capacity may be less affected by blood loss.

Pulmonary. Pulmonary changes include increased ventilation largely as a result of a progesterone-stimulated increase in tidal volume. Normal $Paco_2$ levels are 27 to 32 mm Hg, and the accompanying respiratory alkalosis results in a normal pregnant serum bicarbonate level of 18 to 31 mEq/L. Arterial pH is unchanged. The hyperventilation also results in a small increase in Pao_2 levels to between 104 and 108 mm Hg in early pregnancy, but at term the Pao_2 has fallen to between 90 and 100 mm Hg. Functional residual capacity is also decreased by the encroaching uterus and this, together with increased oxygen consumption by the mother, places her at increased risk for the rapid development of hypoxia following any apneic episode. Maintenance of adequate arterial oxygenation is therefore vital for the injured pregnant patient.

Laboratory tests. The white blood cell (WBC) count peaks during the third trimester to between 12,000 and 18,000/mm^3. Labor induces a further increase to 25,000/mm^3. Because an acute hemorrhage also induces a moderate leukocytosis, and abdominal trauma a pronounced increase in WBC,

confusion may exist between the pregnant state and trauma changes, making interpretation difficult. Other laboratory changes include elevation of clotting factors and serum fibrinogen, reduced prothrombin and plasma thromboplastin times, a fall in the serum albumin to between 2.2 and 2.8 g/dl, and a drop in serum protein levels by 1.0 g/dl. Levels of creatinine and serum urea nitrogen fall to almost one half the nonpregnant levels, and glycosuria is common.

Radiography. Other changes that must be taken into account when evaluating the pregnant trauma victim include a 4- to 8-mm widening of the symphysis pubis by the seventh month, and widening of the sacroiliac joint spaces.

Severity of injuries

All pregnant patients with major injuries will require admission to a hospital with surgical and obstetric facilities. In this group of patients, maternal mortality rate is of the order of 24% and the severity of maternal injuries usually determines fetal outcome. Fetal mortality rate in the severely injured mother may be as high as 61%, while in mothers admitted in hemorrhagic shock fetal mortality will be even higher, at 80%.[2]

Unfortunately, although major maternal injuries are predictive of poor fetal outcome, the same cannot be said for minor maternal injuries that may also be associated with significant fetomaternal hemorrhage. Kissinger and colleagues found that maternal physiologic and laboratory parameters failed to accurately predict fetal outcome.[11] On the other hand, the Injury Severity Score (ISS) did differ significantly between patients whose pregnancies were viable (ISS = 6.2) and those whose pregnancies were nonviable (ISS = 21.6). Although any fetal injury can occur, the most common are skull fractures and intracranial hemorrhage.

Lethal placental or direct injury can occur even in the absence of significant maternal injury.[12,13] In one series, in about 50% of cases other injuries to the mother, excluding injuries related to the pregnancy, were minor. Whether or not the mother is wearing a seat belt seems to be crucial in determining the extent of maternal injuries. Agran and colleagues reported a series of nine fetal deaths in mothers who were not using seat belts.[14] Evidence of fetal distress was not always apparent at the time of initial evaluation and in all fetal deaths placental abruption was documented. The injury mechanism was generally impact with the steering wheel. In another study Wolf examined, retrospectively, pregnancy outcome in relation to the use of seat belts.[15] Unrestrained pregnant women drivers were 1.9 times more likely to have a low birth-weight baby and 2.3 times more likely to give birth within 48 hours after the motor vehicle crash. Although a trend for an increased risk of fetal deaths was observed among unrestrained women, too few fetal deaths occurred to make a conclusive statement.

Allied to the increased risk from a failure to use seat belts are possible socioeconomic factors. Emerick showed that traumatic infant deaths were more likely to occur if any of the following factors were present: low maternal age, out-of-hospital birth, unwed mother, late or no prenatal care, low birth weight, and poor maternal education.[16]

Initial management (obstetric and anesthetic)

Pregnant patients of 20 weeks' gestation or greater should not be placed in the supine position unless a spinal injury is suspected. Uterine compression of the vena cava reduces venous return to the heart, decreases cardiac output, and exacerbates existing shock. In addition, experimental evidence suggests that prolonged vena caval obstruction may result in abruptio placentae.[17] The pregnant patient should therefore be transported and evaluated on her left side. If a spinal injury is suspected and the patient is on a backboard, the right hip should be elevated and the uterus displaced manually to the side. Alternative means of relieving aortocaval compression using a human wedge have also been described.[18]

In the primary assessment of the patient, the ABCs (airway, breathing, circulation, and hemorrhage control) should be followed the same as for the nonpregnant patient. Supplementary oxygen should be administered at the outset. A team approach to the pregnant trauma patient is essential, and the primary goal is stabilization of the mother who will attempt to maintain her own homeostasis even at the expense of the fetus. An assessment of the intravascular volume status is essential. Because of the increased intravascular volume and the rapid contraction of the uteroplacental circulation shunting blood away from the fetus, the pregnant patient can, as outlined above, lose up to 30% of her blood volume before tachycardia, hypotension, and other signs of hypovolemia occur. Thus, although the mother's condition and signs are stable, the fetus may be deprived of vital perfusion. Large-bore intravenous catheters should be placed peripherally and also centrally if required. Crystalloid fluid resuscitation and early type-specific blood are required to maintain the normal hypervolemic state. Vasopressors may be needed to maintain the normal maternal blood pressure; ephedrine should be used as the first line of defense. Crystalloid volume replacement should be in a ratio of 3 ml of fluid to every 1 ml of estimated blood loss until blood becomes available.

Lactated Ringer's solution is the crystalloid of choice because the administration of 0.9% sodium chloride can result in a hyperchloremic acidosis exacerbating the already present lactic acidosis. If ventilatory support is required, the mother should be cautiously hyperventilated to produce a $Paco_2$ similar to the pregnant state.

Initial laboratory studies should include a complete blood count, platelet count, and coagulation profile. The latter should include a prothrombin time, partial thromboplastin time, and fibrinogen. Blood should be typed and cross-matched if appropriate and blood chemistry and urine analysis also performed. The importance of the initial investigations is to establish baseline values, which must be interpreted in the light of the anticipated pregnancy changes. In particular, changes in WBC may be difficult to interpret. A significant rise in leukocyte count following severe abdominal trauma may suggest a ruptured liver or spleen. With the former the leukocyte count averages 24,000 cells/mm^3, while a count of 19,000 cells/mm^3 can be expected with a splenic injury.[1] As outlined above, labor itself can cause a leukocyte count of the order of 25,000 cells/mm^3.

In patients who are unconscious or who have sustained serious abdominal trauma, a nasogastric tube should be inserted. Aspiration of blood necessitates surgical exploration. Patients with suspected cribriform plate fracture should have an orogastic tube placed. A rectal examination should be undertaken to ascertain the presence of blood in the rectum and to assist in the exclusion of urethral injury, following which a urinary catheter should be inserted. Urine output should be maintained at least at 0.5 ml/kg/hr.

Fetal evaluation. Fetal evaluation should be undertaken early in the assessment. Fetal status can be used to assess the effect of maternal resuscitation, in that following adequate maternal resuscitation the fetus may not show any signs of distress. On the other hand, unsuccessful maternal resuscitation may be reflected by continued fetal distress. This is because the uteroplacental unit is highly dependent on an adequate maternal perfusion pressure and because in the healthy uteroplacental unit, functional reserve does not exist. However, oxygen consumption by the fetus does not decrease until levels of oxygen delivery to the fetus are severely compromised, at which time blood flow will be preferentially distributed to the fetal heart, brain, and adrenals.[19]

Abdominal trauma

Abdominal trauma can be categorized into blunt or penetrating, while the latter can be further subdivided into gunshot and knife wounds. Different patterns of injury are seen when knife wounds are in the lower as opposed to the upper abdomen.

Blunt abdominal trauma. Motor vehicle accidents account for approximately 40% of cases, followed by falls (30%) and direct assaults (20%).[7,20,21] Maternal mortality associated with motor vehicle accidents was reported in 1991 by the American College of Obstetricians and Gynecologists (ACOG) to be 7.2%, whilst fetal mortality was 14.7%.[22] Current ACOG recommendations are that pregnant women should wear three-point-restraint seat belts with the lap belt placed across the lap and not over the uterine fundus. Blunt trauma usually results in solid organ damage to the liver, spleen, kidneys or pancreas. Hollow organs such as the gastrointestinal tract are usually involved at points of fixation such as the cecum, hepatic or splenic flexures, duodenum, and anorectal junction.

Management (obstetric and anesthetic). Management of blunt abdominal trauma includes maternal stabilization and close cardiovascular monitoring. Cardiovascular decompensation does not occur until 25% to 30% of blood volume is lost; therefore, crystalloid requirements may be up to 50% greater than that calculated for the nonpregnant trauma patient. If the combination of lateral tilt and crystalloid resuscitation fails to provide stabilization, the patient may need blood without delay. In dire emergencies, O-negative blood may be required. The use of military antishock trousers (MAST) is no longer recommended in the Advanced Trauma Life Support course.[2] In pregnant patients, MAST suits carry an additional disadvantage in that inflation of the abdominal compartment may cause the enlarged uterus to compress the inferior vena cava with a resultant decrease in venous return.

Following the initial primary survey and maternal stabilization, a secondary assessment should be conducted. This secondary survey should follow the same pattern as in the nonpregnant patient (i.e., head-to-toe examination). In addition, examination should include an assessment of uterine irritability, fundal height, uterine tenderness, and fetal heart tones and movement. Pelvic examination should identify pelvic bone abnormalities, vaginal bleeding, injuries to the lower reproductive tract, and an assessment of the integrity of fetal membranes. Uterine contraction may suggest early labor, whilst tetanic contraction accompanied by vaginal bleeding suggests premature separation of the normally implanted placenta. Amniotic fluid in the vagina, with a pH of 7 to 7.5, suggests ruptured chorioamniotic membranes. If blood is coming from the cervical os, an obstetrician should be consulted immediately.

Fetal heart rate is best determined by a Doppler stethoscope or portable ultrasound so as not to confuse fetal tachycardia with maternal tachycardia. Portable ultrasound has the advantage of allowing direct fetal heart visibility, thus facilitating a more certain assessment of fetal viability. Ultrasound also allows assessment of gestational age, fetal presentation, amniotic fluid volume, and placental integrity. However, a normal-appearing placenta assessed on ultrasound does not rule out placental abruption. If delivery of the fetus is to be considered, it would be important to determine the biparietal diameter, abdominal circumference, and femur length so that by using established normograms, gestational age and estimated fetal weight can be determined.

Radiologic evaluation of the pregnant trauma patient should proceed the same as for the non-pregnant patient. Adverse fetal effects from the small radiation dose are rare and should not preclude radiologic evaluation even in the first trimester if indicated. If necessary the maternal abdomen can be shielded for radiographs of the chest and cervical spine. Computed tomography (CT) has been used in evaluation of both head and abdominal trauma; it has a radiation exposure less than conventional radiographs with no demonstrable adverse fetal effects. Unnecessary duplication of films should be avoided.

Diagnosis of intraperitoneal bleeding or perforation of an organ or viscus can be difficult because the usual signs of peritoneal irritation are not as pronounced in the pregnant trauma patient. The closed technique of four-quadrant pericentesis and culdocentesis is no longer used and has been replaced by diagnostic peritoneal lavage (DPL) (Buschbaum). In the pregnant patient, positioning of the DPL catheter may be difficult when the uterus is significantly enlarged. Ultrasound guidance of catheter insertion may be useful. Indications and contraindications for, and interpretation of, DPL are shown in Boxes 15-1 and 15-2, respectively. Because of its approximately 95% rate of accuracy, DPL is highly specific for the presence of significant intraabdominal trauma. If doubt exists despite a negative DPL, laparotomy should be performed.

Organ rupture. Hepatic and/or splenic rupture may occur in up to 25% of patients following blunt abdominal trauma after a motor vehicle accident. Hepatic rupture is not always associated with hypotension or shock. The presenting features may be sudden-onset upper abdominal pain referred to the shoulders, and/or nausea and fever. Serum transaminase levels are grossly elevated, often 10 times normal, and the prothrombin time may be prolonged. If hepatic rupture is suspected, DPL should be performed but diagnosis may need to be

---

BOX 15-1   INDICATIONS AND CONTRAINDICATIONS FOR DIAGNOSTIC PERITONEAL LAVAGE

Indications:
    Peritoneal signs
    Altered mental status
    Unexplained shock
    Multiple severe trauma
    Major thoracic injuries
    Osseus damage to lower rib cage
Contraindications:
    Advanced third trimester pregnancy
    Previous abdominal surgery

BOX 15-2   INTERPRETATION OF DIAGNOSTIC PERITONEAL LAVAGE AFTER BLUNT TRAUMA PERFORMED WITH 1 L RINGER'S LACTATE SOLUTION

Positive (any one indicates need for surgical exploration):
    Grossly bloody lavage fluid
    Red blood count > 100,000 cells/mm^3
    White blood count > 175 cells/mm^3
    Amylase concentration > 175 μ/dl
    Lavage fluid in Foley catheter
Indeterminate (repeat lavage):
    Red blood count > 50,000 cells/mm^3
    White blood count > 100 cells/mm^3
    Amylase concentration > 75 μ/dl

From Rothenberger DA, et al: *J Trauma* 1978; 18(3):173-179.

---

made by serial CT if necessary. Surgery should be undertaken by both a general surgeon and an obstetrician. Surgical procedures include hepatic lobe resection or hepatic artery ligation and the use of diagnostic hepatic arteriography in hemodynamically stable patients offers the option of selective embolization of the hepatic segmental vascular tree.

Splenic rupture may be associated with hypotension, positive peritoneal lavage, or an elevated maternal leukocyte count. Pain may be upper abdominal, generalized, or referred to the shoulder tip. At exploratory laparotomy it is important to identify the splenic artery and vein and not to simply clamp at or near the splenic hilum because the latter could result in damage to the tail of the pancreas. Unlike hepatic trauma, with a splenic rupture the spleen should be removed.

Uterine rupture is usually associated with pelvic fracture, although in a small percentage of cases it may follow direct trauma. Uterine rupture may present with hypotension, absent fetal heart tones, or gross hematuria if the posterior wall of the bladder is involved. Vaginal bleeding is usually present but is not always heavy. Immediate exploration should·be performed and evaluation of the rupture and integrity of the broad ligaments undertaken. Following evacuation of the fetus and membranes, the ruptured area is repaired. If repair is not possible, a hysterectomy should be performed.

Pelvic fractures. Pelvic fractures are associated with lower abdominal trauma and are of great concern. They may be associated with fetal injury or death, placental abruption, and injury to the maternal bladder, urethra, or birth canal. Pelvic fractures are classified as *(i)* minor avulsions, *(ii)* isolated rami fracture, and *(iii)* pelvic ring fractures. The most common fracture involves the anterior half of the pelvic ring involving the pubic rami. A valuable tool for acute evaluation is computed tomography, and the majority of patients with a pelvic fracture can be delivered vaginally.

Because of the cushioning effect of the amniotic fluid and the protective effect of the elastic uterine tissue, injury to the fetus occurs only rarely following blunt abdominal trauma. However, fetal skull fractures have been reported and may well be due to fetal skull entrapment between the maternal sacral promontory and the lap belt if placed over the fundus.

Pelvic fractures commonly result in injury to the maternal bladder or urethra, and injuries to these organs may also occur in advanced pregnancies. Lack of urine following insertion of a Foley catheter is highly suggestive of bladder injury. A cystogram will demonstrate extravasation into the retroperitoneal or intraperitoneal space. An inability to pass a Foley catheter should suggest urethral damage, and temporary drainage can be provided by insertion of a suprapubic cystotomy. Macroscopic or microscopic hematuria is considered suggestive of urinary tract trauma, and the amount of hematuria bears no correlation to either the extent or location of injury. If direct renal trauma is suspected, a drip intravenous pyelogram with CT will reveal the site of bleeding and/or trauma. Minor renal injuries can be managed conservatively, while major injuries with extensive extravasation of urine require immediate exploration through a midline incision.

Placental abruption. Placental abruption is the leading cause of fetal death and may be delayed up to 24 to 48 hours after the traumatic event, necessitating continued fetal monitoring. The diagnosis of abruptio placentae must be made on clinical grounds, and management of mild degrees remains controversial with observation often appropriate. The use of non–stress tests and ultrasound is suggested for the detection of mild degrees of abruption. Indications for prompt delivery include heavy vaginal bleeding, coagulopathy, and fetal distress. Continuous fetal monitoring for at least 48 hours has been recommended by Higgins, while Goodwin recommended observation of only 3 hours in patients who lack obstetric findings on initial presentation.[23,24]

Fetomaternal hemorrhage. Fetomaternal hemorrhage may result in fetal anemia, fetal distress, exanguination, and eventual fetal death.[25] Isoimmunization may also occur if the mother is Rh-negative. As little as 0.01 ml of Rh-positive blood will sensitize 70% of Rh-negative patients; therefore, the presence of fetomaternal hemorrhage in a Rh-negative mother should warrant Rh immunoglobulin therapy. Rose evaluated the incidence of fetomaternal hemorrhage following trauma and demonstrated an incidence of 28% (9 of 32 patients) and concluded that a Kleihauer-Betke analysis should be performed to detect the presence of fetal red cells in maternal circulation.[25] The mean volume transfused from the fetus was 16 ml. The test is conducted as follows. Adult hemoglobin from the maternal red cell is eluted through the cell membrane by an acid washout, but fetal hemoglobin is resistant to removal. After staining, fetal cells stain red and their numbers are compared with the number of adult ghost cells. A positive test is an indication for prolonged fetal monitoring. A negative test does not exclude minor degrees of fetomaternal hemorrhage that are capable of sensitizing the Rh-negative mother. Therefore all pregnant Rh-negative trauma patients should be considered for Rh immunoglobin therapy unless the injury is minor or remote from the uterus. In cases of doubt or established fetomaternal hemorrhage in Rh-negative mothers, a dose of 300 μg anti-D immunoglobin will suppress the immune response to 15 ml of transfused fetal blood cells. Immunoglobin therapy should be instituted within 72 hours of injury. Not all authors agree with the value of the Kliehauer-Betke test. Towery et al found the test to have a sensitivity of 56%, a specificity of 71%, and an accuracy of 27% after blunt injury.[26]

Thirty percent of cases of blunt abdominal injury are as a result of a fall. In these cases fetal outcome is usually good and all that is required is serial abdominal examination and non–stress testing. Assault secondary to domestic or nondomestic violence appears to be on the increase and will require involvement of auxiliary support such as the social services.

Penetrating abdominal injury. Penetrating abdominal injury is usually a result of a gunshot wound or knife injury. The stage of the pregnancy will strongly influence which organs are injured. In advanced pregnancy, penetrating injury below the uterine fundus will result in a lower likelihood of intraabdominal organ injury. If the uterus is involved in penetrating trauma, fetal injury may occur in 59% to 89% of cases, with a fetal mortality rate of 41% to 71%. Penetrating injury above the uterine fundus in an advanced pregnancy often damages multiple loops of bowel compressed into the upper abdomen. In one review, nonuterine intraabdominal damage was reported in 19% of cases with involvement in decreasing order of the small bowel, liver, colon, and stomach.

Gunshot wounds. If a bullet enters the uterus, the dense uterine musculature markedly reduces its velocity and the bullet remains imbedded in the uterus. Fetal death and injury may result from direct injury or indirect injury to the membranes, cord, or placenta. Entry and exit wounds must be identified and radiographs should be taken to localize the bullet if it has not exited. Radiography cannot be used to predict the extent of fetal injury, but ultrasound may be useful to evaluate the fetal biophysical status. Some gunshot wounds to the abdomen have been self-inflicted in an attempt to terminate the pregnancy.[27] In two cases, conservative management of the wounds was undertaken.[27] Current consensus is that even in hemodynamically stable patients, immediate surgical exploration is warranted via a vertical midline or paramedian incision. If the uterus and surrounding adnexa are injured, the problem is whether or not to perform a cesarean section. If a bullet has entered the uterus there is a high chance of fetal injury. If the fetus is dead and bleeding can be controlled, a cesarean section need not be performed. However, if the fetus is alive and near term, cesarean delivery and uterine repair is the usual course of action. When the fetus is beyond 24 weeks but not near term, three indications for cesarean section have been established: (1) fetal hemorrhage (2) uteroplacental insufficiency (3) infection. Cesarean hysterectomy should be performed if uterine injury is extensive with bleeding, hypotension, or significant injury to the parametria or uterine vessels. When the fetus is alive and cesarean delivery has not been performed, tocolytic therapy may be required postoperatively. Because of the cardiovascular side effects of the β-sympathomimetic agents, caution should be exercised in their use. These side effects may interfere with interpretation of maternal vital signs because ritrodrine and terbutaline can cause hypotension, tachycardia, widening of the pulse pressure, cardiac arrhythmias, myocardial ischemia, and pulmonary edema. The primary fetal side effect is tachycardia, which might also interfere with fetal evaluation. As such the preferred tocolytic agent should be magnesium sulfate, although in an animal model $MgSO_4$ has been shown to worsen the hemodynamic response to hemorrhage, in comparison to ritodrine.

Knife wounds. In the United States knife wounds are less common than gunshot wounds and they have a better prognosis because they are not accompanied by the shock waves and cavitation of gunshot wounds. In addition, the likelihood of visceral injury with stab wounds is much lower than gunshot wounds because during a stabbing an organ can slide away from the advancing blade and only about 50% of nonpregnant patients who are stabbed require surgical repair. In pregnancy, the "sliding effect" is lost to some extent; also, stab wounds of the upper abdomen may involve small bowel more frequently because of upper abdominal gastrointestinal compression in advanced pregnancy. Compared with gunshot wounds, stab wounds also result in a lower mortality (1.4% vs. 12.5%).

Whether or not to explore all abdominal stab wounds is controversial, because up to 30% of cases are not accompanied by peritoneal penetration.[9] As such, Cornell introduced the fistulogram in which, following wound cleaning, a catheter is placed into the wound and 75 ml of water-soluble contrast injected rapidly.[9] Subsequent radiographs demonstrate penetration of the peritoneal cavity. The large gravid uterus also influences the site of injury in that more than two thirds of anterior abdominal wounds, comprising 90% of all wounds, are in the upper abdomen, placing the bowel at risk.

Lower abdominal wounds. With sufficient force the uterus will be damaged and the surgeon must decide whether to explore the abdomen. Peritoneal lavage can be used to determine severe uterine bleeding in a stable patient. The major uterine vessels, which are lateral, may be far from the site of penetration, and close monitoring of the gravida together with a negative DPL can be used to rule out this injury. Urinary bladder injury can be ruled out following insertion of a Foley catheter or retrograde cystogram. However, if any doubts exist in the diagnosis of the extent of injury, an exploratory laparotomy should be undertaken. The use of amniocentesis to determine uterine bleeding should be regarded with caution because a negative amniocentesis does not rule out concealed maternal or fetal bleeding.

If the knife penetrates the uterus, fetal injury is likely and the surgeon must then decide whether or not delivery is appropriate. The same considerations for surgical delivery for gunshot wounds apply to knife wounds, and both a neonatologist and pediatric surgeon should be present at delivery.

Upper abdominal wounds. Many authorities believe that all pregnant patients with an upper abdominal stab wound should be explored. This is because the signs of peritoneal irritation are reduced, the results of peritoneal lavage are less satisfactory, and the likelihood of bowel penetration is higher especially in advanced pregnancies. With left-sided stab wounds, laceration of the diaphragm may also allow herniation of the colon, stomach, or small bowel into the thoracic cavity with the potential for strangulation. Although such patients may be initially asymptomatic, generalized abdominal pain, fever, and respiratory distress subsequently develop and result in a mortality rate of 10% to 20%, increasing significantly to 25% to 66% if strangulation and sepsis occur. At laparotomy, thorough evaluation of the diaphragm must be undertaken.

Head trauma

Central nervous system (CNS) trauma is the major contributor to mortality in 60% to 75% of major injuries. The incidence of nonfatal CNS or peripheral nerve injuries with or without permanent sequelae is not known.

Minor head injury. Superficial injuries to the scalp and face are common. If there is no history of severe impact, skull fracture, or loss of consciousness, the laceration may be managed by simple debridement and suturing. Any change in neurologic condition should be accompanied by a neurologic consultation.

Severe head injury. Major facial fractures, penetrating skull injuries, depressed skull fractures, CSF leakage, and unconsciousness suggest severe neurologic injury. Once stabilized, skull radiographs and a CT can be performed, the latter to identify an intracranial mass lesion and to differentiate edema, contusion, and intracerebral hematoma. Management includes securing the airway, oxygenation, hyperventilation, fluid resuscitation, and control of external hemorrhage. Immobilization of the cervical spine should be undertaken as part of the primary management. Once the existence of spinal fractures has been ruled out, the patient may be tilted with a roll placed under the backboard. Subsequent management of the severely head-injured pregnant patient is undertaken along the same lines as in the nonpregnant patient, but the left lateral tilt position must be maintained to avoid supine hypotension and maximize uteroplacental perfusion. External fetal heart rate monitoring should be maintained throughout the initial recovery period, and delivery of the fetus is not necessary unless the patient is beyond 24 weeks' gestation and there is evidence that the mother or fetus is near death. A schematic overview of management of trauma patients is described in Box 15-3.

Burns

Minor burns complicate 1 in 250 pregnancies, although this rate may be an underestimate because of underreporting. There is no evidence that pregnancy alters the incidence or the etiology of thermal injuries, compared with the nonpregnant state. Management of the burns patient depends on the size and severity (partial or full thickness) of the burn.

The "rule of nines," though developed for the nonpregnant patient, is used to assess the surface area involved. Presumably, the abdominal surface area in late pregnancy would account for a larger percentage of the total body surface area, com-

---

BOX 15-3 SCHEMATIC OVERVIEW OF MANAGEMENT OF TRAUMA PATIENTS

Primary survey
Patients are assessed, and life-threatening conditions are identified and managed
  Airway maintenance with cervical spine control
  Breathing and ventilation
  Circulation with hemorrhage control
  Disability: Neurologic evaluation
       Alert
       Responds to vocal stimuli
       Responds to painful stimuli
       Unresponsive
  Exposure/environmental control: Undress patient but prevent hypothermia

Resuscitation
  Airway
  Breathing/Ventilation/Oxygenation
  Circulation
  Urinary and Gastric catheters
  Monitoring ABGs, respiration rate, end-tidal CO_2, oximetry, blood pressure
  Transfer requirements

Radiologic examination
Secondary survey
The secondary survey begins after primary survey (ABCs) has been completed, resuscitation initiated, and ABCs reassessed. The secondary survey is a head-to-toe evaluation.
  History
  Physical examination (head to toe)

Constant reevaluation
Definitive care including appropriate interhospital transfer
Documentation and legal considerations

---

pared with the nonpregnant state. Pregnancy does not appear to have any direct effect on maternal survival. However, controversy exists concerning when to deliver the fetus. Some authors have recommended immediate delivery of second- and third-trimester fetuses in patients whose burns exceed 50% of body surface area. Criticism of these papers is that small numbers of patients were evaluated and retrospectively compared with nonpregnant patients. In addition, it had been speculated that some of the poor maternal-fetal outcome in the burns patients may reflect insufficient fluid resuscitation resulting in hypovolemia and fetal hypoxia.

Burn management should be the same as for the burned nonpregnant patient, and should include oxygenation, chest radiography if smoke inhalation is suspected, arterial blood gases, and blood and laboratory tests. A Foley catheter should be immediately inserted and fluid resuscitation, which is crucial to management, should be initiated according to the percentage of burns and adjusted in relation to serial chemistry and electrolytes. Urine output should be maintained close to 100 ml/hr. Greatest losses occur during the first 12 hours.

Stillbirth or preterm labor and delivery, which usually ensue within the first few days, are often associated with an unstable mother. Prostaglandin levels are increased in the burn trauma patient and this may be related to hypovolemia, hypoxia, and decreased uteroplacental perfusion. All of these may contribute to an increase in the incidence of preterm labor, and the subsequent use of tocolytic agents may aggravate the maternal condition. Beta-sympathomimetic agents are associated with hypotension, increased capillary permeability, and possibly increased fluid requirements. Magnesium sulfate, on the other hand, is associated with a transient vasodilation. In our view, in the face of preterm labor, indomethacin is the safest tocolytic agent until the maternal condition stabilizes.

Perimortem cesarean delivery

Cardiopulmonary resuscitation should begin immediately after a cardiac arrest occurs, and in the nonpregnant patient the best cardiac output is obtained in the supine position. Even in the supine position the best cardiac output is about 30% of the normal output. Placing the pregnant patient in the supine position produces aortocaval compression and reduces venous return to the heart. On the other hand, tilting the patient causes a loss of direct force during external cardiac compression. Therefore, if resuscitation effects are not immediately successful, the infant must be delivered by perimortem section without delay. Delivery by cesarean section should begin within 4 minutes of the cardiac arrest, and cardiopulmonary resuscitation (CPR) should be continued during and after the procedure.[28] The need for sterility should be a low priority, and a classical uterine incision should be used. Attempts at delivery should be made at any time after maternal death if signs of fetal life are documented.

Because cesarean delivery is associated with increased blood loss, it should not be performed on the unstable parturient in whom a cardiac arrest has not yet occurred because this may result in a poorer outcome. Also, if CPR is successful, it is better not to perform cesarean section even if fetal distress is present but first to determine the impact of in utero resuscitation.

Conclusion

The approach to the pregnant trauma patient is team-orientated. Not only is it essential to involve an obstetrician but it is also very important to involve a general surgeon, a pediatrician, and in cases requiring resuscitation and surgery, an anesthesiologist.

ORTHOPEDIC PROBLEMS
Kyphoscoliosis

Kyphoscoliosis is a bony deformity of the spine characterized by either excessive posterior (kyphosis) or lateral (scoliosis) curvature. In approximately 80% of cases, the cause is unknown (idiopathic scoliosis). Other unusual causes include tuberculosis, osteoporosis, neuromuscular disease (poliomyelitis, cerebral palsy), or connective tissue disorders such as Marfan syndrome, Morquio syndrome, or Ehlers-Danlos syndrome. In the United States, the prevalence of scoliosis in adults between 25 and 74 years of age was reported to be 8.3% between 1971 and 1975.[29] The prevalence of scoliosis increases with age among women but not among men. Women have about twice the prevalence as men (10.7% vs. 5.6%).

Patients with untreated kyphoscoliosis have an increased risk of developing respiratory failure and premature death.[30] Kyphoscoliosis causes a reduction in lung volumes that can sometimes be quite severe.[31,32] Airway resistance when related to lung volume is nearly normal, however. There is also an inequality of ventilation and perfusion due to airway closure in dependent regions[33] and a decrease in the size of the pulmonary vascular bed.[34] The lungs are also partially compressed by the altered rib cage, resulting in atelectasis. Gas exchange abnormalities occur, but their severity does not correlate well with the degree of thoracic deformity.[34] The combination of kyphosis and scoliosis is also worse than either abnormality alone. A spectrum of breathing abnormalities has also

been identified during sleep in patients with kyphoscoliosis.[35] All patients who are hypoxemic during sleep are also hypercapnic in the daytime, and the decrease in SaO_2 with sleep is related to hypoventilation.[36]

Scoliosis and pregnancy incidence. The incidence of kyphoscoliosis in pregnancy ranges from 1 in 1471 to 1 in 12,000.[37] Scoliosis patients have more premature births than expected but rates of other adverse reproductive events are not increased.[38] In a review of the literature, Betz and colleagues found the obstetric complication rate in patients with scoliosis to be 1 in 4000 pregnancies.[39] These investigators also examined the effects of scoliosis on pregnancy and delivery in 175 women and found the cesarean section rate to be half the national average.

Pathophysiology. There are conflicting reports of the effects of pregnancy on the risk of progression of the curve in a scoliotic patient.[40] Those with stable curvatures did not progress in one report, whereas those with unstable scoliosis demonstrated progression.[41] Berman concluded that those who were at greater risk of curvature progression had a prepregnancy curve greater than 25 degrees.[42] Other authors have not found that curve stability influences progression.[39]

Respiratory complications during pregnancy in patients with kyphoscoliosis have been reported.[43,44] Increased breathlessness with no serious cardiorespiratory problems was encountered in 17% of patients in one series.[44] As a rule, patients with severe restrictive lung disease with a vital capacity less than 1 L should be advised to avoid pregnancy or consider therapeutic abortion.

Obstetric and anesthetic management. Maternal mortality and morbidity will be related to the degree of cardiorespiratory compromise in the patient. Mortality will be considerably increased if the vital capacity is less than 1.25 L. However, pregnancy may progress normally if the prepregnant lung volumes exceed 50% of predicted.[42,43] Parturients with a pronounced kyphoscoliosis should have an anesthetic consultation at the earliest possible time. Ideally, these patients are followed routinely at least every 2 months, at which time vital capacity, forced expiratory volume, oxygen saturation, and electrocardiography should be performed. If hypoventilation is suspected, an arterial blood gas should be performed.

Monitoring of fetal development, in conjunction with the cardiorespiratory impact of the pregnancy on the kyphoscoliotic state, is indicated. If maternal health deteriorates, fetal lung maturation tests may become necessary and early delivery given consideration. Cesarean section may be indicated in cases of abnormal pelvis, malpresentation, or ineffective labor.

Anesthetic management for labor and delivery should include epidural analgesia with a low concentration of bupivacaine and opiate by continuous infusion. For cesarean section, epidural anesthesia may again be indicated especially if there is associated respiratory problems. Both epidural and spinal anesthesia may be difficult because of distortion of the spinal column and epidural space. Proper placement of an epidural catheter may also be difficult. In extremely difficult case, a continuous spinal anesthesia may be considered. However, in certain cases, during regional anesthesia the patient may not tolerate positioning in the lateral tilt position. General anesthesia may then be necessary to facilitate both proper control of the airway and adequate ventilation. In such cases with disturbed gas exchange, an arterial line would be appropriate. Proper postoperative analgesic management can be achieved via an epidural catheter or spinal catheter if one has been inserted for the cesarean section.

In summary, the incidence of kyphoscoliosis in pregnancy is relatively high. Premature birth rates are higher than in the normal population. The risk of progression of the abnormal curve in scoliotic patients appears low. However, women with unstable scoliosis at the time of pregnancy may demonstrate progression of the curve. Respiratory complications have been reported but are not generally serious unless severe restrictive lung disease is present, in which case pregnancy should be avoided or termination considered. Continuation of the pregnancy requires close monitoring, anesthetic consultation, and time to undertake regional anesthesia.

Surgically corrected orthopedic problems

Surgical correction of kyphoscoliosis has usually been achieved over the past 30 years by the insertion of a metal rod such as a Harrington, Luque or Cotrell-Doubousset rod. The kyphoscoliosis is usually idiopathic, and scoliotic curvatures exceeding 20 degrees that require treatment are up to 7 times more frequent in women.[45,46] As those women with idiopathic scoliosis enter childbearing age, it is not uncommon for them to present to the obstetric department especially for operative delivery, their cesarean section rate being twice that seen in normal women.[47]

The anesthetic implications of scoliosis have been described earlier in this chapter. After surgical correction, cardiorespiratory pathophysiology is either arrested or even improved.[48] In obstetric anesthesia the primary consideration is the feasibility of regional anesthesia for delivery. Instrumentation with a rod poses little impediment to access to the spinal canal, because it is placed overlying the transverse processes. However, it is the healed spinal fusion, usually facilitated with an autologous graft from the iliac bone, that poses the greatest problem for conducting a regional procedure. In preparation for the above graft, the spinous processes are removed and the laminae decorticated as far as the facet joints bilaterally, which are also destroyed. The anesthesiologists' usual tactile landmarks are therefore obliterated, and attempts to penetrate to the interlaminar space may become random so as to avoid healed bone graft.

The likelihood of successful lumbar regional placement depends on the extent of the fusion that can be obtained from the patient records and radiographs. On examination, the cutaneous scar extends slightly beyond the fusion and the spinal processes, if palpable, demonstrate an area not involved. In general, fusions usually stop at L4.[48] Rates of successful epidural placement vary, depending on the level of fusion. In 12 cases, Hubbert was only able to successfully locate the space in 42% (5 cases), despite multiple attempts at both the lateral and the midline approach.[49] Crosby and Halpern succeeded in 6 of 8 patients, one of which required multiple attempts.[50] Daley et al had a much higher success rate of 94% (16 out of 18 cases), although 29% required three or more attempts.[51] In this series, failure to enter the vertebral canal occurred only if the fusion extended to L3 or lower.

Even if the epidural space can be identified, concern has been raised over the ability of local anesthetic solution to spread normally.[46] Scarring may disrupt the epidural space, and although some have reported normal onset time (2 to 4 minutes), Daley et al noted that 58% of Harrington rod patients had either increased local anesthetic requirements or patchy blockade.[51] Others have reported dural puncture in small series of patients.[49,50] Recently, Pascoe et al reported a case of attempted epidural anesthesia in a parturient with a Harrington rod insertion, in whom the block could not be extended beyond the T10 level.[52] Adequate anesthesia was provided by means of a subarachnoid block. The epidural anesthesia had been attempted with 3% 2-chloroprocaine, and the spinal block was provided by 10 mg of tetracaine in 5% dextrose with a 22-gauge Sprotte needle inserted at L4-L5. The brief duration of the 2-chloroprocaine was of benefit in that it permitted the safe administration of a different regional anesthetic.

Considering the problems with lumbar epidural anesthesia, Kardash et al felt the choice of subarachnoid block at the L5-S1 interspace offered distinct advantages.[53] By using the lowest available lumbar interspace, the chance of success at the first attempt is greatly increased. Second, the clear end-point of cerebrospinal fluid (CSF) eliminates equivocal identification of the epidural space. Third, spread of local anesthetic solution should be more reliable, and finally, the L5 S1 space is the widest in the spine. When using hyperbaric solutions it may be necessary to employ a degree of Trendelenburg tilt, depending on the degree of correction of the spinal curvature abnormality. In his case report, Kardash used 15 mg bupivacaine 0.75% in 8.25% dextrose and placed the patient in a 15-degree Trendelenburg tilt for 5 minutes.

For vaginal delivery, an epidural catheter could be placed at the L5-S1 level; this would be considerably less traumatic than attempted insertion at the midlumbar level.

In summary, it is essential that obstetricians be encouraged to send patients with previous spinal surgery to the anesthesia department for consultation well before the expected date of delivery. The various options for analgesia in labor and operative delivery can then be adequately discussed. One consideration when opting for epidural anesthesia is that there is an increased likelihood of a dural puncture with subsequent headache, which requires an epidural blood patch. Provision of such a blood patch may be extremely difficult.

Achondroplasia

Achondroplasia, characterized by abnormal endochondral bone formation, is inherited as an autosomal dominant genetic condition with spontaneous mutation in 80% of cases. The condition is rare, with an approximate incidence of 4 in 100,000, and it is the most common cause of dwarfism. Females are more frequently affected, and fertility rates are low. However, a number of cases have been reported in which pregnancy progresses to term, and in view of the bony abnormalities of the pelvis and the likelihood of cephalopelvic disproportion, most deliver by cesarean section.

Anesthetic management. Although many patients with achondroplasia will request regional anesthesia, some authors have cautioned against the use of epidural anesthesia because the abnormal spinal anatomy in these cases may increase the risks of patchy blocks, dural puncture, or spinal cord trauma.[54,55] This, combined with a lack of dosage guidelines, have led to a reluctance to use regional anesthesia. However, the advantages of regional anesthesia must be weighed against the disadvantages of general anesthesia in an achondroplastic patient who is also pregnant.[56] The shortened skull base, due to

premature occipital fusion, may cause limited atlanto-occipital extension. The narrow foramen magnum and possible atlanto-axial instability may render attempts at neck extension hazardous; in later years the development of spinal stenosis and exaggerated lumbar lordosis and possible scoliosis may cause technical difficulties with epidural anesthesia.

Mather in 1966 described a case of intubation difficulty in a male achondroplastic patient,[56] and several authors have found that smaller than expected tracheal tubes were usually necessary.[57,58] However, not all investigators have experienced intubation difficulties[59,60] in pregnant achondroplastic patients, and it may be that pregnant women in their third or fourth decade represent a subgroup that has survived the deformity-related risks of earlier life but has not yet acquired those of the fifth decade and beyond. In a recent report by McArthur, preoperative airway assessment indicated a Mallampati Class I airway, and radiographs of the cervical spine undertaken in full neck extension and flexion reassured the author who proceeded with an uneventful general anesthetic.[61] In this report, McArthur also experienced problems with the placement of an automated noninvasive blood pressure cuff in that the arm of the patient was short and thick-set. The only cuff that could be fitted resulted in inaccurately high systolic readings, and a direct arterial pressure line was required.

The published literature contains five case reports describing the use of epidural anesthesia for cesarean section in achondroplastic dwarfs.[59,62-65] Difficulty with catheter insertion was experienced in two cases. One of these was complicated by dural puncture and the other by epidural vein cannulation. However, all five patients had a successful epidural block. In one, it was necessary to insert the epidural needle above the patient's pronounced lordotic lumbar spine.[65] In all but one of the cases a very small epidural dose was required to achieve an adequate level of surgical anesthesia. In all cases careful epidural titration with small incremental doses is essential, and it would seem prudent to use a fast-onset agent such as lidocaine to facilitate early detection of the achieved sensory level.[66] In one case the slow onset of 0.5% bupivacaine may have contributed to excessive dosing and a very high epidural block.[63] Use of a test dose containing epinephrine is also controversial because the volume of test dose should be reduced to 1 ml, which in a standard solution of 1:200,000 would only contain 5 μg of epinephrine. Preparation of a separate solution containing epinephrine 15 μg/ml would seem more appropriate, in addition to carefully monitoring the patient after each administered increment.

To date there have been no detailed reports on the use of spinal anesthesia for cesarean section in the pregnant achondroplastic patient. As one would expect a narrower spinal canal and exaggerated spinal curvature in these patients, spread of a subarachnoid solution could be highly unpredictable.

In summary, the decision to choose general or epidural anesthesia in these patients would depend to a large extent on the technical ability of the anesthesiologist. Although the fear of a difficult intubation may be less than previously thought, wherever possible regional anesthesia would seem to be the preferred technique. Because no dosage guidelines are available and most case reports indicate a lower than usual epidural dose requirement, the block must be established with small increments and sufficient time allowed for each dose to take effect.

Osteogenesis imperfecta

Pathophysiology and clinical features. Osteogenesis imperfecta (OI) is an inherited disease of connective tissue that affects bone, sclera, and the inner ear. The genetic defect that leads to this disorder is thought to be explained by mutations within the genome that encodes for type 1 collagen, specifically type I procollagen.[67] Expression ranges from mild osteoporosis to the classic clinical stigmata characterized by multiple bone fractures, blue sclera, and middle ear deafness. The heterogeneity of OI is responsible for four clinical entities.[68] Type I, or osteogenesis imperfecta tarda levis, is the most prevalent, occurring with a frequency of 1 in 28,000 live births. Type II, or perinatal lethal form, is associated with a stillborn infant or early neonatal death. Type III OI is usually manifested by progressive skeletal deformities in the first and second decades of life. The blue sclera is less intense than in type I and may be normal. Type IV patients have normal sclera.

The functional immaturity of cells in OI is not limited to bone and connective tissue. Pathologic evaluation has demonstrated decreased collagen on a uterus that ruptured during spontaneous vaginal delivery.[69] There have also been reports of dysfunctional platelet aggregation and prolonged bleeding.[70,71] In addition, a hypermetabolic state with hyperthermia has been reported, and these patients may be at increased risk of developing malignant hyperthermia when exposed to general anesthesia, though this has not been reported in clinical practice.[72,73]

Genetic counseling requires an accurate family history to at least three generations and a review of all phenotypic diagnostic studies such as ultrasound, as well as radiographic and genotypic data obtained by collagen and/or DNA linkage analysis.

Only types I and IV are of importance to the obstetric anesthetist, because type II is perinatally fatal and type III patients usually die in childhood from severe kyphoscolosis. Types I and IV are both autosomally dominant and both have short stature and dentinogenesis resulting in easily broken teeth. Fractures in type I, the most common of the four, are generally nondeforming, while those of type IV tend to cause long-bone and thoracic deformities.

Anesthetic management. When managing anesthesia, care must be taken with the teeth because of the propensity for broken or dislodged teeth. Care must also be taken when moving the patient to and from the operating table, and pressure areas should be well padded. An automated arterial pressure cuff, if overinflated, may cause a fractured humerus. Suxamethonium-induced fasciculations may also cause fractures. Hyperextension of the neck must be avoided.

Because there is a tendency for these patients to develop hyperthermia (though not of a malignant type), the temperature should be monitored closely.[74] If thoracic deformities are severe they may be associated with significant mechanical disease including a reduced vital capacity, decreased chest-wall compliance, and hypoxemia from ventilation-perfusion mismatch. Therefore, an increased F_{IO_2} and decreased tidal volumes are recommended.[75] Unusual bleeding caused by platelet abnormalities may require platelet transfusion. Increased serum thyroxin concentrations associated with increased oxygen consumption occur in at least 50% of patients.[76]

Cho and colleagues reported a case of general anesthesia in a parturient with OI.[75] Although the procedure was successful, hyperthermia (38° 7) did occur, and it responded to cooling by blanket and cold intravenous solutions. General anesthesia was used because the patient refused a regional procedure. Conduction block is preferred because it avoids the necessity for tracheal intubation, it makes the development of hyperthermia less likely, and it facilitates the detection of thyroid storm. For cesarean section either spinal or epidural anesthesia may be used. In two case reports, epidural anesthesia was used successfully, although there is the possibility of technical difficulty if there has been a previous fracture of the lumbar spine.[77]

Backache

Because of various changes that take place during pregnancy, some preexisting orthopedic problems may deteriorate. As the uterus enlarges anteriorly, progressive lordosis becomes common as a compensatory posture, shifting the center of gravity over the lower extremities. Because of the hormone relaxin, there is increased mobility of the sacroiliac, sacrococcygeal, and pubic joints during pregnancy. Backache is a common problem in parturients; it is usually related to anterior sacroiliac joint dysfunction.[78] Minor backache may follow excessive strain when bending, lifting, or walking. Severe backache associated with radiating leg pain can restrict activity. However, it is interesting to note that pain due to herniated lumbar disk is not common in pregnancy. Both LaBan et al[79] and Crawford[80] described the incidence of acute herniated lumbar disk disease during pregnancy to be in 1 in 10,000 parturients.

Mild backache can be treated by avoiding stress and strain or by using a lightweight maternity girdle. Severe acute backache requires orthopedic consultation, and depending on the cause, treatment can vary from analgesics to heat compression to complete bedrest. Occasionally, parturients can have severe pelvic pain, which may be related to relaxation of symphysis pubis, lumbosacral joints, and pelvic ligaments. Application of a wide belt at the level of iliac spine to bring the symphysis pubis together has been used to treat the pain. In severe cases, parturients may need prolonged bed rest or even treatment with local anesthetic and steroid injection in the sacroiliac joint. Usually back pain associated with pregnancy will not change the mode of delivery. If vaginal delivery is selected, proper pain relief becomes an essential part of the labor and delivery. Parturients with severe back pain or an associated prolapsed disk should visit with the anesthesiologist for consultation before the expected date of delivery. During the visit the patient should be thoroughly examined in regard to the source and type of pain. Any sensory and motor deficits are noted carefully in the consultation chart. The neurologist's notes or investigation results are also charted, if available. Following this the patient is consulted for an anesthetic plan for vaginal delivery or cesarean section. Regional anesthesia, either spinal or epidural, should not be contraindicated in the majority of these patients. In a large series from Canada, Ong observed that complications from regional anesthesia in these patients were infrequent (19 in 10,000) and in all cases reported, the problems resolved within 72 hours.[81] Peng et al suggested that injection of 1.0 ml of 0.5% bupivacaine bilaterally into the interspinous space near the lamina will reduce the incidence of backache.[82] In the presence of a herniated lumbar disk there is some evidence of delayed onset[83] or occasionally absence of an-

esthesia at the site of damaged intervertebral disks. This might be related to adhesions or scarring resulting from the healing process following intervebral disk injury, which may limit the spread of local anesthetics in the epidural space.

Back pain occurring in the days after delivery has been reported in 30% to 45% of women receiving epidural analgesia during labor.[84,85] However, in an interview study of 155 women who had singleton deliveries, Grove found that back pain occurred in 40% women who delivered without epidural anesthesia and that the back pain was gone within 6 days after delivery.[86] MacArthur et al, in a postal questionnaire study of more than 11,000 deliveries, showed that new-onset long-term backache occurred in 19% of women who received epidural anesthesia for vaginal delivery and 10% of women who did not.[87] Long-term backache was defined as backache of at least 6 weeks' duration beginning within 3 months of delivery. However, the response rate in MacArthur's study was only 19% and the study required voluntary reporting of back pain that occurred 1 to 9 years previously. In a study with less recall bias, Russell et al, using either postal questionnaire or phone interview, found a 12% incidence of new-onset postpartum back pain in women who delivered without epidural anesthesia and an 18% incidence in women who had epidural anesthesia.[88] In this study, 1015 women were included, with a 68% response rate. In addition, data were collected within 18 months of delivery. The most recent study from Breen et al looked at the incidence of back pain 1 to 2 months postpartum in a group of 1042 women who delivered a singleton infant.[89] Parturients were interviewed 12 to 48 hours following delivery and 2 months later by questionnaire. Breen found that the incidence of postpartum back pain in women who received epidural anesthesia was equivalent to those who did not (44% vs. 45%). Breen and colleagues found that postpartum backache was associated with a history of back pain, younger age, and greater body weight. In the Breen study there was a 26% incidence of new-onset back pain, of which 6.5% was reported to be severe. New-onset postpartum back pain was found to be associated with greater body weight and shorter stature. No association was found between postpartum back pain and epidural anesthesia, number of attempts at epidural placement, duration of second stage of labor, mode of delivery, or birth weight.

In summary, regional anesthesia is the preferred method in parturients with backache. In addition, the importance of early antenatal assessment and counseling of the patient by the department of anesthesia cannot be overemphasized.

REFERENCES

1. Buchsbaum HJ: Accidental injury during pregnancy. *Contemp Ob Gyn* 1982; 20:27.
2. Alexander RH, Proctor HJ: *Trauma in Pregnancy: Advanced Trauma Life Support Course for Physicians*, ed 5, The American College of Surgeons, 1993, pp 283-292.
3. Rothenberger D, Quattlebaum FW, Perry JF, et al: Blunt maternal trauma: A review of 103 cases. *J Trauma* 1978; 18(3):173.
4. Stuart GC, Harding PG, Davies EM: Blunt abdominal trauma in pregnancy. *Can Med Assoc J* 1980; 122:901.
5. Pearlman MD, Tintinalli JE, Lorenz RP: Blunt trauma during pregnancy. *N Engl J Med* 1990; 323:1609.
6. Pearlman MD, Tintinalli JE, Lorenz RP: A prospective controlled study of outcome after trauma during pregnancy. *Am J Obstet Gynecol* 1990; 162:1502.
7. Esposito TJ, Gens DR, Smith LG, et al: Trauma during pregnancy—a review of 79 cases. *Arch Surg* 1991; 126:1073.
8. Pearlman MD, Tintinallo JW: Evaluation and treatment of the gravida and fetus following trauma during pregnancy. *Gynecol Clin North Am* 1991; 18(2):371.
9. Kuhlmann RS, Cruikshank DP: Maternal trauma during pregnancy. *Clin Obstet Gynecol* 1994; 37(2):274.
10. Whitehead EM, Smith M, Dean Y, et al: An evaluation of gastric emptying times in pregnancy and the puerperium. *Anaesthesia* 1993; 48:53.
11. Kissinger DP, Rozycki GS, Morris JA, et al: Trauma in pregnancy—predicting pregnancy outcome. *Arch Surg* 1991; 126:1079.
12. Farmer DL, Adzick NS, Crombleholme WR, et al: Fetal trauma: relation to maternal injury. *J Pediatr Surg* 1990; 25(7):711.
13. Lane PL: Traumatic fetal deaths. *J Emerg Med* 1989; 7(5):433.
14. Agran PF, Dunkle DE, Winn DG, et al: Fetal death in motor vehicle accidents. *Ann Emerg Med* 1987; 16(12):1355.
15. Wolf ME, Alexander BH, Rivara FP, et al: A retrospective cohort study of seatbelt use and pregnancy outcome after a motor vehicle crash. *J Trauma* 1993; 34(1):116.
16. Emerick SJ, Foster LR, Campbell DT: Risk factors for traumatic infant death in Oregon, 1973 to 1982. *Pediatrics* 1986; 77:518.
17. Reed NE, Teteris NJ, Essig GF: Inferior venal caval obstruction syndrome with electrocardiographically documented fetal bradycardia. *Obstet Gynecol* 1970; 36:462.
18. Goodwin AP, Pearce AJ: The human wedge: A manoeuvre to relieve aortocaval compression during resuscitation in late pregnancy. *Anaesthesia* 1992; 47(5):433.
19. Iwamoto HS: Cardiovascular responses to reduced oxygen delivery: Studies in fetal sheep at 0.55-0.7 gestation, in Gluckman P, Johnson MB, Nathaniely P, (eds): *Advances in Fetal Physiology.* vol 8: Research in Perinatal Medicine. Ithaca, NY, *Perinatology Press,* 1980, p 55.
20. Rothenberger D, Quattlebaum FW, Perry JF, et al: Blunt maternal trauma: A review of 103 cases. *J Trauma* 1978; 18:173.
21. Crosby WM, Costiloe JP: Safety of lap-belt restraint for pregnant victims of automobile collisions. *N Engl J Med* 1971; 284:632.
22. Automobile passenger restraints for children and pregnant women. *ACOG Technical Bulletin,* 1991; 151:1.
23. Higgins SD, Garite TJ: Late abruptio placenta in trauma patients: Implications for monitoring. *Obstet Gynecol* 1984; 63(3):10S.
24. Goodwin TM, Breen MT: Pregnancy outcome and fetomaternal hemorrhage after non-catastrophic trauma. *Am J Obstet Gynecol* 1990; 162(3):665.
25. Rose PG, Strohm PL, Zuspan FP: Fetomaternal hemorrhage following trauma. *Am J Obstet Gynecol* 1985; 153:844.
26. Towery R, English TP, Wisner DW: Evaluation of pregnant women after blunt injury. *J Trauma* 1993; 35:735.
27. Buchsbaum HJ, Staples PP Jr: Self-inflicted gunshot wound to the pregnant uterus: Report of two cases. *Obstet Gynecol* 1985; 65(3):32S.
28. Katz VL, Dotters DJ, Droegemueller W: Perimortem cesarean delivery. *Obstet Gynecol* 1986; 68:571.
29. Carter OD, Haynes SG: Prevalence rates for scoliosis in US adults: Results from the first National Health and Nutrition Examination Survey. *Int J Epidemiol* 1987; 16:537.
30. Pehrsson K, Bake B, Larsson S, et al: Lung function in adult idiopathic scoliosis: A 20 year follow up. *Thorax* 1991; 46:474.
31. Bergofsky EH: Respiratory failure in disorders of the thoracic cage. *Am Rev Respir Dis* 1979; 119:643.
32. Weber B, Smith JP, Briscoe WA, et al: Pulmonary function in asymptomatic adolescents with idiopathic scoliosis. *Am Rev Respir Dis* 1975; 111:389.
33. West JB: Pulmonary pathophysiology, in *Pulmonary Pathophysiology.* Baltimore, Williams & Wilkins, 1978, p 92.
34. Rochester DF, Findley LJ: The lungs and neuromuscular and chest wall diseases, in Murray JF, Nadel JA (eds): *Textbook of Respiratory Medicine.* Philadelphia, WB Saunders, 1988.
35. Mezon BL, West P, Israels J, et al: Sleep breathing abnormalities in kyphoscoliosis. *Am Rev Respir Dis* 1980; 122:617.
36. Midgren B, Petersson K, Hansson L, et al: Nocturnal hypoxaemia in severe scoliosis. *Br J Dis Chest* 1988; 82:226.
37. Kopenhager T: A review of 50 pregnant patients with kyphoscoliosis. *Br J Obstet Gynaecol* 1977; 84:585.
38. Visscher W, Lonstein JE, Hoffman DA, et al: Reproductive outcomes in scoliosis patients. *Spine* 1988; 13:1096.
39. Betz RR, Bunnell WP, Lambrecht ME, et al: Scoliosis and pregnancy. *J Bone Joint Surg [Am]* 1987; 69:90.
40. King TE: Restrictive lung disease in pregnancy, in Nierderman MS (ed): *Clinics in Chest Medicine: Pulmonary Disease in Pregnancy,* vol 13, 1992; p 607.
41. Blount WP, Mellencamp D: The effect of pregnancy on idiopathic scoliosis. *J Bone Joint Surg [Am]* 1980; 62:1083.
42. Berman AT, Cohen DL, Schwentker EP: The effects of pregnancy on idiopathic scoliosis. A preliminary report on eight cases and a review of the literature. *Spine* 1982; 7:76.
43. Sawicka EH, Spencer GT, Branthwaite MA: Management of respiratory failure complicating pregnancy in severe kyphoscoliosis: A new use for an old technique? *Br J Dis Chest* 1986; 80:191.
44. Siegler D, Zorab PA: Pregnancy in thoracic scoliosis. *Br J Dis Chest* 1981; 75:367.
45. Rogala E, Drummond DS, Gurr J: Scoliosis: Incidence and natural history. *J Bone Joint Surg [Am]* 1978; 60:173.
46. Feldstein G, Ramanathan S: Obstetrical lumbar epidural anesthesia in patients with previous posterior spinal fusion for kyphoscoliosis. *Anesth Analg* 1985; 64:83.
47. Cochran T, Irstam L, Nachemson A: Functional changes in patients with adolescent idiopathic scoliosis treated by Harrington rod fusion. *Spine* 1983; 8:576.
48. Winter RB: Posterior spinal fusion in scoliosis: Indications, technique and results. *Orthop Clin North Am* 1979; 10:787.
49. Hubbert CH: Epidural anaesthesia in patients with spinal fusion (correspondence). *Anesth Analg* 1985; 64:843.
50. Crosby ET, Halpern SH: Obstetric epidural anaesthesia in patients with Harrington instrumentation. *Can J Anaesth* 1989; 36:693.

51. Daley MD, Rolbin SH, Hew EM, et al: Epidural anaesthesia for obstetrics after spinal surgery. *Reg Anesth* 1990; 15:280.

52. Pascoe HF, Jennings GS, Marx GF: Successful spinal anesthesia after inadequate epidural block in a parturient with prior surgical correction of scoliosis. *Reg Anesth* 1993; 18:191.

53. Kardash K, King BW, Datta S: Spinal anaesthesia for Caesarean section after Harrington instrumentation. *Can J Anaesth* 1993; 40:667.

54. Allanson JE, Hall JG: Obstetric and gynecologic problems in women with chondrodystrophies. *Obstet Gynecol* 1986; 67:74.

55. Bancroft GH, Lauria JI: Ketamine induction for cesarean section in a patient with acute intermittent porphyria and achondroplastic dwarfism. *Anesthesiology* 1983; 59:143.

56. Mather JS: Impossible direct laryngoscopy in achondroplasia. *Anaesthesia* 1966; 21:244.

57. Mayhew JF, Katz J, Miner M, et al: Anaesthesia for the achondroplastic dwarf. *Can Anaesth Soc J* 1986; 33:216.

58. Walts LF, Finerman G, Wyatt GM: Anaesthesia for dwarfs and other patients of pathological small stature. *Can Anaesth Soc J* 1975; 22:703.

59. Cohen SE: Anesthesia for cesarean section in achondroplastic dwarfs. *Anesthesiology* 1980; 52:264.

60. Kalla GN, Fening E, Obiaya MO: Anaesthetic management of achondroplasia. *Br J Anaesth* 1986; 58:117.

61. McArthur RD: Obstetric anaesthesia in an achondroplastic dwarf at a regional hospital. *Anaesth Intensive Care* 1992; 20:376.

62. Waugaman WR, Kryc JJ, Andrews MJ: Epidural anesthesia for cesarean section and tubal ligation in an achondroplastic dwarf. *J Am Assoc Nurse Anesthetists* 1986; 54:436.

63. Brimacombe JR, Caunt JA: Anaesthesia in a gravid achondroplastic dwarf. *Anaesthesia* 1990; 45:132.

64. Wardall GJ, Frame WT: Extradural anaesthesia for caesarean section in achondroplasia. *Br J Anaesth* 1990; 64:367.

65. Carstoniu J, Yee I, Halpern S: Epidural anaesthesia for caesarean section in an achondroplastic dwarf. *Can J Anaesth* 1992; 39:708.

66. Rodney GE, Callander CC, Harmer M: Spondyloepiphyseal dysplasia congenita: caesarean section under epidural anaesthesia. *Anaesthesia* 1991; 46:648.

67. Carlson JW, Harlass FE: Management of osteogenesis imperfecta in pregnancy: A case report. *J Reprod Med* 1993; 38:228.

68. Sillence DO, Senn A, Danks DM: Genetic heterogenicity in osteogenesis imperfecta. *J Med Genet* 1979; 16:101.

69. Young BK, Gorstein F: Maternal osteogenesis imperfecta. *Obstet Gynecol* 1968; 31:461.

70. Hathaway WE, Solomons CC, Ott JE: Platelet function and pyrophosphates in osteogenesis imperfecta. *Blood* 1972; 39:500.

71. Siegle B, Friedman I, Swartz A: Hemorrhagic disease in osteogenesis imperfecta: Study of platelet function defect. *Am J Med* 1957; 22:315.

72. Humbert JR, Solomons CC, Ott J: Increased oxidative metabolism by leukocytes of patients with osteogenesis imperfecta and their relatives. *J Pediatr* 1971; 78:648.

73. Solomons CC, Myers DN: Hyperthermia of osteogenesis imperfecta and its relationship to malignant hyperthermia, in Gordon RA, Britt BA, Kalow W, eds: *Malignant Hyperthermia*. Springfield, Il, Charles C Thomas, 1973, pp 319-330.

74. Bullard JR, Alpert CC, James WF Jr: Anesthetic management of a patient with osteogenesis imperfecta undergoing Cesarean section. *J South Carolina Med Assoc* 1977; 73:417.

75. Cho E, Dayan SS, Marx GF: Anaesthesia in a parturient with osteogenesis imperfecta. *Br J Anaesth* 1992; 68:422.

76. Libman R: Anesthetic considerations for the patient with osteogenesis imperfecta. *Clin Orthop Rel Res* 1981; 159:123.

77. Cunningham AJ, Donnelly M, Comerford J: Osteogenesis imperfecta: Anesthetic management of a patient for cesarean section: A case report. *Anesthesiology* 1984; 61:91.

78. Mantle MJ, Greenwood RM, Currey HLF: Backache in pregnancy. *Rheumatol Rehabil* 1977; 16:94.

79. LaBan MM, Perrin JCS, Latimer FR: Pregnancy and the herniated lumbar disc. *Arch Phys Med Rehabil* 1983; 64:319.

80. Crawford JS: Some maternal complications of epidural analgesia for labour. *Anaesthesia* 1985; 40:1219.

81. Ong BY: Paresthesias and motor dysfunction after labor and delivery. *Anesth Analg* 1987; 66:18.

82. Peng ATC, Behar S, Blancato LS: Reduction of postlumbar puncture backache by the use of field block anesthesia prior to lumbar puncture. *Anesthesiology* 1985; 63:227.

83. Benzon HT, Braunchweig R, Molloy RE: Delayed onset of epidural anesthesia in patients with back pain. *Anesth Analg* 1981; 60:874.

84. Massey Dawkins CJ: An analysis of the complications of extradural and caudal block. *Anaesthesia* 1969; 24:554.

85. Crawford JS: Lumbar epidural block in labor: A clinical analysis. *Br J Anaesth* 1971; 44:66.

86. Grove LH: Backache, headache and bladder dysfunction after delivery. *Br J Anaesth* 1973; 45:1147.

87. MacArthur C, Lewis M, Knox FG, et al: Epidural anaesthesia and long-term backache after childbirth. *Br Med J* 1990; 301:9.

88. Russell R, Groves P, Taub N: O'Dowd J, Reynolds F: Assessing long-term backache after childbirth. *Br Med J* 1993; 306:1299.

89. Breen TW, Ransil BJ, Groves PA, et al: Factors associated with back pain after childbirth. *Anesthesiology,* 1994; 81(1):29.

16 Malignant Hyperthermia

Stephen Longmire, Wesley Lee, and Jim Pivarnik

INCIDENCE

Since malignant hyperthermia (MH) was first recognized by Denborough in 1960,[1] very few cases have been documented during pregnancy. Estimates of the incidence of MH crises range from 1 in 5000 anesthetics in the pediatric population to 1 in 50,000 in the general population.[2] A recent review by Ørding in Denmark suggests that fulminant crises are now very rare (1 in 220,000 anesthetics), while less severe, "abortive" reactions may occur as often as 1 in 16,000 anesthetics.[3] Given a mean frequency of 1 in 50,000, and a cesarean section rate of approximately 25%[4] in the United States, one might expect hundreds, if not thousands, of MH episodes in pregnant patients. Yet, in reviewing the world literature for this chapter, we found only 12 documented cases.[5-15]

Indeed, Crawford questioned whether or not MH even occurred in pregnancy as late as 1972. In a *Lancet* editorial he postulated that pregnancy might confer some special protective effect against MH,[16] since many known MH-susceptible patients routinely underwent cesarean sections under all forms of anesthesia. Since Crawford's editorial, controversy has reigned about MH in pregnancy. In this chapter we attempt to clarify some of the issues and provide what we believe is a rational approach to the management of the MH-susceptible parturient.

NORMAL METABOLIC CHANGES ASSOCIATED WITH PREGNANCY

The physiologic and metabolic changes associated with pregnancy are presented in Table 16-1 to provide a basis for comparing the changes seen during MH.

DEFINITION AND PATHOPHYSIOLOGY OF MALIGNANT HYPERTHERMIA

Malignant hyperthermia is a genetically transmitted syndrome in which calcium metabolism in the sarcoplasmic reticulum of skeletal muscle is deranged. This derangement results in dramatic increases in anaerobic and aerobic metabolism; excessive heat, carbon dioxide, and lactate production; muscle contracture; and eventual death if left untreated. It is initiated by exposure of susceptible muscle to certain "triggering agents," which include potent volatile anesthetics, succinylcholine, or a combination of the two. Thus, a genetically susceptible individual may undergo numerous exposures to triggering agents before experiencing a reaction.

Recent work has documented that the "MH gene" is located on human chromosome 19, between two DNA markers (D19S9 and BCL3). This region of chromosome 19 is approximately 20 million base pairs long, and contains genes for glucose phosphate isomerase (GPI) and the so-called ryanodine receptor (RYR). The ryanodine receptor is the calcium release channel in the sarcoplasmic reticulum of skeletal muscle, and has been shown to be defective in MH-susceptible swine. The genetic linkage group containing the GPI and RYR genes is conserved across species. The discovery by McCarthy et al that the MH-susceptibility locus cosegregates with this region in both humans and swine validated the porcine MH syndrome as an appropriate model for human malignant hyperthermia. These authors state that "a mutation in the RYR gene is responsible for susceptibility to MH."[63]

The work of McCarthy's team is very exciting, since it not only establishes the location of the gene responsible for MH-susceptibility, but also offers hope of a new screening diagnostic test requiring only a sample of the subject's DNA! Such samples are routinely obtained using buccal swipes and/or blood samples—methods that are clearly less risky than those for obtaining muscle biopsies now. This team is currently attempting to develop and type markers for the RYR gene and its mutants.

Following exposure to triggering agents, altered calcium metabolism within the sarcolemma of skeletal muscle results in profound disturbances in intracellular organelle function. Mitochondria begin actively taking up excess intracellular calcium, and fail to supply adequate amounts of adenosine triphosphate (ATP). Despite the dramatic increases in metabolism, there is only a threefold increase in oxygen consumption during an MH crisis, which represents only one sixth of the normal aerobic

Table 16-1 Late third trimester changes in physiologic variables[17-22]

Variable	Change from nonpregnant value*
Minute ventilation	↑30%-40%
Alveolar ventilation	↑60%-70%
Tidal volume	↑25%-30%
Respiratory rate	NC
Total lung capacity	↓5%-10%
Vital capacity	NC
Residual volume	↓15%-20%
Metabolic rate ($ml\ O_2\ min^{-1}$)	↑20%-30%
Metabolic rate ($ml\ O_2\ kg^{-1}\ min^{-1}$)	NC
Respiratory quotient ($\dot{V}_{CO_2}/\dot{V}_{O_2}$)	↑ slightly or NC
Pa_{O_2}	↑ ± 4 mm Hg
$P\bar{v}_{O_2}$	NC
Pa_{CO_2}	↓ ± 9 mm Hg
$P\bar{v}_{CO_2}$	↓ ± 9 mm Hg
$a[HCO_3^-]$	↓ ± 4 mEq L^{-1}
$\bar{V}[HCO_3^-]$	↓ ± 3 mEq L^{-1}
apH	↑ ± 0.04 units
$\bar{V}pH$	↑ ± 0.04 units
Aerobic capacity ($ml\ O_2\ min^{-1}$)	↑ slightly or NC
Aerobic capacity ($ml\ O_2\ kg^{-1}\ min^{-1}$)	↓ slightly or NC
Maximum voluntary ventilation	↓ 5%-10%
Creatine kinase (term, prelabor)	NC
Creatine kinase (post-partum day 1)	↑ ± 300%
Creatine kinase (1 wk postpartum)	NC

*NC = no change.

capacity of muscle during vigorous exercise. On the other hand, lactate production is much greater than during exercise, and may occur in response to the ATP deficiency, which is needed for sarcolemmal calcium pumps as homeostatic mechanisms within the muscle attempt to restore the normal balance of intracellular and extracellular calcium.[24] Contracture, which is a sustained contraction no longer dependent on depolarization of the motor end-plate, develops as the intracellular calcium concentration increases above 5×10^{-5} mol L^{-1},[25] and may progress to irreversible rigor if the intracellular ATP concentration decreases to less than one half its normal resting concentration. Further damage to the cell membrane occurs as ATP stores are exhausted, resulting in loss of intracellular contents such as potassium and myoglobin.[24]

CLINICAL MANIFESTATIONS

From the above discussion, it follows that the clinical manifestations of this destructive hypermetabolic state should include increased serum lactate levels, increased P_{CO_2}, and a mixed respiratory metabolic acidosis. In spontaneously breathing patients, tachypnea is present. Since the crisis is occurring in skeletal muscle, venous blood chemistries are more indicative of the severity and progression of the crisis than are arterial chemistries.[25] Skeletal muscle rigidity, hyperkalemia, tachycardia, heart block (secondary to hyperkalemia), and hypertension may occur alone or in combination. Only late in the course of the crisis does significant temperature elevation occur. Rhabdomyolysis resulting in myoglobinemia and myoglobinurea is proportional to the severity and duration of the crisis. The destruction of muscle tissue releases tissue thromboplastin into the circulation, which may result in disseminated intravascular coagulation.

Since no cases of MH crisis occurring during labor have been documented, there are no reports of the fetal effects of such a crisis. However, we can reasonably speculate that it would result in profound fetal acidosis, impaired uteroplacental exchange (secondary to maternal sympathetic hyperactivity), and fetal hypoxia. In all of the case reports of MH crisis occurring during cesarean section, neonatal outcome has been good, with Apgar scores of 4 or greater at 1 minute and 7 or greater at 5 minutes.[5-15]

DIAGNOSIS

The diagnosis of MH is unfortunately not as straightforward as the above discussion of clinical signs might suggest. Indeed, short of a documented full-blown crisis (which is very rare), the only way to definitively diagnose MH susceptibility is the caffeine-halothane contracture test.[26] This requires a fresh muscle biopsy specimen, and the test itself is technically difficult and available only at regional MH centers. It therefore is not a practical tool for diagnosis during a suspected crisis.

Patients exhibiting unexplained tachycardia, hypertension, muscle rigidity, tachypnea, central venous hypercarbia, lactic acidosis, and/or rapidly increasing body temperature under anesthesia should be presumed to be having a crisis, and should be treated immediately as outlined below. It must be emphasized that an isolated tachycardia may be the only presenting symptom, so that once other causes for tachycardia are ruled out, further investigation for MH should be carried out. The current recommended approach is to obtain central venous blood gas analysis, electrolytes, and creatine phosphokinase (CPK) levels. Although CPK levels do not typically peak until 18 to 24 hours following the crisis, they are frequently elevated initially.[26] A mixed metabolic and respiratory acidosis with a base deficit of greater than 5 mEq L^{-1} and PCO_2 greater than 55 to 60 mm Hg should be considered diagnostic in the absence of other causes.[25] Once the suspicion of MH is raised, exposure to all triggering agents should be terminated immediately, and an alternative technique employed, since survival is inversely proportional to the total dose of the triggering agent(s).[23]

Other laboratory studies helpful in establishing the diagnosis and severity of a crisis include determinations of serum lactate levels, plasma myoglobin, urine myoglobin, fibrin degradation products, and plasma free hemoglobin. A quick test for myoglobinurea is the urine "dipstick" for blood, as the reagent will react to either hemoglobin or myoglobin. Obstetric patients undergoing cesarean section often have small amounts of blood in their urine following insertion of the urinary catheter and surgical manipulation of the bladder, so the usefulness of this test may be limited in this population.

TRIGGERING AGENTS

Any potent inhalational anesthetic agent may trigger an episode of MH, but halothane seems to be the most potent.[23,25] This may be due to halothane's intrinsic property of depolarizing the sarcolemmal membrane. (Twenty minutes of exposure to halothane reduces the resting membrane potential of the sarcolemma by 7 to 15 mV.[27]) The combination of halothane and succinylcholine is a particularly potent trigger.

Other agents incriminated as possible triggers include ketamine and phencyclidine, nitrous oxide, cyclopropane, amide local anesthetics, digoxin, calcium, fever, stress, exercise, hypercarbia, sympathomimetic drugs, parasympatholytic drugs, ergot preparations, and iodinated radiographic contrast media. Because the data concerning each of these supposed triggers are controversial, we shall go over the current status of each below.

Ketamine and phencyclidine have each been associated with febrile responses in normal subjects, and ketamine occasionally with temperature elevations in MH-susceptible individuals. Although ketamine has reportedly been safely used in MH-susceptible individuals,[23] the best current advice seems to be to avoid ketamine when possible. If it is not possible, then it should be administered with close monitoring and care should be taken to ensure that no other triggering agents are given concomitantly.

Nitrous oxide was once considered capable of triggering MH on the basis of four reported cases in children.[23,25] The diagnosis of MH was supported by laboratory evidence (blood gas analysis) in only one of these cases, however, and it seems unlikely that nitrous oxide is by itself a triggering agent. A combination of light nitrous oxide anesthesia, fever, or stress, may result in triggering.

There is a single case report of MH during cyclopropane anesthesia for cesarean section.[8] This case is interesting in that the fetus was delivered 20 minutes following anesthetic induction. The mother was then given ergometrine, 0.25 mg intravenously, and 10 minutes later her first symptoms developed. From this case report we cannot determine whether the triggering agent responsible for the development of the crisis was cyclopropane, ergometrine, the combination of the two, or the combination of both agents plus the intense sympathetic activity known to accompany either agent.

Amide local anesthetics were formerly considered potential triggering agents since they may increase calcium efflux from the sarcoplasmic reticulum. This largely theoretical prohibition has proved unwarranted, since the concentrations required are far greater than those associated with clinical use, and lidocaine, mepivacaine, and bupivacaine have all been used safely to provide anesthesia and analgesia to MH-susceptible patients.[28] In 1985, the Malignant Hyperthermia Association of the United States (MHAUS) removed amide local anesthetics from the list of triggering agents.[29]

During animal investigations even supratoxic concentrations of digoxin, calcium, or hypercarbia failed to induce MH in purebred swine.[25] It therefore seems highly unlikely that they could trigger an episode in such a genetically heterogeneous species as humans.

Fever alone may trigger MH,[30] provided the temperature is greater than 41° C,[25] but it is quite rare in humans as the sole trigger for an episode. The association of fever with MH episodes during cesarean section is interesting, though. In two of the case reports reviewed for this chapter, the patients had either established fever and chorioamnionitis, or were diagnosed to have chorioamnionitis by placental culture following delivery.[9,13] Although fever itself was not the sole agent responsible in these two cases, it probably contributed to the development of MH in each. The anesthetics used were nitrous oxide/oxygen plus succinylcholine in the first case, and spinal tetracaine in the second. Spinal anesthesia for vaginal delivery in a third MH-susceptible patient (also using tetracaine) was associated with an increase in CPK from 1,605 to 2,390 IU, but this patient had been in labor for nearly 5½ hours prior to the block.[5]

Stress and exercise have been proposed as possible triggers for MH in humans, since they certainly are in purebred swine. Confusing this issue are reports from as early as the 1930s of a strange syndrome of cardiovascular collapse and sudden death in otherwise healthy young athletes undergoing strenuous exercise. This syndrome, called exercise-induced anaphylaxis, was subsequently shown to be an allergic/anergic phenomenon completely unrelated to MH.[31-36] If stress is a trigger for MH in humans, it seems that it must be accompanied by other triggering factors for a crisis to result. Evidence for stress as a triggering "agent" in human MH stems largely from observations that the longer surgery continues during a crisis, the more severe the crisis, and the higher the mortality of MH.[2] The observation that MH-susceptible individuals tested higher for anxiety levels than nonsusceptible individuals in the State-Trait Anxiety Inventory, and that the results of the inventory correlated significantly with muscle biopsy results, provides further anecdotal evidence for stress as a factor in human MH.[37]

Sympathomimetic drugs have long been considered to be triggers for MH, because crises are accompanied by profound sympathetic hyperactivity. However, this sympathetic hyperactivity is now believed to be a "normal" response to an extremely stressful disturbance of homeostasis. Animal studies of sympathomimetic drugs as triggering agents for MH have yielded conflicting results. Alpha-adrenergic agents (phenylephrine) were capable of inducing MH, alpha-adrenergic antagonists modified thermal and pressure responses during a crisis, and beta-adrenergic agents altered the glycolytic changes in MH. Beta-adrenergic antagonists (propranolol) decreased myocardial oxygen consumption, but only in large doses, which then resulted in impaired myocardial performance and increased myocardial lactate production. Finally, infusions of norepinephrine that resulted in serum concentrations several-fold higher than those known to occur during MH were incapable of inducing an attack in swine that were later easily induced by exposure to halothane and succinylcholine.[25] Gronert et al[25] point out that there are likely to be differences in the response to sympathomimetic drugs between humans and swine, since the former rely primarily on evaporative heat loss through sweating, whereas the latter are incapable of sweating, and rely on radiant loss from the skin and evaporative losses via the respiratory tract. Alpha-adrenergic-induced vasoconstriction could have caused decreased heat loss sufficient to trigger an attack in swine by blocking this radiant loss mechanism.

Parasympatholytic drugs (atropine, scopolamine, glycopyrrolate, and meperidine) may func-tion as "partial triggers" in human MH by a mechanism analogous to that of alpha-adrenergic agents in swine.[23] That is, they block heat loss by obtunding sweating, allowing heat build-up that then functions in concert with other triggering factors to precipitate or exacerbate a crisis. Indeed, the aunt of the patient who developed elevated CPK levels during spinal anesthesia herself developed rigidity and died during labor in 1943. The "anesthetic" employed was "twilight sleep" (scopolamine/meperidine).[5] In contrast, meperidine has been used without apparent adverse effect in many of the cases reporting different methods of management of the MH-susceptible parturient in labor.[38] Given the possible risks of decreased heat loss induced by meperidine, and the fact that other nonparasympatholytic narcotics are now available, it seems wise to avoid meperidine in MH-susceptible individuals, particularly in the presence of fever.

Ergot preparations are probably best avoided as well, since they decrease muscle perfusion by inducing vasoconstriction.[38,39] This can only result in further worsening the lactic acidosis. No data are currently available regarding the use of prostaglandins in MH-susceptible parturients, but maternal administration of prostaglandins commonly leads to mild temperature elevation. Febrile morbidity is reported to be less common with intramuscular 15-methyl-$F_{2\alpha}$ (carboprost) when compared to prostaglandin E_2 suppositories.[40] Maternal arterial desaturation has also been observed from use of prostaglandin 15-methyl $F_{2\alpha}$ for uterine atony.[41] This is particularly interesting since dantrolene, as a uterine muscle relaxant, may potentially predispose parturients to postpartum atony.[13] Oxytocin appears to be a safe alternative.

There is a single case report of a fatal episode of MH apparently triggered by intravenous iodinated contrast media given for intravenous pyelograms.[42]

OTHER ASSOCIATED SYNDROMES

Ever since the identification of MH as a genetically transmitted syndrome, there have been attempts to correlate MH susceptibility with other musculoskeletal syndromes. Particularly prominent have been investigations of the association between the muscular dystrophies and MH, and between the neuroleptic malignant syndrome (NMS) and MH.

The discovery of the MHS gene on chromosome 19, and of the fact that it is inherited in an autosomal dominant pattern with 100% penetrance, has forced a reevaluation of traditional views of the relationships between MH susceptibility and other syndromes. The *apparent* penetrance of MH has been estimated to be 0.33, because only about one third of MH-susceptible patients actually experience a malignant hyperthermic crisis even when anesthetized with known triggering agents.[2] The only reasonable explanation for these conflicting observations is that more than a single genetic or environmental factor must be present to *trigger* the malignant hyperthermic reaction in MH-susceptible individuals. Thus, even though the loci of the genes for MHS and other syndromes may not lie on the same chromosome, the risk of *triggering* a crisis in someone who has muscular dystrophy *and* a mutation of the RYR gene may still be higher than it is in someone who has only the mutation of the RYR gene responsible for MH susceptibility.[63,64]

Duchenne muscular dystrophy, an X-linked muscular dystrophy, has historically been associated with an increased risk of MH susceptibility. Though it is now proved that inheritance of the two syndromes is independent, it seems prudent to consider patients with Duchenne dystrophy as MH-susceptible unless proved otherwise by *in vitro* contracture testing.[43]

Myotonic dystrophy is associated with a higher incidence of obstetric complications, which include polyhydramnios, preterm labor, higher cesarean section rates, postpartum hemorrhage, and neonatal deaths.[44,45] Myotonic syndromes (myotonia congenita, myotonic dystrophy) are all characterized by delayed relaxation following voluntary contraction[46,47] and may be easily mistaken for MH in the operating room, since succinylcholine induces rigidity rather than relaxation in both cases. This rigidity may be prolonged in the case of myotonia, and is not reversible by treatment with nondepolarizing neuromuscular blocking drugs, whereas procainamide or prednisone will reverse the contracture. Potent halogenated agents also reverse myotonic contracture (at the expense of profound cardiac depression), but these worsen MH-induced contracture. In vitro contracture testing has not demonstrated any increased risk of MH susceptibility among patients with myotonic syndromes as compared with normal subjects.[48]

Patients with myotonia requiring surgery are probably best managed by a combination of general anesthesia and infiltration of muscles surrounding the operative site with local anesthetics to reduce the percussion myotonia. Although myotonic patients respond normally to nondepolarizing neuromuscular blocking drugs in the absence of myotonic contractures, neither neuromuscular blocking drugs nor regional nerve blocks are effective when contractures develop.[48] Awake fiberscopic tracheal intubation is the method of choice for protecting the airway in myotonic patients with full stomachs. Careful attention must be paid to postoperative pulmonary function, since myotonic patients are more prone to the development of apnea following exposure to any central nervous system (CNS) depressant. Since steroids are beneficial in reducing myotonic contractions, and since myotonic patients may also suffer adrenocortical insufficiency as a consequence of their disease, it is probably wise to administer steroids to cover the stress of the perioperative period.

Camann and Johnson[49] recently reported their management of a pregnant patient with myotonia dystrophica with the use of epidural anesthesia. This patient initially underwent an exploratory laparotomy at 28 weeks' gestation, and later that same day developed fetal distress, requiring an emergency cesarean section. Anesthesia for the first operation was provided with 2% lidocaine with 1:200,000 epinephrine and sufentanil; and for the second with 3% 2-chloroprocaine. Although the neonate was not successfully resuscitated, the mother exhibited no shivering or myotonia throughout and following either procedure. The authors pointed out the need for careful attention to providing a thermoneutral environment for myotonic patients, and suggested that the use of epidural sufentanil may also have helped to prevent the development of shivering and myotonia.

Neuroleptic malignant syndrome, first recognized in 1959, is a syndrome of hyperpyrexia, skeletal muscle rigidity, autonomic instability, and rhabdomyolysis induced by potent neuroleptic agents. First thought to represent a variant of MH, it is now clear that NMS is mediated by a disruption of CNS dopamine metabolism, rather than by skeletal muscle calcium metabolism. Current estimates of the incidence of NMS are 0.5% to 1% of all patients exposed to neuroleptic agents, with a mortality of up to 30% in severe cases. Triggering agents for NMS include thioxanthenes, butyrophenones, phenothiazines, and other central dopaminergic antagonists. Acute withdrawal of central dopaminergic agonists such as levodopa and amantadine has also been associated with the development of NMS.[50-54]

The clinical presentation of NMS is similar in many ways to that of MH, but it should be remembered that NMS usually develops over 24 to 72 hours, whereas MH develops much more rapidly—usually within minutes to a few hours of exposure to a triggering agent. Neuroleptic malignant syndrome is most likely to develop shortly after the initiation of neuroleptic therapy, or after an increase in the dosage of a neuroleptic agent. While dantrolene therapy reduces the hyperthermia of both NMS and MH, the altered consciousness often associated with NMS frequently responds only to therapy with central dopaminergic agonists such as bromocriptine. Further, MH is a genetically transmitted, autosomal dominant syndrome, and, as such, susceptibility to MH would seem irreversible. Neuroleptic malignant syndrome, however, may be triggered in otherwise normal patients upon one exposure to neuroleptic agents, but not triggered by later exposure to the same agents.[54] Finally, although there are reports of patients testing positive for MH-susceptibility with in vitro contracture tests following recovery from NMS, it has not been substantiated that they are at greater risk than the general population for MH susceptibility.[43]

Obstetric and anesthetic management. Prior to the introduction of dantrolene in 1979, the mortality associated with an episode of MH was as high as 80%, but it is now expected that nearly all patients who receive appropriate monitoring and therapy will survive. No other drug or combination of drugs has proved as effective as dantrolene in the treatment of MH. Any location where anesthetics are administered should stock, as a minimum, sufficient quantities of dantrolene for at least the first loading dose.[2,23,55,56]

Therapy of MH is first directed toward terminating exposure to all triggering agents and ensuring adequate oxygenation and ventilation to compensate for the greatly increased metabolic rate. The anesthetic breathing circuit and machine should be changed out immediately for one that has not been exposed to halogenated agents. The new machine should be stocked with fresh soda lime, since the carbon dioxide absorption cannister is frequently exhausted by the large quantity of carbon dioxide produced by the patient. Several large-bore intravenous catheters should be inserted and sufficient chilled fluids administered to ensure a diuresis of at least 2 ml kg hr^{-1}. As mentioned earlier, central venous blood chemistries are of greater value in guiding therapy than arterial blood chemistries, since they represent the effluent from the affected areas (the skeletal muscle beds).[23] The electrocardiogram should be monitored for the development of ventricular dysrhythmias, which may be treated with procainamide, although most dysrhythmias will resolve soon after initiating dantrolene therapy. The patient's core and skin temperatures should be continuously monitored during the crisis, and at least hourly following its resolution for a period of 24 to 36 hours. It is helpful to insert an arterial catheter for continuous monitoring of the blood pressure, and a urinary catheter to monitor urine output and urinary excretion of myoglobin.

Initial laboratory studies are shown in Box 16-1.

Although simply terminating exposure to all triggering agents within the first 10 minutes of administration frequently aborts the crisis, most MH investigators still recommend treatment with dan-

---

BOX 16-1   RECOMMENDED LABORATORY ANALYSES DURING MALIGNANT HYPERTHERMIA*

Central venous blood gas analysis
Arterial blood gas analysis
Central venous electrolytes
  (Na^+, **K^+**, Cl^-, HCO_3^-)
Serum glucose
Central venous CPK
  and isoenzymes—immediately and every 12 hours
Hemoglobin or hematocrit
Fibrinogen and fibrin degradation products
Plasma myoglobin
Urine myoglobin
Urine pH

---

*Essential studies shown in **boldface** type.

---

trolene if there is any evidence of a mixed metabolic and respiratory acidosis. The initial loading dose is 2.4 mg kg^{-1} intravenously, and this dose may be repeated every 15 minutes until the muscle rigidity is reversed, the cardiac rhythm is stabilized, the temperature is stabilized, or a total dose of 10 mg kg^{-1} is given.[56] Very rarely is it required to give more than two doses initially. Profound metabolic acidosis may be controlled by administration of sodium bicarbonate, but it must be emphasized that the definitive therapy is dantrolene and the acidosis will resolve once a therapeutic level of dantrolene (>3 μg ml^{-1}) is achieved.

Active cooling of the patient is indicated for temperatures exceeding 39.5° C, but to avoid the risk of inducing hypothermia, this should be terminated once the temperature falls below this value.

The Malignant Hyperthermia Association of the United States maintains a 24-hour hotline to assist practitioners with the diagnosis and management of MH crises (Fig. 16-1). The association also offers a number of educational materials and posters outlining emergency therapy.

Following resolution of the immediate crisis, the patient should be continuously monitored in an intensive care unit setting for 24 to 36 hours to ensure against the redevelopment of symptoms. Many authors recommend that a second dose of 2.4 mg kg^{-1} of dantrolene be given 12 hours after the first to further protect against recrudescence.[57] It must be emphasized that therapy of MH does not end once the crisis is over and the patient is discharged. Since MH is a genetically transmitted disease, all blood relatives of the patient should be advised of their risks and afforded the opportunity to be tested for susceptibility as indicated.

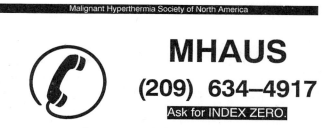

Fig. 16-1 MHAUS hotline. Call 24 hours a day for information on management of MH crisis.

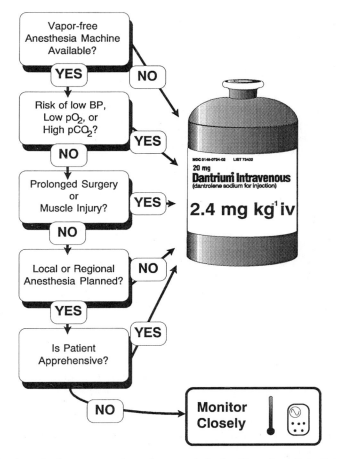

Fig. 16-2 Indications for intravenous dantrolene prophylaxis. (Data from Britt BA: *Can Anaesth Soc J* 1984; 31:61.)

Indications for prophylactic administration of dantrolene

The issue of whether or not to prophylactically administer datrolene to MH-susceptible parturients is currently very controversial. About the only real concensus that exists now is that oral dantrolene should *not* be used as prophylaxis against MH. Dantrolene is absorbed poorly when administered orally, even in nonpregnant patients, and achieving therapeutic blood levels requires several days and is not predictable. Given the impaired gastric emptying of parturients, it is even less likely that therapeutic levels can be achieved by this route of administration.

Figure 16-2 depicts current guidelines regarding *intravenous* prophylactic administration of dantrolene. Note the requirement for a "vapor-free" anesthetic apparatus if administration of dantrolene is not elected.

Pharmacologic effects of dantrolene

The structure of dantrolene is shown in Fig. 16-3. It is highly lipid-soluble, but poorly water-soluble. It is supplied in glass ampules containing 20 mg dantrolene sodium with 3 g mannitol and sufficient sodium hydroxide to raise the pH to 9 to 10. It must be reconstituted in 60 ml sterile water prior to administration. The final concentration is therefore 0.3 mg ml^{-1} (so the initial loading dose using this dilution is 0.8 ml kg^{-1}).

Dantrolene works by uncoupling excitation-contraction at the sarcoplasmic reticulum. Its exact mechanism and site of action have not been discovered. Its elimination half-life following intravenous administration is 12 hours, with therapeutic concentrations maintained for 5 hours following administration. It undergoes both oxidative and reductive metabolism in the liver and is excreted in both bile and urine. Several of its metabolites are also active.[56,57]

The most prominent complaint following dantrolene administration in conscious patients is weakness. Dantrolene has a ceiling effect that produces 75% twitch depression and diminishes grip strength by about 40%. This level of weakness is not sufficient to compromise protective airway reflexes or ventilation. Although it is completely devoid of CNS effects, many patients complain of dizziness.

Adverse effects of dantrolene include possible hepatocellular damage (although this has recently been questioned), profound myocardial depression when given in the presence of verapamil,[58,59] prolongation of neuromuscular blockade by vecuronium,[60] and possible uterine atony.[13] Regarding this last effect, it is interesting to note that though the patient involved had other risk factors for the development of postpartum uterine atony (chorioamnionitis, magnesium sulfate therapy, prolonged labor), the development of atony did not occur until after the administration of dantrolene and required hysterectomy to control hemorrhage.

Two studies have documented dantrolene's lack of adverse effects on the fetus and newborn. The first used a sheep model and intravenous dantrolene.[61] The second studied humans given oral dantrolene prophylaxis, although the authors pointed out that they failed to achieve maternal serum levels in the protective range. The mean maternal serum concentration was 0.99 mg ml^{-1}, and

the mean cord blood concentration was 0.68 mg ml^{-1}. No adverse effect of dantrolene sodium was detected by extensive evaluation of the fetus and neonate.[62]

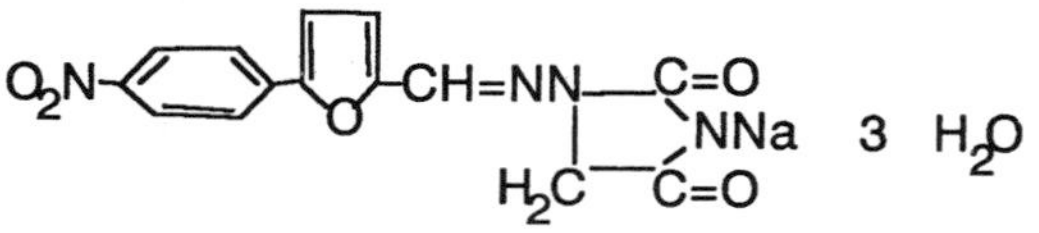

Anesthetic management of susceptible parturients

Since all pregnant patients are considered to have full stomachs, it is recommended that the routine prophylaxis employed at the reader's institution against acid aspiration be given to all MH-susceptible patients. This usually includes the administration of an H$_2$ blocking drug (cimetidine or ranitidine), a particulate-free oral antacid, and, in some cases, metoclopramide. Although not contraindicated in MH, metoclopramide is contraindicated in patients with NMS, since it blocks central dopamine transmission.

For labor. Intravenous narcotics (including meperidine), inhalational analgesia (using Entonox, 50% N$_2$O/50% O$_2$),* epidural analgesia, and spinal anesthesia have all been used to provide analgesia for MH-susceptible patients in labor. In the case of spinal anesthesia reported, however, the patient developed an increased CPK level following institution of the block, so it is questionable whether this technique was truly without deleterious effects.[5,38,39]

Since stress may play a role in the genesis of MH in humans undergoing operative procedures, and since labor is certainly a stress-inducing phenomenon, it seems prudent to ensure that the patient is as comfortable as possible throughout her labor. The best method available today is carefully managed epidural analgesia. These patients should receive a generous preload (1-2 L) to reduce the risk of hypotension and the need for ephedrine, and they should be monitored intensively during labor to detect early signs of MH.[33] MH-susceptible parturients should be monitored throughout labor, delivery, and for several hours thereafter following the ASA's Standards for Basic Intraoperative Monitoring. This includes continuous electrocardiogram, axillary temperature, pulse oximetry, and frequent blood pressure determinations. The urine should be checked periodically, and if it becomes reddish-brown, should be sent for myoglobin determination. Continuous fetal monitoring is also indicated, since changes in the fetal heart rate pattern may indicate the development of maternal acidosis.

Bupivacaine, lidocaine, or 2-chloroprocaine may be used to initiate and maintain the block. All solutions should be epinephrine-free, and the test

$$O_2N-\langle\ \rangle-\overset{O}{\underset{O}{\bigcirc}}-CH=NN-\underset{\underset{C=O}{|}}{\overset{C=O}{\underset{H_2C}{}}}NNa \quad 3\ H_2O$$

Fig. 16-3 Dantrolene sodium (mol wt 399).

---

*This technique is not recommended at Brigham and Women's Hospital.—*Editor*

dose should also probably not contain epinephrine in these patients. There is currently no data available regarding the safety of local anesthetic/narcotic combinations (such as bupivacaine/fentanyl) in this setting. Given the importance of avoiding sudden changes in blood pressure and heart rate, it is particularly important to use small (3-5 ml) incremental doses when initiating, redosing, or extending the block. There is some merit to the suggestion that the block should be slowly brought up to a level of T6 and maintained there, in case an urgent cesarean section becomes necessary. (The rationale for this is that the chances of hypotension when extending the block from T6 to T4 are less than when extending from T10 to T4 over a short period of time.) If this is done, the patient must clearly be monitored very closely, and there may be some interference with the progress of labor. Adequate left uterine displacement must be assured throughout the course of labor and delivery to avoid the development of maternal acidosis.

Preblock laboratory evaluations should include hemoglobin (or hematocrit), platelet count, serum electrolytes, and CPK level as a baseline. Determination of bleeding time or a thromboelastrogram may be indicated because platelet dysfunction has been reported in MH patients. This latter point is controversial, however, since the platelet defect in MH has not been well characterized.[25]

Medications that are contraindicated are (1) beta-mimetic drugs such as ritodrine and terbutaline; (2) anticholinergic drugs such as scopolamine; and (3) ergot preparations.[38,39] Oxytocin is safe as an adjunct for labor. No intramuscular injections should be given unless absolutely necessary, since they alter CPK values.

Hypotension is to be avoided, because if left untreated or undertreated it will result in the development of maternal and fetal acidosis. Labor and delivery personnel should be continually vigilant to prevent even subtle degrees of aortocaval compression. Ephedrine is the vasopressor of choice in MH-susceptible parturients. If ephedrine is contraindicated or ineffective, *small* doses (50 μg) of phenylephrine may be used. Continuous infusions of low-dose vasopressors or intramuscular doses of vasopressors are to be avoided, since either may interfere with cutaneous heat loss.

In patients who refuse epidural analgesia or in whom it is contraindicated, narcotic analgesia is the second choice. In this setting butorphanol, 2 to 4 mg intravenously, produces moderate sedation and analgesia without impairing heat loss via sweating. Nalbuphine may also be used, but it results in less sedation and analgesia. Small doses of fentanyl (1-3 μg kg^{-1}) produce profound analgesia of 1 or 2 hours' duration with little risk of neonatal depression, but repeated doses may have cumulative effects. Meperidine (0.5-1 mg kg^{-1}) has been used without apparent adverse effect in MH-susceptible patients in labor, but it may impair sweating and decrease normal heat loss. Meperidine is contraindicated in the presence of maternal fever.

Finally, inhalation of 50% nitrous oxide* in oxygen has been reported to be safe in MH-susceptible patients in labor, provided it is administered from a "vapor-free" machine (an anesthesia machine that has never been used to administer potent halogenated agents). This is usually not very practical in obstetric suites in the United States, since few are equipped with such an apparatus. It may, however, prove beneficial during the second stage of labor in the delivery room.

For forceps- or vacuum-assisted vaginal delivery. The same basic considerations apply here as for labor, except that low spinal anesthesia ("saddle block") is a possibility. Once again, care must be taken to ensure a generous preload prior to the institution of the block, and epinephrine-containing solutions should be avoided. Hyperbaric lidocaine or bupivacaine may be used, but the level of the block should be kept low to avoid hypotension.

Bilateral pudendal block using 2-chloroprocaine or lidocaine may be used, but it rarely affords the same quality of anesthesia as epidural or saddle block. In such cases, supplementation with 50% nitrous oxide in oxygen* often proves very beneficial. A vapor-free machine must be used if one selects this technique.

As a last resort, general anesthesia may be employed for forceps-assisted vaginal delivery, following the guidelines discussed below.

For cesarean section. Once again the technique of choice is a slowly titrated epidural anesthetic. Bupivacaine 0.5%, lidocaine 2%, or 2-chloroprocaine 3% may be used so long as they are epinephrine-free. A generous preload of 2 L is required to reduce the risk of hypotension. Adequate sacral as well as thoracic levels must be assured to avoid nausea. Should peritoneal traction result in significant discomfort, a large volume of dilute local anesthetic (50 ml 0.5% lidocaine or 1.0% 2-chloroprocaine, but not bupivacaine) may be instilled into the peritoneal cavity by the surgeon. This usually remedies the discomfort within 2 or 3 minutes if the level of the epidural block is otherwise adequate. An alternative is to administer fentanyl, 1-3 μg kg^{-1} intravenously. If dantrolene is given, uterine atony may result, and *cal-*

---

*Not used at Brigham and Women's Hospital.—*Editor*

cium will not reverse this effect of dantrolene. Ergot preparations are contraindicated. If severe, such atony may necessitate hysterectomy to control hemorrhage.[13]

Provided that the patient is not febrile, and the cesarean section and anesthetic are reasonably stress-free, it is acceptable to closely monitor MH-susceptible patients receiving epidural anesthesia without administering prophylactic dantrolene.[56] If the patient appears stressed, is febrile, or has had a prolonged labor, it is probably safer to administer dantrolene. Because of the long time required to achieve therapeutic levels following oral administration, and the unpredictable absorption, it is no longer recommended to administer dantrolene orally for MH prophylaxis.

Spinal anesthesia for cesarean section in MH-susceptible patients has been associated with a crisis in one case in which there was a history of prolonged labor and chorioamnionitis.[13] It is also associated with a higher incidence of hypotension than is epidural anesthesia, and on these grounds it is less preferable than epidural anesthesia for cesarean section in MH-susceptible individuals. Agents employed include lidocaine, bupivacaine, or tetracaine (each epinephrine-free). Oxygen should be administered from a vapor-free machine throughout the procedure. Small doses of ephedrine may be used to correct hypotension, and it is preferred to correct hypotension early, using a small dose of ephedrine, rather than to wait and then need a larger dose.

General anesthesia is the method of last resort. Additional personnel must be present, both to assist with the preparation of dantrolene and to resuscitate the neonate. Intravenous dantrolene prophylaxis should be administered (2.4 mg kg^{-1}) before the induction of anesthesia. A "vapor-free" anesthesia machine or a non–rebreathing circuit must be used to administer the anesthetic.

Strong consideration must be given to the advantages of awake fiberoptic-guided tracheal intubation prior to induction!

Awake fiberoptic-guided tracheal intubation prior to induction of general anesthesia avoids the need for rapid-sequence induction and intubation, which requires high doses of nondepolarizing muscle relaxants. This significantly reduces the risk of failed tracheal intubation! Adequate topical anesthesia of the oropharynx is essential, and moderate sedation should be provided to permit the patient to cooperate for this procedure. Induction of general anesthesia, using thiopental 4 mg kg^{-1}, follows verification of the placement of the endotracheal tube.

In cases where awake fiberoptic-guided tracheal intubation is not feasible, rapid sequence induction and intubation is required. Cricoid pressure is applied following preoxygenation. An intubating dose of a nondepolarizing muscle relaxant is then administered, followed by thiopental 4 mg kg^{-1}. Some practitioners prefer to have the patient hold up a forearm while administering the nondepolarizing muscle relaxant, and to wait until the patient's forearm begins to fall before administering the thiopental. The rationale behind this practice is that the onsets of muscle relaxation and loss of consciousness are better synchronized, reducing the period of apnea prior to achieving good intubating conditions. Proper placement of the endotracheal tube is then verified.

With either of the above techniques of intubation/induction or induction/intubation, anesthesia is maintained using a mixture of 50% oxygen and 50% nitrous oxide at high fresh gas flow rates. Anesthesia may be supplemented with fentanyl or alfentanil (although either will result in neonatal depression). Muscle relaxation is very rarely needed, since dantrolene alone frequently provides sufficient relaxation for cesarean delivery under general anesthesia. If absolutely necessary, additional relaxation can be provided using *very small, carefully titrated doses* of a nondepolarizing muscle relaxant.

At the conclusion of the case, reversal of neuromuscular blockade with the use of glycopyrrolate and neostigmine is not contraindicated, but the patient must be carefully monitored for signs of prolonged blockade following the concomitant use of dantrolene and nondepolarizing neuromuscular blocking drugs.

Succinylcholine is absolutely contraindicated, as are halothane, enflurane, isoflurane, desflurane, and sevoflurane.

Triggering agents like succinylcholine and inhalation anesthetics should be avoided during cesarean under general anesthesia in case of MH history, to prevent possible triggering of MH-susceptible neonate.

SUMMARY

In this chapter we have seen that MH is fortunately a rare event during pregnancy, with only 12 cases reported in the literature. Pregnancy, however, is not a rare event among MH-susceptible patients, so we must all be aware of the latest information about MH, and ever vigilant to avoid missing its clinical features.

Significant reductions in mortality have been achieved following the introduction of dantrolene therapy, but for further reductions to occur, greater efforts to recognize the variable presentations of this syndrome are necessary. Management of a crisis in the obstetric setting involves a team effort among obstetricians, anesthesiologists, and neonatologists. Further investigations of the effects of pregnancy on MH-susceptibility in humans are desperately needed and may well shed light on its pathophysiology in nonpregnant individuals as well.

REFERENCES

1. Denborough MA, Lovell RRH: Anaesthetic deaths in a family. *Lancet* 1960; 2:45.
2. Britt BA, Kalow W: Malignant hyperthermia: A statistical review. *Can Anaesth Soc J* 1970; 17:293.
3. Ørding H: Incidence of malignant hyperthermia in Denmark. *Anesth Analg* 1985; 64:700.
4. Phelan JP, Clark SL: *Cesarean Delivery.* New York, Elsevier, 1988, p 14.
5. Wadhwa RK: Obstetric anesthesia for a patient with malignant hyperthermia susceptibility. *Anesthesiology* 1977; 46:63.
6. Litarczek G, Bentia L, Ghiga R: Maligne hyperthermie: Bericht uber einen mit Procaininfusion erfolgreich behandelten Fall. *Anaesthetist* 1978; 27:566.
7. Augustyniak B, Uszynski M: Opis przypadku niewyjasnionej goraczki w okresie pooperacyjnym-zespo hipertermii zosliwej? *Ginekol Pol* 1979; 50:969.
8. Lips FJ, Newland M, Dutton G: Malignant hyperthermia triggered by cyclopropane during cesarean section. *Anesthesiology* 1982; 56:144.
9. Cupryn JP, Kennedy A, Byrick RJ: Malignant hyperthermia in pregnancy. *Am J Obstet Gynecol* 1984; 150:327.
10. Gibbs JM: Unexplained hyperpyrexia during labour (letter). *Anaesth Intensive Care* 1984; 12:375.
11. Marin Ruiz R, Zepeda J: Hiperpirexia maligna. Informe de un caso. *Ginecol Obstet Mex* 1983; 51:317.
12. Kiwitt A, Pingel E: Ein Fall von Maligner Hyperthermie in der operativen Geburtshilfe. *Zentralbl Gynakol* 1985; 107:966.
13. Weingarten AE, Korsh JI, Neuman GG, et al: Postpartum uterine atony after intravenous dantrolene. *Anesth Analg* 1987; 66:269.
14. Thomas A, Leopold U, Winklerr H: Maligne Hyperthermie bei Paramyotonia congenita. *Anaesthesiol Reanim* 1988; 13:295.
15. Houvenaeghel M, Achilli-Cornesse E, Jullian-Papouin H, et al: Dantrolene oral chez une parturiente atteinte de myotonie de Steinert et sensible à l'hyperthermie maligne. *Ann Fr Anesth Reanim* 1988; 7:408.
16. Crawford JS: Hyperpyrexia during pregnancy. *Lancet* 1972; 1:1244.
17. Bonica JJ: Maternal respiratory changes during pregnancy and parturition. *Clin Anesth Parturition Perinatal* 1973; 10:2.
18. Lotgering FK, Gilbert RD, Longo LD: Maternal and fetal responses to exercise during pregnancy. *Physiol Rev* 1985; 65:1.
19. Pivarnik JM, Lee W, Spillman T, et al: Maternal respiration and blood gases during aerobic exercise performed at moderate altitude. *Med Sci Sports Exerc* 1992; 24:868.
20. Pivarnik JM, Lee W, Clark SL, et al: Unpublished data, 1990.
21. McMurray RG, Mottola MF, Wolfe LA, et al: Recent advances in understanding maternal and fetal responses to exercise. *Med Sci Sports Exerc* 1993; 25:1305.
22. Isherwood DM, Ridley J, Wilson J: Creatine phosphokinase (CPK) levels during pregnancy: A case report and a discussion of the value of CPK levels in the prediction of possible malignant hyperpyrexia. *Br J Obstet Gynaecol* 1975; 82:346.
23. Gronert GA: Malignant hyperthermia. *Anesthesiology* 1980; 53:395.
24. Heffron JJA: Malignant hyperthermia: Biochemical aspects of the acute episode. *Br J Anaesth* 1988; 60:274.
25. Gronert GA, Mott J, Lee J: Aetiology of malignant hyperthermia. *Br J Anaesth* 1988; 60:253.
26. Ørding H: Diagnosis of susceptibility to malignant hyperthermia in man. *Br J Anaesth* 1988; 60:287.
27. Gallant EM, Godt RE, Gronert GA: Role of plasma membrane defect of skeletal muscle in malignant hyperthermia. *Muscle Nerve* 1979; 2:491.
28. Paasuke RT, Brownell AKW: Amide local anesthetics and malignant hyperthermia. *Can Anaesth Soc J* 1986; 33:126.
29. MHAUS Professional Advisory Committee adopts new policy statement on local anesthetics. *MHAUS Communicator* 1985; 3(4).
30. Fuchs F: Thermal inactivation of the calcium regulatory mechanism of human muscle actomyosin: A possible factor in the rigidity of malignant hyperthermia. *Anesthesiology* 1975; 42:584.
31. Sheffer AL, Austen KF: Exercise-induced anaphylaxis. *J Allergy Clin Immunol* 1980; 66:106.
32. Kaplan AP, Natbony SF, Tawil AP, et al: Exercise-induced anaphylaxis as a manifestation of cholinergic urticaria. *J Allergy Clin Immunol* 1981; 68:319.
33. Buchbinder EM, Bloch KJ, Moss J, et al: Food-dependent, exercise-induced anaphylaxis. *JAMA* 1983; 250:2973.
34. Sheffer AL, Austen KF: Exercise-induced anaphylaxis. *J Allergy Clin Immunol* 1984; 73:699.
35. Grant JA, Farnam J, Lord RAA, et al: Familial exercise-induced anaphylaxis. *Ann Allergy* 1985; 54:35.
36. Sheffer AL, Tong AKF, Murphy GF, et al: Exercise-induced anaphylaxis: A serious form of physical allergy associated with mast cell degranulation. *J Allergy Clin Immunol* 1985; 75:479.
37. Smith RJ: Preoperative assessment of risk factors. *Br J Anaesth* 1988; 60:317.
38. Douglas MJ, McMorland GH: The anaesthetic management of the malignant hyperthermia susceptible parturient. *Can Anaesth Soc J* 1986; 33:371.
39. Willatts SM: Malignant hyperethermia susceptibility: Management during pregnancy and labour. *Anaesthesia* 1979; 34:41.
40. American College of Obstetricians and Gynecologists: Methods of midtrimester abortion. *ACOG Technical Bulletin.* Washington, DC, ACOG, 1987.
41. Hankins GD, Berryman GK, Scott RT, et al: Maternal arterial desaturation with 15-methyl prostaglandin F2-alpha for uterine atony. *Obstet Gynecol* 1988; 72:367.
42. Mozley PD: Malignant hyperthermia following intravenous iodinated contrast media: Report of a fatal case. *Diagn Gynecol Obstet* 1981; 3:81.
43. Brownell AKW: Malignant hyperthermia: Relationship to other diseases. *Br J Anaesth* 1988; 60:303.
44. Webb D, Muir I, Faulkner J, et al: Myotonia dystrophica: Obstetric complications. *Am J Obstet Gynecol* 1978; 132:265.
45. Alberts MJ, Roses AD: Myotonic muscular dystrophy. *Neurol Clin* 1988; 3:1.
46. Jozefowicz RF, Griggs RC: Myotonic dystrophy. *Neurol Clin* 1988; 3:455.
47. Barchi RL: Myotonia. *Neurol Clin* 1988; 3:473.
48. Azar I: The response of patients with neuromuscular disorders to muscle relaxants: A review. *Anesthesiology* 1984; 61:173.
49. Camann WR, Johnson MD: Anesthetic management of a

parurient with myotonia dystrophica: A case report. *Reg Anaesth* 1990; 15:41.

50. Parikh AM, Camara EG: Neuroleptic malignant syndrome. *Am Fam Physician* 1988; 37:296.

51. Guzé BH, Baxter LR II: Neuroleptic malignant syndrome. *N Engl J Med* 1985; 313:163.

52. Kellam AMP: The neuroleptic malignant syndrome, so-called: A survey of the world literature. *Br J Psych* 1987; 150:752.

53. Levenson JL: Neuroleptic malignant syndrome. *Am J Psychiatry* 1985; 142:1137.

54. Susman VL, Addonizio G: Recurrence of neuroleptic malignant syndrome. *J Nerv Ment Dis* 1988; 176:234.

55. Ellis FR: The diagnosis of MH: Its social implications (editorial). *Br J Anaesth* 1988; 60:251.

56. Britt BA: Dantrolene (review article). *Can Anaesth Soc J* 1984; 31:61.

57. Harrison GG: Dantrolene: Dynamics and kinetics. *Br J Anaesth* 1988; 60:279.

58. Saltzman LS, Kates RA, Corke BC, et al: Hyperkalemia and cardiovascular collapse after verapamil and dantrolene administered in swine. *Anesth Analg* 1984; 63:473.

59. Lynch C, Durbin CG, Fisher NA, et al: Effects of dantrolene and verapamil on atrioventricular conduction and cardiovascular performance in dogs. *Anesthesiology* 1986; 65:252.

60. Driessen JJ, Wuis EW, Gielen JM: Prolonged vecuronium neuromuscular blockade in a patient receiving orally administered dantrolene. *Anesthesiology* 1985; 62:523.

61. Craft JB, Goldberg NH, Lim M, et al: Cardiovascular effects and placental passage of dantrolene in the maternal-fetal sheep model. *Anesthesiology* 1988; 68:68.

62. Shime J, Gare D, Andrews J, et al: Dantrolene in pregnancy: Lack of adverse effects on the fetus and newborn infant. *Am J Obstet Gynecol* 1988; 159:831.

63. McCarthy TV, Healy JMS, Lehane M, et al: Recent developments in the molecular genetics of malignant hyperthermia: Implications for future diagnosis at the DNA level. *Acta Anaesth Belgica* 1990; 41:107.

64. Mortier W: Malignant hyperthermia: Relation to other diseases. *Acta Anaesth Belgica* 1990; 41:120.

65. Abovleish E, Abbovd T, Lechevalieor Jeval: Rocuronism (ORG 9426) for cesarean section. *Br J Anaesth* 1994; 73:336.

17 Hematologic Disease

Gerard M. Bassell and Douglas V. Horbelt

Obstetric hemorrhage remains of continuing importance as a cause of maternal and fetal morbidity and mortality. In fact, after a progressive decline in maternal deaths in the United Kingdom from antepartum and postpartum hemorrhage during the preceding three triennial periods, an upward trend occurred during the latest triennium.[1]

Apart from mechanical causes of bleeding, a variety of hematologic diseases can be associated with significant blood loss during the peripartum period. A sudden onset of hemorrhage can result in significant, even fatal, blood loss before arrival in the labor and delivery suite. Yet, even if obstetric bleeding occurs within the hospital, it is an unfortunate fact that frequently the attending medical and nursing personnel do not possess the expertise to diagnose and manage the event.

In few other medical emergencies is interdisciplinary collaboration as important as in the management of peripartum hemorrhage. If outcome is to be successful, the obstetrician, anesthesiologist, and pathologist (blood banker) must play active and coordinated roles. The recognition that an episode of acute bleeding is occurring must set into motion a predetermined effort that includes identification of the etiology of the hemorrhage, assessment of the volume of blood being lost, diagnosis of any accompanying or developing bleeding diathesis, and institution of appropriate therapy based initially on clinical assessment and later on information provided by the laboratory.

Knowledge of the hematologic diseases commonly encountered in pregnant women is an absolute requirement if diagnosis and therapy are to be expeditious since rapid diagnosis and institution of therapy are the hallmarks of success. Forestalling excessive consumption of coagulation factors removes one of the causes of a bleeding diathesis. To this end, familiarity with the causes of hemorrhage in obstetrics and delineation of a plan of management that includes early consultation with blood bank personnel and possibly hematologists can minimize the likelihood of a fatal outcome.

CONGENITAL DISORDERS OF HEMOSTASIS

Inherited abnormalities of the coagulation process are relatively rare. The major coagulopathies should be identifiable by specific historical questioning. Usually, how a person has fared during dental or other surgical procedures is an excellent indicator of the presence or absence of a congenital defect. The events surrounding a previous labor are not as good an indicator because of the changes in the concentrations of coagulation factors that usually accompany term pregnancy.[2] A family history of a bleeding disorder can also signal the possibility of a congenital coagulopathy. Although most of these disorders are inherited with autosomal or sex-linked distribution, penetrance of the characteristic can vary. And, since coagulation factors are present at levels several times greater than needed for normal clotting, even a 50% decrease may not be clinically evident.

Almost all coagulation factors, including Factor XIII (clot stabilization factor),[3] can be deficient.[4,5] Fortunately, in women, only a few clotting factor deficiencies are of clinical importance.[6-8] If the presence of a defect is known before surgery or vaginal delivery, specific factor replacement to a prescribed level can be undertaken and maintained for as long as is indicated.

von Willebrand's disease

von Willebrand's disease is the most prevalent coagulation disorder to affect women of childbearing years with an incidence in the general population of $1:10,000$.[9] It is a family of disorders that, apart from type IIB, are inherited in an autosomal recessive manner with variable penetrance. von Willebrand factor helps protect platelet Factor VIII against proteolysis *in vivo*. Thus, patients with von Willebrand's disease display a pattern of bleeding similar to that found in disorders of platelet function (i.e., mucosal and gingival bleeding, menorrhagia, intestinal hemorrhage, and epistaxis). Blood loss tends to occur immediately after trauma such as delivery or surgery.[10,11]

323

Management of bleeding

Bleeding associated with von Willebrand's disease is usually treated with infusion of cryoprecipitate unless responsiveness to DDAVP (desmopressin acetate) has previously been demonstrated (usually in *mild* type I or type IIA with Factor VIII levels > 5%).[12,13] If DDAVP is indicated, the initial dose is 0.3 μg/kg infused over 15 to 30 minutes. This line of therapy is also useful in Factor VIII deficiency. If cryoprecipitate treatment is chosen either because of associated hypofibrinogenemia or known lack of responsiveness to DDAVP, 6 to 10 units are given initially. Until a specific diagnosis for hemorrhage is made, fresh frozen plasma (FFP) should be administered in addition to cryoprecipitate.[14] In the absence of clinical deterioration, coagulation profiles should be rechecked every 6 to 8 hours. Adjustments can then be made to the fresh frozen plasma and cryoprecipitate doses based on measurements of specific coagulation factors.

Anesthetic management considerations

The major anesthetic risk to women with von Willebrand's disease is bleeding into the epidural space during regional block, and subsequent hematoma formation with the potential for permanent neurologic damage. If a full evaluation of hemostasis can be performed and any abnormal measurements corrected by the administration of cryoprecipitate, conduction block can be administered for labor analgesia or cesarean section. It must be remembered, however, that depletion of coagulation factors can occur during labor or in the postpartum period, so the coagulation profile should be repeated every 3 to 4 hours during regional block and any abnormalities treated.

For labor analgesia, epidural block (preferably by continuous infusion) using the lowest concentration of local anesthetic that produces adequate analgesia and preserves motor function can be used. Here, the addition of narcotic analgesics to the anesthetic solution can facilitate a major reduction in the local anesthetic concentration. This makes retention of lower limb motor function throughout labor more likely. Similarly, the addition of epinephrine to the local anesthetic used either for subarachnoid or epidural block for cesarean section should be avoided so that an early evaluation of the legs can be made in the postanesthesia recovery room. If attention is paid to these points, regional analgesia/anesthesia should be a relatively safe technique in women with the disease.

On occasion, there will be insufficient time either to perform the required laboratory investigations or to correct coagulation abnormalities before analgesia or anesthesia is required. Under these circumstances, labor analgesia can be provided by intravenous narcotics and local perineal infiltration at delivery. The effectiveness of the latter can be improved by the addition of intravenous low-dose ketamine (5–10 mg aliquots up to a total dose of 50 mg), and/or nitrous oxide in oxygen (up to 50%) by spontaneous ventilation.* Care must be taken to maintain continual communication with the parturient under these circumstances to ensure that the technique does not result in unconsciousness with the associated risk of regurgitation and aspiration of gastric contents. The parturient receiving nitrous oxide by mask must also be discouraged from hyperventilating excessively since detrimental effects on uteroplacental blood flow and oxygen provision to the fetus can result[15] (Fig. 17-1). Block of the pudendal nerves should be avoided since hematoma formation due to lacerations of the pudendal arteries or other nearby vessels can be produced relatively easily when the ability to coagulate is impaired.

If general anesthesia is indicated either for cesarean section or for complicated obstetric maneuvers (e.g., rotation or midforceps delivery) that cannot be performed safely under the analgesic techniques just described, care must be taken to perform laryngoscopy and intubation of the trachea carefully and gently. Failure to do this can result in production of expanding hematomas of the airway that can cause severe compromise of respiration intraoperatively or in the postanesthetic period. As is usual in obstetrics, an endotracheal tube at least one size smaller than that which would be used in a nonpregnant woman of similar bodily habitus should be used.

Christmas disease

Christmas disease is a deficiency of Factor IX that, like classic hemophilia (Factor VIII deficiency), is inherited as a sex-linked recessive trait. Although the genetic abnormality affects only males, female carriers can experience a variable degree of factor deficiency with an associated mild bleeding diathesis. The defect in coagulation occurs in the intrinsic pathway and is demonstrated in the laboratory by a prolonged partial thromboplastin time (PTT) with a normal prothrombin time (PT) and bleeding time.

As with other deficiencies of vitamin K-dependent Factors (II, VII, IX and X), therapy consists of ensuring adequate levels of the vitamin for procoagulant production by a healthy liver, and administration of FFP (10–20 ml/kg) for short-term enhancement of circulating levels.[16] The effective-

---

*This is not used in our institution—*Editor.*

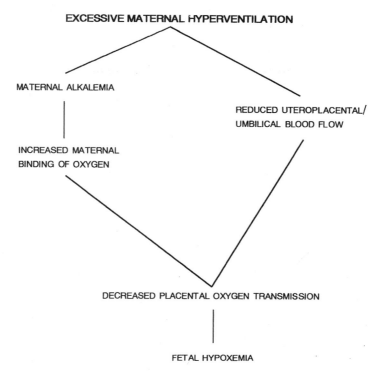

Fig. 17-1 Effects of maternal hyperventilation on the fetus. Maternal alkalosis, by moving the hemoglobin/oxygen dissociation curve to the left, restricts movement of oxygen across the placenta. Reduced blood inflow to the placenta further impairs fetal oxygenation. The end result can be a hypoxic-acidotic fetus.

ness of the latter approach should be reassessed every 6 to 8 hours during labor, particularly if an epidural catheter has been placed after the initial dose of FFP.

Other coagulation factor deficits

Deficiencies of specific clotting factors may be revealed either in an immediate or delayed fashion. A frequent occurrence is incisional bleeding or development of a deep hematoma or hemarthrosis. If these are the presenting signs, a coagulation factor deficiency is easily suspected. Usually, however, the presentation is nonspecific enough to render the diagnosis difficult.

Women in whom such deficiencies are suspected but who have not experienced blood loss should not receive intramuscular injections or aspirin/nonsteroidal antiinflammatory agents. The latter drugs can themselves impair hemostatic ability and make the likelihood of hemorrhage greater. And, after the successful resolution of a bleeding episode, a full hematologic evaluation should be performed so that a complete diagnosis can be made and future bleeding situations anticipated and potentially avoided by the administration of deficient factors before any planned surgery or vaginal delivery.

Genetic and family planning considerations are specific to each inherited disorder.

In the case of male fetuses with potential hemophilia A (Factor VIII) disease, or female fetuses whose parents could produce a homozygote state of hemophilia A, there are specific concerns about intrapartum bleeding.[17] When suspected, consideration should be given to delivering these infants by cesarean section with extraction of the infant performed in an extremely gentle fashion through an adequate hysterotomy. In theory, this would reduce the risk of spontaneous intracranial or other bleeding episodes.

If a congenital defect of coagulation is suspected, several sample tubes of blood should be collected (number and type dictated by the hematology laboratory) before beginning nonspecific fresh frozen plasma therapy. This provides laboratory specimens that have not been influenced by the administration of exogenous clotting factors. An important consideration is that hereditary absence or depletion of a specific clotting factor can, by causing hemorrhage, result in reduction of the concentration of factors not otherwise affected by the congenital defect. This can produce a picture of consumptive coagulopathy rather than that of a specific inherited disorder. So, as replacement therapy continues, periodic assessment of the co-agulation profile may reveal hereditary defects—with their future clinical implications—even though the initial clinical picture was one of con-sumptive coagulopathy.

ACQUIRED DISORDERS OF HEMOSTASIS
Disorders not produced by coagulation factor consumption

Idiopathic thrombocytopenic purpura
Incidence. Idiopathic or immune thrombocyto-penic purpura (ITP) is a syndrome characterized by a reduced platelet count, increased peripher-al destruction of platelets, and augmented plate-let production as evidenced by increased circu-lating megathrombocytes (and higher numbers of megathrombocytes in the bone marrow).[18] An acute form exists mostly limited to children fol-lowing a viral infection. The chronic form usually manifests in patients 20 to 40 years of age. The female to male ratio is 3 : 1, and this combined with the age distribution produces an incidence of preg-nancy complicated by ITP of 1 to 2/10,000.[19]

Pathophysiology. Chronic ITP is an insidious disease in which easy bruising and petechiae are initial symptoms. The presenting complaint may be menorrhagia or epistaxis. The diagnosis may have been made and therapy instituted before labor or even before pregnancy. The pregnant state itself usually does not change the clinical course of ITP and, as long as medical treatment does not include hormonal or immunosuppressive therapy, no changes in management are usually indicated.[20]

Drug therapy usually begins with oral pred-nisone (1–2 mg/kg/day).[21] The dose is reduced un-til the platelet count stabilizes at 75,000 to 100,000/mm³. Splenectomy may be necessary even during pregnancy to control platelet destruc-tion, and evaluation for accessory spleens and their removal should be undertaken at that time. Immu-nosuppressive therapy (e.g., vinca alkaloids, cyclo-phosphamide) should be reserved for only the most refractory cases during pregnancy, and their usage should be limited if possible to the second and third trimesters after organogenesis has been com-pleted.[22,23] Platelet transfusions are only effective for a matter of hours; thus, their use is indicated only when severe bleeding occurs or when surgery is planned. Immunoglobulins and plasmapheresis are also used in life-threatening or anticipated sur-gical situations. Danazol (Danocrine) has been re-ported to have an effect on ITP but its role in therapy, especially during pregnancy, remains to be defined.[24]

Obstetrical management. Patients with low platelet counts should begin to receive steroids at around 37 weeks of gestation in order to increase their platelet numbers and to produce an effect on the fetal platelet count. The antibody responsible for ITP is an immunoglobulin G (IgG) gamma globulin that can traverse the placenta and produce fetal thrombocytopenia.[25] Corticosteroid adminis-tration during the several weeks before delivery at-tempts to treat both mother and fetus.[26] Some au-thorities prefer betamethasone or dexamethasone over prednisone during pregnancy since placental enzymes inactivate the major portion of a pred-nisone dose that is presented to the placental cir-culation. Although there are well-defined benefits to prenatal steroid therapy, the drugs do pose the risk of fetal adrenal suppression and an increased incidence of maternal hypertension, preeclampsia, or postpartum psychosis.

Some women may not have a low platelet count determined until the intrapartum period when pe-techiae, hemorrhage, or other indications of a co-agulation defect occur. In that event, standard labo-ratory studies including PT, PTT, platelet count, se-rum fibrinogen concentration, serum fibrin degra-dation products (FDP), or fibrin split products (FSP) should be performed. The abnormality in ITP is limited to a decreased platelet count with other measures of coagulability being within their normal ranges. Idiopathic thrombocytopenic pur-pura is, therefore, a diagnosis of exclusion. The differential diagnosis comprises all other causes of thrombocytopenia, including drug reactions; sepsis; disseminated intravascular coagulopathy (DIC); myeloproliferative disorders such as leuke-mia, sarcoidosis, and other autoimmune diseases; tuberculosis; and acquired immunodeficiency syn-drome (AIDS).[27] The diagnosis of ITP is supported by the presence of IgG antibody to platelets. Un-fortunately, this test is not readily available and even if it is, it may not be able to be performed and completed before delivery. If other possible causes for ITP can be excluded, and if the remain-ing coagulation studies (PT, PTT, FSP, fibrinogen) are normal, then the patient should be managed as if ITP were the diagnosis. Considerations are then directed toward maternal and fetal management.

Maternal considerations. The maternal conse-quence of ITP is hemorrhage. The ability to con-trol bleeding relates to the platelet count and plate-let function. Patients are not at greater risk for ab-ruptio placentae or placenta previa than the gen-eral pregnant population.[28] Nor are they at more risk for postpartum hemorrhage from uterine bleeding since myometrial contractions produce mechanical hemostasis without a significant con-tribution from platelets. Rather, bleeding compli-cations are usually associated with surgical inci-sions (episiotomy), postoperative surgical sites, and lacerations of the birth canal. If a surgical or abdominal delivery is anticipated, platelets should be maintained above 50,000/mm^3. From the maternal standpoint, platelet counts between 30,000 and 50,000/mm^3 are acceptable for spontaneous vaginal delivery without incision or laceration. Platelet counts below 20,000/mm^3 should be augmented by platelet transfusion, particularly if surgical intervention is anticipated.[29] The survival of donor platelets may be severely limited (3 to 6 hours), so coordination and timing of the surgical event must be considered. Postdelivery levels must also be measured and augmented if necessary, depending on postpartum hemostasis and incisional integrity. The definitive diagnosis of ITP can then be carried out in the period after delivery with subsequent institution of long-term medical treatment.

Fetal/neonatal consideration. Idiopathic thrombocytopenic purpura or the possible diagnosis of ITP represents a potential risk to the fetus.[30] Thrombocytopenia may result from placentally transmitted maternal antibody.[31] Means of assessing fetal status have included estimations based on maternal platelet concentration, whether or not a splenectomy had been performed; fetal scalp blood sampling to measure fetal platelet numbers; and assays for quantitative measurements of maternal antibodies. The major fetal risk is intracranial bleeding with neurologic sequelae or death. Neonatal thrombocytopenia caused by maternal ITP is self-limiting. The infant's platelet count is usually normal by 1 month of age. Nonetheless, in the interim the newborn should be observed closely for signs of hemorrhage.

Intrapartum management considerations. Management choices are contingent upon availability of the more sophisticated antibody tests and the availability of fetal scalp sampling for platelet estimation. Currently, there are a number of proposed regimens:

1. If the maternal platelet count is 100,000/mm^3 or greater and the spleen is in situ, a vaginal delivery is attempted.
2. If the platelet count is less than 100,000/mm^3 or a splenectomy has been performed, cesarean section is indicated.
3. All patients are delivered vaginally except when there are other obstetric indications for abdominal delivery.
4. All women are delivered by cesarean section irrespective of their platelet count.
5. A fetal scalp blood platelet count is measured. If it is 50,000/mm^3 or greater, vaginal delivery is attempted.
6. Cesarean section is indicated when the fetal scalp blood platelet count is less than 50,000/

mm^3. This regimen assumes that an abdominal delivery will be gentler than a vaginal, thereby reducing the likelihood of birth trauma-induced fetal hemorrhage in the face of fetal thrombocytopenia.
7. All women with high antiplatelet antibodies are delivered by cesarean section.

Perhaps the most reasonable alternative is to deliver all afflicted women by cesarean section. Idiopathic thrombocytopenic purpura does not occur frequently, and the more sophisticated laboratory testing may not be readily available in a community hospital setting.

In summary, ITP occurs most commonly in women in the childbearing age group. It usually presents as less-than-life-threatening bleeding or as a history of abnormal bleeding or bruising. From the obstetric viewpoint, the diagnosis should be considered before pregnancy and hopefully before labor and delivery. It is, however, a disease that can present during labor and for which alternative, more catastrophic etiologies must be excluded before appropriate therapy can be instituted.

Anesthetic management. The choice of anesthetic technique in parturients with ITP depends in large part on the mode of presentation. The proposed method of delivery, gestational age of the fetus, associated or coincident obstetric complications, coagulation status, history of recent or current hemorrhage, and other significant medical history are all factors that influence the choice of anesthetic method.

Circulating platelet numbers and their efficacy are the main determinants of the safety of regional block for women with ITP. Placement of a needle in the epidural or subarachnoid space carries with it the risk of vascular perforation with consequent bleeding into the spinal canal. In the normal course of events, such bleeding is limited by coagulation processes and there are no untoward sequelae. When the ability to form a clot is impaired by thrombocytopenia, for example, volumes of blood and clot large enough to compress nerve tissue and decrease neural conduction can leak into the spinal canal. Unless the diagnosis is made rapidly and surgical decompression achieved with dispatch, permanent and potentially devastating nerve damage can ensue.

Recognition of this complication may be delayed by the effectiveness of the regional block itself since it is impossible to identify the onset of neurologic impairment when conduction analgesia is present in the area supplied by the affected nerves. Prevention of this hazard requires diligence in assessing coagulation whenever abnormalities are a possibility. Recommendations about minimal acceptable platelet concentrations abound with little evidence to support the use of one regimen over another. However, especially in this disorder, platelet effectiveness must be assessed as well. The traditional clinical method of assessing platelet functionality has been the bleeding time. Although the test can be performed rapidly and interpreted easily, its accuracy and reliability is doubtful when accomplished as it usually is in most hospitals. To be meaningful, the test must be performed with extreme care and consistency by experienced personnel. The template method of bleeding time estimation has proven to be the most reliable in providing reproducible results.[32] Even in those women in whom platelet numbers have risen to 100,000/mm^3 or more as a result of therapy, bleeding time should be assessed before placing a regional block to reassure the anesthesiologist that the platelets are functioning adequately. Recently a laboratory test has been developed that holds great promise for the evaluation of the coagulation system including assessment of platelet function. The whole blood viscoelastic coagulogram has been used to assess clotting ability in normal pregnant women[33] and in a parturient with thrombocytopenia.[34] In the latter situation, regional block was made possible in a gravida in whom the technique would otherwise have been contraindicated on the basis of low platelet numbers by the demonstration of adequate platelet function. Unfortunately, the equipment required for this procedure is not widely available.

As a general rule, if platelet numbers are deemed to be adequate, bleeding time is within normal limits, and there is no active hemorrhage, conduction block (subarachnoid or epidural) can be employed provided no other contraindications are present. Epidural analgesia for labor and vaginal delivery, and either epidural or spinal anesthesia for cesarean section, are the preferred choices. If, however, coagulation is abnormal or there is concurrent bleeding and general anesthesia for an urgent cesarean section becomes necessary, the anesthesiologist must ensure that attempts at laryngoscopy are extremely gentle. Endotracheal intubation should be performed with a smaller sized, well-lubricated tube to minimize the likelihood of producing an airway hematoma that could compromise laryngotracheal caliber during the anesthetic or following extubation. Emergence from anesthesia and removal of the endotracheal tube must also be performed in a smooth and atraumatic manner. In addition, excellent muscle relaxation must be provided during either a regional or general anesthetic for cesarean section if the delivery is to be achieved in a gentle fashion thereby avoiding appreciable trauma to the infant.

Hemolytic anemias. The hemolytic anemias are classified as either inherited or acquired. The former are further subdivided into structural or enzymatic abnormalities. Acquired hemolytic anemias are divided into those caused by (1) antibodies, (2) physical or infectious agents, (3) abnormalities of structure (paroxysmal nocturnal hemoglobinuria), or (4) fragmentation syndromes (microangiopathic hemolytic anemia).[35]

The family of inherited hemoglobinopathies characterized by "sickling" of red blood cells includes true sickle cell anemia (homozygous, hemoglobin SS), sickle cell trait (heterozygous, hemoglobin AS), sickle-hemoglobin C disease (hemoglobin SC), sickle thalassemia (hemoglobin S-β Thal), and other, much rarer forms. "Sickling" is the hypoxia-induced conformational change produced in red cells that contain a significant amount of hemoglobin S. The resultant shape interferes with the cells' ability to traverse the microcirculation in the usual unhindered manner of discoid cells, and the affected cells are unable to carry oxygen. The end result of a severe sickling episode can be tissue ischemia and necrosis together with a hemolytic crisis.

Parturients with sickle cell anemia have often received multiple blood transfusions to raise their concentration of normal hemoglobin. In recent years, blood used for this purpose has increasingly frequently been buffy coat poor, washed red blood cells with a much lower potential for provoking a recipient antibody response. Despite this, difficulty in crossmatching blood can still be encountered and plans should be made as far in advance of delivery as possible to have adequate amounts of blood available.

In addition, there is frequently a history of previous exposure to large doses of narcotic analgesics for the severe pain commonly associated with the disease. There is, therefore, the potential for narcotic addiction or, at the least, an increased requirement for analgesia. In the past, it was sometimes believed that regional block brought with it the risk of desaturation of hemoglobin, as well as subsequent sickling due to sympathetic block-induced pooling of blood in the peripheral circulation. Current opinion holds that flow through the peripheral vasculature is enhanced by sympathetic block and, therefore, desaturation is unlikely unless severe hypotension is allowed to occur. Because of the safety and effectiveness of well-conducted regional block, and since narcotic requirements are likely to be extremely high in these women, epidural block is recommended for labor analgesia in affected parturients. Spinal or epidural anesthesia are appropriate choices for cesarean section. In those circumstances when general anesthesia may be indicated (e.g., severe fetal distress) safety can be enhanced and the potential for a sickle crisis reduced by maintaining a warm environment, augmenting intravascular volume with crystalloid solutions, administration of a high inspired oxygen fraction, and monitoring arterial oxygen saturation with a pulse oximeter. Although unproved, it is possible that the decrease in blood viscosity resulting from intravenous "preload" in preparation for regional block or general anesthesia can reduce the potential for "sludging" and desaturation in small peripheral blood vessels.

The mild form of the disease, sickle cell trait, is the one most commonly encountered in the labor suite. Clinical evidence of its existence is rarely present, and women with sickle cell trait usually undergo delivery without hematologic complications. Severe hypoxia or acidosis can provoke sickling in these women, however, and the precautions taken for gravidae with homozygous sickle cell disease should be maintained.

Women with acquired hemolytic anemia usually exhibit jaundice, cholelithiasis, and splenomegaly in addition to the clinical anemia. Patients may present with abdominal, back, and limb pain. There is associated pallor, jaundice, and profound prostration, and a tachycardia that represents a cardiac response to anemia.

Autoimmune hemolytic anemia is a disease in which the Coombs' test is positive. It can be subdivided into cases caused by warm-reactive antibodies and those caused by cold-reactive antibodies. Warm-reactive antibodies are usually of the IgG type and most often react against some component of the Rh system. Since IgG antibodies can cross the placenta, there is some potential for the production of anemia in the fetuses of women with this form of the disease. There are conflicting reports concerning the influence that this may have on increasing perinatal mortality. Autoimmune hemolytic anemias of the warm antibody type are associated with hemolytic malignancies, systemic lupus erythematosus, viral illnesses, and drugs such as penicillin and methyldopa. Cold-reactive antibodies are of the IgM type. They are usually anti-I or anti-i. Most often, they are associated with mycoplasma infections, infectious mononucleosis, and lymphoreticular neoplasms. Autoimmune hemolytic anemia has been reported to be exacerbated by pregnancy.[36]

Other forms of red cell destruction besides hereditary and acquired hemolytic anemia can develop during pregnancy. Infections with malaria, the TORCH agents (toxoplasmosis, rubella, cytomegalovirus, and herpes simplex virus), and *Clostridium perfringens* can produce hemolysis. Many drugs, chemicals, and venoms can also be responsible. Lastly, red cell life span can be shortened by thermal injury or exposure to ionizing radiation thereby increasing markedly the rate of hemolysis.

Irrespective of the cause of hemolysis, acute therapy should be directed primarily toward maintaining maternal oxygen-carrying capacity and correcting any cardiovascular compromise. The lifespan of transfused red cells may be reduced considerably by the precipitating disease process, yet the risks to the fetus of impaired maternal oxygenation mandate early and frequent blood transfusion to maintain the mother's hemoglobin concentration. The additional cardiac work load imposed by severe anemia can result in rapid deterioration of maternal cardiac status. Therefore, monitoring of central venous pressure or pulmonary artery occluded (wedge) pressure during transfusion is recommended.

Disorders resulting from coagulation factor consumption

Coagulopathies that occur during pregnancy are usually the result of massive consumption of coagulation factors.[37] Although the concentrations of clotting factors normally present are much greater than those required to secure hemostasis during uncomplicated obstetrics, in some instances that buffer can be very rapidly overcome. Under those circumstances, the body's ability to replace coagulation factors is overwhelmed by their utilization rate. Such extraordinary consumption can lead to DIC and may be precipitated by infection, hemorrhage, preeclampsia, or obstetric events such as abruptio placentae, placenta previa, and ruptured uterus.[38] A discussion of the diagnosis and management of DIC appears later in this chapter.

INTRAPARTUM HEMORRHAGE

Therapeutic choices. The timely recognition that blood loss is becoming excessive is essential to the favorable resolution of obstetric bleeding. If such realization occurs early in the clinical course of a hemorrhagic state, diagnosis of the cause and institution of specific therapy can reduce the likelihood of progression to a consumptive coagulopathy (Fig. 17-2). Sometimes, accurate evaluation of the volume of blood loss is difficult. "A little oozing" from the vaginal vault may not truly represent the extent of uterine bleeding. Even if it does, its continuation over many hours can represent significant blood loss although no dramatic, massive bleeding event has occurred. Establishment of large-bore venous access with associated fluid resuscitation should begin contemporaneously with attempts to diagnose the source of hemorrhage.[39]

Once the presence of more than expected blood loss has been recognized, the first consideration should be toward assessment of the state of the uterus. Tone should be assessed manually and, if uterine relaxation is present, attempts to establish

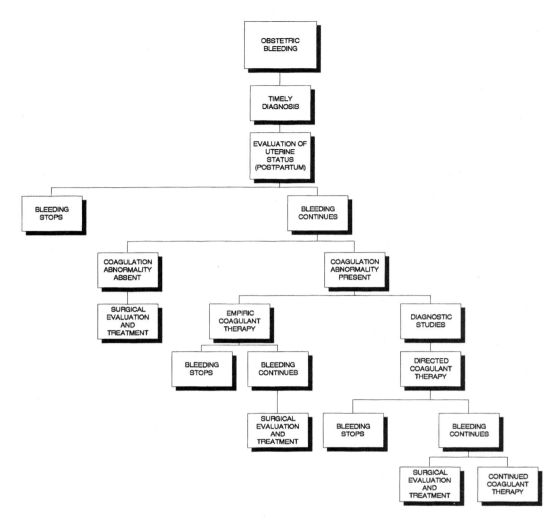

Fig. 17-2 Management of obstetric hemorrhage. A rational approach to the diagnosis and therapy of obstetric bleeding. Attention is drawn to the importance of beginning empiric coagulant therapy (e.g., cryoprecipitate, fresh frozen plasma) whenever a clotting abnormality is suspected. Such treatment should begin while laboratory tests of coagulation are pending.

contractions should ensue. Initially, these include uterine massage and the administration of intravenous oxytocin by dilute infusion. If these maneuvers fail to produce the desired degree of uterine activity, ergot preparations such as methylergonovine (Methergine) (0.2 mg) can be administered by the intramuscular route provided there is no concurrent hypertension.

15-Methyl prostaglandin $F_{2\alpha}$ (carboprost, Hemabate) has also been shown to be an effective uterotonic drug in the face of postpartum hemorrhage. In the past, the suppository or gel (Prostin 15-M) was used for this purpose by direct application to the uterus. With the availability of the parenteral preparation, the deep intramuscular route is preferred with an initial dose of 250 µg.

The intramyometrial and intravenous routes have also been employed, although the latter is not an approved method of administration. The dose can be repeated every 15 to 30 minutes, if required, up to a total dose of 2 mg. The effectiveness of this agent is not without cost, however. Pulmonary side effects that include bronchospasm and resultant hypoxemia are possible, particularly when larger, frequent doses are employed.[40] Continued atony may necessitate surgical intervention (vide infra).

Once adequate uterine contractions have been established, it is important to evaluate the effect on continuing blood loss. Preferably, this assessment should be performed by a single individual who is an experienced member of the obstetric team and who has the ongoing charge of tallying both the total blood loss and the rate of bleeding. Most often, these assessments will be performed visually with additional information provided by weighing surgical sponges, gauze swabs, and towels. At this stage, progressive blood loss is an indication for formal examination of the uterus and birth canal with adequate analgesia provided by the anesthesia team.

An examination under anesthesia during peripartum hemorrhage should include a thorough evaluation of the uterus. The cavity should be free of placental fragments. The uterine wall should be in the correct position to rule out a partial or complete uterine inversion.[41] Reduction of an inverted uterus can usually be accomplished with gentle pressure in a cephalad direction with the myometrium relaxed by concurrent administration of a low concentration (up to 0.75 minimum alveolar concentration [MAC]) of a volatile anesthetic. Once recovery of the correct anatomic configuration has been achieved, careful assessment of the uterine wall should be carried out to exclude rupture.[42]

Once the body of the uterus has been evaluated, attention is directed to the cervix and vagina. The cervix is inspected circumferentially for sources of bleeding.[43] The vagina is evaluated in a similar fashion. Lacerations should be observed for hemostasis following repair. In the vagina, lacerations should be closed in such a manner as to obliterate any potential space that could harbor a hematoma. Tissues surrounding the birth canal are extremely distensible and can accommodate clots of a size sufficient to consume large quantities of coagulation factors, thereby resulting in a bleeding diathesis.

Hematoma formation can be an insidious source of blood loss since often no actual bleeding is seen.[44] The traumatic events of vaginal birth, with or without operative intervention, can result in development of hematomas. Bleeding into the tissues surrounding the vagina can produce collections of blood around the vaginal vault or vulvar area or can extend retroperitoneally and affect pelvic structures. The only effective therapy for hematomas is incision, drainage, securing hemostasis, and either closure over a drain or allowance of healing by secondary intent.

Occasionally, intraabdominal hemorrhage can produce signs of shock together with some vaginal bleeding. Evaluation of the abdomen should be a part of the general assessment of any woman with peripartum bleeding. Exhaustion from labor, excessive sedation, or the presence of regional block can mask the signs and symptoms of intraperitoneal bleeding. If intraabdominal bleeding is

---

BOX 17-1   BRANCHES OF THE INTERNAL ILIAC (HYPOGASTRIC) ARTERY*

Anterior division
  Parietal branches   Obturator artery
                                   Internal pudendal artery
                                   Inferior gluteal artery
  Visceral branches   Uterine artery
                                   Vesical arteries
                                   Hemorrhoidal arteries
                                   Vaginal artery

Posterior division
  Parietal branches   Iliolumbar artery
                                   Lateral sacral artery
                                   Superior gluteal artery

---

*Tributaries of the internal iliac artery. The posterior division is not responsible for visceral blood flow and is not usually ligated to control blood loss from pelvic organs.

---

suspected, however, the status of the peritoneal cavity should be assessed by all means available including ultrasound and/or paracentesis.

Packing has long been used to control surgical hemorrhage. Although packing the uterus can provide initial control of bleeding, the presence of a foreign body within the uterine cavity inhibits its ability to contract, thereby interfering with the major hemostatic mechanism.[45] In addition, blood can pool above a pack and give observers the false impression that bleeding has been controlled.

Once a careful examination has been concluded and repairs made, any incremental major blood loss is an indication for surgical intervention. The primary blood supply of the pelvis is the internal iliac (hypogastric) artery, which has two divisions: posterior and anterior[46] (Box 17-1). The posterior division has only parietal branches. These are the lateral sacral, the iliolumbar, and the superior gluteal arteries. The anterior division has six visceral and three parietal branches. The visceral branches are the uterine, superior vesical, inferior vesical, middle rectal, vaginal, and obliterated umbilical arteries (Fig. 17-3). The parietal branches are the obturator, internal pudendal, and inferior gluteal arteries. These vessels anastomose with the blood supply of the colon, with the aortic circulation, and with the ovarian artery. Collateral perfusion of the pelvis is well developed, particularly during pregnancy.

Vascular ligation at various points in the pelvic circulation has been described frequently. Because of the rich collateral circulation, interruption of a single vessel is unlikely to produce ischemia and organ death. It will, however, promote hemostasis by reducing organ pulse pressure.[47] This lower

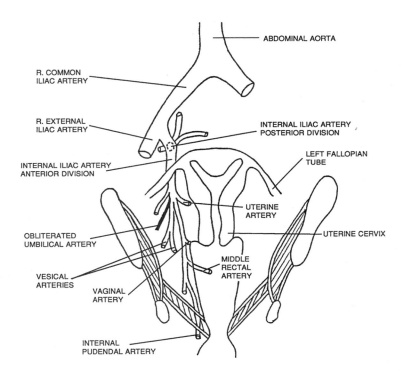

Fig. 17-3 Pelvic arterial circulation. Collateral circulation is well developed, so ligation of branches of the hypogastric artery is unlikely to prejudice organ viability.

pressure increases the probability that the mechanical and coagulation factors that usually produce hemostasis can have their desired effect. The main vessels to consider ligating are the uterine, hypogastric, and ovarian arteries.

The uterine artery can be ligated by identifying the isthmus of the body of the uterus and placing a suture ligature (0 or 1) superficially into the uterus passing from anterior to posterior, and then placing the same ligature lateral to the vessels in the broad ligament to encircle both the artery and the veins of the lateral aspect of the uterus.[48] This must be done bilaterally. Accurate placement decreases uterine perfusion pressure without necessitating a retroperitoneal dissection to identify the hypogastric artery. This procedure does not affect the perfusion of any other pelvic organ. It is intended to control uterine bleeding and is ineffective if bleeding arises from an area outside that supplied by the uterine artery.

Hypogastric artery ligation decreases perfusion of all pelvic organs. Usually only the anterior division is ligated. This is performed by entering the retroperitoneal space lateral to the infundibulopelvic ligament and superior to the round ligament. The psoas muscle is identified and medial to it lies the common iliac artery. The ureter usually crosses the artery at its bifurcation and stays with the sheet of peritoneum as the retroperitoneal space is de-

veloped. The common iliac artery divides into the external and internal iliac arteries. Approximately 4 to 5 cm from the origin of the internal iliac artery, its posterior branch leaves and runs dorsally. Because of its course, this artery can be difficult to identify and significant blood loss can accompany dissection carried out to free it. Distal to its usual location is the preferred site of ligation of the anterior division of the hypogastric artery. A long, blunt, curved instrument is used to dissect carefully under the vessel. Attention must be directed to avoiding the hypogastric vein, which lies medial and posterior to the artery. A tie is then placed under the vessel and secured.[49] This is repeated with a second tie. The artery is not cut. Again, these procedures must be performed bilaterally to produce the desired effect.

On some occasions, the contribution of the ovarian arteries to uterine bleeding is great enough to warrant their ligation. This is performed at the level of the ovarian ligament and not at the infundibulopelvic ligament. Care must be taken to avoid the fallopian tubes when placing ties around the vasculature inferior to the tubes. This method of ligature placement should preserve perfusion of the ovary and tube while producing the desired effect of reducing uterine pulse pressure.

Each surgical procedure performed to decrease hemorrhage should have its effectiveness evaluated. Use of the low lithotomy position allows a qualified observer to perform such an assessment at each stage of the surgical procedure. If vascular ligation does not produce demonstrable improvement in the rate of blood loss, hysterectomy is the only further option.

Anesthetic management. The request for urgent anesthetia in a woman with concurrent hemorrhage is one of the most difficult clinical situations faced by the anesthesiologist in the obstetric suite. Although such occurrences are rarely predictable, planning for the eventuality will reduce the likelihood of disaster. All parturients admitted to the labor suite and all women admitted to the antepartum ward with a diagnosis of vaginal bleeding should be interviewed by anesthesiology personnel and an anesthetic history should be recorded and promulgated. This simple exercise reduces the incidence of unpleasant surprises at the time of urgent anesthetic induction.

Active hemorrhage is one of the few absolute contraindications to regional block in obstetrics. The possibility of an associated coagulopathy and the inability to augment intravascular volume safely render the technique unsafe. A history of recent hemorrhage excludes spinal or epidural analgesia only if abnormalities of coagulation exist or blood volume is still depleted and cannot be corrected in time to place a regional block safely. It has been suggested that spinal anesthesia can be used even in the face of clotting abnormalities as long as a very small-bore needle (25-gauge or smaller) is used for placement of the block. The theory operative here is that any perforation of vessels within the spinal canal by this type of needle will be so tiny as to make the risk of bleeding into the epidural space inconsequential. There is no evidence either to support or disprove this contention.

Requirements for intravenous volume augmentation demand even more stringent adherence when there has been recent major blood loss. Whenever possible, central venous pressure measurements should guide intravenous "preload" since the degree of volume depletion caused by recent hemorrhage is difficult to determine otherwise.

Often, however, the request for an anesthetic will be part of the overall management of excessive intrapartum bleeding after vaginal delivery. Hemorrhage from a partially adherent placenta can necessitate intrauterine manual examination and evacuation that would be intolerable to the patient in the absence of effective analgesia. In addition, a degree of myometrial relaxation can be indicated, particularly if there is an associated partial or complete uterine inversion. If delivery has been accomplished with no analgesia or with the aid of a pu-

dendal block or local perineal infiltration, extensive repairs of lacerations of the birth canal or evacuation of sidewall hematomas may be impossible without the provision of adequate pain relief. In these situations, local anesthetic infiltration may be only partially effective and, since the injection is made around actively bleeding areas, the complications of intravascular drug placement are likely. The responsibility for providing safe, effective analgesia and adequate surgical conditions, then, devolves upon the anesthesiologist.

Under these circumstances, the primary rule is *assess the clinical situation.* A complete appraisal must include a discussion with the obstetrician about the management plan. The anesthetic requirements for removal of a retained placenta are obviously vastly different from those for exploratory laparotomy and planned vascular ligation. In fact, relatively brief procedures such as manual exploration of the uterus can often be performed with intravenous analgesia (ketamine, 5–10 mg; fentanyl, 25–50 μg; midazolam, 1.25–2.5 mg) with the parturient retaining consciousness and protective airway reflexes yet having adequate pain relief for the procedure. More complex surgical intervention will require general anesthesia.

There is no role for mask *anesthesia* in obstetrics. The risks of regurgitation and aspiration are heightened by pregnancy hormones and by the mechanical effects of the enlarging uterus and its contents. In addition, labor pain and narcotic analgesics used to treat it reduce gastric emptying further.[50] Therefore, the use of adequate means to protect the maternal airway during general anesthesia is mandatory. These include performance of a rapid-sequence induction with cricoid pressure and passage of a cuffed endotracheal tube. If hemorrhagic hypotension is present, intravenous injection of sodium thiopental as part of a rapid-sequence technique can worsen the clinical situation by producing myocardial depression. Under these circumstances, small doses of ketamine (0.5–0.7 mg/kg) or diazepam (50–75 μg/kg) are usually sufficient to produce unconsciousness and allow protection of the airway. Following anesthetic induction, intravenous narcotic anesthesia will reduce the likelihood of myometrial depression, which can produce worsening of any uterine bleeding.

Disseminated intravascular coagulopathy

Hemostasis depends on the presence of clotting factors in adequate amounts and their successful completion of a coagulation cascade when activated or stimulated. The result of this is a solid seal of any breach in the intravascular space. The coagulation mechanism may initiate either the intrinsic cascade, which uses Factors XII, XI, X, IX, V, platelets, and Factors II and I, or the extrinsic cascade, which relies on tissue thromboplastin, Factors VII, V, X, platelets, and Factors II and I (Table 17-1). Each of the procoagulant factors (precursors) is usually present in 2 to 10 times the amount needed for coagulation and, once consumed, is able to be replaced in a healthy individual within 24 to 48 hours. Pregnancy increases the concentration of some factors, especially fibrinogen, as much as 50% above nonpregnant levels as further assurance of hemostatic effectiveness during parturition.

If the coagulation cascade is initiated in the intravascular space, anticoagulation and possibly fibrinolytic systems begin to function in an attempt to prevent clot formation within the bloodstream. Antithrombin III inhibits activated Factors II, IX, X, and XI. Plasma protein C and its coenzyme protein S inactivate Factors V and VIII after they have been activated. If fibrin forms in the blood, the plasminogen activating system cleaves it into fibrin degradation (split) products (FDPs or FSPs). These end products of fibrin breakdown possess anticoagulant properties of their own that contribute to further inhibition of the clotting cascade.

The equilibrium between coagulation activity and anticlotting mechanisms allows blood to remain liquid within the intravascular space yet have the almost instantaneous ability to produce a solid clot when injury to a blood vessel occurs. Imbalance from whatever the source can result in a coagulopathy or a fibrinolytic abnormality that can be life-threatening.

The most common imbalance of coagulation encountered during the peripartum period is DIC. This syndrome can be caused by a number of different diseases or physiologic states (Box 17-2). It can be encountered in many obstetric situations including abruptio placentae, amniotic fluid embolism, dead fetus syndrome, gram-negative septicemia, and preeclampsia/eclampsia (HELLP syndrome). It also has had a reported association with saline-induced midtrimester abortions.

The pathophysiology of DIC revolves around a precipitating event that initiates the coagulation mechanism. Subsequent consumption and destruction of clotting factors overcome the body's ability to replace them. Tissue thromboplastin (e.g., abruptio placentae), endothelial cell damage (e.g., HELLP), or hypotensive-acidemic states (e.g., gram-negative shock) may initiate the events. Treatment is directed at stopping or counteracting the precipitating event and providing supportive therapy until the patient can replace the clotting factors necessary for adequate coagulation.

Disseminated intravascular coagulopathy in obstetric processes has a component of intravascular fibrin formation that activates the plasminogen system and produces fibrin degradation products. There is also vascular occlusion, which manifests as decreased perfusion of capillary beds and in signs of microangiopathic hemolytic anemia (presence of increased numbers of circulating schistocytes). The consumptive component first drops the platelet count to thrombocytopenic levels. Next, plasma clotting factors are consumed, with Factors V and VIII dropping below a functional level first. However, all factors, including fibrinogen, can fall below the levels necessary for adequate coagulability.

The clinical presentation of DIC is usually several manifestations of hemorrhage such as petechiae, ecchymoses, and bleeding from venipunc-

Table 17-1 Human coagulation factors

Factor number	Common name
I	Fibrinogen
II	Prothrombin
III	Tissue thromboplastin
IV	Calcium
V	Proaccelerin
VII	Proconvertin
VIII	Antihemophilic factor
IX	Christmas factor
X	Stuart-Prower factor
XI	Plasma thromboplastin antecedent factor
XII	Hageman factor
XIII	Fibrin stabilizing factor

BOX 17-2 CLINICAL ENTITIES ASSOCIATED WITH DISSEMINATED INTRAVASCULAR COAGULOPATHY

Obstetric complications (abruptio placentae, amniotic fluid embolism, HELLP syndrome, dead fetus syndrome, gram-negative septicemia)
Pulmonary embolism
Malignancy
Heat stroke
Snake bite
Autoimmune diseases (systemic lupus erythematosus, sarcoidosis)
Burns
Massive trauma
Liver disease
Myocardial infarction
Transfusion reaction
Allergic reaction

ture or operative sites. Other sites of potential hemorrhage are the uterus, mucous membranes, gastrointestinal tract, renal system, or central nervous system. Confusion, difficulty in oxygenation, and hematuria are usually late complications.

Whenever excessive bleeding occurs, the patient's ability to coagulate should be evaluated. A complete assessment requires laboratory support and time and therefore should be initiated as soon as an untoward bleeding episode is identified. Pending receipt of the results of these investigations, fluid and red blood cell resuscitation is undertaken. In addition, a sample of the patient's blood should be placed in a clean glass (clot) tube and retained by the bedside or taped to a nearby wall. The tube should be viewed frequently and the time taken to produce a solid clot measured. Once a clot has formed, its firmness can be assessed and any early lysis identified. This simple bedside maneuver provides valuable information that can direct empiric administration of blood products until the results of laboratory tests are available.

The "standard" coagulation profile includes PT, PTT, serum fibrinogen, platelet count, and presence of FSPs. Defects or deficiencies in major coagulation factors produce an elevated PTT (normally 24 to 36 sec) with other measures remaining within normal limits. If the clot tube result or laboratory profile is abnormal, replacement of basic coagulation factors should be undertaken. Fresh frozen plasma (15–25 ml/kg) is administered initially. This represents 4 to 7 units each containing 200 to 225 ml. Although this is a relatively large fluid and colloid load, the plasma contributes to the restoration of systemic blood pressure and cardiac output as well as to the correction of any coagulation deficit. Central venous pressure and pulmonary status should be monitored. If fluid overload occurs once hemorrhage has been corrected, it can be managed in the usual fashion with diuretics, oxygen, and positive end-expiratory pressure ventilation as indicated. Depending on the clinical situation, approximately half the original dose of fresh frozen plasma should be repeated every 6 to 12 hours until the exact defect and specific replacement therapy can be identified.

Once the results of coagulation studies have been received, specific replacement therapy can be initiated. Fibrinogen levels below 150 mg/dl should be corrected to at least this level. Cryoprecipitate is a useful product for this purpose. Each unit can be expected to raise serum fibrinogen concentration by approximately 10 mg/dl. The usual initial dose of 6 to 10 units will, therefore, produce a 60 to 100 mg/dl augmentation in blood fibrinogen level.

Thrombocytopenia, a major feature of DIC, is treated by platelet transfusion. Each unit should increase the platelet count by $10,000/mm^3$. Transfusions usually consist of 8 to 10 pooled units contained in approximately 250 ml of fluid. The platelet count should be kept at $50,000/mm^3$ or greater when active bleeding is present or if a surgical procedure is planned. Further fresh frozen plasma can be administered, depending on the PT and PTT measurements, but it must be remembered that these tests are only accurate if the serum fibrinogen level is greater than 100 mg/dl.

The syndrome of DIC is an active, not a static process, and serial determinations are necessary to ensure that factor replacement is rational and adequate. It is important to remember that the successful treatment of DIC depends on arresting the precipitating event and allowing the patient to recover her own thrombotic/thrombolytic equilibrium. Often, clotting factor, platelet, and red cell transfusions must be repeated frequently and in large volume over many hours or even days until the gap between consumption and recovery is narrowed.

Disseminated intravascular coagulopathy in obstetrics is usually an acute event associated with active, sometimes massive, blood loss. In more chronic instances of the syndrome, intravascular thrombosis plays a more central role. Under this circumstance, heparin therapy may be indicated. This may occur in the dead fetus syndrome, particularly if the fetus has been dead *in utero* for 4 weeks or longer. Heparin therapy may return the coagulation factor levels to normal over a period of several days, after which delivery can be accomplished with a reduced risk of hemorrhage. If active bleeding is present, heparin can be expected to accentuate it. Its use should be avoided, therefore, in the management of acute, hemorrhagic DIC.

CONCLUSION

Whenever hematologic disease is encountered in pregnancy, the obligations of the attending physicians are to identify the impact on maternal and fetal well-being and the conduct of parturition. With the majority of such diseases, hemorrhage is a potential complication and additional responsibilities are to replace deficient factors and assess the clinical response to therapy. It must be remembered that any hemorrhage can have more than one etiology, and an exhaustive effort must always be made to find other clinical or mechanical reasons for continuing blood loss. Specific factor replacement therapy can only be effective when mechanical causes have been treated effectively. From the anesthesiologist's viewpoint, hematologic diseases influence the choice of anesthetic technique since deficiencies in coagulability can increase the risk of both regional and general anesthesia.

REFERENCES

1. Hibbard BM, Anderson MM, Drife JO, et al: *Report on Confidential Enquiries into Maternal Deaths in the United Kingdom 1988-1990*. Her Majesty's Stationery Office, London, 1994, pp 34-42.
2. Fletcher AP, Alkjaersig NK, Burstein R: The influence of pregnancy upon blood coagulation and plasma fibrinolytic enzyme function. *Am J Obstet Gynecol* 1979; 134:743.
3. Kitchens CS, Newcomb TF: Factor XIII. *Medicine* 1979; 58:413.
4. Greenwood RJ, Rabin SC: Hemophilia-like postpartum bleeding. *Obstet Gynecol* 1967; 30:362.
5. Voke J, Letsky E: Pregnancy and antibody to factor VIII. *J Clin Path* 1977; 30:928.
6. Philips LL, Little WA: Factor V deficiency in obstetrics. *Obstet Gynecol* 1962; 19:507.
7. Purcell G, Nossel HL: Factor XI (PTA) deficiency: Surgical and obstetric aspects. *Obstet Gynecol* 1970; 35:69.
8. Saidi P, Siegelman M, Mitchell VB: Effect of factor XII deficiency on pregnancy and parturition. *Thromb Hemostas* 1979; 41:523.
9. Bloom AL: The von Willebrand syndrome. *Semin Hematol* 1980; 17:215.
10. Evans PC: Obstetric and gynecologic patients with von Willebrand's disease. *Obstet Gynecol* 1971; 38:37.
11. Lipton RA, Ayromlooi J, Coller BS: Severe von Willebrand's disease during labor and delivery. *JAMA* 1982; 248:1355.
12. Weiss HJ, Rogers T: Correction of the platelet abnormality in von Willebrand's disease by cryoprecipitate. *Am J Med* 1972; 53:734.
13. Cohen S, Goldiner PL: Epidural analgesia for labor and delivery in a patient with von Willebrand's disease. *Reg Anesth* 1989; 14:95.
14. Perkins HA: Correction of the hemostatic defects in von Willebrand's disease. *Blood* 1967; 30:375.
15. Levinson G, Shnider SM, deLorimier AA, et al: Effects of maternal hyperventilation on uterine blood flow and fetal oxygenation and acid-base status. *Anesthesiology* 1974; 40:340.
16. Spector I, Corn M: Laboratory tests of hemostasis: The relation to hemorrhage in liver disease. *Arch Intern Med* 1967; 119:577.
17. Levine PH: The clinical manifestations and therapy of hemophilia A and B, in Coleman RW, Hirsch J, Marder VJ, et al (eds): *Hemostasis and Thrombosis*. Philadelphia, Lippincott, 1982, p 85.
18. Burstein SA, Harker LA: Quantitative platelet disorders, in Bloome AL, Thomas DP (eds): *Haemostasis and Thrombosis*. Edinburgh, Churchill-Livingstone, 1981, pp 279-300.
19. Wintrobe MM, Lee G, Bogs DR, et al (eds): Immunologic platelet destruction, in *Clinical Hematology*. Philadelphia, Lea & Febiger, 1981, pp 1092-1110.
20. Kessler I, Lancet M, Borenstein R, et al: The obstetrical management of patients with immunologic thrombocytopenic purpura. *Int J Gynecol Obstet* 1982; 20:23.
21. Carloss HW, McMillan R, Crosby WH: Management of pregnancy in women with immune thrombocytopenic purpura. *JAMA* 1980; 244:2756.
22. Ahn YS, Byrnes JJ, Harrington WJ, et al: The treatment of idiopathic thrombocytopenia with vinblastine-loaded platelets. *N Engl J Med* 1978; 20:1101.
23. Nicholson HO: Cytotoxic drugs in pregnancy. *J Obstet Gynaecol Br Commonw* 1968; 75:307.
24. Ahn YS, Harrington WJ, Simon SR, et al: Danazol for the treatment of idiopathic thrombocytopenic purpura. *N Engl J Med* 1983; 308:1396.

25. Scott JR, Cruikshank DP, Kochenour NK, et al: Fetal platelet counts in the obstetric management of immunologic thrombocytopenic purpura. *Am J Obstet Gynecol* 1980; 136:495.
26. Goodhue PA, Evans TS: Idiopathic thrombocytopenic purpura during pregnancy. *Obstet Gynecol* 1963; 18:671.
27. Horger EO III, Keane MWD: Platelet disorders in pregnancy. *Clin Obstet Gynecol* 1979; 22:843.
28. Laros RK Jr, Sweet RL: Management of idiopathic thrombocytopenic purpura during pregnancy. *Am J Obstet Gynecol* 1975; 122:182.
29. Cines DB, Dusak B, Tomaski A, et al: Immune thrombocytopenic purpura and pregnancy. *N Engl J Med* 1982; 306:826.
30. Kernoff L, Malan E, Gunston K: Neonatal thrombocytopenia complicating autoimmune thrombocytopenia in pregnancy. *Ann Intern Med* 1979; 90:55.
31. Kohler PF, Farr RS: Elevation of cord maternal IgG immunoglobulins: Evidence for an active placental IgG transport. *Nature* 1966; 210:1070.
32. Kumar R, Ansell JE, Canoso RT, et al: Clinical trial of a new bleeding time device. *Am J Clin Pathol* 1978; 70:642.
33. Steer PL, Krantz HB: Thromboelastography and sonoclot analysis in the healthy parturient. *J Clin Anesth* 1993; 5:419.
34. Steer PL: Anaesthetic management of a parturient with thrombocytopenia using thromboelastography and sonoclot analysis. *Can J Anaesth* 1993; 40:84.
35. Dacie JV: The haemolytic anaemias. *The Hereditary Haemolytic Anaemias*, ed 3. New York, Churchill Livingstone, 1985, pp 4-6, vol 1.
36. Hurd WW, Miodovnik M, Stys SJ: Pregnancy associated with paroxysmal nocturnal hemoglobinuria. *Obstet Gynecol* 1982; 60:742.
37. Bick RL: Disseminated intravascular coagulation and related syndromes: Etiology, pathophysiology, diagnosis, and management. *Am J Hematol* 1978; 5:265.
38. Beller FK, Uszynski M: Disseminated intravascular coagulation in pregnancy. *Clin Obstet Gynecol* 1974; 17:250.
39. Hayashi RH: Heading off disaster in postpartum hemorrhage. *Contemp Obstet Gynecol* 1982; 20:91.
40. Hankins GDV, Berryman GK, Scott RT, et al: Maternal arterial desaturation with 15-methyl prostaglandin $F_{2\text{-alpha}}$ for uterine atony. *Obstet Gynecol* 1988; 72:367.
41. Herbert WNP: Complications of the immediate puerperium. *Clin Obstet Gynecol* 1982; 25:219.
42. Spaulding LB, Gallup DG: Current concepts of management of rupture of the gravid uterus. *Obstet Gynecol* 1979; 54:437.
43. Graber EA, O'Rourke JJ: Postpartum cervical laceration. *Obstet Gynecol* 1957; 10:247.
44. Pieri RJ: Pelvic hematomas associated with pregnancy. *Obstet Gynecol* 1958; 12:249.
45. Lucas WE: Postpartum hemorrhage. *Clin Obstet Gynecol* 1980; 23:637.
46. Clemente CD: Anatomy: *A Regional Atlas of the Human Body*, ed 2. Baltimore, Urban & Schwartzenberg, 1981, p 333.
47. Burchell RC: Physiology of internal iliac artery ligation. *J Obstet Gynaecol Br Commonw* 1968; 75:642.
48. O'Leary JL, O'Leary JA: Uterine artery ligation for control of postcesarean section hemorrhage. *Obstet Gynecol* 1974; 43:849.
49. Mattingly RF, Thompson JD (eds): *Operative Gynecology*. Philadelphia, JB Lippincott, 1985, pp 50-55.
50. Murray FA, Erskine JP, Fielding J: Gastric secretion in pregnancy. *J Obstet Gynaecol Br Emp* 1957; 64:373.

18 Erythroblastosis Fetalis

Richard B. Clark, J. Gerald Quirk, Jr., and H. Breckenridge Collins

Erythroblastosis fetalis (EBF) is an immune-mediated hemolytic disease of the fetus characterized by the presence of nucleated red cells (erythroblasts) in the fetal circulation. It is also frequently called isoimmunization or alloimmunization, since hemolysis is caused by maternal antibodies directed against fetal red cell antigens. Although hemolysis can be caused by many red cell antigens and can lead to EBF, the antigens of the Rh system are most commonly responsible. In the 55 years since the Rh antigen was discovered, great progress has been made in our understanding and management of EBF, resulting in an impressive decrease in perinatal morbidity and mortality. Perhaps the most significant advance has been the use of Rh immune globulin (RHIG) to prevent alloimmunization in Rh-negative women. A recent estimate of the incidence of EBF due to Rh disease is 10.6 cases per 10,000.[1] This chapter will review the pathophysiology of EBF, using the Rh antigen system as a prototypical example; it will also present the management strategies used by obstetricians and anesthesiologists to provide optimal outcome in these high-risk pregnancies.

THE Rh BLOOD GROUP SYSTEM

Rhesus* antigen was discovered and first described by Landsteiner and Wiener in 1940.[2] The Rh system, however, refers to a group of antigens (of which the Rhesus, or LW, antigen is one) that are inherited as a complex. A controversy still exists surrounding the appropriate nomenclature for the system as a whole (Table 18-1). In the United States, the nomenclature and theories of inheritance of the various antigens in the Rh system first proposed by Fisher followed by Race have been the most popular.[3] This system continues to be useful as more specific information about the genetics of the Rh system has been discovered. It is now apparent that the antigen complex is comprised of

a series of at least three membrane-associated proteins that are homologous but distinct. Two of these proteins, C and E, have immunologically distinguishable isoforms, designated c and e, respectively. There is no apparent isoform for the principal protein D. The rhesus gene locus on chromosome 1 consists of two adjacent homologous structural genes designated RhCcEe and RhD.[4] Rarely, neither gene is inherited; in this case, none of the three proteins are present on the red cell. This circumstance is designated as Rh_{null}. Red cells lacking any Rh protein have abnormal membranes, which results in hemolytic anemia.[5]

It is the presence of D that confers Rh-positive antigen status to the individual. Since the antithetical antigen for D has never been found and no antibody with an anti-D specificity has ever been discovered, it is the absence of D that confers Rh-negative status to an individual. According to the Fisher-Race hypothesis, the antigens are inherited in two sets of three. Conceptually this still works, although it might be more accurate to state that a form of the RhCcEe gene is inherited from each parent, and an RhD gene may or may not be inherited, depending on the parents' genotype for D. We will continue to use the Fisher-Race nomenclature in this chapter.

Approximately 45% of Rh-positive individuals are homozygous for D, which means they have inherited a D-containing haplotype from each of their parents. The remainder of Rh-positive individuals are heterozygous, which means they have inherited a D-containing haplotype from one parent and a non–D-containing haplotype from the other. By definition, an Rh-negative individual has inherited a haplotype from each of the parents lacking the D gene.

The individual sets of three (or haplotypes) are found in the general population with a varying frequency (Table 18-1). Certain haplotypes such as [C,D,e] are found commonly in Caucasian populations. Conversely, the haplotype [c,D,e] is found in highest frequency in the black population. The highest rate of haplotypes lacking the RhD gene is found in the Basque population, which is thought to be the genetic source of Rh-negative status.

---

*Rhesus comes from classical mythology; he was the son of the muse Euterpe and a Thracian ally of Troy. The French naturalist Jean B. Audebert in 1798 gave the scientific name *Simia rhesus* to what is now commonly known as the rhesus monkey. The scientific name was later changed to *Macaca mulatta*.

Table 18-1 Rh alleles, their antigenic determinants and frequencies*

Allele	Associated antigenic determinants		Approximate allele frequency in americans of different descent†		
	Race and Sanger	Weiner	Western European	African	Oriental
R^1	D,C,e	Rh$_0$, rh′, ,rh′,hr″	0.45	0.10	0.55
r	c,e	hr′, hr″	0.37	0.15	0.10
R^2	D,c,E	Rh$_0$, hr′, rh″	0.14	0.10	0.35
R^0	D,c,e	Rh$_0$, hr′, hr″	0.02	0.60	Low
$r″$	c,E	hr′, rh″	0.01	Low	Low
$r′$	C,e	rh′, hr″	0.01	Low	Low
R^z	D,C,E	Rh$_0$, rh′, rh″	Low	Low	Low
R^y	C,E	rh′, rh″	Low	Low	Low

*From Giblett ER: Blood groups and blood transfusion, in Braunwald E, Isselbacher KJ, Petersdorf RG, et al (eds): *Harrison's Principles of Internal Medicine,* ed 11. New York, McGraw-Hill, 1987. Used by permission.
†Low frequency means less than 0.01. Individuals of African descent have other alleles not listed here, thus accounting for failure of their frequencies to total 1.0.

As alluded to earlier, the Rh blood group system is actually much more complex than the system envisioned by Race and Sanger. There are known to be at least 40 other antibodies that delineate other Rh antigenic determinants. One such antigen is D^u, or D variant, which is usually protective against immunization to a D-positive fetus when present in the mother. Fetomaternal incompatibility for these other Rh antigens, as for the antigens listed in Table 18-1, can result in alloimmunization of the mother, thus placing her fetus at variable risk of developing EBF. However, from a clinical point of view we are concerned more with D antigen since it is the most frequently encountered and most immunogenic of the proteins in the Rh system. It is important to note that, in contrast to the A and B major blood group antigens, the Rh antigen is expressed only on the red cell membrane glycocalyx; it is not expressed on other cell membranes such as vascular endothelium or fibroblasts. Importantly, it is expressed on the fetal red cell surface from approximately 4 weeks' gestation.[6]

ETIOLOGY OF ALLOIMMUNIZATION

Immunization occurs when an individual is exposed to antigens that are not recognized as originating from "self." In the case of blood group antigens, non–self antigens can be introduced primarily in two ways: transfusion and fetal-to-maternal hemorrhage. Since the immune reaction generates antibodies against those non–self, or "other" antigens, the term alloimmunization is applied. A later transfusion or subsequent pregnancy (being genetically dissimilar to the mother) can be thought of as an allograft to the mother, which may incite a secondary immune response.

Before the discovery of the Rh antigen blood group system, incompatible blood transfusion was an important cause of Rh alloimmunization. With the discovery of the Rh antigen and the introduction of pretransfusion crossmatching, the incidence of Rh immunization decreased to a limited degree. Transfusion-initiated immunization remains an important source of EBF caused by the other blood group systems listed in Table 18-2, however.

Levine and Stetson described in 1939 the presence of atypical antibodies in the blood of pregnant women who had delivered stillborn macerated fetuses.[7] They postulated that maternal immunization was the result of a fetal antigen inherited from the father but lacking in the mother. Their conjecture was correct, for it is now known that there are many red cell surface antigens that fetuses can inherit from the father that are capable of eliciting an immune response in the mother. If the mother produces an IgG antibody against that antigen, and if that antigen is expressed on fetal red blood cells, the fetus may develop an acquired hemolytic anemia. Table 18-2 presents red cell surface antigens expressed on fetal red blood cells that are associated with a risk of developing EBF.

In 1948, Wiener suggested that transplacental hemorrhage of fetal Rh-positive red blood cells into the maternal circulation was a cause of Rh immunization.[8] Subsequent work confirmed this theory.[9] Approximately 50% of mothers show evidence of transplacental hemorrhage following delivery of an ABO-compatible baby. Indeed, 5% to 15% of women will show evidence of transplacental hemorrhage in the second month of pregnancy. The "gold standard" test for identification of fetal cells in the maternal circulation is the Kleihauer-Betke test.[10] In this technique, a peripheral blood smear is washed in acid-citrate buffer (pH 3.3) resulting in elution of hemoglobin from adult red blood cells ("red cell ghosts"). At pH 3.3, fetal hemoglobin is not eluted from fetal red blood cells (Fig. 18-1). Recently, flow cytometry has also been

Table 18-2 Antibodies causing hemolytic disease in the fetus or infant (HDN)

Blood group system	Antigens related to HDN	Severity of HDN	Proposed management
Rh	D	Mild to severe	Amniotic fluid studies
	C	Mild to moderate	Amniotic fluid studies
	c	Mild to severe	Amniotic fluid studies
	E	Mild to severe	Amniotic fluid studies
	e	Mild to moderate	Amniotic fluid studies
Lewis		Not a proven cause of HDN*	
I		Not a proven cause of HDN	
Kell	K	Mild to severe with hydrops fetalis	Amniotic fluid studies
	k	Mild to severe	Amniotic fluid studies
Duffy	Fy^a	Mild to severe with hydrops fetalis	Amniotic fluid studies
	Fy^b	Not a cause of HDN	
Kidd	Jk^a	Mild to severe	Amniotic fluid studies
	Jk^b	Mild to severe	Amniotic fluid studies
MNSs	M	Mild to severe	IgG titers, amniotic fluid studies if high
	N	Mild	Expectant
	S	Mild to severe	Amniotic fluid studies
	s	Mild to severe	Amniotic fluid studies
Lutheran	Lu^a	Mild	Expectant
	Lu^b	Mild	Expectant
Diego	Di^a	Mild to severe	Amniotic fluid studies
	Di^b	Mild to severe	Amniotic fluid studies
Xg	Xg^a	Mild	Expectant
P	$PP_1P^k(Tj^a)$	Mild to severe	Amniotic fluid studies
Public antigens	Yt^a	Moderate to severe	Amniotic fluid studies
	Yt^b	Mild	Expectant
	Lan	Mild	Expectant
	En^a	Moderate	Amniotic fluid studies
	Ge	Mild	Expectant
	Jr^a	Mild	Expectant
	Co^a	Severe	Amniotic fluid studies
Private antigens	Co^{a-b}	Mild	Expectant
	Batty	Mild	Expectant
	Becker	Mild	Expectant
	Berrens	Mild	Expectant
	Biles	Moderate	Amniotic fluid studies
	Evans	Mild	Expectant
	Gonzales	Mild	Expectant
	Good	Severe	Amniotic fluid studies
	Heibel	Moderate	Amniotic fluid studies
	Hunt	Mild	Expectant
	Jobbins	Mild	Expectant
	Radin	Moderate	Amniotic fluid studies
	Rm	Mild	Expectant
	Ven	Mild	Expectant
	$Wright^a$	Severe	Amniotic fluid studies
	$Wright^b$	Mild	Expectant
	Zd	Moderate	Amniotic fluid studies

From American College of Obstetricians and Gynecologists: Management of isoimmunization in pregnancy. *Technical Bulletin* no. 148, Washington, DC, Oct 1990. Used by permission.

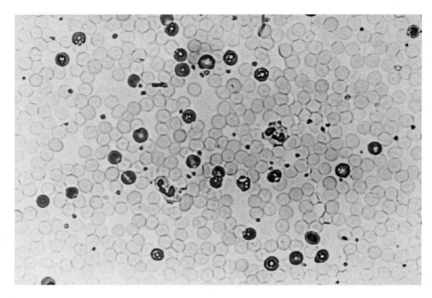

Fig. 18-1 Kleinhauer-Betke test. Peripheral blood smear from a pregnant woman following a placental abruption. The smear was prepared according to the Kleihauer-Betke method and Wright stained. The dark staining red blood cells are of fetal origin; the "ghosts" are maternal red blood cells.

used to identify fetal cells in the maternal circulation, with good results.[11] In general the volume of fetal blood found in the maternal circulation is less than 0.2 ml. In 65% of cases where transplacental hemorrhage can be documented, the volume of fetal red blood cells found in the maternal circulation is less than 0.1 ml. Fewer than 1% of women will have more than 5 ml of fetal red blood cells in their circulation; however, 2 to 3 women per 1,000 will have more than 30 ml.[12] A history of antepartum hemorrhage, preeclampsia, cesarean section, external version, and postpartum hemorrhage correlates with the volume of fetal red blood cells in the maternal circulation. Transplacental hemorrhage is known to occur following amniocentesis at any stage of pregnancy. With the use of ultrasound to localize the placenta prior to amniocentesis, this incidence is considered to be approximately 2% to 3%.[13] In addition, abortion in the first and second trimesters of pregnancy has been associated with detectable fetomaternal hemorrhage.

Relatively small amounts of Rh-positive red blood cells are needed to elicit the primary immune response. It has been shown in experiments using Rh-negative male volunteers that an infusion of 1 ml of Rh-positive red blood cells will result in the immunization of approximately 15% of volunteers, and 40 ml of Rh-positive red blood cells will immunize about one third of Rh-negative individuals; however, transfusions of as much as 250 mL of Rh-positive red blood cells will immunize only 65% to 70% of Rh-negative individuals.[14] In sharp contrast, the secondary immune response (the immune response seen *in vivo* with a second Rh-positive pregnancy in an alloimmunized individual) can be provoked with as little as 0.1 to 0.5 ml of Rh-positive fetal red blood cells. Although the Rh-negative mother carrying an Rh-positive fetus is at risk for immunization at any time during her pregnancy, the time of greatest risk is during the third stage of labor following separation of the placenta. Any fetal red blood cells in the endometrial cavity may find their way into the maternal circulation through the gaping maternal venous sinuses at the placental implantation site. If present in large enough numbers these fetal red blood cells will elicit a primary immune response, which generally takes up to 8 to 9 weeks to develop. However, that response may not be detectable with standard serologic methods for up to 6 months. Because this is a classic primary immune response, the initial antibody produced is an IgM. When the patient conceives again and carries an Rh-positive fetus, the anamnestic response elicited requires much less antigen. The small amount of fetal blood that normally finds its way into the maternal circulation early in pregnancy is capable of eliciting this response, and the antibody produced is an IgG capable of crossing the placenta. Once the antibodies find their way to the fetal compartment, the only cell surfaces containing Rh antigen to which

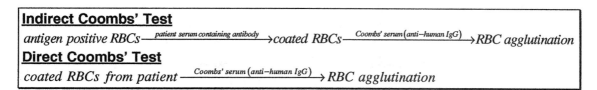

Indirect Coombs' Test

antigen positive RBCs —— *patient serum containing antibody* —→ *coated RBCs* —— *Coombs' serum (anti–human IgG)* —→ *RBC agglutination*

Direct Coombs' Test

coated RBCs from patient —— *Coombs' serum (anti–human IgG)* —→ *RBC agglutination*

Fig. 18-2 Coombs' tests.

Table 18-3 Approximate risk of Rh isoimmunization*

Rh isoimmunization	Risk (%)
Husband D negative, baby D negative	0
Husband D positive, homozygous ABO compatible	16
Husband D positive, homozygous ABO incompatible, ABO of baby unknown	7
Baby D positive, ABO incompatible	2
Husband D positive, heterozygous ABO compatible	8
Husband D positive, heterozygous ABO incompatible, ABO and Rh of baby unknown	3.5

*From Bowman JM, Friesen P: Rh isoimmunization, in Goodwin JW, Godden JO, Chance AW (eds): *Perinatal Medicine: The Basic Science Underlying Clinical Practice.* Baltimore, Williams & Wilkins, 1976, p 100. Used by permission.

these antibodies will adsorb are the fetal red blood cells.

Although all Rh-negative women delivering Rh-positive babies are at risk for Rh isoimmunization, only a fraction of these women will become alloimmunized[15] (Table 18-3). Several factors affect that risk, such as (1) the mother may be anergic to the rhesus antigen; (2) the volume of transplacental hemorrhage that occurs at delivery may be too small; and (3) there may be ABO incompatibility between the mother and the fetus. If the volume of transplacental hemorrhage is small enough, insufficient antigen will gain access to the maternal circulation to elicit the primary immune response. The risk of Rh immunization developing as the result of an ABO-compatible Rh-positive pregnancy is approximately 16% (Table 18-3). However, with an ABO-incompatible Rh-positive pregnancy, that risk decreases to approximately 2%. Fetomaternal hemorrhage of ABO-incompatible blood results in complement-mediated intravascular hemolysis of the fetal cells with sequestration of these cell fragments in the maternal liver. Compared with the spleen, there are far fewer potential antibody-forming immunocytes in the liver. As a result, for a given volume of fetal-to-maternal hemorrhage, the risk of alloimmunization is diminished. ABO compatibility issues are important when one is counseling a patient whose prophylactic RHIG was omitted.

The laboratory methodology for identifying the patient who is Rh alloimmunized is the indirect Coombs' test (Fig. 18-2). In that test, the pregnant woman's plasma is mixed with type 0, Rh-positive red blood cells. If the mother's plasma contains antibodies that recognize the Rh antigen, they will adsorb to these red blood cells. To this mixture is added Coombs' serum (goat anti-human IgG). If the red cells are coated with the anti-D there will be agglutination by Coombs' serum, which constitutes a positive indirect Coombs' test. The titer for the indirect Coombs' test is the reciprocal of the weakest dilution of maternal serum that will produce agglutination.

PREVENTION OF ALLOIMMUNIZATION

Since 1968 Rh immune globulin has been licensed for use in the prevention of maternal immunization to the D antigen. This prevention strategy is based on the knowledge that active immunization to an antigen may be prevented by the presence of passively acquired antibody to that antigen.[16] Nine studies published between 1968 and 1971 were reviewed in a meta-analysis by Bennebroek Gravenhorst, showing a typical odds ratio of 0.11 (95% confidence interval 0.08–0.15) for development of D immunization following postpartum RHIG administration.[17] Subsequent work has shown antepartum administration of RHIG also to be useful in the reduction of the incidence of alloimmunization. Currently recommended prophylaxis regimens are summarized in Table 18-4 for D-negative D^u-negative pregnant women. At delivery, cord blood should be obtained for fetal blood typing; RHIG is given within 72 hours to mothers of D or D^u positive newborns. If the newborn appears anemic or a risk for larger-than-normal fetomaternal hemorrhage is present, a Kleihauer-Betke or similar test should be done on the mother's blood to ensure that an adequate amount of RHIG is given. The standard 300-μg dose of RHIG will cover a hemorrhage of 15 cc packed fetal red cells (30 cc whole fetal blood). If for some reason postpartum RHIG administration is omitted, it should still be offered up to 14 days after delivery, because there are data that suggest some continuing benefit even with delayed administration.[18]

Postpartum administration of RHIG will not protect the small proportion of women who have a fetomaternal hemorrhage during pregnancy that is unanticipated. In 1979 a summarization of 11 studies reported that 262 of 30,155 women had become immunized during their first pregnancy (0.87%), most apparently from fetomaternal hemorrhage occurring after 28 weeks. Data suggest that routine antepartum administration of RHIG at 28 weeks may further reduce the remaining Rh immunization rate to 0.06%.[17] This is the current practice in the United States.[19]

PATHOGENESIS OF ERYTHROBLASTOSIS FETALIS

The severity of EBF can be classified as mild, moderate, and severe (Table 18-5). Three fourths of fetuses with EBF will have either mild or moderate disease and are not at risk for the development of fetal hydrops or stillbirth. Approximately 25% of fetuses with EBF will have the severe disease, and approximately half again of these fetuses are at risk for developing fetal hydrops before 34 weeks' gestation. The severity of the hemolytic disease experienced by the fetus is the result of several factors, including the amount of maternal IgG anti-D produced, the binding constant of this IgG, the efficiency of transport of this IgG across the placenta,[20,21] and, importantly, the ability of the fetus to respond by producing more fetal red blood cells without developing hepatocellular dysfunction and portal hypertension.

Erythropoiesis begins in the human embryo in the third to fourth week of gestation, and by the eighth to ninth week active erythropoiesis can be demonstrated in extramedullary sites, especially the liver and spleen. As the third trimester approaches, bone marrow becomes the predominant site of erythropoiesis, and by term, red cell production ceases in extramedullary sites. The primary pathologic defect in the Rh-positive fetus of the Rh-immunized mother is a shortened red cell half-life. As a result, extramedullary erythropoiesis continues to occur in the liver and spleen. If extramedullary hematopoiesis in the liver is sufficient in magnitude that it alters liver function and

Table 18-4 Rh immunoglobin prophylaxis*

Situation	Recommended dose
Threatened abortion	300 μg IM, repeat q 12 weeks†
Spontaneous abortion, <13 weeks	50 μg IM
Spontaneous abortion, >13 weeks	300 μg IM
Ectopic pregnancy, <13 weeks	50 μg IM
Ectopic pregnancy, >13 weeks	300 μg IM
Amniocentesis	300 μg IM
Percutaneous umbilical blood sampling	300 μg IM
Chorionic villus sampling	300 μg IM
External cephalic version	300 μg IM
Antepartum prophylaxis	300 μg IM
Delivery	Dependent on cord blood Rh type and Kleihauer-Betke test

*From American College of Obstetricians and Gynecologists: Prevention of D isoimmunization. *ACOG Technical Bulletin* no. 147. Washington, DC, 1990.
†Bowman JM: Hemolytic disease (erythroblastosis fetalis), in Creasy RK, Resnick R (eds): *Maternal-Fetal Medicine: Principles and Practice,* ed 3. Philadelphia, WB Saunders, 1993, p 736.

Table 18-5 Severity of erythroblastosis fetalis

	Mild	Moderate	Severe
Percent (%) of affected Fetuses/newborns	50	20–30	25
Degree of anemia	None to mild	Mild to moderate	Severe
Bilirubin metabolism	Indirect remains < 20 mg/dL (<16 mg/dL if premature)	Indirect exceeds neonatal Binding and metabolic capacities	Same as moderate
Evidence of hydrops	None	None	Ascites, pleural effusion, pericardial effusion, and/or scalp edema

liver macroarchitecture,[22] then the following pathologic entities arise: (1) fetal liver production of albumin (or alpha-fetoprotein in early pregnancy) decreases, resulting in decreased intravascular oncotic pressure, (2) destruction of the macroarchitecture results in portal and umbilical venous hypertension, and (3) the combination of portal and umbilical hypertension and decreased intravascular oncotic pressure results in the ascites and anasarca characteristic of the hydropic fetus. Moise et al have provided support for this theory of development of hydrops.[23]

Others have argued that anemia leading to congestive heart failure and increased venous pressure may be an important event in the ultimate development of fetal hydrops.[24] It has also been demonstrated recently that cardiac output index is increased in alloimmunized fetuses, the result of increased stroke volume.[25] This difference could not be explained on the basis of greater heart rate, larger valve diameters, or small fetuses. In addition, the fetal hematocrit did not appear to correlate with the calculated cardiac output indices. Copel et al suggested that though there is no significant relationship between hematocrit values and cardiac output, extremely compromised fetuses may demonstrate diminished cardiac function as a terminal finding. At this time, few feel that cardiac failure initiates hydrops, but it may well be a late event in the evolution of hydrops fetalis. The hepatic damage theory of pathogenesis of hydrops is probably the most reasonable explanation; it explains the poor relationship between the degree of anemia found in many fetuses and the degree of hydrops.

Those fetuses only mildly affected require no intervention, have minimal or no anemia at birth, and do not experience significant hyperbilirubinemia in the neonatal period (indirect bilirubin < 20 mg/dL for term infants, 15–18 mg/dL for preterm infants). Moderate disease does not require obstetric intervention. This is because unconjugated bilirubin produced in utero is removed from the fetus by the placenta. But if moderate disease is untreated in the neonatal period, icterus gravis, kernicterus, and frequently death will occur. After birth the bilirubin concentration exceeds the neonate's albumin-binding capacity. The newborn's ability to conjugate and excrete bilirubin is inadequate both from the hepatic dysfunction from EBF and the normal delay of glucuronyl transferase activity appearance. In addition, mild to moderate anemia will be present. Exchange transfusion is performed in the early neonatal period to correct these problems. Approximately 85% of the fetal red cells will be removed, along with about 50% of the unconjugated bilirubin, when a double-volume (160 mL/kg body weight) exchange transfusion technique is used.[26]

MONITORING AND MANAGEMENT OF THE Rh-ALLOIMMUNIZED PREGNANCY

Obstetricians caring for patients immunized for the Rh antigen or other antigens (Table 18-2) must be able to predict the severity of EBF in these fetuses. In the absence of an ability to modify prenatal care, fully 25% of these pregnancies will result in hydropic or stillborn fetuses. In years past, great emphasis was placed on the Rh-alloimmunized patient's obstetric history. Patterns could be identified that predicted to a limited degree the risk of severe EBF in the index pregnancy. At the present time, in the United States we depend less on the woman's history; most of our patients have low parity (this fact also contributes to the decreased incidence of hemolytic disease of the newborn [HDN]). In addition, it is known that a woman carrying her first pregnancy following immunization has a risk of 8% to 10% of delivering a hydropic fetus, which could not be predicted by her history.

At the first prenatal visit, all patients are screened with blood type, Rh-antigen type, and an indirect Coombs' test to detect antibodies directed against red blood cell antigens. In those who are Rh-negative and not alloimmunized, the indirect Coombs' test is repeated at 28 weeks and RHIG is given to prevent immunization in the third trimester. At delivery, RHIG is administered again if the newborn is Rh-positive.

If the patient is found to be alloimmunized to a red cell antigen, she is followed closely with serial indirect Coombs' titers until that titer reaches a critical level. At our institution, that titer is 1:16 for anti-D antibodies; no cases of hydrops fetalis or stillbirths have been identified at or below this level. For antibodies directed against red blood cell antigens other than anti-D that are known to cause EBF, we establish that the antibody is of the IgG subclass, since IgM antibodies do not cross the placenta and thus cannot cause EBF. Consideration is also given to paternity; history may reveal that the father of this pregnancy has had Rh-negative children, suggesting him to be heterozygous, or even that he is Rh-negative if he is a new partner for the patient.

Once a critical titer is reached, we then follow the patient with serial amniocentesis and ultrasound. Currently, a method for determining fetal RhD status is under investigation. This technique uses the polymerase chain reaction to amplify the Rh locus on chromosome 1, such that the presence or absence of the RhD gene can be ascertained.[4] Use of this technology may in the future allow selection of only Rh-positive fetuses for further evaluation and intervention. However, until validation and wider availability of this technique is achieved, the Liley method of amniotic fluid evaluation will remain the standard for assessment of disease severity in all pregnancies with elevated anti-D titers.

Once a patient has passed critical anti-D titer, antenatal corticosteroids are given to enhance fetal pulmonary maturation if 24 weeks' gestation has been achieved, in anticipation of potential preterm delivery. We give 12 mg betamethasone IM initially, followed by repeat dose in 24 hours.

The amniotic fluid is assayed in a semiquantitative fashion for bilirubin; using a spectrophotometer the change in optical density at 450 nm (ΔOD_{450}) is measured.[27] It has been known for over 30 years that bilirubin, a normal constituent of amniotic fluid, is found in elevated concentrations in amniotic fluid in pregnancies complicated by EBF. In 1961, Liley described the spectrophotometric measurement of bilirubin in amniotic fluid (the ΔOD_{450}).[28] His method of measuring bilirubin in amniotic fluid and of interpreting the result continues to be used worldwide by most centers today. While it is challenging to perform the chloroform extraction method he devised, it is reliable and predictive relative to other possible techniques.[29] In normal pregnancies, the concentration of bilirubin in amniotic fluid decreases from the 23rd week of gestation until term.

Based on a retrospective analysis of over 100 Rh-alloimmunized pregnancies, Liley was able to divide his spectrophotometric graph into three zones. Subsequent modifications have been made to extend its use for pregnancies below 27 weeks' gestation[5] (Fig. 18-3). Readings in zone I indicated mild or no hemolytic disease; in this group of fetuses approximately 10% required exchange transfusions in the neonatal period. Readings in zone II indicate variable disease, the severity of which increased as the ΔOD_{450} rose. Readings in zone III identified fetuses with severe hemolytic disease in whom hydrops and fetal death would likely occur within 7 to 10 days. Single ΔOD_{450} readings in the

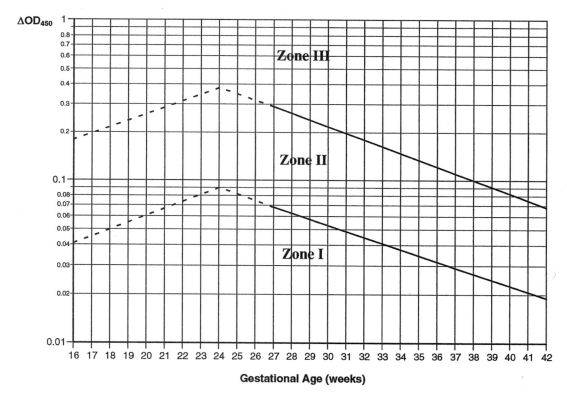

Fig. 18-3 Modified Liley graph. The solid lines represent boundaries from Liley's original data; the dotted lines represent extrapolated boundaries. (Modified from American College of Obstetricians and Gynecologists: Management of isoimmunization in pregnancy. Technical Bulletin no. 148, Washington DC, Oct 1990; and Bowman JM: Hemolytic disease (erythroblastosis fetalis), in Creasy RK, Resnick R (eds): *Maternal-Fetal Medicine: Principles and Practice,* ed 3. Philadelphia, WB Saunders, 1993, p 724.)

second trimester of pregnancy are poor predictors of ultimate perinatal outcome. For that reason, multiple amniocenteses for measurement of ΔOD_{450} are performed throughout pregnancy. It is our experience and the experience of others that observing the slope of the line connecting each reading gives a reasonably accurate prediction of the severity of Rh disease. A rising slope to the line is associated with increased risk of hydrops. In general, amniotic fluid examinations are repeated at intervals of 7 to 28 days, depending on the ΔOD_{450} reading. A ΔOD_{450} in zone I will result in repeat amniocentesis in 4 weeks. A reading in the lower half of zone II will be followed with a repeat amniocentesis in 2 weeks unless this represents an unfavorable trend. Readings in the upper half of zone II will be repeated in 1 week and values in zone III will result in either intrauterine transfusion (see below) or premature delivery, depending on gestational age and the state of fetal lung maturation.

If a rise into Liley zone III or upper zone II occurs, or if hydrops is diagnosed, fetal transfusions are performed. Current estimates of procedure-related fetal loss rates with fetal transfusion are 0.8% for intravascular and 3.5% for intraperitoneal.[5] These risks combined with our neonatal survival rates lead us to deliver rather than transfuse after 34 weeks. However, many factors are weighed in deciding whether to deliver the fetus prematurely or perform a fetal transfusion. These include estimated fetal weight, assessment of fetal lung maturity, results of fetal biophysical testing, technical ease of transfusion, and fetal response. A number of protocols have been developed, incorporating serology, amniocentesis, percutaneous umbilical blood sampling, and intrauterine transfusion to obtain the lowest perinatal morbidity and mortality while avoiding needless invasive procedures or intervention.[30,31] Incorporation of RhD typing by PCR will likely soon occur.

Intrauterine fetal transfusion

A major advance in the treatment of severe EBF was Liley's introduction in 1963 of intrauterine intraperitoneal transfusion.[32] In the last decade, numerous reports of intravascular transfusion of these fetuses have been published.[33,34] In a recent excellent review of Rh isoimmunization, Bowman has described in detail his methods and experiences of performing both fetal intraperitoneal and intravascular transfusions.[5]

Type-specific or O-negative blood with hematocrits of 85% to 90% is used for transfusion. If time allows, cells may be irradiated; potentially this may reduce the risk of graft versus host disease mediated by the few intermixed lymphocytes.

Intraperitoneal fetal transfusion. Intraperitoneal fetal transfusion (IPT) depends on the ability of fetal subdiaphragmatic lymphatics to effect uptake into the fetal circulation of intact red blood cells placed in the fetal peritoneal cavity. As originally described by Liley, proper placement of the infusion needle for fetal IPT was assessed by x-ray examination and fluoroscopy.[32] Subsequently, Hobbins and co-workers[35] described a technique using real-time ultrasound to guide placement of the transfusion needle and monitor the fetus during IPT. Several investigators have since modified Hobbins' approach and described their experience using real-time ultrasound for fetal IPT.[36]

With ultrasound guidance, an 18- to 16-gauge spinal needle is introduced into the fetal peritoneal cavity; the position of the needle tip within the peritoneal cavity is confirmed, and infusion of red cells is begun. The volume infused is calculated according to the following formula:

$$\text{Volume (cc)} = (\text{Weeks' Gestation} - 20) \times 10$$

This quantity of transfusion should not lead to significantly elevated intraperitoneal pressure, which could compress the intraabdominal portion of the umbilical vein and cause fetal distress.[5] The fetal heart rate is monitored throughout the transfusion by ultrasound. Red blood cells injected into the peritoneal cavity are absorbed intact into the fetal circulation via subdiaphragmatic lymphatics. In the absence of fetal hydrops, about 10% to 15% of the injected blood cells will be absorbed every 24 hours after the transfusion. If a repeat transfusion is to be performed, the second IPT generally occurs 7 to 10 days following the first transfusion. Subsequent transfusions occur at about 4-week intervals, since the amount of fetal cells available to be hemolyzed has been drastically reduced. Finally, the fetus is delivered usually between 33 and 35 weeks' gestation.

Direct intravascular transfusion. Direct transfusion of blood into the fetal circulation using fetoscopic control of insertion of a needle was introduced by Rodeck and co-workers in 1981.[33] Subsequently, many investigators have reported their experience with direct infusion of blood into the fetal umbilical vein under real-time ultrasound control. Although technically more difficult to perform, direct intravascular transfusion (IVT) offers several advantages over IPT: (1) fetal blood type and hematocrit are obtained, thus avoiding unnecessary transfusions; (2) posttransfusion hematocrits document adequate transfusion volumes; and (3) direct injection of blood into the intravascular compartment avoids the vagaries of blood absorption from the peritoneal cavity.[37] Furthermore, recent series suggest a lower fetal loss rate for IVT compared to IPT (0.8% vs. 3.5%).[5,38]

Again, the procedure is performed under local anesthesia supplemented by intravenous sedation, allowing for maternal comfort and decreased fetal activity. If the fetus is active or if fetal limbs obstruct the site of insertion of the umbilical cord into the placenta or the umbilicus, we have paralyzed the fetus with curare (3 mg/kg estimated fetal weight) or pancuronium (0.3 mg/kg estimated fetal weight) by intramuscular injection into the upper outer aspect of the fetal thigh in a sterile fashion under ultrasound guidance 30 minutes before the transfusion[39] (see below). We do not routinely administer antimicrobials or tocolytics. Under sterile conditions, the obstetrician introduces a 22-gauge spinal needle, keeping the tip in continuous view with a real-time ultrasound transducer held in the other hand. The needle is inserted into the umbilical cord either adjacent to its insertion at the placenta or at the umbilical ring. Blood is aspirated and confirmed to be fetal, based on red blood cell indices (mean corpuscular volume > 100 fL); an initial hematocrit is checked. Blood as described above is transfused at a rate of ~10 ml/min. It is important to see the turbulent flow of blood within the fetal vessel. Inadvertent injection of blood into Wharton's jelly in the cord could result in vascular occlusion. The volume of blood to be infused at the time of transfusion is computed from the following formula (EFW, estimated fetal weight; Hct, hematocrit):

$$\text{Volume (cc)} = \frac{110 \, (EFW \text{ in kg}) \, (Hct_{desired} - Hct_{initial})}{Hct_{unit}}$$

The total volumes vary from 10 to 40 mL of packed red blood cells; recent data suggest that final hematocrits should be limited to 50% to 55%,[40] and that umbilical pressure increases should be avoided.[41] The fetal heart rate is monitored by real-time ultrasound throughout the procedure. Further transfusions are carried out when it is calculated that the donor hemoglobin concentration will fall into the 8–9 g/dL range, which in general is 12 to 20 days. Some investigators have introduced the needle tip for IVT under ultrasound control into the hepatic portion of the fetal umbilical vein. Others have inserted the needle tip into the umbilical vein adjacent to its insertion into the placenta.[39]

Anesthetic management

The anesthetic care of the mother and her fetus compromised by EBF follows basic principles. Maintenance of uterine blood flow, transplacental gas exchange, and a relatively normal acid base state would seem to be even more important than in the nonaffected infant. Fetal complications may include anemia, prematurity, signs of fetal distress, and acidosis.[42] If labor ensues and vaginal delivery is planned, the fetus should be stressed as little as possible and fetal oxygenation should be maintained.[43] Segmental lumbar epidural analgesia approaches the ideal anesthetic technique. The block may be extended to include the perineum for delivery. Lumbar epidural anesthesia is also very useful for cesarean section, if generous fluid loading and left uterine displacement are employed to prevent maternal hypotension, a possible cause of fetal compromise. Prompt treatment with vasopressor may be necessary in the presence of a drop in baseline maternal pressure. A routine fetal heart rate monitoring is important during the induction of epidural anesthesia. General anesthesia may be administered with good results if the mother refuses epidural anesthesia or there is a contraindication[43]; it may be necessary in the presence of severe fetal distress. Because of the reduced number of drugs given when employing epidural anesthesia, it seems preferable; in addition, possible complications such as hypoxemia, aspiration, and hypertension, which can occur with general anesthesia, are avoided. Since there is a high incidence of hypotension from spinal anesthesia for cesarean section (especially for elective section), spinal would seem a less desirable choice than epidural or general anesthesia.[44] We deliver many of our patients with EBF by cesarean section, and we commonly use lumbar epidural anesthesia. The amide compounds are said to cause less maternal hypotension, but they result in higher fetal blood levels. 2-Chloroprocaine undergoes rapid maternal metabolism, with subsequent low fetal levels.[42]

Anesthesia personnel can be of great help when intrauterine transfusion or percutaneous umbilical blood sampling is performed. This is often done in the operating room, with maternal intravenous sedation (monitored anesthesia care). Maternal vital signs such as blood pressure, heart rate, respiratory rate, and oxygen saturation are regularly recorded. Frequent reassurance is given. The mother remains awake but is lightly sedated with narcotic drugs. Local anesthesia is given by the obstetrician for the abdominal puncture. Meperidine and diazepam have most frequently been used for sedation, but we have also employed fentanyl. Even though diazepam and fentanyl do not have FDA approval for obstetrics, the frequency of their use makes this indication acceptable. We have not used midazolam, although others have.[42] Since the gestation period is past the time of organogenesis, there should be little concern about developmental anomalies.[43] These medications relieve maternal anxiety and reduce fetal movement.

A very important aspect of fetal intervention that is necessary for these procedures is reduction in fetal movement, a problem that can compound the obstetrician's attempts at performing definitive procedures (guided by a sense of touch and a constantly changing image on the ultrasound screen) deep within the mother's abdomen. Tranquilizers given to the mother may not provide adequate fetal relaxation. Since muscle relaxants do not readily cross the placenta (as do narcotics and tranquilizers), the relaxant must be injected directly into the fetus if it is to have an effect. Curare was used earlier to decrease fetal movement.[45] Seeds et al used 0.5 mg pancuronium intramuscularly with good results.[46] Bernstein et al performed 12 intrauterine transfusions using atracurium 0.2 to 0.4 mg/kg intravenously through the umbilical vein. The higher dose produced better results. All fetuses were immobilized for the duration of the procedure, and fetal activity returned 20 to 130 minutes later.[47] Vecuronium was used by Daffos et al. For karyotyping and magnetic resonance imaging in an infant of 32 weeks' gestation.[48] The drug was given through the umbilical vein at a dose of 0.1 mg/kg (0.2 mg for an estimated fetal weight of 2 kg.) Fetal movement disappeared within a few seconds and resumed 2 hours later. Leveque and colleagues have also studied vecuronium in alloimmunized pregnancies.[49] In theory, vecuronium would appear to be the least desirable relaxant for immobilizing the fetus since it is metabolized by the liver, an organ likely to be compromised in EBF. Other relaxants are hydrolyzed (atracurium) or excreted by the kidney and the liver (curare, pancuronium). Recently, Weiner and Anderson assessed the effect of pancuronium on umbilical artery wave-form indices.[50] Though the authors described a significant decline in systolic/end diastolic ratio, resistance index, and pulsatility index as a consequence of percutaneous blood sampling and intravascular transfusion, fetal paralysis did not alter the magnitude of the decline in the indices. Moise et al administered pancuronium to fetuses by funipuncture, and developed a formula involving the hematocrit to adjust the dose.[51]

CONCLUSION

The incidence of severe fetal hydrops has decreased significantly as a result of recent advances in obstetric management. However, peripartum and intrapartum management of these severely compromised infants will always remain a major challenge to the perinatologist and the anesthesiologist.

REFERENCES

1. Chavez GF, Mulinare J, Edmonds LD: Epidemiology of Rh hemolytic disease of the newborn in the United States. *JAMA* 1991; 265(24):3270.
2. Landsteiner K, Wiener AS: Agglutenable factor in human blood recognized by immune sera for rhesus blood. *Proc Soc Exp Biol Med* 1940; 43:223.
3. Race RR, Sanger R: *Blood Groups in Man,* ed 6. Oxford, Blackwell Scientific, 1975.
4. Bennett PR, Le Van Kim C, Colin Y, et al: Prenatal determination of fetal RhD type by DNA amplification. *N Engl J Med* 1993; 329(9):607.
5. Bowman JM: Hemolytic disease (erythroblastosis fetalis), in Creasy RK, Resnick R (eds): *Maternal-Fetal Medicine: Principals and Practice,* ed 3. Philadelphia, WB Saunders, 1993, p 713.
6. Bowman JM: Maternal alloimmunization and fetal hemolytic disease, in Reece EA: *Medicine of the Fetus & Mother,* p. 1154.
7. Levine P, Stetson ER: Unusual cases of intra-group agglutination. *JAMA* 1939; 113:126.
8. Wiener AS: Diagnosis and treatment of anemia of the newborn caused by occult placental hemorrhage. *Am J Obstet Gynecol* 1948; 56:717.
9. Chown B: Anemia from bleeding of the fetus into the maternal circulation. *Lancet* 1954; 1:1213.
10. Kleihauer E, Braun H, Betke K: Demonstration von fetalem Hamoglobin in den Erythrocyten eines Blutausstrichs. *Klin Wochenschr* 1957; 35:37.
11. Bayliss KM, Kueck BD, Johnson ST, et al: Detecting fetomaternal hemorrhage: A comparison of five methods. *Transfusion* 1991; 31(4):303.
12. Bowman JM, Pollock JM, Penston LE: Fetomaternal transplacental hemorrhage during pregnancy and after delivery. *Vox Sang* 1986; 51:117.
13. Bowman JM, Pollock JM: Transplacental fetal hemorrhage after amniocentesis. *Obstet Gynecol* 1985; 66:749.
14. Bowman JM: Hemolytic disease (erythroblastosis fetalis), in Creasy RK, Resnick R (eds): *Maternal-Fetal Medicine: Principles and Practice,* ed 2. Philadelphia, WB Saunders, 1989, p 613.
15. Bowman JM, Friesen P: Rh isoimmunization, in Goodwin JW, Godden JO, Chance AW (eds): *Perinatal Medicine: The Basic Science Underlying Clinical Practice.* Baltimore, Williams & Wilkins, 1976, p 92.
16. Bowman JM: Hemolytic disease (erythroblastosis fetalis), in Creasy RK, Resnick R (eds): *Maternal-Fetal Medicine: Principles and Practice,* ed 3. Philadelphia, WB Saunders, 1993, p 734.
17. Bennebroek Gravenhorst J: Rhesus isoimmunization, in Chalmers I, Enkin M, Keirse MJNC (eds): *Effective Care In Pregnancy and Childbirth,* vol I. New York, Oxford University Press, 1989, p 566-567.
18. Samson D, Mollison PL: Effect on primary Rh-immunization of delayed administration of anti-Rh. *Immunology* 1975; 28:349.
19. American College of Obstetricians and Gynecologists: Management of isoimmunization in pregnancy. *Technical Bulletin* no. 147, Washington, DC, Oct 1990.
20. Economides DL, Bowell PJ, Seligner M, et al: Anti-D concentrations in fetal and maternal serum and amniotic fluid in rhesus allo-immunised pregnancies. *Br J Obstet Gynaecol* 1993; 100(10):923.
21. Dooren MC, Engelfriet CP: Protection against Rh D-haemolytic disease of the newborn by a diminished transport of maternal IgG to the fetus. *Vox Sang* 1993; 65(1):59.
22. Nicolini U, Nicolaidis P, Tannirandorn Y, et al: Fetal liver

dysfunction in Rh alloimmunization. *Br J Obstet Gynaecol* 1991; 98(3):287.

23. Moise KJ, Carpenter RJ, Hesketh DE: Do abnormal Starling forces cause fetal hydrops in red blood cell alloimmunization? *Am J Obstet Gynecol* 1992; 167(4):907.

24. Phibbs RH, Johnson P, Tooley WH: Cardiorespiratory status of erythroblastotic newborn infants. II. Blood volume, hematocrit and serum albumin concentration in relation to hydrops fetalis. *Pediatrics* 1974; 53:13.

25. Copel JA, Grannum PA, Green JJ, et al: Fetal cardiac output in the isoimmunized pregnancy: A pulsed Doppler echocardiographic study of patients undergoing intravascular intrauterine transfusion. *Am J Obstet Gynecol* 1989; 161:361.

26. Gartner LM, Lee K-S: Jaundice and liver disease (unconjugated hyperbilirubinemia), in Fanaroff AA, Martin RJ (eds): *Neonatal-Perinatal Medicine: Diseases of the Fetus and Infant,* ed 5. St. Louis, Mosby, 1992, p 1093.

27. Albright GA, Ferguson JE, Joyce TH, et al: *Anesthesia in Obstetrics: Maternal, Fetal, and Neonatal Aspects,* ed 2. Boston, Butterworths, 1986, p 540.

28. Liley AW: Liquor amnii analyses in the management of the pregnancy complicated by Rhesus sensitization. *Am J Obstet Gynecol* 1961; 82:1359.

29. Spinnato JA, Ralston KK, Greenwell ER, et al: Amniotic fluid bilirubin and fetal hemolytic disease. *Am J Obstet Gynecol* 1991; 165(4):1030.

30. American College of Obstetricians and Gynecologists: Management of isoimmunization in pregnancy. *Technical Bulletin* no. 148, Washington, DC, Oct 1990.

31. Copel JA, Grannum PA, Green JJ, et al: Fetal cardiac output in the isoimmunized pregnancy: A pulsed Dopplerechocardiographic study of patients undergoing intravascular intrauterine transfusion. *Am J Obstet Gynecol* 1989; 161:361.

32. Liley AW: Intrauterine transfusion of foetus in haemolytic disease. *Br Med J* 1963; 2:1107.

33. Rodeck CH, Holman CA, Karnicki J, et al: Direct intravascular fetal blood transfusion by fetoscopy in severe Rhesus isoimmunization. *Lancet* 1981; 1:625.

34. Berkowitz RL, Chitkara U, Wilkins IA, et al: Intravascular monitoring and management of erythroblastosis fetalis. *Am J Obstet Gynecol* 1988; 158:783.

35. Hobbins JC, Davis CD, Webster J: A new technique utilizing ultrasound to aid in intrauterine transfusion. *J Clin Ultrasound* 1976; 4:135.

36. Larkin RM, Knochel JQ, Lill TG: Intrauterine transfusions: New techniques and results. *Clin Obstet Gynecol* 1982; 25:303.

37. Berkowitz RL, Chitkara U, Goldberg JD, et al: Intrauterine intravascular transfusions for severe red blood cell isoimmunization: Ultrasound-guided percutaneous approach. *Am J Obstet Gynecol* 1986; 155:574.

38. Weiner CP, Wenstrom KD, Sipes SL, et al: Risk factors for cordocentesis and fetal intravascular transfusion. *Am J Obstet Gynecol* 1991; 165:1020.

39. Berkowitz RL, Chitkara U, Wilkins LA, et al: Technical aspects of intravascular transfusions. *Am J Obstet Gynecol* 1987; 157:4.

40. Welch R, Rampling MW, Anwar A, et al: Changes in hemorheology with fetal intravascular transfusion. *Am J Obstet Gynecol* 1994; 170(3):726.

41. Hallak M, Moise KJ, Hesketh DE, et al: Intravascular transfusion of fetuses with rhesus incompatibility: Prediction of fetal outcome by changes in umbilical venous pressure. *Obstet Gynecol* 1992; 80(2):286.

42. James FM, Wheeler AS, Dewan DM: *Obstetric Anesthesia: The Complicated Patient,* ed 2. Philadelphia, FA Davis, 1988; p 301.

43. Shnider S, Levinson G: *Anesthesia for Obstetrics,* ed 2. Baltimore, Williams & Wilkins, 1987; p 446.

44. Clark RB, Thompson DS, Thompson C: Prevention of spinal hypotension associated with cesarean section. *Anesthesiology* 1976; 45:670.

45. de Crespigny L, Robinson HP, Quinn M, et al: Ultrasound-guided fetal blood transfusion for severe Rhesus isoimmunization. *Obstet Gynecol* 1985; 66:529.

46. Seeds JW, Corke BC, Spielman FJ: Prevention of fetal movement during invasive procedures with pancuronium bromide. *Am J Obstet Gynecol* 1986; 155:818.

47. Bernstein HH: Use of atracurium besylate to arrest fetal activity during intrauterine intravascular transfusions. *Obstet Gynecol* 1988; 72:813.

48. Daffos F, Forestier F, MacAleese J, et al: Fetal curarization for prenatal magnetic resonance imaging. *Prenat Diagn* 1988; 8:311.

49. Leveque C, Murat I, Toubas F, et al: Fetal neuromuscular blockade with vecuronium bromide: Studies during intravascular intrauterine transfusion in isoimmunized pregnancies. *Anesthesiology* 1992; 76:642.

50. Weiner CP, Anderson TL: The acute effect of cordocentesis with or without fetal curarization and of intravascular transfusion upon umbilical artery waveform indices. *Obstet Gynecol* 1989; 73:219.

51. Moise KJ, Deter RL, Kirshon B, et al: Intravenous pancuronium bromide for fetal neuromuscular blockade during intrauterine transfusion for red-cell alloimmunization. *Obstet Gynecol* 1989; 74:905.

19 Autoimmune Disease

Martha A. Hauch and Bruce B. Feinberg

It has been long thought that autoimmune reactions are harmful to the host. However, it is now well recognized that autoimmunity is essential to normal ongoing immune surveillance. Autoimmune disease occurs when the regulation of this normal surveillance system is disturbed. Clinically, these diseases are typically chronic, multisystemic inflammatory diseases, whose courses range from benign to fatal. Generally, no cures are available, but medical therapies are useful in ameliorating clinical symptoms.

Interestingly, women are more susceptible than men to autoimmune diseases, particularly in their reproductive years. For this reason an understanding of these disease processes during pregnancy is essential to ensure satisfactory maternal and neonatal outcomes.

When evaluating a patient with a collagen vascular disease it is important to consider the natural history of the disease process, the impact of pregnancy on the disease, and the impact of the disease on the pregnancy. Patients with autoimmune diseases who are considering pregnancy should be counseled about the risks and potential outcomes to themselves and their fetuses. Should pregnancy be undertaken, optimal care involves a team approach, using the skills of a rheumatologist, obstetrician, anesthesiologist, and neonatologist to provide the best perinatal outcome. This chapter discusses the medical, obstetric, and anesthetic considerations of the various autoimmune disorders seen in pregnancy.

RHEUMATOID ARTHRITIS

Rheumatoid arthritis (RA) is an autoimmune, chronic inflammatory disorder, systemic in nature, though usually characterized by synovial joint inflammation. It is the most common systemic rheumatic disease. It affects females three times more often than males and has a peak onset in the fourth decade of life. Rheumatoid arthritis is thought to complicate 1 in 1000 to 2000 pregnancies.[1]

Etiology

The precise etiology of RA remains unknown. First-degree relatives as well as identical twins of patients with RA have a high concordance for the disease, suggesting an immunogenetic predisposition. Virtually all patients who develop RA carry a "susceptibility" epitope associated with the third hypervariable region of the HLA-DR β chain, although many normal patients carry this epitope as well.[2] Interestingly, some HLA-DR genotypes seem to protect against the development of RA.[3]

Evidence suggests that RA may result from prior Epstein-Barr virus (EBV) infection. Antibodies against EBV glycoprotein gp110 cross react with the susceptibility epitope on DR β chains. Therefore, EBV gp110 may trigger an autoimmune response by molecular mimicry in susceptible patients.[4]

Some RA patients demonstrate antibodies to heat shock proteins purified from *Mycobacterium tuberculosis* and *Escherichia coli*. These heat shock proteins are also expressed on synovial cells in response to infection and may lead to T cell proliferation and local inflammation.[5]

Macrophage cytokines are abundantly expressed in cell cultures of rheumatoid synovitis.[6] GM-CSF may initiate RA in susceptible patients because it induces MHC expression on Ag-presenting cells.[7]

Pathophysiology

The disease is characterized by selective, usually symmetrical inflammation of the synovial joints. Rheumatoid factors, a family of immunoglobulins with antibody specificity for the Fc region of human IgG, is present in 90% of patients with classic RA, although it may be seen in other connective tissue disorders and nonrheumatic diseases. The predominant rheumatoid factor is IgM, while IgG and IgA are less commonly detected. The interaction of rheumatoid factors with normal IgG leads to the formation of immune complexes that activate the complement system. The subsequent production of anaphylatoxins and chemoattractants initiates a series of nonspecific immune responses, which ultimately leads to local tissue destruction.

Clinical manifestations

Many RA patients report an insidious onset of the disease. Thirty five percent of seropositive individuals present with constitutional symptoms 1 to 9 months before joint symptoms.[8] The most commonly affected joints are metacarpophalangeal joints, the proximal interphalangeal joints, and the wrists. Inflammation of the distal interphalangeal joint is distinctly unusual. Other peripheral joints including the elbows, shoulders, knees, ankles, and feet are involved to varying degrees. Thoracic, lumbar, and sacral vertebral joints are rarely affected. Lumbar tenderness is reported in 15% of patients, but limitation of motion is not generally observed. Cervical spine disease, however, is reported in 45% of seropositive patients and 37% of seronegative patients; it may have neurologic consequences as a result of atlantoaxial subluxation and separation at the atlantoodontoid articulation.

Extraarticular manifestations of RA occur in those patients with the highest titers of rheumatoid factors. Rheumatoid nodules are the common extraarticular manifestation, occurring in 20% of patients. They occur primarily in pressure-sensitive areas such as the elbows. Systemic granulomas may be found in the lungs. These pulmonary lesions occasionally cavitate and erode into the pleural space, resulting in pneumothorax or bronchopleural fistulas. Granulomas may also be found in the myocardium, coronary arteries, valves, and the aortic root. The most life-threatening manifestation of rheumatoid arthritis is a coronary vasculitis characterized by thrombosis of small nutrient arteries. Peripheral neuropathies are common in Felty's syndrome (rheumatoid arthritis, lymphadenopathy, and keratoconjunctivitis sicca).

Diagnosis

As noted above, the onset and course of rheumatoid arthritis is highly variable and often insidious. Since there is no specific serologic marker for rheumatoid arthritis, the diagnosis of RA may be quite difficult. The American Rheumatism Association 1987 revised diagnostic criteria for rheumatoid arthritis reportedly has a 90 sensitivity and specificity for the diagnosis. Overlap of symptoms and findings with other related disorders such as systemic lupus erythematosus may require alterations in diagnosis and treatments.

Treatment

Treatment is directed towards pain relief, reduction of inflammation, and preservation of function. Physical therapy and aspirin or nonsteroidal antiinflammatory agents are the mainstays of initial therapy. If the disease persists beyond 6 weeks and symptoms are not subsiding with this therapeutic regimen, second-line agents should be administered to prevent irreversible progression of cartilage damage and joint destruction. These include antimalarials, sulfasalizine, gold salts, penicillamine, levamisole, glucocorticoids, methotrexate, and cytotoxic agents such as cyclophosphamide and azathioprine (see below). Additional treatments such as plasma- or lymphoplasmapheresis are costly and not of proven benefit. Occasionally, corrective orthopedic surgical intervention is required.

Effect of pregnancy on rheumatoid arthritis

There is no well-documented impairment of fertility in patients with rheumatoid arthritis and no evidence to support the therapeutic termination of pregnancy. In fact, most studies report that pregnancy induces clinical remission of rheumatoid arthritis. Hench first reported that rheumatoid arthritis improved in 24 of 30 pregnancies.[9] More recently, Persellin similarly identified remission of symptoms in 74% of RA patients in the first trimester, 20% in the second trimester, and 5% in the third trimester.[10] This amelioration of RA, including extraarticular manifestations, was further confirmed by Klipple and Cecere, who reported that 70% of RA patients in pregnancy experienced considerable improvement.[11]

The basis for clinical remission of symptoms in pregnancy is unclear. Hench proposed that increased levels of cortisol were responsible, though follow-up studies by others demonstrated that increased cortisol did not account for all cases of symptomatic improvement.[12] Although epidemiologic and immunologic evidence suggested female sex hormones such as estrogen in mitigating the course of RA, Bijlsma demonstrated that estrogens were not able to alleviate the symptoms of RA.[13] Furthermore, Jara-Quezada found no difference in serum estradiol levels between RA patients and normal controls.[14] In a study by Unger, two thirds of patients had clinical improvement of their disease during pregnancy. These patients had elevated levels of pregnancy-associated α_2 glycoprotein, thereby implicating this protein in the remission of RA in pregnancy.[15] Recently, Nelson demonstrated that amelioration of RA during pregnancy is associated with a disparity in HLA class II antigens between mother and fetus, suggesting that the maternal immune response to paternal HLA antigens may have a role in the pregnancy-induced remission of rheumatoid arthritis.[16] Not all patients have symptomatic improvement during pregnancy. Neely noted that up to 38% of patients have either no change in status or a worsening of their disease.[17] Occasionally, the disease may first present during pregnancy. If a specific pregnancy has not produced amelioration of the disease process, it is unlikely that a subsequent pregnancy will do so.

Despite the clear clinical improvement seen during pregnancy, unfortunately many of these patients exhibit an exacerbation of their disease process in the postpartum period. Most reports[10,11] found that 90% of patients experienced a postpartum exacerbation of their disease, usually within 6 to 8 months postpartum. The mechanism theory for these postpartum relapses is speculative. Thompson noted that increased postpartum levels of agalactosyl IgG coincide with a burst in Il-6 activity, postulating that changes in IgG glycoforms may be related to postpartum exacerbations of RA.[18] Nelson also demonstrated a rapid postpartum rise in IgG glycosylation, associated with symptomatic relapses. Alternatively, Silver postulated an immunosensitization theory whereby exposure to the fetus's paternal HLA peri-delivery might represent a risk factor for disease causation.[19] Quinn observed that increased disease activity postpartum correlated with a rise in IgM rheumatoid factor and a fall in pregnancy-associated α_2 glycoprotein.[20]

One often overlooked aspect of rheumatoid arthritis and pregnancy is the physical and psychological problems and constraints of coping with neonatal care during a postpartum flare. Patients should be made aware of the likelihood of postpartum relapses of arthritic symptoms so that appropriate support systems can be put in place.

Effect of rheumatoid arthritis on pregnancy

No particular maternal effects have been described. Specifically, there does not appear to be an increased incidence of preeclampsia in these patients. From a fetal perspective, there is no increase in miscarriage or stillbirths in women with rheumatoid arthritis.[21] Although a case of intrauterine growth retardation secondary to vasculitis associated with severe extraarticular rheumatoid arthritis has been reported, in general one can expect normal perinatal outcomes for patients with rheumatoid arthritis.

The most significant fetal risks come not from the disease itself but from the medications used for treatment.

Medications

Salicylates are the drugs of choice in treating rheumatic diseases in pregnancy. The second-line agents are the nonsteroidal antiinflammatory drugs (NSAIDs).

Aspirin is not known to be teratogenic in humans.[22,23] Many of the important side effects of salicylates result from their inhibition of prostaglandin synthesis. There have been reports of prolonged gestation and prolonged labor in patients using aspirin.[24] Other reports have suggested maternal and neonatal hemostatic abnormalities leading to increased blood loss during labor and delivery, as well as neonatal petechiae, intraventricular hemorrhage, cephalohematoma, and prolonged bleeding after circumcision.[25,26] It has therefore been recommended that salicylates be discontinued 10 to 14 days before the expected date of delivery. In addition, prostaglandins are important in controlling the smooth muscle of the ductus arteriosus, and prostaglandin inhibitors may result in preterm closure of the ductus as well as pulmonary hypertension.[27,28] Salicylates cross into breast milk, and women taking chronic high doses of aspirin may have potentially dangerous levels of salicylate in their breast milk.[29] In general, NSAIDs are weak acids and therefore do not achieve high concentrations in breast milk. Caution in their use due to lack of information rather than known adverse outcome.[23]

Gold salts have been shown to be efficacious in the treatment of rheumatoid arthritis. Gold is highly protein bound and therefore crosses the placenta poorly. No known teratogenic effects have been documented with gold therapy; however, due to the ameliorating affects of pregnancy on rheumatoid arthritis, most authors do not recommend the use of gold during pregnancy.[30-32] Small quantities of gold have been detected in breast milk.

Penicillamine is occasionally used in the treatment of rheumatoid arthritis. It has been successfully used in pregnancy in the treatment of Wilson's disease without severe sequelae.[33,34] Penicillamine does cross the placenta, and two cases of fetal connective tissue abnormalities have been reported.[35,36] Therefore, because of the generally mild course of rheumatoid arthritis in pregnancy, the use of penicillamine is not recommended.

Steroid therapy is not usually required during pregnancy because of the usual improvement of disease. A detailed discussion of steroid use in pregnancy appears in the section on systemic lupus erythematosus.

Obstetric and anesthetic management

Obstetric management. As previously noted, patients with rheumatoid arthritis may expect a generally uncomplicated prenatal course. Medications should be limited to the less toxic agents unless the disease process is unusually severe. In patients with vascular disease, close attention must be paid to fetal growth. In general, a vaginal delivery at term may be expected. Many patients experience a postpartum exacerbation of disease, peaking between 4 to 6 weeks postpartum.[37]

Anesthetic considerations. Predelivery anesthetic consultation for the patient with rheumatoid arthritis is essential because of the disease's widespread organ involvement. In addition to taking a careful history (including medications, previous complications, and hospitalization) a thorough physical examination, especially concentrating in the areas listed below, is mandatory.

Inflammation of the synovial joints of the airway is a common occurrence for which the anesthesiologist must look. In particular, the temporomandibular joint may be ankylosed, making it impossible for the patient to open her mouth adequately for intubation. Involvement of the cricoarytenoid joint may result in an edematous constriction of the glottis. To make matters worse, cervical spine disease is common and may result in a severe flexion deformity of the neck along with atlantoaxial instability, possibly resulting in spinal cord damage with neck extension.[38] A recent onset of hoarseness or change in voice quality may indicate involvement of the larynx, and symptoms of neck pain may indicate cervical spine involvement and should be included in one's review of systems.[39] The anesthesiologist can avoid potential problems with endotracheal intubation by having the patient open her mouth so the uvula and tonsillar pillars can be visualized, and by having her extend her neck. The patient with severe limitations should probably have her airway secured (with fiberoptic assistance) before an operative delivery.

In addition to involvement of airway joints, inflammation may also be present in the hip, knee, and lumbar intervertebral joints. Deformities in these areas will therefore limit spine and hip flexion and abduction. If these limitations are present, the anesthesiologist should warn the patient that proper positioning for a regional anesthetic may be difficult or even impossible. Severe hip disease may warrant vaginal delivery with special stirrups, no stirrups, or at times it even preclude the use of stirrups.[40] A recent retrospective review of 76 pregnancies in 51 patients with juvenile rheumatoid arthritis (JRA) revealed that JRA was associated with a higher frequency of cesarean delivery, with bilateral hip prosthesis as the main reason.[41]

A thorough examination of the patient's heart and lungs may detect arthritic involvement of these organs. Restrictive lung disease created by kyphosis of the spine, inflammatory fixation of the ribs, and the presence of rheumatoid pleural effusions is complicated by the presence of a large gravid uterus. This restrictive process may result in a markedly reduced functional residual capacity and thus a diminished ability of the patient to push during the second stage of labor secondary to diminished oxygen reserves. The presence of severe restrictive disease may also contraindicate a high level of sensory blockade with a regional technique since this would further compromise respiratory effort. Predelivery pulmonary function testing may alert the obstetric team to these possible problems. Cardiac disease may be noted by the presence of a pericardial effusion (listen for a rub or distant heart sounds), valvular and conduction defects (detected by auscultation and electrocardiogram [ECG] abnormalities), or cardiomyopathy (presence of a third heart sound, ECG, and echo abnormalities).

Because of occasional peripheral nerve involvement, especially in those patients with Felty's and Sjögren's syndromes, a thorough examination to detect the presence of sensory deficits should be performed. These deficits should be documented, because these patients may later receive a regional anesthetic.

Finally, certain medications taken by the patient may dictate choice of anesthetic technique for delivery. Ingestion of aspirin results in interference of platelet function for up to 10 days, so recent ingestion probably warrants obtaining a bleeding history if a regional anesthetic is contemplated. In addition, steroid use may result in adrenal suppression, and recent ingestion dictates giving the patient a full supplementation to cover her adrenal function. In addition, osteoporosis secondary to steroid treatment dictates careful positioning of these patients at all times during labor and delivery to avoid fractures. Nonsteroidal antiinflammatory drugs have been associated with hepatotoxicity, so baseline serum glutamic oxaloacetic transaminase (SGOT) and serum glutamic pyruvic transaminase (SGPT) levels should be documented before delivery.[42] Adverse drug reactions to gold include extensive skin eruptions, oral ulcers, membranous glomerulopathy, agranulocytosis, aplastic anemia, and renal damage with proteinuria.[43] Thorough evaluation of dermal integrity, complete blood cell (CBC) count with differential, blood urea nitrogen (BUN), creatinine, and urinalysis should be performed on the parturient receiving gold therapy.

Anesthetic management of the parturient with rheumatoid arthritis thus depends greatly on the degree of multiorgan involvement. Epidural anesthesia avoids the risk of intubation, but in the patient with severe joint contractures a limited range of motion may limit its ability to be successfully administered. As mentioned earlier, peripheral neuropathies may exist in these patients and while they do not contraindicate the use of regional anesthesia, these deficits should be documented before initiation of conduction blockade. In addition, normal clotting studies should be verified prior to placement of a regional anesthetic.

The patient with severe airway abnormalities warrants special care. A large intravascular or subarachnoid injection of local anesthetic intended for the epidural space may result in seizures or a total spinal blockade and loss of the airway. Needless to say, this would be catastrophic in the patient who may be impossible to ventilate or intubate in the usual manner because of rheumatoid involvement of her airway. Because of rapid, and at times unpredictable, spread of anesthesia, spinal anesthesia for cesarean delivery in the patient with severe airway disease is not advised. If epidural anesthesia is performed for cesarean delivery, the level must be raised cautiously with only 3 to 4 mL of local anesthetic at a time with the anesthesiologist continuously on the lookout for signs and symptoms of subarachnoid or intravascular injection. It is probably safest in the patient with severe airway involvement to secure the airway before cesarean delivery. This is most effectively done with fiberoptic awake intubation. Under no circumstances should a parturient with a compromised airway be delivered by cesarean section using the usual emergent rapid-sequence general anesthetic induction, since it may result in loss of the airway and maternal death. An abdominal wall field block with local infiltration is a much safer alternative for these patients.

Regardless of anesthetic technique, a large-bore intravenous catheter should be placed during early labor, since these patients may experience increased blood loss secondary to aspirin therapy and have the expected baseline anemia of pregnancy. Patients with extensive cardiorespiratory involvement may require invasive monitoring especially if regional anesthesia is planned. Sachs et al were able to manage the labor of a parturient with restrictive pericarditis secondary to long-standing juvenile rheumatoid arthritis under epidural anesthesia with the aid of a Swan-Ganz catheter.[44] In patients with more severe constrictive pericarditis, pericardiectomy was reported to be successful during pregnancy.[45]

Depending on the degree of spine and cardiorespiratory involvement, postoperative pain relief may be achieved with a variety of methods. If an epidural or subarachnoid catheter was placed preoperatively, it may be used postoperatively to deliver epidural or intrathecal narcotics with or without a low concentration of local anesthetic. The patient whose hematologic or anatomic problems contraindicate regional anesthesia may be managed with a patient-controlled device to deliver intravenous narcotic pain relief.

SYSTEMIC LUPUS ERYTHEMATOSUS

Systemic lupus erythematosus (SLE) is a chronic disease that may affect many organ systems. The disease has a strong female preponderance and may present at any age. It is believed that SLE complicates approximately 1 in 1600 to 5000 pregnancies and that over 80% of cases occur in women during their childbearing years.[46-48]

Systemic lupus erythematosus is an autoimmune disease in which antigen-antibody complexes in serum and autoantibodies are present in excess and may be deposited in tissues. The etiology of this increased antibody production is not known. The clinical manifestations and criteria for classification have been recently reviewed.[31,48,49,50] In pregnancy, the most common clinical manifestations are arthralgias/arthritis, fever, skin lesions, and renal disease.[46]

Pathophysiology and effect of pregnancy on systemic lupus erythematosus

The natural course of SLE in both the pregnant and nonpregnant state is variable. The exacerbation of lupus during pregnancy may be difficult to diagnose since no clear consensus exists as to the definition of a flare. Many studies have reported that pregnancy increases the risk of SLE exacerbation. Unfortunately, the definition of exacerbation is not uniform and the variation in exacerbation rates is wide. In addition, many of these studies have been retrospective and have used patients as their own controls.[46,51-53]

In contrast, Lockshin et al[54] in a prospective case-control study showed no significant increase in exacerbation of SLE with pregnancy. These findings have been supported by Mintz and Rodriguez-Alvarez,[55] who reported on 102 pregnancies and noted no significant difference in disease activity in pregnant SLE patients compared with SLE controls. In a prospective analysis, Lockshin[56] reported that if all potential manifestations of lupus flare are included, less than 25% of pregnancies are associated with flare. If only lupus-specific abnormalities are included, the risk of flare in pregnancy is less than 13%. In addition, no increase in exacerbation rates were noted postpartum. Because pregnancy-induced exacerbation is relatively uncommon, prophylactic prednisone therapy is not recommended.[56]

Other investigators have suggested that the risk of lupus exacerbation in pregnancy was related to the degree of clinical activity at conception.[57,58] Hayslett and Lynn,[57] in a retrospectively collected series of 65 pregnancies, observed 46 patients with clinical signs of lupus nephropathy. They reported a 35% exacerbation rate in patients whose disease process had been quiescent in the 6 months prior to conception, and a 48% exacerbation rate in those patients whose disease was active at conception. The most severe exacerbations occurred in patients with active disease, and the most common manifestations of exacerbation in this study were hypertension, proteinuria, and declining renal function.

The relationship between pregnancy and lupus nephropathy is still under investigation. In 57% to 80% of patients, evidence of lupus nephritis antedates pregnancy.[55,59] The influence of pregnancy on the underlying course of nephropathy remains controversial, but there is a high probability of an uncomplicated course if the nephritis is in remission before conception.[57,58,60] A small but significant chance of permanent renal dysfunction exists, but this risk may be consistent with that of the general SLE population.

Findings such as hypertension and proteinuria may be due to preeclampsia rather than a lupus flare. It is difficult to differentiate between a lupus flare and preeclampsia, but the diagnosis may be crucial because of different management. A lupus flare is managed medically with glucocorticoids and possibly immunosuppressive agents, while severe preeclampsia is an indication for delivery. If a determination is unable to be made, a renal biopsy should be considered.

Effect of systemic lupus erythematosus on pregnancy

There is no known effect of SLE on conception rates. Fertility is not known to be affected, except possibly in those patients with severe renal insufficiency. In addition, termination of pregnancy is not known to influence the subsequent clinical course of the disease.[51,61,62]

The incidence of spontaneous abortion is higher in women with SLE than in controls. Abortion rates in SLE are reported to occur in 7% to 40% of pregnancies.[55,59,61-63] The lymphotoxic antibodies found in some patients with SLE may be an immunologic mediator of spontaneous abortion, and placental vascular abnormalities have also been proposed.[64]

In patients who exhibit clinical remission at the onset of pregnancy, the fetal survival is excellent. In contrast, fetal survival is markedly reduced in patients with active disease at conception.[57,58,65] In combined series, the overall fetal survival is reported to be 76% in those patients with lupus documented prior to conception.[59] The rate of fetal loss increases with increasing renal dysfunction.[57] A high rate of fetal wastage was noted in those patients in whom the onset of SLE was concurrent with gestation. In this circumstance, fetal wastage approaches 40% to 45%.[58,64] The incidence of stillbirth has been reported as 17% to 22%.[55,63]

Prematurity is a significant perinatal problem occurring more frequently in patients with SLE.[45,54,55,63,66] Mintz et al[55,67] report an almost 50% incidence of prematurity in patients with SLE

and the rate of prematurity was noted to be highest among those patients with active disease. Other investigators have not reported a higher-than-expected rate of prematurity.[57]

Intrauterine growth retardation has been reported to occur in 23% of lupus pregnancies.[55] This incidence may be higher in those patients with hypertension and renal disease.[59]

Isolated complete congenital heart block (CHB) is occasionally seen in infants whose mothers have SLE. The presence of CHB has been strongly associated with the presence of Anti-Ro (SSA) antibody. Anti-Ro (SSA) and Anti-La (SSB) are antibodies directed toward nonnuclear histone antigens; they are found in 25% to 30% of patients with SLE.[68] These antibodies freely cross the placenta, but their precise role in the development of CHB remains to be elucidated. Most infants born with CHB are born to mothers with Anti-Ro, but many of these women have no evidence of collagen vascular disease.[69] Conversely, the presence of Ro does not confer an overwhelming risk of CHB, and it has been estimated to occur in 1 in 20 to 32 women with SLE and Anti-Ro.[68,70] Titers of Ro are not clearly related to the development of CHB, and discordance for CHB between twins suggests that other factors must be involved.[71] Congenital heart block is a permanent disorder, and in the absence of other cardiac anomalies it is associated with a 5% mortality.[55] Autopsy findings suggest that immunoglobulins may be deposited in cardiac tissue resulting in myocarditis, calcium deposits, endocardial fibroelastosis, and conduction defects.[72] There have been several attempts to treat CHB in utero with plasmapheresis and/or steroid therapy, but the heart rate has remained consistently bradycardic.[73-75]

Transient neonatal lupus is characterized by skin rash and serologic and hematologic abnormalities. Most manifestations of neonatal lupus resolve within 6 to 12 months postpartum. The maximal risk of neonatal lupus in a study by Lockshin was thought to be 1 in 3. For gravid women with SLE and anti-Ro, the risk of life-threatening neonatal lupus occurs in fewer than 1 in 38 pregnancies.[68] Discordance in neonatal lupus has been described in twin gestations. Prophylactic therapy for mothers was believed unnecessary because of the transient nature of neonatal lupus and the infrequency of severe manifestations of the disease.[68]

The etiology of fetal compromise in patients with SLE has been attributed to several factors. Small placental size, placental infarction, and decidual vasculopathy have been reported, as has the deposition of immunoglobulin and complement in trophoblastic tissue.[64,76,77]

Various immunologic abnormalities have been identified in pregnant patients with SLE. The lupus anticoagulant[78-81] and anticardiolipin[82-84] are antibodies to phospholipids that are found in 5% to 20% of patients with SLE. They have also been reported in a substantial number of patients without known collagen vascular disease.[78] These antibodies to phospholipids may be manifested by a biologic false positive test for syphilis, or by a prolonged activated partial thromboplastin time (aPTT) that fails to correct when mixed with normal plasma. The antibodies are related but independent, and any one individual may possess one or several of them. There is an increased perinatal risk associated with the presence of these autoantibodies.[78-81,83,84] The presence of anticardiolipin is thought to be the most sensitive and specific indicator of poor fetal outcome,[74,82,84] and maternal thrombocytopenia is correlated with its presence.[79] Lupus anticoagulant is paradoxically associated with thrombosis in 25% to 75% of patients.[85,86] Thrombosis of the deep veins, peripheral arteries, and retinal vessels have been reported as have pulmonary embolism, cerebrovascular events, placental thrombosis, and infarction.[76,78]

The treatment of patients with these autoantibodies remains controversial and is based primarily on uncontrolled studies. Prednisone and aspirin may be of benefit to those patients with lupus anticoagulant. Therapeutic success depends on suppression of lupus anticoagulant and normalization of the aPTT.[80,81,87] In addition, there are reports of good pregnancy outcome in patients with lupus anticoagulant who do not receive therapy.[88] Lockshin has reported that prednisone therapy may actually worsen fetal outcome.[89] Until a randomized controlled trial is undertaken, the issue of therapy remains controversial.

No clear benefit has been reported from therapy in patients with an isolated anticardiolipin.

Obstetric and anesthetic management

Obstetric management. Obstetric management of the gravida is best accomplished by a team approach involving rheumatologists, obstetricians, anesthesiologists, and pediatricians.

Prepregnancy counseling is essential in informing the prospective parturient about the potential risks and complications of pregnancy. As previously mentioned, pregnancy should be attempted when lupus has been quiescent over the previous 6 months. Initial laboratory evaluation should include antinuclear antibodies (ANA), complement levels, Anti-Ro, Anti-La, anticardiolipin, and lupus anticoagulant as well as a baseline evaluation of renal function (BUN/creatinine/24-hour urine for total protein and creatinine clearance). Accurate gestational dating is crucial; should there be any doubt, a first-trimester ultrasound is indicated.

Patients should be seen regularly by the rheumatologist as well as by the obstetrician. Assessment of ANA, complement levels, and renal function should be undertaken every 4 to 6 weeks. More frequent evaluation may be required in patients with active disease. Complement, an acute phase reactant, normally rises during pregnancy and following serial levels may be helpful in monitoring SLE activity. A fall in C3, C4, and CH50 has been associated with an exacerbation of SLE.[90,91] Other authors find complement levels not particularly helpful.[57] Recently, Devoe and Loy[92] have suggested that complement levels may be helpful in monitoring fetal outcome. A fetal echocardiogram at 20 weeks' gestation is useful in those pregnancies with Anti-Ro antibodies or in any patient suspected of having an infant with CHB. Patients should be followed with monthly ultrasounds after 25 weeks' gestation to assess fetal growth.

Because of the increased risk of stillbirth, regular assessment of fetal well-being should begin at 28 weeks' gestation. In the absence of any evidence of compromise, fetal assessment should be performed weekly until 34 to 36 weeks' gestation and twice a week thereafter. Delivery at term is indicated. A nonstress test is the usual first study followed by a contraction stress test or biophysical profile if fetal well-being cannot be documented. It has been suggested that in patients with antiphospholipid antibodies, monitoring may be warranted at an earlier gestational age; however, intervention is rarely undertaken because of the risk of death from prematurity.[79] Ideally, the fetus will be delivered at term unless there are some other obstetric or medical indications for preterm or abdominal delivery. One baby aspirin per day is generally recommended to reduce the risk of superimposed preeclampsia.

Drug therapy in systemic lupus erythematosus

Steroids. Corticosteroids are the mainstay of therapy in the pregnant patient with SLE. We recommend the lowest dose required to control the symptoms of SLE. Steroids are not known to be teratogenic in humans. Prednisone is metabolized by placental 11-β-ol-dehydrogenase to an inactive 11-keto metabolite so that only small amounts reach the fetus.[93,94] Dexamethasone and betamethasone cross the placenta more easily.[95,96] Both methylprednisolone and hydrocortisone are useful for intravenous therapy, but methylprednisolone has fewer mineralocorticoid effects and therefore may be preferable. As previously mentioned, stress doses should be utilized during labor and delivery as well as in the immediate puerperium.

The use of steroids in pregnancy may be associated with glucose intolerance as well as poor fetal growth.[97] Infants born to mothers chronically receiving steroids should be monitored for adrenal suppression, although this is a rare complication of steroid therapy.

Immunosuppressive agents. Azathioprine (Imuran) is occasionally necessary in a patient with severe disease. Azathioprine is a 6-mercaptopurine derivative and readily crosses the placenta. It has not been proven to be teratogenic in humans.[29,30] Chronic azathioprine therapy has been associated with neonatal lymphopenia and decreased fetal growth.[98,99] Little is known about the long-term effects of this agent.

Cyclophosphamide is teratogenic when given in the first trimester and should not be used in a pregnancy destined to continue.

Although unusual, the use of the immunosuppressive drugs may result in serious side effects in the mother, including visual disturbances, retinopathy, peripheral myopathy and neuropathy, cardiomyopathy, aplastic anemia, and thrombocytopenia.

Antimalarial agents. Antimalarial therapy has been associated with chromosomal damage in lymphocyte cultures, and a strong affinity for deposition in the fetal mouse retinal epithelium has been reported.[100,101] This has not been demonstrated in humans, but there are several isolated reports of vestibulocochlear dysfunction in the offspring of patients with SLE maintained on chloroquine.[102] In addition, there have been reports of good pregnancy outcomes without known adverse fetal effects in patients maintained on chloroquine phosphate, and some authors maintain that the risk of pregnancy loss with flare outweighs the risk of the medication.[103]

Anesthetic considerations. The anesthetic management of the pregnant patient with SLE will be influenced by the extent of various end-organ involvement and current medications the patient is receiving. As detailed in the obstetric section, SLE has the ability to damage every major organ in the body, and those effects of special concern to the anesthesiologist will now be discussed in detail.

Recurrent noninfectious pharyngitis and oral ulcers are common, and acute airway closure secondary to inflammation, fortunately uncommon, has also been reported.[104,105]

One of the most serious consequences of SLE is the involvement of the cardiorespiratory system. A cardiomyopathy may stem from direct involvement of the cardiac muscle, resulting in myocarditis and possibly congestive heart failure, or it may be secondary to chronic hypertension, coronary artery disease, endocarditis, or uremia, all of which may be end results of SLE. The most common cardiac manifestation of SLE is pericarditis, with or without a significant pericardial effusion, which may present as acute heart failure. Patients with cardiac involvement have been suggested to be more prone to the development of preeclampsia. On physical examination the anesthesiologist should listen for the presence of a friction rub (evidence of pericarditis), murmurs (evidence of possible endocarditis, also known as Libman-Sacks disease), or a third heart sound (evidence of congestive heart failure). The most common ECG abnormality observed in SLE patients is a nonspecific T-wave change.[106] An echocardiogram may also be useful to evaluate valvular function and the presence of an effusion. Valvular abnormalities may be detected in up to 25% of patients with echocardiography; they are, however, rarely significant.[48] A pulmonary history may reveal a history of hemoptysis and/or shortness of breath that may indicate the presence of pleural effusions, pulmonary infarcts, or a pulmonary vasculitis. Recurrent atelectasis can result in the "shrinking lung syndrome."[48] On physical examination, one should be alerted to the presence of rales (indicating congestive heart failure) or a pleural rub (indicating an effusion or pneumonitis). An arterial blood gas sample from the patient with severe lung involvement may show severe hypoxemia, and pulmonary function testing usually reveals a restrictive pattern with a decreased vital capacity and diffusion abnormality.

Other manifestations include diaphragmatic dysfunction secondary to phrenic neuropathy, interstitial pneumonitis, and pulmonary angiitis with hemorrhage and pulmonary hypertension.[48]

Since one of the leading causes of death in these patients is renal failure, the anesthesiologist should look for the presence of mild to severe hypertension with or without BUN, creatinine, or albumin abnormalities. The patient with severe renal failure may likely be receiving dialysis treatment. Clotting studies, which may be abnormal secondary to the patient's renal disease should be assessed.

Another common organ to be involved in a variety of ways is the central nervous system (CNS). Patients may present with peripheral sensory neuropathies, foot drop, transverse myelitis, seizures, atypical migraine, Guillain-Barré syndrome or pseudotumor.[48,106] Though the mechanism is unknown, certain drugs such as nonsteroidal inflammatory medications can cause aseptic meningitis in patients with lupus.[48] Behavioral changes including depression, paranoia, mania, and schizophrenia frequently have been reported along with cognitive dysfunction, all thought to be a result of vascular abnormalities.[48] The most common lupus-related abnormality of the CNS is microfocal scarring associated with intimal changes in small arterioles; this is probably responsible for primary, lupus-related encephalopathy.[107,108] Arteritis of the larger vessels may occasionally result in stroke or intracranial hemorrhage. Movement disorders such as chorea, athetosis, and hemiballismus may also be present.

As mentioned in the obstetric section, the SLE patient may present with a variety of hematologic abnormalities. To reiterate, the presence of lupus anticoagulant may result in a prolongation of the PTT, and rarely the prothrombin time (PT), secondary to its reaction with phospholipids used in the test.[109] However, there is no correlation between the coagulation tests and clinical hemorrhage, and more often than not, the presence of lupus anticoagulant is usually associated with thrombosis and not bleeding.[110] In addition, anticardiolipin antibodies may be detected in SLE patients as well, often in conjunction with thrombocytopenia and a prolonged bleeding time. The presence of these antibodies may also be associated with venous and/or arterial thromboses. To assess clinical significance, if any, a bleeding time may be performed if there are any abnormalities in the PT or PTT. Because of the increased frequency of thrombotic events in patients with lupus anticoagulant or anticardiolipin antibody, these women may present in labor having been previously placed on long-term anticoagulant therapy. Until coagulation parameters normalize, regional anesthesia is contraindicated.[111] In addition, antibodies associated with SLE may react with Factors VIII, IX, and XI, leading to bleeding, and thrombocytopenia may be present.[112] Because of the presence of these antibodies, crossmatching the patient's blood may be difficult and should be anticipated. Incidentally, it should also be noted that the presence of lupus anticoagulant and/or anticardiolipin antibody may be seen in perfectly healthy patients. Certain medications (procainamide most commonly, but also quinidine and chlorpromazine) and neoplastic tumors are associated with "drug-related SLE" and the presence of lupus anticoagulant.[48,113] Drug-related SLE usually subsides within 4 to 6 weeks after the drug is discontinued, and the clinical manifestations are usually mild compared with primary SLE.

The presence of arthritis in the proximal joints of the hands, wrists, and knees (along with Raynaud's phenomenon) may pose a problem in obtaining intravenous access or in positioning the patient for a regional anesthetic. Deformities due to tendon disease with contractures may also exist. However, there is no bony erosion in SLE and the spine is not affected.

Reported gastrointestinal manifestations include peritonitis, pancreatitis, protein-losing enteropathy, and ischemic bowel disease.[48] In addition, 30% of patients have abnormalities in liver function tests as well.

Appropriate anesthetic management of the patient will depend on the presence or absence, and the extent, of various end-organ disease. Obviously, coagulation abnormalities, if real, preclude regional anesthesia. For those patients who have had thrombotic complications related to the antiphospholipid antibodies, a variety of different anticoagulant regimens may be used.[114] The presence of severe cardiorespiratory complications warrants the placement of invasive monitoring. Medications known to depress cardiac, respiratory, or renal function should be avoided or judiciously administered. Communication between perinatologists, pediatricians, anesthesiologists, and the patient cannot be overemphasized.

The use of bleeding time has significantly decreased throughout the country, and in the majority of centers, it is not performed. Thromboelastogram may be a better indicator for the coagulation profile.

MYASTHENIA GRAVIS

Myasthenia gravis is a rare neuromuscular disorder characterized by weakness and fatigability of skeletal muscles. The underlying defect is a decrease in the number of available acetylcholine receptors at neuromuscular junctions, due to an antibody-mediated autoimmune attack. How the autoimmune response is initiated and maintained is not completely understood; however, the thymus appears to play a role in this process with as many as 10% of patients having thymic tumors (thymomas).

Myasthenia gravis has a prevalence rate of approximately 1 in 10,000 to 50,000. The disease affects both sexes, but in those who develop the disease before 40 years of age, females are affected 2 to 3 times more frequently than males. The peak onset of myasthenia gravis in women is at 20 to 30 years of age. Women with myasthenia gravis have a higher incidence of other autoimmune disorders such as rheumatoid arthritis, autoimmune thyroiditis, and SLE.

Cardinal features include weakness and fatigability of muscles. The weakness increases during repeated use and may improve following rest or sleep. The course of myasthenia is quite variable, with exacerbations and remissions occurring particularly in the first few years after onset of the disease. A typical clinical presentation includes diplopia and ptosis as initial complaints. Other facial muscle weakness may occur, producing difficulty in chewing, speech, and swallowing. Approximately 85% of patients eventually exhibit generalized limb muscle weakness, which is usually proximal and often asymmetric. On occasion, weakness of respiration or swallowing may become severe enough to require respiratory assistance.

The diagnosis is supported by a positive Tensilon test. A negative acetylcholine receptor antibody finding is not unusual, because only about 50% of patients with weakness confined to the ocular muscles will have detectable acetycholine receptor antibodies. Ten percent to 20% of patients with overall clinical evidence of myasthenia gravis have no detectable antibody in their serum. Treatment modalities are usually limited to the use of cholinesterase inhibitors, thymectomy, steroid/cytotoxic immune suppressive agents, and plasmapheresis. Most patients are maintained on acetylcholinesterase inhibitors, the most common of which is neostigmine. At physiologic pH, neostigmine is ionized and therefore does not cross the placenta well. Furthermore, it is not a known teratogen. Doses of neostigmine must be adjusted in pregnancy because of increased volume of distribution and increased clearance.

Effect of pregnancy on myasthenia gravis

With regard to pregnancy, roughly one third of the patients with myasthenia gravis improve during pregnancy, one third remain the same, and one third have worsening of their symptoms. Therapeutic abortion does not alter the symptoms. In patients who have had multiple pregnancies, the course of myasthenia in previous pregnancies does not reflect the course of a subsequent pregnancy. There are some reports that suggest a slightly higher risk of prematurity and/or premature labor in patients with myasthenia. A potentially problematic time for myasthenic patients is often during labor and delivery. The uterus itself is smooth muscle so that it is independent of acetylcholine receptors. However, during the second stage of labor when voluntary efforts at fetal expulsion are required, the patient may tire quickly and not be able to aid in voluntary expulsive efforts. Forceps or vacuum-assisted extraction is often recommended for the final stages of labor. Although the incidence of preeclampsia is not increased in the myasthenic patient, if the patient does have preeclampsia concomitantly, one should avoid using magnesium sulfate since this drug decreases the amount of transmitter liberated at the motor nerve terminal. This diminishes the depolarizing action of acetylcholine at the endplate and depresses excitability of the muscle fiber.

With respect to fetal considerations, no congenital malformations or other neonatal injury have been attributed to maternal treatment with cholinesterase inhibitors. This is also true of cortico-steroid therapy. In addition, prednisone crosses the placenta very poorly. With regard to thymectomy, in one retrospective review patients who were thymectomized had a more stable course than non-thymectomized patients. There was no difference in the development of neonatal myasthenia gravis between these populations. Plasmapheresis has been used during pregnancy without any apparent adverse affects to the fetus. Other neonatal considerations include neonatal myasthenia gravis, which is a transient weakness occurring in approximately 15% to 20% of children born to myasthenic mothers. Occurrence of neonatal myasthenia cannot be predicted by the course of severity of the disease in the mother, by the presence or absence of thymectomy, or by the level of maternal anticholinesterase receptor antibodies. In fact, some mothers in complete remission occasionally may have neonates with transient myasthenia gravis. There is some evidence that mothers who have had one child with neonatal myasthenia gravis are at an increased risk for having a second child developing the same symptoms.

There are rare reports of congenital malformations in children of mothers with myasthenia gravis who have not received corticosteroids or other immunosuppressant drugs. These may include arthogryposis, hypognathism, polydactyly, and hypogammaglobinemia. These congenital anomalies are so infrequent that they may well not be attributed to myasthenia gravis alone.

There appears to be no absolute contraindications to the use of any of the commonly used medications in myasthenic mothers who are breast-feeding.

In general, patients with minimal symptoms who are well controlled with either anticholinesterase inhibitors or steroids do quite well in pregnancy. It is essential to continue medications throughout pregnancy with attention to dosage increase with advancing gestational age. The pediatric unit should be notified before delivery regarding the potential for neonatal myasthenia gravis. An ultrasound for fetal survey at 20 weeks is desirable.

Anesthetic considerations. Anesthetic management of the pregnant patient with myasthenia gravis begins with a careful history and physical examination of the patient before she arrives on the labor floor.

In taking a history from the patient, a list of medications and dosages is essential to obtain since many of these have significant anesthetic interactions. One of the mainstays of treatment for this disease is the administration of quaternary ammonium compounds, which are used to inhibit cholinesterase activity. The most common anticholinesterase drug is neostigmine (Prostigmin), with a duration of 2 to 3 hours. Intravenous neostigmine, 0.5 mg, is equivalent to 1.5 mg subcutaneous neostigmine or 0.7 mg intramuscular neostigmine or 15 mg oral neostigmine. For the longer-acting (4-6 hours) cholinergic drug pyridostigmine (Mestinon), equivalent doses to those of neostigmine are 2.0 mg intravenously, 3.0 mg intramuscularly, and 60 mg orally. Most authorities recommend the use of intramuscular injections during labor, but others maintain this is unnecessary and advocate intravenous injection to provide less fluctuations in clinical symptoms.[115] However, intravenous administration of anticholinesterase drugs has been reported to cause premature labor, so they should be administered carefully.[116] It should also be noted that anticholinesterases potentiate vagal responses and that vagolytic agents should be immediately available.[117] When given parenterally, as during labor, the ratio of oral to parenteral dosage is 30:1.[118]

Symptoms of excess cholinergic medication are secondary to its muscarinic effects; they include abdominal cramps, diarrhea, nausea, vomiting, and increased salivary and tear duct secretions. Life-threatening side effects, referred to as "cholinergic crisis," produce muscle weakness and respiratory failure. These effects may be mistaken for a myasthenic crisis; the two can be differentiated by the administration of edrophonium (Tensilon). The patient's muscle strength is first assessed subjectively (by observing chewing, swallowing, and grip strength) and objectively (measurement of vital capacity) and then reassessed 30 to 90 seconds after a test dose of 1 to 2 mg of edrophonium is administered intravenously.[119] In overmedicated patients, muscle strength either does not change or it may slightly deteriorate, as opposed to patients having a myasthenic crisis in which dramatic improvement in muscle strength is seen. Because it acts rapidly and has a short duration of action, the edrophonium test can be repeated within 10 minutes if results are equivocal. When the edrophonium test indicates myasthenic crisis, the cautious intravenous administration of neostigmine or pyridostigmine can be tried, keeping in mind their potential to increase uterine tone and contractility. Neostigmine, 0.3 mg, or 1.2 mg pyridostigmine should be initially administered, and subsequent doses of half those amounts should be given 3 to 5 minutes apart if needed.[119] Because edrophonium may produce increased oropharyngeal secretions and further weakness of striated muscles, the testing location should be equipped for airway resuscitation. The anesthesiologist should also be aware that atropine, used to reduce the muscarinic side effects of the anticholinesterases, may mask those side effects that signal excessive dosage.[120]

On physical examination, the patient with myasthenia gravis should be examined for the presence of ptosis, which may be seen even if she is receiving anticholinesterase therapy. Inquiry should be made into chewing and swallowing difficulties, blurred vision, difficulties with clear or loud speaking, or shortness of breath during rest or exercise. Hemoglobin and serum electrolytes may be abnormal if the patient has bulbar weakness sufficient to compromise adequate nutrition.[121] Symptoms of respiratory compromise, especially if occurring at rest, warrant pulmonary function testing, which will give the anesthesiologist further insight into the severity of the patient's disease and help to predict the need for peripartum ventilatory assistance. Electrocardiographic testing is recommended because myocardial lesions have been described in these patients.[119,121] Sensory changes both in involved or uninvolved muscle groups are frequently present in myasthenia gravis. Common complaints include lower back pain, headache, ocular pain, and paresthesias of the face, lips, tongue, and extremities.[119] These obviously should be noted before the administration of any anesthetic agent. Since the incidence of hyperthyroidism is frequently associated with myasthenia gravis, any symptoms of thyroid dysfunction warrant thyroid function testing.

In terms of management for delivery, the anesthesiologist and obstetrician should first be aware that respiratory compromise in the myasthenic patient may render her more susceptible to the depressant effects of narcotic drugs, barbiturates, tranquilizers, and volatile anesthetic agents. It is not clear in the literature whether myasthenic patients have a true increased sensitivity to these drugs. Regardless, all depressant medications should be given judiciously.

Since uterine smooth muscle is not involved in the myasthenic process, vaginal delivery is the most common route of delivery. Because of its ability to eliminate the stress response to pain and the need for systemic (and potentially respiratory depressing) medication, regional analgesia is usually preferred.[122,119,115,121] Although low spinal anesthesia had been recommended in the past to avoid high blood levels of local anesthetic, no evidence of increased sensitivity of the neuromuscular junction to local anesthetics in myasthenia gravis patients has been found.[119,122] Both Rolbin et al[121] and Coaldrake and Livingstone[115] have reported no difficulty in myasthenic patients receiving epidural lidocaine doses of 320 to 400 mg. Because plasma cholinesterase enzyme activity may be decreased in myasthenia gravis patients, amide-type local anesthetics are theoretically thought to be a safer choice when used in large quantities, as with epidural anesthesia.[123,119,121,124] Tetracaine has been reported to be safe for use in spinal anesthesia, perhaps because of the relatively small dose required.[121]

Vital capacity measurements and/or continued observation for the development of bulbar weakness should be made throughout the course of labor.[115,121] Because of the emotional and physical stresses of labor, additional anticholinesterase therapy may be required.

The anesthesiologist should also be aware of certain medications frequently administered during labor that may be contraindicated in myasthenic patients (Box 19-1). Calcium is the most effective agent for reversing antibiotic-induced weakness in almost all cases.[120] The anesthesiologist should also be aware that the patient may be receiving chronic steroid treatment as well and therefore may require stress doses of steroids throughout labor. Plasmapheresis may lead to a pronounced reduction in circulating antiacetylcholine receptor antibodies with dramatic improvement in symptoms. It should be noted that improvement lasts for only several days to 3 months, however.[117]

If it is electively determined that the patient requires cesarean delivery, regional anesthesia is rec-

---

BOX 19-1 DRUGS CONTRAINDICATED IN THE PATIENT WITH MYASTHENIA GRAVIS

Antibiotics
Gentamycin
Kanamycin
Streptomycin
Neomycin
Polymyxin
Colistin
Tetracycline
Lincomycin

Cardiac drugs
Quinidine
Propranolol

Beta mimetics
Ritodrine
Terbutaline

Tocolytics
Magnesium sulfate

Others
Quinine
Penicillamine
Lithium salts

---

ommended provided the patient does not have signs of bulbar or respiratory muscle involvement that would warrant protection of the airway via endotracheal anesthesia. Good results have been reported using epidural anesthesia with 2% lidocaine with and without epinephrine 1:200,000.[115,121] If general anesthesia is required, an awake endotracheal intubation or induction and intubation under sodium thiopental (if the patient is very weak) may be performed. For intubation, 30 to 50 mg of succinylcholine may be used if needed.[121] Should intraoperative muscle relaxation be required, 1 to 3 mg doses of curare are recommended. The anesthesiologist should be aware that myasthenia gravis patients are highly sensitive to nondepolarizing relaxants and that even small doses will result in rapid, exaggerated effects. Involved myasthenic muscles are more sensitive to depolarizing agents, and yet uninvolved myasthenic muscles are resistant to their effects, leading some to avoid the use of them entirely.[119,124] In addition, due to the presence of anticholinesterase medication, the duration of action of depolarizing agents may be unpredictably prolonged.[119,121] The abnormal response of the myasthenic gravis patient to muscle relaxants is seen even in patients with localized ocular myasthenia and during remission. However, avoidance of intermediate-acting relaxants such as atracurium and vecuronium may not be necessary, because of their rapid elimination.[124] The use of volatile agents may also potentiate the neuromuscular blockade of any muscle relaxant used. The depth of general anesthesia should be kept at the lightest level compatible with adequate amnesia and analgesia. Infiltration of the skin or regional nerve blocks may be useful to decrease postoperative pain medication requirements.[119] Postoperative analgesia with low-dose bupivacaine has been reported.[115] Epidural anesthesia with bupivacaine and morphine for both primary anesthesia and postoperative pain control has been reported for thymectomy with no depression of ventilatory response to CO_2 and hypoxia.[125] Reversal of neuromuscular blockade with incremental intravenous doses of neostigmine, 0.5 mg, or pyridostigmine, 1.0 mg, and extubation is considered "proper," provided the patient's disease was well controlled preoperatively. A twitch monitor should be used at all times throughout the operation to assess degree of blockade. Factors thought predictive of the need for postoperative mechanical ventilation are (1) duration of myasthenia; (2) history of chronic respiratory disease for >six years; (3) pyridostigmine dosage greater than 750 mg/day; and (4) vital capacity less than 2.9 L.[126] Either of the first two factors by themselves or any combination of two or more factors predicts this need. Since pharyngeal and neck muscles may have a delayed recovery despite the presence of a sustained tetanic stimulation, patients should be able to lift their head for 5 seconds and demonstrate an inspiratory force $\geq$ 25 cm H_2O prior to extubation.

Because postpartum exacerbations have been reported to be sudden and devastating, the mother should be watched closely during her postpartum convalescence.[123] This is often a time for wide swings in anticholinesterase requirements, and close measurements of vital capacity and other observations of muscle strength must be frequently assessed.

PROGRESSIVE SYSTEMIC SCLEROSIS

Progressive systemic sclerosis (PSS) or scleroderma is an uncommon rheumatic disorder characterized by the excessive production of connective tissue and by vascular changes consisting of proliferation of the intima and fibrosis of the adventitia in small vessels.

The spectrum of disease varies from peripheral cutaneous symptoms to widespread cutaneous and systemic involvement. A unique form of PSS is the CREST syndrome, which is manifested by calcinosis, Raynaud's phenomena, esophageal dysfunction, sclerodactyly, and telangiectasis.

Overall, the disease has a 3:1 female to male ratio with a 10:1 female preponderance in the reproductive age groups.[127] The peak age of onset is in the third to fifth decade of life, making PSS fairly uncommon in pregnancy.

Pathophysiology and effect of pregnancy on progressive systemic sclerosis

Progressive systemic sclerosis is a disease characterized by exacerbations and remissions; therefore, the exact effect of pregnancy on the disease process is difficult to ascertain. Black and Stevens,[127] in a review of 101 pregnancies, reported the development of disease in 9 pregnancies, the progression of disease in 30 pregnancies, the remittance of disease in 11 pregnancies, and a stable disease course in 34 pregnancies. The disease rate in the remaining 17 patients was not known.

Renal disease is the primary cause of maternal death in pregnancies complicated by PSS. Renal disease in PSS is primarily a vascular phenomenon and occurs an average of 3.2 years after the onset of disease.[128] In a series reported by Steen et al,[129] renal crisis occurred in 17% of pregnant patients with diffuse cutaneous PSS, but this was not statistically significant when compared with nonpregnant PSS controls. Renal disease may present any time during pregnancy, but it usually occurs in the third trimester and may appear abruptly in patients with previously documented normal renal function.

Accelerated refractory hypertension is the most common manifestation of renal disease,[130] but microangiopathic hemolytic disease and progressive renal failure have also been reported.[131-133]

Effect of progressive systemic sclerosis on pregnancy

The effect of PSS on fertility is controversial.[134,135] Several studies have suggested an increased risk of spontaneous abortion in women with PSS,[134,135] but other investigators have not found an increase in miscarriage rates.[129]

Most reports on PSS in pregnancy are retrospective and uncontrolled; however, an increased risk of stillbirth and prematurity have been reported.[131,136] More recent reports have not noted these findings but do document an increased incidence of small-for-gestational-age infants at term.[129]

The cutaneous changes in PSS involve a decrease in subcutaneous fat and an increase of collagen. Most skin changes occur in the upper extremities, thorax, neck, and face. The abdomen is not usually involved. The skin is usually able to accommodate pregnancy and it heals in an uneventful fashion.[137] One case of obstructive uropathy in a patient with PSS and a twin gestation has been reported.[138]

Xerostomia and esophageal fibrosis may affect nutrition as well as aggravate the usual gastrointestinal discomforts of pregnancy. Pulmonary fibrosis, cardiac disease, and renal disease are quite unusual but are frequently associated with poor maternal and fetal outcome.

Obstetric and anesthetic management

Obstetric management. In patients with known renal, cardiac, or pulmonary disease, pregnancy termination should be offered, and patients who desire to continue pregnancy should be counseled as to the potential serious risks. In patients who desire to continue pregnancy, baseline assessment of renal function, including a 24-hour urine collection, is indicated. Meticulous attention to blood pressure and renal status must be maintained throughout pregnancy. In addition, the pregnancy should be monitored for fetal growth and fetal well-being. A vaginal delivery at term may be anticipated unless other obstetric or medical indications for preterm or abdominal delivery become apparent. Failure to progress in labor has been described secondary to connective tissue changes in the cervix.[139]

Anesthetic considerations. As detailed above, PSS may involve multiple organs that may produce a wide variation of symptoms and physical restrictions. Appropriate anesthetic management will be dictated by the type and extent of end-organ disease. Certain organ involvements of special interest to the anesthesiologist are listed in Table 19-1.

If a vaginal delivery is planned, the patient may be managed with a regional anesthetic, although ligament and joint involvement may preclude proper positioning for placement. If successful, the resultant peripheral vasodilation is helpful in preventing and/or treating vasospasm secondary to Raynaud's phenomenon. One should be aware that the patient may be taking nifedipine, alpha-adrenergic blockers (prazosin, phenoxybenzamine hydrochloride) or centrally acting drugs (methyldopa, reserpine) for treatment of long-standing vasospasm. Warming of the labor room and use of warm intravenous fluids should be employed for the patient regardless of method of delivery. In addition, if regional anesthesia is chosen, smaller doses of local anesthetics are recommended since prolonged sensory blockade with both amide and ester local anesthetics have been reported in patients with PSS.[143,144]

General anesthesia carries a greater than normal increased risk of aspiration for the parturient. Because of lower esophageal sphincter tone and decreased intestinal motility, these patients often present with reflux and/or esophageal stricture. Up to 50% of patients with radiographic evidence of reflux may be asymptomatic. The risk of aspiration is compounded in the sclerodermatous parturient who has a compromised airway secondary to limited oral opening. Inability to open the mouth is usually secondary to changes in the perioral soft tissues but may be due to temporomandibular joint dysfunction in some patients.[140]

Laryngeal edema has also been reported.[145] Endotracheal intubation, if needed, is best facilitated under awake fiberoptic laryngoscopy; under direct vision one can avoid telangiectasias, which may bleed profusely if traumatized.[143] There is a possibility of problems with preoxygenation by mask secondary to oral contractures preventing an adequate seal. Regardless of choice of anesthetic, the use of oral antacids, glycopyrrolate, and metoclopramide are recommended as precautionary aspiration treatment.

Because of the wide extent of organ-system involvement, extensive laboratory evaluation is required in addition to a thorough history and physical examination. Serum electrolytes, BUN/creatinine, CBC, urinalysis, ECG, and, depending on the extent of respiratory impairment, room air arterial blood gas, chest x-ray examination, and pulmonary function tests should be obtained prior to the patient presenting for delivery. Depending on these findings, a rational decision regarding anesthetic options and the need for invasive monitoring can be made.

Table 19-1 Organ involvement in progressive systemic sclerosis

Extraarticular manifestations of PSS	Anesthetic considerations[140-142]
Skin	
Sclerotic skin	Difficult venous access
Vasoconstriction	Vasospasm
Telangiectasis	Difficult blood pressure monitoring
Ulcers	
Cutaneous calcinosis	Airway compromise
	Joint immobility
	Fragile skin
Gastrointestinal	
Smooth muscle atrophy	$\uparrow$ Risk of aspiration
Lower esophageal sphincter incompetence	$\uparrow$ PT, $\uparrow$ bleeding
Malabsorption of vitamin K	
Pulmonary	
Interstitial fibrosis	Hypoxemia
Fibrosis	Restrictive lung disease
Chest wall/ diaphragm sclerosis	Pulmonary hypertension
	Cor pulmonale
	Pleural effusion
Cardiac	
Myocardial fibrosis	Atrioventricular block
Conduction fiber atrophy	Arrhythmias
	Restrictive cardiomyopathy
	Angina
	Pericardial effusion
Renal	
Arteriolar fibrosis	Hypertension
	Proteinuria
	Anemia
	Renal failure
Nervous system	
Vasa nervorum atrophy	Mononeuritis multiplex

ANKYLOSING SPONDYLITIS

Ankylosing spondylitis is a rheumatic disease characterized by inflammation of the apophyseal, sacroiliac, and costovertebral joints of the spine. The disease has a peak onset at 15 to 29 years of age and may occur in women of childbearing age. The primary sites of involvement in pregnant women are the cervical spine and pubic symphysis. Peripheral arthritis has been reported.

Pathophysiology and effect of pregnancy on ankylosing spondylitis

In general, pregnancy does not improve the symptoms of ankylosing spondylitis. In a retrospective review involving 156 cases, Ostensen and Husby[146] reported that ankylosing spondylitis was unchanged in 40% of patients, improved in 30%, and worsened in 30%. In a prospective study by the same authors,[147] symptoms were improved in only those patients with ulcerative colitis or psoriasis. In addition, Ostensen and Husby[146] reported that most patients will experience a temporary flare in the first 6 months postpartum.

Effect of ankylosing spondylitis on pregnancy

Most patients with ankylosing spondylitis have uncomplicated pregnancies and give birth to normal healthy children. Low back pain may be especially bothersome in the second and third trimesters but a vaginal delivery at term may be anticipated unless other obstetric or medical problems become apparent. In a retrospective study of 87 pregnancies in patients with ankylosing spondylitis, 12% of offspring aged 18 years or older developed the disease.[148]

Anesthetic management. Although ankylosing spondylitis does not appear to dramatically alter the course of pregnancy or fetal well-being, the disease does mandate several anesthetic considerations for patient management during labor and delivery. Primary concerns involve possible cardiorespiratory dysfunction, airway difficulties, and arthritic changes, making regional anesthesia potentially impossible.

A small percentage of patients with ankylosing spondylitis develop proximal aortitis. Fibrotic degeneration may lead to the development of aortic insufficiency and/or destruction of the atrioventricular bundle and heart block.[149] Occasional involvement of the mitral valve is noted as well. However, although reports of severe cardiac complications presenting early do exist, most complications are seen in patients who have had the disease at least 15 to 30 years.[150] Nonetheless, a baseline ECG and auscultation for murmurs is warranted.

Respiratory complications result primarily from costovertebral joint ankylosis, producing fixation of the thoracic cage. Diffuse pulmonary fibrosis, cyst formations, or secondary amyloidosis may also be present.[150] In addition, the pregnant patient's gravid uterus will produce further diminutions in lung volumes, and thus the term patient may present with severe restrictive lung disease. Pulmonary function testing should be considered especially if any symptoms of shortness of breath or dyspnea on exertion are elicited. Patients with severe respiratory disease may not be candidates for high levels of regional anesthesia because of their already compromised lung volumes.

Perhaps of most concern to the obstetric anesthesiologist is the possible occurrence of airway abnormalities in these patients. Cervical spine involvement may range from slightly decreased limitation of neck movement to complete neck fusion, usually in the flexed position. If the duration of disease is 16 years or more, 75% of patients develop cervical ankylosis and have a high risk of cervical fractures.[151] Loss of normal flexibility with increasing osteoporosis predisposes the spine to fracture, usually at the C5-6 and C6-7 levels, even after relatively minor trauma.[149] Salathé and Johr report a case of C7 quadriplegia as a result of emergency endotracheal intubation in a patient with unsuspected ankylosing spondylitis.[151] Because of the danger of undiagnosed fractures, some experts advise that every patient suffering from ankylosing spondylitis have preoperative spine radiographs even though visualization of low cervical fractures may be difficult if not impossible.[150,151] Any patient with a cervical spine injury is at risk for dislocation with any neck movement, and tracheal intubation if needed is probably best achieved with either awake retrograde or fiberoptic intubation.[144]

In addition to cervical spine restrictions, involvement of the temporomandibular joints and cricoarytenoid arthritis may also result in airway difficulties. Limited mouth opening as a result of temporomandibular ankylosis is reported to occur in 10% to 40% of patients, depending on duration of the disease.[150] Cricoarytenoid arthritis may make the vocal cords more susceptible to trauma and/or result in vocal cord fixation.[150,151] The patient should be questioned for any signs of dysphagia, hoarseness, or dyspnea.

Ossification of interspinous ligaments and formation of bony bridges between the vertebrae in addition to restriction in lumbar flexion may make the placement of a spinal or epidural anesthetic impossible. The anesthesiologist should also be aware that spinal cord compression, cauda equina syndrome, focal epilepsy, vertebrobasilar insufficiency, and peripheral nerve lesions have all been described in association with the disease.[150] Obviously these patients should all be questioned and examined for any limitations in spine movement and/or presence of existing neurologic impairment before initiation of an anesthetic. Although ankylosing spondylitis may limit motion of the pelvic joints, it is usually not believed to be a hindrance to vaginal delivery.[152]

A thorough list of medications should be obtained, since drug management may include treatment with NSAIDs. Severe side effects of these medications include renal disease, gastrointestinal bleeding, and thrombocytopenia (indomethacin). There is no demonstrated benefit from corticosteroids in the management of spinal disease in ankylosing spondylitis.[153]

In summary, an anesthetic plan should be carefully constructed for the patient with ankylosing spondylitis especially if severe cardiorespiratory or spine involvement is present. The anesthesiologist should be aware that the pregnant patient with a difficult airway poses an even greater risk for aspiration and hypoxemia because of her full stomach and decreased lung volumes. These patients are probably best managed with an awake intubation if an operative delivery is required.[150] Invasive monitoring is warranted in the presence of severe cardiorespiratory disease. Patients without airway involvement and with signs and symptoms of only minimal spine disease may be managed with regional anesthesia for either vaginal or cesarean delivery.

POLYMYOSITIS AND DERMATOMYOSITIS

Polymyositis is a rare inflammatory disease that affects primarily proximal striated muscle in a symmetrical fashion. When the muscular findings are associated with dermatologic changes, the disease is termed dermatomyositis.

Pathophysiology

The muscular changes are characterized by weakness, and the dermatologic change most often seen is that of an erythematous rash with a violaceous component over the eyelids.[31] In addition, pulmonary fibrosis, pneumonitis, cardiac inflammation, Raynaud's phenomenon, and peripheral arthritis may occur. Renal involvement is rare. Laboratory findings may include a leukocytosis and elevated muscle enzymes. The disease is distinctly uncommon.[154,155] There is a female preponderance of 2:1. The disease has a bimodal age of onset with peaks at 1 to 14 years of age and 40 to 60 years of age.[154] Fertility has been reported to be decreased in patients after the onset of disease.[155]

The outcome of pregnancy varies with the age of onset of disease and the degree of disease activity. In a retrospective review of 10 pregnancies in 5 patients with childhood polymyositis/dermatomyositis, the rate of exacerbation in pregnancy was 40% and pregnancy outcome was quite good.[155] In 8 pregnancies in 5 patients with adult onset polymyositis/dermatomyositis under steroid therapy, 16% of pregnancies conceived with inactive disease had an exacerbation. The two pregnancies conceived with active disease had no change in symptoms. This group of adult onset disease antedating pregnancy had an overall fetal loss rate of 37.5%.[155] In patients with inactive disease, most pregnancies not ending in miscarriage proceed to term. In those patients with acute disease, the overall fetal loss rate was 33%, with only 47% of patients proceeding to term.[155] No obvious placental explanation for the fetal losses has been found, and newborns are not known to be affected by the disease.

Obstetric and anesthetic management

Obstetric management. Pregnancy should be planned when the disease is in remission. Given the high fetal wastage in patients with adult onset polymyositis/dermatomyositis, antepartum surveillance is indicated. Vaginal delivery may be anticipated.

Anesthetic considerations. Anesthetic considerations will depend on the degree of cardiorespiratory involvement. An ECG should be obtained during consultation, since myocardial fibrosis may lead to conduction defects and/or an inflammatory cardiomyopathy. Dysphagia due to weakness of the striated muscles of the pharynx may render the patient more susceptible to aspiration of secretions and/or gastric contents. Weakness of the proximal muscles occurs, usually in the lower extremities initially, and should be documented before initiation of an anesthetic agent. Patients may have joint involvement typical of rheumatoid arthritis or SLE that may render the placement of a regional anesthetic or endotracheal tube technically difficult. As mentioned earlier, pulmonary fibrosis and/or pneumonitis may be present, and a thorough respiratory history and examination should be performed.

Because some patients with dermatomyositis have demonstrated a myasthenic response to neuromuscular blockers, caution in the use of these drugs has been advocated.[156] Flusche and others have reported prolonged neuromuscular blockade with vecuronium in a patient with polymyositis as well, even though no abnormality of neuromuscular transmission was found on electromyogram.[157] Atypical cholinesterase activity has also been reported in these patients.[158]

IMMUNE THROMBOCYTOPENIC PURPURA

Immune (idiopathic) thrombocytopenic purpura (ITP) is the most common autoimmune disorder in women of reproductive age.

Thrombocytopenia may be noted incidentally on routine prenatal screening, or the patient may present with bleeding complications. In the obstetric literature, thrombocytopenia is generally defined as a platelet count of less than 100,000/mm^3. Immune thrombocytopenic purpura is a diagnosis of exclusion in patients with isolated thrombocytopenia and a bone marrow showing normal or increased megakaryocytes. The peripheral blood smear may show an increase in platelet size.

The thrombocytopenia in ITP is the result of clearance of antibody-coated platelets by the reticuloendothelial system, primarily the spleen. The maternal antiplatelet antibody is a 7S gamma globulin that attaches to glycoproteins on the surface of maternal platelets. These antibodies are primarily IgG; they cross the placenta by Fc-mediated active transport and they have been noted to cause thrombocytopenia in 50% to 70% of infants.[159,160] There is a poor correlation between maternal platelet count, antibody status, and fetal platelet count.[161]

Immune thrombocytopenic purpura has been associated with other rheumatic diseases. About 5% to 20% of patients with SLE will exhibit thrombocytopenia. Thrombocytopenia also has been reported in rheumatoid arthritis and Sjögren's syndrome. The antibodies produced in ITP are antiplatelet antibodies but they may be associated with other antibodies such as anticardiolipin and Anti-Ro.[162,163] In patients with other rheumatic diseases, it is critical to review medication history because both gold and penicillamine may suppress platelets.

The aim in the treatment of ITP is to decrease antiplatelet antibody production and to decrease the clearance of antibody-coated platelets. The mainstay of medical therapy is the use of corticosteroids. Steroids are thought to work by decreasing antiplatelet antibody production by the reticuloendothelial system. In addition, they interfere with the interaction between antiplatelet antibodies and the platelet surface. It is also believed that they decrease the clearance of antibody-coated platelets by macrophages in the spleen and liver.[164] The most commonly used drug is prednisone, which crosses the placenta poorly and therefore the fetal effects of transplacentally acquired antiplatelet antibody are not ameliorated.[165] If no response in maternal platelet count is seen within 21 days, another mode of therapy should be considered.

In nonpregnant patients who fail to respond to steroids, splenectomy is the next line of treatment. Removing the spleen removes a large source of antibody production as well as a reservoir of macrophages. Splenectomy is usually not performed in pregnancy but if it must be performed, it should be done in the second trimester. Recently, intravenous gamma globulin has been used to treat patients with ITP. Immunoglobulin G is thought to block the Fc receptor in macrophages.[166] Following intravenous IgG therapy, platelet count usually begins to increase by 48 hours and is maximally elevated at approximately 6 days of therapy.[165,167] The response usually lasts 1 to 4 weeks.

Obstetric management. From a *maternal* viewpoint, the greatest risk of ITP in pregnancy revolves around bleeding from a placental previa or from a placental abruption, or at the time of deliv-

ery. Standard medical therapy including the use of steroids or IV immunoglobulin are not contraindicated during pregnancy. Generally therapy is instituted for patients with platelet counts consistently less than 70,000. Additional therapies including cytotoxic agents must be individually tailored to a given pregnancy in consultation with the hematology department. More difficult is the management of the fetus. Unfortunately, the fetal platelet count is not predictable on the basis of maternal platelet count, antibody titer, or clinical course of disease. This is especially true in patients who have previously undergone splenectomy. Some authors have advocated the change from prednisone to beta methasone at 37 weeks' gestation in an effort to affect fetal platelet count.[163] Fetuses with thrombocytopenia are theoretically at risk of increased hemorrhagic complications. This has previously led some physicians to advocate cesarean section for all patients with ITP, but the benefit of cesarean section in these cases has not been clearly demonstrated. Other authors have advocated the measurement of fetal platelets performed via fetal scalp sampling in early labor to be used in the prediction of the fetal platelet count. If this count were to exceed 50,000 per mm^3, this was used as the basis for selection of route of delivery in these patients. For example, a count greater than 50,000 per mm^3 could be delivered vaginally, and less than 50,000 per mm^3 would require cesarean section because of the theoretic concerns of fetal hemorrhagic morbidity.[168] The main question is, what is the true risk for the fetus of severe thrombocytopenia and fetal morbidity? Burrows and Kelton performed a recent metaanalysis in a 10-year period from 1980 to 1990, reviewing all reports concerning ITP in pregnancy.[169] In this analysis, the important factors must be stated up front. First, there is a consistent "worse case" reporting bias to the literature. Specifically, reports with few patients in them (less than 10 patients) compared with large reports tended to describe poor fetal outcome. The second potential source of bias was the timing of the fetal platelet count. It is recognized that platelet counts in the neonate may fall significantly after delivery, specifically several days after delivery. This may be important for further management of the neonate; however, it is less important in making decisions concerning the type of delivery. Results of their analysis indicate that the risk of severe thrombocytopenia leading to poor outcome in infants born to mothers with ITP is much lower than generally has been appreciated. In the group from which the fetal platelet sample was obtained, there were no major morbidity events in infants delivered vaginally or by cesarean section. The fetal platelet sample is defined as a platelet count obtained from the cordocentesis, an umbilical vein sample, and/or a scalp sample, verified by neonatal platelet immediately after birth. There were five adverse outcomes in neonates with low platelet counts after birth. However, this was not related to the type of delivery. Statistically there was no correlation to morbidity, whether birth was vaginal or by cesarean section.

Fetal scalp sampling has been reported as successful by some investigators, while others believe the procedure is unreliable and often leads to erroneous information and inappropriate intervention. In particular, the platelets may often clump, resulting in a falsely low platelet count and thus a clinical decision for a cesarean section.

SUMMARY

Maternal recommendations at Brigham and Women's Hospital (Boston):

1. Monthly platelet counts, if they remain greater than 70,000. If the platelets fall below 70,000, medical therapy including prednisone and/or IV-Ig may be instituted in consultation with a hematologist.
2. If necessary, further therapy such as cytotoxic therapy should be deferred until consultation with a hematologist.
3. Intrapartum, if the platelet count remains above 70,000, no specific precautions are necessary. If the mother's platelet count is below 50,000, one should consider notifying the blood bank for possible short-term platelet transfusion.

Fetal Recommendations:

1. There is no test or maneuver that can predict neonatal thrombocytopenia. Maternal platelet count and the measurement of maternal platelet IgG have not been shown to be useful predictors of neonatal thrombocytopenia.

    We do not currently recommend cordocentesis. The measurement of antiplatelet IgG has been shown to be a very poor predictor of neonatal thrombocytopenia. Specifically, it has been reported to have a sensitivity of 22% and a positive predictive value of 25%.

    Fetal scalp sampling typically is associated with unsuccessful attempts and/or erroneously low results (due to platelet clumping) that leads to the wrong clinical decision (i.e., cesarean section). Therefore, we do not routinely recommend fetal scalp sampling.
2. We recommend avoidance of a difficult forceps delivery or a prolonged second stage of labor in these patients. A cesarean delivery in this situation may be more prudent.

3. Pediatricians should be notified early regarding maternal ITP because neonatal platelet counts may drop precipitously following delivery.

Anesthetic considerations. The anesthetic management of the parturient with ITP will depend on the severity of her disease. Manifestations may range from simply a subclinical decrease in platelet count seen on routine laboratory screening to a patient presenting with petechiae, bleeding gums, and retinal hemorrhages. In severe cases a patient may present with life-threatening internal bleeding and/or intracranial hemorrhage.

Mothers with mild disease and a normal bleeding time pose no special anesthetic considerations. However, those with abnormal bleeding times,* whether or not platelet count is normal, should not be considered for regional anesthesia because they may be prone to epidural hematoma from persistent venous oozing. Analgesia may be provided to these women in the form of intravenous narcotic drugs, given intermittently or via a patient-controlled device. It should also be recognized that these mothers are at increased risk for airway bleeding. Therefore, intubation, if needed, must be done with care and the patients must be observed closely following extubation for signs of bleeding leading to airway obstruction. Avoidance of nasal endotracheal intubation and atraumatic airway instrumentation is essential, because mucosal hemorrhage is a definite concern when platelet counts decrease below $50,000 \times 10^3/mm^3$. The anesthetic management of the mother who presents with a normal bleeding time despite a low platelet count ($<100,000/mm^3$) is controversial, since some anesthesiologists believe regional anesthesia is contraindicated and others do not. Most experts recommend avoidance of epidural catheter placement in patients with platelet counts $<50,000 \times 10^3/mm^3$ or if a platelet count of $<100,000 \times 10^3/mm^3$ is accompanied by a prolonged bleeding time.[170,171] Thromboelastography is also a rapidly developing tool to aid in the diagnosis of true platelet dysfunction.[172] In controversial cases, additional factors such as maternal risk for general anesthesia (should it be needed), alternative pain relief options, and fetal well-being should be considered before making a decision.

If platelet transfusion is deemed necessary, the anesthesiologist should realize that platelet sur-

---

*The use of bleeding time is controversial, and most hematologists and anesthesiologists are staying away from this test.—*Editor*

vival is decreased in patients with ITP as a result of platelet destruction; it has been reported to be as short as 48 to 230 minutes after administration.[173] Because of this, preoperative transfusion should be planned as close to surgery as possible. Use of single-donor plateletpheresis may reduce transmission of hepatitis, exposure to platelet alloantigens, and the incidence of febrile reactions.[174] While a decrease in bleeding time will no doubt be seen following platelet administration, regional anesthesia is still thought to be contraindicated in these patients because of the transient nature of the improvement.

Those mothers already receiving steroid therapy, or within the last 6 months, should be maintained on full-dose coverage peripartum.

AUTOIMMUNE HEMOLYTIC ANEMIA

Autoimmune hemolytic anemia has been reported in pregnancy. In this disease process, the patient develops autoantibodies to the antigens on her red blood cells. These antibodies are primarily divided into two classes: the warm reacting antibodies and the cold antibodies. Warm antibodies are primarily of the IgG subtype and may cross the placenta. Warm antibodies are associated with hematologic malignancies, SLE, viral infections, and drug ingestion. Cold antibodies are primarily of the IgM subtype and therefore do not cross the placenta. Cold antibodies are associated with mycoplasma infections and infectious mononucleosis. A positive direct Coomb's test is the most commonly used test to detect an antibody. Both cold and warm antibodies, alone and in combination, have been reported in pregnancy.

Anesthetic management. The anesthesiologist should be aware that transfusion therapy may be complicated in these patients because the autoantibody is directed to a component of the Rh locus that is present on the erythrocytes of essentially all potential donors.[175] In emergencies, the least incompatible cells available should be used for transfusion. In patients with severe cold agglutinin disease, the cool operating room may cause agglutination to occur with resultant acrocyanosis, Raynaud's phenomenon, purpura, acryl gangrene, or immune complex nephritis. This may then lead to hemolysis and may cause severe anemia, hemoglobinuria, and renal failure.[176] Preoperative plasmapheresis, intraoperative forced air surface warming, and warming of all intravenous solutions are effective techniques in preventing this cascade of events.

SUMMARY

From the amount of information presented in this chapter, it is obvious that when pregnancy occurs in the patient with an autoimmune disease numerous problems in the areas of medical, obstetric, and anesthetic management may arise. These problems may be minor or life-threatening, depending on the degree of end-organ involvement by the disease and the course of pregnancy, which is also often altered by the disease. In addition, the pregnancy itself often influences the course of the disease. It is only with close cooperation and communication between the expectant mother and her obstetrician, internist, and anesthesiologist that her autoimmune disease and pregnancy both can be safely managed.

REFERENCES

1. Hollingsworth JW, Resnick R: Rheumatologic and connective tissue disorders, in Creasy RK, Resnick R (eds): *Maternal-Fetal Medicine: Principles and Practice.* Philadelphia, WB Saunders, 1989, pp 1057-1072.
2. Nepon GT, Byers P, Seyfried C, et al: HLA genes associated with rheumatoid arthritis: Identification of susceptibility alleles using specific oligonucleotide probes. *Arthritis Rheum* 1989; 32:15.
3. Larsen BA, Alderice CA, Hawkins D, et al: Protective HLA-DR phenotypes in rheumatoid arthritis. *J Rheumatol* 1989; 16:455.
4. Roudier J, Petersen J, Rhodes GH, et al: Susceptibility to rheumatoid arthritis maps to a T-cell epitope shared by the HLA-Dw4 DR beta-1 chain and the Epstein-Barr virus glycoprotein gp 110. *Proc Natl Acad Sci USA* 1989; 86:5104.
5. Gaston JS, Life PF, Bailey LC, et al: In vitro responses to a 65-kilodalton mycobacterial protein by synovial T cells from inflammatory arthritis patients. *J Immunol* 1989; 143:2494.
6. Firestein GS, Xu WD, Townsend K, et al: Cytokines in chronic inflammatory arthritis. I. Failure to detect T cell lymphokines (IL-2 and IL-3) and presence of macrophage colony-stimulating factor (CSF-1) and a novel mast cell growth factor in rheumatoid synovitis. *J Exp Med* 1988; 168:1573.
7. Morrissey PJ, Bressler L, Park LS, et al: Granulocyte-macrophage colony-stimulating factor augments the primary antibody response by enhancing the function of antigen-presenting cells. *J Immunol* 1987; 139:1113.
8. Masi AT, Maldanado-Cocco JA, Kaplan SB, et al: Prospective study of the early course of rheumatoid arthritis in young adults: Comparison of patients with and without rheumatoid factor positivity at entry and identification of variables correlating with outcome. *Semin Arthritis Rheum* 1976; 5:299.
9. Hench PG: The ameliorating effect of pregnancy and jaundice on chronic atrophic (infectious rheumatoid) arthritis, fibrositis and intermittent hydrarthrosis. *Proc Mayo Clin* 1938; 13:161.
10. Persellin RH: The effect of pregnancy on rheumatoid arthritis. *Bull Rheum Dis* 1977; 27:922.
11. Klipple GL, Cecere FA: Rheumatoid arthritis and pregnancy. *Rheum Dis Clin North Am* 1989; 15:213.
12. Oskensen M, Aune LB, Husley G: Effect of pregnancy and hormonal changes on the activity of rheumatoid arthritis. *Scand J Rheumatol* 1983; 12:69.
13. Bijlsma JW, Van Den Brink HR: Estrogens and rheumatoid arthritis. *Am J Reprod Immunol* 1992; 28:231.
14. Jara-Quezada L, Graef A, Lavalle C: Prolactin and gonadal hormones during pregnancy in systemic lupus erythematosus. *J Rheumatol* 1991; 18:349.

15. Unger A, Kay A, Griffin AJ, et al: Disease activity and pregnancy associated alpha-2-glycoprotein in rheumatoid arthritis during pregnancy. *Br Med J* 1983; 286:750.

16. Nelson JL, Hughes KA, Smith AG, et al: Maternal-fetal disparity in HLA Class II alloantigens and the pregnancy-induced amelioration of rheumatoid arthritis. *N Engl J Med* 1993; 329:466.

17. Neely NT, Persellin RH: Activity of rheumatoid arthritis during pregnancy. *Tex Med* 1977; 73:59.

18. Thompson SJ, Hitsumoto Y, Zhang YW, et al: Agalacto-syl IgG in pristane-induced arthritis. Pregnancy affects the incidence severity of arthritis and the glycosylation status of IgG. *Clin Exp Immunol* 1992; 89:434.

19. Silver RM, Branch DW: Autoimmune disease in pregnancy. *Ballieres Clin Obstet Gynaecol* 1992; 6:565.

20. Quinn C, Mulpeter K, Casey EB, et al: Changes in levels of IgM RF and alpha 2 PAG correlate with increased disease activity in rheumatoid arthritis during the puerperium. *Scand J Rheumatol* 1993; 22:273.

21. Spector TD, Silman AJ: Is poor pregnancy outcome a risk factor in rheumatoid arthritis? *Ann Rheum Dis* 1990; 49:12.

22. Slone D, Heinonen OP, Kaufman D, et al: Aspirin and congenital malformations. *Lancet* 1976; 1:1373.

23. Byron MA: Prescribing in pregnancy: Treatment of rheumatic diseases. *Br Med J* 1987; 294:236.

24. Lewis RB, Shulman JD: Influence of acetyl-salicylic acid: An inhibitor of prostaglandin synthesis on the duration of human gestation and labour. *Lancet* 1973; 11:1159.

25. Stuart M, Gross SJ, Elrad H, et al: Effect of acetyl salicylic-acid ingestion on maternal and neonatal hemostasis. *N Engl J Med* 1982; 307:909.

26. Rumack CM, Guggenheim MA, Rumack BH, et al: Neonatal intracranial hemorrhage and maternal use of aspirin. *Obstet Gynecol* 1981; 5:5256.

27. Manchester O, Margolis H, Sheldon RE: Possible association between maternal indomethacin therapy and primary pulmonary hypertension of the newborn. *Am J Obstet Gynecol* 1976; 126:467.

28. Goudie BM, Dossetor JFB: Effects on the fetus of indomethacin given to suppress labor. *Lancet* 1979; 2:1187.

29. Goldsmith DP: Neonatal rheumatic disorders: View of the pediatrician. *Rheum Dis Clin North Am* 1989; 15:287.

30. Gabbe SG: Drug therapy in autoimmune disease. *Clin Obstet Gynecol* 1983; 26:635.

31. Urowitz MD, Gladman DD: Rheumatic disease in pregnancy, in Burrow GN, Ferris TF (eds): *Medical Complications During Pregnancy,* ed 3. Philadelphia, WB Saunders, 1988, pp 499-525.

32. Ostenson M, Husby G: Antirheumatic drug treatment during pregnancy and lactation. *Scand J Rheumatol* 1985; 14:1.

33. Lyle WH: Penicillamine in pregnancy. *Lancet* 1978; 1:606.

34. Scheinberg IH, Sternlieb I: Pregnancy in penicillamine treated patients with Wilson's disease. *N Engl J Med* 1977; 296:54.

35. Solomon L, Abram G, Dinner M, et al: Neonatal abnormalities associated with D-penicillamine treatment during pregnancy. *N Engl J Med* 1977; 296:54.

36. Mjolnerod IK, Demmerud SA, Rasmussen K, et al: Congenital connective tissue defect probably due to penicillamine treatment during pregnancy. *Lancet* 1971; 1:673.

37. Persellin RH: The effect of pregnancy on rheumatoid arthritis. *Bull Rheum Dis* 1977; 27:922.

38. Keenan MA, Stiles CM, Kaufman RL: Acquired laryngeal deviation associated with cervical spine disease in erosive polyarticular arthritis. *Anesthesiology* 1983; 58:441.

39. White RH: Perioperative evaluation of patients with rheumatoid arthritis. *Semin Arthritis Rheum* 1985; 14:287.

40. Thurnau GR: Rheumatoid arthritis. *Clin Obstet Gynecol* 1983; 26:558.

41. Ostensen M: Pregnancy in patients with a history of juvenile rheumatoid arthritis. *Arthritis Rheum* 1991; 34:881.

42. Person D: Juvenile rheumatoid arthritis: Anesthetic and surgical considerations. *AORN J* 1986; 44:439.

43. Ruddy S, Roberts WN: Rheumatoid arthritis, in Lichtenstein LM, Fauci AS (eds): *Current Therapy in Allergy, Immunology, and Rheumatology,* ed 3. Toronto, BC Decker, 1988, p 110.

44. Sachs BP, Lorell GH, Mehrez M, et al: Constrictive pericarditis and pregnancy. *Am J Obstet Gynecol* 1986; 154:156.

45. Das DB, Gupta RP, Sukamar P, et al: Pericardiectomy: Indications and results. *J Thorac Cardiovasc Surg* 1973; 66:58.

46. Estes D, Larson DL: Systemic lupus erythematosus and pregnancy. *Clin Obstet Gynecol* 1965; 8:307.

47. Hollingsworth JW, Resnick R: Rheumatologic and connective tissue disorders, in Creasy RK, Resnick R (eds): *Maternal-Fetal Medicine: Principles and Practice,* Philadelphia, WB Saunders, 1989.

48. Mills JA: Systemic lupus erythematosus. *N Engl J Med* 1994; 330:1871.

49. Tan EM, Cohen AS, Fries JF, et al: The 1982 revised criteria for the classification of systemic lupus erythematosus arthritis and rheumatism. *Arthritis Rheum* 1982; 25:1271.

50. Syrop CH, Varner MW: Systemic lupus erythematosus. *Clin Obstet Gynecol* 1983; 26:547.

51. Zulman JI, Talal N, Hoffman GS, et al: Problems associated with the management of pregnancies in patients with systemic lupus erythematosus. *J Rheumatol* 1980; 7:37.

52. Zurier RB, Argyros TG, Urman JD, et al: Systemic lupus erythematosus: Management during pregnancy. *Obstet Gynecol* 1978; 51:178.

53. Garsentstein M, Pollak VE, Karik RM: Systemic lupus erythematosus and pregnancy. *N Engl J Med* 1962; 276:165.

54. Lockshin MD, Reinitz E, Druzin ML, et al: Lupus pregnancy case control prospective study demonstrating absence of lupus exacerbation during or after pregnancy. *Am J Med* 1984; 77:893.

55. Mintz G, Rodriguez-Alvarez E: Systemic lupus erythematosus. *Rheum Dis Clin North Am* 1989; 15:255.

56. Lockshin MD: Pregnancy does not cause systemic erythematosus to worsen. *Arthritis Rheum* 1989; 32:665.

57. Hayslett JP, Lynn RI: Effect of pregnancy in patients with lupus nephropathy. *Kidney Int* 1980; 18:207.

58. Jungers P, Dougados M, Pelissier C, et al: Lupus nephropathy and pregnancy: Report of 104 cases in 36 patients. *Arch Intern Med* 1982; 142:771.

59. Hayslett JP, Reece EA: Systemic lupus erythematosus in pregnancy. *Clin Perinatol* 1985; 12:539.

60. Bobrie G, Liote F, Houillier P, et al: Pregnancy in lupus nephritis and related disorders. *Am J Kidney Dis* 1987; 9:339.

61. Mor-Yosef S, Navot D, Rabinowitz R: Collagen diseases in pregnancy. *Obstet Gynecol Surv* 1984; 39:67.

62. Fraga A, Mintz G, Orozco J, et al: Sterility and fertility rates, fetal wastage and maternal morbidity in systemic lupus erythematosus. *J Rheumatol* 1974; 1:293.

63. Fine LG, Barnett EV, Danovitch GM, et al: Systemic lupus erythematosus in pregnancy. *Ann Intern Med* 1981; 94:667.

64. Abramowski CR, Vegas ME, Swinehart G, et al: Decidual vasculopathy of the placenta in lupus erythematosus. *N Engl J Med* 1980; 303:668.

65. Houser MT, Fish AJ, Tagatz GE, et al: Pregnancy and systemic lupus erythematosus. *Am J Obstet Gynecol* 1980; 138:409.
66. Devoe LD, Taylor R: Systemic lupus erythematosus in pregnancy. *Am J Obstet Gynecol* 1979; 135:473.
67. Mintz G, Niz J, Gutierrez G, et al: Prospective study of pregnancy in systemic lupus erythematosus: Results of multidisciplinary approach. *J Rheumatol* 1986; 13:732.
68. Lockshin MD, Bonfa E, Elkon K, et al: Neonatal lupus risk to newborns of mothers with systemic lupus erythematosus. *Arthritis Rheum* 1988; 31:697.
69. Scott SS, Maddison PJ, Taylor PV, et al: Connective tissue disease, antibodies to ribonucleoprotein and congenital heart block. *N Engl J Med* 1983; 309:209.
70. Ramsey-Goldman R, Hom R, Deng JS, et al: Anti-SS-A antibodies and fetal outcome in maternal systemic lupus erythematosus. *Arthritis Rheum* 1986; 29:1269.
71. Harley JB, Kaine JL, Fox OF, et al: Ro (SSA) antibody and antigen in a patient with congenital complete heart block. *Arthritis Rheum* 1985; 28:132.
72. Litsey SE, Noonan JA, O'Connor WN, et al: Maternal connective tissue disease and congenital heart block: Demonstration of immunoglobulin in cardiac tissue. *N Engl J Med* 1985; 312:98.
73. Buyon JP, Swersky SH, Fox HE, et al: Intrauterine therapy for presumptive fetal myocarditis with acquired heart block due to systemic lupus erythematosus: Experience in a mother with predominance of SS-B (La) antibodies. *Arthritis Rheum* 1987; 30:44.
74. Bierman FZ, Baxi L, Jaffe I, et al: Fetal hydrops and congenital complete heart block: Response to maternal steroid therapy. *J Pediatr* 1988; 112:646.
75. Herreman G, Galezowski N: Maternal connective tissue disease and congenital heart block. *N Engl J Med* 1985; 312:1329.
76. Hanly JG, Gladman DD, Rose TH, et al: Lupus pregnancy: A prospective study of placental changes. *Arthritis Rheum* 1988; 31:358.
77. Guzman J, Avalos E, Ortiz R, et al: Placental abnormalities in systemic lupus erythematosus: In situ deposition of antinuclear antibodies. *J Rheumatol* 1987; 14:924.
78. Lubbe WF, Liggins GC: Lupus anticoagulant and pregnancy. *Am J Obstet Gynecol* 1985; 153:322.
79. Druzin ML, Lockshin M, Edersheim TG, et al: Second trimester fetal monitoring and preterm delivery in pregnancies with systemic lupus erythematosus and/or circulating lupus anticoagulant. *Am J Obstet Gynecol* 1987; 157:1503.
80. Lubbe WF, Butler WS, Palmer SJ, et al: Lupus anticoagulant in pregnancy. *Br J Obstet Gynecol* 1984; 91:357.
81. Branch WB, Scott JR, Kochenour NK, et al: Obstetric complications associated with lupus anticoagulant. *N Engl J Med* 1985; 313:1321.
82. Lockshin MD, Druzin ML, Goli S, et al: Antibody to cardiolipin as a predictor of fetal distress or death in pregnant patients with systemic lupus erythematosus. *N Engl J Med* 1985; 313:152.
83. Lockshin MD, Qamar T, Druzin ML, et al: Antibody to cardiolipin lupus anticoagulant and fetal death. *J Rheumatol* 1987; 14:259.
84. Harris EN, Asherson RA, Gharavi AE, et al: Thrombocytopenia in SLE and related autoimmune disorders: Association with anticardiolipin antibody. *Br J Haematol* 1985; 59:227.
85. Mueh JR, Herbst KD, Rappaport SI: Thrombosis in patients with the lupus anticoagulant. *Ann Intern Med* 1980; 92:156.
86. Jungers PL, Liote F, Dautzenberg MD, et al: Lupus anticoagulant and thrombosis in systemic lupus erythematosus. *Lancet* 1984; 1:574.
87. Lubbe WF, Palmer SJ, Butler WS, et al: Fetal survival after prednisone suppression of maternal lupus anticoagulant. *Lancet* 1983; 1:1361.
88. Stafford-Brady FJ, Gladman DD, Urowitz MB: Successful pregnancy in systemic lupus erythematosus with an untreated lupus anticoagulant. *Arch Intern Med* 1988; 148:1647.
89. Lockshin MD, Druzin ML, Qamar T: Prednisone does not prevent recurrent fetal death in women with antiphospholipid antibody. *Am J Obstet Gynecol* 1989; 160:439.
90. Buyon JP, Cronstein BN, Morris M, et al: Serum complement values (C3 and C4) to differentiate between systemic lupus activity and pre-eclampsia. *Am J Med* 1986; 81:194.
91. Tozman ECS, Urowitz MB, Gladman DD: Systemic lupus erythematosus and pregnancy. *J Rheumatol* 1980; 7:624.
92. Devoe LD, Loy GL: Serum complement levels and perinatal outcome in pregnancies complicated by systemic lupus erythematosus. *Obstet Gynecol* 1984; 63:796.
93. Beitins IZ, Bayard F, Ances IG: The transplacental passage of prednisone and prednisolone in pregnancy near term. *J Pediatr* 1972; 81:936.
94. Blandford AT: In vitro metabolism of prednisolone, dexamethasone, betamethasone and cortisol by the human placenta. *Am J Obstet Gynecol* 1977; 127:264.
95. Ballard PL, Granbeg P, Ballard RA: Glucocorticoid levels in maternal and cord serum after prenatal betamethasone therapy to prevent respiratory distress syndrome. *J Clin Invest* 1975; 56:15.
96. Osathanondh R, Tulchinsky D, Kamali H: Dexamethasone levels in treated pregnant women and newborn infants. *J Pediatr* 1977; 90:617.
97. Reinisch JM, Simon NG, Karwo WG, et al: Prenatal exposure to prednisone in humans and animals retards intrauterine growth. *Science* 1978; 202:436.
98. Cote CJ, Meuwissen HJ, Pickering RJ: Effects on the neonate of prednisone and azathioprine administered to the mother during pregnancy. *J Pediatr* 1974; 85:324.
99. Scott JR: Fetal growth retardation associated with maternal administration of immunosuppresive drugs. *Am J Obstet Gynecol* 1977; 128:668.
100. Neille WA, Panayi GS, Duthie JJ, et al: Action of chloroquine phosphate in rheumatoid arthritis. II. Chromosome damaging effect. *Ann Rheum Dis* 1973; 32:547.
101. Ullberg S, Lindquist NG, Sjostrand SE, et al: Accumulations of chorioretinotoxic drugs in the foetal eye. *Nature* 1970; 227:1257.
102. Maltz GJ, Nanuton RF: Ototoxicity of chloroquine. *Arch Otolaryngol* 1968; 88:50.
103. Parke AL: Antimalarial drugs and pregnancy. *Am J Med* 1988; 85:30.
104. Burge SM, Frith PA, Juniper RP, et al: Mucosal involvement in systemic and chronic cutaneous lupus erythematosus. *Br J Dermatol* 1989; 121:727.
105. Raz E, Bursztyn M, Rosenthal T, et al: Severe recurrent lupus laryngitis. *Am J Med* 1992; 92:109.
106. Steinberg AD: Systemic lupus erythematosus, in Wyngaarden JB, Smith LH, Lloyd H Jr (eds): *Cecil Textbook of Medicine.* Philadelphia, WB Saunders/Harcourt Brace Jovanovich, 1988, p 2011.
107. Richardson EP Jr, Systemic lupus erythematosus, in Vinken PJ, Bruyn GW (eds): *Neurological Manifestations of Systemic Diseases. Part II. of Handbook of Clinical Neurology,* vol 39, Amsterdam, North-Holland, 1980; 273.
108. Hanly JG, Walsh NMG, Sangalang V: Brain pathology in systemic lupus erythematosus. *J Rheumatol* 1992; 19:732.
109. Malinow AM, Rickford WJK, Mokriski BLK, et al: Lupus anticoagulant: Implications for obstetric anaesthetists. *Anaesthesia* 1987; 42:1291.

110. Espinoza LR, Hartmann RC: Significance of the lupus anticoagulant. *Am J Hematol* 1986; 22:331.
111. Lowson SM: Lupus anticoagulant: Implications for the obstetric anaesthesiologist. *Anaesthesia* 1987; 43:508.
112. Abouleish E: Obstetric anesthesia and systemic lupus erythematosus. *Middle East J Anesthesiol* 1988; 9:435.
113. McNeil HP, Chesterman CN, Krilis SA: Immunology and clinical importance of antiphospholipid antibodies. *Adv Immunol* 1991; 49:193.
114. Branch DW, Silver RM, Blackwell JL, et al: Outcome of pregnancies in women with antiphospholipid syndrome: An update of the Utah experience. *Obstet Gynecol* 1992; 80:614.
115. Coaldrake LA, Livingstone P: Myasthenia gravis in pregnancy. *Anaesth Intensive Care* 1983; 11:254.
116. McNall PG, Jafarnia MR: Management of myasthenia gravis in the obstetrical patient. *Am J Obstet Gynecol* 1965; 92:518.
117. Baraka A: Anesthesia and myasthenia gravis. *MEJ Anesth* 1993; 12:9.
118. Pitkin RM: Autoimmune diseases in pregnancy. *Semin Perinatol* 1977; 1:161.
119. Foldes FF, McNall PG: Myasthenia gravis: A guide for anesthesiologists. *Anesthesiology* 1962; 23:837.
120. Engel WK, Festoff BW, Patten BM, et al: Myasthenia gravis. *Ann Intern Med* 1974; 81:225.
121. Rolbin SH, Levinson G, Shnider SM, et al: Anesthetic considerations for myasthenia gravis and pregnancy. *Anesth Analg* 1978; 57:441.
122. Usubiaga JE, Wikinski JA, Morales RI: Interaction of intravenously administered procaine, lidocaine and succinylcholine in anesthetized subjects. *Anesth Analg* 1967; 46:39.
123. Plauche WC: Myasthenia gravis. *Clin Obstet Gynecol* 1983; 26:592.
124. Baraka A: Anaesthesia and myasthenia gravis. *Can J Anaesth* 1992; 39:476.
125. Saito Y, Sakura S, Takatori, et al.: Epidural anesthesia in a patient with myasthenia gravis. *Acta Anesthesiol Scand* 1993; 37:513.
126. Leventhal SR, Orkin FK, Hirsh RA: Prediction of the need for postoperative mechanical ventilation in myasthenia gravis. *Anesthesiology* 1980; 53:26.
127. Black CM, Stevens WM: Scleroderma. *Rheum Dis Clin North Am* 1989; 15:193.
128. Humphreys MH, Alfrey AC: Vascular diseases of the kidney, in Brenner BM, Rector FC Jr (eds): *The Kidney,* ed 3. Philadelphia, WB Saunders, 1986, pp 1193-1196.
129. Steen VD, Conte C, Day N, et al: Pregnancy in women with systemic sclerosis. *Arthritis Rheum* 1989; 32:151.
130. Scarpinato L, Mackenzie AH: Pregnancy and progressive systemic sclerosis: Case report and review of the literature. *Cleve Clin Q* 1985; 52:207.
131. Spellacy WN: Scleroderma and pregnancy. *Obstet Gynecol* 1964; 23:297.
132. Ballou SD, Morley JJ, Kushner I: Pregnancy and systemic sclerosis. *Arthritis Rheum* 1984; 27:295.
133. Palma A, Sanchez-Palencia A, Armas JR, et al: Progressive systemic sclerosis and nephrotic syndrome: An unusual association resulting in postpartum acute renal failure. *Arch Intern Med* 1981; 141:520.
134. Giordano M, Valentini G, Lupoli S, et al: Pregnancy and systemic sclerosis. *Arthritis Rheum* 1985; 28:23.
135. Silman A, Black CM: Increased incidence of spontaneous abortion and infertility with scleroderma before disease onset: A controlled study. *Ann Rheum Dis* 1988; 47:441.
136. Slate WB, Graham AR: Scleroderma in pregnancy. *Am J Obstet Gynecol* 1968; 101:335.
137. Goplervo CP: Scleroderma. *Clin Obstet Gynecol* 1983; 26:587.
138. Moore M, Saffran JG, Baraf HSB, et al: Systemic sclerosis and pregnancy complicated by obstructive uropathy. *Am J Obstet Gynecol* 1985; 153:593.
139. Bellucci MJ, Coustan DR, Plotz RD: Cervical scleroderma: A case of soft tissue dystocia. *Am J Obstet Gynecol* 1984; 150:891.
140. Weisman RA, Calcaterra TC: Head and neck manifestations of scleroderma. *Ann Otol* 1978; 87:332.
141. Siegel RC: Scleroderma. *Med Clin North Am* 1977; 61:283.
142. Bulkley BH, Ridolfi RL, Salyer WR, et al: Myocardial lesions of progressive systemic sclerosis: A cause of cardiac dysfunction. *Circulation* 1976; 53:483.
143. Thompson J, Conklin K: Anesthetic management of a pregnant patient with scleroderma. *Anesthesiology* 1983; 59:69.
144. Eisele JH, Reitan JA: Scleroderma, Raynaud's phenomenon, and local anesthetics. *Anesthesiology* 1971; 34:386.
145. Calcaterra TC: Laryngeal and pharyngeal edema of obscure origin. *Arch Otolaryngol* 1972; 96:341.
146. Ostensen M, Husby G: Ankylosing spondylitis and pregnancy. *Rheum Dis Clin North Am* 1989; 15:241.
147. Ostensen M, Husby G: A prospective clinical study of the effect of pregnancy on rheumatoid arthritis and ankylosing spondylitis. *Arthritis Rheum* 1983; 26:1155.
148. Ostenson M, Romberg O, Husby G: Ankylosing spondylitis and motherhood. *Arthritis Rheum* 1982; 25:140.
149. Pirlo AF, Herren AL: Ankylosing spondylitis: Case report and review of literature. *Anesthesiol Rev* 1978; 5:13.
150. Sinclair JR, Mason RA: Ankylosing spondylitis: The case for awake intubation. *Anaesthesia* 1984; 39:3.
151. Salathé M, Johr M: Unsuspected cervical fractures: A common problem in ankylosing spondylitis. *Anesthesiology* 1989; 70:869.
152. Heckman JD, Sassard R: Musculoskeletal considerations in Pregnancy. *J Bone Joint Surg* 1994; 76:1720.
153. Korn JH: Ankylosing spondylitis, in Lichtenstein LM, Fauci AS (eds): *Current Therapy in Allergy, Immunology and Rheumatology.* Toronto, BC Decker, 1988, p 134.
154. Rosenzweig BA, et al: Primary idiopathic polymyositis and dermatomyositis complicating pregnancy: Diagnosis and management. *Obstet Gynecol Surv* 1989; 44:162.
155. Gutierrez G, Pagnino R, Mintz G: Polymyositis/dermatomyositis and pregnancy. *Arthritis Rheum* 1984; 27:291.
156. Wylie WD, Churchill-Davidson HC: *A Practice of Anaesthesia,* ed 5. Philadelphia, WB Saunders, p 744.
157. Flusche G, Sargon-Unger J, Lambert DH: Prolonged neuromuscular paralysis with vecuronium in a patient with polymyositis. *Anesth Analg* 1987; 66:188.
158. Eielsen O, Stovner J: Dermatomyositis, suxamethonium action and atypical plasmacholinesterase. *Can Anaesth Soc J* 1978; 25:63.
159. Kagan R, Laros RK: Immune thrombocytopenia. *Clin Obstet Gynecol* 1983; 26:537.
160. Laros RK, Sweet RL: Management of idiopathic thrombocytopenia purpura during pregnancy. *Am J Obstet Gynecol* 1975; 122:182.
161. Scott JR, Rote NS, Cruikshank DP: Antiplatelet antibodies and platelet counts in pregnancies complicated by autoimmune thrombocytopenic purpura. *Am J Obstet Gynecol* 1983; 145:932.
162. Harris EN, Chan JK, Asherson RA, et al: Predictive value of the anticardiolipin antibody test. *Arch Intern Med* 1986; 146:2153.
163. Watson R, Kang JE, May M, et al: Thrombocytopenia in the neonatal lupus syndrome. *Arch Dermatol* 1988; 124:56.

164. Martin JM, Morrison JC, Files JC: Autoimmune thrombocytopenic purpura: Current concepts and recommended practices. *Am J Obstet Gynecol* 1984; 150:86.

165. Karpatkin M, Porges RF, Karpatkins: Platelet counts in infants of women with autoimmune thrombocytopenia: Effect of steroid administration to the mother. *N Engl J Med* 1981; 305:936.

166. Besa EC, MacNub MN, Solar AJ, et al: High-dose intravenous IgG in the management of pregnancy in women with idiopathic thrombocytopenia purpura. *Am J Hematol* 1985; 18:373.

167. Tchernia G, Dreyfus M, Laurian Y, et al: Management of autoimmune thrombocytopenia in pregnancy: Response to infusion of immunoglobulins. *Am J Obstet Gynecol* 1984; 148:225.

168. Scott JR, Cruikshank DP, Kochenour NK, et al: Fetal platelet counts in the obstetric management of immunologic thrombocytopenic purpura. *Am J Obstet Gynecol* 1980; 136:495.

169. Burrows RF, Keilton JG: Pregnancy in patients with idiopathic thrombocytopenic purpura: Assessing the risks for the infants at delivery. *Obstet Gynecol Surv* 1993; 48:781.

170. Schindler M, Gatt S, Isert P, et al.: Thrombocytopenia and platelet defects in preeclampsia: Implications for regional anesthesia. *Anaesth Intensive Care* 1990; 18:169.

171. Rolbin SH, Abbott D, Musclow E, et al.: Epidural anesthesia in pregnant patients with low platelet counts. *Obstet Gynecol* 1988; 6:918.

172. Steer PL: Anaesthetic management of a parturient with thrombocytopenia using thromboelastography and sonoclot analysis [letter]. *Can J Anaesth* 1993; 40:84.

173. Angiulo JP, Temple JT, Corrigan JJ, et al: Management of cesarean section in a patient with idiopathic thrombocytopenic purpura. *Anesthesiology* 1977; 46: 145.

174. Kitzmiller JL: Autoimmune disorders: Maternal, fetal, and neonatal risks. *Clin Obstet Gynecol* 1978; 21:385.

175. Schreiber AD: Autoimmune hemolytic anemia, in Lichtenstein LM, Fauci AS (eds): *Current Therapy in Allergy, Immunology and Rheumatology.* Toronto, BC Decker, 1988, pp 280-284.

176. Beebe DS, Bergen L, Palahniuk RJ: Anesthetic management of a patient with severe cold agglutinin hemolytic anemia utilizing forced air warming. *Anesth Analg* 1993; 76:1144.

20 The Diabetic Parturient

Sanjay Datta and *Michael F. Greene*

The prognosis for diabetic women and their offspring has improved steadily and dramatically since the introduction of insulin. In the first two decades of this century, half of the diabetic women attempting to carry pregnancies to term died, and half of the offspring of the surviving women died. As we enter the last decade of the century, the incidence of maternal mortality has become so small that it is difficult to measure. However, significant morbidity such as hypoglycemia, diabetic ketoacidosis, hypertension, and exacerbations of nephropathy and retinopathy still occur with greater frequency during pregnancy. Perinatal mortality is now less than one tenth of what it was when insulin was introduced, but is still twice that for the general population. As the absolute magnitudes of the risks fall, it is important not to become complacent and to understand the pathophysiology of the potential complications that await the unwary. Optimizing outcome furthermore requires close communication among internist, obstetrician, anesthesiologist, and pediatrician.

PATHOPHYSIOLOGY

Several pathophysiologic processes that affect both mother and fetus will ultimately govern the obstetric and anesthetic management of the diabetic parturient and are discussed in this section.

Uteroplacental insufficiency

Placental insufficiency is one of the most important pathophysiologic changes that can be influenced by the anesthetic technique and can directly impact on neonatal well-being.

Placental perfusion. Placental abnormalities have been observed even in association with mild, well-controlled gestational diabetes. Nylund et al compared uteroplacental blood flow in the last trimester of pregnancy in 26 diabetic gravidas to that of 41 healthy nondiabetic pregnant women.[1] They used intravenous indium 113 and recorded the radiation over the placentas with a computer-linked gamma camera. They found a 35% to 45% decrease in uteroplacental blood flow index in diabetic women. Although the blood flow index further decreased with higher blood glucose, there

was no statistically significant difference in the flow between the gestational diabetic patients and the patients whose diabetes antedated their pregnancies. Bjork and Persson[2] observed enlarged villi with a concomitant reduction of the intervillous space. This may help to explain the increased density of the placenta of diabetic women and decreased placental blood flow.

Respiratory physiology. Hemoglobin A_{1c} (Hb A_{1c}) is a glycosylated hemoglobin species. Its concentration is proportional to the level of blood glucose for the 6 weeks prior to its measurement. Determinations of levels of Hb A_{1c} have been used clinically for some time to assess the degree of glycemic control among diabetic patients. Concentrations among diabetic women may be two to three times higher than nondiabetic individuals. Beyond being a useful clinical tool, the glycosylation of hemoglobin has physiologic implications for oxygen transport. Madsen and Ditzel[3] have shown that as the percentage of glycosylated hemoglobin rises, the amount of oxygen, molecule for molecule, carried by hemoglobin falls (Fig. 20-1). The avidity with which the oxygen is bound is also changed. The affinity of hemoglobin for oxygen is normally modulated by binding with 2,3-diphosphoglycerate (2,3-DPG) so that in the presence of 2,3-DPG the P_{50} rises (i.e., the oxygen is less firmly bound). Bunn et al[4] demonstrated that Hb A_{1c} changes its P_{50} only minimally in the presence of 2,3-DPG. Madsen and Ditzel[3] have also observed that the P_{50} is inversely correlated with the concentration of Hb A_{1c} (Fig. 20-2). The displacement of oxygen from native hemoglobin that is facilitated by 2,3-DPG binding is also associated with the acceptance of a proton (H^+) by the deoxygenated hemoglobin (the Bohr effect) and thus contributes to the buffering capacity of blood. Hemoglobin A_{1c} with its more tightly bound oxygen will release the oxygen less well at areas of reduced oxygen tension, such as the placental bed. Diabetic patients who are chronically poorly controlled will have high levels of Hb A_{1c} that will carry less oxygen and release it less well in the periphery.

The effects of chronic hyperglycemia on the oxygen-carrying properties of maternal hemoglo-

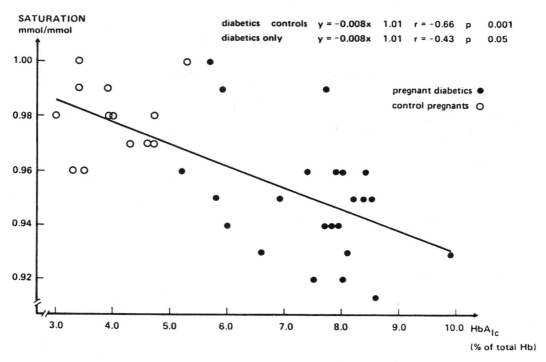

Fig. 20-1 Correlation between Hb A_{1c} and arterial oxygen saturation in diabetic women. (From Madsen H, Ditzel J: *Am J Obstet Gynecol* 1982; 143:421-424. Used by permission.)

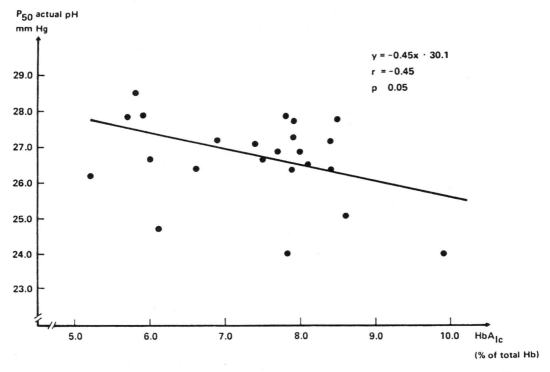

Fig. 20-2 Correlation between Hb A_{1c} and P_{50} at actual pH in diabetic women. (From Madsen H, Ditzel J: *Am J Obstet Gynecol* 1982; 143:421-424. Used by permission.)

bin discussed above are exacerbated by the fetal effects of acute maternal hyperglycemia. Fetal hyperinsulinemia increases the oxygen requirement of the fetus. This is true regardless of how the fetus is rendered hyperinsulinemic. Fetal hyperinsulinemia can be induced experimentally through maternal administration of sulfonylureas[5] or by direct infusion of insulin in chronically catheterized fetuses.[6,7] This occurs most commonly in routine clinical care through maternal hyperglycemia. Although the diabetic mother may be relatively insulin deficient, her fetus is endocrinologically intact. Maternal hyperglycemia is noticed promptly by the fetus since glucose rapidly crosses the placenta to reach concentrations approximately equal to those in the mother. The fetus responds by pouring out insulin from its pancreas. Fetal oxygen consumption rises in direct proportion to the insulin concentration, resulting in falls in both venous and arterial oxygen contents (Fig. 20-3, A and B). Oxygen supply is unable to keep pace with demand, resulting in a progressive rise in the arteriovenous oxygen difference between the umbilical artery and vein (Fig. 20-3, C). Thus, through different mecha-

nisms, acute and chronic hyperglycemia contributes to fetal hypoxia and acidosis.

Diabetic ketoacidosis

One of the major causes of fetal mortality and morbidity in diabetic parturients is diabetic ketoacidosis (DKA); fetal loss has been reported to be as high as 50%.[8] With modern management, however, maternal mortality is so rare that the rate of mortality from DKA is impossible to estimate accurately. There are several causes than can induce diabetic patients to ketoacidosis: (1) inadequate insulin therapy in the face of an otherwise minor illness; (2) omission of the insulin doses in the presence of gastroenteritis because of the parturients' concern about the possibility of an insulin reaction due to associated anorexia, nausea, and vomiting; (3) pump malfunction in patients receiving continuous subcutaneous insulin; and (4) tocolytic therapy with β-sympathomimetic agents, with or without concomitant glucocorticoid therapy.

Pathophysiology. DKA occurs in the presence of both a relative or absolute deficiency of insulin and a relative or absolute increase in the major counter-regulatory hormone, glucagon. The com-

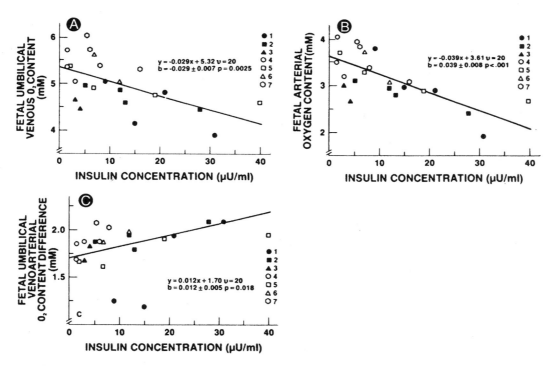

Fig. 20-3 The association between fetal plasma insulin concentration and fetal arterial oxygen content (**A**), fetal venous oxygen content (**B**), and fetal umbilical venoarterial oxygen content difference (**C**). Shown is the regression line as determined by analysis of covariance. Also shown are the regression equations and the slopes with their standard errors and *P* values. Data from seven animals are represented by the symbols shown in the figure. (From Milley JR, Rosenberg AA, Philipps AF, et al: *Am J Obstet Gynecol* 1984; 149:673. Used by permission.)

bined state of hypoinsulinemia and hyperglucogonemia is associated with increased hepatic glucose production and decreased peripheral glucose utilization, ultimately causing severe hyperglycemia. In addition, β-stimulation, either through exogenous β-mimetic agents or endogenous epinephrine release due to stress, inhibits insulin-induced glucose transport into peripheral tissues. The resulting hyperglycemia can cause osmotic diuresis and dehydration, characteristic of DKA. Potassium and sodium concentrations are decreased because of osmotic diuresis.

Uncontrolled diabetes will activate the β-oxidative enzymes in the liver, which metabolize free fatty acids to ketone bodies. β-Hydroxybutyrate and acetoacetate will decrease the maternal pH and stimulate the respiratory center. Because of acidosis, intracellular potassium is decreased as it is replaced by hydrogen ions, total body potassium is thus depleted. Loss of maternal fluid volume will decrease cardiac output and blood pressure and may ultimately leads to cardiovascular collapse and shock.

Effect on the fetus. Fetal heart rate (FHR) during maternal DKA is frequently associated with the development of nonreassuring FHR patterns. These patterns, however usually resolve with treatment of the maternal metabolic disorder without obvious neonatal sequelae. Most obstetricians suggest delaying fetal intervention until the mother is metabolically stabilized.

Clinical features. Classical presentations include (1) anorexia, (2) nausea, (3) vomiting, (4) polyuria, (5) polydypsia, (6) tachycardia, and (7) abdominal pain or muscle cramps. If severe, the picutre could include (1) Kussmaul hyperventilation, (2) signs of volume depletion (e.g., hypotension and oliguria), (3) lethargy to coma, (4) normal-to-cold body temperature, and (5) fruity odor may be noticeable on the patient's breath.

Diabetic parturients can develop ketoacidosis with blood glucose as low as 200 mg/dl. Presence of ketones, loss of maternal areterial pH of less than 7.30 and anion gap will confirm the diagnosis.

Treatment
Volume replacement. Volume replacement should include two intravenous lines, one for rapid fluid infusion and a second for insulin therapy. Initial treatment should be with normal saline at a rate of 15 to 20 ml/kg/hr, 400 ml/m²/hr, or approximately 1 L/h for the first 2 hours of the resuscitation. This will rapidly replete the intravascular volume, improving general tissue perfusion, permitting excretion of glucose in the urine, and slowing potassium wasting in the urine. A Foley catheter should be placed early

in the resuscitation to accurately monitor urine output. Fluid therapy should be reduced in the third and subsequent hours to 7.5 ml/kg/hr according to the clinical situation and urine output. This will prevent hypoglycemia and provide substrate to suppress lipolysis and ketogenesis. As the blood glucose level comes down to 300 to 250 mg/dl, the intravenous fluid solution should be changed to 5% glucose in water. Bicarbonate is only indicated if the maternal pH is less than 7.10. Because of excessive potassium loss, potassium may have to be replaced; hence, extra cellular potassium concentrations should be measured frequently. Intravenous fluids should be continued until all nausea and vomiting have resolved, bowel sounds are present, and the patient is able to tolerate adequate quantities of fluids by mouth.

Patient management with severe DKA does require a setting in which the patient can be monitored with a 1:1 nurse/patient ratio.

Hypertension

Hypertension and/or preeclampsia are common problems among diabetic gravidas. We have recently reported the incidence and impact of this problem among our patient population at Brigham and Women's Hospital.[9] We observed that 29.8% of all pregnancies were associated with a hypertensive disorder. Since only 6% of the patients were known to have hypertensive disorders antedating pregnancy, the majority of these patients had pregnancy-induced hypertension. Hypertension was the major cause of premature delivery, accounting for one third of all premature births (Table 20-1). In addition to the usual degree of hemodynamic fragility associated with severe preeclampsia, many of these patients with longstanding nephropathy have low serum albumin levels and very low colloid oncotic pressures. This makes them particularly vulnerable to pulmonary edema if they are vigorously volume-loaded in preparation for regional anesthesia.

Table 20-1 Prematurity and hypertensive complications by White's class

White's class	Prematurity (%) (<37 weeks)	Hypertensive complications (%)
B	20.4	17.5
C	17.4	23.1
D	25.7	30.7
F	52.5	66.1
R	30.5	25.0
All classes combined	26.2	29.8

Defective epinephrine and growth hormone responses in Type I diabetes

Hirsch and colleagues observed counterregulatory hormone responses to hypoglycemia in Type I diabetic and control patients. The diabetic individuals exhibited normal increment in plasma growth hormone (GH), norepinephrine, and cortisol, but blunted or absent responses in plasma epinephrine and glucagon when hypoglycemia was severe (<40 mg/dl).[10] Hence, it can be emphasized that two counterregulatory hormones that are important for glucose homeostasis may be reduced in Type I diabetic patients. The clinical implications of the phenomenon in diabetic parturients is not known; however, one must be vigilant about the clinical parameters of hypoglycemia in diabetic parturients undergoing cesarean section, especially under general anesthesia.

Impaired cardiac adjustment

Airaksinen and colleagues made an interesting observation by using echocardiography to assess, in diabetic patients, the adaptation of the heart to an increase of blood volume during pregnancy.[11] The mean duration of diabetes was 14 years, and 6 of these 17 patients had microvascular complications. The authors observed a slightly smaller left ventricle in diabetic patients, compared with the control group in the basal state. The pregnancy-induced increase in left ventricular size, stroke volume, and heart rate were observed to be less in dia-

betic parturients. The authors suggested that normal hemodynamic adjustments to pregnancy were impaired in diabetic parturients. The blunted increases of stroke volume and heart rate were associated with the reduced resting cardiac output in diabetic pregnant women. The mechanisms of these changes are not well understood; however, the factors that might be involved are (1) preclinical diabetic cardiomyopathy, and (2) subclinical autonomic neuropathy. Anesthetic implications of these changes might be important. Judicious volume expansion and use of epidural anesthesia for cesarean section might be preferred.

Stiff joint syndrome

Stiff joint syndrome is a rare condition consisting of juvenile-onset diabetes, nonfamilial short stature, and joint contractures.[12] If there is a suggestion of stiff joint syndrome, the patient should have flexion-extension radiographs taken of the cervical spine. Limited atlanto-occipital extension might make intubation difficult, and awake tracheal intubation with or without fiberoptic bronchoscopy may be necessary. A "prayer sign," which is defined by the patient's inability to approximate the palmar surfaces of the phalangeal joints despite maximal effort, secondary to diabetic stiff joint syndrome, may be beneficial for the anesthesiologist (Fig. 20-4) to detect patients with associated involvement of the atlanto-occipital joint.

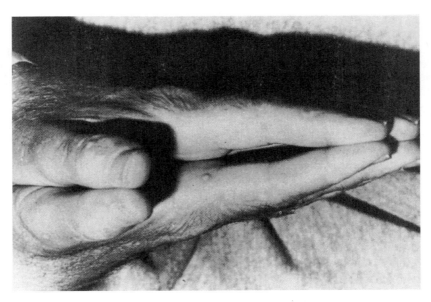

Fig. 20-4 The patient is unable to approximate the palmar surfaces of the phalangeal joints despite maximal effort (a "prayer sign"), secondary to diabetic stiff joint syndrome, which may also involve the atlanto-occipital joint. (From Hogan K, Rusy D, Springman SR: *Anesth Analg* 1988; 67:1162. Used by permission.)

Diabetic scleredema

Diabetic scleredema is synonymous with stiff joint syndrome. Eastwood reported a case of anterior spinal artery syndrome after administration of epidural anesthesia for cesarean section in a parturient with stiff joint syndrome. The cause of the complication was unclear; however, the possible mechanisms, as suggested by the authors, were (1) rigid epidural space because of pathologic changes in the connective tissues and ligaments, which made the epidural space less compliant; (2) diminished arterial supply to the spinal cord due to the increased pressure in the noncompliant epidural space because of the high volume of the local anesthetic agent (35 ml) used in this case; and (3) preexisting microvascular disease.

METABOLIC AND OBSTETRIC CONSIDERATIONS

It is clear that no single medical or obstetric intervention for diabetic gravidas has been as important in improving their prognosis as improved metabolic control. Early pregnancy is often associated with some degree of anorexia, nausea, and vomiting, which result in a decreased calorie intake. For diabetic women who take a fixed daily dose of insulin, this can frequently lead to hypoglycemic episodes in the first trimester. Many diabetic women will recognize early pregnancy by the increased frequency of insulin reactions. As pregnancy progresses through the second trimester, placental production of human placental lactogen, which antagonizes the action of insulin, rises. This causes a dramatic increase in insulin requirements to levels 150% and 200% of the prepregnancy requirements. Frequently requirements are noted to peak around 36 weeks and decrease slightly toward term. Trying to adjust to the constantly changing insulin requirement during pregnancy can be a difficult and frustrating experience for a patient. Just when she thinks she has the right dose, it changes. At Brigham and Women's Hospital, we usually see patients weekly during pregnancy to help them with their glycemic control.

Insulin therapy

There has been considerable discussion regarding the best insulin regimen for achieving optimal glycemic control in pregnancy. The majority of patients will achieve adequate control with a conventional "split-mix" regimen of regular- and intermediate-acting insulin. Some patients seem to do better if the evening dose is broken into two injections, one regular dose before dinner and one intermediate dose before bed.

Ultralente given once or twice daily with premeal doses of regular insulin has become some-what more popular recently. Continuous subcutaneous insulin infusion (CSII) via pump is a labor-intensive method of insulin therapy that requires a very motivated patient. Supplies are expensive, pumps can malfunction, and it is not clear that this method offers significant advantages for large numbers of patients.[13,14] No one of these regimens is clearly superior to any other. Some patients do better with one method than another, and experimentation is helpful. Oral hypoglycemic agents are not appropriate during pregnancy.

Blood glucose monitoring

More important than the precise regimen according to which the insulin is administered is monitoring the results. Any serious effort at achieving euglycemia must include self-monitoring of home capillary blood glucose. It is very unusual to have a patient who cannot be taught to test her own blood sugar level. We ask patients to test their glucose level four times daily; fasting and 2 hours after each meal. The patients are given forms to record their glucose values and they are reviewed at each weekly visit. We aim for fasting values below 105 mg/dL and 2-hour postprandial values of 140 mg/dL or less. We obtain a Hb A_{1c} determination at the first prenatal visit and monthly thereafter.

Congenital anomalies

The first published documentation that poor glycemic control in the first trimester could lead to an increased incidence of congenital anomalies came from the Joslin Clinic. Miller[15] demonstrated that women with Hb A_{1c} concentrations of greater than 8.5% in the first trimester had a 22% risk of major congenital anomaly, while this risk was only 3.3% when Hb A_{1c} was less than 8.5%. Subsequently, Fuhrmann et al[16] have shown that strenuous efforts at rigid control, including frequent hospitalization, can reduce the incidence of congenital anomalies in a diabetic population.

The multicentered National Institute of Child Health and Development (NICHD) Diabetes in Early Pregnancy (DIEP) project was designed to examine the relationship between early metabolic control and major congenital malformations. The investigators have recently completed their study and have begun to present the findings. They found an increased risk of major anomalies among infants of diabetic mothers as compared with nondiabetic controls. They were unable, however, to document any increase in the incidence of major anomalies among the infants of the 350 diabetic parturients that related to increasing level of Hb A_{1c} in the first trimester.[17] Patients were recruited into the study before conception or within 21 days

Table 20-2 Major malformations according to first-trimester Hb A_1 level*

SD above mean	Percentage†	Major malformations	No major malformations	Percentage‡	Risk ratio (95% confidence interval)
≤ 6	≤ 9.3	6	187	3.1	1.0
6.1-9.0	9.4-11.0	9	134	6.3	2.0 (0.7-5.4)
9.1-12.0	11.1-12.7	6	70	7.9	2.5 (0.9-7.4)
12.1-15.0	12.8-14.4	9	18	33.3	10.7 (4.8-23.8)
>15.0	>14.4	5	7	41.7	13.4 (5.5-32.5)

*Joslin Clinic data through 12/31/90.
†Hb A_1 as a percentage of total hemoglobin.
‡Major malformations as a percentage of all pregnancies progressing beyond the first trimester.

Table 20-3 Spontaneous abortions according to first-trimester Hb A_1 level*

SD above mean	Percentage†	Spontaneous abortions	Continuing pregnancies	Percentage‡	Risk ratio (95% confidence interval)
≤ 6	≤ 9.3	31	193	13.8	1.0
6.1-9.0	9.4-11.0	18	143	11.2	0.8 (0.5-1.4)
9.1-12.0	11.1-12.7	23	76	23.2	1.7 (1.03-2.7)
12.1-15.0	12.8-14.4	13	27	32.5	2.4 (1.3-4.2)
>15.0	>14.4	7	12	36.8	2.7 (1.3-5.5)

*Joslin Clinic data through 12/31/90.
†Hb A_1 as a percentage of total hemoglobin.
‡Spontaneous abortions as a percentage of all registered pregnancies.

of conception. It seems likely that such a self-selected group would be in relatively good control during the first trimester. The failure of the project to find a relationship between degree of control and anomalies is probably due to the fact that the study population was rather homogeneous, with few patients in poor metabolic control available for study.

We have recently completed another large study of the relationship between first-trimester glycosylated levels of Hb A_1 and the risk for fetal malformation at the Joslin Clinic; in this, we again observed a strong relationship[18] (Table 20-2). It appears from the very carefully done DIEP study with its own nondiabetic concurrent controls that even well-controlled diabetic women have a greater incidence of malformed infants than do nondiabetic women. The risk for major malformation, however, does not vary over a broad range of glycemic control but rises sharply with very poor control.

Spontaneous abortion

There has been considerable debate as to whether diabetic women in general have an increased incidence of spontaneous abortion. Several studies have indicated that diabetic women with high Hb A_{1c} values in the first trimester are at increased risk

for spontaneous abortion.[19] Recently published data from the DIEP confirm the increased risk of spontaneous abortion associated with poor first trimester metabolic control.[20] Data from the Joslin Clinic[18] also show a significant relationship between first-trimester Hb A_{1c} and the risk for spontaneous abortion (Table 20-3).

Macrosomia

Macrosomia has long been recognized as an important complication of maternal diabetes. According to the classic Pedersen hypothesis, maternal hyperglycemia produces fetal hyperglycemia and thus fetal hyperinsulinemia. The hyperinsulinemia acts as an anabolic stimulus, leading to enhanced accretion of fat, bone, and muscle mass. In support of this hypothesis, Sosenko has documented that macrosomic fetuses of diabetic women have high C peptide levels and are at risk for neonatal hypoglycemia.[21] Attempts to correlate a variety of indices of glycemic control (e.g., mean daily glucose levels, Hb A_{1c}) with risk for macrosomia have had limited success.[22-25] Furthermore, case reports abound documenting the fact that some patients can be in excellent glycemic control by all known parameters and yet deliver remarkably macrosomic fetuses.[26] Macrosomic fetuses are at substantial risk for birth trauma.[27]

BOX 20-1   MODIFIED WHITE'S CLASSIFICATION OF DIABETES IN PREGNANCY

Gestational Diabetes Mellitus Noninsulin Requiring (GDMNI): Abnormal carbohydrate tolerance during pregnancy only not requiring insulin.

Gestational Diabetes Mellitus Insulin Requiring (GDMI): Abnormal carbohydrate tolerance during pregnancy only requiring insulin.

Class A: Abnormal carbohydrate tolerance in the nonpregnant state identified prior to the present pregnancy that does not require insulin either prior to or during the pregnancy.

Class B: Onset of insulin-requiring diabetes after 20 years of age, with duration of less than 10 years.

Class C: Onset of insulin-requiring diabetes between ages 10 and 20 with duration of less than 20 years, or duration 10 to 20 years regardless of age of onset.

Class D: Onset of insulin-requiring diabetes prior to age 10 years, or duration greater than 20 years regardless of age of onset, or insulin-requiring diabetes with chronic hypertension, or insulin-requiring diabetes with benign retinopathy.

Class F: Insulin-requiring diabetes with diabetic nephropathy (proteinuria of greater than 500 mg in a 24-hour urine collection).

Class R: Insulin-requiring diabetes with proliferative retinopathy.

Class T: Insulin-requiring diabetes with renal transplant.

Class H: Insulin-requiring diabetes with coronary artery disease.

Classification

In 1949 Priscilla White proposed the classification of diabetes in pregnancy that later came to bear her name.[28] It was based on criteria that could be identified at the time of the patient's first prenatal visit, including age of onset, duration of diabetes, and presence or absence of microvascular or macrovascular complications. She attempted to correlate these classes with pregnancy outcome, hoping to provide guidelines for the management of the pregnancy and a basis for counseling the patient regarding her prognosis. The system has been modified to add gestational diabetes, which White did not specifically recognize, and renal transplants, which did not previously exist. Other classes have been dropped, such as class E with calcified pelvic vessels on x-ray studies. Several of the classes are not substantially different from one another in many respects, but the modified White's classification system is still useful (Box 20-1).

Gestational diabetes

The hormonal changes of advancing gestation antagonize insulin action, as discussed above. It should not be a surprise then that some women who begin pregnancy with marginal carbohydrate tolerance will become frankly intolerant as pregnancy advances. Since undiagnosed and untreated gestational diabetes of significant degree can result in obstetric complications, women should be screened for gestational diabetes. The method of screening has become a controversial issue. There are several historic risk factors that dispose toward

---

BOX 20-2   RISK FACTORS FOR GESTATIONAL DIABETES

Maternal age 30 years or greater
Family history of diabetes mellitus
Obesity
Previous delivery of macrosomic infant
Previous near-term stillbirth

---

gestational diabetes (Box 20-2). Anyone with any of these risk factors or anyone who spills glucose into the urine at any time should be screened biochemically. Controversy exists as to whether screening by historic risk factors is adequate or whether all pregnant women should be screened biochemically. It has been shown that if a large population is screened biochemically, only one half the patients with abnormal carbohydrate tolerance would have been detected through screening by history. Would this 50% detection rate be essentially all of the people with significant disease and therefore adequate? Approximately half of all deliveries in the United States now involve women having their first babies. These women are not eligible for two of the five criteria listed in the box. Some argue that 50% detection is inadequate and that the only way to deal with the problem is through universal biochemical screening. There is evidence that universal screening coupled with an aggressive approach to insulin therapy in gestational diabetes can reduce the incidence of macrosomia and the necessity for operative delivery due to that macrosomia.[29] However, there has not been a series to date that demonstrates universal screening can reduce the perinatal mortality rate. This is partly due to the fact that the perinatal mortality rate is so low, and a huge study would be necessary that would be very difficult to complete. Currently, the position of the American College of Obstetricians and Gynecologists (ACOG) is that initial screening by history followed up with biochemical testing is appropriate. The position of the American Diabetes Association is that all patients should be screened biochemically.

The issues of how and when to screen are considerably less controversial. A 50-g oral glucose load followed by a single blood glucose test 1 hour after the load should be done at 24 to 28 weeks' gestation. A glucose loading test (GLT) value of 140 mg/dL or more should be followed with a 100-g 3-hour oral glucose tolerance test (GTT). The upper limits of normal for the GTT are: fasting, 105 mg/dL; 1 hour, 190 mg/dL; 2 hours, 165 mg/dL; and 3 hours, 145 mg/dL. Two or more abnormal values define gestational diabetes.

Patients with abnormal glucose tolerance should be placed on appropriate diets and have their blood glucose levels checked regularly. If they normalize their glucose levels on diet alone, then they can be managed as normal obstetric patients. If the fasting glucose levels are in excess of 105 mg/dL or the postprandial levels are greater than 120 mg/dL, the patient should start insulin therapy and be managed as a diabetic patient.

Antenatal monitoring for fetal well-being

The incidence of unexpected near-term demise has been reduced dramatically in the past decade; this is at least partly attributable to careful monitoring. The nonstress test (NST) is the standard, with the oxytocin challenge test (OCT) or contraction stress test (CST) used to evaluate the nonreactive NST in all diabetic parturients. We routinely begin weekly NST at 32 weeks and perform them twice weekly from 36 weeks until delivery. Although some authors have reported an unacceptable incidence of loss using this scheme,[30] we have had only 2 losses of nonmalformed singletons in the third trimester among our last 578 consecutive patients with diabetes antedating pregnancy. It has been proposed that the biophysical profile[31] and Doppler umbilical flow velocity analysis[32] be integrated into the care of these patients, but there is neither much experience nor any motivation to substitute these techniques with the NST. The NST is inexpensive to perform, and it is fast and reliable.

Lung maturity testing

It has been known for some time that the lungs of infants of diabetic mothers (IDM) mature less rapidly than those of nondiabetic women. Furthermore, these infants tend to develop respiratory distress syndrome (RDS) at lecithin/sphingomyelin (L/S) ratios that would indicate maturity for infants of nondiabetic women. To avoid RDS in these patients, a variety of strategies have been tried. Bringing more of the patients closer to term prior to elective delivery is most important. Before electively delivering a diabetic parturient at less than 39 weeks' gestation, fetal lung maturity should be assessed. The presence of a relatively high concentration of phosphatidylglycerol (PG) in the amniotic fluid as demonstrated by thin-layer chromatography in the standard assay is a reliable indicator of maturity. Unfortunately it is a very conservative estimator and only 50% of PG-negative fetuses will develop RDS. We prefer to use a combination of the L/S ratio and quantitation of saturated phosphatidylcholine (SPC) to predict lung maturity. In practice, any IDM with an SPC of greater than 1000 µg/dL and/or an L/S ratio of 3.5 or greater is extremely unlikely (risk <1/260) to develop RDS.

Route and timing of delivery

The route and timing of delivery for diabetic gravidas have always been matters of concern. Prior to the early 1970s the major concern was to avoid late intrauterine demise. Early deliveries, however, were associated with neonatal morbidity and mortality from RDS. Improved glycemic control and electronic assessment of fetal well-being reduced the risk of late demise. Fetal lung maturity testing methods permitted obstetricians to assure lung maturity prior to elective delivery. The decline in perinatal mortality due to late demise and RDS has permitted attention to focus on remaining sources of morbidity and mortality. Chief among these are macrosomia and its associated high incidences of operative delivery and birth trauma. Although the risks for shoulder dystocia and subsequent birth injury increase with increasing birth weight in the general population, these risks are magnified among IDM.[27] It has been suggested that this may be due to the body habitus of the IDM with unusually broad shoulders in relation to the head size.[33]

A variety of strategies have been suggested to minimize the risk of traumatic delivery among IDM. These have included earlier delivery of infants projected to be macrosomic at term and prophylactic cesarean section for macrosomic babies. Unfortunately, earlier delivery is associated with an increased risk for multiple minor morbidities in the nursery, including hyperbilirubinemia and feeding difficulties even after lung maturity has been assured. Attempts to induce labor earlier in pregnancy will also encounter less favorable cervical conditions and result in a higher than necessary cesarean section rate. The major challenges, then, in planning the deliveries of diabetic women are: (1) to minimize the exposure to risk of a late intrauterine demise; (2) to minimize intrapartum fetal distress and recognize and treat it promptly if it occurs; (3) to minimize the risks of traumatic birth injury, RDS, and other sources of neonatal morbidity and mortality; (4) to minimize the cesarean section rate; and (5) to meet the parents' expectations for the birthing experience to the greatest possible extent.

Elective deliveries are planned between 38 and 40 weeks' gestation for all women with insulin-requiring diabetes antedating pregnancy. An ultrasound examination is performed prior to delivery to estimate the fetal weight. If the fetal weight is estimated to be less than 4000 g, a pelvic delivery is planned. If the fetus is estimated to weigh more than 4000 g, a cesarean delivery is planned unless the patient has a history of a previous uncomplicated pelvic delivery of a baby of more than 4000 g. Every effort is made to await a favorable cervical examination prior to the induction of labor.

OBSTETRIC AND ANESTHETIC MANAGEMENT
Management of labor and delivery

A patient scheduled for induction of labor is given one-third her usual morning dose of intermediate-acting insulin, and no regular insulin. Blood glucose levels are monitored hourly during labor via finger sticks and a reflectance meter on the labor floor. If the blood glucose goes above 120 mg/dL, an intravenous infusion of regular insulin is used to bring the blood glucose level within normal limit. It is particularly important during labor to maintain a normal blood glucose level because hyperglycemia will magnify the degree of acidosis caused by any degree of hypoxemia that may occur. To avoid the accidental infusion of a large volume of glucose-containing intravenous fluid, the main line is always a non–glucose-containing solution. A 5% glucose-containing solution is "piggybacked" into the main line via an infusion pump at 125 mL/hr. Immediately postpartum the insulin requirement drops dramatically so that for a brief period it is usually less than the prepregnancy dose. On the first postpartum day, the patient should be given one half the prepregnancy dose of intermediate-acting insulin with regular insulin as necessary.

All laboring patients should be electronically monitored continuously with liberal use of scalp pH sampling when necessary. Prophylactic antibiotics are not routinely used for patients undergoing cesarean section with intact membranes and without labor. If a patient has been in labor or has had ruptured membranes prior to cesarean section, then prophylaxis is indicated. A single dose of intravenous antibiotic given at the time of cord clamping has been shown to be effective in series of nondiabetic patients. Whether a more extensive program including second and third doses of antibiotic offers any greater efficacy in diabetic parturients is unknown. Similarly, it is not obvious that the more expensive third-generation cephalosporins offer any advantage over cephazolin or even ampicillin.

Anesthetic mancgement for labor and vaginal delivery. Moderate pain of early labor can be relieved with small doses of narcotic drugs (e.g., butorphanol or nalbuphine). The main problem with larger doses of systemic medication is maternal and neonatal respiratory depression. Prolonged labor and decreased uteroplacental perfusion associated with maternal hemodynamic changes due to intravenous narcotics may result in fetal acidosis. Fetal acidosis subsequently can alter the placental transfer of the drugs, affect the perinatal homeostasis, and ultimately potentiate the depressant effects of these drugs. Pain and anxiety associated with natural childbirth may further decrease the placental perfusion as a result of increased catecholamine concentrations.[34] Paracervical block can also cause fetal hypoxia because of umbilical and uterine arterial vasoconstriction. Reduced placental perfusion as well as deranged buffering capacity will affect IDM significantly more than it will infants of normal parturients. Epidural analgesia is associated with a few obvious advantages: (1) it will reduce maternal endogenous catecholamine release and indirectly will increase placental blood flow; (2) it will reduce the maternal lactic acid production and hence fetal acidosis,[35] and (3) it will provide excellent pain relief during the first stage as well as during the second stage especially if forceps delivery is necessary. Induction of epidural analgesia might be started with 0.25% bupivacaine and a continuous infusion of 0.125% 0.0625% bupivacaine with 2 μg/mL of fentanyl (8-10 mL/hr) can be used during the first stage. For forceps delivery, dense perineal anesthesia might be necessary; this can be provided by an adequate dose of 3% 2-chloroprocaine. Fetal heart rate tracing before induction and throughout the epidural analgesia should be monitored carefully. If there is associated preeclampsia, then determinations of clotting parameters will be essential for these patients before the use of regional analgesia. In the absence of epidural analgesia, spinal anesthesia may be necessary in case of forceps delivery. This technique will provide good perineal relaxation and hence less chance of birth trauma; this is especially important for delivery of a large baby. Hyperbaric lidocaine (1.5%) or bupivacaine (0.75%) can be used. A separate intravenous line for the rapid infusion of nondextrose solution to prevent hypotension may be necessary, since maternal hypotension should be treated aggressively in these patients.

Anesthetic management for cesarean section. Anesthesia for cesarean section requires special attention for diabetic parturients. Hemodynamic alterations are more dramatic during cesarean section compared with vaginal delivery because of (1) higher sympathetic blockade, and sympathetic tone might also alter in long-standing diabetic patients; and (2) aortocaval compression by the gravid uterus accentuates the problem of hypotension, especially when associated with high sympathetic block.

In 1977 Datta and Brown compared spinal and general anesthesia for cesarean section in healthy and diabetic parturients (Table 20-4).[36] Infants delivered of diabetic women receiving spinal anesthesia were significantly more acidotic than the infants of parturients who had general anesthesia. This difference was not apparent in healthy individuals. This acidosis was mixed (respiratory and metabolic) and related to both maternal diabetes and to maternal hypotension. In a subsequent study they observed maternal and neonatal acid base values following epidural anesthesia in diabetic parturients[37] (Table 20-4); there was a 60% incidence of neonatal acidosis (umbilical artery pH of 7.20 or less). Interestingly, the fetal acidosis related to

both the severity of maternal diabetes and to the presence of maternal hypotension. The umbilical artery pH was always higher than 7.20 in the absence of maternal hypotension. In both studies, the authors used 5% dextrose with lactated Ringer's solution for acute volume expansion and treated maternal hypotension when systolic blood pressure dropped below 100 mm Hg.

The mechanism responsible for fetal acidosis in diabetic parturients remains unclear, but multiple complex factors might be associated with this observation: (1) the human placenta has been observed to produce lactate in vitro, especially under conditions of hypoxia,[38] and the lactate concentration can further increase in the presence of excess glycogen, as occurs in diabetic pregnancy; (2) elevated fetal blood glucose has been shown to be associated with fetal acidosis. Swanstrom and Bratteby observed a significant correlation between blood glucose concentration and base deficit in infants with low 1-minute Apgar scores.[39] More recently, in a randomized controlled study of maternal intravenous fluid administration with or without dextrose in healthy parturients having abdominal delivery, Kenepp et al observed significantly lower umbilical artery pH values in infants of mothers who received glucose infusion.[40] It is possible that hypoxia following maternal hypotension might produce fetal lactic acidemia in the presence of hyperglycemia as a result of acute volume expansion of dextrose. To investigate this hypothesis, Kitzmiller et al observed the effect of acute hyperglycemia in monkey fetuses subjected to acute maternal hypoxia.[41] The control group of monkeys received the same volume of normal sa-

Table 20-4 Effect of maternal hypotension on neonatal acid base status in diabetic parturients

	No hypotension	Hypotension
Spinal anesthesia ($n = 15$)[32]		
Umbilical artery		
pH	7.24 ± 0.02*	7.16 ± 0.01†
Po_2 (mm Hg)	19 ± 2	16 ± 2
Pco_2 (mm Hg)	65 ± 3	71 ± 4
Base deficit (mEg/L)	4.35 ± 0.88	8.25 ± 1.74†
	$n = 9$	$n = 6$
Epidural anesthesia ($n = 16$)[33]		
Umbilical artery		
pH	7.26 ± 0.02	7.16 ± 0.01†
Po_2 (mm Hg)	25 ± 2.5	18 ± 1.3†
Pco_2 (mm Hg)	52 ± 2	65 ± 3†
Base deficit (mEq/L)	5 ± 1.2	10 ± 0.6†
	$n = 6$	$n = 10$

*Mean ± standard error.
†$P < 0.05$.

line and underwent the same duration of hypoxia. Hyperglycemic fetuses showed several interesting clinical findings: (1) a greater reduction in arterial oxygen tension and content than controls, even in the presence of similar maternal arterial oxygen partial pressure in each group; and (2) severe metabolic acidosis (umbilical artery pH 7.06) compared with a modest reduction of umbilical artery pH (7.23) in normoglycemic fetuses. Carson et al in an animal model observed that chronic infusion of insulin directly into the sheep fetus increased fetal glucose uptake and oxidative utilization of glucose, and surprisingly reduced arterial oxygen content.[7] They suggested that hyperinsulinemia can increase oxygen consumption and that fetal hyperglycemia and hyperinsulinemia might result in reduced fetal oxygenation in pregnancies complicated by uncontrolled diabetes. Datta et al[42] reevaluated acid base status in 10 rigidly controlled insulin-dependent diabetic mothers and in 10 healthy nondiabetic control women, all having spinal anesthesia for cesarean section (Table 20-5). They used dextrose-free Ringer's lactate solution for volume expansion before induction of anesthesia, and hypotension (systolic blood pressure <100 mm Hg) was prevented by aggressive treatment with ephedrine. No significant differences were observed in acid base values between the infants of the two groups. It was concluded that if maternal diabetes is well controlled, non–dextrose-containing intravenous solution is used for acute volume expansion, and maternal hypotension is prevented by aggressive use of ephedrine, then spinal anesthesia can be used safely for diabetic parturients having cesarean section. The other disadvantage of the use of acute volume expansion of dextrose-containing solution is neonatal hypoglycemia. Soler and Malins reported an incidence of over 40% of neonatal hypoglycemia when the mean maternal blood glucose level at delivery exceeded 130 mg/dL.[43] Beside the usual advantages of regional anesthesia, another advantage that might be theoretically important is related to the better regulation of glucose homeostasis.[44] This might be due to less of an increase in the plasma catecholamine and serum cortisol concentrations during epidural anesthesia, compared with general anesthesia. Although both spinal and epidural anesthesia if properly performed can be used in these patients with good neonatal outcome, we prefer epidural anesthesia in most severe cases (e.g., classes F and R), especially if there is any sign of fetal compromise.

Because there are some suggestions of abnormal hemodynamic adjustments in diabetic patients, one has to be more cautious in hydrating these patients, especially those with severe diabetes, because of the possibility of preclinical diabetic cardiomyopathy and autonomic neuropathy. Epidural anesthesia may be preferable over spinal anesthesia because of slower onset and less cardiovascular instability. Although these problems are rare in patients with diabetic stiff joint syndrome (diabetic scleredema), one has to check the airway as well as the movement of the atlantooccipital joint. If epidural anesthesia is used, one should avoid the use of a large volume of local anesthetic at any one time.

At Brigham and Women's Hospital, the local anesthetic of choice in such a situation has been 0.5% bupivacaine with 50 μg of fentanyl. The level of anesthesia is usually brought up slowly to control the maternal blood pressure and thus uteroplacental perfusion. Otherwise for spinal anesthesia one can use hyperbaric bupivacaine 0.75% with 10 μg of fentanyl, and for epidural anesthesia 2% lidocaine with epinephrine 1:200,000 or 3% 2-chloroprocaine. For general anesthesia, 10 mg of metoclopramide intravenously should be given at least 30 to 45 minutes before the surgery. This will reduce the intragastric volume since diabetic patients are associated with increased gastric stasis.

Diabetic patients associated with severe preeclampsia or parturients with diabetic nephropathy with superimposed hypertension might pose a special challenge to the anesthesiologist. Invasive monitoring to determine the fluid status as well as

Table 20-5 Effect of strict control of maternal blood glucose, nondextrose solution for volume expansion, and prevention of maternal hypotension on neonatal acid base status in diabetic parturients*†

Umbilical artery ($n = 20$)	No hypotension (diabetic) ($n = 10$)	No hypotension (control) ($n = 10$)
pH	7.27 ± 0.01	7.30 ± 0.01
Po_2 (mm Hg)	20 ± 2	22 ± 2
Pco_2 (mm Hg)	56 ± 2	50 ± 2.5
Base deficit (mEg/L)	4 ± 1	3 ± 0.7

*From Datta S, Kitzmiller JL, Naulty JS, et al: *Anesth Analg* 1982; 61:662. Used by permission.
†Values represent mean ± standard error.

the cardiovascular function might be necessary. Infusion of colloid occasionally may be required; oxygen saturation monitoring and urine output determination should be essential parts of the monitoring system.

Diabetic ketoacidosis is the major cause of fetal morbidity and mortality and it represents a major obstetric emergency. Cesarean section may be necessary because of severe fetal distress; the anesthetic of choice will depend on maternal condition. If the patient is unconscious, general anesthesia may be indicated; otherwise spinal anesthesia (a small amount of local anesthetic is needed) or epidural anesthesia with 3% 2-chloroprocaine (short half-life) may be used with proper maintenance of maternal blood pressure.

After either vaginal or abdominal delivery insulin management must be carefully regulated. Lev-Ran noted a drop in insulin requirement to zero for 1 to 2 days in 11 of 12 patients undergoing cesarean section. Hypoglycemia appeared in 3 of these patients.[45] A steep rise in blood glucose levels followed this temporary drop in insulin requirement.

Neonatal resuscitation

Active neonatal resuscitation is quite often necessary because of the complex nature of the maternal disease. Therefore, a neonatologist should attend both vaginal and abdominal deliveries of infants of diabetic parturients, and birth should take place in a hospital with access to facilities for neonatal intensive care. Infants of diabetic mothers have an increased risk of RDS. However, the incidence of RDS recently has declined throughout the country. Serious RDS must be differentiated from milder and more transient (48 hours) tachypnea of the newborn, which may be due to retained fetal lung fluid. The diagnosis of RDS will be made by (1) clinical signs including grunting, retractions, and a respiratory rate of more than 60 per minute; (2) an x-ray finding of diffuse reticulogranular patterns; and (3) an increased oxygen requirement to maintain Pao_2 at 50 to 70 mm Hg for more than 48 hours without other causes of respiratory problems. With the advent of modern ventilatory support, including high frequency ventilation and surfactant therapy, the survival rate of RDS infants has increased dramatically. The presence of high hematocrit can also be a major problem in these infants; in its extreme, this condition can produce thrombosis, especially in the renal veins. Hyperbilirubinemia and hypocalcemia can also develop more frequently in these infants.

Finally, a high incidence of complex congenital anomalies still remains a major problem, because these defects may make resuscitative measures more complex.

CONCLUSION

Management of diabetic parturients and their babies may pose special challenges to the perinatal team. Close communication between the perinatologist, anesthesiologist, and neonatologist is essential for good maternal and neonatal outcome.

REFERENCES

1. Nylund L, Lunell NO, Lewander R, et al: Uteroplacental blood flow in diabetic pregnancy: Measurements with indium-113m and a computer linked gamma camera. *Am J Obstet Gynecol* 1982; 144:298.
2. Bjork O, Persson B: Placental changes in relation to the degree of metabolic control in diabetes mellitus. *Placenta* 1982; 3:367.
3. Madsen H, Ditzel J: Changes in red blood cell oxygen transport in diabetic pregnancy. *Am J Obstet Gynecol* 1982; 143:421.
4. Bunn HF, Briehl RW, Larrabee P, et al: The interaction of 2,3-diphosphoglycerate with various human hemoglobins. *J Clin Invest* 1970; 49:1088.
5. Phillipps AF, Dubin JW, Raye JR: Fetal metabolic response to endogenous insulin release. *Am J Obstet Gynecol* 1981; 139:441.
6. Milley JR, Rosenberg AA, Philipps AF, et al: The effect of insulin on ovine fetal oxygen extraction. *Am J Obstet Gynecol* 1984; 149:673.
7. Carson BS, Philipps AF, Simmons MA, et al: Effects of sustained insulin infusion upon glucose uptake and oxygenation of ovine fetus. *Pediatr Res* 1980; 14:147.
8. Drury MI, Greene AT, Stronge JM: Pregnancy complicated by clinical diabetes mellitus: A study of 600 pregnancies. *Obstet Gynecol* 1977; 49:519.
9. Greene MF, Hare JW, Krache M, et al: Prematurity among insulin-requiring diabetic gravid women. *Am J Obstet Gynecol* 1989; 161:106.
10. Hogan K, Rusy D, Springman SR: Difficult laryngoscopy and diabetes mellitus. *Anesth Analg* 1988; 67:1162.
11. Hirsch BR, Shamoon H: Defective epinephrine and growth hormone responses in Type I diabetes are stimulus specific. *Diabetes* 1987; 36:20.
12. Airaksinen KEJ, Ikaheimo MJ, Slmea PI, et al: Impaired cardiac adjustment to pregnancy in Type I diabetes. *Diabetes Care* 1986; 9:376.
13. Kitzmiller JL, Younger MD, Hare JW, et al: Continuous subcutaneous insulin therapy during early pregnancy. *Obstet Gynecol* 1985; 66:601.
14. Coustan DR, Reece EA, Sherwin RS, et al: A randomized clinical trial of the insulin pump vs. intensive conventional therapy in diabetic pregnancies. *JAMA* 1986; 255:631.
15. Miller E, Hare JW, Cloherty JP, et al: Elevated maternal hemoglobin A_{1c} in early pregnancy and major congenital anomalies in infants of diabetic mothers. *N Engl J Med* 1981; 304:1331.
16. Fuhrmann K, Reicher H, Semmler K, et al: Prevention of congenital malformations in infants of insulin dependent diabetic mothers. *Diabetes Care* 1983; 6:219.
17. Mills JL, Knopp RH, Simpson JL, et al: Lack of relation of increased malformation rates in infants of diabetic mothers to glycemic control during organogenesis. *N Engl J Med* 1988; 318:671.
18. Greene MF: Prevention and diagnosis of congenital anomalies in diabetic pregnancies. *Clin Perinatol* 1993; 20:533.
19. Miodovnik M, Lavin JP, Knowles JC, et al: Spontaneous abortion among insulin-dependent diabetic women. *Am J Obstet Gynecol* 1984; 150:372.

20. Mills JL, Simpson JL, Driscoll SG, et al: Incidence of spontaneous abortion among normal women and insulin-dependent diabetic women whose pregnancies were identified within 21 days of conception. *N Engl J Med* 1988; 319:1617.

21. Sosenko IR, Kitzmiller JL, Loo SW, et al: The infant of the diabetic mother: Correlation of increased cord C-peptide levels with macrosomia and hypoglycemia. *N Engl J Med* 1979; 301:859.

22. Widness JA, Schwartz HC, Thompson D, et al: Glycohemoglobin (HbA$_{1c}$): A predictor of birth weight in infants of diabetic mothers. *J Pediatr* 1978; 92:8.

23. Adashi EY, Pinto H, Tyson JE: Impact of maternal euglycemia on fetal outcome in diabetic pregnancy. *Am J Obstet Gynecol* 1979; 133:268.

24. O'Shaughnessy R, Russ J, Zuspan FP: Glycosylated hemoglobins and diabetes mellitus in pregnancy. *Am J Obstet Gynecol* 1979; 135:783.

25. Miller JM: A reappraisal of "tight control" in diabetic pregnancies. *Am J Obstet Gynecol* 1983; 148:158.

26. Knight G, Worth RC, Ward JD: Macrosomy despite a well-controlled diabetic pregnancy. *Lancet* 1983; 2:1431.

27. Acker DB, Sachs BP, Friedman EA: Risk factors for shoulder dystocia. *Obstet Gynecol* 1985; 66:762.

28. White P: Pregnancy complicating diabetes. *Am J Med* 1949; 7:609.

29. Coustan DR, Imarah J: Prophylactic insulin treatment of gestational diabetes reduces the incidence of macrosomia, operative delivery, and birth trauma. *Am J Obstet Gynecol* 1984; 150:836.

30. Miller JM, Horger EO: Antepartum heart rate testing in diabetic pregnancy. *J Reprod Med* 1985; 30:515.

31. Golde SH, Montoro M, Good-Anderson B, et al: The role of nonstress tests, fetal biophysical profile, and contraction stress tests in the outpatient management of insulin-requiring diabetic pregnancies. *Am J Obstet Gynecol* 1984; 148:269.

32. Landon MB, Gabbe SG, Bruner JP, et al: Doppler umbilical artery velocimetry in pregnancy complicated by insulin-dependent diabetes mellitus. *Obstet Gynecol* 1989; 73:961.

33. Modanlou HD, Komatsu G, Dorchester W, et al: Large-for-gestational-age neonates: Anthropometric reasons for shoulder dystocia. *Obstet Gynecol* 1982; 60:417.

34. Shnider SM, Abboud T, Artal R, et al: Maternal endogenous catecholamine decrease during labor after epidural anesthesia. *Am J Obstet Gynecol* 1983; 147:13.

35. Pearson JF: The effect of continuous lumbar epidural block on maternal and fetal acid-base balance during labor and at delivery, in Doughty A (ed): *Proceedings of the Symposium on Epidural Analgesia in Obstetrics.* London, HK Lewis, 1968, p 26.

36. Datta S, Brown WU: Acid-base status in diabetic mothers and their infants following general or spinal anesthesia for cesarean section. *Anesthesiology* 1977; 47:272.

37. Datta S, Brown WU, Ostheimer GW, et al: Epidural anesthesia for cesarean section in diabetic parturients: Maternal and neonatal acid-base status and bupivacaine concentration. *Anesth Analg* 1981; 60:574.

38. Gabbe SG, Deiner DLM, Greep RO: The effects of hypoxia on placental glycogen metabolism. *Am J Obstet Gynecol* 1972; 114:540.

39. Swanstrom S, Bratteby LE: Metabolic effects of obstetric regional analgesia and of asphyxia in the newborn infant during the first two hours after birth. *Acta Paediatr Scand* 1981; 70:791.

40. Kenepp NB, Shelley WC, Gabbe SG, et al: Fetal and neonatal hazards of maternal hydration with 5% dextrose before caesarean section. *Lancet* 1980; 1:1150.

41. Kitzmiller JL, Phillippe M, VonOeyen P, et al: Effect of glucose on fetal acidosis in rhesus monkeys. *XI European Congress of Perinatal Medicine.* Rome, Cic Editione Internationale, 1988.

42. Datta S, Kitzmiller JL, Naulty JS, et al: Acid-base status of diabetic mothers and their infants following spinal anesthesia for cesarean section. *Anesth Analg* 1982; 61:662.

43. Soler NG, Malins JM: Diabetic pregnancy: Management on the day of delivery. *Diabetologia* 1978; 15:441.

44. Lund J, Stjernstrom H, Jorfeldk L, et al: Effects of extradural analgesia on glucose metabolism and gluconeogenesis: Studies in association with upper abdominal surgery. *Br J Anaesth* 1986; 58:851.

45. Lev-Ran A: Sharp temporary drop in insulin requirement after cesarean section in diabetic patients. *Am J Obstet Gynecol* 1974; 120:905.

21 Pregnancy-Induced Hypertension

Theodore G. Cheek and *Philip Samuels*

The past 20 years have seen many advances in the management of preeclampsia-eclampsia that include improved precision in maternal and fetal monitoring, a broader understanding of maternal pathophysiology and hemodynamics, the benefits and limitations of crystalloid and colloid infusion, and increasing evidence for the safety and advantages of epidural anesthesia. Although the etiology of this often misunderstood disorder remains elusive, obstetricians and anesthesiologists continue their efforts to clarify the dynamics of this disease and improve maternal-fetal outcome. This chapter will review the assessment and care of the preeclamptic patient during the puerperium, discuss monitoring criteria for both mother and fetus, and describe a clinical approach to obstetric and anesthetic management. There are several suggested methods for managing preeclampsia, but we present the approach that we have found to be successful in a large-volume setting with an above-average incidence of preeclampsia.

THE DISORDER

Preeclampsia-eclampsia is unique to human pregnancy. A suitable animal or in vitro model has yet to be devised, making the disorder fundamentally difficult to study. With improved trophoblast tissue culture techniques, new investigation should be forthcoming in this area. The classic diagnosis of preeclampsia is based on a triad of increased blood pressure accompanied by proteinuria and/or edema. There must be an increase in systolic blood pressure of at least 30 mm Hg over the baseline and/or an increase in diastolic blood pressure of at least 15 mmHg over the baseline that persists between two blood pressure determinations taken at least 6 hours apart. A blood pressure reading greater than 140/90 after 20 weeks' gestation indicates a presumptive diagnosis. Page and Christianson prefer to use mean arterial pressure for the diagnosis of preeclampsia.[1] These authors suggest an elevation in mean arterial pressure of 20 mmHg above baseline, or an absolute mean arterial pressure greater than or equal to 105 mmHg is sufficient to diagnose pregnancy-associated hypertension.

In a nonpregnant individual, urinary excretion of up to 0.25 g of protein may be normal. In pregnancy, urinary excretion of up to 0.3 g of protein daily is a normal finding because of increased glomerular filtration, renal plasma flow, and capillary permeability. In preeclampsia, urinary protein should exceed 0.3 g in 24 hours or have a concentration greater than 0.1 g/L in a random specimen.

Edema as a diagnostic sign of preeclampsia is, at best, imprecise and subjective. Lower extremity swelling is common during normal gestation. The first sign of impending preeclampsia is often a rapid weight gain that occurs before increased edema is noted. Patients at risk for preeclampsia or those with mild preeclampsia should have their weights checked frequently. Edema of preeclampsia will usually involve the upper and lower extremities.

Preeclampsia is usually classified as either mild or severe in order to simplify the often complex and confusing array of symptoms. Both maternal and fetal criteria are used to classify preeclampsia as severe. Maternal criteria include systolic blood pressure greater than or equal to 160 mmHg and/or diastolic blood pressure greater than or equal to 110 mm Hg on at least two occasions at least 6 hours apart; greater than 5 g of proteinuria in 24 hours or persistent 4+ proteinuria on dipstick; increased liver function indices (excluding alkaline phosphatase, which is also produced by the placenta) or epigastric pain (both signs of liver capsule stretching due to hepatic engorgement); unrelenting headache and/or scotoma (signs of cerebral edema); hyperreflexia with clonus (signs of central nervous system irritability); thrombocytopenia; oliguria (evidence of renal vascular spasm and poor perfusion); and pulmonary edema. Fetal criteria include intrauterine growth retardation and oligohydramnios. In general, diagnosis of a patient with severe preeclampsia warrants delivery in a timely fashion, and is the definitive cure.

The diagnosis of eclampsia is made when signs of preeclampsia are accompanied by convulsion and/or coma. Eclampsia can develop in the presence of either mild or severe preeclampsia. With improved treatment, maternal and perinatal mortality associated with eclampsia has decreased. Nonetheless, a careless or missed diagnosis can result in life-threatening consequences. For example, a patient that is 28 weeks pregnant with a growth-retarded fetus is brought to the emergency room in status epilepticus. The pregnancy may go unnoticed while the patient undergoes a time-consuming battery of diagnostic and therapeutic procedures. The treatment for this patient should be magnesium sulfate, appropriate blood pressure control, maternal and fetal monitoring, and delivery!

Certain groups of patients are at high risk for developing preeclampsia during gestation. These include adolescent and elderly primigravidae; women with chronic hypertension; patients with underlying renal disease of any etiology; patients with sickle cell anemia and other hemoglobinopathies; and women with systemic lupus erythematosus and related collagen vascular diseases.[2]

Sutherland showed that there is a familial tendency toward preeclampsia.[3] In his study, the incidence of preeclampsia was 15% in mothers of preeclamptic women, but only 4% in mothers-in-law of the same patients. Any patient deemed to be at increased risk for developing preeclampsia should be monitored closely throughout the third trimester of pregnancy for any warning signs or symptoms.

PATHOPHYSIOLOGY

Although of unknown etiology, the hallmark of preeclampsia is vasospasm that produces pathologic changes seen in organ systems throughout the body. These changes may be related to disruption and damage to three major cell types—endothelial cells, platelets, and trophoblasts. Cell damage may release vasoactive amines and other substances that act locally or throughout the body. Prostaglandins appear to play a role in both the symptoms and possibly the etiology of preeclampsia. This evidence has been reviewed in detail by Friedman.[4]

Decreased elasticity and narrowing of vessels leads to increased total peripheral resistance seen in preeclampsia. Pollak and Nettles have shown narrowed retinal arterioles on fundoscopic examination correlate with narrowed vessels in renal biopsy specimens from severely preeclamptic women.[5] Suggested mechanisms for the observed narrow vessels include changes in (1) the intrinsic nature of blood vessels; (2) plasma concentrations of circulating vasoactive substances; or (3) sensitivity of blood vessels to normal concentrations of circulating vasoactive substances. Zuspan[6] and later Talledo[7] have shown that in patients with preeclampsia there is increased sensitivity to plasma

concentrations of epinephrine and norepinephrine, respectively. Gant et al report most convincingly that preeclamptic patients have increased sensitivity to circulating vasoactive substances.[8] In normal pregnancy, women lose their sensitivity to angiotensin II, a potent vasoconstrictor produced in the liver. In contrast, patients destined to become preeclamptic do not lose their sensitivity to this substance. This can be demonstrated weeks before signs and symptoms of overt preeclampsia develop.

The role of prostaglandins in preeclampsia remains controversial. Thromboxane A_2, a potent vasoconstrictor, and prostacyclin, a potent vasodilator, are both prostaglandin metabolites. Decreased concentrations of prostacyclin have been found in the umbilical cords of infants born to mothers with preeclampsia[9] and in the serum of preeclamptic women.[10] It appears that the ratio of thromboxane A_2 to prostacyclin is increased in preeclampsia, favoring vasospasm and platelet aggregation.[4]

Many changes are seen in the kidney in the preeclamptic patient. In preeclampsia, the filtration fraction (glomerular filtration/renal plasma flow) is often decreased and is attributed to glomerular capillary endotheliosis, a lesion distinct to preeclampsia. In this lesion, glomerular capillary cells are edematous, a condition that attenuates blood filtration.

Proteinuria results from increased permeability of damaged renal glomeruli, capillaries, and tubules. Many proteins that are normally filtered and reabsorbed by renal tubule cells are poorly reabsorbed in the presence of cell injury. Vasospasm is also associated with proteinuria.[11] The combination of these events leads to the waxing and waning of proteinuria, often seen in the hospitalized preeclamptic patient and first described by Chesley.[12] Conversely, urate clearance decreases in the preeclamptic patient, resulting in the well-recognized increase in serum uric acid concentration seen in preeclampsia. These changes appear to occur earlier than the changes seen in glomerular filtration rate. Urate is filtered by the glomeruli and actively secreted by tubular cells. Because urate clearance often decreases before proteinuria develops, it is felt that tubular damage is most responsible for this change.

Activation of the coagulation cascade appears to occur in preeclampsia, even when there is no clinical evidence of coagulopathy. The late development of coagulopathy probably occurs because there is a great increase in clotting factors and in procoagulants during a normal pregnancy. The only factors that do not increase during pregnancy are factors V, XI, and XIII. Denson has shown that the ratio of factor VIII antigen to factor VIII activity, normally 1:1, is increased in preeclampsia,[13] a change that provides presumptive evidence for consumption of procoagulants. Fibrin degradation products are present in the plasma of preeclamptic patients and gives further evidence of a mild consumptive coagulopathy. A slight fall in platelet count is seen early in the course of preeclampsia but does not become clinically evident until well into the course of the disease; this usually remains unnoticed unless serial platelet counts are followed. A decreased platelet count is probably the result of increased platelet aggregation and destruction. This may be associated with the previously mentioned increase in ratio of thromboxane A_2 to prostacyclin, because thromboxane A_2 stimulates platelet aggregation.

During pregnancy, characteristic changes occur in the blood vessels of the placental bed that include an increase in spiral artery diameter[14] and replacement of endothelial lining by trophoblasts.[15] This occurs in the decidual portion of the spiral arterioles and extends outward as pregnancy continues and may reach the distal portion of the radial arteries. In preeclampsia, trophoblast invasion is limited to the decidual portion of the arterioles, which are 40% narrower than their counterparts in the nonpreeclamptic patient. In addition, acute atherosis may occur in some spiral and basal arterioles.[16] Kitzmiller and Benirschke found components of complement in atherotic decidual vessels in preeclampsia, suggesting an immune-mediated etiology of this lesion.[17] Placental infarctions are also common in preeclampsia and usually occur in areas supplied by atherotic vessels.

OBSTETRIC CARE OF THE PREECLAMPTIC PATIENT

It is common obstetric practice to hospitalize and closely monitor all patients with a diagnosis of preeclampsia. Because the course of preeclampsia can change rapidly, there is rarely a place for outpatient management of this disorder. Proper care includes frequent assessment of blood and urine parameters as well as close surveillance of physical signs and symptoms.

Inpatient management of the preeclamptic patient

Once the patient is admitted, she is kept at bed rest and is followed with frequent blood pressure determinations, daily weights, and twice weekly determinations of creatinine clearance, total protein excretion in the urine, serum uric acid, and platelet counts. Fetal nonstress tests and ultrasound determinations of amniotic fluid adequacy should be performed once or twice weekly, depending on the severity of the disease and the gestational age of the fetus. An anesthesia and pediatric consultation should be obtained shortly after admission.

The decision to deliver a patient is based on either maternal or fetal indications. Maternal indications include any of the previously cited criteria that classify the disease process as severe preeclampsia.

Fetal indications for delivery are based on abnormal fetal testing or evidence of fetal maturity. A nonreactive nonstress test (evidence of some degree of fetal compromise) should be followed up with either a contraction stress test or biophysical profile. The contraction stress test requires sufficient oxytocin to mimic labor as well as observation of fetal heart rate patterns in response to contractions. Three uterine contractions in 10 minutes without fetal heart rate decelerations related to the contractions is considered a negative test and is presumptive evidence of fetal well-being. Three consecutive contractions followed by a "late" deceleration is evidence of uteroplacental insufficiency, and delivery is indicated. Any other permutation is considered an "equivocal" test and requires a repeat or alternative test based on the gestational age of the fetus and the clinical situation.

The biophysical profile consists of fetal evaluation by ultrasound that includes evidence of fetal muscle tone, fetal breathing motion, fetal movement, and amniotic fluid adequacy combined with results of the nonstress test.[18] Each observation is assigned a score of either 2 or 0, based up published criteria. In a sense, it is like an in utero APGAR score to determine fetal well-being. A score equal to or greater than 8 is considered normal and a score equal to or less than 4 is considered evidence of fetal compromise. A score of 6 indicates that the test needs to be extended to 2 hours or should be repeated within 24 hours.

If either the contraction stress test or the biophysical profile is abnormal, delivery should be accomplished in a timely fashion. Other fetal indications for delivery include oligohydramnios or intrauterine growth retardation (fetal growth less than the 5th percentile) at a viable gestational age. If the fetus is close to term gestation, the obstetrician should attempt to induce labor as soon as maternal conditions are optimal.

Obstetric conduct of labor and delivery

Once the decision is made to proceed with delivery, the obstetrician, anesthesiologist, and pediatrician should establish a plan of action and a time frame in which to work. If at all possible, a vaginal delivery should be attempted. During labor, the clinical course of the mother and fetus should be continuously evaluated, and the physician team should be prepared to intervene with operative delivery at any time.

If the mother's cervix is already somewhat dilated, amniotomy should be performed and internal fetal heart rate and uterine contraction monitors should be applied before oxytocin induction is begun. In this way, the fetus and uterus are sensitively monitored and optimal uterine contractions obtained using the smallest amount of oxytocin possible. If the cervix is unfavorable, oxytocin can be administered using external fetal monitors. Some physicians now use prostaglandin E_2 gel to ripen the cervix.[19] A dose of 0.5 mg is instilled into the cervix, or 2 mg is placed in the posterior vaginal fornix where it causes mild contractions but is most active locally on cervical stroma. This is much less than the 20-mg dose used to initiate therapeutic abortion. Although prostaglandin E_2 has not gained approval for this indication by the FDA, it is widely used by obstetricians. Since its use in preeclampsia is controversial, we do not recommend its routine use, but to date, we have not observed ill effects from the medication in a dose of 0.5 mg.

If a long labor is anticipated, it is important the mother and fetus are carefully monitored as outlined below. Oxytocin is endogenously produced in the hypothalamus and is secreted by the paraventricular nuclei of the posterior pituitary. Its structure is similar to that of antidiuretic hormone, ADH, also released from the neurohypophysis. Oxytocin, if used for extended periods or if used in doses above 20 mU/min, can exert an ADH-like effect. If a decreased urine output occurs, it may be difficult to determine if it is preeclampsia related or caused by oxytocin. In this situation, evaluation of serum and urine electrolytes and central venous pressure can be helpful.

If the maternal condition rapidly deteriorates despite intensive medical management with an unfavorable cervix, or in the case of a premature infant with malpresentation, primary cesarean section is preferred over vaginal delivery. If a cesarean section is anticipated, the anesthesiologist should be informed as soon as the decision is made and laboratory parameters of coagulation (discussed below) evaluated. Usually, a low transverse cesarean section is performed. If, however, there is malpresentation and the fetus is very premature, or if oligohydramnios is present and the lower uterine segment is not well developed, a vertical uterine incision (either corporosegmental or classical) may be necessary. Both of these uterine incisions carry a greater inherent blood loss and a longer operating time than the low transverse approach.

Initial predelivery assessment

Once a decision has been made to deliver, the obstetrician and anesthesiologist should work together to devise a rational and efficient plan of management for the patient. In this way efforts are not duplicated and plans are implemented in a time-efficient manner. The anesthesiologist should be involved early in the treatment of preeclampsia because of his or her expertise in pain control, airway management, and hemodynamic monitoring, and because the pathophysiology and therapy of pregnancy-induced hypertension will significantly alter the conduct of anesthesia. Indeed, there is increasing evidence that maternal and fetal protection from preeclampsia-induced risks can be obtained from establishing analgesia early in the course of labor.

First the anesthesiologist should learn the obstetrician's plan for delivery and determine the need for further monitoring and medical therapy within the time available. Vaginal delivery is optimal for these patients. If the disease process is severe and the patient's cervix is unfavorable, a primary cesarean section is usually indicated.

Except in cases of severe fetal distress or maternal hemorrhage, there is usually sufficient time to establish adequate antiseizure therapy with magnesium, evaluate urinary output, obtain appropriate laboratory studies, initiate antihypertensive drugs, and provide adequate monitoring of the mother and fetus. The extent of monitoring and further therapy will be determined by the severity of the disease.

Laboratory studies. Laboratory studies should include hemoglobin, hematocrit, BUN, creatinine, uric acid, and type and screen. A coagulation profile should be obtained that includes prothrombin time, partial thromboplastin time, fibrinogen concentrations, and platelet count. If there is a clinical suspicion of coagulopathy, fibrin split products and a thromboelastography study, if possible, should be obtained. If there is decreased urine output, electrolytes should also be obtained. If the patient shows signs of severe preeclampsia, liver enzymes (including LDH) should be obtained to determine if the HELLP syndrome is present (discussed below).

Blood should be crossmatched if unusual maternal antibodies are present, hemoglobin is less than 11.0 gm%, and cesarean section is likely. If coagulation abnormalities are present, blood should be crossmatched and the blood bank should be informed that fresh frozen plasma or cryoprecipitate may be required. Platelet transfusion is rarely helpful in the management of thrombocytopenia because the half-life of transfused platelets in a preeclamptic patient is very short. If the platelet count less than or equal to $40,000/\mu L$ and a cesarean section is planned, we recommend platelet infusion as the skin incision is made. In this way, platelets should remain effective long enough to promote intraoperative hemostasis.

Coagulation profile: issues in patient management. Presence of coagulopathy has long been considered a contraindication to regional block because of the fear of epidural or spinal hematoma. However, the laboratory values and clinical findings that limit use of regional block are not agreed upon. The most common coagulation disorder in preeclampsia is a decrease in platelet number or function.[20,21] In general, laboratory evidence of coagulopathy is found in about 10% of preeclamptic patients and in 30% of severe preeclamptic patients.[22] Clinically significant coagulopathy is found in about 15% of severe preeclamptic patients and less than 5% of mild preeclamptic patients. The decrease in platelet count is thought to be due to an increase in platelet turnover with inadequate time to release enough new platelets from megakaryocytes in the bone marrow to compensate for the increased destruction. Evidence for a thrombocyte immune disorder was found by Samuels et al,[23] who have shown that preeclamptic individuals have a similar antiplatelet antibody profile to patients with immune thrombocytopenic purpura. The disorders differ in that neonatal platelet counts are not depressed in preeclampsia.

Rasmus et al.[24] retrospectively examined 2929 consecutive parturients and found 24 had platelet counts less than 100,000/μl (mean = 64,000, range = 18,000–90,000/μl). Fourteen of these thrombocytopenic patients received regional block and none had sequelae of spinal hematoma. These authors also reviewed the literature and found no reports of spinal or epidural hematoma in thrombocytopenic parturients receiving regional block, except one patient with spinal ependymoma. These authors did not ignore the potential risk of regional block in the presence of thrombocytopenia but questioned the teaching that platelet counts below 100,000/μl preclude regional anesthesia. An increased bleeding time has been associated with a decreased platelet count.[25] Some authorities believe the bleeding time is a reliable means of measuring platelet function. However, recent reviews of the subject have concluded that bleeding time is not a useful indicator of the risk of hemorrhage.[26] A current editorial in *Lancet* concluded that there was little evidence to support the use of the bleeding time as a diagnostic test in individual patients before using regional anesthesia techniques.[27] In our practice we rarely use the bleeding time.

In an emergency when there is little time for return of laboratory studies and regional block is well advised, we recommend a thorough patient history and examination for signs of bleeding from puncture sites, observation of test tube clot formation, and bedside use of activated clotting time, ac-cepting 145 seconds or less as criteria to allow the block. In carefully selected patients in whom regional block has a distinct advantage (difficult airway or obesity) we have occasionally utilized regional block in the presence of platelet counts of 50,000/μl. In 10 years of experience and more than 1000 epidural blocks in preeclamptic patients, we have observed no sequelae of epidural bleeding with the above criteria. Alternative coagulation studies such as "Sonoclot"[28] or the thromboelastogram have been suggested as effective methods to ensure clot formation. Although early studies have been promising, the technology and/or trained staff are not routinely available in many hospitals.

Prevention. Wallenburg[29] and others have demonstrated that aspirin, 60 mg a day, effectively decreases the risk of preeclampsia by inhibition of thromboxane production but not prostacyclin. The use of aspirin prophylaxis for preeclampsia is now increasing. It appears to be most useful in patients with a history of recurrent preeclampsia, as well as in those with a history of chronic hypertension, renal disease, and collagen vascular disease who are at increased risk of developing preeclampsia. The published reports are encouraging, but use of aspirin has the potential to lead to overuse and abuse because the medication is readily available. Any obstetrician can label a teenage primigravida as being at increased risk for preeclampsia and place her on low-dose aspirin. Current investigation in a large population (n = 1985) has shown that although aspirin significantly lowers the risk of preeclampsia, the benefits of this effect are outweighed by the increase in incidence of abruptio placenta from 0.1% to 0.7%.[30] Routine aspirin prophylaxis is not recommended at the present time.[31]

Although it is labeled as "innocuous," small doses of aspirin can decrease platelet function for over a week. Some anesthesiologists question whether epidural block should be performed in these aspirin-treated patients without first performing a bleeding time to assess platelet function.

Benigni et al[32] studied the effect of 60-mg oral doses of aspirin daily on 17 pregnant women from 12 weeks to term, compared with 16 pregnant control subjects. At 28 weeks' gestation, bleeding times were 6.2 ± 1.8 and 4.17 ± 1.2 in the aspirin group and controls, respectively. We believe bleeding time is not necessary in parturients receiving prophylactic low-dose aspirin.

Oxygen delivery. Normal tissue oxygen delivery is usually 4 to 5 times that of tissue oxygen consumption. In preeclampsia, recent evidence indicates tissue oxygen extraction is 30% less than in normal pregnancy (normal O_2 extraction ratio = 0.29, preeclampsia = 0.2). Belfort et al.[33] studied oxygen consumption and delivery in 32 women with severe preeclampsia. Both oxygen consumption and extraction were significantly reduced in the face of decreased O_2 delivery when compared with historical normal controls. These patients also failed to show a progressive increase in arterial-mixed venous oxygen difference in response to increased tissue oxygen requirements. The authors suggest this is associated with vasospasm-based regional hypoxia and may offer a further explanation for widespread organ ischemia. The authors found improvement in oxygen delivery/extraction associated with magnesium therapy (decrease in afterload) and increased intravenous fluid.

Monitoring. The present and potential risk imposed by preeclampsia requires increased and more frequent surveillance of both the fetus and mother. Continuous electronic fetal monitoring is necessary. Uteroplacental insufficiency, intrauterine growth retardation, and oligohydramnios are common in the severely preeclamptic patient. Oligohydramnios results in an increased frequency of variable (umbilical cord compression) decelerations. Doppler blood flow studies have shown that uterine blood flow can be diminished in the severely preeclamptic patient.[34] This can result in intrauterine growth retardation and uteroplacental insufficiency manifest on the fetal monitor as late decelerations, a finding that may necessitate emergency cesarean section.[35] If the patient is in labor, or an induction of labor is being attempted, amniotomy should be performed as early as possible and a direct scalp clip should be applied to the fetus. Simultaneously, an intrauterine pressure transducer should be placed into the uterine cavity. In this way, subtle signs of fetal distress can be detected, often obviating the need for truly emergency cesarean sections. Before amniotomy is feasible, continuous external fetal monitoring should be performed. The preeclamptic uterus is very sensitive to oxytocin, and hyperstimulation and fetal distress due to uteroplacental insufficiency are possible complications of induction of labor.

Maternal urine output and protein excretion are important indicators of the severity of preeclampsia. For the patient who is hospitalized at bed rest for mild preeclampsia, a 24-hour urine collection should be performed at least twice weekly to assess creatinine clearance and total protein excretion. In pregnancy, up to 0.3 g of protein excretion is considered normal. When 24-hour protein excretion exceeds 5 g in a preeclamptic patient, the disease is reclassified as severe.

Once the decision is made to deliver the patient either by oxytocin induction or cesarean section, a bladder catheter should be placed early in the course to assess renal perfusion and maternal response to fluid therapy. Meticulous assessment of intake and output is important because a substantial percentage of severely preeclamptic patients become oliguric during the puerperium.

Hypertension is an important symptom of preeclampsia and is thought to be due to severe vasospasm.[36] Early studies indicate that during a normal pregnancy, the patient loses her sensitivity to angiotensin II. Patients destined to become preeclamptic patients do not lose this sensitivity to angiotensin II.[37] The resultant vasospasm, when severe, can lead to organ ischemia, and when associated with severe hypertension it can result in potential cerebral hemorrhage and pulmonary edema. The use of an automated blood pressure monitor equipped with oscillometric or Doppler technology is recommended, and this will decrease the need for an arterial cannula. A recent study pointed out that oscillometric blood pressure measurements (such as Dinamap) compared with auscultatory methods are associated with underrecording diastolic blood pressure by as much as 15 mm Hg in severe preeclampsia.[38] Mean blood pressure obtained from oscillometry, however, did not differ widely with that calculated from auscultation. Arterial cannulation is usually indicated when frequent blood gas analysis is required, such as in the presence of pulmonary edema or in the use of mechanical ventilation, or when continuous infusion of rapid-acting vasodilators such as nitroprusside or nitroglycerin are employed.

Invasive central venous and pulmonary artery catheters in preeclampsia provide a sensitive and useful method to assess maternal volume requirements or determine cardiac ventricular function and vascular resistance. Many investigators have attempted to describe the hemodynamic profile of severe preeclampsia.[39-44] Unfortunately, some disagreement among these studies exists because measurements were often made after fluid and vasodilator therapy. Recently, 45 parturients with severe preeclampsia were studied invasively before therapy and compared with historical controls.[45] These investigators found heart rate and cardiac output (CO) normal, mean arterial pressure (MAP) and systemic vascular resistance (SVR) increased, central venous pressure (CVP) low to normal and poorly correlated with pulmonary artery capillary wedge pressure (PCWP) (which was usually normal), pulmonary artery pressure decreased, and left ventricular function increased or normal (Figs. 21-1 to 21-3). Table 21-1 compares the most recent hemodynamic data from normal and preeclamptic patients at various times during parturition.

Several investigators have recommended pulmonary artery catheterization in patients with severe preeclampsia[39,42,46-48] and have maintained

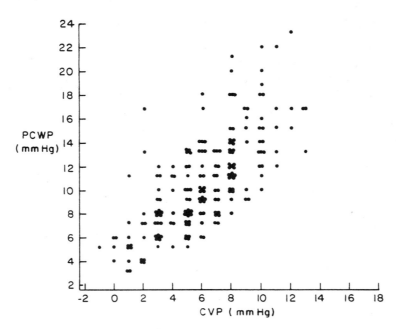

Fig. 21-1 Relationship between CVP and PCWP in women with severe pregnancy-induced hypertension before therapy. Patients with same data values are represented by a single point. (From Cotton DB, Lee W, Huhta JC, et al: *Am J Obstet Gynecol* 1988; 158:523-529. Used by permission.)

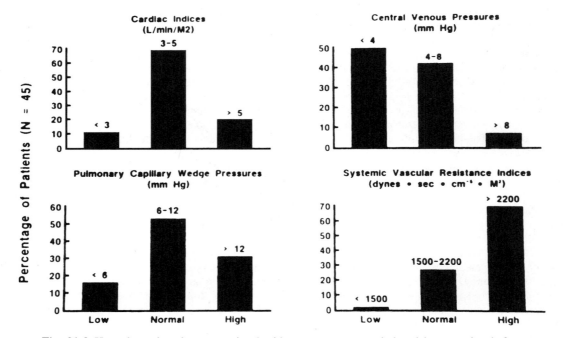

Fig. 21-2 Hemodynamic subsets associated with severe pregnancy-induced hypertension before therapy in 45 subjects. (From Cotton DB, Lee W, Huhta JC, et al: *Am J Obstet Gynecol* 1988; 158:523-529. Used by permission.)

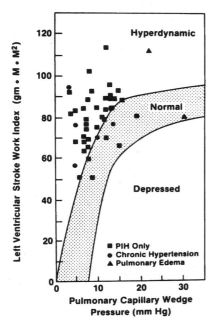

Fig. 21-3 Left ventricular function curve from 45 women with severe pregnancy-induced hypertension (PIH) before therapy. Patients with same data values are represented by a single point. (From Cotton DB, Lee W, Huhta JC, et al: *Am J Obstet Gynecol* 1988; 158:523-529. Used by permission.)

that in the presence of left ventricular dysfunction, CVP may not accurately reflect fluid replacement or left ventricular function. This recommendation is not widely followed because the vast majority of severe preeclamptic patients have excellent left ventricular function and usually demonstrate fair agreement between CVP and PCWP. The discrepancies in CVP and PCWP reported in severe preeclampsia are in most cases an accurate reflection of decreased CVP and an expected increased left ventricular filling pressure caused by increased afterload and not usually evidence of left ventricular failure.[45] However, individual parameters may vary, depending on severity of disease, degree of fluid and vasodilator therapy, and the duration of severe hypertension and its effects on the left ventricle. The intensity of monitoring required in severe preeclampsia should be individualized and not routinely consigned to a standing protocol applied to all parturients with severe hypertension. We are aware of two maternal deaths and several cases of severe morbidity that were associated with Swan-Ganz catheter placement. Because most preeclamptic-eclamptic patients have adequate left ventricular function and normal pulmonary artery pressures, one must weigh the risks of pulmonary artery catheterization against the usefulness of any

additional information obtained beyond that of an antecubital long-line CVP.

Maternal conditions for which we believe a pulmonary artery catheter is well advised are listed in Table 21-2. Our indications for CVP monitoring before the induction of anesthesia are less stringent and include the presence of diastolic pressure greater than 105 mm Hg after the initiation magnesium therapy, visual changes, signs of central nervous system irritability, epigastric pain, oliguria, and when patients are receiving antihypertensive agents other than magnesium. Our technique of choice is an antecubital vein drum catheter placed at the bedside with simultaneous pressure wave and ECG monitoring. This allows the clinician to recognize correct placement by assurance of a right atrial wave-form and the avoidance of or therapy for arrhythmias. A chest x-ray film should be obtained to assure correct placement. An alternative popular approach is the use of external or internal jugular cannulation. However, central venous monitoring from the neck may increase the incidence of certain complications such as carotid cannulation and pneumothorax and in our institution it is chosen if an antecubital site is unusable.

The need for central venous monitoring in severe preeclampsia if general anesthesia is planned is less well defined in the literature. However, the possibility of severe hypovolemia superimposed on any form of anesthesia may result in unstable blood pressure and further organ hypoperfusion, and we recommend the same monitoring standards regardless of the planned anesthetic. In our practice approximately half of severe preeclamptics receive a long-line CVP and 2% to 5% receive pulmonary artery catheters.

We have found that the CVP line not only is useful to the anesthesiologist during delivery but also aids the obstetrician in fluid management during the postpartum period. In the immediate postpartum period, the autotransfusion of uterine involution may produce an increase in functional blood volume and relative fluid overload intensified by a markedly increased systemic vascular resistance. The CVP removes much of the guesswork that was once involved in managing these patients; it is usually left in place until the patient begins a spontaneous diuresis. This usually occurs 24 to 36 hours after delivery.

Intravenous fluid management. Preeclamptic patients require a reliable means of intravenous drug administration provided by at least an 18-gauge indwelling catheter. Intravenous fluids should not consist of dextrose in water alone because of the danger of water intoxication. When oxytocin is administered in doses of greater than 20 milliunits mU/min or when infused for more

Table 21-1 Comparison of hemodynamic measurements in normal nonpregnant, normal pregnant, and severely preeclamptic women

	Normal nonpregnant* (11-13 wks postpartum) (n = 10)	Normal pregnancy* (36-38 wks gestation) (n = 10)	Severe PIH before delivery† (n = 45)	Severe preeclampsia before delivery‡ (n = 41)	Severe preeclampsia with pulmonary edema§ (n = 8)
MAP (mm Hg)	86.4 ± 7.5	90.3 ± 5.8	138 ± 3	130 ± 2	136 ± 3
CVP (mm Hg)	3.7 ± 2.6	3.6 ± 2.5	4 ± 1	4.8 ± 0.4	11 ± 1
PCWP (mm Hg)	6.3 ± 2.1	7.5 ± 1.8	10 ± 1	8.3 ± 0.3	18 ± 1
CO (L/min)	4.3 ± 0.9	6.2 ± 1	7.5 ± 0.23	8.4 ± 0.2	10.5 ± 0.6
SVR (dyne·cm·sec^{-3})	1530 ± 520	1210 ± 266	1496 ± 64	1226 ± 37	964 ± 50
PVR (dyne·cm·sec^{-3})	119 ± 47	78 ± 22	70 ± 5	65 ± 3	71 ± 9
LVSWI (g·m·m^{-2})	41 ± 8	48 ± 6	81 ± 2	84 ± 2	87 ± 10

MAP = mean arterial pressure; CVP = central venous pressure; PCWP = pulmonary capillary wedge pressure; CO = cardiac output, SVR = systemic vascular resistance; PVR = pulmonary vascular resistance; LVSWI = left ventricular stroke work index; PIH = pregnancy-induced hypertension.
*Data from 10 normal pregnancies at 36 to 38 weeks' gestation and 11 to 13 weeks' postpartum. (Adapted from Clark SL, et al: Central hemodynamic assessment of normal term pregnancy. *Am J Obstet Gynecol* 1989; 161:1439-1442.)
†Results from 45 patients with severe pregnancy-induced hypertension (PIH) near time of delivery. (Adapted from Cotton DB, et al: Hemodynamic profile of severe pregnancy-induced hypertension. *Am J Obstet Gynecol* 1988; 158:523-529.)
‡Data from 41 patients with severe preeclampsia but no pulmonary edema shortly before delivery. (Adapted from Mabie WC, et al: The central hemodynamics of preeclampsia. *Am J Obstet Gynecol* 1989; 161:1443-1448.)
§Measurements from 8 patients with pulmonary edema superimposed on severe preeclampsia shortly before delivery. (Adapted from Mabie WC, et al: The central hemodynamics of preeclampsia. *Am J Obstet Gynecol* 1989; 161:1443-1448.)

Table 21-2 Conditions that indicate pulmonary artery catheterization in severe preeclampsia or eclampsia: symptoms and therapy

---

1. Pulmonary edema
   a. Cardiogenic or left ventricular failure (Rx: afterload reduction or inotropes)
   b. Increased systemic vascular resistance (Rx: afterload reduction)
   c. Non–cardiogenic-volume overload (Rx: diuretics, fluid restriction)
   d. Decreased colloid oncotic pressure (Rx: 25% albumin, fluid restriction)
2. Oliguria unresponsive to modest fluid load (500–1000 ml IV)
   a. Low preload (Rx: crystalloid infusion)
   b. High systemic vascular resistance with low cardiac output (Rx: afterload reduction)
   c. Selective renal artery vasoconstriction (Rx: vasodilation??)
3. Severe hypertension unresponsive or refractory to therapy
   a. High systemic vascular resistance (Rx: vasodilators)
   b. Increased cardiac output (Rx: decreased preload-NTG or beta blocker)
4. Persistent arterial desaturation; unable to distinguish between cardiac or noncardiac origin

---

Modified from Clark SB, Cotton DB: Clinical indications for pulmonary artery catheterization in patients with severe preeclampsia. *Am J Obstet Gynecol* 1988; 158:453-458.

than 24 hours, an antidiuretic hormone (ADH) effect is seen. Balanced salt solutions, such as normal saline or lactated Ringer's solution, are recommended. Rapid infusions of dextrose-containing solutions especially before delivery are associated with neonatal hypoglycemia[49] and should be avoided. This is especially true if the mother is carrying a fetus with intrauterine growth retardation, where there are less hepatic glycogen stores. However, 7 to 10 g of glucose per hour in the form of dextrose 5% in 0.45 normal saline is not associated with neonatal hypoglycemia and will supply some metabolic needs of the mother. This is important if a long induction is anticipated because it avoids ketosis in the mother.

The amount and type of intravenous fluid recommended in severe preeclampsia is a subject of continuing debate that originates with a conflict of therapeutic goals between the need to maintain or improve organ (kidney, liver, brain, and placenta) perfusion in the face of intense vasoconstriction and to avoid pulmonary edema, a well-known risk in this disease. Pulmonary edema in severe preeclampsia has been attributed by some investigators to a decreased gradient between colloid os-

motic pressure (COP) and PCWP[50,51] and is usually associated with a COP of less than 13 mm Hg. Normal COP values for term pregnancy compared with severe preeclampsia are reported as 22 ± 0.7 mm Hg and 17.9 ± 0.7, respectively.[52]

Kirshon et al[53] attempted to maintain COP at 17 mm Hg or greater with albumin and intravenous fluid in 15 patients with severe preeclampsia before vasodilator therapy. Using a formula that allows 1 gr of albumin per 100 ml estimated blood volume to exert 4.5 mm Hg oncotic pressure, they infused large volumes of albumin (some exceeded 85 g) and fluid and administered furosemide if PCWP exceeded 15 mm Hg. They were successful in avoiding abrupt decreases in maternal blood pressure and acute fetal distress after antihypertensive therapy. However, postpartum, they observed a dramatic overall increase in PCWP that often required furosemide (as much as 210 mg) to maintain PCWP less than 15 mm Hg. Although no patient developed pulmonary edema, they concluded that aggressive correction of COP was not indicated unless COP values were very low (less than 12 mm Hg) or a prolonged negative COP to PCWP gradient existed. Other investigators have suggested the use of serial COP measurements as a simple and inexpensive means to identify patients at risk for pulmonary edema.[54] We do not routinely measure COP in preeclampsia.

Early in the management of severe preeclampsia it is our practice to restrict hourly intravenous fluid to 75 to 125 mL/hr. After the initial assessment, requirements for fluid therapy are based on clinical signs of poor perfusion such as decreased urine output, decreased CVP or PCWP, increased SVR, and normal CO. Fluid is restricted in the presence of signs of hypervolemia such as increased CVP or PCWP and normal SVR, or in the presence of decreased CO or signs of impending pulmonary edema. In our opinion it is physiologically irrational to routinely restrict fluid or apply aggressive fluid therapy in severe pregnancy-induced hypertension, and that it is instead best to approach fluid therapy in moderation based on the patient's individual need.

Although the obstetric literature does not agree as to the value of volume expansion in the therapy of preeclampsia,[53,55-57] this issue should not be confused with the need for plasma volume expansion before anesthesia, particularly epidural block. Misunderstanding of this issue is due in part to the fact that in some institutions, there is still an unwarranted hesitation to use conduction anesthesia.

It has been shown that between 1 and 2 L of balanced salt solution are required before induction of regional block for cesarean section in healthy parturients[58,59] to avoid a pronounced decrease in blood pressure. Intravascular blood volume, though variable in preeclampsia, is decreased from 15% to 35%[60,61] and tends to be inversely proportional to the severity of the disease as reflected in central venous measurements.[62]

Central venous monitoring before anesthesia is rarely required in the presence of mild preeclampsia. However, vasodilation induced by drugs or regional block in the presence of severe uncorrected hypovolemia may result in an abrupt decrease in peripheral resistance and a profound decrease in systemic perfusion pressure. It is important to ensure adequate blood volume in order to maintain organ perfusion during induction of anesthesia. Sudden hypotension can lead to decreased uterine perfusion and a relative uteroplacental insufficiency leading to fetal distress. This can be effectively avoided with central venous or pulmonary artery pressure monitoring before induction of anesthesia, whereby partial correction of the volume deficit may be accomplished before and during induction of anesthesia.

Joyce et al.[62] evaluated the effects of fluid loading in preeclampsia on CVP before epidural anesthesia. They found that the highest diastolic blood pressures (greater than 110 mm Hg) were associated with the lowest CVP measurements (-1 to -4 cm H_2O) and that these patients required 750 ml Plasmanate and 2 L of lactated Ringer's to achieve a CVP of 6 cm H_2O. In an attempt to increase CVP to 6 cm H_2O, one patient received 4 L of crystalloid and experienced mild pulmonary edema. These investigators later reported that this therapy resulted in postpartum increase of CVP to 16 to 18 cm H_2O and was associated with rare but troublesome pulmonary edema. They subsequently limited crystalloid to 75 ml/hr, infused 50 to 100 g 25% salt-poor albumin, and effectively increased CVP, improved urine output, and protected against significant decreases in blood pressure following epidural block. Postpartum CVP values did not exceed 12 cm H_2O.

We believe it is ill advised to attempt to increase CVP to 6 to 8 cm H_2O in all preeclamptic patients before the induction of regional block since this may occasionally result in fluid overload. Rather it is sufficient to convert a negative CVP to a positive pressure (2 to 3 cm H_2O) to avoid hypotension following epidural block. When diastolic blood pressure is less than 100 mm Hg, only 1 to 2 L of isotonic balanced salt solution without glucose is usually necessary. It is our practice in severe preeclampsia, with diastolic blood pressure greater than 100 mm Hg and CVP of 0 or less, to infuse no more than 1 L of normal saline and 25 to 50 g of 25% salt-poor albumin over 30 to 45 minutes before the induction of epidural block,

with a goal of CVP of 2 to 3 cm H_2O. Further fluid infusion is determined by changes in CVP following the block-induced sympathectomy.

In the rare patient who shows clinical evidence of a severe early coagulopathy, fresh frozen plasma can be infused in place of albumin if a cesarean section is being planned. Realizing that in the face of frank disseminated intravascular coagulopathy the half-life of labile clotting factors is very short, one should infuse the FFP as close to the time of surgery as possible.[63]

After experience with more than 350 cases of preeclampsia receiving this regimen, we have had no cases of pulmonary edema associated with a moderate approach to anesthetic fluid preload. The argument that there is not sufficient time to institute the above therapy before anesthesia is usually without foundation; with few exceptions the argument indicates either poor planning on the part of the obstetrician in not notifying the anesthesiologist in a timely manner, or the anesthesiologist's delay of patient evaluation until the last minute. These patients deserve the same meticulous preoperative care extended to the high-risk hypertensive emergency in the main operating room.

Epidural block, hypotension, and the fetus. There are those who still object to the use of epidural block in severe preeclampsia and eclampsia because they fear severe maternal hypotension will cause placental hypoperfusion and fetal deterioration. A recent *Williams Obstetrics* text[64] states: "Conduction anesthesia has been avoided in women with severe preeclampsia and eclampsia because of concern for sudden, severe hypotension produced by splanchnic blockade and in turn, the dangers from pressor agents or large volumes of intravenous fluid given to try to correct the hypotension so induced." This argument persists despite the fact that there are no human or animal studies to support the suggestion that epidural block in preeclampsia is associated with either a deterioration of intervillous blood flow or fetal oxygen exchange in the presence of moderate fluid loading before anesthesia, and despite the knowledge that uterine displacement and rapid correction of blood pressure are strictly practiced after induction of anesthesia. Indeed, controlled studies show that if significant maternal hypotension can be avoided, uteroplacental blood flow does not deteriorate but moderately increases following epidural block in preeclampsia.[65] In addition, plasma concentrations of circulating catecholamines decrease[66] and the development of eclampsia may be prevented,[67] thus providing for satisfactory intrauterine oxygen exchange.

Studies have shown that after modest prehydration and strict assurance of left uterine displacement, epidural block for cesarean section was associated with no greater hypotension than was general anesthesia.[68,69] The latter, in fact, frequently caused serious and difficult-to-control maternal hypertension on induction, intubation, and emergency[70,71] (Fig. 21-4A). In the presence of modest decreases in blood pressure following epidural block, CO and other cardiovascular parameters were maintained or favorably influenced[44,72] (Figs. 21-4B and 21-5).

In a retrospective study, Moore et al[69] reviewed the records of 285 women who met the criteria for the diagnosis of pregnancy-induced hypertension. Of these, 185 delivered vaginally and 100 required cesarean section. Twenty three percent (68) of all patients had severe hypertension. The purpose of the study was to determine whether fetal or maternal morbidity was altered in patients with pregnancy-induced hypertension who received epidural anesthesia, and to compare fetal and mater-

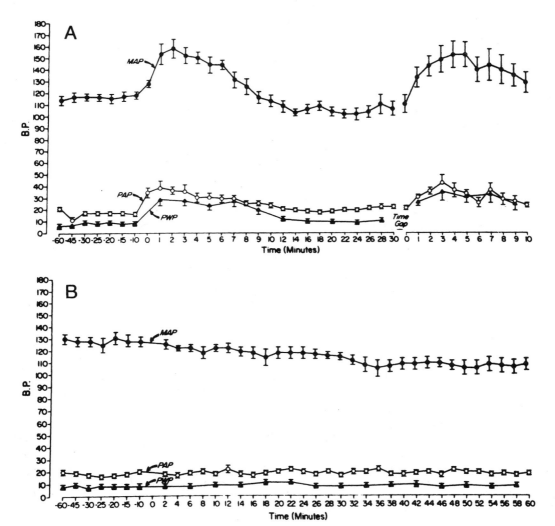

Fig. 21-4 A, Mean and SE of MAP, pulmonary artery pressure (PAP), and PCWP of eight preeclamptic patients who underwent cesarean section under thiopental and nitrous oxide (40%) anesthesia. Values before induction of anesthesia are indicated by −60 to −10. The start of induction is indicated by the first 0. The second 0 refers to the start of suction and extubation. The time gap refers to the time elapsed between the completion of the first 30 minutes of anesthesia and the start of suction and extubation. **B,** Mean and SE of MAP, PAP, and PCWP of nine preeclamptic patients who underwent cesarean section under epidural anesthesia. Values before epidural injection of bupivacaine at 0 minutes are indicated as −60 to −10 and values during epidural analgesia as 2 to 60. (From Hodgkinson R, Husain FJ, Hayashi RH: *Can Anaesth Soc J* 1980; 27:389-394. Used by permission.)

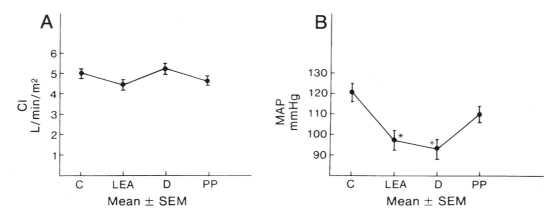

Fig. 21-5 A, Cardiac index (CI) fro severe preeclamptic patients before anesthesia *(C)*, after lumbar epidural anesthesia *(LEA)*, at delivery *(D)*, and 2 hours postpartum *(PP)*. Data expressed as mean ± SEM. Statistical significance at $p \leq 0.05$. **B,** MAP from severe preeclamptic patients before anesthesia *(C)*, after lumbar epidural anesthesia *(LEA)*, at delivery *(D)*, and 2 hours postpartum *(PP)*. Data expressed as mean ± SEM. Statistical significance at $p \leq 0.05$. (From Newsome LR, Bramwell RS, Curling PE: *Anesth Analg* 1986; 65:31-36. Used by permission.)

Table 21-3 Cesarean section in preeclampsia: epidural vs. general anesthesia*

	Epidural		General		P
	n	**%**	**n**	**%**	
Deliveries	85		15		—
Hypotension	11	13	4	27	NS
Hypertension	0		10	67†	—

*Adapted from Moore TM, Key TC, Reisner LS, et al: *Am J Obstet Gynecol* 1985; 152:404-412.
†Despite prophylaxis with sodium nitroprusside in five patients.

nal outcomes among patients who delivered with either epidural, general, or local anesthesia. Forty-seven subjects with severe hypertension received either CVP or pulmonary artery (PA) pressure catheters. Of the women who delivered vaginally, 116 received epidural anesthesia and 69 received local anesthesia. The incidence of hypotension defined as systolic pressure of 100 mm Hg or less or diastolic pressure of 50 mm Hg or less was 7% in the epidural group and 6% in the local anesthesia group. There was no difference in Apgar scores or umbilical cord blood gas values between the two neonatal groups. Of the women who underwent cesarean section, 85 received epidural analgesia and 15 received general anesthesia. The incidence of hypotension was 12% and 27% in the epidural and general anesthesia groups, respectively.

In contrast, blood pressure during induction in the general anesthesia group ranged from 170/100 to 240/120 in 5 patients despite aggressive treatment with sodium nitroprusside (Table 21-3). These patients were at risk for cerebral hemorrhage

and pulmonary edema, though no cardiovascular or neurologic sequelae were noted postoperatively. Neonatal Apgar scores less than 7 and umbilical cord pH <7.20 were lower in the general anesthesia group (Table 21-4).

Jouppila et al[65] prospectively studied uterine intervillous blood flow in 9 women with severe preeclampsia who received epidural block. All patients received 500 mL lactated Ringer's solution and were kept in 15-degree left lateral tilt. Eight of 9 women had increases in intervillous blood flow following epidural block. One patient who gave birth to a 2200-g newborn at 39 weeks' gestation had a decrease in intervillous blood flow from 72 to 68 mL/min/dL after epidural block and no fetal distress. Mean increase in group intervillous blood flow was from 196 ± 120 mL/min/dL to 320 ± 183 mL/min/dL following epidural block. These same investigators found a 35% reduction in intervillous blood flow after induction of elective general anesthesia in 10 patients who received 4 mg/kg thiopental and 1 mg/kg succinylcholine for tracheal intubation.[73]

Other investigators using the same methodology in pregnancy-induced hypertension found no change in intervillous blood flow following epidural block.[74] Details of the technique, limitations, and reliability of the measurements with intravenous xenon 133 have been described by Rekonen et al.[75] Although a mechanism for improved blood flow after epidural block is unknown, it is suggested that myometrial spiral arteries remain abnormally narrow in preeclampsia[76] and that they retain receptor site activity in response to circulating catecholamines (Fig. 21-6). Abboud[66] has

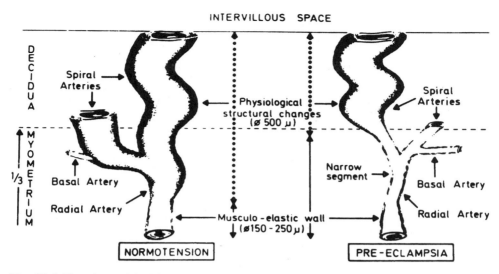

Fig. 21-6 The placental bed in normal and preeclamptic pregnancy. In preeclampsia the physiologic changes in the uteroplacental bed do not extend beyond the deciduomyometrial junction, leaving a constricting segment between the parent radial artery and the decidual portions. This area may retain sensitivity to circulating catecholamines. (Adapted from Brosens IA: *Clin Obstet Gynaecol* 1977; 4:573-593.)

Table 21-4 Cesarean section neonatal outcome (severe preeclampsia)*

	Epidural		General		*P* value
	n	%	n	%	
Deliveries	85		15		
Intensive care	25	29	9	60	0.05
5 minute Apgar <7	6	7	8	53	0.001
Cord pH	7.28	± 0.07	7.16	± 0.18	0.001
Cord pH <7.20	3	4	8	53	0.001

*Adapted from Moore TM, Key TC, Reisner LS, et al: *Am J Obstet Gynecol* 1985; 152:404-412.

shown that circulating catecholamines are significantly increased in preeclampsia compared with normal parturients and that lumbar epidural block decreases maternal sympathoadrenal activity in preeclampsia.

Fetal distress is one of the most common indications for rapid delivery in preeclampsia. The safety of epidural block in the presence of fetal distress has been questioned because even in women who have a fluid preload and continuous uterine displacement before block induction, occasional hypotension (systolic BP <100 mm Hg or a decrease in systolic BP >20%) does occur.

The question is: In the presence of fetal distress, if maternal hypotension develops and is rapidly corrected with further fluid infusion, positioning, and intravenous ephedrine, is there then a deterioration in the intrauterine environment leading to a decrease in fetal pH or Po$_2$? Brizgys et al[77]

reviewed 35 cases of fetal distress in women receiving epidural block. Those women who became hypotensive received rapid correction of blood pressure over 1 to 2 minutes with increased intravenous fluid infusion, increased uterine displacement, and intravenous ephedrine. Neonatal Apgar scores and umbilical cord blood gas values were compared between normotensive and transiently hypotensive mothers who received rapid hemodynamic correction. Mean cord blood gas values for pH and Po$_2$ were decreased compared with neonates of the normal controls, but there was no difference in blood gas values between distressed neonates of the normotensive mothers and those of the rapidly treated hypotensive mothers. This study provides evidence that during epidural block in the presence of fetal distress, rapidly corrected maternal hypotension is not associated with further intrauterine fetal deterioration.

The clinician will bear in mind that sustained maternal hypotension under any circumstance but particularly in the presence of preeclampsia represents a potentially life-threatening condition to the fetus. This requires close continuous monitoring and maintenance of maternal hemodynamics during major conduction block as well as continuous fetal heart rate monitoring to ensure fetal well-being.

In view of widespread favorable clinical experience and investigation cited above, it is the author's opinion that lumbar epidural block is the *preferred method* for analgesia for labor and vaginal delivery and for anesthesia for cesarean section in most patients with pregnancy-induced hypertension. Epidural block can provide complete analgesia and can afford a restful labor without the need for sedation. It does not incur neonatal depression, and it provides ideal obstetric conditions for spontaneous vaginal, operative vaginal, or cesarean delivery. Maternal physiology is stabilized,[78] and the risk of maternal aspiration is greatly reduced because the mother remains awake. In addition to the above benefits, it is apparent that epidural block placed early in the course of labor decreases the need for emergency induction of general anesthesia and thereby protects the mother from such life-threatening conditions as the loss of ability to ventilate or pulmonary and cerebral hypertension seen during laryngoscopy. For a favorable outcome, anesthesia should be administered by a qualified anesthesiologist. The mother and fetus should receive continuous monitoring, and epidural block is avoided when standard contraindications exist.

From a psychological standpoint, epidural anesthesia for cesarean section has the advantage of allowing the mother to view the neonate shortly after delivery. In severely preeclamptic patients, the fetus is often premature and is admitted to the intensive care nursery. At the same time, the mother is severely hypertensive and not always stable. Hence, mother and baby are often separated for several days. With the patient awake during cesarean delivery, she has the opportunity to see the neonate. Often this allays much anxiety and allows a smoother immediate postoperative course.

The use of epidural analgesia and its advantages in the management of the severe preeclamptic patient has been concisely reviewed elsewhere by several authorities in the fields of anesthesia and obstetrics.[79]

ANALGESIA AND ANESTHESIA

The following section will outline an approach to pain relief for labor, spontaneous vaginal delivery, operative vaginal delivery, and anesthesia for cesarean section in the presence of preeclampsia. In our practice every effort is made to use continuous lumbar epidural analgesia for either labor and vaginal delivery and anesthesia for cesarean section.

Labor analgesia

When the obstetrician is committed to delivery the anesthesiologist is contacted, the patient's condition assessed, and consent for anesthesia is obtained. Since rapid delivery is more likely in preeclampsia because of increased uterine activity or deterioration of the maternal or fetal condition, analgesia is started earlier than in normal labor. Whether labor is spontaneous or induced, epidural analgesia is usually initiated when the patient first experiences discomfort. Most patients receive no narcotics or sedatives during labor. A coagulation profile is obtained before proceeding with anesthesia. In the rare case in which a full profile is not available, we accept a bedside activated coagulation time of less than 145 seconds, evidence of good clot formation, and assurance of no other clinical signs of abnormal coagulation (petechiae, bleeding from puncture sites). Patients with blood pressure exceeding 140/90 mm Hg receive magnesium sulfate, which is continued throughout labor and delivery. An initial bolus of 4 to 6 g of magnesium sulfate (8 to 10 mL of 50% magnesium sulfate in 100 to 250 mL of normal saline) is administered over 30 to 45 minutes. This is followed by a continuous infusion of 2 g/hr. Electronic fetal monitoring (preferably internal) and one-on-one nursing monitoring are also required. If preeclampsia is severe or eclampsia is present a urinary catheter and a central line (usually CVP) are inserted. A modest fluid preload of 500 mL balanced salt solution is infused. If preeclampsia is severe, fluid is infused to a CVP of 2 to 4 cm H_2O. Crystalloid infusion is limited to 1000 mL and if more fluid is required, colloid in the form of 25% salt-poor albumin is infused in quantities rarely exceeding 50 mL.

Heller[80] and later Dror[81] have reported the use of 1:200,000 and 1:400,000 epinephrine combined with local anesthetics in preeclampsia of varied severity. Maternal hemodynamic response showed neither pronounced maternal hypertension, hypotension, or cardiac dysrhythmia. One subject who received 130 μg epidural epinephrine experienced a transient tachycardia of 130 beats per minute. Fetal heart rate monitored continually revealed no abnormalities. The cardiovascular effect of epidural epinephrine/local anesthesia combinations in nonpregnant subjects is a greater reduction of systemic vascular resistance than is seen with non–epinephrine-containing solutions.[82] This is attributed to absorption of small amounts of epinephrine that cause beta agonist effects in the cardiovascular system. Other investigators[83] have shown epidural epinephrine does not alter intervillous blood flow in normal parturients. Costin et al[84] and Alahuta et al[85] argue against the use of epinephrine in local anesthetic agents because they observed decreased umbilical blood velocity and decreased fetal pulsatility index in renal and middle cerebral arteries during Doppler studies in humans. Marx believes epidural epinephrine is contraindicated in preeclampsia.[86]

Another theoretical argument against the use of epinephrine-containing solutions is the possibility of transient decrease in uterine blood flow following accidental intravenous injection.[87] Currently, our clinical experience and most available data indicate the incidence is low for adverse reactions to epinephrine-containing local anesthetics when injected into the epidural space in preeclampsia.

We avoid epinephrine in the test dose and rely on early CNS signs of intravascular local anesthetic injection of lidocaine 1.5% to 2% and slow incremental injection of the therapeutic. When epidural placement is clear, epinephrine 1:400,000 is added to epidural local anesthetic for further therapeutic injections. Initially the anesthesiologist seeks to block only a T10 sensory level with 6 to 12 mL of lidocaine 1.5% or bupivacaine 0.25%. Uterine displacement of 15 degrees or more is assured and a maternal decrease in systolic pressure greater than 25% or less than 100 mm Hg or deterioration in fetal heart rate is treated with further intravenous infusion of balanced salt solution or colloid and incremental doses of intravenous ephedrine (5-mg increments). Oxygen 50% or greater by face mask is usually administered. Once the block has been established, a level higher and denser than normal labor is sought. This is done by reinjection with 10 to 12 mL of 0.375% bupivacaine with a goal of a solid T8-T6 sensory level to cold. The advantages of this approach include assurance of adequate analgesia for immediate operative vaginal or cesarean delivery; prevention of precipitous delivery associated with intracerebral bleeds in the preterm and small neonate; and less maternal hypotension when the level of block is rapidly elevated. Such a dense block is unlikely to interfere with second-stage labor as the fetal size is often small and uterine activity is usually increased. In cases where second-stage labor is slightly prolonged under epidural block, recent evidence shows that neonatal Apgar scores and blood gases are not affected.[88]

Total maternal body clearance of lidocaine is reported to be slightly prolonged in women with preeclampsia.[89] Maternal local anesthetic toxicity is avoided by using continuous infusion epidural analgesia with dilute anesthetic concentrations, low dose epidural fentanyl supplementation, appropriate test doses, and slow incremental epidural injection.

Subarachnoid block for vaginal delivery

Smith et al[90] have shown that a modified subarachnoid block to T10 sensory level can safely provide analgesia for vaginal delivery in the presence of preeclampsia. Sudden maternal hypotension is usually not great if the level does not exceed T10, uterine displacement is assured, and adequate intravenous infusion of balanced salt solution precedes the block. Recommended doses include hyperbaric bupivacaine or tetracaine 4 to 6 mg or hyperbaric lidocaine 35 to 50 mg. The risk of postspinal headache can be decreased by using small-gauge needles (25- to 29-gauge) or needles with noncutting points such as Whitacre or Sprotte.

Other methods of analgesia for labor

If epidural block is contraindicated or refused by the patient, other less effective alternatives for analgesia are available. Narcotics, if used, should be given early in labor and in small doses to minimize neonatal depression. Although narcotics provide analgesia, they have no anticonvulsant and little antihypertensive effects. Tranquilizers, often given with narcotics, are administered sparingly because there are no drugs available to antagonize their effects. Phenothiazines, often given with narcotics to decrease the associated nausea, should also be administered sparingly because they theoretically lower seizure threshold. Late first-stage and second-stage analgesia can be supplemented with 30% to 40% nitrous oxide, which will also provide supplemental oxygen and incur minimal cardiovascular depression and negligible neonatal effects. At delivery, bilateral transvaginal pudendal block added to inhaled nitrous oxide will allow most forceps deliveries and either Silastic or Maalstrom vacuum extraction. Local infiltration will allow episiotomy for vaginal delivery. Small amounts of enflurane (0.4% to 0.6%) combined with inhaled nitrous oxide will improve analgesia.

If maternal hypertension is well controlled, a satisfactory alternative to inhalation analgesia for delivery is low-dose (0.25 mg/kg) intravenous ketamine not exceeding 0.75 mg/kg before delivery. This will provide 2 to 5 minutes of intense analgesia usually sufficient to allow forceps or vacuum delivery. Techniques of inhalation analgesia do not require endotracheal intubation if precautions are taken to ensure continued maternal consciousness and sustained airway reflexes.

The advantages of inhalation/intravenous analgesia techniques include simplicity and speed, which make them appropriate for precipitous delivery or when maternal or fetal conditions do not allow time for major conduction block. These techniques do not provide ideal obstetric conditions because pain relief is often incomplete and precipitous delivery is more likely with the attendant risks of cerebral hemorrhage. Also, incomplete pain relief is associated with exacerbations of hypertension in the preeclamptic patient with its associated risks.

In the rare event that general anesthesia is required for vaginal delivery, the techniques described below under anesthesia for emergency cesarean section should be followed. Every effort should be made to avoid severe maternal hypertension during rapid sequence induction of general anesthesia.

Anesthesia for nonemergent cesarean section

Urgent but not emergent cesarean section in patients with preeclampsia-eclampsia is characterized by failure to progress, failed induction, previous vertical uterine scar or hysterotomy, prolonged rupture of membranes with the development of severe chorioamnionitis, or an unripe cervix in the presence of worsening preeclampsia. The vast majority of these patients are candidates for epidural block, which can be initiated in three steps. In mild preeclampsia prehydration is accomplished with 1 to 2 L of balanced salt solution. In severe preeclampsia, intravenous fluid is infused to ensure that a CVP of 2 to 4 cm H_2O and no more than 1 L of balanced salt solution is given. If further prehydration is required, 25 to 50 mL of 25% salt-poor albumin is used.

Epidural block is initiated to a T10 level using 6 to 10 mL of 0.5% bupivacaine or 1.5% lidocaine. Sufficient time is allowed for maternal response and stabilization after partial sympathectomy. With incremental injections of local anesthetic, the level is gradually (over 20 minutes) elevated to a T4-T2 sensory level. Fentanyl 50 to 75 µg or meperidine 50 mg is usually added to the local anesthetic mixture. Fifteen degrees left uterine displacement is maintained, and significant hypotension is treated with intravenous ephedrine in 5-mg doses. A decrease in CVP below 2 cm H_2O is treated with further infusion of balanced salt solution or colloid as indicated. It is not uncommon following delivery to observe sudden, asymptomatic decreases in blood pressure lasting several minutes. Unless accompanied by maternal discomfort or early signs of hypoperfusion (dizziness, nausea, pallor, or sustained tachycardia) these episodes are often not treated. At the conclusion of surgery it is our practice to administer 4 to 5 mg of epidural morphine to provide sustained postoperative analgesia while the patient is monitored on the labor floor for 24 hours. In an institution where close monitoring of the vital signs is possible, epidural morphine will be the ideal way to take care of postoperative pain relief. However, in institutions where ideal supervision is not possible, PCA may be the second best choice.

Anesthesia for emergency cesarean section

Emergency cesarean section in preeclampsia-eclampsia is most often done for fetal distress. In our practice, these patients usually have a functioning epidural catheter that was placed earlier in labor. With some exceptions, the absence of an epidural catheter in this population is considered an error in patient management either in the obstetrician not contacting the anesthesiologist with sufficient dispatch or in an unnecessary delay on the anesthesiologist's part. The presence of uteroplacental insufficiency or fetal distress are not in themselves contraindications to epidural block.

Often there is time to initiate epidural block when results of a fetal scalp blood sample are being obtained and analyzed. If a functioning epidural catheter is in place and a T8-T6 sensory level is present, the block level and density can be elevated adequately by slowly injecting (over 3 to 5 minutes) a full cesarean section dose of 18 to 22 mL of lidocaine 1.5% or 15 to 20 mL of 2 chloroprocaine 3%. This will usually produce an adequate T4-T2 sensory level within 5 to 8 minutes. Unless the epidural was "topped up" within the last 10 minutes, a full volume dose will usually be required. Epinephrine 1:400,000 and fentanyl 50 to 75 µg or meperidine 50 mg can also be included in the injectate.

If an epidural catheter is not in place or is not functioning properly, some clinicians believe general anesthesia is then indicated. We usually prefer initiation of spinal block instead of general anesthesia because of the many maternal risks (described below) and in particular because of the significant airway changes associated with disease. If preeclampsia is not severe, hyperbaric subarachnoid lidocaine 5% (70 to 80 mg), bupivacaine 0.75% (12 to 15 mg), or tetracaine 0.5% (9 to 11 mg) are recommended reliable doses to obtain a T4 sensory level. The addition of 25 µg fentanyl and 0.15 to 0.25 mg morphine to the local anesthetic solution will improve the quality of the block and allow for prolonged postoperative analgesia. Subarachnoid block in severe preeclampsia may be associated with sudden and profound hypotension related to sympathetic block and severe blood volume contraction. Although past wisdom has advised against spinal block in severe untreated pre-eclampsia, we are inclined to use subarachnoid anesthesia in selected cases if rapid modest hydration can be obtained and if continuous maternal blood pressure monitoring and small doses (5 mg) of intravenous ephedrine are used to provide a stable hemodynamic environment. The reader is cautioned that the risks of this approach must be balanced against the equal if not greater risks of a hurried "crash" induction of general anesthesia. Indications for general anesthesia include very severe fetal distress such as a sustained bradycardia in the absence of an indwelling epidural catheter, maternal refusal of regional block, and standard contraindications to regional block such as uncorrected hypovolemia, severe coagulopathy, and septicemia.

Problems of general anesthesia in preeclampsia

In addition to the usual precautions for general anesthesia in pregnancy (such as the need for left uterine displacement until delivery, avoidance of hyperventilation, and the prevention of pulmonary aspiration), there are special problems that increase anesthetic risk associated with preeclampsia-eclampsia. These include edema of the upper airway, severe hypertensive response to laryngoscopy, and the interaction of magnesium with general anesthesia, especially muscle relaxants. In severe preeclampsia, magnesium therapy and other respiratory depressant medications may increase the susceptibility to hypoventilation and hypoxia compounded by an increased alveolar arterial blood gas gradient often seen in this disease. Kambam et al[91] have shown that in preeclampsia, the P_{50} of the maternal oxyhemoglobin dissociation curve is shifted left from a normal of about 30 mm Hg to less than 25 mm Hg. These effects that predispose to maternal hypoxia indicate that supplemental high-flow oxygen administration is required throughout labor and delivery or cesarean section and into the recovery period.

Airway edema. There are numerous reports in the literature describing severe airway edema associated with preeclampsia complicating intubation.[92-94] This requires a special attention to the airway examination before induction of general anesthesia in preeclampsia. Hoarseness, a high pitched or stridorous voice, and small stature mean that a small (5–6 mm) endotracheal tube may be necessary.

Of equal importance, a decision must be made as to whether awake intubation is required. If on examination the uvula is not visualized, hyoid-mental distance of less than 3 cm is found, the jaw opening is limited, a short neck is evident, or a re-ceding jaw or buck teeth are present, the anesthesiologist must avoid a rapid sequence induction and ensure that the airway is protected with a cuffed endotracheal tube while the patient is conscious before surgery starts. This almost always requires both oropharyngeal topical anesthesia with some sedation and time.

Hypertensive response to general anesthesia. The induction of general anesthesia for cesarean section is designed to provide sufficient maternal hypnosis/analgesia and avoid newborn depression. The maternal hemodynamic response to 4 mg/kg thiopental, 1.5 mg/kg succinylcholine, and two thirds minimum alveolar concentration of a potent inhalation drug is usually associated with an increase in heart rate and blood pressure that often lasts until delivery. This hypertensive response is particularly severe in the presence of preeclampsia and is difficult to control.[68-71] The pulmonary and cerebral hypertension seen at both induction and emergence further predisposes the mother to the two most common causes of maternal death in preeclampsia: cerebral hemorrhage and pulmonary edema.[95]

Intravenous hydralazine titrated in 5-mg increments is widely used to control hypertension in preeclampsia[96] and is not associated with decreased uterine blood flow. This drug is not very useful as an antihypertensive agent before emergency induction of general anesthesia because of the latency of onset (10 to 15 min). Nitroprusside,[97] nitroglycerin,[98] and trimethaphan[99] have been advocated for rapid perioperative treatment of maternal hypertension, but precise control is often difficult. A frequent response to vasodilator therapy in preeclampsia is reflex tachycardia, widened pulse pressure, and minimal decrease in mean blood pressure. Moore et al reported a 50% increase in mean arterial pressure during laryngoscopy in preeclamptic patients despite aggressive use of nitroprusside.[69] Trimethaphan may offer some advantages over other rapid-acting vasodilators because there is little change in cerebral blood flow or intracranial pressure during trimethaphan-induced hypotension and because fetal transfer is unlikely because of high molecular weight.[100] Prolonged neuromuscular paralysis from succinylcholine was reported in one parturient after 1700 mg of Arfonad.[101] However, this is an extremely rare occurrence combined with an unusual dose of trimethaphan. Another side effect of trimethaphan that may be important in this condition is pupillary dilation. The relative advantages and pitfalls of vasodilator therapy are discussed in some detail elsewhere.[99]

More recently the use of preoperative narcotics or beta blockers have been advocated to attenuate this response. Lawes et al. recently reported successful attenuation of the hypertensive response to laryngoscopy with the use of 200 μg fentanyl and 5 mg droperidol administered before rapid sequence induction in severe preeclampsia.[71] Although this combination of medications appears to effectively control hypertension during induction, it is preferable to avoid drugs that predispose an already compromised fetus to further depression.

The use of beta-adrenergic receptor blockers such as labetalol may provide effective protection from the hypertensive response to endotracheal intubation while avoiding adverse neonatal effects.

Ramanathan compared the maternal hemodynamic response to general anesthesia induction with and without labetalol antihypertensive therapy.[102] Intravenous labetalol 20 mg followed by increments of 10 mg up to a maximum of 1 mg/kg resulted in moderate reductions in maternal mean arterial pressure and heart rate with attenuation of the hypertensive response to laryngoscopy and intubation (Fig. 21-7). Excessive hypotension with general anesthesia and usual blood loss did not occur. Neonatal heart rate, blood pressure, plasma glucose, Apgar scores, and umbilical blood gases did not differ between the group receiving labetalol and

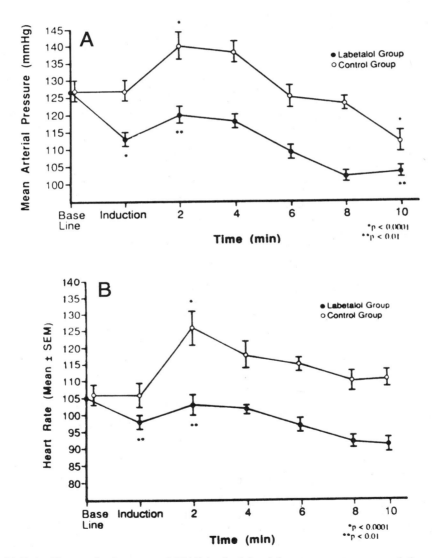

Fig. 21-7 A, Changes in the maternal MAP in the labetalol pretreatment group and the control group: preeclampsia. **B,** Changes in the maternal mean heart rate in the labetalol pretreatment group and the control group: preeclampsia. (From Ramanathan J, Siba BM, Mabie WC, et al: *Am J Obstet Gynecol* 1989; 159:650-654. Used by permission.)

the group receiving no therapy. Morgan et al showed labetalol in doses of less than 0.5 mg/kg decreased maternal blood pressure and increased uteroplacental blood flow in the hypertensive baboon models.[103] However, the same authors observed a decrease in uterine blood flow at doses of 1 to 2 mg/kg of labetalol. Chronic oral labetalol therapy (100 to 200 mg three times a day) from 20 to 38 weeks' gestation until birth effectively lowers maternal blood pressure and is not associated with adverse neonatal effects.[104] In higher doses, labetalol has been associated with neonatal adrenergic blockade.[105] There are isolated reports of marked hypotension following 10 mg of labetalol in severe preeclampsia. Although this is rare, it may be a response of compromised myocardium to negative inotropic effects of labetalol. In our practice, labetalol has replaced trimethaphan as an acute antihypertensive of choice in preeclampsia. We usually give a small initial intravenous dose of 5 mg to assess hemodynamic response before progressing to larger doses. Esmolol is not as widely used for acute blood pressure control because of increased placental passage compared with labetalol; a study in fetal sheep[106] also showed beta-adrenergic blockade and hypoxemia. Although we rarely use this drug, the benefits of ultrashort onset and offset of beta-blockade with esmolol may outweigh the reported risks in selected cases. Oral nifedipine, an effective antihypertensive in severe preeclampsia,[107] is not routinely used in our practice for acute preoperative blood pressure control.

Before rapid sequence induction for emergency cesarean section in preeclampsia, we attempt to decrease diastolic blood pressure to less than 105 mm Hg with intravenous labetalol 5 to 20 mg. Intravenous trimethaphan 1 to 4 mg may be combined with further incremental doses of labetalol to provide an effective blood pressure reduction. Other methods used to prevent hypertension at intubation include an adequate induction dose of thiopental (4 mg/kg), intravenous lidocaine (100 mg) 3 to 5 minutes before induction, and intravenous fentanyl (6 μg/kg). This amount of intravenous fentanyl before fetal delivery may be associated with neonatal respiratory depression and may require ventilatory support followed by naloxone reversal. The problem is minor if a pediatrician is present and has been informed that the mother received a narcotic agent.

Ketamine, to our knowledge, has not been studied in a controlled manner as an induction agent for general anesthesia in preeclampsia. It is associated with hypertension in intravenous doses of 0.75 to 1.0 mg and is not a first-line choice as an induction agent.

Magnesium sulfate. Magnesium sulfate is the anticonvulsant therapy for preeclampsia most widely used in the United States. Blood levels are estimated by monitoring deep tendon reflexes. Absence of deep tendon reflexes may indicate magnesium levels of 10 mEq/L or higher; these are associated with organ toxicity ranging from lengthened PR and QS intervals, sinoatrial and atrioventricular block, respiratory depression, and cardiac arrest. Blood levels should be monitored frequently if the patient is oliguric, if deep tendon reflexes disappear, or if the patient appears to have labored breathing. If the cesarean section is emergent, the presence of deep tendon reflexes can assure the anesthesiologist that the serum magnesium level is usually less than 10 mEq/L.

Magnesium causes increased sensitivity to all muscle relaxants especially nondepolarizing blockers.[108] It is well advised to avoid nondepolarizing muscle relaxants entirely and to use succinylcholine exclusively for relaxation. A defasciculation dose of 3 mg of intravenous curare may result in rapid paralysis of the patient and is to be avoided.[109] A full dose of 100 mg or 1.5 mg/kg intravenous succinylcholine (whichever is greater) is injected at induction to provide relaxation and airway visualization. Thereafter, small increments of 5 to 10 mg are administered intravenously as indicated. Routine neuromuscular blockade monitoring should be mandatory.

Because of the natural decrease in muscle tone that occurs in pregnancy and the presence of maternal therapeutic magnesium levels, muscle relaxants are rarely required after induction of general anesthesia in preeclampsia. We recommend avoidance of further muscle relaxants if possible and administration of a "real" postdelivery anesthetic after delivery of the fetus that consists of two thirds minimum alveolar concentration of a potent inhalation drug until closure, 65% to 70% nitrous oxide after fetal delivery, and short-acting intravenous narcotics such as fentanyl.

Strict extubation criteria in the patient include consciousness, eyes wide open, response to command, and ability to lift her head off the pillow for greater than five seconds. Even if these criteria are met, the decision threshold for continued postoperative ventilation after general anesthesia should be low for patients receiving magnesium.

HELLP syndrome

In 1982, Weinstein[110] reported a syndrome in pregnancy characterized by *he*molysis, elevated *l*iver enzymes, and *l*ow *p*latelet count (HELLP), and he described it as a severe consequence of pregnancy-induced hypertension. The obstetric management and definition of HELLP has generated debate in the literature. Although traditionally the HELLP syndrome has been considered synonymous with severe preeclampsia, there is some evidence that it might be a freestanding syndrome.[111] The diagnosis of hemolysis is based on elevated LDH and decreased haptoglobin. There may or may not be evidence of hemolysis on the peripheral smear, depending on the severity of the disorder. To diagnose liver dysfunction, transaminases must be elevated. They are not elevated to the degree one sees in hepatitis, but they are usually in the range of 100 to 500 IU/L. Alkaline phosphatase is not used to diagnose liver dysfunction because the placenta produces an abundance of this enzyme and it is normally elevated during pregnancy. Bilirubin may or may not be elevated in the HELLP syndrome, and thrombocytopenia is diagnosed by platelet count. Management plans should not be based solely on a depressed platelet count without any other signs of HELLP or preeclampsia. Burrows and Kelton have shown that an isolated platelet count between 100,000 and 150,000/μL is not an uncommon finding in late pregnancy.[112] Of the patients in their study, 75% had normal platelet counts within 3 days following delivery without any maternal or fetal sequelae.

One problem is that laboratory evidence of HELLP may develop before there are any signs of hypertension and proteinuria in the patient.[113] If unrecognized, the HELLP syndrome can be misdiagnosed as immune thrombocytopenic purpura, mild hepatitis, or even cholecystitis.[114]

The classic teaching has been that delivery should be accomplished as soon as the diagnosis of HELLP syndrome is made. We and others have followed selected patients expectantly if the fetus is remote from term.[115] In our most dramatic case, a patient was referred at 28 weeks because there was a fear of dwarfism in the fetus. A review of the patient's previous ultrasound reports and history revealed the fetus was experiencing symmetric intrauterine growth retardation. Laboratory parameters showed evidence of the HELLP syndrome. She was hospitalized and followed expectantly. She did not develop hypertension until 31 weeks' gestation, and she did not develop evidence of severe preeclampsia (except for a diminished platelet count) until 33 weeks' gestation when she underwent primary cesarean section and delivered a viable infant with minimal neonatal morbidity. Van Dam et al. suggest that patients can be followed expectantly as long as they do not show signs or laboratory parameters of active disseminated intravascular coagulopathy.[115]

Severe complications can result from the HELLP syndrome and in the majority of cases, di-

agnosis is an indication for delivery. Sibai et al. surveyed the outcome of a large series of women with HELLP syndrome.[116,117] HELLP syndrome developed in 18.9% of 2331 patients with severe preeclampsia. De novo DIC occurred in less than 5% of HELLP patients, but the overall rate of DIC was 21%. Hysterectomy was higher in this group as was laparotomy for intraabdominal bleeding. Abruptio placenta occurred in 16%, acute renal failure in 8%, severe ascites in 8%, and pulmonary edema or effusion in 12%. Four patients had severe laryngeal edema, and two sustained hypoxic brain damage due to airway control difficulty. There were five maternal deaths of which 4 were HELLP related. Three of these were due to diffuse hypoxic encephalopathy and one to multiple organ failure.

Duffy[118] reported the anesthetic management of four parturients with HELLP or HELLP-like symptoms. Two patients received epidural block, the first had an initial platelet count of 184,000/μL that later decreased to 66,000/μL accompanied by severe hemolysis and subsequent adult respiratory distress syndrome. The second patient did not show symptoms of HELLP until after epidural block was placed and an isolated platelet count of 74,000/μL was obtained following observation of a puncture site that would not clot. Neither patient showed evidence of epidural hematoma, and both recovered. Two patients did not receive regional block, one because of an initial misdiagnosis of infectious hepatitis, the second because of a platelet count of 77,000/μL.

The problem for the anesthesiologist is that the HELLP syndrome may occasionally be misdiagnosed or missed completely since clear physical symptoms such as hypertension, hyperreflexia, and edema may be absent on the patient's hospital admission. Thus, platelet count, coagulation profile, and liver function studies may not be immediately available to the anesthesiologist. In addition to coagulopathy and hemolysis-anemia, these patients are also at risk for hemorrhage, liver rupture, adult respiratory distress syndrome, acute renal failure, and postpartum jaundice. In clinical practice, it is rare for the HELLP syndrome to remain undiagnosed before anesthesia is requested. However, the anesthesiologist must maintain a high index of suspicion and when in doubt, a coagulation profile and platelet count should be obtained. Placement of early epidural infusion before severe drop of platelet count may be advantageous in this group of patients. Sibai[116] recommends aggressive blood volume expansion to prevent acute renal failure especially if DIC is present. Hemorrhage of hepatic origin is rare but requires aggressive surgery when diagnosed.

Postpartum considerations

Approximately 30% of preeclamptic mothers who develop eclampsia do so in the postpartum period. The patient remains at risk for this for at least 48 hours and up to 1 week. The peak period for postpartum eclampsia is usually within the first 8 hours, and the condition may occur as an epidural block dissipates.[67] Postpartum preeclamptic patients should receive continuous monitoring in an intensive care setting for at least 24 hours. Antihypertensive and anticonvulsant therapy are continued during this time. Magnesium infusion is usually continued for 24 hours after delivery. Diuretics should be considered if large amount of intravenous fluids were administered before delivery and diuresis is not brisk in the first 24 hours postpartum. The need for diuresis is indicated in the presence of a sustained high CVP (greater than 10 cm H_2O) or with high left ventricular filling pressures in the face of a normal cardiac output and normal blood pressure. It is well advised to continue postoperative analgesia with either epidural infusion of low concentration bupivacaine (0.125%) or intravenous or epidural narcotics. This may avoid the intense vasoconstriction associated with postoperative pain and hypothermia.

Obstetric and anesthetic management of the patient with eclampsia

When a pregnant woman develops tonic-clonic seizures, the immediate diagnosis is eclampsia until proved otherwise. Most eclampsia occurs after 28 weeks' gestation, but there are several conditions in which eclampsia can occur earlier. These include multiple gestation, coexistant hydatidiform mole, uncontrolled chronic hypertension, and systemic lupus erythematosus. The seizures may be single or multiple leading to status epilepticus, and they should be treated in the same way as seizures of any other cause. The most important goals are to stop the convulsion, ensure an adequate protected airway, and prevent aspiration. While magnesium sulfate is the drug of choice for eclamptic seizures, any parenteral anticonvulsant agent may be used. If a pregnant woman arrives in the emergency room with seizures, treatment should not be delayed until magnesium can be found; alternatives such as diazepam, phenytoin, or phenobarbital, readily available in virtually all emergency rooms, should be administered immediately. Because many anticonvulsant agents are respiratory depressants, it is important to have the ability to provide ventilatory support in the event the patient hypoventilates following an intravenous dose of anticonvulsant drug.

The treatment of eclampsia is delivery, but it is a disservice to both mother and fetus if operative intervention is initiated before the mother has received adequate medical therapy. Many fetuses will experience a transient bradycardia following maternal tonic/clonic seizure. If there are no signs of placental abruption, the bradycardia will often resolve spontaneously. Immediate delivery following seizure is rarely required and predisposes the unprepared mother to a number of obstetric and anesthetic risks that can be avoided with appropriate monitoring and timely therapy. We agree with the recommendations of Sibai et al[119] that except in the most dire emergencies, a minimum of 2 hours should be allowed for maternal stabilization before induction of labor or abdominal delivery. Initial recommendations include an immediate slow intravenous infusion of 4 g magnesium sulfate over 15 to 20 minutes, followed by an intravenous pump infusion of 1 to 2 g/hr.

Immediate laboratory assessment of maternal hemoglobin/hematocrit and coagulation profile should be obtained. Fetal gestational age is established and assurance obtained that anesthesia and pediatric neonatal support personnel are readily available. It is our practice to establish central venous access as soon as possible in most of our eclamptic patients and to initiate antihypertensive therapy if indicated. There is increasing evidence that early use of computed tomography (CT) may facilitate the timely diagnosis and treatment of cerebral pathology, especially hemorrhage, in eclamptic patients.[120] It is our recent experience that the use of CT scanning combined with diagnostic changes in patient consciousness and motor function will allow neurosurgical intervention that may be life-saving in the presence of impending or ongoing cerebral hemorrhage.

Eclampsia is not synonymous with cesarean section. If the patient is stabilized and the cervix is inducible, oxytocin induction should be attempted. Conversely, if the patient continues to have breakthrough seizures despite intensive medical therapy or if the cervix is long and closed, a primary cesarean section is appropriate. Also, if fetal distress occurs or the patient experiences placental abruption, an urgent cesarean section may be required. The presence of eclampsia does not contraindicate the use of epidural block for labor or for cesarean section. Moodley et al[121] reported 67 eclamptic patients who received epidural block as the anesthetic of choice for vaginal delivery and cesarean section without any increase in patient morbidity. Indeed, during the time epidural block was functional, no seizures occurred, but following recovery from the block the incidence of convulsions increased.[67] Guidelines for the use of epidural block or general anesthesia in the presence of eclampsia are similar to those for patients with severe preeclampsia; these are covered in detail in those sections of this chapter. If uterine atony is encountered following delivery, oxytocin can be given both by intravenous infusion or bolus. Ergot alkaloids should be used with caution because they can precipitate hypertensive crisis. The use of prostaglandin $E_{2\alpha}$, and its derivatives has not been investigated in enough detail in the presence of eclampsia, and its use should be guided by clinical indication and judgment. Postoperatively, it is important to maintain adequate urine output and assess clotting parameters frequently. As with preeclamptic patients, magnesium infusion should continue for at least 24 hours after delivery.

Neonatal considerations

The neonate of a preeclamptic patient is at greater risk of prematurity, asphyxia, drug depression, meconium aspiration, and being small for gestational age. Prolonged in utero exposure to magnesium sulfate can also lead to flaccidity at birth. A person skilled at neonatal resuscitation should be present at delivery, and intensive care is usually required to avoid or treat problems frequently seen in this population, including respiratory distress (due to prematurity), hypoglycemia, hypocalcemia, temperature instability, and poor feeding. Koenig and Christensen have recently observed that neutropenia is common in the neonate born to the preeclamptic mother.[122] This can be mistaken for sepsis in the newborn and may lead to unnecessary antibiotic therapy. On the other hand, this neutropenia can place the newborn at increased risk of sepsis in the neonatal period.

CONCLUSIONS

Preeclampsia was once a disorder that carried a high maternal and perinatal morbidity and mortality rate in this country. It is still a major cause of perinatal morbidity and mortality in third world nations. Significant advances in anesthetic and obstetric care, including invasive and noninvasive maternal hemodynamic monitoring of the mother, rational fluid replacement, increased use of regional anesthesia, and a large array of available pharmaceuticals (including magnesium sulfate), have made maternal mortality an exceedingly rare occurrence and have greatly decreased maternal morbidity. Advances in fetal monitoring and in the care of the newborn that is premature or small for gestational age have greatly diminished neonatal morbidity and mortality. Anesthesiologists, obstetricians, and neonatologists must continue to work together and devise and test new surveillance and therapeutic modalities so that we can further reduce the impact of this once feared and still misunderstood disorder on both mother and baby.

REFERENCES

1. Page AW, Christianson R: The impact of mean arterial blood pressure in the middle trimester upon the outcome of pregnancy. *Am J Obstet Gynecol* 1976; 125:740.
2. Sibai BM, Gordon T, Thom E, et al: Risk factors for preeclampsia in healthy nulliparous women: A prospective multicenter study. *Am J Obstet Gynecol* 1995; 172:642.
3. Sutherland A, Cooper DW, Howie PW: The incidence of severe preeclampsia amongst mothers and mothers-in-law of preeclamptics and controls. *Br J Obstet Gynaecol* 1981; 88:785.
4. Friedman SA: Preeclampsia: A review of the role of prostaglandins. *Obstet Gynecol* 1988; 71:122.
5. Pollak VE, Nettles JB: The kidney in toxemia of pregnancy: A clinical and pathologic study based on renal biopsies. *Medicine* 1960; 39:469.
6. Zuspan FP, Nelson GH, Ahlquist RP: Epinephrine infusions in normal and toxemic pregnancies. I. Nonesterified fatty acids and cardiovascular alterations. *Am J Obstet Gynecol* 1964; 90:88.
7. Talledo OE, Chesley LC, Zuspan FP: Renin-angiotensin system in normal and toxemic pregnancies. III. Differential sensitivity to angiotensin II and norepinephrine in toxemia of pregnancy. *Am J Obstet Gynecol* 1968; 100:218.
8. Gant NF, Daley GL, Chand S: A study of angiotensin II pressor response throughout primigravid pregnancy. *J Clin Invest* 1973; 52:2682.
9. Remuzzi C, Marchesi D, Zoja C: Reduced umbilical and placental vascular prostacyclin in severe preeclampsia. *Prostaglandins* 1980; 20:105.
10. Bussolino F, Benedetto C, Massobrio M, et al: Maternal vascular prostacyclin activity in preeclampsia (letter). *Lancet* 1980; 2:702.
11. Chesley LC, Markowitz I, Wetchler BB: Proteinuria following momentary vascular constriction. *J Clin Invest* 1939; 18:51.
12. Chesley LC: Hypertension in pregnancy: Definitions, familial factor, and remote prognosis. *Kidney Int* 1980; 18:234.
13. Denson KWE: The ratio of factor VIII-related antigen and factor VIII biological activity as an index of hypercoagulability and intravascular clotting. *Thromb Res* 1977; 10:107.
14. Ramsey EM, Harris HWS: Comparison of uteroplacental vasculature and circulation in the rhesus monkey and man. *Contributions to Embryology* No. 261. Carnegie Institution of Washington 1966; 38:59.
15. Brosens IA, Robertson WB, Dixon HG: The role of the spiral arterioles in the pathogenesis of preeclampsia. *Obstet Gynecol Annu* 1972; 1:171.
16. Zeek PM, Assali NS: Vascular changes in the decidua associated with eclamptogenic toxemia. *Am J Clin Pathol* 1950; 20:1099.
17. Kitzmiller JL, Benirschke K: Immunofluorescent study of placental vessels in preeclampsia. *Am J Obstet Gynecol* 1973; 115:248.
18. Platt LD, Walla CA, Paul RH, et al: A prospective trial of the fetal biophysical profile versus the nonstress test in the management of high-risk pregnancies. *Am J Obstet Gynecol* 1985; 153:624.
19. MacKenzie IZ, Castle B, Bellinger J: Transfer of prostaglandins to the fetus after prostaglandin E2 vaginal pessary administration. *Am J Obstet Gynecol* 1989; 161:920.
20. Kelton JG, Hunter DJS, Neame P: A platelet function defect in preeclampsia. *Am J Obstet Gynecol* 1985; 65:107.
21. de Boer K, Leconder I, ten Kate JW, et al: Placenta-type plasminogen activator inhibitor in preeclampsia. *Am J Obstet Gynecol* 1988; 158:518.
22. De Boer K, ten Cate JW, Sturk A, et al: Enhanced throm-

bin generation in normal and hypertensive pregnancy. *Am J Obstet Gynecol* 1989; 160:95.

23. Samuels P, Main EK, Tomaski A, et al: Abnormalities in platelet antiglobulin tests in preeclamptic mothers and their neonates. *Am J Obstet Gynecol* 1987; 107:109.

24. Rasmus KT, Rottman RL, Kotelko DM, et al: Unrecognized thrombocytopenia and regional anesthesia in parturients: A retrospective review. *Obstet Gynecol* 1989; 73:934.

25. Ramanathan J, Sibai BM, Vu T, et al: Correlation between bleeding times and platelet counts in women with preeclampsia undergoing cesarean section. *Anesthesiology* 1989; 71:188.

26. Channing-Rogers RP, Levin: A critical review of the bleeding time. *Semin Thromb Hemost* 1990; 16:1.

27. The bleeding time (editorial): *Lancet* 1991; 337:1447.

28. Goldstein R, Sinatra R, Hines R, et al: An evaluation of pregnancy associated coagulopathies utilizing the sonoclot coagulation analyzer. *Society for Obstetric Anesthesia and Perinatology Handbook,* Scientific Session G2, Seattle, May 1989.

29. Wallenburg HCS, Dekker GA, Makovitz JW, et al: Low dose aspirin prevents pregnancy induced hypertension and preeclampsia in angiotensin sensitive primigravidae. *Lancet* 1986; 1:1.

30. Sibai BM, Caritis SN, Thom E, et al: Prevention of preeclampsia with low-dose aspirin in healthy, nulliparous pregnant women. *New Engl J Med* 1993; 329:1213.

31. Zuspan FP, Samuels P: Preventing preeclampsia (editorial). *New Engl J Med* 1993; 329:1265.

32. Benigni A, Gregorini G, Frusca T, et al: Effect of low-dose aspirin on fetal and maternal generation of thromboxane by platelets in women at risk for pregnancy induced hypertension. *N Engl J Med* 1989; 321:357.

33. Belfort MA, Anthony J, Saade GR, et al: The oxygen consumption/oxygen delivery curve in severe preeclampsia: Evidence for a fixed oxygen extraction state. *Am J Obstet Gynecol* 1993; 169:1448.

34. Ducey J, Schulman H, Farmakides G: A classification of hypertension in pregnancy based on doppler velocimetry. *Am J Obstet Gynecol* 1987; 157:860.

35. Schifrin BS: Fetal heart rate patterns following epidural anesthesia and oxytocin infusions during labour. *J Obstet Gynaecol Br Commonw* 1972; 79:332.

36. Hankins GDV, Wendel GD, Cunningham FG: Longitudinal evaluation of hemodynamic changes in eclampsia. *Am J Obstet Gynecol* 1984; 150:506.

37. Gant NJ Jr, Chad C, Whalley PJ, et al: The nature of pressor responsiveness to angiotensin II in human pregnancy. *Obstet Gynecol* 1974; 43:854.

38. Quinn M: Automated blood pressure measurement devices: A potential source of morbidity in preeclampsia. *Am J Obstet Gynecol* 1994; 170:1303.

39. Benedetti T, Cotton DB, Read JC, et al: Hemodynamic observations in severe preeclampsia with a flow-directed pulmonary artery catheter. *Am J Obstet Gynecol* 1980; 136:465.

40. Rafferty TD, Berkowitz RL: Hemodynamics in patients with severe toxemia during labor and delivery. *Am J Obstet Gynecol* 1980; 138:263.

41. Phelan JP, Yurth DA: Severe preeclampsia. I. Peripartum hemodynamic observations. *Am J Obstet Gynecol* 1982; 144:17-22.

42. Groenendijk R, Trimbos JB, Wallenberg HC: Hemodynamic measurements in preeclampsia: Preliminary observations. *Am J Obstet Gynecol* 1984; 150:232.

43. Clark SI, Greenspoon JS, Aldahl D, et al: Severe preeclampsia with persistent oliguria: Management of hemodynamic subsets. *Am J Obstet Gynecol* 1986; 154:490.

44. Newsome LR, Bramwell RS, Curling PE: Severe preeclampsia: Hemodynamic effects of lumbar epidural anesthesia. *Anesth Analg* 1986; 65:31.

45. Cotton DB, Lee W, Huhta JC, et al: Hemodynamic profile of severe pregnancy-induced hypertension. *Am J Obstet Gynecol* 1988; 158:523.

46. Gibbs CP: Anesthetic management of the high risk gravida, in WN Spellacy (ed): *Management of the High Risk Pregnancy.* Baltimore, University Park Press, 1976, pp 209-226.

47. Clark SL, Cotton DB: Clinical indications for pulmonary artery catheterization in the patient with severe preeclampsia. *Am J Obstet Gynecol* 1988; 158:453.

48. Gibbs CP: Pulmonary artery catheterization in severe preeclampsia. *Am J Obstet Gynecol* 1989; 162:1089.

49. Kenepp NB, Kumar S, Shelley WC, et al: Fetal and neonatal hazards of maternal hydration with 5% dextrose before cesarean section. *Lancet* 1982; 1:1150.

50. Henderson DW, Vilos GA, Milne KJ, et al: The role of Swan-Ganz catheterization in severe pregnancy-induced hypertension. *Am J Obstet Gynecol* 1984; 148:570.

51. Cotton DB, Gonik B, Dorman K, et al: Cardiovascular alterations in severe pregnancy induced hypertension: Relationship of central venous pressure to pulmonary capillary wedge pressure. *Am J Obstet Gynecol* 1985; 151:762.

52. Benedetti TJ, Carlson RW: Studies of colloid osmotic pressure in pregnancy induced hypertension. *Am J Obstet Gynecol* 1979; 135:308.

53. Kirshon B, Moise KJ, Cotton DB, et al: Role of volume expansion in severe preeclampsia. *Surg Gynecol Obstet* 1988; 167:367.

54. Yeast JD, Halberstadt C, Meyer BA, et al: The risk of pulmonary edema and colloid osmotic pressure changes during magnesium therapy. *Am J Obstet Gynecol* 1993; 169:1566.

55. Assali NS, Vaughn DL: Blood volume in preeclampsia: Fantasy or reality. *Am J Obstet Gynecol* 1977; 129:355.

56. Seghal NN, Hitt JR: Plasma volume expansion in the treatment of preeclampsia. *Am J Obstet Gynecol* 1980; 138:165.

57. Gallery EDM, Deprado W, Gyory AZ: Antihypertensive effect of volume expansion in pregnancy associated hypertension. *Aust N Z J Med* 1981; 11:20.

58. Wollman SB, Marx GF: Acute hydration for prevention of hypotension of spinal anesthesia in parturients. *Anesthesiology* 1968; 29:374.

59. Caritis SN, Abouleish E, Edelstone MD, et al: Fetal acid-base state following spinal or epidural anesthesia for cesarean section. *Obstet Gynecol* 1980; 56:610.

60. Soffronoff EC, Kaufmann BM, Connaughton JF: Intravascular volume determination and fetal outcome in hypertensive diseases of pregnancy. *Am J Obstet Gynecol* 1977; 127:4.

61. Hays PM, Cruikshank DP, Dunn LJ: Plasma volume determination in normal and preeclamptic pregnancies. *Am J Obstet Gynecol* 1985; 151:958.

62. Joyce TH III, Debnath KS, Baker EA: Preeclamsia: Relationship of CVP and epidural anesthesia. *Anesthesiology* 1979; 51:S 297.

63. Roberts JM, Taylor RN, Musci TJ, et al: Preeclampsia: An endothelial cell disorder. *Am J Obstet Gynecol* 1989; 161:1200.

64. Cunningham FG, MacDonald PC, Gant NF: *Williams Obstetrics,* ed 18, Norwalk, Conn., Appleton & Lange, 1989, p 686.

65. Joupilla P, Joupilla R, Hollmen A, et al: Lumbar epidural analgesia to improve intervillous blood flow during labor in severe pre-eclampsia. *Obstet Gynecol* 1982; 59:158.

66. Abboud T, Artal R, Sarkis F, et al: Sympathoadrenal

activity, maternal, fetal and neonatal responses after epidural anesthesia in the preeclamptic patient. *Am J Obstet Gynecol* 1982; 144:915.

67. Merrell DA, Koch MA: Epidural anesthesia as an anticonvulsant in the management of hypertensive and eclamptic patients in labour. *South Afr Med J* 1980; 58:875.

68. Hodgkinson R, Husain FJ, Hayashi RH: Systemic and pulmonary blood pressure during cesarean section in parturients with gestational hypertension. *Can Anaesth Soc J* 1980; 27:389.

69. Moore TR, Key TC, Reisner LS, et al: Evaluation of the use of continuous lumbar epidural anesthesia for hypertensive pregnant women in labor. *Am J Obstet Gynecol* 1985; 152:404.

70. Connell H, Dalgleish JG, Downing JW: General anesthesia in mothers with severe preeclampsia/eclampsia. *Br J Anaesth* 1987; 59:1375.

71. Lawes EG, Downing JW, Duncan PW, et al: Fentanyl-droperidol supplementation of rapid sequence induction in the presence of severe pregnancy induced and pregnancy aggravated hypertension. *Br J Anaesth* 1987; 59:1381.

72. Graham C, Goldstein A: Epidural analgesia and cardiac output in severe preeclampsia. *Anaesthesia* 1980; 35:709.

73. Jouppila P, Kuikka J, Jouppila R et al: Effect of induction of general anesthesia for cesarean section on intervillous blood flow. *Acta Obstet Gynecol Scand* 1979; 58:249.

74. Husemeyer RP, Crawley JCW: Placental intervillous blood flow measured by inhaled ^{133}Xe clearance in relation to induction of epidural analgesia. *Br J Obstet Gynaecol* 1979; 86:426.

75. Rekonen A, Luotola H, Pitkanen H, et al: Measurement of intervillous and myometrial blood flow by an intravenous ^{133}Xe method. *Br J Obstet Gynaecol* 1976; 83:723.

76. Brosens IA: Morphological changes in the utero-placental bed in pregnancy hypertension. *Clin Obstet Gynecol* 1977; 4:573.

77. Brizgys RV, Dailey PA, Shnider SM, et al: The incidence and neonatal effects of maternal hypotension during epidural anesthesia for cesarean section. *Anesthesiology* 1987; 67:782.

78. Gutsche BB: Obstetric anesthesia, why? in Joyce TH III (ed): *Clinics in Perinatology,* vol 9, 1982, pp 215-224.

79. Gutsche BB editor: Expert's Opine: The role of epidural anesthesia in preeclampsia. *Surv Anesthesiol* 1986; 30:304.

80. Heller PJ, Goodman C: Use of local anesthetics with epinephrine for epidural anesthesia in preeclampsia. *Anesthesiology* 1986; 65:224.

81. Dror A, Abboud TK, Moore J, et al: Maternal hemodynamic responses to epinephrine containing local anesthetics in mild preeclampsia. *Reg Anaesth* 1988; 13:107.

82. Bonica JJ, Akamatsu TJ, Berges PU, et al: Circulatory effects of peridural block. II. Effects of epinephrine. *Anesthesiology* 1971; 34:514.

83. Albright GA, Jouppila R, Hollmen AI, et al: Epinephrine does not alter human intervillous blood flow during epidural anesthesia. *Anesthesiology* 1981; 54:131.

84. Costin M, Milliken R, et al: Epinephrine is unsafe in the preeclamptic patient. *Anesthesiology* 1987; 66:99.

85. Alahuta S, Rasanen J, Jouppila P, et al: Uteroplacental and fetal circulation during extradural bupivacaine-adrenaline and bupivacaine for cesarean section in hypertensive pregnancies with chronic fetal asphyxia. *Br J Anaesth* 1993; 71:348.

86. Marx GF: Editorial comment. *Obstet Anesth Dig* 1994; 14:22.

87. Hood DD, Dewan DM, James FM III: Maternal and fetal effects of epinephrine in gravid ewes. *Anesthesiology* 1986; 64:610.

88. Chestnut DH, Vandewalker GE, Owen CL, et al: The influence of continuous epidural bupivacaine analgesia on the second stage of labor and method of delivery in nulliparous women. *Anesthesiology* 1987; 66:774.

89. Ramanathan J, Bottorff M, Jeter JN, et al: The pharmacokinetics and maternal and neonatal effects of epidural lidocaine in preeclampsia. *Anesth Analg* 1986; 65:120.

90. Smith BE, Cavanaugh D, Moya F: Anesthesia for vaginal delivery in the patient with toxemia of pregnancy. *Anesth Analg* 1966; 45:853.

91. Kambam JR, Handte RE, Brown WU, et al: Effect of normal and preeclamptic pregnancies on the oxyhemoglobin dissociation curve. *Anesthesiology* 1986; 65:426.

92. Heller PJ, Scheider EP, Marx GF: Pharyngolaryngeal edema as a presenting symptom in preeclampsia. *Obstet Gynecol* 1983; 62:523.

93. Jouppila R, Jouppila P, Hollmen A: Laryngeal oedema as an obstetric anesthesia complication. *Acta Anaesth Scand* 1980; 24:97.

94. Brock-Utne JG, Downing JW, Seedat F: Laryngeal oedema associated with preeclamptic toxemia. *Anaesthesia* 1977; 32:556.

95. Fox EJ, Sklar GS, Hill CH, et al: Complications related to the pressor response to endotracheal intubation. *Anesthesiology* 1977; 47:524.

96. Cotton DB, Gonik B, Dorman KF: Cardiovascular alterations in severe pregnancy-induced hypertension seen with intravenously given hydralazine bolus. *Surg Gynecol Obstet* 1985; 161:240.

97. Shoemaker CT, Meyers M: Sodium nitroprusside for control of severe hypertensive disease of pregnancy: A case report and discussion of potential toxicity. *Am J Obstet Gynecol* 1984; 149:171.

98. Hood DD, Dewan DM, James FM III, et al: The use of nitroglycerin in preventing the hypertensive response to tracheal intubation in severe preeclampsia. *Anesthesiology* 1985; 63:329.

99. Gutsche BB, Cheek TG: Anesthetic considerations in preeclampsia-eclampsia, in Shnider SM, Levinson G (eds): *Anesthesia for Obstetrics.* Baltimore, Williams & Wilkins, 1993, pp 305-336.

100. Sosis M, Leighton B: In defense of trimethaphan for use in preeclampsia. *Anesthesiology* 1986; 64:657.

101. Poulton TJ, James FM III, Lockridge O: Prolonged apnea following trimethaphan and succinylcholine. *Anesthesiology* 1979; 50:54.

102. Ramanathan J, Sibai BM, Mabie WC, et al: The use of labetalol for attenuation of the hypertensive response to endotracheal intubation in preeclampsia. *Am J Obstet Gynecol* 1989; 159:650.

103. Morgan MA, Silavin SA, Dormer KJ, et al: Effects of labetalol on uterine blood flow and cardiovascular hemodynamics in the hypertensive gravid baboon. *Am J Obstet Gynecol* 1993; 168:1574.

104. Pickles CJ, Symonds EM, Pipkin FB: The fetal outcome in a randomized double-blind controlled trial of labetalol versus placebo in pregnancy-induced hypertension. *Br J Obstet Gynaecol* 1989; 96:38.

105. Klarr JM, Bhatt-Mehta V, Donn SM: Neonatal adrenergic blockade following single-dose maternal labetalol administration. *Am J Perinatol* 1994; 11:91.

106. Eisenach JB, Castro MI: Maternally administered esmolol produces fetal beta dadrenergic blockade and hypoxemia in sheep. *Anesthesiology* 1989; 71:718.

107. Fenakel K, Fenakel G, Appleman Z, et al: Nifedipine in

the treatment of severe preeclampsia. *Obstet Gynecol* 1991; 77:331.

108. Ghoneim MM, Long JP: Interaction between magnesium and other neuromuscular blocking agents. *Anesthesiology* 1970; 32:23.

109. Devore JS, Asrani R: Magnesium sulfate prevents succinylcholine-induced fasciculations in toxemic parturients. *Anesthesiology* 1980; 52:76.

110. Weinstein L: Syndrome of hemolysis, elevated liver enzymes and low platelet count: A severe consequence of hypertension in pregnancy. *Am J Obstet Gynecol* 1982; 142:159.

111. Vegna G, Leone S, Sorrentino M, et al: New issues for nosografic setting of "HELLP" syndrome. *Acta Eur Fertil* 1989; 20:99.

112. Burrows, RF, JG Kelton: Incidentally detected thrombocytopenia in healthy mothers and their infants. *New Engl J Med* 1988; 319:142.

113. Baca L, Gibbons RB: The HELLP syndrome: A serious complication of pregnancy with hemolysis, elevated levels of liver enzymes and low platelet count. *Am J Med* 1988; 85:590.

114. Duffy BL, Watson RI: The HELLP syndrome mimics cholecystitis. *Med J Aust* 1988; 148:473.

115. Van Dam PA, Renier M, Baekelandt M, et al: Disseminated intravascular coagulation and the syndrome of hemolysis, elevated liver enzymes, and low platelets in severe preeclampsia. *Obstet Gynecol* 1989; 73:97.

116. Sibai B, Ramadan MK, Usta I, et al: Maternal morbidity and mortality in 442 pregnancies hemolysis, elevated liver enzymes and low platelet (HELLP). *Am J Obstet Gynecol* 1993; 169:1000.

117. Sibai BM, Taslimi MM, El-Nazer A, et al: Maternal-perinatal outcome associated with the syndrome of hemolysis, elevated liver enzymes and low platelets in severe preeclampsia-eclampsia. *Am J Obstet Gynecol* 1986; 155:501.

118. Duffy BL: HELLP syndrome and the anesthetist. *Anaesthesia,* 1988; 43:223.

119. Sibai BM, McCubbin JH, Anderson GD, et al: Eclampsia. I. Observations from 67 recent cases. *Obstet Gynecol* 1981; 58:609.

120. Richards AM, Moodley J, Graham DI, et al: Active management of the unconscious eclamptic patient. *Br J Obstet Gynaecol* 1986; 93:554.

121. Moodley J, Naicker RS, Mankowitz E: Eclampsia: A method of management. *South Afr Med J* 1983; 63:530.

122. Koenig JM, Christensen RD: Incidence, neutrophil kinetics, and natural history of neonatal neutropenia associated with maternal hypertension. *N Engl J Med* 1989; 321:557.

22 Preterm Labor and Delivery

Andrew M. Malinow and *Lindsay S. Alger*

Prematurity is the leading cause of perinatal morbidity and mortality in the United States, accounting for as many as 85% of the neonatal deaths in structurally normal infants.[1] Preterm delivery has assumed even greater importance as advances in the fields of neonatology, infectious disease, genetics, and pediatric surgery have reduced morbidity from other causes. In addition to the increased risk of immediate complications such as respiratory distress syndrome (RDS), intraventricular hemorrhage, patent ductus arteriosus, and necrotizing enterocolitis, many of the survivors will be permanently handicapped. Preterm infants subsequently demonstrate lower IQ scores and a higher incidence of neurologic abnormalities, learning disabilities, chronic pulmonary disease, and visual defects.[2-4] More than $2 billion in health care costs are associated annually with preterm birth. Although developed countries have seen a steady decline in the neonatal mortality rate over the past 20 years, it is disheartening to realize this improvement has been accomplished without any significant reduction in the delivery of very low birth weight infants.[5]

DEFINITIONS AND INCIDENCE

Preterm labor is defined as regular uterine contractions productive of cervical change (dilation or effacement) before 37 completed weeks of gestation from the first day of the last menstrual period.[6] Since pregnancies terminating before 20 weeks of gestation are considered abortions, the terms preterm labor and preterm birth assume a lower gestational limit of 20 weeks. This lower limit is somewhat arbitrary. Consequently, many obstetricians are willing to diagnose and treat, somewhat earlier in gestation, preterm labor in patients who otherwise satisfy the definition.

Since gestational age is often difficult to ascertain, many statistics refer to birth weight of between 500 and 2499 g. However, this results in the inclusion of many term infants with growth retardation and the exclusion of preterm infants who are large for gestational age. The very low birth weight infant is defined as weighing less than 1500 g. This typically corresponds to a gestational age of less than 32 weeks.

The incidence of preterm birth is dependent on many factors and varies from one country to another, one community to another, and one institution to another. Racial differences have been noted as well. In the United States, 9% to 10% of deliveries are before term.[7] Because the diagnosis of preterm labor is harder to define and does not uniformly result in preterm birth, preterm labor rates are unavailable, although they are undoubtedly greater than those for preterm birth.

RISK FACTORS

The mechanism of term labor remains incompletely defined. It is not surprising, therefore, that the cause of preterm labor is only partially understood. Risk factors associated with prematurity may be grouped under five headings (Box 22-1): maternal characteristics,[8-19] socioeconomic factors,[8,9,20] past reproductive history,[21-29] current pregnancy complications, and genital tract infections.[1,7,30-45] In more than one third of all cases no risk factor can be identified and the cause is unknown.

Identification of the pregnancy at risk will heighten antenatal vigilance for signs of preterm labor. Prompt diagnosis allows for aggressive obstetric management, including pharmacologic therapy. Although the decisions to initiate pharmacologic therapy as well as the timing and route of delivery are mainly obstetric, implications for the anesthesiologist may be complex. The following discussion outlines active obstetric management and profiles the desired and undesired effects of the many drugs commonly used by perinatologists. Anesthetic management of the parturient in preterm labor involves decisions that may depend solely on previous obstetric management. Anesthetic consideration of this high-risk pregnancy must include analysis of possible interactions of drug therapy and evaluation of fetal well-being in order to select the best technique for labor and delivery as well as for cesarean section. Early communication between the perinatologist, neonatologist, and anesthesiologist will provide opportunity

---

BOX 22-1 **RISK FACTORS FOR PREMATURITY AND PRETERM LABOR**

Maternal characteristics

Age: <15 or >40 years and nulliparous
Race: Black (highest risk)
Weight: Underweight for height (especially, prepregnancy weight <50 kg)
Drug use: Nicotine (especially, >20 cigarettes/ day), ethanol (controversial), cocaine, narcotics (controversial)
Social factors:
    Stress: Work related, psychosocial
    Sexually active (coitus) after 20 weeks' gestation (controversial)

Socioeconomic factors

Social class:
    Public clinic patients
    Late registrants to or no antenatal care
Occupation: Physically demanding job (e.g., laborer)
Marital status: Single mother (especially white women)

Reproductive history

Previous preterm birth:
    One: Up to 35% chance of preterm labor
    Two or more: Up to 70% chance of preterm labor
Previous abortion: Second-trimester spontaneous abortion, but not first-trimester therapeutic abortion
Uterine abnormality:
    Uterine malformation or septum
    Diethylstilbestrol (DES) exposure
    Intramural or submucosal leiomyoma
    Asherman's syndrome
    Cervical incompetence

Current pregnancy

Inadequate weight gain during pregnancy
Unexplained elevated maternal serum alpha-fetoprotein
Uterine distention:
    Multiple gestation (increased risk with each additional fetus)
    Monozygous twins more than dizygous twins
    Polyhydramnios: 30% to 40% incidence
Fetal abnormality:
    Congenital anomalies (genetic or environmental)
    Intrauterine growth retardation
Antepartum hemorrhage:
    Placenta previa
    Abruptio placentae
    Other pregnancy-related causes
Maternal illness:
    Severe disease or trauma, demanding obstetric intervention and delivery
    Coexisting illness (e.g., asthma; collagen vascular disease (lupus anticoagulant); coronary, hepatobiliary, or endocrine disease; surgical abdomen; systemic infection; asymptomatic bacteriuria
Genital tract infections:
    Intrauterine infection (clinically apparent or occult chorioamnionitis
    Lower genital tract colonization
    Neisseria gonorrhea, group B streptococci, *Chlamydia trachomatis, Gardnerella vaginalis,* etc.

Miscellaneous factors

Retained intrauterine device
Premature rupture of membranes
Inaccurate dates (by obstetrician)

---

for joint, efficient planning of delivery, should it become inevitable.

OBSTETRIC AND ANESTHETIC MANAGEMENT
Obstetric management

Diagnosis of preterm labor. To make the diagnosis, the physician must determine whether the patient is truly in labor and, equally important, whether the pregnancy is truly preterm. Frequency, regularity, duration, or discomfort of contractions does not readily distinguish true preterm labor from false labor. Perhaps half of all women presenting preterm with regular uterine contractions are in false labor, since they appear to be effectively treated by placebo. Evidence of cervical change must be documented before initiating

therapy to prevent unnecessary pharmacologic intervention with its attendant expense and side effects.[46] Fortunately, awaiting cervical change does not jeopardize the likelihood of successful tocolysis.[47]

Patients with intact membranes who present with little or no cervical change are observed at bedrest, avoiding the dorsal supine position. Intravenous hydration (500 mL bolus of a physiologic salt solution) is initiated because it may improve uterine blood flow and reduce myometrial activity. Failure of the maternal plasma volume to expand appropriately during pregnancy may actually be a factor in initiating preterm labor. In a study of 22 women with preterm labor or premature rupture of membranes, almost 60% had plasma volumes measuring less than 3 standard deviations

(SD) below the mean of normal pregnant women.[48] In addition, should it become necessary to use tocolytic drugs, conservative hydration may counteract the vasodilatory effects of these agents, thus preventing a possible reduction in uteroplacental perfusion. Interestingly, no prospective controlled trials are available to support the efficacy of this approach.[49]

External tocographic and fetal heart rate monitoring is begun. The cervix is assessed for change by the same examiner at regular intervals. If progressive cervical effacement or dilation is documented or if the cervix is at least 2 cm dilated or 80% effaced on initial evaluation, a diagnosis of labor is made. The most frequently used definitions of preterm labor also stipulate a contraction frequency of at least four in 20 minutes or six to eight in 1 hour, since it is unusual for cervical change to occur when the interval between contractions is greater than 10 minutes.

A determination of fetal age must be made while proceeding with the above maneuvers. It is inappropriate to maintain a term but growth-retarded fetus in an adverse intrauterine environment. Although ideally obtained earlier in gestation, ultrasound evaluation performed on admission is still useful and is noninvasive. If there is still doubt about the prematurity of the fetus, amniocentesis can be helpful. Although amniocentesis cannot distinguish a term from a preterm fetus, it can establish pulmonary maturity and therefore identify those fetuses unlikely to benefit from further labor inhibition. In addition, some institutions routinely obtain amniotic fluid specimens to analyze for evidence of infection. Amniotic fluid glucose levels, leukocyte counts, Gram's stains, leukocyte esterase determinations, interleukin-6 levels, and serum C-reactive protein all have been suggested as useful tests for diagnosing occult chorioamnionitis.[45] However, there are no randomized, prospective studies demonstrating that knowledge of occult intra-amniotic infection improves management resulting in better maternal or neonatal outcomes. Labor inhibition is unlikely to be successful in cases of true chorioamnionitis.

Active obstetric management. Once the diagnosis of preterm labor is established, a complete history and physical examination and appropriate laboratory tests are necessary to determine whether any maternal or fetal conditions exist that may contraindicate treatment (Box 22-2). For example, severe preeclampsia, chorioamnionitis, or fetal distress generally warrant delivery. Labor inhibition beyond 35 weeks is usually not indicated unless there is uncertainty regarding gestational age.[50] Attempts to achieve any further reduction in morbidity after this time is not cost effective, although

---

BOX 22-2 CONTRAINDICATIONS TO THE INHIBITION OF PRETERM LABOR

Absolute contraindications
Fetal death
Nonviable fetus (congenital anomaly)
Chorioamnionitis
Complications requiring immediate delivery (fetal, maternal)

Relative contraindications
Advanced cervical dilation (>4 cm)
Vaginal bleeding (placenta previa, abruptio placentae)
Preeclampsia or eclampsia
Fetal distress
Intrauterine growth retardation

---

individual cases may benefit from delaying labor until 37 weeks' gestation.[51]

There are few absolute contraindications to the use of tocolytic drugs (Box 22-2). While several conditions are associated with increased risk, analysis of relative risk must be made. If the risks of preterm delivery appear to outweigh those of tocolysis, then inhibition of labor may be cautiously undertaken with careful monitoring of both mother and fetus. Even selected patients with preeclampsia may be candidates for tocolysis in order to gain an additional 48 hours, during which time corticosteroids may be administered to promote pulmonary maturation. When severe bleeding results from placenta previa or placental abruption, use of any agent that will promote cardiovascular instability is contraindicated. However, in milder forms, tocolysis may actually serve to decrease further bleeding by preventing further placental separation.[52,53] Maternal conditions such as diabetes or coexisting cardiac disease may influence the selection of tocolytic agent since the beta-adrenergic agonists, in contrast to magnesium sulfate or indomethacin, may exacerbate certain existing abnormalities.

Once the cervix is greater than 4 cm dilated, the chances of successfully prolonging pregnancy by initiating tocolysis are greatly reduced and it is likely that the fetus will deliver with high systemic levels of drug present. When dealing with a very preterm fetus where a week longer in utero may improve perinatal outcome, an attempt at tocolysis may be warranted even with advanced cervical dilation. To achieve optimal results, the obstetrician must avoid using fixed protocols and instead assess and treat each patient individually.

Finally, it must be remembered that any attempts to inhibit labor may be sabotaged by the obstetri-

---

BOX 22-3 PHARMACOLOGIC AGENTS USED IN TREATMENT OF PRETERM LABOR

Tocolytic agents
Beta-adrenergic agonists: terbutaline, ritodrine
Magnesium sulfate
Prostaglandin synthetase inhibitors
Calcium-channel blockers

Steroids

Antibiotics

---

cian's failure to identify a treatable condition. In particular, urine and cervico-vaginal specimens should be routinely obtained for culture, in particular, to rule out possible group B streptococcus (GBS) colonization. Although preliminary reports suggests that empiric antibiotic treatment of women in preterm labor improves the chances of successfully prolonging pregnancy,[45,54,55] it is generally recommended that antibiotic therapy be reserved for a proven infection. However, until the results of the genital tract cultures become available, it is reasonable to protect the woman in active preterm labor from possible GBS infection by treating her with ampicillin or penicillin.[56]

Pharmacologic treatment of preterm labor. There are a variety of effective tocolytic agents currently in use (Box 22-3). Ethanol was widely used into the 1970s to treat preterm labor by suppressing posterior pituitary secretion of oxytocin and directly inhibiting myometrial activity. Intravenous ethanol has been supplanted by more effective drugs with fewer side effects. The pharmacologic agents now used to inhibit labor act at different points in the smooth muscle contraction pathway. There are also differences among these drugs in the spectrum and in the severity of associated side effects. It is difficult to compare their efficacies; none is universally successful. Although multiple studies support the contention that tocolytic agents reduce the frequency of preterm birth and low birth weight, it has been difficult to demonstrate a beneficial effect of treatment on perinatal mortality.

Beta-adrenergic agonists. The smooth muscle-relaxing properties of the beta-adrenergic agonists result from their interaction with beta$_2$-receptor sites on the outer membrane of myometrial cells. The agonist-receptor complex activates the enzyme adenyl cyclase, causing an increase in the intracellular concentration of cyclic adenosine monophosphate (cAMP).[57] Cyclic adenosine monophosphate activates a protein kinase that decreases the intracellular concentration of calcium and prevents the actin-myosin interaction necessary for smooth muscle contraction. In addition, the trophoblast increases progesterone production in response to cAMP.[58] Progesterone inhibits transmission of impulses between myometrial cells by reducing gap junction formation.

A meta-analysis of the data from 890 women participating in 16 methodologically acceptable controlled trials of beta-adrenergic agonists demonstrates an unequivocal effect of these agents in delaying delivery and reducing the frequency of preterm birth and low birth weight.[59] However, the impact of these agents on the incidence of preterm delivery remains controversial. A recent randomized, placebo-controlled study in over 700 women conducted by the Canadian Preterm Labor Investigators Group found that the use of ritodrine had no significant beneficial effect on perinatal mortality or the frequency of prolongation of pregnancy to term.[60]

The agents in current use were selected because they predominantly affect beta$_2$-receptors, but all beta-adrenergic agonists have both beta$_1$ and beta$_2$ effects. Thus, the efficacy of a given agent is generally limited by the severity of its associated cardiovascular side effects. Ritodrine and terbutaline are the agents most commonly used in this country. Ritodrine is the only beta-agonist approved for parenteral use in preterm labor in the United States. However, a large body of literature supports the safety and efficacy of the use of terbutaline and, in many institutions, it remains the agent of choice. In individual studies, differing efficacies have been reported but available data do not consistently indicate superior efficacy or safety for any one of these drugs.

Continuing exposure to beta-agonists results in down regulation and desensitization of tissues. For example, in sheep after 24 hours of infusion the ability of ritodrine to inhibit contractions is substantially reduced.[61] This effect may be dose related and may be minimized by limiting total drug exposure.

Maternal side effects of the beta-adrenergic agonists are varied, due to the widespread distribution of beta-adrenergic receptors (Box 22-4). Cardiovascular alterations are most common and pronounced. Stimulation of vascular beta$_2$-receptors produces vasodilation, minimal hypotension, and a compensatory tachycardia in almost all patients. At least one third of women will complain of palpitations. Systolic blood pressure and pulse pressure may increase due to increased cardiac output, but the falls in systemic vascular resistance and diastolic blood pressure are greater, resulting in a slight reduction in mean arterial pressure.[62] In

---

BOX 22-4 MATERNAL SIDE EFFECTS OF BETA-ADRENERGIC TOCOLYTIC THERAPY

Anemia
Arrhythmias
Chest pain
Elevated hepatic transaminase levels
Glucose intolerance
Hypokalemia
Mycocardial ischemia
Nausea
Palpitations
Paralytic ileus
Pulmonary edema
Rash
Restlessness, agitation
Tremor

---

most cases the heart rate and pulse pressure return to pretreatment values with continued treatment.

The residual beta$_1$ activity inherent in all of these agents results in direct cardiac effects as well.[63,64] Cardiac arrhythmias occur, most commonly premature ventricular and atrial contractions.[65,66] Up to 60% of patients on ritodrine complain of chest pain.[67] Furthermore, electrocardiographic changes such as ST segment depression, T wave flattening, or inversion and prolongation of the QT interval suggest that myocardial ischemia may result from the use of these agents. However, it is not always clear whether these alterations represent true myocardial ischemia or result instead from tachycardia and hypokalemia. Isoenzyme confirmation of myocardial damage has not been documented.[68,69] In animal studies, metoprolol, a beta$_1$-selective adrenergic blocker, inhibits ritodrine-induced increases in cardiac work without disturbing labor.[70,71] Concomitant beta$_1$-selective adrenergic antagonist therapy might therefore reduce the incidence of side effects from ritodrine therapy.

Pulmonary edema, a potentially serious side effect, is reported in a small percentage of women treated with these agents. In the literature detailing early experience with beta-adrenergic agonists, pulmonary edema had been reported in up to 5% of women treated with intravenous therapy.[72] The incidence of pulmonary edema in these women today is probably much lower since a decade of experience has identified risk factors for the development of this complication, including multiple gestation, fluid overload, anemia, and prolonged duration of maternal tachycardia. Pulmonary edema is unlikely to develop within the first 24

hours of therapy. In initial reports the majority of cases occurred in patients receiving corticosteroids as well. However, steroids used today have little mineralocorticoid activity; also, their apparent association with the development of pulmonary edema may be coincidental since pulmonary edema does occur in the absence of steroid therapy.

In the majority of these cases there was no evidence of left ventricular failure on echocardiography or by right ventricular catheterization.[73,74] The exact mechanism for the generation of pulmonary edema remains unclear. Aldosterone levels are increased during pregnancy, peaking in the third trimester.[75,76] Beta-adrenergic stimulation further increases aldosterone as well as renin and antidiuretic hormone secretion.[77] Increased sodium resorption with decreased renal blood flow and urine output occurs. Large volumes of intravenous hydration may then decompensate an already fragile, hyperdynamic cardiac state. In the final analysis, fluid overload appears to be the principal mechanism for pulmonary edema.[78] The wide disparity between institutions in the incidence of pulmonary edema suggests that it is largely dependent on differences in administration protocols of fluid and tocolytic drugs. Strict surveillance of fluid therapy and use of the smallest effective dose of beta-adrenergic agonist for the shortest period of time should minimize the risk of pulmonary edema.

There have been reports of normal to low pulmonary capillary wedge pressure pulmonary edema in these patients, which suggests a picture of increased pulmonary vascular permeability.[79] There is little evidence, though, for the theory of direct beta-adrenergic pulmonary toxicity (i.e., pulmonary capillary leakage).[79] In fact, there is evidence that direct beta-adrenergic stimulation decreases pulmonary vascular permeability.[80,81] Beta-adrenergic agonist therapy does lead to a decrease in serum albumin and protein concentrations.[79] A decrease in the colloid oncotic pressure/hydrostatic pressure gradient may lead to low or normal pulmonary capillary wedge pressure pulmonary edema.[79] In clinical doses, ritodrine causes a decrease in hypoxic pulmonary vasoconstriction,[82] further compounding any preexisting pulmonary shunt flow. Arterial hypoxemia may be severe and out of proportion to the radiographic picture.

Women receiving beta-adrenergic agonists are likely to become anemic. Initially, there is a fall in hematocrit as the patient placed at bedrest mobilizes third-space fluid into the intravascular space. Intravenous hydration and stimulation of the renin-angiotensin-aldosterone system results in further volume expansion and dilutional anemia. There is an average 15% fall in hematocrit. This must be considered when observing patients with vaginal bleeding who are receiving tocolytic therapy so the degree of hemorrhage is not misinterpreted. Peripartum blood loss will result in diluted red cell mass in the case of failed tocolysis with subsequent delivery. Possible transfusion requirement should incorporate this knowledge.

Maternal metabolic effects resulting from beta-adrenergic receptor stimulation include hyperglycemia and increased insulin levels.[83] There is commonly a transient, modest increase in blood glucose levels that rarely exceeds 180 mg/dL, and is thus of little consequence. Glucose levels peak 3 to 6 hours after the initiation of therapy, returning to baseline within 24 hours without treatment. Exogenous insulin is usually unnecessary.[84] The insulin-dependent diabetic patient who is inadequately monitored rarely develops ketoacidosis, but this can be avoided by simultaneous administration of insulin via a calibrated infusion pump.[85] The increased lactate produced by glycogenolysis is usually insufficient to produce acidosis. Serum liver transaminase levels are infrequently elevated.[86]

Transient hypokalemia occurs as a result of redistribution of potassium from the extracellular to the intracellular compartment.[83] On average, levels fall to a nadir of 2.7 mEq/L but urinary excretion and total potassium remain unchanged.[84] There are no reports of adverse effects of serum hypokalemia. Potassium supplementation is unnecessary, since potassium levels return to normal without therapy within 24 hours.

The symptoms women most often complain of include anxiety with feelings of restlessness and agitation, tremor, palpitations, or chest tightness. Nausea, bloating, and rarely, paralytic ileus may develop.[87] Rash is infrequently encountered.

Fetal and neonatal side effects depend on which beta-adrenergic agonist is used (since they cross the placenta to varying degrees) and the interval from discontinuation to delivery. Although fetal levels are lower than maternal levels, both ritodrine and terbutaline cause fetal tachycardia. As a consequence of maternal hyperglycemia, these agents may cause neonatal hyperinsulinemia and hypoglycemia. Hypocalcemia, ileus, hypertension, and death have been reported with the use of isoxsuprine in two retrospective studies, but this agent is no longer used.[88,89] Periventricular-intraventricular hemorrhage has been reported to occur more frequently in neonates exposed to beta-adrenergic agents,[90] but others have not observed this.[91] There are no reports of adverse long-term effects in children exposed to these agents in utero.[92,93]

Possible routes of delivery, depending on which agent is selected, include oral, intravenous, intra-

muscular, or subcutaneous. The intravenous route has been preferred in most studies for initial therapy. The patient is instructed to avoid the direct supine position and encouraged to remain on her side or in left lateral tilt position. Baseline maternal heart rate, blood pressure, and respiratory rate are obtained. Fetal heart rate and uterine activity are continuously monitored. During therapy, these parameters are reassessed every 15 to 30 minutes until a maintenance dose has been established and then every hour for the duration of intravenous administration.

Therapy is instituted via a calibrated intravenous infusion pump using fluids low in sodium. Half-strength normal saline may be used initially, followed by 5% dextrose in water in the absence of significant hyperglycemia. Current practice is to employ a continuous infusion, but there is some evidence that intermittent pulsatile administration of small intravenous boluses requires less drug and shorter duration of therapy and may be more effective.[94] With standard therapy, the infusion rate is initially set at the lowest recommended for the selected agent. The dosage is increased every 10 to 20 minutes until contractions are more than 10 minutes apart. At this point, the infusion rate is increased less frequently until there are fewer than four contractions per hour. If maternal heart rate is greater than 140 beats/min or other unacceptable side effects develop, dosage is reduced. It is rarely necessary to discontinue the drug.

Once effective tocolysis has been achieved, the infusion rate may be tapered as long as uterine activity remains inhibited. Depending on the difficulty encountered in initially inhibiting contractions, intravenous infusion is maintained for an additional 12 to 24 hours. The patient may then be switched to oral therapy and the infusion discontinued 30 minutes later (though there is still some question as to the efficacy of oral beta agonists for preventing recurrence of labor). If recurrent contractions do not permit switching to oral therapy, then long-term intravenous tocolysis for weeks may be necessary or an alternative agent can be selected.[95] Terbutaline can also be administered subcutaneously by an infusion pump capable of delivering a constant basal rate with periodic supplementary boluses as necessary.[96] This modality enables the patient to continue parenteral therapy without requiring hospitalization.

Magnesium sulfate. The exact mechanism by which magnesium sulfate acts to inhibit myometrial contractility is not entirely certain. Magnesium competes with calcium for entry into the cell at depolarization. By activating adenyl cyclase, magnesium increases cAMP levels, which further reduces intracellular calcium.[97] In addition, magnesium indirectly promotes calcium uptake by the sarcoplasmic reticulum by stimulating calcium-dependent adenosine triphosphatase (ATPase). Increased urinary excretion of calcium also decreases its availability. The end result is that less intracellular free calcium is available to participate in the actin-myosin interaction of smooth muscle contraction.[98]

Magnesium also acts at the neuromuscular junction, decreasing the release of acetylcholine and decreasing the postjunctional membrane potentials generated by acetycholine-receptor interaction.[99,100] This is one mechanism for magnesium toxicity, which leads to striated muscle paresis (especially muscles of respiration) and also potentiation of neuromuscular relaxants, especially the nondepolarizing drugs (e.g., curare or pancuronium).

The normal serum magnesium level during pregnancy is 1.8 to 3 mg/dL. Magnesium levels of 5 to 8 mg/dL are necessary to inhibit uterine activity, but levels as high as 11 mg/dL do not guarantee labor inhibition.[101] Magnesium has been compared to ritodrine and terbutaline and has been found to be equally effective with fewer adverse side effects.[102,103] For this reason, magnesium sulfate may be the intravenous tocolytic of choice in patients with diabetes mellitus, hyperthyroidism, or coexisting cardiac disease. Magnesium has also been effective in patients with advanced cervical dilatation.[104] Long-term intravenous magnesium sulfate therapy has been employed for as long as 13 weeks after tocolysis with intravenous ritodrine failed.[101] The use of magnesium sulfate in combination with a beta-adrenergic agent may produce better results than using either agent alone.[106] Combination therapy is controversial since side effects may be increased. However, long-term intravenous tocolysis with combined terbutaline and magnesium sulfate for periods as long as 123 days has been reported to be safe and to have acceptable side effects in a group of 1000 women.[107] Still, most practitioners prefer to substitute, rather than add, an alternative drug should the initially chosen agent fail to inhibit labor.[108] Regardless of which drug is initially employed, the alternative drug will be successful in 50% to 60% of cases.[102,109]

Maternal side effects of magnesium sulfate are varied (Box 22-5). Magnesium sulfate causes peripheral vasodilation. After bolus administration, most women experience uncomfortable warmth and a flushing sensation. Nausea, headache, and lethargy are not uncommon. Dizziness, chest tightness, palpitations, and visual symptoms secondary to ocular muscle paresis can occur. Cardiovascular side effects are minimal when compared with

---

BOX 22-5   MATERNAL SIDE EFFECTS OF MAGNESIUM SULFATE THERAPY

Warmth, flushing, headache
Nausea, dizziness
Transient hypotension
Electrocardiographic changes: widened QRS, increased PR interval
Depressed deep tendon reflexes
Muscle weakness
Respiratory depression
Cardiac arrest

---

beta-adrenergic agonist therapy. A mild maternal tachycardia and reduction in mean arterial pressure may be associated with bolus infusion, but these changes are transient.[110] Pulmonary edema has been reported in patients who have received corticosteroids.[104] Therapeutic maternal serum levels of magnesium are associated with maternal electrocardiographic changes such as a widened QRS complex and prolonged PR interval.

Magnesium levels of 18 mg/dL result in respiratory arrest, and levels exceeding 25 mg/dL can produce cardiac arrest.[97] However, deep tendon reflexes are lost at levels exceeding 12 mg/dL. Therefore, as long as deep tendon reflexes are present, the patient is not at immediate risk for the more serious complications. Calcium gluconate is an effective intravenous antidote. Magnesium must be used with caution in patients with renal failure to prevent excessive levels from accumulating; it is contraindicated in patients with myasthenia gravis or heart block.

Several investigators, though not all, have observed some decrease in fetal heart rate variability without evidence of neonatal compromise in patients receiving magnesium for the treatment of preeclampsia or preterm labor.[111,112] In one study, administration of magnesium resulted in nonreactive nonstress test results and cessation of fetal breathing movements in a significant proportion of fetuses; it also significantly reduced overall biophysical profile scores in the majority of fetuses.[113] A decrease in baseline fetal heart rate was also observed. These changes are probably the result of pharmacologic central nervous system depression.

Neonatal depression manifested as flaccidity, hyporeflexia, respiratory depression requiring assisted ventilation, and a weak or absent cry has occasionally been reported following prolonged intravenous therapy with high doses close to delivery. These infants are clinically improved within 24 to 36 hours. In the majority of neonates, there is no significant alteration in neurologic state or

Apgar score.[114] Demineralization of fetal long bones may occur if therapy exceeds 7 days.[115]

In patients with normal renal function, an intravenous loading dose of 6 g magnesium sulfate is administered over 20 minutes followed by an initial maintenance dose of 4 g/hr by constant infusion. Serum magnesium levels normally do not reach therapeutic levels immediately after a 4-g bolus, and high constant infusion rates may be necessary to do so.[116] If there is no initial response, the infusion rate is gradually increased by 0.5 g every 30 minutes until tocolysis is achieved or to a maximum dose of 6 g/hr. Women can be maintained on high doses for a relatively short period of time before the serum magnesium level exceeds the recommended threshold of 8 mg/dL and the infusion dose must be tapered. Before each increase in dosage, the patient's deep tendon reflexes are checked. Serum magnesium levels are ascertained frequently. Once uterine contractions are successfully inhibited, the maintenance dose is tapered as uterine activity permits, to as low as 2 g/hr. The infusion is maintained at this rate for 12 to 24 hours. If there is no recurrence of labor, then intravenous therapy is discontinued and oral beta-adrenergic agonist agents are substituted. The large doses of oral magnesium that would be needed to maintain tocolysis would be impractical to administer.

Prostaglandin synthetase inhibitors. Prostaglandins, particularly PGF_2 and PGE_2, play a dual role in the production of preterm labor. These compounds are integral to the final pathway of smooth muscle contraction.[117] They promote the production of myometrial gap junctions. Prostaglandin F_2 stimulates entry of calcium in the cell and its release from the sarcoplasmic reticulum.[118] At the same time, PGE_2 induces biochemical changes in cervical collagen that facilitate cervical dilation.

A group of enzymes collectively called prostaglandin synthetases act to convert free arachidonic acid to prostaglandin. Indomethacin, when administered orally or rectally, acts specifically and reversibly to inhibit the cyclooxygenase enzyme necessary for conversion of arachidonic acid. The most extensively studied of the prostaglandin synthetase inhibitors, indomethacin, abolishes spontaneous contractions when added to human myometrial strips.[119]

Currently, indomethacin appears to be the most effective oral tocolytic agent available. Two prospective, randomized trials and several retrospective studies totaling 600 patients have uniformly reported successful labor inhibition and delay in delivery.[97] Indomethacin has arrested labor in women who failed to respond to beta-agonists.[120] It is usually administered as a loading dose of 50 to 100 mg via rectal suppository followed by 25 mg orally every 6 hours. Although indomethacin inhibits the synthesis of all classes of prostanoids, including prostaglandins, prostacyclins, and thromboxanes, few maternal side effects have been reported with its use for tocolysis.

Blockage of the cyclooxygenase pathway will decrease the production of thromboxane A_2, decreasing platelet aggregatory properties. Indomethacin has a transient effect on platelets, in contrast to the 7- to 10-day antiplatelet effect of aspirin.[121] It can be assumed that tests of platelet function, including bleeding time, will reflect the antiplatelet effects of indomethacin. In one study of 20 patients, the bleeding time was doubled after taking indomethacin, although the prothrombin time and activated partial thromboplastin time remained unchanged.[122] Postpartum hemorrhage due to inhibition of myometrial contraction and perhaps platelet inactivation has been reported, but it is uncommon.[123] Drug rash has been observed.[123] Gastrointestinal side effects such as nausea are minimal and can be reduced by giving the drug with meals or as a rectal suppository. Indomethacin use should be avoided in the presence of maternal infection, bleeding disorders, or renal or peptic ulcer disease.

Indomethacin crosses the term placenta freely, but initial animal studies suggested that early in gestation there is minimal transfer. As the use of indomethacin has increased in recent years, the presumed safety of its administration before 32 weeks has been called into question. A recent study in human fetuses has found that placental passage of indomethacin is independent of gestational age.[124] In the fetus the patency of the fetal ductus arteriosus is maintained by circulating prostaglandins. There are case reports of narrowing of the fetal ductus arteriosus and persistent fetal circulation or primary pulmonary hypertension, especially when indomethacin was used for prolonged periods in high doses or close to term.[125-127] A study using echocardiography to examine the fetal heart during indomethacin tocolysis found transient ductal constriction in 7 of 14 fetuses receiving therapy for less than 72 hours.[128] Tricuspid regurgitation also developed in three fetuses. These changes occurred as early as 26 ½ weeks of gestation. In all cases, effects were reversible within 24 hours of discontinuing therapy. Similar results from another group of investigators prompted them to recommend fetal echocardiographic surveillance when prostaglandin synthetase inhibitors are used.[129] The constricting effects of indomethacin may be augmented by the concomitant administration of betamethasone.[130] Postnatally, the opposite problem can arise with failure of the ductus arteriosis to respond to indomethacin or oxygen, resulting in a patent ductus arteriosis. Once the ductus has responded to the effects of indomethacin in utero, its ability to respond again is limited[131] and therefore the chance that surgical ligation will be necessary is increased for these infants.[132]

Oligohydramnios, thought to be secondary to a decrease in fetal urine excretion, has been described following long-term indomethacin use.[133,134] In a series of 17 patients treated with a variety of nonsteroidal antiinflammatory drugs, but predominantly indomethacin, 14 (82.3%) demonstrated a decrease in amniotic fluid while none of 10 control patients receiving other tocolytic agents did so.[135] Oligohydramnios did not develop until at least 5 days of therapy had been completed, and it was generally reversible within 1 week of discontinuing treatment. Infants delivered shortly after indomethacin exposure also exhibit lower urine output.[132] Rarely, long-term indomethacin treatment may lead to neonatal renal failure and irreversible renal damage with cystic dilation of developing nephrons.[136]

Gastrointestinal complications, especially an increased incidence of necrotizing enterocolitis, occur in neonates exposed to indomethacin in utero.[132,137] Indomethacin reduces mesenteric blood flow,[138] disrupts autoregulation of oxygen consumption in the terminal ileum,[139] and, in mice, increases the likelihood of bowel necrosis following temporary ischemia.[140] Increased incidences of neonatal intracranial hemorrhage and periventricular leukomalacia have also been reported.[132,141] Finally, a greater incidence of respiratory distress and bronchopulmonary dysplasia has been described in a population where glucocorticord administration was uncommon.[142]

Since these serious complications are generally not seen with the use of other tocolytic agents, indomethacin should not be used as a first-line drug for tocolysis. It should be reserved for situations in which the clinician feels the risks of delivery outweigh the risks of indomethacin use. In addition, because these complications appear to be more likely after prolonged administration, and especially when there has been a short interval between discontinuation of therapy and delivery, substitution of an alternative agent as soon as possible is appropriate.

Calcium-channel blockers. Calcium-channel blockers inhibit the influx of calcium ions through voltage-dependent, calcium-selective cell membrane channels. Smooth muscle contractility is inhibited as a result of the reduction in cytoplasmic free calcium. Various calcium-channel blockers have been studied, but nifedipine has fewer side effects on cardiac conduction, does not alter serum electrolytes, is more specific in its tocolytic properties, and has been the agent most extensively studied in humans.[143-146] At least 10 studies, including three randomized, prospective investigations, have found nifedipine to be effective for tocolysis.[147-151] In all of the studies that have compared nifedipine to a beta-mimetic drug such as ritodrine or to magnesium sulfate, nifedipine has been at least as successful in stopping preterm contractions.[152-154] Nifedipine has the added advantage that it does not induce tachyphylaxis.[155] Nifedipine can easily be administered by the oral route. Therapeutic doses range from 10 to 30 mg orally every 4 to 8 hours. Over 90% of an oral dose of nifedipine is absorbed with onset of action in less than 20 minutes.[156,157] Absorption is 100% after sublingual administration (first breaking the capsule), and the onset of action is only 3 to 5 minutes, making this the preferred route if nifedipine is selected for initial tocolysis. An initial 10-mg sublingual dose may be followed by repeated doses at 20-minute intervals up to three times if contractions persist. Oral therapy is then begun.

Headache, nausea, flushing, a modest increase in heart rate, and a fall in diastolic blood pressure can occur secondary to vasodilation. Current evidence indicates that nifedipine does not adversely affect uterine blood flow in pregnancy.[158,159] Vascular relaxation is less pronounced in normotensive subjects, and studies in pregnant women have not found significant elevations in maternal heart rate with oral nifedipine.[146,147,159] Side effects reported in isolated cases include heartburn, dyspnea, chest pain or tightness, nervousness, constipation, diarrhea, and hepatotoxicity.[156,157,160] Side effects rarely lead to discontinuation of therapy.

Caution should be exercised if nifedipine is given to a woman receiving magnesium therapy. Combination therapy has been reported to cause an unexpected degree of hypotension in a preeclamptic patient[161] as well as suspected neuromuscular weakness.[162] Other authors have described the concurrent use of these two agents without adverse effects.[163,164] Because of increased hepatic blood flow, nifedipine may affect serum levels of digoxin, theophyline, phenytoin, quinidine, and other drugs.[156] The relatively long half-life of nifedipine might cause uterine atony unresponsive to routine uterine stimulants in a woman who has delivered despite tocolytic therapy. Theoretically, calcium therapy might decrease the degree of postpartum uterine atony in such cases.

Nifedipine crosses the placenta but does not appear to be teratogenic.[165] There has been no evidence of fetal compromise or long-term adverse effects in children.[143,147,149,164] Fetal heart rate, umbilical artery Doppler flow studies, and birth weight are unaffected.[149,158,159]

Miscellaneous agents. Diazoxide, an antihypertensive agent, has been used successfully to inhibit labor in humans, but it may cause significant hypotension and it has diabetogenic effects. Similarly, aminophylline and progestogens have tocolytic properties, but none of these agents has demonstrated superiority to any of the agents listed above and thus they have not gained popularity.

Early experimental data have indicated new directions for future study in the development of tocolytic therapy. In the human uterus, increasing sensitivity to oxytocin and an increase in oxytocin receptor concentrations parallel gestational maturation.[166] Atosiban, an oxytocin analogue (antagonist) currently under study, seems to be a potent in vitro inhibitor of oxytocin-induced contractility in human pregnant myometrium,[167] and initial clinical trials are promising.[168] Nitric oxide is a potent endogenous smooth-muscle relaxant acting by increasing levels of cyclic guanosine monophosphate. Glyceryl trinitrate, a nitric oxide donor, has been used successfully as a uterine relaxant for breech extraction[169] and more recently when administered transdermally via a skin patch; it has proved to be a noninvasive, well-tolerated, tocolytic agent for preterm labor.[170] Since only small numbers of pregnant women have been studied, both drugs must be considered experimental.

Role of glucocorticoids. The beneficial effect of antenatal corticosteroid therapy on fetal pulmonary maturation was first reported in 1972. Evidence from more than 25 studies, including at least 12 randomized controlled trials, and a recent meta-analysis support the conclusion that corticosteroid administration is associated with significant reductions in respiratory distress syndrome (RDS), intraventricular hemorrhage (IVH), necrotizing enterocolitis (NEC) and neonatal death for infants delivered between 28 and 34 weeks' gestation.[171-174] Although there is not a clear decrease in the incidence of RDS in infants born at 24 to 28 weeks, recent studies show the severity is reduced and, more importantly, that there is a clear reduction in mortality and the incidence of IVH in this group.[175] Despite this evidence, concern for potential complications such as maternal hypoglycemia, infection, and impaired wound healing as well as increased neonatal sepsis, adrenal suppression, and impaired fetal growth has limited the use of steroids in many institutions.[176,177] To address these issues, in March of 1994 the National Institute of Child Health and Human Development and the Office of Medical Applications of Research of the National Institutes of Health convened a consensus conference on the effect of corticosteroids for fetal maturation on perinatal outcomes. The consensus panel made the following recommendations, which are also endorsed by the American College of Obstetricians and Gynecologists Committee on Obstetric Practice.[178,179]

· The benefits of antenatal corticosteroid administration to fetuses at risk of preterm delivery vastly outweigh the potential risks. In addition to a reduction in the risk of RDS, these benefits include a substantial reduction in mortality and IVH. There is no convincing evidence that steroid therapy increases the risk of neonatal infection or adrenal suppression, and follow-up studies of children up to 12 years of age do not show a risk of adverse neurodevelopmental outcome.[171,178,180]

· All women between 24 and 34 weeks of pregnancy at risk for preterm delivery are candidates for antenatal corticosteroid treatment.

· Fetal race, gender, and the availability of surfactant should not affect the decision to treat with steroids. Antenatal administration of corticosteroids acts additively with postnatal administration of surfactant to reduce RDS. Furthermore, surfactant replacement appears to have little, if any, impact on the incidence of IVH or PDA. Any patient eligible for tocolysis should also be eligible for treatment with antenatal corticosteroids.

· Treatment consists of two doses of 12 mg of betamethasone, intramuscularly, given 24 hours apart, or 4 doses of 6 mg of dexamethasone, intramuscularly, given 12 hours apart. These agents are virtually identical in biological activity; they both cross the placenta and have little or no mineralocorticoid activity.

· Optimal benefits begin 24 hours after initiating therapy and last 7 days, but treatment for less than 24 hours is still associated with significant reductions in neonatal mortality. Therefore, corticosteroids should be given unless immediate delivery is anticipated.

The consensus panel also recommended that steroids be used in women with preterm premature rupture of membranes at less than 30 to 32 weeks' gestation in the absence of chorioamnionitis because of the high risk of IVH early in gestation. However, the Committee on Obstetric Practice believes that further research is required before steroids can be recommended in this group. Another area in which additional research is needed is in the benefits and risks of repeated courses of steroids at 7-day intervals in women who remain at risk for preterm delivery. The use of thyroid-releasing hormone to accelerate fetal lung maturity has been described but is currently considered experimental.[181]

Intrapartum management. When labor progresses despite maximal therapy or the patient presents in advanced labor precluding successful labor inhibition, decisions must be made as to how best to accomplish delivery. Ideally, delivery should occur at a facility equipped to care for the infant since transferring the neonate postdelivery reduces the chances of a successful outcome.[182] As recently as 10 years ago, infants less than 26 weeks' gestation were largely thought to be previable. However, more recent studies indicate that in selected hospitals 20% to 50%[1,183-185] of infants delivered at 24 to 25 weeks' gestation survive and are no more likely to develop major handicaps than infants born at 26 to 28 weeks' gestation.[183,186] These survival rates are likely to continue to improve with recent introduction of the use of exogenous pulmonary surfactants at neonatal resuscitation. Since a 2-week error in gestational dating is not uncommon, it is recommended that all neonates estimated to be at 24 weeks or greater be provided intensive care until it is determined that the infant is previable or has major anomalies.

All tocolytic medications should be discontinued immediately once it has been determined that successful labor inhibition is impossible. The infant born with high levels of these agents may be depressed, and the side effects of these drugs can complicate resuscitative efforts. Fetal distress is relatively common during preterm labor, perhaps because placental dysfunction plays a role in the development of such labors. Respiratory distress syndrome and intracranial hemorrhage are more likely to develop in infants asphyxiated at birth. Thus, continuous fetal heart rate monitoring is perhaps more valuable for the extremely preterm infant than for infants at term. It allows prompt diagnosis of asphyxia and significantly reduces neonatal mortality in the fetus weighing less than 1500 g.[187] Interpretation may be slightly more difficult since the variability is somewhat reduced in the very preterm infant and the baseline heart rate may be higher. However, heart rates above 170 beats/min require further investigation. Fetal scalp blood sampling should be performed any time there is a suggestion of fetal compromise.

Both prolonged and precipitous labor should be avoided and oxytocin use carefully monitored. Vaginal examinations should be kept to a minimum because the preterm infant is especially vulnerable to infection. A traumatic delivery is poorly tolerated by the preterm infant, but this does not mean

that cesarean section is the preferred route of delivery. For the infant presenting vertex, cesarean delivery after the onset of labor does not prevent central nervous system bleeding, and there is insufficient evidence to recommend its routine use.[188-190] Possible advantages of vaginal delivery include (1) more complete expression of amniotic fluid from the fetal lungs; (2) rapid chest decompression at delivery, facilitating lung expansion and the intake of the first breath; and (3) increased placental transfusion at birth. However, should a prolonged induction in the presence of a rigid unyielding cervix be required, cesarean delivery may be preferable.

Proponents of elective outlet forceps delivery believe that this method protects the fragile preterm head. In general, it is doubtful that forceps produce less trauma.[191,192] Currently available forceps were not designed for the very low birth weight infant. Studies on the use of the vacuum extractor in the very low birth weight infant are unavailable, but potential risks argue against its use. A single study reporting the use of the vacuum for delivery of 61 infants with birth weights between 1500 and 2499 g found this method to be safe, but the relatively small number of infants do not permit any definite conclusions.[193] Although routine episiotomy to reduce resistance and shorten the second stage of labor is often recommended, at this time there is insufficient data to suggest that a liberal episiotomy will improve perinatal outcome in the preterm infant. Personnel trained in the resuscitation of the preterm infant should be present at the delivery with all necessary equipment ready for immediate use.

No prospective, randomized controlled trials have been conducted to determine whether the preterm breech infant should be abdominally delivered. While several retrospective reports suggest that cesarean delivery is the safest route for the fetus weighing less than 1500 g, these studies have been plagued by confounding variables.[194-196] Other reports have demonstrated no such advantage.[188,197] Until the results of appropriately designed studies become available, the majority of obstetricians believe it is prudent to abdominally deliver the infant with an estimated gestational weight of between 800 and 1500 g. Although head entrapment is most likely to occur in the infant weighing less than 800 g, the decision of whether the increased maternal morbidity associated with cesarean delivery is justified for these infants must be determined individually at each institution, as well as for each pregnancy. External version under tocolysis to convert the preterm breech to a cephalic presentation may be feasible on occasion, but there is insufficient experience to recommend this approach. Since external version would usually be considered only in situations where labor inhibition has been unsuccessful, the likelihood of success would be considerably hindered.

Before proceeding with surgery, major congenital anomalies should be excluded by careful sonographic evaluation. Knowledge of such anomalies may influence both the decision of whether operative intervention is warranted and the choice of uterine incision. The type of uterine incision selected is also dependent on whether or not there is a well-developed lower uterine segment. In many cases, a transverse incision may be feasible, but it is inconsistent to subject the mother to surgery to avoid fetal trauma, only to have the fetal head trapped by an unyielding incision in a poorly developed lower segment.

Cesarean delivery has been recommended for all preterm twin gestations in which twin A is non-vertex, despite the lack of controlled trials to support this recommendation.[198] Fetal heart rate monitoring allows continuous assessment of the well-being of both infants simultaneously. Should fetal distress occur in either infant, immediate cesarean delivery can always be performed. It would seem reasonable that the same consideration for vaginal breech delivery given the singleton be accorded to the twin fetus. The phenomenon of locked twins is extremely rare, occurring in 1 in 1000 twin gestations,[199] and intrapartum sonography can be used to anticipate its occurrence. The obstetrician must be prepared to proceed immediately with cesarean delivery if this diagnosis is suspected.

Vaginal delivery is planned if twin A presents vertex and twin B breech. Three different methods of delivering the second twin have been successfully employed: (1) Immediately after delivery of twin A, external version (with or without sonographic guidance) may be attempted. This procedure may be facilitated by short-term intravenous tocolysis. (2) Total breech extraction may be performed either immediately or in the event that external version attempts are unsuccessful. There is evidence fo suggest that breech extraction as the initial approach decreases the chances of requiring a cesarean delivery for the second twin following failed attempts at external version. (3) The patient may be allowed to continue labor, with twin B delivered as an assisted breech. Although some obstetricians prefer to perform a cesarean delivery, there is little evidence that this will improve outcome for twin B.[200] In any event, an anesthesiologist should be in attendance at all twin deliveries. Rarely, following delivery of twin A, contractions cease and the use of tocolysis, cerclage, and anti-

biotics may permit considerable delay of delivery of twin B (by as much as 114 days).[201]

Preterm rupture of the membranes. Rupture of the fetal membranes occurring between 20 and 37 completed weeks of gestation is called preterm rupture of membranes. Uterine contractions may or may not be present. Thirty percent of preterm deliveries are directly attributable to membrane rupture. Although many of the conditions associated with preterm labor are also associated with preterm rupture of the membranes, it is often impossible to identify the specific etiology in a given patient. A history of preterm rupture of the membranes places a patient at greatest risk since one out of five subsequent pregnancies will be similarly affected.[202]

Initial management. At the time of admission, a sterile speculum examination is performed to (1) confirm the diagnosis, (2) obtain culture specimens from the cervix, (3) provide an estimate of cervical dilation, effacement, and position, and (4) exclude gross prolapse of the umbilical cord. To reduce the risk of infection, digital examination is avoided until it has been decided to proceed with labor and delivery.[203] If sufficient amniotic fluid is present in the vaginal vault, an aliquot may be obtained for pulmonary maturity assessment. The lecithin-to-sphingomyelin (L:S) ratio and phosphatidylglycerol results obtained are usually accurate, although the L:S ratio may be altered by the presence of blood or meconium and, rarely, bacterial contamination may influence phosphatidylglycerol results. In general, the results of these tests do not alter management for the fetus of less than 33 or 34 weeks' gestation, although they may indicate which women are candidates to receive steroids.

Ultrasound examination is useful for assessing fetal age and presentation, and in confirming a decreased volume of amniotic fluid. The role of amniocentesis in preterm rupture of the membranes for determining occult amniotic fluid infection remains undefined. Other indicators of chorioamnionitis such as maternal fever, maternal or fetal tachycardia, uterine tenderness, contractions, foul vaginal discharge, or a leukocytosis with a left shift in the polymorphonuclear leukocyte differential should be sought.[204]

Subsequent management. Management of preterm rupture of the membranes is made particularly difficult because prevention of the two major complications associated with the condition, infection and prematurity, requires divergent management plans. The longer the latent period from membrane rupture to the onset of contractions, the greater the maternal and fetal infectious morbidity and mortality,[205,206] although this is not as striking in preterm rupture as it is in postdate rupture.[207] Aggressive management with early delivery would reduce these risks. However, to minimize the risks of prematurity, a conservative management plan that allows the fetus to remain in utero as long as possible is indicated. The majority of perinatal deaths in cases of premature rupture of the membranes are due to RDS, not neonatal sepsis.

When membranes rupture before 24 weeks' gestation, the chance of a successful pregnancy outcome is low, but intact survivors do occur.[208,209] Therefore, either immediate pregnancy termination or expectant management is acceptable, depending on the patient's wishes. The latter option does entail the risk (approximately 3.5%) of developing fetal pulmonary hypoplasia or compression deformities (e.g., clubfeet).[210]

There is no general concensus of opinion as to how to manage the patient between 24 and 34 weeks' gestation; policies advocating pharmacologic tocolysis, expectant management, or induction of labor each have their proponents. In our practice, patients are placed on strict bed rest, and monitoring is initiated for evidence of uterine contractions, fetal distress (daily nonstress tests), or sepsis. Variable fetal heart rate decelerations may indicate an occult cord prolapse. Even without prolapse, umbilical cord compression secondary to oligohydramnios is more common with ruptured membranes.[211] If a nonstress test is reactive and there is no evidence of labor or infection, then the parturient is observed. Should contractions supervene during the initial 48 hours of observation, as may be expected in approximately half of patients, tocolytic agents are instituted provided there is no contraindication. These agents are discontinued 48 hours after membrane rupture. Whether prolonging tocolysis beyond 48 hours might improve outcome for the very preterm infant of less than 28 weeks' gestation (where the problems of prematurity are paramount) has not been determined. Since preterm rupture of membranes is associated with an increased risk of placental abruption, any report by the patient of vaginal bleeding is carefully evaluated.[212]

For most institutions, any time before 34 weeks' gestation the complications of prematurity outweigh the risks of infection and therefore a policy of expectant management with close observation for evidence of infection is justified.[213] Lung maturity does not mean fetal maturity. A preterm infant without RDS may still develop serious complications such as necrotizing enterocolitis, intracerebral bleeding, or hyperbilirubinemia. In addition, there is a small possibility that leakage will stop, amniotic fluid will reaccumulate, and the patient may be discharged home with "resealed" membranes.[214]

After 34 weeks' gestation, neonatal survival rates are excellent and the risk of cord prolapse and infection assume greater importance. If the cervix is favorable, labor induction is generally advisable,[215] although some investigators believe that continued expectant management is preferable even at term.[216] Induction attempts in the presence of an unfavorable cervix may result in a high incidence of cesarean delivery. Delaying induction of labor for a period of at least 24 hours might provide time for further pulmonary maturation and cervical ripening (whether spontaneous or promoted by prostaglandin application), thus improving the chances for successful vaginal delivery.

Multiple studies have concluded that prophylactic antibiotics reduce the incidence of maternal puerperal infectious morbidity following preterm rupture of the membranes. Whether or not they reduce neonatal infectious morbidity is unsettled. Recent studies suggest that antibiotic administration may prolong the latent period as well as decrease neonatal infectious complications.[45,217-220] Evidence is mounting in support of the use of prophylactic ampicillin, pending cervical culture results, specifically to prevent early onset group B beta-hemolytic streptococcal infection in the neonate.[221] However, adverse effects on perinatal outcome, such as a higher incidence of neonatal necrotizing enterocolitis[222] and the emergence of resistant enterobacteriaceae resulting in fatal perinatal sepsis,[223] have been reported following antenatal antibiotic use. There is general agreement that prophylactic antibiotics are indicated in the event of a cesarean delivery.

Once a diagnosis of chorioamnionitis is made, delivery should be accomplished expeditiously in all cases, preferably by the vaginal route. Cesarean delivery is reserved for the usual obstetric indications since perinatal outcome is not improved and maternal morbidity is increased when infection is the sole indication for this procedure. Unless delivery is imminent, broad-spectrum antibiotics in high doses should be started immediately. Should variable fetal heart rate decelerations occur, saline amnioinfusion may be useful in abolishing this pattern by restoring fluid volume and relieving cord compression.[224] Other investigators have used amnioinfusion to administer antibiotics or restore fluid volume in the nonlaboring patient, but this approach is currently investigational.[225,226]

Anesthetic management

The high incidence of operative vaginal and cesarean deliveries of the preterm fetus necessitates efficient obstetric anesthesia management.[227,228] In addition, provision of obstetric analgesia can be in itself an integral part of intrauterine resuscitation of the distressed fetus. Choice of appropriate anesthetic technique and agents may actually decrease intrapartum maternal and fetal complications.

Anesthetic management must include consideration of associated medical, obstetric, and social conditions (see Box 22-1) as well as possible drug interactions between anesthetic and maternal drug therapy (see Box 22-3). Once the diagnosis of preterm labor is made, the anesthesiologist must be prepared for obstetric intervention. Inhibition of labor for preterm pregnancy is far from an exact science. The anesthesiologist is often presented with a patient requiring emergency induction of anesthesia who may be already receiving a variety of potent systemic medications to inhibit preterm labor.

Anesthetic implications of the pharmacologic treatment of preterm labor

Ethanol. The use of intravenous ethanol as a tocolytic agent has essentially disappeared. The anesthesiologist may never again be faced with the problem of an acutely intoxicated parturient. The memory of such "drunken" patients still lives in the minds of many obstetric anesthesiologists and, therefore, deserves mention. Alterations in mental status, respiratory depression, lactic acidosis, hyperthyroidism or hypothyroidism, hypertension, and increased gastric volume and acidity are all seen in intoxicated patients.[229] The vomiting patient with less than optimal laryngeal reflexes is at high risk for possible aspiration and pneumonitis. The routine use of nonparticulate antacids, metoclopramide, and H_2-receptor antagonists should be part of aspiration prophylaxis. Minimum alveolar concentration (MAC) is decreased in the intoxicated patient. Cumulative depressant effects of ethanol with anesthetic agents must be expected.[229] Even the patient recovering from anesthesia after delivery must be vigilantly observed for effects of intoxication. As with any intoxicated patient, disturbances in fluid and electrolyte balance should be corrected.[230]

Beta-adrenergic agonist. The anesthesiologist dealing with the parturient who has received a beta-adrenergic agent within the prior 24 hours has several concerns. Serum glucose and potassium levels and hematocrit should be evaluated. An electrocardiogram may be helpful in evaluating the patient symptomatic with chest pain and in detecting arrhythmias.

Tachycardia and pulmonary edema may compound difficulties in clinically estimating intravascular volume status and may necessitate invasive monitoring of right-sided or bilateral cardiac filling pressures. Empiric prophylactic intravenous hydration prior to regional anesthesia increases the risk of pulmonary edema, although preload reduction with the sympathectomy of regional anesthesia may be beneficial to the parturient with pulmonary edema.[231]

It has been theorized that intravenous ritodrine infusion may enhance the deleterious cardiovascular effects of aortocaval compression.[232] Especially in patients who need higher doses of ritodrine to effect tocolysis, displacing the gravid uterus in the preterm pregnant patient seems to ameliorate these cardiovascular effects.[232]

Epidural anesthesia in the gravid ewe model receiving intravenous ritodrine therapy showed no deleterious effect on maternal arterial pressure or cardiac index.[233] In this study, only a midthoracic level of sensory anesthesia was induced, but there is little reason to believe that extension of sensory anesthesia to upper thoracic levels would cause further acute cardiac decompensation. As opposed to "single-shot" spinal anesthesia, continuous catheter techniques of epidural or spinal anesthesia may be a superior choice for abdominal delivery of the parturient in whom sudden vasodilation or a large volume of intravenous fluid would lead to hemodynamic compromise. Incremental dosing via catheter to induce anesthesia would allow time for the anesthesiologist and mother to adjust to the hemodynamic effects of regional anesthesia. The need for pressor therapy or intravenous fluid volume could reasonably be minimized. Even incremental intravenous titration of ephedrine might worsen the cardiac profile in the presence of severe maternal tachycardia. In the case of extreme hypotension, consideration should be given to pressor therapy using dilute intravenous phenylephrine (Neo-Synephrine) infusion.

Fetal considerations often necessitate emergency abdominal delivery and therefore general anesthesia may be required. Sympathomimetic agents that might worsen severe maternal tachycardia, such as ketamine, should be avoided. Atropine, glycopyrrolate, and pancuronium should be used with caution. Halothane, in comparison with enflurane and isoflurane, sensitizes the myocardium to catecholamines,[234] possibly leading to arrhythmia, it is best avoided. Laryngoscopy and intubation is often associated with tachycardia and hypertension. Adjuncts such as intravenous low-dose narcotics, lidocaine, or low doses of beta-adrenergic blocking agents[235] have all been used to blunt these cardiovascular effects, especially in the parturient with preeclampsia. Possible fetal effects must be considered before routine use of these agents.

Magnesium sulfate. Magnesium sulfate potentiates both depolarizing and especially nondepolarizing neuromuscular relaxants.[236] Administration of curare before an intubation dose of succinylcholine may lead to unexpected respiratory difficulty. The dose of succinylcholine needed for intubation should not be decreased, since the extent of magnesium sulfate potentiation is variable.[237,238] During maintenance of anesthesia, the need for additional neuromuscular relaxation should be guided by a neuromuscular blockade monitor. Estimating the volume of prophylactic intravenous hydration needed before induction of regional anesthesia, with its resultant vasodilation, is complicated in parturients receiving magnesium therapy, for reasons similar to those previously discussed with beta-adrenergic agonist therapy.

Induction of epidural anesthesia in the general ewe model receiving magnesium sulfate does not worsen maternal cardiac output or uteroplacental perfusion.[239] However, a slightly exaggerated maternal hypotensive response may accompany induction of epidural anesthesia.[239]

In the clinical situation, the anesthesiologist may therefore need to administer a vasopressor. In the gravid ewe model receiving intravenous magnesium sulfate and made hypotensive with induction of epidural anesthesia, intravenous ephedrine increased maternal cardiac output, uteroplacental blood flow, fetal pH, and blood oxygen concentration.[240] While it is as effective a vasopressor as ephedrine, intravenous phenylephrine increased uterine vascular resistance and was associated with a decreased fetal pH.

Perhaps because of a decrease in the blood levels of circulating stress catecholamines, epidural anesthesia will further exacerbate any episode of hemorrhagic hypotension, hastening fetal deterioration.[241] If regional anesthesia is chosen for delivery, then any significant vaginal hemorrhage (e.g., partial placental abruption) or acute sudden hemorrhage at operative delivery should prompt an aggressive response by the anesthesiologist to maintain maternal circulating intravascular volume.

Prostaglandin synthetase inhibitor. The effects of indomethacin on platelet function are well documented. However, it is obvious that vast numbers of regional anesthetics (as well as nerve blocks) have been administered without reports of adverse sequelae in patients with rheumatologic or orthopedic disease who have ingested drugs with antiplatelet effects similar to indomethacin. Few reports detailing this experience are in the literature.[242,243]

Calcium-channel blockers. Calcium-channel blockers have a wide variety of anesthetic interactions. The dose of calcium-channel blocker necessary to inhibit preterm labor is rarely associated with impairment of atrioventricular conduction and hypotension. Although of the calcium-channel blockers nifedipine has the fewest side effects on cardiac conduction, it does have the potential for vasodilation and hypotension.[244] A moderate reflex tachycardia is sometimes seen soon after therapy is initiated.

It should be noted that in the isolated rat heart model (already perfused with magnesium sulfate), nifedipine as well as verapamil lead to a dose-dependent increase in cardiac depression.[245] Such combination drug therapy in a patient presenting for anesthesia should, therefore, heighten the anesthesiologist's concern for maternal hypotension. An exaggerated hypotensive response might also be anticipated in the parturient on a calcium-channel blocker receiving a volatile anesthetic.[246]

In one study, nifedipine administered immediately after birth abolished methylergometrine-induced uterine contraction without leading to qualitatively increased hemorrhage.[247] Contractions induced by uterine stimulant had already occurred, and calcium-channel blockers had not been given chronically. Chronic antepartum administration or the use of other calcium-channel blockers may not act similarly. A variety of uterine stimulants, including oxytocin, methergine, 15-methyl-$PGF_{2\alpha}$, and calcium chloride, should be immediately available for use in a patient who delivers shortly after failed tocolysis with calcium-channel blockers. Availability of banked compatible blood components as well as large-bore intravenous access should be ensured predelivery.

Antibiotics. Many institutions will institute antibiotic therapy, especially in a parturient with premature rupture of membranes who is delivered abdominally. Most antibiotic regimens use ampicillin or a cephalosporin, both of which are devoid of neuromuscular blocking potential. Use of other antibiotics with possible potentiation of neuromuscular relaxants,[248] especially in the parturient receiving magnesium sulfate, demands the use of a neuromuscular blockade monitor for efficient administration of neuromuscular blocking drugs for general anesthesia.

Anesthetic implications for neonatal outcome. Appropriate selection of anesthetic technique and agents may potentially benefit the preterm, and sometimes distressed, fetus.

Labor and vaginal delivery. The preterm fetus has less protein-binding capacity than does a term fetus; this leads to increased circulating free drug concentration. In addition, the preterm fetus cannot metabolize and excrete drug as efficiently as can a term fetus. The preterm fetal blood-brain barrier is thought to be more permeable to circulating drug. Circulating maternal stress-related catecholamines decrease uteroplacental perfusion.[249] The preterm fetus is sensitive to decreases in uteroplacental perfusion and may rapidly develop fetal asphyxia.[250] The fetal response to possible asphyxia increases cerebral blood flow and therefore cerebral exposure to maternally administered drug. Induction of epidural analgesia and thereby decreasing maternal stress while maintaining maternal arterial pressure will benefit uteroplacental perfusion.[251] It is for these reasons that epidural analgesia or combined spinal epidural for labor and delivery is thought to be superior compared with the use of sedatives and/or narcotics. Preliminary data have indicated that epidural analgesia is at least as safe for the fetus as administering no anesthesia in labor and/or using local infiltration or pudendal block at delivery.[252] Vaginal delivery of the preterm fetus may necessitate a generous episiotomy, whether or not forceps are used, to decrease extracranial pressure and to better control delivery. Epidural analgesia or low spinal anesthesia will provide excellent perineal anesthesia at delivery and will facilitate atraumatic delivery.

Local anesthetic. Choice of local anesthetic for epidural anesthesia may be of some importance to fetal outcome. Data are generated mainly from gravid ewe models. Caution must be used before experimental analysis can be used to conclusively support clinical application.

Bupivacaine is an amide local anesthetic with a low fetal-to-maternal plasma concentration ratio secondary to its relatively high (90%) protein binding.[253] Lidocaine, with lower protein binding (60%),[254] will present a relatively larger anesthetic load to the fetus. Gestational age does not seem to alter fetal pharmacokinetics or pharmacodynamics of lidocaine.[255] However, the asphyxiated preterm fetus is more sensitive than the asphyxiated term fetus to the depressant effects of lidocaine.[256,257] Ion trapping of local anesthetic by an acidotic fetus will greatly increase the fetal-to-maternal plasma concentration ratio.[258] 2-Chloroprocaine, rapidly hydrolyzed in maternal and fetal plasma, will expose the acidotic fetus to a smaller level of local anesthetic. Therefore, 2-chloroprocaine is our preferred local anesthetic to intensify and/or extend epidural anesthesia to facilitate operative vaginal or abdominal delivery of the distressed preterm fetus.

"Single-shot" spinal anesthesia with lidocaine produces fetal drug levels 15% to 30% of those measured after epidural anesthesia.[259] The small amount of local anesthetic needed for "single shot"

spinal anesthesia for vaginal delivery (e.g., 35 mg of hyperbaric 5% lidocaine) allows the choice of local anesthetic to be made independent of fetal considerations.

Cesarean delivery. Cesarean delivery of the nondistressed fetus can be done under regional anesthesia, if time permits. The choice of local anesthetic for epidural anesthesia in the nondistressed fetus is not an issue. Approximately 18 to 22 mL of 2% lidocaine with epinephrine or 0.5% bupivacaine with epinephrine will provide surgical anesthesia in 20 to 30 minutes. Spinal anesthesia for cesarean delivery, whether "single shot" (e.g., 10 to 12 mg of hyperbaric 0.75% bupivacaine) or via a catheter, is an alternative to epidural anesthesia. A significant percentage of parturients given spinal anesthesia will have hypotensive episodes after induction.[260,261] Prompt treatment of maternal hypotension has been shown to make such episodes inconsequential to fetal outcome in the term fetus.[260,261] This may not be the case during abdominal delivery of the distressed preterm fetus. Therefore, meticulous attention to hydration and pharmacologic support of maternal blood pressure must be practiced. Vast experience of successful outcome with spinal anesthesia for abdominal delivery of the preterm fetus makes it an excellent method of surgical anesthesia.

Drugs used for the induction and maintenance of general anesthesia can potentially anesthetize the preterm infant; the induction to delivery time and the uterine incision to delivery time (as always) should be minimized. A retrospective study of almost 4000 babies born by cesarean delivery under general or regional (mainly epidural) anesthesia analyzed neonatal outcome according to 1- and 5-minute Apgar scores, the need for oxygen by mask, the need for tracheal intubation, and neonatal death.[262] Cord blood analysis was not reported. It was concluded that preterm neonates (all types of maternal anesthesia) had a two to five times higher incidence of a 1-minute Apgar score of 0 to 4 than did term neonates. The estimated relative risk of a 1-minute Apgar score of 0 to 4 for neonates born under general anesthesia was three times greater, compared with regional anesthesia regardless of the gestational age. There was significant improvement in 5-minute Apgar scores, and there was no difference in neonatal mortality. It is known that fetal lambs have a lower MAC to halothane and isoflurane than do lambs 24 hours or older.[263,264] Newborn sensitivity to general anesthetics may manifest as low Apgar scores. It is logical to believe that immediate neonatal ventilation, oxygenation, and therefore elimination of anesthetic would lead to significant improvement in 5-minute Apgar scores. This practice must be emphasized in the resuscitation of the "depressed" preterm neonate, although it will be true for any newborn.

After nonparticulate antacid treatment, uterine displacement, and appropriate denitrogenation, rapid sequence induction of anesthesia is begun with intravenous thiopental (4 mg/kg). Intravenous ketamine (1 mg/kg) is an acceptable alternative induction agent except in the preeclamptic parturient or perhaps those women with certain coexisting neurologic or cardiac disease. Ketamine is thought to better maintain redistribution of cardiac output to the central nervous system in the distressed fetal lamb.[265] Intubation is facilitated with 1 to 1.5 mg/kg of intravenous succinylcholine. Light anesthesia should be avoided, since increased maternal catecholamine production may decrease uteroplacental perfusion. Two-thirds MAC of any of the volatile agents is then given. Maternal inspired oxygen concentration should be at least 50%. In term gestations undergoing elective cesarean delivery, fetal Po_2 will not rise above 50 mm Hg after maternal Po_2 has reached 300 mm Hg.[266] Some anesthesiologists will deliver up to 100% oxygen to the mother during abdominal delivery of a distressed fetus. After delivery, the volatile agent can be discontinued, nitrous oxide concentration is increased, and supplemental intravenous narcotic drugs are given. Additional neuromuscular relaxant (succinylcholine or a nondepolarizing agent) is titrated intravenously as monitored by peripheral neuromuscular blockade.

Hyperventilation should be avoided. Respiratory alkalosis increases maternal oxygen-hemoglobin affinity. Hyperventilation via intermittent positive pressure ventilation decreases uteroplacental blood flow. The net result is decreased maternal oxygen presentation to the fetoplacental unit.[267]

Special situations

Breech presentation (singleton or twin). Delivery of a breech fetus (singleton or even second twin), whether by cesarean or vaginal delivery, may demand uterine relaxation for internal podalic version or full breech extraction or to facilitate delivery of a trapped aftercoming head.

Beside general anesthesia, acute uterine relaxation can be achieved by other medications. In the past, inhalation of amyl nitrate in 100% oxygen via a closed-circuit breathing was often advocated to relax the uterus. Many anesthesiologists are now administering nitroglycerin (either an intravenous bolus dose or a sublingual spray) to quickly achieve transient uterine relaxation.[268-270] Although there are few clinical studies even attempting to show the efficiency of nitroglycerin,[268] anecdotal reports have been published.[269,270] Doses of nitroglycerin (50 to 100 mg IV or 400 μg sub-

lingual metered dose spray) can be administered. Both the anesthesiologist and obstetrician must remain in constant communication as to the timing of each dose and the desired uterine effects. The anesthesiologist should be ready to support maternal blood pressure if maternal hypotension is seen.

The complete perinatal team should be aware that deep-inhalation anesthesia may be needed to relax the uterus should nitroglycerin therapy fail.

The parturient should be forewarned that emergency induction of general anesthesia may be necessary even after induction of regional anesthesia. It is our practice to readminister nonparticulate antacid to all parturients with breech or twin gestation on arrival in the delivery room. One hundred percent inspired oxygen is administered by mask to denitrogenate and avoid delay of rapid sequence induction should general anesthesia become necessary. Rapid sequence induction of general anesthesia can be accomplished with intravenous pentothal and intubation facilitated by intravenous succinylcholine. High inspired concentrations of volatile anesthetic is then given until delivery. Maternal blood pressure is supported with fluid and pressor therapy. At delivery, the volatile anesthetic agent is discontinued, and the patient is kept anesthetized until placental extraction and surgical repair is accomplished.

Cervical (Dührssen's) incisions are sometimes made in an attempt to free a trapped aftercoming head.[271] Careful observation of maternal blood loss per vaginum as well as maternal vital signs should be made. Occult hemorrhage into the pelvis may suddenly lead to maternal cardiovascular decompensation out of proportion to the observed blood loss per vaginum. A high index of suspicion and effective communication with the obstetrician may avoid maternal morbidity.

Chorioamnionitis. The incidence of blood aspirated via epidural needle or catheter is less than 10%.[272] The incidence of occult vein laceration as detected by precordial Doppler monitor after epidural air test dose is over 40%.[273] The use of regional anesthesia in the febrile parturient raises the question of possible hematogenous contamination of the epidural or subarachnoid space. However, most, if not all, parturients with a diagnosis of chorioamnionitis will be treated with intravenous antibiotics. An effective blood level of antibiotic is therefore possible before regional anesthesia is considered. Also, the degree of pyrexia in a parturient does not correlate well with the presence of bacteremia.[274] Clinical evaluation of the parturient should be made regarding the possibility of sepsis or other signs of systemic debilitation. The presence of ongoing antibiotic therapy is noted. It is our practice to offer epidural or spinal anesthesia to parturients with diagnosed chorioamnionitis who are not overtly septic, who are receiving antibiotics, and who are without other contraindications to regional anesthesia.

SUMMARY

Early induction of epidural analgesia is our technique of choice in providing first stage of labor analgesia. Subsequent conversion to provide anesthesia for vaginal or abdominal delivery can be readily accomplished, using 3% 2-chloroprocaine if the fetus becomes distressed. Spinal anesthesia is an excellent alternative to epidural anesthesia for elective or urgent cesarean delivery as long as maternal hypotension is promptly treated. General anesthesia can be safely achieved for abdominal delivery of a seriously distressed fetus or if immediate delivery (e.g., prolapsed fetal part) is indicated. Previously informed pediatric staff should be present and available for immediate neonatal evaluation and possible resuscitation at the delivery of any preterm fetus regardless of route of delivery or type of maternal anesthesia.

Recognition of gravidae at risk as well as prompt diagnosis and treatment of preterm labor are of major concern to the perinatologist. The consequences of preterm delivery are draining for the family and the community, and the emotional and financial costs of initial and long-term medical care can be staggering. Once delivery becomes inevitable, the anesthesiologist is often faced with a distressed fetus and/or a parturient receiving multiple pharmacologic therapy. Early communication of the obstetric and anesthetic plan to the entire perinatal care team, as well as to the parturient and her family, is obligatory to the best care for the high-risk pregnancy.

REFERENCES

1. Cooper RL, Goldenberg RL, Creasy RK, et al: A multicenter study of preterm birth weight and gestational age specific mortality. *Am J Obstet Gynecol* 1993; 168:78.
2. Kitchen W, Yu VYH, Orgill AA, et al: Infants born before 29 weeks gestation: Survival and morbidity at 2 years of age. *Br J Obstet Gynaecol* 1982; 89:887.
3. Astbury J, Orgill A, Bajuk B, et al: Determinants of developmental performance of very low-birthweight survivors at 1 and 2 years of age. *Dev Med Child Neurol* 1983; 25:709.
4. McCormick M: The contribution of low birthweight to infant mortality and childhood morbidity. *N Engl J Med* 1985; 312:82.
5. Lee K-S, Paneth N, Gartner L, et al: Neonatal mortality: An analysis of the recent improvement in the United States. *Am J Public Health* 1980; 70:15.
6. Anderson ABM: Pre-term labour: Definition, in Anderson ABM, et al (eds): *Proceedings of the Fifth Study Group of the Royal College of Obstetricians and Gynaecologists.* London, Royal College of Obstetricians and Gynaecologists, 1977.

7. Monthly Vital Statistics Report: *Advance Report on Final Natality Studies,* 1991, 40(Suppl):8.
8. Frederick J, Anderson ABM: Factors associated with spontaneous preterm birth. *Br J Obstet Gynaecol* 1976; 83:342.
9. Baird D: Epidemiologic patterns over time, in Reed DM, Stanley J (eds): *The Epidemiology of Prematurity,* Baltimore, Md, Urban and Schwarzenberg, 1977, p 3.
10. Hardy JB, Mellits ED: Relationship of low birthweight to maternal characteristics of age, education and body size, in Reed DM, Stanley FJ (eds): *The Epidemiology of Prematurity.* Baltimore, Md, Urban and Schwarzenberg, 1977, p 105.
11. *Report of the Secretary's Task Force on Black and Minority Health.* Publ No. 0-487-637 (QL3), vol 6, US Dept of Health and Human Services, Hyattsville, Md., 1988.
12. Meyer MB, Tonascia JA: Maternal smoking, pregnancy complications and perinatal mortality. *Am J Obstet Gynecol* 1977; 128:494.
13. MacGregor SN, Keith LG, Chasnoff IJ, et al: Cocaine use during pregnancy: Adverse perinatal outcome. *Am J Obstet Gynecol* 1987; 157:686.
14. Mamelle N, Laumon B, Lazar P: Prematurity and occupational activity during pregnancy. *Am J Epidemiol* 1984; 119:309.
15. Murphy J, Dauncey M, Newcombe R, et al: Employment in pregnancy: Prevalence, maternal characteristics, perinatal outcome. *Lancet* 1984; 1:1163.
16. Newton RW, Hunt L: Psychosocial stress in pregnancy and its relation to low birthweight. *Br Med J* 1984; 288:1191.
17. Lobel M, Dunke-Schetter C, Scrimshaw PC: Prenatal maternal stress and prematurity: A prospective study of socioeconomically disadvantaged women. *Health Psychol* 1992; 11:32.
18. Wagner NN, Butler JC, Sanders JP: Prematurity and orgasmic coitus during pregnancy: Data on a small sample. *Fertil Steril* 1976; 27:911.
19. Naeye RL: Coitus and associated amniotic-fluid infections. *N Engl J Med* 1979; 301:1198.
20. Katreider DF, Kohl S: Epidemiology of preterm delivery. *Clin Obstet Gynecol* 1980; 23:17.
21. Keirse MJNC, Rush RW, Anderson ABM: Risk of preterm delivery in patients with previous pre-term delivery and/or abortion. *Br J Obstet Gynaecol* 1978; 85:81.
22. Bakketeig LS, Hoffman HJ: The epidemiology of preterm birth: Results from a longitudinal study in Norway, in Elder MG, Hendricks CH (eds): *Preterm Labor.* London, Butterworths International Medical Reviews, 1981, p 17.
23. Rush RW: Incidence of pre-term delivery in patients with previous pre-term delivery and/or abortion. *S Afr Med J* 1979; 56:1085.
24. Linn S, Schoenbaum SC, Monson RR, et al: The relationship between induced abortion and outcome of subsequent pregnancies. *Am J Obstet Gynecol* 1983; 146:136.
25. Heinonen PK, Saarikoski S, Pystnen P: Reproductive performance of women with uterine anomalies. *Acta Obstet Gynaecol Scand* 1982; 61:157.
26. Kaufman RH, Nolles K, Adam E, et al: Upper genital tract abnormalities and pregnancy outcome in diethylstilbestrol-exposed progeny. *N Engl J Med* 1985; 313:1322.
27. Muran D, Gillieson J, Walters JH: Mycomas of the uterus in pregnancy: Ultrasonographic follow-up. *Am J Obstet Gynecol* 1980; 138:16.
28. Forssman L: Posttraumatic intrauterine synechiae and pregnancy. *Obstet Gynecol* 1965; 26:710.
29. Crenshaw MC, Jones DED, Parker RT: Placenta previa: A survey of 20 years' experience with improved perina-

tal survival by expectant therapy and cesarean delivery. *Obstet Gynecol Surv* 1973; 28:461.

30. MacGillivary I, Campbell DM, Samphier M, et al: Preterm deliveries in twin pregnancies in Aberdeen. *Acta Genet Med Gemellol (Roma)* 1982; 31:207.

31. Abrams B, Newman V, Key T, et al: Maternal weight gain and preterm delivery. *Obstet Gynecol* 1989; 74:577.

32. Wenstrom KP, Sipes SL, Williamson RA, et al: Prediction of pregnancy outcome with single versus serial maternal serum x-fetoprotein tests. *Am J Obstet Gynecol* 1992; 167:1529.

33. Kirbinen P, Jouppila P: Polyhydramnion: A clinical study. *Ann Chir Gynaecol Fenniae* 1978; 67:117.

34. Turnbull AC: Aetiology of preterm labour, in Anderson ABM, et al (eds): *Proceedings of the Fifth Study Group of the Royal College of Obstetricians and Gynaecologists.* London, Royal College of Obstetricians and Gynaecologists, 1977, p 56.

35. Kincaid-Smith P: Bacteriuria and urinary infection in pregnancy. *Clin Obstet Gynecol* 1968; 11:533.

36. Romero R, Oyarzun E, Mazor M, et al: Meta-analysis of the relationship between asymptomatic bacteriuria and preterm delivery/low birthweight. *Obstet Gynecol* 1989; 73:576.

37. Tatum HJ, Schmidt FH, Jain AK: Management and outcome of pregnancies associated with Copper-T intrauterine contraceptive device. *Am J Obstet Gynecol* 1976; 126:869.

38. Edwards LE, Barrada MI, Hamann AA, et al: Gonorrhea in pregnancy. *Am J Obstet Gynecol* 1978; 132:637.

39. Regan JA, Chao S, James LS: Premature rupture of membranes, preterm delivery, and group B streptococcal colonization of mothers. *Am J Obstet Gynecol* 1981; 141:184.

40. Minkoff HL, Grunebaum AN, Schwarz RH, et al: Risk factors for prematurity and premature rupture of membranes: A prospective study of the vaginal flora in pregnancy. *Am J Obstet Gynecol* 1984; 150:965.

41. Martin DH, Koutsky L, Eschenbach DA, et al: Prematurity and perinatal mortality in pregnancies complicated by maternal *Chlamydia trachomatis* infection. *JAMA* 1982; 247:1585.

42. Alger LS, Lovchik JC, Hebel JR, et al: The association of *Chlamydia trachomatis, Neisseria gonorrhea* and group B streptococci with preterm rupture of membranes and pregnancy outcome. *Am J Obstet Gynecol* 1988; 159:397.

43. Remington JT, Klein JO: *Infectious Diseases of the Fetus and Newborn Infant,* ed 2. Philadelphia, WB Saunders, 1983, p 102.

44. McDonald HM, O'Loughlin JA, Jolley P, et al: Prenatal microbiological risk factors associated with preterm birth. *Br J Obstet Gynaecol* 1992; 99:190.

45. Gibbs RS, Romero R, Hillier SL, et al: A review of premature birth and subclinical infection. *Am J Obstet Gynecol* 1992; 166:1515.

46. Stamilio D, Shlossman P, Manley J, et al: Tocolysis for preterm contractions without cervical change does not improve perinatal outcome. SPO Abstract No. 568. *Am J Obstet Gynecol* 1995; 172:415.

47. Utter GD, Dooley SL, Tamera RK, et al: Awaiting cervical change for the diagnosis of preterm labor does not compromise the efficacy of ritodrine tocolysis. *Am J Obstet Gynecol* 1990; 163:882.

48. Goodlin RC, Quaife MA, Dirkson JW: The significance, diagnosis, and treatment of maternal hypovolemia as associated with fetal/maternal illness. *Semin Perinatol* 1981; 5:163.

49. Pircon RA, Strassner HT, Kirz DS, et al: Controlled trial of hydration and bed rest versus bed rest alone in the evaluation of preterm contractions. *Am J Obstet Gynecol* 1989; 161:775.

50. Korenbrot CC, Aalto LH, Laros RK: The cost effectiveness of stopping preterm labor with beta-adrenergic treatment. *N Engl J Med* 1984; 310:691.

51. Konte JM, Holbrook RH Jr, Laros RK, et al: Short-term neonatal morbidity associated with prematurity and the effect of a prematurity prevention program on expected incidence of morbidity. *Am J Perinatol* 1986; 3:283.

52. Henderson CE, Goldman B, Divon MY: Ritodrine therapy in the presence of chronic abruptio placentae. 1992; 80:510.

53. Sampson MB, Lastres O, Tomasi AM, et al: Tocolysis with terbutaline sulfate in patients with placenta previa complicated by premature labor. *J Reprod Med* 1984; 29:248-50.

54. McGregor JA, French JI, Reller LB, et al: Adjunctive erythromycin treatment for idiopathic preterm labor: Results of a randomized, double-blinded, placebo-controlled trial. *Am J Obstet Gynecol* 1986; 154:98.

55. Morales WJ, Angel JL, O'Brien WF, et al: A randomized study of antibiotic therapy in idiopathic preterm labor. *Am J Obstet Gynecol* 1988; 72:829.

56. Group B streptococcal infections in pregnancy. *ACOG Tech Bull No. 170,* July 1992.

57. Roberts JM: Current understanding of pharmacologic mechanisms in the prevention of preterm labor. *Am J Obstet Gynecol* 1988; 72:829.

58. Caritis SN, Hirsch RP, Zeleznik AJ: Adrenergic stimulation of placental progesterone production. *J Clin Endocrinol Metab* 1983; 86:959.

59. King JF, Grant A, Keirse MJNC, et al: Beta-mimetics in preterm labour: An overview of the randomized controlled trials. *Br J Obstet Gynaecol* 1988; 95:211.

60. The Canadian Preterm Labor Investigators Group: Treatment of preterm labor with the beta-adrenergic agonist ritodrine. *N Engl J Med* 1992; 327:308.

61. Caritis SN, Chiano JP, Moore JJ, et al: Myometrial desensitization after ritodrine infusion. *Am J Physiol* 1987; 253:E410.

62. Bieniarz J: Cardiovascular effects of beta-adrenergic agonists, in Anderson ABM, et al (eds): *Proceedings of the Fifth Study Group of the Royal College of Obstetricians and Gynaecologists.* London, Royal College of Obstetricians and Gynaecologists, 1977.

63. Benedetti TJ: Maternal complications of parenteral beta sympathomimetic therapy for premature labor. *Am J Obstet Gynecol* 1983; 145:1.

64. Hadi HA, Abdulla AM, Fadel HE, et al: Cardiovascular effects of ritodrine tocolysis. *Obstet Gynecol* 1987; 70:608.

65. Hosenpud JD, Morton MJ, O'Grady JP: Cardiac stimulation during ritodrine hydrochloride tocolytic therapy. *Obstet Gynecol* 1983; 62:52.

66. Merkatz IR, Peter JB, Barden TP: Ritodrine hydrochloride: A beta-mimetic agent for use in preterm labor. II. Evidence of efficacy. *Obstet Gynecol* 1980; 56:7.

67. Taylor ES: Angina pectoris. *Obstet Gynecol Surv* 1981; 36:14.

68. Hendricks SK, Keroes J, Katz M: Electrocardiographic changes associated with ritodrine-induced maternal tachycardia and hypokalemia. *Am J Obstet Gynecol* 1986; 154:921.

69. Ying Y-K, Tejani NA: Angina pectoris as a complication of ritodrine hydrochloride therapy in premature labor. *Obstet Gynecol* 1982; 60:385.

70. Gerritse R, Reuwer PJHM, Pinas IM, et al: Cardiovascular effects of ritodrine are blocked by metoprolol in the anesthetized dog. *Arch Int Pharmacodyn* 1985; 278:97.

71. Strigl R, Pfeiffer U, Aschenbrenner G, et al: Influence of the beta-1 selective blocker, metoprolol, on the development of pulmonary edema in tocolytic therapy. *Obstet Gynecol* 1986; 67:537.

72. Eggleston MK: Management of preterm labor and delivery. *Clin Obstet Gynecol* 1986; 29:230.

73. Finley J, Katz M, Rojas-Perez M, et al: Tocolysis: An echocardiographic study. *Obstet Gynecol* 1984; 64:787.

74. Philipsen T, Erikson PS, Lynggard F: Pulmonary edema following saline-ritodrine infusion in premature labor. *Obstet Gynecol* 1981; 58:304.

75. Wesley LC: Renin, angiotensin and aldosterone. *Obstet Gynecol Ann* 1974; 3:235.

76. Lammintusta R, Erkkolla R: Renin-angiotensin-aldosterone system and sodium in normal pregnancy: A longitudinal study. *Acta Obstet Gynecol* 1977; 56:221.

77. Grospietsch G, Fenske M, Firndt J, et al: The renin-angiotensin-aldosterone system: Antidiuretic hormone levels and water balance under tocolytic therapy with fenoterol and verapamil. *Int Gynecol Obstet* 1980; 17:590.

78. Armson CA, Samuels P, Miller F, et al: Evaluation of maternal fluid dynamics during tocolytic therapy with ritodrine hydrochloride and magnesium sulfate. *Am J Obstet Gynecol* 1992; 167:758.

79. Pisani J, Rosenow EC: Pulmonary edema associated with tocolytic therapy. *Ann Intern Med* 1989; 110:714.

80. Persson GA, Erjefalt I: Vascular antipermeability effects of beta-receptor agonists and theophylline in the lung. *Acta Pharmacol Toxicol* 1979; 44:216.

81. Berthiaume Y, Staub NC, Matthay MA: Beta-adrenergic agonists increase lung liquid clearance in anesthetized sheep. *J Clin Invest* 1987; 79:335.

82. Conover WB, Benumof JL, Key TC: Ritodrine inhibition of hypoxic pulmonary vasoconstriction. *Am J Obstet Gynecol* 1983; 146:652.

83. Cano A, Tovar I, Parilla JJ, et al: Metabolic disturbances during intravenous use of ritodrine: Increased insulin levels and hypokalemia. *Obstet Gynecol* 1985; 65:356.

84. Young DC, Toofanian A, Leveno KJ: Potassium and glucose concentrations without treatment during ritodrine tocolysis. *Am J Obstet Gynecol* 1983; 145:105.

85. Mordes D, Kreutner K, Metzger W, et al: Dangers of intravenous ritodrine in diabetic patients. *JAMA* 1982; 248:973.

86. Lotgering FK, Huikeshoven FJM, Wallenburg HCS: Elevated serum transaminase levels during ritodrine administration. *Am J Obstet Gynecol Reprod Biol* 1981; 11:317.

87. Robertson PA, Herron M, Katz M, et al: Maternal morbidity associated with isoxsuprine and terbutaline tocolysis. *Eur J Obstet Gynecol Reprod Biol* 1981; 11:317.

88. Brazy JE, Pupkin MJ: Effects of maternal isoxsuprine administration on preterm infants. *J Pediatr* 1979; 94:444.

89. Freysz H, Willard D, Lehr A, et al: A long-term evaluation of infants who receive a beta-mimetic drug while in utero. *J Perinat Med* 1977; 5:94.

90. Groome LJ, Goldenberg RL, Cliver SP, et al: Neonatal periventricular-intraventricular hemorrhage after maternal B-sympathomimetic tocolysis. *Am J Obstet Gynecol* 1992; 167:873.

91. Laros RK Jr, Kitterman JA, Heilbron D, et al: Outcome of very low birth weight infants exposed to B-sympathomimetics in utero. *Am J Obstet Gynecol* 1991; 164:1657.

92. Epstein MF, Nicols E, Stubblefield PG: Neonatal hypoglycemia after beta-sympthomimetic tocolytic therapy. *J Pediatr* 1979; 94:449.

93. Hadders-Algra M, Touwen BCL, Huisjes HJ: Long-term follow-up of children prenatally exposed to ritodrine. *Br J Obstet Gynaecol* 1986; 93:156.

94. Spatling L, Fallenstein F, Schneider H, et al: Bolus tocolysis: Treatment of preterm labor with pulsatile administration of beta-adrenergic agonist. *Am J Obstet Gynecol* 1989; 160:713.

95. Hill WC, Katz M, Kitzmiller JL, et al: Continuous long-term intravenous beta-sympathomimetic tocolysis. *Am J Obstet Gynecol* 1985; 152:271.

96. Lam F, Gill P, Smith M, et al: Use of the subcutaneous terbutaline pump for long-term tocolysis. *Obstet Gynecol* 1988; 72:810.

97. Caritis SN, Darby MJ, Chan L: Pharmacologic treatment of preterm labor. *Clin Obstet Gynecol* 1988; 31:635.

98. Altura BM, Altura BT: Magnesium ions and contraction of vascular smooth muscles: Relationship to some vascular diseases. *Fed Proc* 1981; 40:2672.

99. Gambling DR, Birmingham CL, Jenkins C: Magnesium and the anaesthetist. *Can J Anaesth* 1988; 35:644.

100. Skaredoff MN, Roaf ER, Datta S: Hypermagnesemia and anesthetic management. *Can Anaesth Soc J* 1982; 29:35.

101. McCubbin JH, Sibai GM, Abdella TM, et al: Cardiopulmonary arrest due to acute maternal hypermagnasaemia (letter). *Lancet* 1981; 1:1058.

102. Hollander DI, Nagey DA, Pupkin MJ: Magnesium sulfate and ritodrine hydrochloride: A randomized comparison. *Am J Obstet Gynecol* 1987; 156:631.

103. Cotton DB, Strassner HT, Hill LM, et al: Comparison of magnesium sulfate, terbutaline and a placebo for inhibition of preterm labor. *J Reprod Med* 1984; 29:92.

104. Elliott JP: Magnesium sulfate as a tocolytic agent. *Am J Obstet Gynecol* 1983; 147:277.

105. Wilkins IA, Goldberg JD, Phillips RN, et al: Long-term use of magnesium sulfate as a tocolytic agent. *Obstet Gynecol* 1986; 67S:38.

106. Hatjis CG, Nelson H, Meis PJ, et al: Addition of magnesium sulfate improves effectiveness of ritodrine in preventing premature delivery. *Am J Obstet Gynecol* 1984; 150:142.

107. Kosasa TS, Busse R, Wahl N, et al: Long-term tocolysis with combined intravenous terbutaline and magnesium sulfate: A 10-year study of 1000 patients. *Obstet Gynecol* 1994; 84:369.

108. Ferguson JE, Hensleigh PA, Kredenster D: Adjunctive use of magnesium sulfate with ritodrine in for preterm labor tocolysis. *Am J Obstet Gynecol* 1984; 148:166.

109. Valenzuela G, Cline S: Use of magnesium sulfate in premature labor that fails to respond to beta-mimetic drugs. *Am J Obstet Gynecol* 1982; 143:718.

110. Cotton DB, Gonik B, Dorman KF: Cardiovascular alterations in severe pregnancy-induced hypertension: Acute effects of intravenous magnesium sulfate. *Am J Obstet Gynecol* 1984; 148:162.

111. Lin CC, Pielet BW, Poon E, et al: Effect of magnesium sulfate on fetal heart rate variability in preeclamptic patients during labor. *Am J Perinatol* 1988; 5:208.

112. Thiagarajah S, Harbert GM, Bourgeois FJ: Magnesium sulfate and ritodrine hydrochloride: Systemic and uterine hemodynamic effects. *Am J Obstet Gynecol* 1985; 153:666.

113. Peaceman AM, Meyer BA, Thorp JA, et al: The effect of magnesium sulfate tocolysis on the fetal biophysical profile. *Am J Obstet Gynecol* 1989; 161:771.

114. Green KW, Key TC, Coen R, et al: The effects of maternally administered magnesium sulfate on the neonate. *Am J Obstet Gynecol* 1983; 146:29.

115. Holcomb WL Jr, Shackelford GD, Petrie RH: Magnesium tocolysis and neonatal bone abnormalities: A controlled study. *Obstet Gynecol* 1991; 78:611.

116. Elliot JP: Magnesium sulfate as a tocolytic agent. *Contemp Obstet Gynecol* Jan 1985:49.

117. Garfield RE, Kannan MS, Daniel EE: Gap junction formation in the myometrium: Control by estrogens, progesterone and prostaglandins. *Am J Physiol* 1980; 238:C81.
118. Liggins GC: Initiation of spontaneous labor. *Clin Obstet Gynecol* 1983; 26:47.
119. Garrioch DB: The effect of indomethacin on spontaneous activity in the isolated human myometrium and on the response to oxytocin and prostaglandin. *Br J Obstet Gynaecol* 1978; 85:47.
120. Wiqvist N, Kjellmer I, Thiringer K, et al: Treatment of premature labor by prostaglandin synthetase inhibitors. *Acta Biol Med* 1978; 37:923.
121. Kolsis JJ, Hernandovich J, Silver MJ, et al: Duration of inhibition of platelet prostaglandin formation and aggregation by ingested aspirin or indomethacin. *Prostaglandins* 1978; 3:141.
122. Lunt CC, Satin AJ, Barth WH, Hankins GDV: The effect of indomethacin tocolysis on maternal coagulation status. *Obstet Gynecol* 1994; 84:820.
123. Reiss U, Atad J, Reuinstein L, et al: The effect of indomethacin in labour at term. *Int J Gynaecol Obstet* 1976; 14:369.
124. Van den Veyver IB, Moise KJ Jr: Prostaglandin synthetase inhibitors in pregnancy. *Obstet Gynecol Surv* 1993; 48:493.
125. Csaba IF, Sulyok E, Erth T: The relationship of maternal treatment with indomethacin to persistence of fetal circulation syndrome. *J Pediatr* 1978; 92:484.
126. Goudie BM, Dossetor JFB: Effect on the fetus of indomethacin given to suppress labor. *Lancet* 1979; 2:1187.
127. Besinger RE, Niebyl JR, Keyes WG, et al: Randomized comparative trial of indomethacin and ritodrine for the long-term treatment of preterm labor. *Am J Obstet Gynecol* 1991; 164:981.
128. Moise KJ, Huhta JC, Sharif DS, et al: Indomethacin in the treatment of premature labor: Effects on the fetal ductus arteriosus. *N Engl J Med* 1988; 319:327.
129. Eronen M, Pesonen E, Kurki T, Ylikorkala O, et al: The effects of indomethacin and B-sympathomimetic agent on the fetal ductus arteriosus during treatment of premature labor: A randomized double-blind study. *Am J Obstet Gynecol* 1991; 164:141.
130. Momma K, Takao A: Increased constriction of the ductus arteriosus with combined administration of indomethacin and betamethasone in fetal rats. *Pediatr Res* 1989; 25:69.
131. Clyman RI, Campbell D, Heymann MA, et al: Persistent responsiveness of the neonatal ductus arteriosus in immature lambs: A possible cause for reopening of patent ductus arteriosus after indomethacin-induced closure. *Circulation* 1985; 71:141.
132. Norton ME, Merrill J, Bruce BAB, et al: Neonatal complications after the administration of indomethacin for preterm labor. *N Engl J Med* 1993; 329:1602.
133. Novy MJ: Effects of indomethacin on labor, fetal oxygenation and fetal development in Rhesus monkesys. *Adv Prostaglandin Thromboxane Res* 1987; 4:285.
134. Dudley DKL, Hardie MJ: Fetal and neonatal effects of indomethacin used as a tocolytic agent. *Am J Obstet Gynecol* 1985; 151:181.
135. Hickok DE, Hollenbach KA, Reilly SF, et al: The association between decreased amniotic fluid volume and treatment with nonsteroidal anti-inflammatory agents for preterm labor. *Am J Obstet Gynecol* 1989; 160:1525.
136. vander Heijden BJ, Carlus C, Narcy F, et al: Persistent anuria, neonatal death, and renal microcystic lesions after prenatal exposure to indomethacin. *Am J Obstet Gynecol* 1994; 171:617.
137. Major CA, Lewis DF, Harding JA, Porto MA, et al: Tocolysis with indomethacin increases the incidence of necrotizing enterocolitis in the low-birth-weight neonate. *Am J Obstet Gynecol* 1994; 170:102.

138. Van Bell F, Van Zwieten PHT, Guit GL, et al: Superior mesenteric artery blood flow velocity and estimated volume flow: Duplex Doppler US study of preterm and term neonates. *Radiology* 1990; 174:165.
139. Meyers RL, Alpan G, Lin E, et al: Patent ductus arteriosus, indomethacin, and intestinal distension: Effects of intestinal blood flow and oxygen consumption. *Pediatr Res* 1991; 29:569.
140. Krasna IH, Kim H: Indomethacin administration after temporary ischemia causes bowel necrosis in mice. *J Pediatr Surg* 1992; 27:805.
141. Baerts W, Fetter WP, Hop WC, et al: Cerebral lesions in preterm infants after tocolytic indomethacin. *Dev Med Child Neurol* 1990; 32:910.
142. Eronen M, Pesonen E, Kurki T, et al: Increased incidence of bronchopulmonary dysplasia after antenatal administration of indomethacin to prevent preterm labor. *J Pediatr* 1994; 124:782.
143. Ulmsten U, Andersson KE, Wingerup L: Treatment of premature labor with the calcium antagonist nifedipine. *Arch Gynecol* 1980; 229:1.
144. Forman A, Andersson KE, Ulmsten U: Inhibition of myometrial activity by calcium antagonists. *Semin Perinatol* 1981; 5:288.
145. Malgaard S, Forman A, Andersson KE: Comparison of the effects of nicardipine and nifedipine on isolated human myometrium. *Gynecol Obstet Invest* 1983; 16:354.
146. Ferguson JE, Dyson DC, Holbrook RH, et al: Cardiovascular and metabolic effects associated with nifedipine and ritodrine tocolysis. *Am J Obstet Gynecol* 1989; 161:788.
147. Read MD, Wellby DE: The use of a calcium antagonist (nifedipine) to suppress preterm labor. *Br J Obstet Gynaecol* 1986; 93:933.
148. Murray C, Haverkamp AD, Orleans M, et al: Nifedipine for the treatment of preterm labor: A historic prospective study. *Am J Obstet Gynecol* 1992; 167:52.
149. Ferguson JE Jr, Dyson DC, Schutz T, et al: Comparison of nifedipine and ritodrine for the treatment of preterm labor. *Am J Perinatol* 1991; 8:365.
150. Bracero LA, Leikin E, Kirschenbaum N, et al: Comparison of nifedipine and ritodrine for the treatment of preterm labor. *Am J Perinatol* 1991; 8:365.
151. Meyer WR, Randall HW, Graves WL: Nifedipine versus ritodrine for suppressing preterm labor. *J Reprod Med* 1990; 35:649.
152. Smith CS, Woodland MB: Clinical comparison of oral nifedipine and subcutaneous terbutaline for initial tocolysis. *Am J Perinatol* 1993; 10:280.
153. Kaul AF, Osathanondh R, Safon LE, et al: The management of preterm labor with the calcium channel-blocking agent nifedipine combined with the B-mimetic terbutaline. *Drug Intell Clin Pharmacol* 1985; 19:369.
154. Glock JL, Morales WJ: Efficiency and safety of nifedipine versus magnesium sulfate in the management of preterm labor: A randomized study. *Am J Obstet Gynecol* 1993; 169:960.
155. Childress CH, Katz VL: Nifedipine and its indications in obstetrics and gynecology. *Obstet Gynecol* 1994; 83:616.
156. Sorkin EM, Clissold SP, Brogden RN: Nifedipine: A review of its pharmacodynamic and pharmacokinetic properties, and therapeutic efficacy, in ischemic heart disease, hypertension and related cardiovascular disorders. *Drugs* 1985; 30:182.
157. Murad F: Drugs used for the treatment of angina: Organic nitrates, calcium-channel blockers, and B-adrenergic antagonists, in Gilman GA, Rall TW, Nies AS, et al (eds): The pharmocologic basis of therapeutics, ed 8. New York, Pergamon Press, 1990, pp 764-783.
158. Mari G, Kirshon B, Moise KJ Jr, et al: Doppler assessment of the fetal and uteroplacental circulation during ni-

fedipine therapy for preterm labor. *Am J Obstet Gynecol* 1989; 161:1514.

159. Pirhonen JP, Erkkola RU, Ekblad UU, et al: Single dose of nifedipine in normotensive pregnancy: Nifedipine concentrations, hemodynamic responses, and uterine and fetal flow velocity waveform. *Obstet Gynecol* 1990; 76:807.

160. Sawaya GF, Robertson PA: Hepatotoxicity with the administration of nifedipine for preterm labor. *Am J Obstet Gynecol* 1992; 167:512.

161. Waisman GD, Mayorga LM, Camera MI, et al: Magnesium plus nifedipine: Potentiation of hypotensive effect in preeclampsia? *Am J Obstet Obstet Gynecol* 1988; 159:308.

162. Snyder SW, Cardwell S: Neuromuscular blockade with magnesium sulfate and nifedipine. *Am J Obstet Gynecol* 1989; 161:35.

163. Barton JR, Hiett AK, Conover WB: The use of nifedipine during the postpartum period in patients with severe preeclampsia. *Am J Obstet Gynecol* 1990; 162:788.

164. Fenakel K, Fenakel G, Appelman Z, et al: Nifedipine in the treatment of severe preeclampsia. *Obstet Gynecol* 1991; 77:331.

165. Briggs GG, Freeman RK, Yaffe SJ: Drugs in pregnancy and lactation, ed 3. Baltimore, Williams & Wilkins, 1990, pp 450-453.

166. Guillon G, Balestre MN, Oberst JM, et al: Oxytocin and vasopressin: Distinct receptors in the myometrium. *J Clin Endocrinol Metab* 1987; 64:1125.

167. Akerlund M, Stromberg P, Hauksson A, et al: Inhibition of uterine contractions of premature labor with an oxytocin analogue: Results from a pilot survey. *Br J Obstet Gynaecol* 1987; 94:1040.

168. Goodwin TM, Paul R, Silver H, et al: The effect of the oxytocin antagonist atosiban on preterm uterine activity in the human. *Am J Obstet Gynecol* 1994; 170:474.

169. Greenspoon JS, Kovacic A: A breech extraction facilitated by glyceryl trinitrate spray. *Lancet* 1991; 338:124.

170. Lees C, Campbell S, Jauniauge E, et al: Arrest of preterm labour and prolongation of gestation with glyceryl trinitrate, a nitric oxide donor. *Lancet* 1994; 343:1325.

171. Avery ME, Aylward G, Creasy RK, et al: Update on prenatal steroids for prevention of respiratory distress. *Am J Obstet Gynecol* 1986; 155:2.

172. Crowley P, Chalmers I, Keirse MJNC: The effects of corticosteroid administration before preterm delivery: An overview of the evidence from controlled trials. *Br J Obstet Gynaecol* 1990; 97:11.

173. Ohlsson A: Treatment of preterm premature rupture of the membranes: A meta-analysis. *Am J Obstet Gynecol* 1989; 160:890.

174. Liggins GC, Howie RN: A controlled trial of antepartum glucocorticoid treatment for prevention of respiratory distress syndrome. *Pediatrics* 1972; 50:515.

175. Garite TJ, Rummey PJ, Briggs GG, et al: A randomized, placebo-controlled trial of betamethasone for the prevention of respiratory distress syndrome at 24 to 28 weeks' gestation. *Am J Obstet Gynecol* 1992; 166:646.

176. Taeusch HW, Frigoletto F, Kitzmiller J, et al: Risk of respiratory distress syndrome after prenatal dexamethasone treatment. *Pediatrics* 1979; 63:64.

177. Mosier HP Jr, Dearden LC, Tanner SM, et al: Disproportionate organ growth in the fetus after betamethasone administration. *Pediatr Res* 1979; 13:486.

178. NIH Consensus Development Panel: Effect of corticosteroids for fetal maturation on perinatal outcomes. *JAMA* 1995; 273:413.

179. ACOG Committee Opinion: Antenatal corticosteroid therapy for fetal maturation. *ACOG Bull No. 147,* Dec 1994.

180. MacArthur G, Howie R, Dezoete J, et al: School progress and cognitive development of 6-year-old children whose mothers were treated antenatally with betamethasone. *Pediatrics* 1982; 70:99.

181. Ballard RA, Ballard PL, Creasy RK, et al: Respiratory disease in very-low-birth weight infants after prenatal thyrotropin-releasing hormone and glucocorticoid. *Lancet* 1992; 339:510.

182. Paneth N, Kiely JL, Wallenstein S, et al: The effect of the choice of place of delivery and hospital level or mortality in all singleton births in New York City. *Am J Dis Child* 1987; 141:60.

183. Milligan JE, Shennan AT, Hoskins EM: Perinatal intensive care: Where and how to draw the line. *Am J Obstet Gynecol* 1984; 148:499.

184. Milner R, Beard R: Limit of fetal viability. *Lancet* 1984; 1:1079.

185. Hack M, Fanaroff AA: Outcomes of extremely-low-birth-weight infants between 1982 and 1988. *N Engl J Med* 1989; 321:1642.

186. Yu V, Orgill A, Bajuk B, et al: Survival and 2-year outcome of extremely preterm infants. *Br J Obstet Gynaecol* 1984; 91:640.

187. Bowes WA, Gabbe SG, Bowes C: Fetal heart rate monitoring in premature infants weighing 1500 gm or less. *Am J Obstet Gynecol* 1980; 137:791.

188. Ahn MO, Cha KY, Phelan JP: The low birth weight infant: Is there a preferred route of delivery? *Clin Perinatol* 1992; 19:411.

189. Malloy MH, Onstad L, Wright E: National Institute of Child Health and Human Development Neonatal Research Network. The effect of cesarean delivery on birth outcome in very low birth weight infants. *Obstet Gynecol* 1991; 77:498.

190. Anderson GD, Bada HS, Shaver DC, et al: The effect of cesarean section on intraventricular hemorrhage in the preterm infant. *Am J Obstet Gynecol* 1992; 166:1091.

191. Schwartz DB, Miodovnik M, Lavin JP: Neonatal outcome among low birthweight infants delivered spontaneously or by low forceps. *Obstet Gynecol* 1983; 62:283.

192. O'Driscoll K, Maegher D, MacDonald D, et al: Traumatic intracranial hemorrhage in firstborn infants and delivery with obstetric forceps. *Br J Obstet Gynaecol* 1981; 88:577.

193. Morales R, Adair CD, Sanchez-Ramos L, et al: Vacuum extraction of preterm infants with birth weights of 1,500-2,499 grams. *J Reprod Med* 1995; 40:127.

194. Goldenberg RJ, Nelson KG: The premature breech. *Am J Obstet Gynecol* 1977; 127:240.

195. Duenhoelter JH, Wells CE, Reisch JS: A paired controlled study of vaginal and abdominal delivery of the low birth-weight breech fetus. *Obstet Gynecol* 1979; 54:310.

196. Main DM, Main EK, Maurer MM: Cesarean section versus vaginal delivery for the breech fetus weighing less than 1500 grams. *Am J Obstet Gynecol* 1983; 146:580.

197. Bodmer B, Benjamin A, MacLean FH, et al: Has use of cesarean section reduced risks of delivery in the preterm presentation? *Am J Obstet Gynecol* 1986; 154:244.

198. Chervenak FA, Johnson RE, Yourcha S: Intrapartum management of twin gestation. *Obstet Gynecol* 1985; 65:119.

199. Khunda S: Locked twins. *Obstet Gynecol* 1972; 39:453.

200. Acker D, Lieberman M, Holbrook RH, et al: Delivery of the second twin. *Obstet Gynecol* 1982; 59:710.

201. Arias F: Delayed delivery of multifetal pregnancies with premature rupture of membranes in the second trimester. *Am J Obstet Gynecol* 1994; 170:1233.

202. Naeye RL: Factors that predispose to premature rupture of the fetal membranes. *Obstet Gynecol* 1982; 60:93.

203. Lewis DF, Major CA, Towers CV, et al: Effects of digital vaginal examinations on latency period in preterm premature rupture of membranes. *Obstet Gynecol* 1992; 80:630.

204. Ohlsson A, Wong E: An analysis of antenatal tests to detect infection in preterm PROM. *Am J Obstet Gynecol* 1990; 162:809.

205. Gunn GL, Mishell DR, Morton DG: Premature rupture of membranes: A review. *Am J Obstet Gynecol* 1970; 106:469.

206. Schreiber J, Benedetti T: Conservative management of preterm rupture of fetal membranes in a low socioeconomic population. *Am J Obstet Gynecol* 1980; 136:92.

207. Johnson JWC, Daikoku NH, Niebyl JR, et al: Premature rupture of the membranes and prolonged latency. *Obstet Gynecol* 1981; 57:547.

208. Taylor J, Garite TJ: Premature rupture of membranes before fetal viability. *Obstet Gynecol* 1984; 64:615.

209. Bengston JM, Van Marter LJ, Barss VA, et al: Pregnancy outcome after premature rupture of the membranes at or before 26 weeks' gestation. *Obstet Gynecol* 1989; 73:921.

210. Garite TJ: Premature rupture of the membranes, in Creasy R (ed): *Maternal Fetal Medicine,* WB Saunders, Philadelphia, 1994, p 628.

211. Rutherford SE, Phelan JP, Smith CV, et al: The four-quadrant assessment of amniotic fluid volume: An adjunct to antepartum fetal heart rate testing. *Obstet Gynecol* 1987; 70:353.

212. Liske S, Panter K, Amankwah K: Abruptio placenta and prolonged premature rupture of membranes. SPO abstract No. 117. *Am J Obstet Gynecol* 1995; 172:295.

213. Nelson LH, Anderson RL, O'Shea M, et al: Expectant management of preterm premature rupture of the membranes. *Am J Obstet Gynecol* 1994; 171:350.

214. Johnson JWC, Egerman RS, Moorhead J: Cases with ruptured membranes that "reseal." *Am J Obstet Gynecol* 1990; 163:743.

215. Mercer BM, Crocker LG, Boe NM, et al: Induction versus expectant management in premature rupture of the membranes with mature amniotic fluid at 32 to 36 weeks: A randomized trial. *Am J Obstet Gynecol* 1993; 169:775.

216. Kappy KA, Cetrulo CL, Knuppel RA, et al: Premature rupture of the membranes: A conservative approach. *Am J Obstet Gynecol* 1979; 134:655.

217. Amon E, Lewis SV, Sibai BM, et al: Ampicillin prophylaxis in premature rupture of the membranes: A prospective randomized study. *Am J Obstet Gynecol* 1988; 59:539.

218. Johnston MM, Sanchez-Ramos L, Vaughn AJ, et al: Antibiotic therapy in preterm premature rupture of membranes: A randomized, prospective, double-blind trial. *Am J Obstet Gynecol* 1990; 163:743.

219. Christmas JT, Cox SM, Andrews W, et al: Expectant management of preterm ruptured membranes: Effects of antimicrobial therapy. *Obstet Gynecol* 1992; 80:759.

220. Ermest JM, Givner LB: A prospective, randomized, placebo-controlled trial of penicillin in preterm premature rupture of membranes. *Am J Obstet Gynecol* 1994; 170:516.

221. Minkoff H, Mead P: An obstetric approach to the prevention of early onset group B beta-hemolytic streptococcal sepsis. *Am J Obstet Gynecol* 1986; 154:973.

222. Owens J, Groome LJ, Hauth JC: Randomized trial of prophylactic antibiotic therapy after preterm amnion rupture. *Am J Obstet Gynecol* 1993; 169:976.

223. McDuffies RS, McGregor JA, Gibbs RS: Adverse perinatal outcome and resistant enterobacteriaceae after antibiotic usage for premature rupture of the membranes and group B streptococcus carriage. *Obstet Gynecol* 1993; 82:487.

224. Nageotte MP, Freeman RK, Garite TJ, et al: Prophylactic intrapartum amnioinfusion in patients with premature rupture of membranes. *Am J Obstet Gynecol* 1985; 153:557.

225. Ogita S, Imanaka M, Matsumoto M, et al: Transcervical amnioinfusion of antibiotics: A basic study for managing premature rupture of membranes. *Am J Obstet Gynecol* 1988; 158:23.

226. Imanaka M, Ogita S, Sugawa T: Saline solution amnioinfusion for oligohydramnios after premature rupture of the membranes. *Am J Obstet Gynecol* 1989; 161:102.

227. Creasy RK: Threatened preterm labor. *Contemp Obstet Gynecol* 1984; 23:26.

228. Gonik B, Creasy RK: Preterm labor: Diagnosis and management. *Am J Obstet Gynecol* 1986; 154:3.

229. Caldwell TB: Anesthesia for patients with behavioral and environmental disorders, in Katz J, Benumof JL, Kadis L (eds): *Anesthesia and Uncommon Diseases,* ed 3. Philadelphia, WB Saunders, 1990, pp 792-922.

230. Fuchs AR, Fuchs F: Ethanol for prevention of preterm birth. *Semin Perinatol* 1981; 5:236.

231. Marks RJ, DeChazol RCS: Ritodrine-induced pulmonary edema in labor: Successful management using epidural anaesthesia. *Anaesthesia* 1984; 24:1012.

232. Park YK, Hidaka A: Effect of left lateral position in maternal hemodynamics during ritodrine treatment in comparison with supine position. *Acta Obstet Gynecol Jpn* 1991; 43:655.

233. Chestnut DH, Pollack KL, Thompson CS, et al: Does ritodrine worsen maternal hypotension during epidural anesthesia in gravid ewes? *Anesthesiology* 1990; 72:315.

234. Johnston R, Eger I, Wilson C: A competitive interaction of epinephrine with enflurane, isoflurane and halothane in man. *Anesth Analg* 1976; 55:709.

235. Ramanathan J, Sibai BM, Mabie WC, et al: The use of labetalol for attenuation of the hypertensive response to endotracheal intubation in preeclampsia. *Am J Obstet Gynecol* 1988; 159:650.

236. Morris R, Giesecke AH: Potentiation of muscle relaxants by magnesium sulfate therapy in the toxemia of pregnancy. *South Med J* 1968; 61:25.

237. Kambam JR, Perry SM, Entman S, et al: Effect of magnesium on plasma cholinesterase activity. *Am J Obstet Gynecol* 1988; 159:309.

238. James MFM, Cork RC, Dennett JE: Succinylcholine pretreatment with magnesium sulfate. *Anesth Analg* 1986; 65:373.

239. Vincent RD, Chestnut DH, Sipes SL, et al: Magnesium sulfate decreases maternal blood pressure but not uterine blood flow during epidural anesthesia in gravid ewes. *Anesthesiology* 1991; 74:77.

240. Sipes, SL, Chestnut DH, Vincent RD, et al: Which vasopressor should be used to treat hypotension during magnesium sulfate infusion and epidural anesthesia? *Anesthesiology* 1992; 77:101.

241. Vincent RD, Chestnut DH, Sipes SL, et al: Epidural anesthesia worsens uterine blood flow and fetal oxygenation during hemorrhage in gravid ewes. *Anesthesiology* 1992; 76:799.

242. Benzion HT, Brunner EA, Vaisrub N: Bleeding time and nerve blocks after aspirin. *Reg Anaesth* 1983; 9:86.

243. Horlocker TT, Wedell DJ, Schroeder DR, et al: Preoperative antiplatelet therapy does not increase the risk of spinal hematoma associated with regional anesthesia. *Anesth Analg* 1995; 80:303.

244. Reves JG, Kissin I, Lell WA, et al: Calcium entry blockers: Uses and implications for anesthesiologists. *Anesthesiology* 1982; 57:504.

245. Kurtzman JL, Thorp JM, Spielman FJ, et al: Do nifedipine and verapamil potentiate the cardiac toxicity of magnesium sulfate? *Am J Perinatol* 1993; 10:450.

246. Laszlo A, Buljubask N, Zsolani B, et al: Interactive effects of volatile anesthetics, vergamil and ryanodine on contractility and calcium homeostasis of isolated pregnant rat myometrium. *Am J Obstet Gynecol* 1992; 167:804.

247. Forman A, Gandrup P, Andersson KE, et al: Effects of nifedipine on spontaneous and methylergometrine-

induced activity post partum. *Am J Obstet Gynecol* 1982; 144:442.

248. Miller RD: Antagonism of neuromuscular blockade. *Anesthesiology* 1976; 44:318.

249. Shnider SM, Wright G, Levinson GL, et al: Uterine blood flow and plasma norepinephrine changes during maternal stress in the pregnant ewe. *Anesthesiology* 1979; 50:524.

250. Bowes WA: Delivery of the very low birth weight infant. *Clin Perinatol* 1981; 8:183.

251. Hollmen AI, Joupilla R, Albright GA, et al: Effect of extradural analgesia using bupivacaine and 2-chloroprocaine on intervillous blood flow during normal labor. *Br J Anaesth* 1982; 54:837.

252. Wright RG, Shnider SM, Thirion A-V, et al: Regional anesthesia for preterm labor and vaginal delivery: Effects on the fetus and neonate. *Anesthesiology* 1988; 69:A654.

253. Thomas J, Long G, Moore G, et al: Plasma protein binding and placental transfer of bupivacaine. *Clin Pharmacol Ther* 1976; 19:426.

254. Covino BG, Scott DB: Pharmacologic considerations, in *Handbook of Epidural Anaesthesia and Analgesia.* Orlando, Grune & Stratton, 1985, pp 57-77.

255. Pedersen H, Santos AC, Morishima O, et al: Does gestational age affect the pharmacokinetics and pharmacodynamics of lidocaine in mother and fetus? *Anesthesiology* 1988; 68:367.

256. Morishima HO, Santos AC, Pedersen H, et al: Effect of lidocaine on asphyxial responses in the maternal and fetal lamb. *Anesthesiology* 1987; 66:502.

257. Morishima HO, Santos AC, Pedersen H, et al: Pharmacodynamics of lidocaine in the asphyxiated premature fetal lamb. *Anesthesiology* 1986; 65:A372.

258. Biehl D, Shnider S, Levinson G, et al: Placental transfer of lidocaine: Effects of fetal acidosis. *Anesthesiology* 1978; 48:409.

259. Kuhnert BR, Philipson EH, Pimental R, et al: Lidocaine disposition in mother, fetus and neonate after spinal anesthesia. *Anesth Analg* 1986; 65:139.

260. Datta S, Alper MH, Ostheimer W, et al: Method of ephedrine administration and nausea and hypotension during spinal anesthesia for cesarean section. *Anesthesiology* 1982; 56:68.

261. Norris MC: Hypotension during spinal anesthesia for cesarean section; does it affect neonatal outcome? *Reg Anaesth* 1987; 12:191.

262. Ong BY, Cohen MM, Pahalniuk RJ: Anesthesia for cesarean section: Effects on neonates. *Anesth Analg* 1989; 68:270.

263. Gregory FA, Wagde JG, Biehl DR, et al: Foetal anesthetic requirements (MAC) for halothane. *Anesth Analg* 1983; 62:9.

264. Bachman R, Biehl DR, Sitar DS, et al: Isoflurane potency and cardiovascular effects during short exposures in the foetal lamb. *Can Anaesth Soc J* 1986; 33:41.

265. Pickering BG, Pahalniuk RJ, Cote J, et al: Cerebral vascular responses to ketamine and thiopentone during foetal acidosis. *Can Anaesth Soc J* 1982; 29:463.

266. Marx F, Mateo CV: Effects of different oxygen concentrations during general anaesthesia for elective cesarean section. *Can Anaesth Soc J* 1987; 18:587.

267. Levinson G, Shnider SM, de Lorimier AA, et al: Effects of maternal hyperventilation on uterine blood flow and fetal oxygenation and acid-base status. *Anesthesiology* 1974; 40:340.

268. Mayer DC, Weeks SK: Antepartum uterine relaxation with nitroglycerin at cesarean delivery. *Can J Anaesth* 1992; 39:166.

269. Greenspoon J, Kovacic A: Breech extraction facilitated by glycerol trinitrate sublingual spray. *Lancet* 1991; 13:124.

270. Rolbin SH, Hew EM, Bernstein A: Uterine relaxation can be life saving. *Can J Anaesth* 1991; 38:939.

271. Pritchard JA, MacDonald PC, Gant NF (eds): *William's Obstetrics,* ed 17. Appleton Lange, 1985, pp 855-866.

272. Crawford JS: *Principles and Practice of Obstetric Anaesthesia,* ed 5. Oxford, Blackwell Scientific Publications, 1984, pp 181-283.

273. Naulty JS, Ostheimer GW, Datta S, et al: Incidence of venous air embolism during epidural catheter insertion. *Anesthesiology* 1982; 57:410.

274. Davies JM, Thistlewood JM, Rolbin SH, et al: Infections and the parturient: Anaesthetic considerations. *Can J Anaesth* 1988; 35:270.

23 Postdate Pregnancy

Bernard Gonik, Amr E. Abouleish, and Ezzat I. Abouleish

Management of the postdate pregnancy is filled with controversy, including disagreement as to its definition and nomenclature. Clinicians frequently use the terms "postdate," "postmature," and "dysmature" interchangeably, which adds to the confusion. Perhaps the most conventional definition of a postdate pregnancy would be that which progresses beyond 294 days (or 42 weeks) after the first day of the last menstrual period (LMP). Inherent in this definition are several limitations. First, there is some biologic variability in the relationship between ovulation, conception, and the LMP. Second, many patients are uncertain of their correct LMP, since this information is only important to the patient in a retrospective manner. Regardless, the estimated date of confinement (EDC) is traditionally calculated by subtracting 3 months from the first day of the LMP and then adding 7 days (Nägele's rule). Criteria usually used in addition to the LMP for establishing accurate dating of the pregnancy are listed in Box 23-1.

INCIDENCE

The incidence of a postdate pregnancy, as defined above, has been estimated to be between 6% and 14%. This value can probably be reduced to its lower limits (approximately 6%) if only patients with early prenatal care and confirmatory ultrasound studies are used to define this condition. Postmaturity occurs in up to one third of all postdate pregnancies. This syndrome, first described by Clifford,[2] can only be diagnosed following delivery. Features of this neonatal condition are listed in Box 23-2.

PATHOPHYSIOLOGY

From a pathophysiologic perspective, postmaturity syndrome is thought to be due to a relative decrease in the relationship between fetal growth and uteroplacental reserve.[3] Also associated with this condition are variable degrees of oligohydramnios and fetal/neonatal hypoxemia.

ETIOLOGY

The etiology of postdate pregnancy, in most circumstances, is not apparent. This is basically due to the fact that we still have a very poor understanding of the normal mechanisms of parturition. Certain clinical conditions have been associated with a minority of these postdate pregnancies, including anencephaly, placental sulfatase deficiency, and fetal adrenal hypoplasia. Figure 23-1 describes the relationship between postdate pregnancies, "true" postdate pregnancies, and postmaturity syndrome.

PERINATAL MORBIDITY AND MORTALITY

The association between postdate pregnancy and an increased perinatal mortality is well accepted (Fig. 23-2). Overall, perinatal mortality increases from 1% to 2% for term gestations to 5% to 7% for those pregnancies beyond 42 weeks. As a general rule, perinatal mortality doubles at 43 weeks' gestation and increases fourfold to sixfold by 44 weeks' gestation.[4]

Breakpoints for neonatal morbidity are less well defined, and morbidity may actually begin to increase before 42 weeks' gestation.[5] Reputed adverse neonatal outcomes associated with postdate pregnancies are listed in Table 23-1. Cumulative morbidity rates range from 20% to 30%, as compared with 5% to 6% in term gestations.[6] Although antenatal testing has been advocated to reduce many of these identified complications, its benefit in this regard remains controversial.

OBSTETRIC AND ANESTHETIC MANAGEMENT
Obstetric management

Given all the confounding definitional and clinical variables associated with the problem of the postdate pregnancy, it is not surprising that there is no consistent approach to the management of this condition. Basic considerations when deciding a management scheme should include

1. Accuracy of dating.
2. Likelihood of a successful induction.
3. Recognition of associated findings increasing fetal risk (i.e., poor past obstetric history, abnormal antepartum testing, fetal macrosomia).

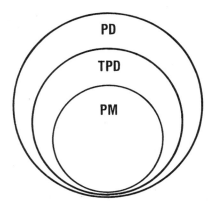

Fig. 23-1 Relationship between postdate pregnancies *(PD)*, "true" postdate pregnancies *(TPD)*, and postmaturity syndrome *(PM)*. Six percent to 14% of all pregnancies are postdates, and 3% to 6% of all pregnancies are true postdates. Postmaturity syndrome is seen in up to one third of all postdate pregnancies (i.e., 2% to 5% of all pregnancies).

BOX 23-1   CRITERIA FOR PREGNANCY DATING

Accurate dating criteria
Known LMP
Known conception date
Early pregnancy testing (human chorionic gonadotropin)
Basal body temperature charting
First-trimester physical examination
First-trimester ultrasound examination
Less accurate dating criteria
Quickening date
Fetal heart beat with Delee-Hillis stethoscope
Second-trimester ultrasound examination

BOX 23-2   POSTMATURITY SYNDROME FEATURES

Peeling skin
Decreased subcutaneous fat
Long nails
Loss of vernix
Meconium-stained placenta, skin
Metabolic disturbances (e.g., hypoglycemia)
Increased perinatal morbidity and mortality

Most clinicians would agree that if a pregnancy is presumed to be beyond 42 weeks and the patient has favorable conditions for induction (i.e., ripe cervix), delivery should be expeditious, preferably by the vaginal route.

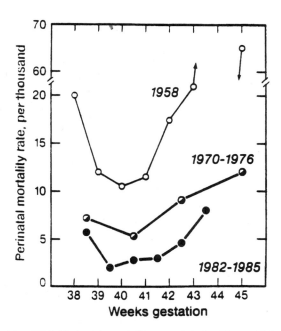

Fig. 23-2 Perinatal mortality associated with postdate pregnancy over three different time periods (1958, 1970-1976, 1982-1985). (Modified from Dyson DC: *J Reprod Med* 1988; 33:262.)

Table 23-1 Adverse neonatal outcomes associated with postdate pregnancy*

Characteristic	Incidence (%)
Forceps delivery	17.0
Cesarean section	17.6
Meconium staining	26.5
Meconium aspiration	1.6
Macrosomia (>4500 g)	2.8
Shoulder dystocia	1.3
Low Apgar score (1 min, <7)	10.2
Perinatal mortality (no. per 1000)	4.9

*Adapted from Eden RD, et al: *Obstet Gynecol* 1987; 69:296.

The controversy regarding management usually centers on the patient with uncertain dating or in whom a low Bishop score (unripe cervix) is noted on pelvic examination. Table 23-2 highlights several recent studies, including antenatal surveillance techniques used and authors' recommendations. Variations in each of the study populations, along with differences in induction methodologies, explain some of the discrepant conclusions. These studies support the fact that there are several acceptable alternatives in the management of these patients.

Fetal surveillance methods. As suggested above, one approach to the otherwise uncomplicated postdate pregnancy involves expectant

Table 23-2 Postdate pregnancy management approaches

Study	Surveillance	Recommendations at 42 weeks
Cardozo et al[7]	Nonstress test, ultrasonography	Expectant
Dyson et al[8]	Nonstress test	Induction
Augensen et al[9]	Nonstress test	Expectant
Witter et al[10]	Fetal monitor, estriol, oxytocin challenge test	Induction
Gibb et al[11]	Fetal monitor, estriol, nonstress test	Expectant
Johnson et al[12]	Biophysical profile	Expectant

management. Given the increased incidence of perinatal morbidity and mortality, fetal surveillance (antenatal testing) is a necessary component of this approach. By strict criteria, testing should be initiated at 42 weeks' gestation, although recent evidence supports antenatal surveillance beginning at the completion of 41 weeks.[5] Recognized techniques (Box 23-3) include the use of fetal movement counts, nonstress testing (NST), contraction stress testing (CST), and biophysical profile testing (BPP). Biochemical markers such as serum estriols or human placental lactogen are no longer commonly used due to poor sensitivity and specificity in predicting adverse neonatal outcome.

Fetal movement count. It has been recognized that regular fetal movements during the second half of pregnancy are a sign of fetal well-being. During normal pregnancy, maximum fetal movements occur in or around the 32nd week and decrease thereafter.[13] Although there is considerable individual variation in the perception of fetal movement, many clinicians incorporate this self-administered antenatal test into their management protocols. The test is inexpensive, noninvasive, and readily available. Reasonable cutoff values for a normal test would be four or more definitive fetal movements per hour, when the patient is postprandial and in an environment that minimizes distraction.

Nonstress testing. Until recently, NST was perhaps the most common method used to confirm a healthy fetal condition. A "reactive" (normal) test is that which demonstrates fetal heart rate (FHR) accelerations during fetal movement. Traditionally, two FHR accelerations within a 10-minute window is considered the end point of the test. In general, the use of the NST on a weekly basis for fetal surveillance is supported by a false negative rate of only approximately 1.4 per 1000. However, recent evidence suggests that a reactive NST is not as reliable an indicator of fetal well-being in the postdate pregnancy. One study reported a fetal death rate of 31/1000 in patients with a reactive NST one week before delivery.[14] It has been observed that the majority of these false negative results relate to the

---

BOX 23-3 ANTEPARTUM TESTING METHODS FOR POSTDATE PREGNANCY

Physical
Fetal movement counts

Ultrasound
Amniotic fluid volume
Biophysical profile scoring

Electronic fetal heart rate
Nonstress testing
Contraction stress testing
Oxytocin
Nipple stimulation

Biochemical markers
Estriol
Human placental lactogen

---

presence of variable or nonspecific decelerations, which are not normally considered in the evaluation of the NST reactivity. Currently proposed management schemes for postdate pregnancy incorporate the NST with other antenatal tests, such as amniotic fluid volume determinations, in an attempt to better identify the at-risk fetus.[15]

Contraction stress testing. The CST is carried out by generating at least three moderately firm uterine contractions over 10 minutes with exogenously administered oxytocin or by nipple stimulation (endogenous oxytocin). A positive (abnormal) test is defined as consistent late decelerations in the FHR with each contraction. The test is based on the principle that "stressing" the fetus with uterine contractions reduces uteroplacental blood flow and predicts marginal degrees of placental insufficiency. Although the CST is more time-consuming and complex in comparison to the NST, clinical studies demonstrate a lower false negative rate with weekly CSTs.[16]

Of the available electronic FHR tests (NST, CST), there still remains a great deal of controversy as to the best method for detecting the compromised fetus.

Biophysical profile. The BPP testing method is based on the assessment of (1) fetal breathing, (2) gross body movements, (3) tone, (4) amniotic fluid volume with the use of real-time ultrasonography, and (5) FHR reactivity (NST). Two points are given for each normal biophysical parameter (maximum 10/10), and a value greater than 8 is considered indicative of fetal well-being. Manning et al[17,18] have examined this relatively new testing system in high-risk pregnancies with findings at least as good as any of the above described techniques (false negative rate <1/1000). Others have specifically shown that BPP scoring is reliable in the expectant management of the postdate pregnancy.[12]

Suggested approach. As indicated above, it is important to recognize that there are many equally acceptable alternatives in the management of the postdate pregnancy. There is a general consensus that each patient should be dealt with on an individual basis. In counseling the patient, specific risks to each approach should be clearly delineated. When induction of labor is chosen, some of these risks include failed induction (and need for cesarean section), hyperstimulation of the uterus, uterine rupture, fetal distress, and chorioamnionitis (particularly if labor is prolonged in the presence of ruptured membranes). Conversely, expectant management has been associated with such complications as fetal macrosomia and traumatic delivery, unexpected fetal demise, and increased antepartum costs (for fetal surveillance).

At our institution, we begin antepartum testing of the otherwise uncomplicated postdate pregnancy at 42 weeks. Patients are routinely questioned about adequacy of fetal movements throughout pregnancy, and fetal movement counts are at times begun at 41 weeks. In the patient with good dating criteria, at 42 completed weeks, and with a favorable cervix, induction is strongly considered. Under these circumstances, the patient is admitted to the hospital for amniotomy and expectant management for up to 12 hours. If prolonged rupture of the membranes is anticipated, the patient will be screened for vaginal colonization with Group B beta-hemolytic streptococci. Empiric antimicrobial prophylaxis may be administered until the screening results are determined. Before transfering to the antepartum unit, external FHR monitoring is performed to document the healthy fetal status. Continuous fetal monitoring is not the rule if all other conditions are favorable. Although the use of early amniotomy in the induction process may be controversial, we believe this approach improves the success of induction and allows us to evaluate the amniotic fluid for the presence of meconium early in the course of labor.

When the patient is at 42 weeks and has an unfavorable cervix for induction, we think two approaches are equally acceptable. If expectant management is selected, the patient is counseled on fetal movement counts and scheduled for more objective antenatal testing such as:

1. Twice-weekly NSTs/weekly amniotic fluid volume assessment
2. Weekly or twice-weekly BPPs
3. Weekly CST and amniotic fluid volume assessment

We define oligohydramnios as a vertical pocket of amniotic fluid of less than 2 cm. This is determined using real-time ultrasonography. The obstetric literature is somewhat confusing in this regard, and data can be found to support cutoff values of 1, 2, or 3 cm for oligohydramnios. As expected, these variations represent a continuum of outcomes, with the larger amniotic fluid pocket cutoffs having less associated neonatal mortality but a higher false positive rate.[19] More sophisticated approaches, such as the calculation of a four-quadrant amniotic fluid volume status, have also been advocated as an adjunct to other forms of antenatal testing.[20] Using this latter approach, most clinicians would consider an amniotic fluid index less than 5 consistent with the diagnosis of oligohydramnios.

If induction is selected under these circumstances, the unfavorable cervix substantially increases the risk of an unsuccessful induction and operative delivery. We therefore usually recommend the use of cervical ripening agents such as vaginal prostaglandin E$_2$ (PGE$_2$) gel.[21] Our pharmacy prepares this preparation by combining a 20-mg PGE$_2$ suppository with 60 cc of sterile surgical lubricant. Six 10-cc syringes are then divided from this mixture (each containing 3.3 mg PGE$_2$) and stored at $-20°$ C until needed. The clinician should have experience in the use of this product for cervical ripening and should be aware of potential side effects such as hyperstimulation. Before placement of the PGE$_2$ gel, the FHR pattern should be assessed. In addition, the patient should not be having regular uterine contractions before PGE$_2$ ripening.

We place the 10-cc gel mixture intravaginally by using a diaphragm. Care should be taken not to insert the PGE$_2$ preparation directly into the cervix since substantially lower doses are needed if this route is used. We continuously monitor the FHR after the procedure, although some centers believe that this is unnecessary in the otherwise low-risk patient. A repeat dose can be given at 4-hour intervals provided the fetal status is confirmed. Standard oxytocin induction, following amniotomy, is usually carried out 4 hours or more after the last PGE_2 application.

Recently, a commercially available intracervical prostaglandin E_2 product (Prepidil Gel, Upjohn Company) has been marketed for cervical ripening. Since it is administered endocervically, a substantially lower dose (0.5 mg) has been formulated. Indications and contraindications are similar to that of the intravaginal prostaglandin preparation.

When the patient's EDC is uncertain, as is frequently the case, expectant management is usually chosen, provided the pregnancy is considered lowrisk. Antenatal testing, as outlined early, is initiated and continued to no more than 44 completed weeks' gestation. If historical and physical examination (or ultrasound) findings are inconsistent, we occasionally perform amniocentesis to confirm pulmonary maturity before deciding on induction.

Intrapartum management of the postdate pregnancy should include continuous FHR monitoring. Up to one third of all postdate fetuses will have meconium staining and/or fetal distress.[15] None of the previously described antenatal testing methods can reliably predict these events. The consistency of meconium does, however, appear to be correlated with amniotic fluid volume (i.e., thicker meconium with less amniotic fluid volume). Recent reports have recommended the prophylactic use of amnioinfusion when oligohydramnios and/or meconium are identified to reduce the incidence of fetal distress, thick meconium staining, and need for operative intervention.[22] This technique is easy to learn and involves the intraamniotic infusion of normal saline through a preexisting intrauterine pressure catheter. Other measures to be considered when the postdate gravida enters the labor and delivery suite include early notification of the pediatrician and consultation with the anesthesiologist.

Anesthetic management

When providing anesthetic care to postdate parturients, one must consider the following possible problems:

1. Uteroplacental insufficiency
2. Oligohydramnios
3. Hyperstimulating and tocolytic agents
4. Thick meconium
5. Macrosomia and shoulder dystocia

First, the uteroplacental blood flow becomes comprised secondary to vascular endarteritis and calcification. Thus, hypotension is less tolerated and should be avoided. Before administering a regional block such as spinal or epidural anesthesia,

prehydration is required. Increased aortocaval compression associated with macrosomia necessitates special attention to left uterine displacement. Hypotension, if it occurs, should be treated promptly with intravenous fluids and administration of 10-mg increments of ephedrine.

Second, umbilical core compression commonly occurs due to oligohydramnios, which can lead to fetal heart rate concerns and an emergent cesarean section. Thus, the availability of an anesthesiologist on a 24-hour basis is important.

Third, hyperstimulation of the uterus may occur during an attempt to induce or augment labor, necessitating the use of a beta$_2$-agonist as a tocolytic agent.[23] This may lead to hypotension and tachycardia,[24] further reducing uteroplacental circulation. The judicious use of phenylephrine may be needed to restore vasomotor tone and cause reflex bradycardia.

Fourth, the frequent meconium staining of amniotic fluid should alert the anesthesiologist to several additional potential problems. Again, reductions in uteroplacental blood flow should be minimized since the subsequent fetal acidosis could increase the risk of meconium aspiration under these circumstances. In addition, the obstetrician will require a controlled delivery environment so that suctioning of the infant's oropharynx can be done upon delivery of the fetal head. A Delee trap suctioning device, attached to wall suction (at a reduced pressure), should be available at the perineum for this purpose. Following delivery, endotracheal suctioning for meconium below the vocal cords is also standard practice in many institutions. This procedure will require a skilled resuscitation team, with each participant's responsibilities prospectively decided. Although under most circumstances positive pressure ventilation should be delayed until after adequate clearing of the pharynx and trachea, the timing of this supportive measure needs to be decided based on other clinical factors, such as degree of neonatal depression at birth and composition of the meconium. It should be recognized that Apgar scores will be artificially lowered during these maneuvers, since a concerted effort is made to suppress spontaneous respirations (and fetal stimulation) to minimize the risk of meconium aspiration. Under these circumstances, it would be prudent to measure umbilical cord blood gases to document the acid base status of the neonate at delivery.

Fifth, macrosomia and shoulder dystocia are important factors that can lead to an operative delivery.[25] Thus, when an epidural technique is used for labor, a bilateral block to a T10 level should be obtained and maintained at all times. The catheter should be well secured with tape. The mortality and morbidity inherent to general anesthesia[26] are unacceptable in an operative patient with a functioning epidural. An adequate sensory and motor block can be achieved within a few minutes using epidural chloroprocaine 3% with a narcotic (i.e., fentanil, 75 μg). Cesarean section or vaginal delivery may then proceed without undue delay.

Because of the variability in length of labor and the possibility of operative vaginal or cesarean delivery, epidural analgesia is the method of choice in postdate pregnancies planned for labor and vaginal delivery. Using an epidural catheter provides versatility in duration as well as excellent quality of analgesia. Recently, the technique of combined spinal epidural (CSE) has been described for labor analgesia. CSE maintains the benefits of epidural catheter technique but also utilizes a single intrathecal dose of narcotics, specifically sufentanil, with or without local anesthetic.

For analgesia for postdate parturients, CSE may provide several advantages over epidural continuous infusion. In normal parturients, intrathecal sufentanil, 10 μg, provides excellent and complete analgesia with very rapid onset for the first stage of labor (cervical dilation less than 5 cm) for 90 to 120 minutes.[28-30] The addition of 2.5 mg bupivacaine with sufentanil used intrathecally will prolong the analgesia to 120 to 180 minutes in the first stage of labor and provide analgesia beyond cervical dilation of 5 cm.[31,32] By using intrathecal sufentanil, the amount of subsequent doses of epidural local anesthetics and narcotics appears to be decreased.[33] Because postdate parturients may have prolonged labors requiring long duration of epidural infusions for analgesia, CSE technique may reduce the total amount of epidural medications required. Finally, by using only intrathecal narcotics, parturients may be allowed to walk in early labor in the presence of a medical assistant, which may promote labor.[34,35]

Although rarely practiced since the introduction of continuous epidural infusion, a "double-catheter" technique (epidural and caudal)[36] has been used to ensure sacral roots block during spontaneous and instrumental vaginal delivery. It is still important to verify sacral analgesia before to vaginal delivery so that there may be no delay in the event operative vaginal delivery is required.

Postdate pregnancies increase the incidence of cesarean delivery because of uteroplacental insufficiency, macrosomia, shoulder dystocia, oligohydramnios, thick meconium, and failure to progress. The anesthetic method of choice for cesarean section is regional anesthesia. If an epidural catheter is not already in place, spinal block is the method of choice. The advantages of spinal anesthesia include a rapid onset, a high success rate, definitive

needle end point location, and intense analgesia. We recommend the use of hyperbaric bupivacaine 0.75% (10 to 12 mg) with the addition of epinephrine (0.2 mg)[37] and preservative-free morphine (0.2 mg)[38,39] for subarachnoid injection to improve the duration and quality of the block and to provide prolonged postoperative analgesia.

An anesthesiologist's presence at the time of delivery is essential for rapid intervention should an operative delivery become necessary or for assistance in neonatal resuscitation.

CONCLUSION

Postdate pregnancy usually is associated with delivery of an infant at high risk; thus continuous monitoring before, during, and after delivery is important. The anesthesiologist must tailor the technique so that there is minimal reduction placental perfusion.

REFERENCES

1. Goldenberg RL, Davis RO, Cutter GR, et al: Prematurity, postdates, and growth retardation: The influence of use of ultrasonography on reported gestational age. *Am J Obstet Gynecol* 1989; 160:462.
2. Clifford SH: Postmaturity with placental dysfunction: Clinical syndrome and pathologic findings. *J Pediatr* 1954; 44:1.
3. Vorherr H: Placental insufficiency in relation to postterm pregnancy and fetal postmaturity. *Am J Obstet Gynecol* 1975; 123:67.
4. McClure-Brown JC: Postmaturity. *Am J Obstet Gynecol* 1963; 85:573.
5. Guidetti DA, Divon MY, Langer O: Postdate fetal surveillance: Is 41 weeks too early? *Am J Obstet Gynecol* 1989; 161:91.
6. Arias F: Predictability of complications associated with prolongation of pregnancy. *Obstet Gynecol* 1987; 70:101.
7. Cardozo L, Fysh J, Pearce M: Prolonged pregnancy: The management debate. *Br Med J* 1986; 293:1059.
8. Dyson DC, Miller PD, Armstrong MA: Management of prolonged pregnancy: Induction of labor versus antepartum fetal testing. *Am J Obstet Gynecol* 1987; 156:928.
9. Augensen K, Bergsjo P, Eikland T, et al: Randomized comparison of early versus late induction of labor in post-term pregnancy. *Br Med J* 1987; 294:1192.
10. Witter FR, Weitz CM: A randomized trial of induction at 42 weeks gestation versus expectant management for post-dates pregnancies. *Am J Perinatol* 1987; 4:206.
11. Gibb DMF, Cardozo LD, Studd JWW, et al: Prolonged pregnancy: Is induction of labour indicated? A prospective study. *Br J Obstet Gynecol* 1982; 89:292.
12. Johnson JM, Harman CR, Lange IR, et al: Biophysical profile scoring in the management of the post-term pregnancy: An analysis of 307 patients. *Am J Obstet Gynecol* 1986; 154:269.
13. Ehrstrom C: Fetal movement monitoring in normal and high risk pregnancy. *Acta Obstet Gynecol* 1979; 80:1.
14. Miyazaki FS, Miyazaki BA: False reactive nonstress tests in postterm pregnancies. *Am J Obstet Gynecol* 1981; 140:269.
15. Eden RD, Gergely RZ, Schifrin BS, et al: Comparison of antenatal testing schemes for the management of the post-date pregnancy. *Am J Obstet Gynecol* 1982; 144:683.

16. Freeman RK: The use of the oxytocin challenge test for anterpartum clinical evaluation of uteroplacental respiratory function. *Am J Obstet Gynecol* 1975; 121:481.

17. Manning FA, Morrison I, Lange IR, et al: Fetal assessment based on fetal biophysical profile scoring: Experience in 12,260 referred high-risk pregnancies. I. Perinatal mortality by frequency and etiology. *Am J Obstet Gynecol* 1985; 151:343.

18. Manning FA, Morrison I, Harman CR, et al: Fetal assessment based on fetal biophysical profile scoring: Experience in 19,221 referred high-risk pregnancies. *Am J Obstet Gynecol* 1987; 157:880.

19. Fisher RL, McDonnell M, Biancolli KW, et al: Amniotic fluid volume estimation in the postdate pregnancy: A comparison of techniques. *Obstet Gynecol* 1993; 81:635.

20. Rutherford SE, Phelan JP, Smith CV, et al: The four-quadrant assessment of amniotic fluid volume: An adjunct to antepartum fetal heart rate testing. *Obstet Gynecol* 1987; 70:353.

21. Rayburn W, Gosen R, Ramadei C, et al: Outpatient cervical ripening with prostaglandin E$_2$ gel in uncomplicated postdate pregnancies. *Am J Obstet Gynecol* 1988; 158:1417.

22. Sadovsky Y, Amon E, Bade ME, et al: Prophylactic amnioinfusion during labor complicated by meconium: A preliminary report. *Am J Obstet Gynecol* 1989; 161:613.

23. Shekarloo A, Mendez-Bauer C, Cook V, et al: Terbutaline (intravenous bolus) for the treatment of acute intrapartum fetal distress. *Am J Obstet Gynecol* 1989; 160:615.

24. Grospietsch G, Walther K: Effects of betamimetics on maternal physiology, in Fuchs F, Stubblefield PG (eds): *Preterm Birth: Causes, Prevention and Management.* New York, McMillan, 1984, pp 173-174.

25. Mannino F: Neonatal complications of postterm gestation. *J Reprod Med* 1988; 33:271.

26. Chervenak JL, Divon MY, Hirsch J, et al: Macrosomia in the postdate pregnancy. *Am J Obstet Gynecol* 1989; 161:753.

27. Endler GC, Mariona FG, Sokol RJ, et al: Anesthesia-related maternal mortality in Michigan 1972-1984. *Am J Obstet Gynecol* 1988; 159:187.

28. Camann WR, Denney RA, Holby ED, et al: A comparison of intrathecal, epidural and intravenous sufentanil for labor analgesia. *Anesthesiology* 1992; 77:884.

29. Honet JE, Arkoosh VA, Norris MC, et al: Comparison among intrathecal fentanyl, meperidine, and sufentanil for labor analgesia. *Anesth Analg* 1992; 75:734.

30. Camann WR, Minzter BH, Denney RA, et al: Intrathecal sufentanil for labor analgesia: Effects of added epinephrine. *Anesthesiology* 1993; 78:870.

31. Abouleish AE, Abouleish EI, Camann WR: Combined spinal-epidural analgesia in advanced labor. *Can J Anaesth* 1994; 41:575.

32. Campbell DC, Camann WR, Datta S: The addition of bupivacaine to intrathecal sufentanil for labor analgesia. *Anesth Analg* 1995; 81:305.

33. Abouleish AE, Camann WR, Holden D, et al: Antinociceptive interaction between intrathecal sufentanil and epidural bupivacaine: Additivity or synergism? *Anesthesiology* 1994; 81:A1144.

34. Collis RE, Baxandall MC, Srikantharajah FD, et al: Combined spinal epidural with ability to walk throughout labor. *Lancet* 1993; 341:727.

35. Camann WR, Abouleish AE: Spinal epidural analgesia and walking throughout labor. *Lancet* 1993; 341:1095.

36. Abouleish E: *Pain Control in Obstetrics.* Philadelphia, JB Lippincott, 1977, p 285.

37. Abouleish E: Epinephrine improves the quality of spinal hyperbaric bupivicaine for cesarean section. *Anesth Analg* 1987; 66:395.

38. Abouleish E, Rawal N, Fallon K, et al: Combined intrathecal morphine and bupivacaine for cesarean section. *Anesth Analg* 1983; 67:370.

39. Abouleish E, Rawal N, Tobon-Randall B, et al: A clinical and laboratory study to compare the addition of 0.2 mg morphine, 0.2 mg epinephrine or their combination to hyperbaric bupivacaine for spinal anesthesia in cesarean section. *Anesth Analg* 1993; 77:457.

24 Emboli in Pregnancy

Jonathan H. Skerman and Warren N. Otterson

EMBOLI IN PREGNANCY

Embolic events still today are one of the leading causes of maternal mortality.[1-7] The clinical presentation, diagnosis, treatment, and prognosis depend on the type of material embolized, the size of the emboli, and the target organs affected. The three types of emboli that can occur during pregnancy are thrombotic, amniotic, and air. Embolic events can occur during both cesarean section and vaginal delivery. Air may be the most frequent embolic material, followed by thromboembolism. Amniotic fluid is the rarest. Both amniotic and air emboli can occur in labor or in association with delivery, and thrombotic emboli occur more commonly in the puerperium. The pulmonary system is the most common target organ, but if a right to left shunt exists any organ can be in jeopardy. This chapter discusses the three types of emboli that may complicate pregnancy, their obstetric significance, and anesthetic management.

THROMBOEMBOLIC DISEASE

Thromboembolic conditions have been well documented since the early 19th century. Dark red patches in the lung or clots in branches of the pulmonary artery were described before Virchow's classic studies were published in 1858.[8] The incidence of thromboembolic events during pregnancy is often clouded by difficulties in making the correct diagnosis. Many epidemiologic studies, particularly in the last decade, confirm a reasonable estimate that the disease is five and a half times more common during pregnancy or in the postpartum period than in nonpregnant women, and thrombosis occurs three to six times more frequently postpartum than antepartum. In addition, the complications associated with this disease entity are three times more frequent in women taking oral contraceptives.[9]

Incidence

There is a very wide range in the reported incidence of deep venous thrombosis during pregnancy. It has been reported as frequently as 0.018 per delivery[10] to 0.00052 per delivery.[11] Other recent reports indicate an incidence of deep venous thrombosis in 0.7 per thousand pregnancies.[12,13] This is further complicated by the reported incidence for fatal pulmonary embolism. In the report on confidential enquiries in maternal death in England and Wales, pulmonary embolism was responsible for the deaths of 12 women per year before or immediately after delivery, or 9.4 per million pregnancies.[2] Even with this rare occurrence it was second only to abortion as the leading cause of maternal death. However, pulmonary embolism and deep venous thrombosis are not easily diagnosed in nonfatal cases, particularly in pregnancy. It is therefore difficult to obtain accurate data for the incidence of nonfatal deep vein thrombosis and pulmonary embolism.

Risk factors include increased maternal age and parity, obesity, cesarean section, prolonged bedrest during pregnancy, estrogen therapy for lactation suppression, blood type other than O, and antithrombin III deficiency.[13,14]

Etiology

The cause of thrombosis is best described in terms of Virchow's classic triad: vessel wall trauma, venous stasis, and alterations in the coagulation mechanism.[8] These factors may contribute to the increased risk of thromboembolism in the pregnant or postpartum patient.

Although vessel injury does not seem to be necessary to initiate thrombosis in the calf veins, it may contribute to the increased incidence of some forms of thrombosis, i.e., increased risk of pelvic thrombophlebitis following cesarean section.[15]

Venous stasis is certainly a risk factor during pregnancy. Venous distensibility increases during the first trimester of pregnancy. Varicose veins, hormonal changes, anemia, toxemia, and the hypercoagulable state have also been implicated. Mechanical compression by the gravid uterus on the inferior vena cava causes venous stasis and is uniformly considered a major factor contributing to deep venous thrombosis. This mechanical obstruction is known to result in increased femoral venous pressure beginning in the early part of the second trimester and continuing until term. Leg vein obstruction was found by Ikard et al,[16] using Doppler ultrasound, to be almost universal in the standing position in the third trimester and to be partly present in the lateral decubitus position as well. The most common sites of deep venous thrombosis are the venous sinuses within the soleus muscles and the valve sinuses in the left iliofemoral segment, which likewise are the most common sites of venous stasis. The left lower extremity is most often involved with antepartum deep venous thrombosis secondary to probable compression of the left common iliac vein where it is crossed by the common iliac artery.[13]

Thrombophlebitis has been described in each trimester, but is more common in patients who are bedridden for complications of pregnancy, such as threatened abortion, premature rupture of the membranes, and pregnancy-induced hypertension.

Pregnancy causes a number of significant alterations in the coagulation mechanism. All trace protein coagulation factors except XI and XIII are increased during pregnancy. Antithrombin III activity falls during pregnancy in patients with hereditary antithrombin III deficiency. Antithrombin III is the major inhibitor of thrombin, Factor Xa, and other proteases, and inhibits coagulation in vivo.[17,18] The incidence of an autosomal dominant antithrombin III deficiency is between 1 in 2000 and 1 in 5000.[19,20] It has been described in two forms, depending on the level of antithrombin III antigen. In classical antithrombin III deficiency the level of antithrombin III antigen is below 50% of normal, whereas in variant antithrombin III deficiency there is a normal antithrombin III antigen level with abnormalities in the molecule that interfere with function. Women with hereditary antithrombin III deficiency are at risk of developing thromboembolism in pregnancy or when taking oral contraceptives. Thromboembolism associated with antithrombin III deficiency tends to occur during the antepartum period.[21]

Fibrinolytic activity is decreased in pregnancy. There is also evidence that the concentration of soluble fibrin-fibrinogen complexes is increased. The increased Factor VIII activity contributes to the stabilization of these complexes. The role played by platelets in the formation of the thrombus is somewhat equivocal; neither the platelet count nor platelet adhesiveness is increased during pregnancy. The decreased number of circulating platelets after delivery is probably related to normal thrombus formation at the placental site. Venous thrombi contain relatively few platelets, and platelets are not believed to be the instigators of the thrombotic process.

Pathophysiology

The most common embolism is pulmonary thromboembolism. This produces complex alterations in the pulmonary mechanics and circulatory function. These changes depend on the quantity and size of the embolus, the site of obstruction, and the presence of preexisting cardiopulmonary disease. A single small embolus may have no effect while a large thrombus may break and shower the lungs with multiple emboli, producing life-threatening bilateral pulmonary dysfunction. With a unilateral pulmonary thromboembolus the right lower lobe is the most frequently affected area. A large embolus may cause fatal obstruction of the pulmonary circulation.

Pulmonary embolism in patients with cardiac disease is often regarded as synonymous with pulmonary infarction. However, this is not always the case. The ratio of infarct to emboli is about 1 in 10. Recurrent pulmonary emboli often result in pulmonary hypertension. Amniotic fluid embolism or fat embolism may present as adult respiratory distress syndrome. Very small emboli pass through to the periphery of the lung. If they do not obstruct a branch of the pulmonary artery, rapid lysis occurs and there are no hemodynamic disturbances and no clinical symptoms. With large or multiple emboli, occlusion of the pulmonary artery affects the performance of the cardiac and respiratory systems secondary to both mechanical alterations and reflex changes.

Since the pulmonary arteries receive the right ventricular output, an embolus in the main pulmonary artery or in its major branches can significantly lower left ventricular output. In patients with limited cardiac reserve the reduction in coronary artery blood flow is poorly tolerated. The right ventricle is comparatively thin-walled and becomes an early target for increased right ventricular pressures. Right coronary blood flow does not seem to decrease during embolization; it may increase secondary to local autoregulation. It might take a longer time to develop right ventricular failure, depending on the preexisting cardiovascular status. With a massive pulmonary embolism of any type, cardiovascular collapse, hypotension, and refractory shock may occur.

Some of the reflex changes from microembolization result in bronchoconstriction and vasoconstriction, but the hemodynamic changes always seem to include an elevation of the right atrial pressure and a lowered cardiac output.[22] These abnormalities are directly related to the extent of embolic obstruction both in patients with previously normal cardiopulmonary systems and in those with prior cardiopulmonary disease.

Respiratory changes include the presence of hypoxemia from an increase in dead space ventilation. The mismatched ventilation/perfusion, bronchoalveolar constriction of terminal airways, and loss of surfactant lead to alveolar atelectasis and the development of regional pulmonary edema, which further contributes to the hypoxemia. Venoarterial shunting and the reduction in cardiac output will augment intrapulmonary shunting and also cause a fall in Pao_2. Bronchoalveolar constriction has been attributed to released humoral factors, including serotonin or histamine, and decreased $Paco_2$. The hypoxemia is not fully corrected by oxygen administration, indicating an intrapulmonary shunt.

Clinical and laboratory diagnosis

Clinical manifestations of pulmonary embolism are nonspecific and the diagnosis is frequently missed, even in patients with segmental or larger vessel occlusion. The presenting signs and symptoms include shortness of breath, chest pain (sometimes described as a dull substernal tightness), apprehension, altered sensorium, cough, hemoptysis, sweating, syncope, and tachycardia. A sudden gasping attempt of the patient to breathe during ventilation may be the first indication of an intraoperative pulmonary embolus. If the patients are grouped by severity, small emboli are associated with a higher incidence of syncope while sudden massive emboli are associated with a higher incidence of pleural pain. The most common physical findings include tachypnea at a rate of 30 to 40 shallow breaths per minute, decreased breath sounds, rales, tachycardia, and pyrexia. Pain, tenderness, swelling, and warmth of the affected limb, including Homans' sign, are also highly significant. A chest x-ray examination may offer confirmatory evidence: diminished vascular markings, diaphragmatic elevation, and pleural effusion. The electrocardiogram (ECG) may show changes consistent with right ventricular failure as well as tachycardia or arrhythmias. However, both chest x-ray film and ECG are frequently normal even in the presence of the pulmonary embolus, and Moser[23] states that their main value is to rule out other causes of chest pain, such as pneumothorax, rib fracture, tumor, infection, or primary cardiac disease.

Ascending venography is the most accurate test for deep venous thrombi. In this technique, radiographic contrast dye is injected into a distal dorsal vein of the foot. During examination the leg must be relaxed and non–weight-bearing, with the patient in approximately a 40-degree incline, which allows gradual filling of the leg veins and prevents layering of the dye. Diagnosis of a venous thrombus requires visualization of a well-defined filling defect in more than one radiographic view. Suggestive evidence includes abrupt termination, absence of opacification, or diversion of flow. False positive studies can occur as a result of poor technique, poor choice of injection site, leg muscle contraction, or with a pathologic condition such as external compression by a popliteal cyst, hematoma, local cellulitis and edema, or muscle rupture. Ascending venography is suboptimal for examining the deep femoral and pelvic veins, since large nonobstructive thrombi can go undetected.

There are well-known systemic side effects of radiologic contrast dye; however, up to 24% of patients also experience muscle pain, leg swelling, tenderness, and erythema.[24] Lowering the concentration of the contrast medium reduces such complications by 70%.[25] Heparinized saline flushing after injection can prevent the uncommon occurrence of clot formation following venography.

Many symptoms mimicking those of deep venous thrombosis, particularly edema and evidence of stasis, can occur in normal pregnancy. The benefit of a definitive diagnosis outweighs the side effects and possible complications of venography. Patients with negative studies thus can avoid the significant hazards of anticoagulation as well as the long-term stigma of a diagnosis of deep venous thrombosis.

Noninvasive tests such as Doppler ultrasound and impedance plethysmography are without risks or complications but are much less sensitive for thrombi below the knee. Changes in Doppler shift occur when normal venous blood flow varies with respiration and maneuvers such as the Valsalva, release of pressure over a distal vein, or squeezing of the muscles. A decrease in amplitude of these shifts can indicate partial venous obstruction while complete occlusion gives no Doppler shift. Doppler ultrasound is most useful in the detection of popliteal, femoral, or iliac thromboses, and it has a sensitivity of 90%.[25] Thrombi that completely occlude proximal veins and those not large enough to obstruct blood flow can escape detection. Because of collateral venous channels, at least 50% of small calf thrombi are missed with Doppler ultrasound.[25] Results can vary with technique, experience, and patient positioning.

Impedance plethysmography uses changes in electrical resistance to measure changes in blood volume within a limb. With inflation of a thigh cuff, blood is retained in the leg. In the absence of venous obstruction, sudden deflation results in immediate outflow of blood and a concomitant sudden increase in electrical resistance. A much slower change is associated with impaired outflow, which indirectly implies venous thrombosis. A sensitivity of 95% and specificity of 98% can be achieved with proximal vein thrombi.[25] As in Doppler ultrasound, detection of calf vein thrombi with impedance plethysmography is unreliable. In pregnancy, compression of the inferior vena cava by the gravid uterus can yield false positive results,[26] and confirmation by venography may be necessary.

Though infrequently used, thermography detects deep venous thrombosis by an increase in skin temperature. Infrared radiation emission is increased when blood flow is diverted to superficial collaterals or when inflammation is present. These changes are more likely to occur with extensive disease. False negative results can occur with early or limited thrombosis.

Fibrinogen scanning with ^{125}I is contraindicated during pregnancy because unbound ^{125}I crosses the placental barrier and enters the fetal circulation. It can collect in the fetal thyroid, which becomes theoretically functional at 10 weeks' gestation, and can produce thyroid damage. It is also contraindicated in lactating women because radioactivity has been detected in breast milk. Because ^{125}I has a half-life of 60.2 days,[27] temporary interruption of lactation is impractical. In nonlactating postpartum patients, ^{125}I-labeled fibrinogen can be used to identify deep venous thrombosis. It has a longer half-life and gives a smaller radiation dose than the previously used [131]I. After intravenous injection, ^{125}I is incorporated like normal fibrinogen into developing thrombi. Sequential scintillation scanning is performed from four hours to seven days later but usually at 24, 48 and 72 hours. With each scan, radioactivity is compared to background precordial values in search of a hot spot. For the lower thigh and calf, accuracy can be as high as 92%.[26] Higher background counts in the femoral artery, bladder, and the overlying muscle mass make detection of thrombi in the common femoral and pelvic veins difficult.

Radionuclide venography using [99mTc] particles is of low risk to the fetus but requires a rapid sequence gamma camera, which may not be available in many institutions. This technique is more than 90% accurate for deep venous thrombosis above the knee.[27]

More accurate for the diagnosis of pulmonary embolus is a combined ventilation/perfusion scan. A mismatch between ventilation and perfusion defects is sufficiently diagnostic of pulmonary vascular occlusion to begin therapy. If the ventilation defects match those seen on the perfusion scan, pulmonary angiography may not be necessary for the absolute diagnosis. The ventilation/perfusion scan can be performed safely during pregnancy, although technetium should be used rather than iodine and uterine shielding is necessary. Pulmonary angiography is usually avoided because of the danger of radiation exposure to the fetus.[23,28] Serious morbidity can occur in 2% to 4% of patients undergoing arteriography.[28]

Obstetric and anesthetic management

Treatment of pulmonary embolism is designed to support cardiopulmonary function and to prevent extension or recurrence of the pulmonary embolism by institution of systemic anticoagulant therapy.[29] Surgical intervention may be indicated in very few selected cases. Oxygen therapy is essential; intubation is usually necessary. The levels of PaO_2 should be maintained at 70 mmHg or above to prevent fetal hypoxia. Morphine is sometimes necessary to relieve pain and anxiety. Fluid status must be monitored closely and pulmonary edema, cardiac failure, or shock must be treated with the necessary drugs as indicated.

The cornerstone of therapy is anticoagulation.[30] After one thromboembolic event there is a 12% risk of repeat thrombosis during the same pregnancy and a 5% to 10% risk of recurrent thromboembolism with subsequent pregnancies.[9,14] The initial anticoagulation should always be induced with intravenous heparin, since its effect is immediate.[9,31,32] Heparin is a large mucopolysaccharide molecule (molecular weight approximately 20,000 daltons). It acts by combining with antithrombin III (heparin cofactor) to inhibit the formation of thrombin. The lack of thrombin prevents the conversion of fibrinogen to fibrin. Heparin also increases the level of activated Factor X inhibitor that again interferes with the production of thrombin from prothrombin. Heparin also inhibits the activation of Factor IX (Christmas factor). Heparin prevents the formation of further thrombi but does not act to lyse clots already present. Heparin has a relatively short half-life of 1.5 hours, and for this reason continuous intravenous administration is the preferred method for heparin therapy. A suggested protocol by Bolan,[9] Hyers,[31] or Hirsh[32] is shown in Box 24-1.

Heparin is not absorbed from the gastrointestinal tract, and intramuscular injection is not advisable because of the risk of hematoma formation at the injection site. In fact, intramuscular injection of any drug should be avoided in a patient on heparin therapy.

Some groups have used low-molecular-weight heparins for treatment as well as for prophylaxis of thromboembolism in pregnancy.[33-35] Bone density scans performed shortly after delivery have shown normal mineral mass.[36] Low-molecular-weight heparins are undoubtly more convenient,

---

BOX 24-1   SUGGESTED PROTOCOL FOR CONTINUOUS HEPARIN THERAPY

---

1. Baseline complete blood cell count (CBC), prothrombin time (PT), partial thromboplastin time (PTT), and platelet count.
2. Loading dose of 5000 U of heparin by intravenous bolus.
3. a. Heparin solution (concentration 100 U/mL): add 50,000 U of heparin to 500 mL of normal saline.
   b. Start therapy at a rate of 1000 U/hr.
      Alternatively 5 to 20 U/kg/hr may be used for initial dose.
   c. Adjust infusion rate to achieve a PTT 2 to 3 times the control.
      Check the PTT after any change in infusion rate and once or twice daily after dosage stabilized.
   d. Control flow of heparin solution with an electronic infusion pump.
4. Check CBC and urinalysis every other day to monitor for occult hemorrhage.

Modified from (1) Bolan JC: Thromboembolic complications of pregnancy. *Clin Obstet Gynecol* 1983; 26:913. (2) Hirsh J, Fuster V: Guide to anticoagluant therapy. Part 1. Heparin. *Circulation* 1994; 89:1449. (3) Hyers TM: Heparin therapy. *Drugs* 1992; 44:738.

---

necessitating once- rather than twice-daily injections. This has considerable implications for patient acceptability, because pregnant women considered to be at high risk of recurrent thromboembolism are taught to inject themselves and may be given thromboprophylaxis for up to 10 months to cover pregnancy and the puerperium. Low-molecular-weight heparins have less hemorrhagic risks, and this may encourage greater use of heparin for thromboprophylaxis if the risk of hemorrhagic complications is perceived to be minimized.[33,35]

The greatest risk with heparin therapy is hemorrhage, which has been noted to be between 4% and 33%.[37] In addition, heparin can result in allergic reactions, alopecia, osteoporosis, and thrombocytopenia. The etiology of the thrombocytopenia is unknown, but it may be related to platelet consumption as reported in "white clot syndrome."[38] Opinions differ regarding the duration of anticoagulant therapy advisable following an acute episode of thromboembolic disease.[33] de Swiet[14] advocates continuing full anticoagulation until 6 weeks after delivery for all patients who had either deep venous thrombosis or pulmonary embolus during pregnancy. Laros and Alger[39] would also continue anticoagulation for the patient with pulmonary embolus, as would Hyers[31] and Hirsh.[32]

Considerable controversy also exists as to which therapeutic agent or regime is preferable for long-term therapy. The standard method in a nonpregnant patient is to initiate anticoagulation with heparin, then to convert gradually to oral anticoagulants.[40] The oral agent most commonly used is sodium warfarin, which acts as a competitive inhibitor of vitamin K in the liver. Warfarin is a small molecule (molecular weight, 1000 daltons) that crosses the placenta readily. In fact, the oral anticoagulants appear to affect the fetus more profoundly than they do the mother, because of immature liver enzyme systems in the fetus. A number of adverse effects from the use of warfarin agents during the first trimester have significant teratogenic potential. Continued warfarin therapy in the late third trimester can cause fetal bleeding either before or after delivery. Other effects secondary to fetal hemorrhage have reportedly resulted from exposure to warfarin during the second and third trimesters. Bonnar[41] reports an overall fetal mortality rate between 15% and 30% in women taking oral anticoagulants during the pregnancy. Because of these adverse effects, most investigators no longer recommend the use of warfarin at any point during pregnancy. Warfarin embryopathy results when Coumadin is administered in the first trimester in 15% to 25% of cases. The most consistent anomalies are degrees of nasal hypoplasia and epiphyseal stapling. Exposure in the second trimester results in a 3% or more incidence of severe central nervous system anomalies.[42]

If the patient is receiving heparin therapy at the time of labor and delivery, the situation is much less hazardous. First, the fetus is not affected by the heparin, so fetal hemorrhage is not a risk factor. Second, the half-life of heparin is short; if delivery is anticipated more than 4 to 6 hours after the last heparin injection, there is no need to reverse the anticoagulant activity. The usual recommendation is simply to stop the heparin as soon as the patient goes into labor or to omit the heparin dose on the morning of induction or elective cesarean section. If an emergency delivery or cesarean section is needed while the heparin is still active, protamine, a heparin antagonist, may be given. Protamine forms a stable salt with heparin, with the result that both drugs lose their intrinsic anticoagulant activity. Each milligram of protamine neutralizes 100 U of heparin. The calculated dose of protamine, up to 50 mg, should be slowly administered intravenously over a 3-minute period. Protamine can also be used if the patient develops hemorrhagic complications from heparin therapy, but it must be used with care and caution because protamine sulphate excess may cause anticoagulation. Needless to say, strict attention to circulatory homeostasis during surgery or delivery is essential if anticoagulation is to be resumed in the postpartum period.

Because of heparin's failure to cross the placenta and its easy reversibility, a number of investigators advocate maintaining the patient on heparin therapy throughout the pregnancy.[31-37] Laros and Alger use 150 to 250 U/kg every 12 hours administered subcutaneously.[39]

A continuous infusion pump has been used in an effort to increase patient compliance with subcutaneous heparin therapy. Although early reports are conflicting, it appears that infusion pump delivery of subcutaneous heparin helps maintain therapeutic levels of anticoagulation in the ambulatory or noncompliant patient.[43]

Thrombolytic therapy must be considered in patients with a massive pulmonary embolus.[44,45] Both urokinase and streptokinase have been used in pregnancy. Urokinase is less antigenic and, in theory, should have fewer side effects.[46] Although an increase in the PTT and fibrin degradation products can be used to follow thrombolytic therapy, the most sensitive measure is the thrombin time.[46] The thrombin time should be no greater than 5 times normal. Nonetheless, the risk of bleeding is always present.

Recombinant tissue plasminogen activator (rt-PA) has a theoretical advantage over streptokinase and urokinase in that it does not induce systemic fibrinolysis. Instead, rt-PA is active when bound to thrombin and is therefore clot-specific.[47] Recombinant tissue plasminogen factor has been used successfully in pregnant women suffering massive pulmonary embolism.[48,49]

The role of surgery in the treatment of thromboembolic disease during pregnancy is also limited. Procedures that have been used include femoral vein or vena cava interruption, and thrombectomy or embolectomy. Femoral vein interruption has been used since 1934, and recently the use of an internal saphenous graft to bypass a thromboembolic region has been reported. Interruption of the vena cava is used to prevent recurrent emboli rising in the lower extremities from reaching the lungs. A number of different procedures have been used for this purpose, including ligation, clipping, plication, and placement of a variety of filters or intraluminal grids,[50] but vena cava interruption is associated with a postoperative mortality between 1% and 10% with a significant risk of long-term morbidity secondary to venous obstruction.

Pulmonary embolectomy is a dangerous procedure but may be life-saving in some patients. The location and extent of the embolus must be confirmed with angiography before surgery; in fact, it has been stated this is the only indication for angiography during pregnancy.[51] Embolectomy should be reserved for the parturient with such massive emboli that she is expected to die before medical therapy would have any effect. Criteria for intervention, according to one investigator, include a systolic blood pressure of less than 90 mm Hg, urine output of less than 20 mL/hr and Pao_2 of less than 60 mm Hg after 1 hour of nonoperative management. The mortality from embolectomy is high (about 80%), and a minimum success during pregnancy has been described.[51]

Anesthetic management

Anesthetic management depends on when the patient develops her thromboembolism because it may occur in the perinatal period, during labor and delivery or cesarean delivery, or postpartum. When thromboembolism has occurred before the time of delivery, the primary problem is providing anesthesia for an anticoagulated patient. When it occurs during labor and delivery the goal is to provide resuscitation, including ventilation and oxygenation (frequently necessitating endotracheal intubation), inotropic support, rapid delivery if indicated, and anticoagulation. The goal of anticoagulation is to prolong the partial thromboplastin time (PTT) 1.5 to 2.5 times normal control. Many fear this significantly increases the risk of regional anesthesia and consider epidural and spinal anesthetics to be contraindicated in anticoagulated patients.[52] Epidural, subdural, and subarachnoid bleeding resulting in spinal cord compression and neurologic dysfunction has been reported with regional anesthetics in anticoagulated patients. Owens[52] reported 33 cases of spinal hematoma following lumbar puncture or spinal anesthesia. Six of the cases were in association with the administration of a regional anesthetic and 27 of the cases involved lumbar puncture for diagnostic or therapeutic purposes. Forty percent (13 patients) had received anticoagulant therapy (heparin, 6; Coumadin, 1; both, 6).

However, regional techniques have been administered to anticoagulated patients without complications. Odoom and Sih[53] reported the results of over 1000 lumber epidural blocks in 950 patients undergoing vascular surgery. All patients received oral anticoagulants preoperatively, and the majority also received intravenous heparin intraoperatively. Ten percent of patients experienced postoperative backache, but no side effects were observed that indicated epidural hemorrhage or hematoma, and no patient developed neurologic complications. They concluded that with adequate precautions, epidural anesthesia can be safely used.

When thromboembolism occurs during labor and delivery in a patient when epidural anesthesia has already been initiated, can the epidural be safely continued? Rao and El-Etr[54] reported their results on 3164 epidural and 847 subarachnoid catheterizations where all patients received intravenous heparin 1 hour after the institution of the regional anesthetic. The activated clotting time (ACT) was maintained at twice the baseline. They reported no incidence of peridural hematoma. Matthews and Abrams[55] also reported similar findings on patients receiving intrathecal morphine before heparinization for cardiac surgery.

As with any anesthetic the risks must be balanced by the benefits to the patient. Although neurologic symptoms associated with regional anesthetics may be rare, the effect of a spinal or epidural hematoma can be catastrophic. There is always the possibility of vascular trauma secondary to needle placement. Phillips et al[56] reported a 3% incidence of trauma (bloody tap) with epidural and spinal procedures, and they noted a 6% incidence when multiple attempts were required. The incidence of epidural vein cannulation has been estimated to be about 1% during epidural procedures.[57] Even in patients receiving low dose ("minidose") heparin there are no case reports or prospective studies that provide assurance that spinal and epidural techniques are safe.[58]

There are some advantages of regional anesthetics in patients with a high risk for thromboembolism. The high incidence of thromboembolism following surgery has been related to blood flow stasis during anesthesia and may therefore be modified by anesthetic technique. Several studies have compared the risk of thromboembolism following general anesthesia with that following epidural or spinal anesthesia in patients undergoing procedures with a high risk of postoperative deep venous thrombosis. In a randomized study by Modig et al,[59] 67% of patients developed proximal deep venous thrombosis and 33% of patients developed pulmonary embolism when total hip replacement was performed with general anesthesia. When epidural anesthesia (continued for 24 hours postoperatively) was used, these incidences were reduced to 13% and 10%, respectively. Similarly, McKenzie et al[60] reported a reduction in the incidence of deep venous thrombosis from 76% to 40% by the use of spinal anesthesia in patients undergoing repair of femoral neck fractures. A similar effect with epidural anesthesia has been reported in patients undergoing open prostatectomy.[61] The benefit of regional anesthesia for thoracic or general surgical procedures has not been conclusively demonstrated.[62] It is also not known if spinal/epidural anesthesia has a protective effect that is additive to other methods such as heparin or dextran prophylaxis.

Several mechanisms have been proposed by which spinal or epidural anesthesia may decrease the incidence of deep venous thrombosis. The major effect is probably reversal of blood flow stasis in the lower limbs due to a reduction in vascular resistance as a result of sympathetic block; there may also be a decrease in blood viscosity due to hemodilution. In contrast to spinal and epidural anesthesia, general anesthesia definitely reduces lower limb blood flow. The second mechanism for the protective effect of spinal/epidural anesthesia is prevention of the hypercoagulable state that may follow general anesthesia.

The recommendations for regional anesthesia techniques in "minidose" anticoagulated parturients are shown in Box 24-2.[58]

Further recommendations include letting the epidural block wear off at intervals to allow for neurologic assessment. Should anticoagulation be instituted following epidural placement, the catheter should be left in place until all systemic anticoagulation is reversed or normalized. After catheter removal, frequent neurologic examinations are necessary to detect early changes indicating hematoma formation. Hematoma diagnosis depends on physical examination, electromyogram, computed tomography, and magnetic resonance imaging studies. Should an epidural hematoma occur, recovery is unlikely without surgical intervention.[63]

Considerations for general anesthesia include careful manipulation of the oral mucosa and gentle endotracheal intubation, avoidance of any type of nasal tube placement, avoidance of neck lines unless absolutely necessary, and close observation of intraoperative and postoperative bleeding.

BOX 24-2   RECOMMENDATIONS FOR REGIONAL ANESTHESIA IN "MINIDOSE" ANTICOAGULATED PARTURIENTS

1. Restrict regional techniques to mothers receiving heparin no more frequently than every 12 hours.
2. Before the initiation of the block, the bleeding profile (ACT or aPTT) must be normal.
3. Use the left lateral position during block placement to reduce aortocaval compression and distention of the epidural veins.
4. Use a midline approach since lateral techniques will more likely lacerate epidural vessels.
5. Abandon the procedure and proceed with an alternate anesthetic if a traumatic tap occurs.

Modified from Writer WDR: Hematologic disease, in James FM, Wheeler AS, Dewan DM (eds): *Obstetric Anesthesia: The Complicated Patient.* Philadelphia, FA Davis, 1988, p 267.

Summary

Physiologic changes in clotting factors and venous flow during pregnancy increase the likelihood of deep venous thrombosis. Factors placing the pregnant patient at a higher risk include previous history of thromboembolic disease, surgery, or bed rest for any reason during the pregnancy. In the high-risk patient (prior pregnancy-associated thromboembolic event that is well documented), prophylactic therapy with low-dose heparin is advised throughout pregnancy and continued for 2 weeks after delivery. Clinical diagnosis of thrombophlebitis or pulmonary embolus is unreliable and should be confirmed objectively before therapy is started. The preferred method of therapy is full anticoagulation followed by subcutaneous heparin for the remainder of the pregnancy and the puerperium, although there is considerable controversy regarding long-term therapy. Fibrinolytic agents have no place in pregnancy, and surgical therapy should be reserved for the severely ill patient. If surgery is indicated for a pulmonary embolus in a pregnant woman, anesthetic technique is based on understanding the pathophysiology of pulmonary hypertension. Anesthetic choice must include a careful consideration of the risks of peridural hematoma formation with regional anesthetics in anticoagulated patients. Should a pulmonary thromboembolism occur during labor and delivery, severe maternal pulmonary and cardiovascular dysfunction may result with concomitant fetal distress. Immediate treatment includes tracheal intubation, ventilation with 100% oxygen, establishment of large-bore intravenous lines, arterial line placement for both blood pressure monitoring and arterial blood gas analysis, rapid infusion of intravenous fluids to maintain a high venous pressure and augment venous return, administration of sodium bicarbonate to treat acidosis, and inotropic support. Massive embolism with shock, hypotension, and hypoxemia may require cardiopulmonary bypass[64] and pulmonary embolectomy.

AMNIOTIC FLUID EMBOLISM

Amniotic fluid embolism is a rare, unpredictable, and unpreventable obstetric catastrophe. It is initiated by entry of amniotic fluid into the maternal circulation and is characterized by the sudden onset of severe dyspnea, tachypnea, and cyanosis during labor, delivery, or the early puerperium.

Amniotic fluid embolism was first reported by Meyer[65] in 1926. It was reported again in an experiment on laboratory animals by Warden in 1927.[66] The importance of this condition and these early studies was not established until 1941, when Steiner and Lushbaugh[67] noted the clinical and pathologic findings of eight women who died suddenly during or just after labor. They performed experimental studies on laboratory animals that produced the same severe disturbances of cardiopulmonary function following the entry of amniotic fluid into maternal circulation. Their study was documented with pathologic findings of pulmonary embolism caused by amniotic fluid particulate matter. Schneider et al[68] in 1968 showed that lethal qualities of human amniotic fluid infused intravenously into dogs was enhanced greatly by the addition of meconium. This description by Steiner and Lushbaugh of a patient with amniotic fluid embolism is classical in its detailed brevity:

> Profound shock coming on suddenly and unexpectedly in a woman who is usually in severe labor or has just finished such a labor, especially if she is an elderly multipara with an excessively large, perhaps dead, fetus and with meconium amniotic fluid, should lead to a suspicion of the possibility. If, also, the shock is introduced by a chill which is followed by dyspnea, cyanosis, vomiting, restlessness and the like and is accompanied by a pronounced fall in blood pressure and a rapid, weak pulse, the picture is more complete. If pulmonary edema now develops quickly in the known absence of previously existing heart disease the diagnosis is reasonably certain.

Their description is complete except for the development of disseminated intravascular coagulopathy in patients surviving the initial pulmonary insult.

Incidence

The incidence of amniotic fluid embolism has been reported to be between 1:8000 to 1:80,000 pregnancies; a more realistic figure is likely between these two extremes.[67,69,70] The mortality rate is very high. Although it is a rare occurrence, it still remains a leading cause of maternal and fetal death. Morgan[71] in 1979 reviewed 272 cases documented in the British medical literature and reported a mortality rate of 86%. From the same study, 25% of the deaths occurred within the first hour of the onset of symptoms, indicating that even with optimum critical care management a high mortality rate persists. All sudden deaths in late pregnancy are not due to amniotic fluid embolism. We must be careful not to let this diagnosis become the wastebasket for cases of unexplained death in labor, especially without confirmation by autopsy.

Etiology

Predisposing factors for amniotic fluid embolism include advanced maternal age, multiple pregnancies, macrosomic fetuses, short duration of labor, and intense contractions often augmented with a uterine muscle stimulant such as oxytocin.[72] Others suggest that fetal demise, meconium staining of amniotic fluid, amniotomy, PIH, cesarean section delivery, abruptio placenta, placenta previa, ruptured uterus, amniocentesis, insertion of an intrauterine pressure catheter, and pregnancy at term with the presence of an intrauterine device are also causative factors. A significant association of amniotic fluid embolism with advanced maternal age has been documented.[71] Amniotic fluid embolism has also been reported following intrauterine injection of hypertonic saline solution to induce abortion.

Amniotic fluid embolus syndrome has been reported in association with a myriad of conditions. These conditions include first- and second-trimester abortion with saline, prostaglandins, and urea, and hysterotomy. It has occurred during labor, at delivery, just after delivery, and one case even developed 32 hours postpartum. Most reported cases of amniotic fluid embolism occur during labor; a pattern of vigorous labor or hypertonic uterine contractions or labor further stimulated by use of oxytocin often has been implicated in the pathogenesis. Evidence for this association (use of an oxytocic) is primarily anecdotal and must be regarded with skepticism. In a review of this subject, Morgan[71] concluded: "In view of the very wide use of accelerated labour and the rarity of amniotic fluid embolism, it must be concluded that there is no direct association between the two." Placental abruption is present in up to 50% of cases and may contribute to the pattern of uterine hypertonus associated with amniotic fluid embolism. In 40% of cases, fetal death is reported before the acute clinical presentation.

In an analysis of data collected in another study,[73] the age range was from 18 to 43 years, with 22 patients 30 years old or older and 12 patients over 35 years of age. The parity of patients ranged from one to eight; the majority of patients were greater than three; however, there were four cases documented in primaparas. The gestational ages of the pregnancies in the patients who subsequently died ranged from 38 to 44 weeks. This of course is excluding those patients who died from amniotic fluid embolism secondary to saline or other fluids injected intraamniotically to induce abortion.

The characteristics of the labor pattern varied. However, it is of interest to note that four patients developed amniotic emboli without evidence of labor occurring. The majority of patients were in various stages of labor either spontaneously or augmented (in 22% labor had been induced and in 11% labor had been augmented with an oxytocic agent). The augmentation or induction of labor was instituted for the usual reasons: ruptured membranes without consistent uterine contractions or postmaturity, in one patient due to pregnancy-induced hypertension and in one patient who was electively induced. In 10%, labor was augmented because of poor progress. Forty-four percent of patients who labored spontaneously had tumultuous and unusually short labors averaging less than 1 hour in duration. No comparably short labors or precipitous deliveries were identified in the patients who received oxytocin stimulation, nor were tetanic contractions reported.

The membranes were documented to be intact in three patients at the time the embolism or onset of symptoms occurred. In most cases studied, the membranes had ruptured either spontaneously or by amniotomy before the onset of symptoms. There is, however, documentation indicating that simultaneous rupture of membranes with onset of symptoms of amniotic fluid embolus and meconium fluid was present in approximately 75% of these patients.[67]

Concerning fetal factors, no clear pattern of fetal presentation, position, or engagement could be ascertained; most cases documented indicate a vertex presentation. There was generally a lack of documentation associating station of the presenting part with onset of symptoms. It could be assumed, since the onset of symptoms occurred just before or during delivery, that the fetal presenting part was engaged.

The size of the infant varied from 5 to 11 pounds, but the data particular to exact weight of all infants were not available. There is a high incidence of fetal deaths and intrapartum death of infants, and of those few infants born alive, a very high percentage die in the neonatal period. In one study of 21 infants for whom information was available, 9 died, 5 intrapartum. Ten live births were recorded in this particular study, but only two infants were documented to have survived. There is a disproportionately large number of stillbirths, and some researchers feel that presence of a dead fetus reduces the strength of the membranes and greatly increases the quantity of particulate matter in the amniotic fluid.[67]

In order for amniotic fluid embolism to occur, the fluid must enter into the maternal circulation. Currently, there are three recognized conditions that must exist for this to result: amniotomy, laceration of endocervical or uterine vessels, and a pressure gradient sufficient to force the fluid into the maternal circulation.

A tear or rent in the membranes such as occurs with amniotomy has been associated with proven embolism.[74] Various sites of entry of amniotic fluid into maternal circulation have been suggested. Laceration of endocervical veins can occur during the normal process of cervical dilation and effacement, although more severe lacerations may occur with a very rapid and tumultuous labor or vigorous cervical manipulation associated with vaginal examination. Uterine vessels can be damaged through surgical procedures such as cesarean section or amniocentesis. Trauma is also responsible for causing damage of the uterine vessels. According to Landing,[75] an abnormal opening of the uterine vessels, either decidual or myometrial, that occurs with uterine rupture, placenta accreta, cesarean section, or retained placenta may provide a portal of entry for amniotic fluid. Abruptio placenta, whether marginal or complete, as well as any degree of placenta previa, could also provide a route of entry. If amniotic fluid finds an open maternal venous sinus, it could be pumped by a vigorous contraction through the disrupted amniotic membrane, with resultant embolization.

Intraamniotic injections of fluid (e.g., hypertonic saline or saline solution or urea) causes a rise in intrauterine pressure that may be greater than that associated with normal labor. Frost[76] in 1967 reported a patient with a hydatidiform mole who died from trophoblastic embolization of the lungs following injection of intraamniotic hypertonic saline. A review of deaths following legal abortions in the United States from 1972 to 1978 revealed that 15 (12%) were due to amniotic fluid embolus; all of these followed intraamniotic injections, and none followed uterine curettage.[77] The clinical symptoms in these patients were the same as in those with embolism occurring at term. This study also revealed gestational age to be a significant factor. No deaths occurred below 12 weeks' gestation, but the mortality was 7.2:100,000 at 21 weeks or more, representing a risk factor 24 times greater after 21 weeks' gestation.[77]

Due to the rarity of the condition combined with the fact that diagnosis is most often made during the postmortem examination, it is difficult to determine a definite cause and effect with this catastrophic obstetric event.

Pathophysiology

The two life-threatening consequences of amniotic fluid embolism, cardiopulmonary collapse and disseminated intravascular coagulation, may occur in sequence or together. The physiology of amniotic fluid embolism results in pulmonary hypertension with a sudden reduction of blood flow to the left heart, decreased left ventricular output, and subsequent peripheral vascular collapse. The sudden development of pulmonary hypertension precipitates acute cor pulmonale and congestive heart failure that thereby cause pulmonary edema. The derangement of the ventilation/perfusion ratio of the lungs produces hypoxemia and tissue hypoxia. Multiple

emboli are usually necessary to cause this acute onset of symptoms.

The toxicity of intravenously infused amniotic fluid appears to vary remarkably, depending on the particulate matter it contains; this is especially true of meconium fluid. The particulate materials found in amniotic fluid and especially in meconium-stained fluid, according to some authors, may account for the cause of sudden death associated with this syndrome.[78] A recent study suggested the presence of a heat-stable pressor agent in meconium, which enhances the cardiopulmonary response to the infusion of autologous amniotic fluid in goats.[79]

Meconium includes shed fetal squamous cells (squames), fetal hairs, vernix caseosa, and mucin. If the severe pulmonary vascular obstruction and cor pulmonale that develop are not immediately fatal, hemorrhage from disseminated intravascular coagulopathy is soon evident. The cause of disseminated intravascular coagulopathy is controversial. Evidence suggests a potent thromboplastic action of amniotic fluid that causes disseminated deposition of fibrin clots and activation of the lysis system. These hemodynamic processes defibrinate the blood,[80] resulting in afibrinogenemia, coagulopathy, and subsequent hemorrhage.[81] The powerful thromboplastin effects of trophoblasts are well established; systemic release of trophoblastic material may play an even greater role in the coagulopathy of amniotic fluid embolism than has been appreciated.

Kitzmiller has shown that amniotic fluid collected during labor, as compared with fluid collected prior to labor, has greater toxicity when infused into rabbits.[81] The particular substance mediating this reaction is still unknown. Prostaglandins and leukotrienes produce many of the hemodynamic and hematologic effects present in patients with amniotic fluid embolism and have been implicated by some researchers.[82] These metabolites of arachidonic acid are present in increased quantities during labor.[83]

Some researchers postulate that an acute anaphylactoid reaction may play a part in the development of the cardiovascular collapse.[84] For a true anaphylactic reaction to occur, sensitization is required, but evidence for this is inconclusive. Stefanini and Turpini[85] noted that an intravenous injection of 15 mL of homologous amniotic fluid in dogs produced no effect, but 1 month later, further administration of a 15 mL aliquot, which had been kept frozen, resulted in hypotension, hypofibrinogenemia, and thrombocytopenia. It was therefore suggested that the animal had become sensitized to amniotic fluid and that this might occur in humans. It is possible that penetration of amniotic fluid into the systemic circulation during the antepartum period causes a state of sensitization in humans, and subsequent entry into the circulation during labor and delivery induces an acute anaphylactic reaction. However, the absence or rarity of pruritus, urticaria, laryngospasm, or wheezing in case reports does not indicate a mast cell-mediated mechanism.

The most significant pathologic findings at autopsy are limited to the lungs. The lungs show gross evidence of pulmonary edema (in 70% of the cases).[86] Alveolar hemorrhage and pulmonary embolism of amniotic fluid materials are present; the presence of embolic particles is essential for diagnosis, but on histologic search, they may be missed because of their small size.[78] They are composed of amorphous debris, epithelial squames, and mucin (from meconium). They tend to lodge in small arteries, arterioles, and capillaries of the lungs.[80] Since uterine trauma is a significant factor in the pathogenesis, signs of uterine laceration or uterine rupture may be evident.[87] Acute right ventricular dilation is usually present. From recent experiences with hemodynamic monitoring during the resuscitation of parturients with amniotic fluid embolism, Clark[88] described a biphasic response to amniotic fluid embolism. The early phase consists of transient (but perhaps intense) pulmonary vasospasm, which probably results from the release of vasoactive substances. This may account for the right heart dysfunction that is often fatal. This phase probably has a duration of less than thirty minutes.[88] Low cardiac output leads to increased ventilation/perfusion mismatch, hypoxemia, and hypotension. This phase probably has a duration of less than 30 minutes.[88] Of interest, right heart function and pulmonary artery pressures are usually close to "normal" by the time that hemodynamic monitoring is begun in humans during resuscitation from amniotic fluid embolism.[88,89] A second phase of left ventricular failure and pulmonary edema often occurs in those women who survive the initial insult.[88,89]

Amniotic fluid elements are sometimes found in uterine vessels and the right side of the heart, and careful evaluation of the other organs may also identify the magnitude of embolization with the finding of particulate matter in the maternal brain, kidneys, liver, and spleen. The hypothalmus is also an area that deserves special evaluation.

Clinical and laboratory diagnosis

In a small percentage of patients the onset of symptoms have begun before labor was clinically evident. The majority of patients develop symptoms during the latter part of the first stage of labor and a lesser number become acute during birth. There have been two cases documented that were associated with delivery of the placenta, and only one

case has been documented to occur as late as 32 hours postpartum. In one series, 45% of cases were associated with placental abruption of varying degrees. Many writers believe this to be one of the primary catalysts in the development of an amniotic fluid embolism.

In a review of obstetric patients who developed amniotic embolism,[71] the most common complications that were already present or developed during delivery are, in order of frequency of occurrence, severe amnionitis, moderate to severe pregnancy-induced hypertension, cephalopelvic disproportion, and traumatic midforceps delivery.

Prodromal symptoms in amniotic fluid embolism are sudden chills, shivering, sweating, anxiety, and coughing followed by signs of respiratory distress, shock, cardiovascular collapse, and convulsions. All patients were conscious during the onset of symptoms. Respiratory difficulty, evidenced by cyanosis, tachypnea, and bronchospasm, frequently culminates in fulminate pulmonary edema. Hypoxemia explains the cyanosis and likely accounts for the restlessness, convulsions, and coma. Reflex tachypnea results from the decreased arterial oxygen saturation, and cardiovascular collapse (heralded by hypotension, tachycardia, and arrhythmia) may end in cardiac arrest.

Convulsions may be an early manifestation of involvement combined with cerebral ischemia and eventually may lead to coma and death. If the patient survives this initial episode, bleeding occurs secondary to disseminated intravascular coagulopathy and uterine atony. In all cases studied, bleeding was never documented as one of the first indications. A definitive diagnosis is usually made at postmortem examination by demonstration of amniotic fluid material in the maternal circulation and the small arteries, arterioles, and capillaries of the pulmonary vessels. In the living patient, diagnosis can be made by identification of lanugo or fetal hair and fetal squames in an aspirate of blood from the right heart.[90] Fetal squames have been recovered in the maternal sputum in some cases.[91] In the past, physicians thought that detection of fetal squamous cells in the pulmonary circulation was pathognomonic of amniotic fluid embolism.[92,93] However, obstetricians have detected fetal squames in the pulmonary circulation of both antepartum and postpartum patients with no clinical evidence of amniotic fluid embolism. Recently, Kobayashi et al[94] described the use of a monoclonal antibody for detection of an amniotic fluid-specific antigen in the maternal circulation of patients with signs and symptoms of amniotic fluid embolism.

Additional diagnostic tools for confirmation of amniotic fluid embolism suspected by the classic clinical picture include (1) chest x-ray, which may show enlarged right atrium and ventricle and prominent proximal pulmonary artery (in massive pulmonary embolism) and pulmonary edema; (2) lung scan, which may demonstrate some areas of reduced radioactivity in the lung field; (3) central venous pressure (CVP), with an initial rise due to pulmonary hypertension and eventually a profound drop due to severe hemorrhage; and (4) measurement of blood coagulation factors. In pregnancy, blood coagulation factors are normally increased. However, with amniotic fluid embolism, evidence of disseminated intravascular coagulopathy ensues with failure of blood to clot, decreased platelet count, decreased fibrinogen and afibrinogenemia, prolonged prothrombin time (PT) and PTT, and presence of fibrin degradation products.

In the differential diagnosis of amniotic fluid embolism, the following entities are to be considered.[95]

1. Thrombotic pulmonary embolism, which is usually caused by a thrombus originating from the lower extremities or pelvic veins, is usually associated with chest pain. However, it generally occurs later in the postpartum period, and it may occur with evidence of venous thrombosis.[96]
2. Air embolism, which may follow a ruptured uterus, blood transfusion under pressure, or manipulation of placenta previa, can occur during labor or cesarean section. It is associated with chest pain, but an important differentiating factor from amniotic fluid embolism is the auscultation of a typical waterwheel murmur over the pericardium.[97]
3. Aspiration of gastric contents into the lungs causes cyanosis, tachycardia, hypotension, and pulmonary edema (similar to amniotic fluid embolism). However, acid aspiration is usually seen in an unconscious patient with loss of the cough reflex,[96] or during induction or emergence from general anesthesia.
4. Eclamptic convulsions and coma in a pregnant patient may resemble this syndrome, but the state of shock in amniotic fluid embolism, as well as the presence of hypertension, proteinuria, and edema[97] in the eclamptic patient differentiate these two conditions.
5. Convulsions from toxic reaction to local anesthetic drugs may be confused with this syndrome. However, the close temporal relationship between the onset of symptoms and administration of the drug[97] is an important differentiating factor. Also, hypertension is usually present in the clinical picture of drug toxicity.
6. Acute left heart failure (seen most commonly in pregnant patients with rheumatic heart dis-

ease) may simulate an amniotic fluid embolism, but the history of previous disease with ECG changes and other clinical symptoms, i.e., cardiac murmur, helps in the diagnosis.
7. A cerebrovascular accident may be considered in the differential diagnosis, but it is distinguished from amniotic fluid embolism by the absence of cyanosis, hypotension, and pulmonary edema. Also, examination of cerebrospinal fluid should help in the diagnosis.
8. Finally, hemorrhagic shock in an obstetric patient, which is usually associated with ruptured uterus, uterine inversion, abruptio placentae, and placenta previa, may lead to the erroneous diagnosis of amniotic fluid embolism. A careful history and physical examination, and the absence of cyanosis and presence of low CVP with hemorrhagic shock, should lead to the correct diagnosis.

Obstetric and anesthetic management

To prevent amniotic fluid embolism, trauma to the uterus must be avoided during maneuvers such as insertion of a pressure catheter or rupture of membranes. Incision of the placenta during cesarean delivery should also be avoided if possible.[71] Since one of the most frequent predisposing factors is considered to be tumultuous labor, excessively strong and frequent uterine contractions should be controlled by administration of intravenous beta-adrenergic drugs[71] or magnesium sulfate. Also, oxytocic drugs, which might precipitate tetanic uterine contractions, should be used appropriately and judiciously.

In most cases, no therapy has proved effective. Whenever unexplained cyanosis and shock develops during labor, a diagnosis of amniotic fluid embolism should be considered.[98] Assuming a diagnosis could be made prior to death, supportive measures should be focused at cardiopulmonary resuscitation, blood volume replacement, and treatment of coagulopathy.

Resuscitation should begin with endotracheal intubation and mechanical ventilation using inspired oxygen concentrations of 50% to 100% delivered by positive pressure and positive end-expiratory pressure (PEEP). With the use of PEEP, functional residual capacity will hopefully increase and if oxygenation improves, as evidenced by pulse oximetry or arterial blood gases, a lowered PEEP setting may be tried. However, high PEEP may produce a decrease in cardiac output due to the effect on the increased intrathoracic pressure and subsequently decreased tissue perfusion. Improved oxygenation will hopefully reduce pulmonary capillary fragility and thereby decrease the severity of pulmonary edema. To date, there has been no documentation in the use of hyperbaric oxygen and some authors think it would be worthwhile in treating the severe tissue hypoxia. To prevent and/or recognize further deterioration, careful monitoring is essential. Placement of an arterial line to monitor arterial blood gases and other pertinent chemistries, as well as a central venous or Swan-Ganz catheter to monitor cardiac status and state of hydration, are of enormous value.

The causes of the development of pulmonary edema have been variably ascribed to vigorous fluid resuscitation, increased pulmonary capillary permeability, and cardiac decompensation due to hypoxia and tachycardia. The severity of pulmonary edema certainly plays an important role in the initial gas exchange abnormality and duration of the aberration.

Currently there is no clear regime of drug therapy to reverse the symptoms and complications of amniotic fluid embolism. Drug therapy and other treatment has been supportive and aimed at improving ventilation/perfusion ratio, maintaining adequate blood pressure, and treating disseminated intravascular coagulopathy.

The drug used to treat pulmonary complications such as bronchospasm and vasoconstriction of pulmonary arterioles is terbutaline, especially if the patient is undelivered with a live fetus. Isoproterenol also relieves pulmonary vasoconstriction and improves cardiac function, although it can cause peripheral vasodilation, which will exacerbate the hypotension. Dopamine may be preferable to isoproterenol, since it improves cardiac function and increases peripheral and renal perfusion unless given in too large a dose, which would decrease renal perfusion. Administration of aminophylline for its bronchodilation and cardiac stimulation effects is controversial, especially because of the tachycardia it produces.

Hydrocortisone in pharmacologic doses up to 2 g/24 hrs reduces pulmonary vasospasm and pulmonary edema and potentiates the cardiac response to catecholamines. In the event of heart failure, digitalization with a rapid-acting agent is recommended.[99] Diuretics can be used if pulmonary wedge pressure is elevated. Indomethacin has been effective in treating severe pulmonary hypertension in laboratory animals and should be considered for use. In a condition with such a high rate of mortality, there would be nothing to lose.

Hypotension should be treated first by left uterine displacement if the patient is undelivered. This can be accomplished easily by insertion of a wedge under the right hip. The vasopressor of choice is ephedrine because it does not decrease uterine perfusion. However, if the fetus has expired or perhaps is already delivered, isoproterenol or dobutamine can be used. The fluid of choice should be lactated Ringer's since its pH is most near that

of blood; the rate of infusion will depend on the CVP values or filling pressures if a Swan-Ganz catheter is in place. If acidosis is present, as evidenced by blood gas values, sodium bicarbonate should be administered.

Treatment of the bleeding diathesis requires blood replacement using fresh whole blood when available, so that the clotting factors so badly needed are intact. Cryoprecipitate and platelet infusions are also required to help combat the coagulopathy. Heparin therapy is controversial; some patients have been documented to survive with its use but there is documentation of survival without using heparin.

Uterine bleeding in a patient already delivered should be controlled by massage and use of intravenous oxytocin. If uterine bleeding is unresponsive to these methods, one should consider exploration for retained placenta or membranes or a search for cervical or uterine lacerations. Methylergonovine is also a strong uterine stimulant and can be given very slowly by intravenous push. The use of prostaglandins (Hemabat) to control hemorrhage is controversial and may cause bronchospasm and/or pulmonary hypertension. The use of aminocaproic acid and aprotinin is not very well documented in the treatment of amniotic embolus, but they can be used when rapid reversal of the lytic state is needed before delivery. Aprotinin (Trasylol) should be the drug of choice if the fetus is still viable since it does not cross the placenta; aminocaproic acid does cross the placenta and it is teratogenic as well.

When amniotic fluid embolism occurs, the accompanying respiratory distress, cardiovascular collapse, and hemorrhagic tendency are contraindications to any regional techniques and if severe shock develops, general anesthetics must be administered with extreme caution. Since immediate delivery is indicated, emergency cesarean section is usually required. These patients are young and typically healthy before the onset of amniotic fluid embolism. Resuscitative measures must be aggressive. Esposito et al[64] reported the successful use of cardiopulmonary bypass and pulmonary artery thromboembolectomy for treatment of postpartum shock caused by amniotic fluid embolism. Large-volume, rapid intravenous infusion devices may be invaluable during resuscitation. The choice of anesthetic agents will depend on the patient's condition, and aggressive cardiopulmonary resuscitation may be all that the anesthesiologist can provide. Anesthetic agents that produce myocardial depression must be avoided.

Summary

Amniotic fluid embolism, although fortunately rare, is one of the most catastrophic situations in obstetrics. The clinical events in this syndrome include cardiopulmonary collapse and disturbances of the clotting mechanism. Although maternal and fetal prognosis is grave, death need not be the inevitable outcome if early diagnosis is followed by prompt and aggressive management. Recently there have been several published cases of patients who survived amniotic fluid embolism.[64,100] Again, Clark has reported two cases of successful pregnancy outcomes in women who survived amniotic fluid embolism in earlier pregnancies.[101,102]

VENOUS AIR EMBOLISM

The phenomenon of air embolism has been recognized as a pathophysiologic condition at least since the time of the Napoleonic Wars, when Baron Larre first observed that cavalry officers suffering saber wounds of the head and neck frequently died not as a result of blood loss but as a result of air bubbles in the right heart and pulmonary circulation.[103] Although the first diagnosed intraoperative air embolus occurred in 1818 during the excision of a supraclavicular tumor,[104] it was not until 1839 that the concept of the "dangerous region" for surgery was promulgated.[105] In those times, when surgery was performed on conscious patients in the sitting position, it was noted that air embolism could occur whenever the surgical site was "above the level of the venous pulsations." Typically, these events were described as an audible hissing sound in the surgical field, followed by the patient's crying out expressing a sense of impending doom. Often, a "lapping" or "murmuring" sound could be heard in the patient's chest just as the vital signs deteriorated and the patient died. Quick-witted surgeons were able to abort these events by simply compressing the incision site or occluding the offending vein, if it could be found.

By 1885, Senn had described the pathophysiology of air entrainment from cranial veins in great detail. He observed that whenever an animal's head was elevated above the level of the heart, air would enter the circulation through an opening in the superior sagittal sinus, and that this process would stop when the head was lowered. Furthermore, he not only noted the presence of air in the heart and pulmonary vessels; he also observed that it could be removed by aspirating through rubber catheters that had been inserted into the right heart via the neck veins.[106]

Incidence

Until recently it was considered highly unlikely that venous air embolism could occur during a cesarean or vaginal delivery. Venous air embolism had been a well-recognized potential complication in abdominal, orthopedic, plastic, urologic, tho-

racic, and head and neck procedures,[107] and had also been noted to develop in neurosurgical cases in the lateral, prone, and supine positions.[108] It was first proposed as a potential danger in pregnancy by Legallois in 1829,[109] and later in 1845 the first case of a fatal air embolism in association with pregnancy was reported. Since that time similar reports by others have followed.[110-114]

The incidence of venous air embolism in pregnancy is not known.[114,115] This is due in part to the difficulty encountered in making the diagnosis. In fatal cases, the reports and autopsy evidence may not be of sufficient detail to allow the diagnosis to be made with certainty. In nonfatal cases, there are no clinical signs and symptoms that are specific for only venous air embolism. Previous attempts at determining the incidence were based on reports of maternal deaths. Klein et al reported 2 deaths in 254,249 live births.[116] Barno and Freeman reported 6 deaths in 559,843 live births.[117] Similar data from England and Wales indicate 7 deaths in approximately 750,000 live births.[118] It might be concluded that the incidence of maternal mortality from venous air embolism is approximately 1:100,000 live births.[115] In the most recently published statistics for maternal deaths in the United States,[1] 25 cases (about 1%) were thought to be due to venous air embolism, although the circumstances of these deaths were not disclosed in detail.

But what is the incidence of venous air embolic events? Studies by Malinow[119] and Fong[120] indicate that although maternal death from venous air embolism may be a rare event, the occurrence of venous air embolism during cesarean section may be more common than previously appreciated. Using a precordial Doppler signal change as evidence of an embolic event, Malinow noted positive Doppler change in 52% (46 of 89) of the women undergoing cesarean section. Fong et al monitored patients with both precordial Doppler and precordial two-dimensional echocardiography and noted a 71% incidence of changes indicating venous air embolism during general anesthesia for cesarean section and a 39% incidence during epidural anesthesia for cesarean section. Only 1 of 129 parturients (0.78%) in Fong's study experienced chest pain, dyspnea, ventricular tachycardia, and hypotension. A 100% correlation between the two detection modes was also demonstrated.

Etiology

For venous air embolism to occur certain conditions must exist. As noted by early experimentation, there must be a vascular access and a gradient between the incisional area and the right heart to promote the movement of air.[121] Gradients as small as 5 cm have been shown to result in the entrainment of large amounts of air (up to 200 ml).[108] Nelson provides the following summary of the physiologic defects that singly or in combination are required for a venous air embolic event:[114]

1. Fixation of the traumatized vein. This prevents normal vascular retraction. The uterine veins, because of their position, course, and fixation, have been assessed the most vulnerable to air embolism.
2. Gravity. Venous drainage secondary to gravitational effect creates a high negative pressure. Such veins when opened will forcibly entrain air.
3. Suction effect of respiration and circulation. The negative intrathoracic pressures generated with inspiration augment venous return to the heart through increased venous negative pressure.
4. Introduction of gas under pressure into the body.

Certain features of pregnancy and parturition make venous air embolism possible:[114,115]

1. The availability of the uterine sinuses to the entrance of air. Air forced into the vagina during pregnancy as may occur with douching, abortion, or insufflation, can result in venous air embolism. In addition, these sinuses can be exposed during low segment cesarean sections, uterine rupture, and placenta previa.
2. Manipulation of the uterus in labor and the puerperium. Uterine manipulation, manual extraction of the placenta, incision of the uterus may all result in the opening of uterine venous sinuses, and possible entrance of air. Malinow et al noted positive Doppler changes occurring 74% at the time of hysterotomy, 2% with the delivery of the baby, 13% with the delivery of the placenta, and 11% during the hysterotomy repair.[119] Fong et al noted a 20% occurrence of venous air embolism by precordial two-dimensional echocardiography with uterine incision, 6% with delivery of the infant, 26% with placental removal, and 34% with uterine closure under epidural anesthesia. Under general anesthesia there was a 10% incidence with uterine incision, 30% with placental removal, and 90% with uterine closure.[120]
3. Negative intraabdominal and uterine venous pressure secondary to positional change. The knee-chest and Trendelenburg positions can create significant negative intraabdominal pressure and increase the gravitational gradient draining the uterine venous sinuses.

4. Douching during pregnancy. Although well-recognized as a hazard it continues to be a popular practice. It creates a situation where air can be forcibly introduced into the vagina with subsequent risk of venous air embolism. Recently a case of a venous air embolism following orogenital sex during pregnancy has also been reported.[121]

In a review of 45 fatal cases and 2 nonfatal cases, the following etiologic factors were noted.[114] The average age was 32 years. Seven of the patients (17%) were delivered by cesarean section with either no labor or incomplete labor. Among the laboring patients who developed venous air embolism, it occurred in 12 patients in the first stage, in 12 patients in the second stage, and in 14 patients in the third stage. The most frequently associated finding was placenta previa, which occurred in 24% of patients. Manual extraction of the placenta was performed 8 times.

Venous air embolism has also been reported in the puerperium. A review of 25 cases occurring within the first day after delivery revealed the following details.[115] The average age of the patients was 32 years. The venous air embolism was delayed from 1 to 6 hours after delivery. Six patients collapsed following uterine irrigation, 3 with packing of the uterus, and 1 with manual exploration of the uterus. In 7 of the patients no specific factor could be determined as the precipitating event. There have also been 10 reported cases occurring after 24 hours. Five of these 10 cases occurred as a result of the knee-chest position, a therapy at that time for retroversion and subinvolution of the uterus in the puerperium. Other factors felt to be associated with the embolic event include "violent jumping in bed" and uterine douching.

Pathophysiology

When air enters the venous system, pulmonary embolism, coronary embolism, and cerebral embolism may all occur, resulting in significant maternal morbidity and/or mortality. The severity of the air embolism will depend on the size of the subject, the patient's general condition, the rate of entrainment of the gas, the type of gas, and the total volume of gas introduced.[114,115,121] Wolffe and Robertson[122] demonstrated that the severity of gas embolism is proportional to body weight and pulmonary artery size. Additional work by Richardson et al[123] indicate that 500 to 600 ml of air (7 ml/kg) administered as a single rapid bolus would be uniformly fatal to humans. The prolonged continuous entrainment of about 1 to 3 ml/kg/min for as long as 1 to 2 minutes could result in a fatal embolism.[114] In the presence of nitrous oxide during general anesthesia, a smaller volume of air could be rapidly doubled and produce a fatal embolism.

It has been proposed that when massive air embolism occurs, the introduced air is collected in the right ventricle, creating an "air trap" between the right ventricle and the pulmonary artery.[124] This "air trap" results in foaming of the blood, loss of valve function, and loss of blood propulsion into the pulmonary inflow tract. Central venous pressures increase and pulmonary artery pressures decrease. Since pulmonary blood flow has ceased, oxygenation is impaired and anoxia results. Left ventricular filling is severely diminished and cardiac output drops to zero. Without immediate intervention, cardiac arrest is inevitable. Boyer and Curry have shown that bronchospasm also accompanies these circulatory changes.[125]

In nonfatal cases, small emboli do not produce the air trap, but they enter the pulmonary circulation and may result in ventilation/perfusion defects.[104] "Paradoxical" embolism has also been described, with patency of the foramen ovale.[126] Once in the left side of the heart, air emboli to the coronary or cerebral circulation is possible.

Clinical and laboratory diagnosis

Signs of venous air embolism may include gasping (spontaneous) respiration, chest pain, increases in CVP, ECG changes, hypotension, changes in heart sounds, cyanosis, and cardiac arrest.[127] Venous air embolism may or may not be present with complaints of chest pain and/or dyspnea, perhaps depending on the venous air volume. Malinow found a significant relationship between unsolicited complaints of chest pain and/or dyspnea during cesarean section and the occurrence of positive Doppler changes. The chest pain was described as retrosternal, heavy, nonradiating, and lasting 5 to 10 minutes. In addition, 20% of the women with Doppler changes complained of dyspnea, and 8 women complained of both chest pain and dyspnea. Chest pain is not associated with the type of anesthesia given or with surgical exteriorization of the uterus for hysterotomy repair.[119]

The concomitant hypoxemia, ventilation/perfusion mismatch, and increased dead space ventilation will be reflected in decreased oxygen saturation by pulse oximetry, and decreased end-tidal carbon dioxide as measured by capnography. These changes can be verified by blood gas analysis.

Since treatment depends on rapid diagnosis and evacuation of the air, an early sensitive method of detection is needed. A precordial ultrasonic Doppler monitor is capable of detecting as little as 0.1 ml of intracardiac air.[128] It has been found that Doppler changes occur in about 50% of all patients undergoing elective cesarean delivery under regional anesthesia. Precordial Doppler monitoring is simple and noninvasive. Fong et al[120] monitored patients with ultrasonic Doppler in the horizontal position simultaneously with two-dimensional echocardiography. There was a 100% correlation between the simultaneous Doppler and echo detection of emboli, which most likely meant that they saw echolucent air emboli and not echodense thromboemboli or amniotic fluid emboli. A recent study by Vartikar et al[129] recommended oxygen saturation monitoring as a routine practice to detect venous air embolism in patients undergoing cesarean section. Venous air embolism was often associated with a decrease in oxygen saturation, and patients who demonstrated the greatest changes in saturation were most likely to show persistent Doppler changes and manifest clinical signs.

The role of precordial Doppler and two-dimensional echocardiography during routine cesarean section for early detection of venous air embolism is still undefined. It has been suggested that precordial Doppler monitoring should be considered for cases at risk for air embolism, such as profound hypovolemia, abruptio placentae, or placenta previa.[111]

Obstetric and anesthetic management

The best management of venous air embolism is prevention. Although there is no study clearly documenting a therapeutic technique for the prevention of this catastrophic event, the elimination of such etiologic factors as uterine irrigation, vaginal insufflation, knee-chest position, and Trendelenberg position during the peripartum period has been suggested.[114,115] It is further suggested that obstetricians avoid placing traction on the uterus and exteriorizing it, since exteriorization and particularly traction probably distend the venous sinuses, increasing the risk of venous air embolism.[114] Fong et al reported that air embolism could occur at any time during a cesarean section, regardless of the anesthetic technique used: before and after uterine incision with the delivery of the baby, with the removal of the placenta, upon uterine closure, and after uterine repair. No significant difference in the formation of air emboli was found between manual extraction and passive separation of the placenta, nor was placenta previa associated with an increased risk.[120]

The foregoing findings and recommendations have since been challenged by Downing et al[130] They claimed that modest head-up patient posture (5 to 10 degrees), did not influence the occurrence of venous air embolism, nor were they able to substantiate the very high incidence of "definite" venous air embolism reported in the previous studies.[119,121,127] Their findings also differed with regard to the distribution of venous air embolism in relation to operative events: the highest incidence of venous air embolism occurred with delivery of the placenta rather than during hysterotomy[119] or uterine closure.[120] Perhaps these findings are to be expected since shortly after placental separation, large uterine sinuses lie open and vulnerable to the entry of air from a now empty uterus.

When venous air embolism does occur, immediate treatment is needed; for this, the following recommendations have been made:[127]

1. Prevent further embolization by placing the patient in reverse Trendelenburg position with a 15-degree left-sided tilt. This position tends to prevent air from entering the right ventricle, therefore allowing easier aspiration from the superior vena cava via a central catheter. By lowering the uterus, the negative pressure gradient in the uterine venous sinuses due to gravity drainage is eliminated. The surgical field should also be flooded with normal saline to reduce and prevent further entrainment of air.
2. Discontinue nitrous oxide and provide 100% oxygen.
3. Start immediate cardiopulmonary resuscitation if cardiovascular collapse occurs.
4. Advance a catheter into the superior vena cava from a central vein or peripheral vein access and aspirate as much air as possible.
5. If neurologic symptoms develop, a computed tomography scan should be done immediately to search for possible paradoxical air embolism. If intraaxial air is present in the brain, hyperbaric oxygen therapy is necessary to reduce the bubble size.

Despite the suggested findings that venous air embolism of low magnitude occurs frequently in cesarean sections, fortunately usually without major associated clinical signs and symptoms of cardiopulmonary compromise, there is little room for complacency. Although lethal venous air embolism is a rare event in obstetrics, even small air bubbles in the circulation threaten patients with a patent foramen ovale, a surprisingly common abnormality.[123] This fact should be borne in mind during cesarean section and the anesthetic management planned accordingly. In patients with known right to left shunts, epidural anesthesia techniques involving the "loss of resistance with air" should be avoided.

Routine monitoring for venous air embolism using Doppler ultrasound would seem wise, especially in patients likely to have a low CVP predisposing them to significant venous air embolism. Beside the ultrasonic Doppler air bubble detector, the hallmark for venous air embolism detection also involves end-tidal capnography as well as helpful verification by air aspiration from a previously placed central venous line (Fig. 24-1).

Patients who are dehydrated due to prolonged labor may be especially at risk, as may patients with compensated hemorrhagic shock. In these latter instances, the use of a multiorifice central venous catheter would seem advisable since this device allows effective removal of air from the central circulation.[131-133]

When the venous air embolism occurs, the anesthetic most likely will have already been chosen and administered. There are no studies that provide conclusive evidence that there is any particular anesthetic technique that should be either avoided or advocated. Epidural and spinal anesthesia without adequate volume preloading of the circulation could in theory predispose the patient to venous air embolism by lowering CVP and increasing the right atrial to uterine "negative" venous pressure gradient. Parturients appear to be at greater risk of clinically significant venous air embolism under general anesthesia,[120] and the reduced risk with regional anesthesia could be attributed to generous volume loading before induction of epidural or spinal anesthesia. In patients under general anesthesia receiving nitrous oxide, small insignificant nondetected air emboli could expand into larger detectable clinically significant emboli[134] because of the solubility characteristics of N_2O. A recent report described treating a venous air embolism that occurred during a cesarean section with hyperbaric oxygen.[135]

Further investigation is needed to determine if nitrous oxide administration with general anesthetics increases the risk of venous air embolism during cesarean section.

Summary

In conclusion, we think that the problem of venous air embolism during cesarean section should be taken at least as seriously as that of pulmonary acid aspiration and failed intubation. Further research efforts are indicated to define more clearly those mothers at particular risk of serious venous air embolism. The contribution of different surgical techniques, intraoperative positions, and anesthetic techniques to the incidence of venous air embolism also requires elucidation. Should a patient develop symptoms of venous air embolism, immediate intervention with possible central line placement and aspiration of the embolized air is

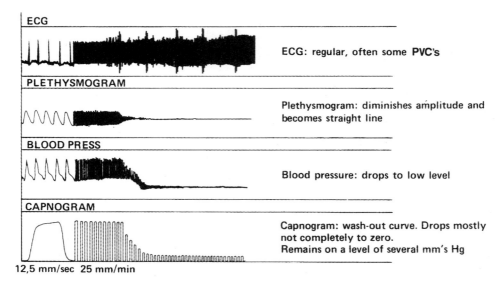

Fig. 24-1 Large venous air embolism. Recovery is usually gradual. Even after a small air embolism, which is not life-threatening, the capnogram does not return to its original level for at least 5 to 10 minutes. Patient is in severe danger! *PVC* = premature ventricular contraction; *blood press* = blood pressure. (Adapted from Smalhout B: *A Quick Guide to Capnography and Its Use in Differential Diagnosis.* Boblingen, Hewlett-Packard GmbH, 1983, p 48.)

required to prevent significant maternal morbidity and mortality.

REFERENCES

1. Koonin LM, Atrash HK, Lawson HW, et al: Maternal mortality surveillance, United States, 1979-1986. Vol 40/SS-1, July 1991. United States Public Health Service. Centers for Disease Control, Atlanta, Ga.
2. Confidential Enquiries into Maternal Deaths in the U.K., 1985-87. Department of Health, London, Her Majesty's Stationery Office, 1991, p 28.
3. Sipes SL, Weiner CP: Venous thromboembolic disease in pregnancy. *Semin Perinatol* 1990; 14:103.
4. Franks AL, Atrash HK, Lawson HW, et al: Obstetrical pulmonary embolism mortality: United States 1970-1985. *Am J Pub Health* 1990; 80:720.
5. Sachs BP, Brown DAJ, Driscoll SC, et al: Maternal mortality in Massachusetts. *N Engl J Med* 1987; 316:667.
6. Gabel HD: Maternal mortality in South Carolina from 1970-1984: An analysis. *Obstet Gynecol* 1987; 69:307.
7. Kaunitz AM, Hughes JM, Grimes DA, et al: Causes of maternal mortality in the United States. *Obstet Gynecol* 1985; 65:605.
8. Sabiston DC: Pathophysiology, diagnosis and management of pulmonary embolism. *Am J Surgery* 1979; 138:384.
9. Bolan JC: Thromboembolic complications of pregnancy. *Clin Obstet Gynecol* 1983; 26:913.
10. Villasanta U: Thromboembolic disease in pregnancy. *Am J Obstet Gynecol* 1965; 93:142.
11. Aaro LA, Juergens JL: Thrombophlebitis associated with pregnancy. *Am J Obstet Gynecol* 1971; 109:1128.
12. Kierkegaard A: Incidence and diagnosis of deep vein thrombosis associated with pregnancy. *Acta Obstet Gynecol Scand* 1983; 62:239.
13. Bergqvist A, Bergqvist D, Hallbrook T: Deep vein thrombosis during pregnancy: A prospective study. *Acta Obstet Gynecol Scand* 1983; 62:443.
14. de Swiet M: Thromboembolism. *Clin Haematol* 1985; 14:643.
15. Tawes RL, Kennedy PA, Harris EJ, et al: Management of deep vein thrombosis and pulmonary embolism during pregnancy. *Am J Surg* 1982; 144:141.
16. Ikard RW, Veland K, Folse R: Lower limb venous dynamics in pregnant women. *Surg Gynecol Obstet* 1979; 132:483.
17. Brandt JT: Current concepts of coagulation. *Clin Obstet Gynecol* 1985; 28:3.
18. Caldwell DC, Williamson RA, Goldsmith JC: Hereditary coagulopathies in pregnancy. *Clin Obstet Gynecol* 1985; 28:53.
19. Rosenberg RD: Actions and interactions of antithrombin and heparin. *N Engl J Med* 1975; 292:146.
20. Thaler E, Lechner K: Antithrombin III deficiency and thromboembolism. *Clin Haematol* 1981; 10:369.
21. Samson D, Stirling Y, Woolf L, et al: Management of planned pregnancy in a patient with congenital antithrombin III deficiency. *Br J Haematol* 1984; 52:173.
22. Staub MC: Pathophysiology of microembolism lung injury. *Anesthesiology Annual Review Lectures* 1983; p 302.
23. Moser KM: Diagnosis and management of pulmonary embolism. *Hosp Pract* 1980; 15:57.
24. Bettman MA, Paulin S: Leg phlebography: The incidence, nature and modifications of undesirable side effects. *Radiology* 1977; 122:101.
25. Markisz JA: Radiologic and nuclear medicine diagnosis, in Goldhaber SZ (ed): *Pulmonary Embolism and Deep Venous Thrombosis.* Philadelphia, WB Saunders, 1985, p 41.
26. Perry PJ, Herron GR, King JC: Heparin half-life in normal and impaired renal function. *Clin Pharmacol Res* 1974; 16:514.

27. Kakkar V: The diagnosis of deep vein thrombosis using the ^{125}I fibrinogen test. *Arch Surg* 1972; 104:152.
28. Ginsberg JS, Hirsh J, Rainbow AJ, et al: Risks to the fetus of radiologic procedures used in the diagnosis of maternal venous thromboemboic disease. *Thromb Haemost* 1992; 61:189.
29. Morris GK, Mitchell JR: Clinical management of venous thromboembolism. *Br Med Bull* 1978; 34:169.
30. Kalimada P, Rashad MN, Murthy BN, et al: Pulmonary embolism: Hemodynamics, diagnosis, prophylaxis and management. *Anesthesiol Rev* 1985; 12:29.
31. Hyers TM: Heparin therapy. *Drugs* 1992; 44:738.
32. Hirsh J, Fuster V: Guide to anticoagluant therapy, Part 1: Heparin. *Circulation* 1994; 89:1449.
33. Greer IA, deSwiet M: Thrombosis prophylaxis in obstetrics and gynaecology. *Br J Obstet Gynaecol* 1993; 100:37.
34. Nelson-Piercy C: Low molecular weight heparin for obstetric thromboprophylaxis. *Br J Obstet Gynaecol* 1994; 101:6.
35. Sturridge F, deSwiet M, Letsky E: The use of low molecular weight heparin for thromboprophylaxis in pregnancy. *Br J Obstet Gynaecol* 1994; 101:69.
36. Dahlman TC: Osteoporotic fractures and the recurrence of thromboembolism during pregnancy and the puerperium in 184 women undergoing thromboprophylaxis with heparin. *Am J Obstet Gynecol* 1993; 168:1265.
37. Salzman JG, Deykin K, Shapiro RM, et al: Management of heparin therapy: A controlled prospective trial. *N Engl J Med* 1975; 292:1046.
38. Edleman WL, Barrett RL, Gladney JD, et al: Heparin-induced white clot syndrome. *J La State Med Soc* 1989; 141:21.
39. Laros RK, Alger LS: Thromboembolism and pregnancy. *Clin Obstet Gynecol* 1979; 22:871.
40. Hirsh J, Fuster V: Guide to anticoagulant therapy, Part 2: Oral anticoagulants. *Circulation* 1994; 89:1469.
41. Bonnar J: Venous thromboembolism and pregnancy. *Baillieres Clin Obstet Gynaecol* 1981; 8:456.
42. LoSasso AM: Pulmonary embolism, in Stoelting RK, Dierdorf SF (eds): *Anesthesia and Co-existing Disease*. New York, Churchill Livingstone, 1983, p 165.
43. Floyd RC, Gookin KS, Hess LW, et al: Administration of heparin by subcutaneous infusion with a programmable pump. *Am J Obstet Gynecol* 1991; 165:931.
44. Spence TH: Pulmonary embolization syndrome, in Civetta JM, Taylor RN, Kirby RR (eds): *Critical Care*. Philadelphia, JB Lippincott, 1988, p 1091.
45. Gal TJ: Causes and consequences of impaired gas exchange, in Benumof J, Saidman L (eds): *Anesthesia and Perioperative Complications*. St Louis, Mosby, 1992, p 203.
46. Fagher B, Ahlgren M, Astedt B: Acute massive pulmonary embolism treated with streptokinase during labor and the early puerperium. *Acta Obstet Gynecol Scand* 1990; 69:659.
47. Bounameaux H, Vermylen J, Collen D: Thrombolytic treatment with recombinant tissue-type plasminogen activator in a patient with massive pulmonary embolism. *Ann Intern Med* 1985; 103:64.
48. Baudo F, Caimi TM, Redaelli R, et al: Emergency treatment with recombinant tissue plasminogen activator of pulmonary embolism in a pregnant woman with antithrombin III deficiency. *Am J Obstet Gynecol* 1990; 163:1274.
49. Flossdorf T, Breulmann M, Hopf HB: Successful treatment of pulmonary embolism with recombinant tissue type plasminogen activator (rt-PA) in a pregnant woman with intact gravidity and preterm labour. *Intensive Care Med* 1990; 16:454.
50. Barnes AB, Kanarek DJ, Greenfield AJ, et al: Vena cava filter placement during pregnancy. *Am J Obstet Gynecol* 1981; 140:707.
51. Alfrey DD, Benumof JL: Pulmonary diseases, in Katz J, Benumof J, Kadis LB (eds): *Anesthesia and Uncommon Diseases*. Philadelphia, WB Saunders, 1981, p 227.
52. Owens EL, Kasten GW, Hessel EA: Spinal subarachnoid hematoma after lumbar puncture and heparinization: A case report, review of the literature, and discussion of anesthetic implications. *Anesth Analg* 1986; 65:1201.
53. Odoom JA, Sih IL: Epidural analgesia and anticoagulation therapy: Experience with one thousand cases of continuous epidurals. *Anaesthesia* 1983; 38:254.
54. Rao TL, El-Etr AA: Anticoagulation following placement of epidural and subarachnoid catheters: An evaluation of neurologic sequelae. *Anesthesiology* 1981; 55:618.
55. Matthews ET, Abrams LD: Intrathecal morphine in open heart surgery. *Lancet* 1980; 2:543.
56. Phillips OC, Ebner H, Nelson AT, et al: Neurologic complications following spinal anesthesia with lidocaine. *Anesthesiology* 1969; 30:284.
57. Bromage PR: *Epidural Anesthesia*. Philadelphia, WB Saunders, 1978, p 229.
58. Writer WDR: Hematologic disease, in James FM, Wheeler AS, Dewan DM (eds): *Obstetric Anesthesia: The Complicated Patient*. Philadelphia, FA Davis, 1988; p 267.
59. Modig J, Burg T, Karlstrom G, et al: Thromboembolism after total hip replacement: Role of epidural and general anesthesia. *Anesth Analg* 1983; 62:174.
60. McKenzie PJ, Wishart HY, Gray I, et al: Effects of anaesthetic technique on deep vein thrombosis: A comparison of subarachnoid and general anaesthesia. *Br J Anaesth* 1985; 57:853.
61. Hendalin H, Mattila MAK, Poikolainen E: The effect of lumbar epidural analgesia on the development of deep vein thrombosis of the legs after open prostatectomy. *Acta Chir Scand* 1981; 147:425.
62. Mellbring G, Dahlgren S, Reiz S, et al: Thromboembolic complications after major abdominal surgery: Effect of thoracic epidural analgesia. *Acta Chir Scand* 1983; 149:263.
63. Janis KM: Epidural hematoma following postoperative epidural analgesia: A case report. *Anesth Analg* 1972; 51:689.
64. Esposito RA, Grossi EA, Coppia G, et al: Successful treatment of postpartum shock caused by amniotic fluid embolism with cardiopulmonary bypass and pulmonary artery thromboembolectomy. *Am J Obstet Gynecol* 1990; 163:571.
65. Meyer JR: Embolia pulmonar amnio-caseosa. *Brazil Med* 1926; 2:301.
66. Warden MR: Amniotic fluid as possible factor in etiology of eclampsia. *Am J Obstet Gynecol* 1927; 14:292.
67. Steiner PE, Lushbaugh CC: Maternal pulmonary embolism by fluid as a cause of obstetric shock and expected deaths in obstetrics. *JAMA* 1941; 117:1245.
68. Schneider CC, Henry MM, Chaplick MJ: Meconium embolism in vivo. *Am J Obstet Gynecol* 1968; 101:909.
69. Liban E, Raz S: A clinicopathologic study of fourteen cases of amniotic fluid embolism. *Am J Clin Path* 1969; 51:477.
70. Abouleish E: Amniotic fluid embolism: Report of a fatal case. *Curr Res Anesth Analg* 1974; 53:549.
71. Morgan M: Amniotic fluid embolism. *Anaesthesia* 1979; 34:20.
72. Courtney LD: Amniotic fluid embolism. *Obstet Gynecol Surv* 1974; 29:169.

73. Anderson DG: Amniotic fluid embolism: A re-evaluation. *Am J Obstet Gynecol* 1967; 98:336.

74. Schenken JR, Slaughter GP, DeMay GH: Maternal pulmonary embolism of amniotic fluid. *Am J Clin Pathol* 1950; 20:147.

75. Landing BJ: The pathogenesis of amniotic fluid embolism. II. Uterine factors. *N Engl J Med* 1950; 243:590.

76. Frost ACG: Death following intrauterine injection of hypertonic saline solution with hydatidiformole. *Am J Obstet Gynecol* 1967; 101:342.

77. Guidotti RJ, Grimes DA, Cates W: Fatal amniotic fluid embolism during legally induced abortion in the United States; 1972-1978. *Am J Obstet Gynecol* 1981; 141:257.

78. Holland AJC: Amniotic fluid embolism. *Anaesthesia* 1968; 23:273.

79. Hankins GDV, Snyder RR, Clark SL, et al: Acute hemodynamic and respiratory effects of amniotic fluid embolism in the pregnant goat model. *Am J Obstet Gynecol* 1993; 168:1113.

80. Russell W, Nicholson J: Amniotic fluid embolism. A review of the syndrome with a report of 4 cases. *Obstet Gynecol* 1965; 26:476.

81. Kitzmiller JL, Lucas WE: Studies on a model of amniotic fluid embolism. *Obstet Gynecol* 1972; 39:626.

82. Azegami M, Mori N: Amniotic fluid embolism and leukotrienes. *Am J Obstet Gynecol* 1986; 155:1119.

83. Karim SN, Devlin J: Prostaglandin content of amniotic fluid during pregnancy and labor. *J Obstet Gynaecol Br Commonw* 1979; 74:230.

84. Dutta D, Bhargava KC, Chakravarti RN, et al: Therapeutic studies in experimental amniotic fluid embolism in rabbits. *Am J Obstet Gynecol* 1974; 106:1201.

85. Stefanini M, Turpini RA: Fibrinogenopenic accident of pregnancy and delivery: Syndrome with multiple etiological mechanism. *Ann NY Acad Sci* 1959; 75:601.

86. Peterson EP, Taylor HB: Amniotic fluid embolism: An analysis of 40 cases. *Obstet Gynecol* 1970; 35:787.

87. Josey WE: Hypofibrinogenemia complicating uterine rupture: Relationship to amniotic fluid embolism. *Am J Obstet Gynecol* 1966; 94:29.

88. Clark SL: New concepts of amniotic fluid embolism: A review. *Obstet Gynecol Surv* 1990; 45:360.

89. Malinow AM: Embolic disorders, in Chestnut DH (ed): *Obstetric Anesthesia: Principles and Practice.* St. Louis, Mosby, 1994, p 722.

90. Lumley J, Owen R, Morgan M: Amniotic fluid embolism: A report of 3 cases. *Anaesthesia* 1979; 34:33.

91. Schaerf RHM, DeCampo T, Avetta J: Hemodynamic alterations and rapid diagnosis in a case of amniotic fluid embolus. *Anesthesiology* 1977; 46:155.

92. Dolyniuk M, Orfei E, Vania H, et al: Rapid diagnosis of amniotic fluid embolism. *Obstet Gynecol* 1983; 61:28S.

93. Lee W, Ginsburg KA, Cotton DB, et al: Squamous and trophoblastic cells in the maternal pulmonary circulation identified by hemodynamic monitoring during the peripartum period. *Am J Obstet Gynecol* 1986; 155:999.

94. Kabayashi H, Ohi H, Terao T: A simple, noninvasive, sensitive method for diagnosis of amniotic fluid embolism by monoclonal antibody TKH-2 that recognizes NeuAc*2-6GalNAc. *Am J Obstet Gynecol* 1993; 168:848.

95. Ziadlourad F, Conklin KA: Amniotic fluid embolism. *Semin Anesth* 1987; 6:171.

96. Abouleish E: Amniotic fluid embolism and disseminated intravascular coagulopathy, in Ezzat A (ed): *Pain Control in Obstetrics.* Philadelphia, JB Lippincott, 1977, p 160.

97. Shnider SM, Moya F: Amniotic fluid embolism. *Anesthesiology* 1961; 22:108.

98. Phillips OC, Weigel JE, McCarthy JJ: Amniotic fluid embolus: Fundamental considerations and a report of cases. *Obstet Gynecol* 1964; 24:431.

99. Mulder JI: Amniotic fluid embolism: An overview and case report. *Am J Obstet Gynecol* 1985; 152:430.

100. Alon E, Atanassoff PG: Successful cardiopulmonary resuscitation of a parturient with amniotic fluid embolism. *Int J Obstet Anesth* 1992; 1:205.

101. Clark SL: Successful pregnancy outcomes after amniotic fluid embolism. *Am J Obstet Gynecol* 1992; 167:511.

102. Sprung J, Cheng EY, Patel S, et al: Understanding and management of amniotic fluid embolism. *J Clin Anesth* 1992; 4:235.

103. Lesky E: Notes on the history of air embolism. *German Med Monthly* 1961; 6:159.

104. Magendie F: Sur l'entree accidentelle de l'air dans les veines, sur la mort subite, qui en est l'effet; sur les moyens de prevenir cet accident et d'y remedier. *J Physiol Experiment Pathol* 1821; 1:190.

105. Amussat JZ: Recherches sur l'introduction accidentale de l'air dans les veines. *Germer Bailliere* (Paris) 1839; p 255.

106. Senn N: An experimental study of air-embolism. *Ann Surg* 1885; 2:197.

107. Albin MS, Babinski MF, Gilbert TJ: Venous air embolism is not restricted to neurosurgery! *Anesthesiology* 1983; 59:151.

108. Albin MS, Carroll RG, Maroon JC: Clinical considerations concerning detection of venous air embolism. *Neurosurgery* 1978; 3:380.

109. Legallois E: Des maladies occasionees par la resorbtion de pus. *J Heb de Med* 1829; 3:166.

110. Merrill DG, Samuels SI, Silverberg GD: Venous air embolism of uncertain etiology. *Anesth Analg* 1982; 61:65.

111. Younker D, Rodriguez V, Kavanaugh J: Massive air embolism during cesarean section. *Anesthesiology* 1986; 65:77.

112. Rofke F: Luftenbolie de Kaiserschnitt. *Zentralbl Gynakol* 1967; 1:22.

113. Davies DE, Digwood KI, Hilton JH: Air embolism during cesarean section. *Med J Aust* 1980; 1:644.

114. Lowenwirt IP, Chi DS, Handwerker SM: Nonfatal venous air embolism during cesarean section: A case report and review of the literature. *Obstet Gynecol Surv* 1994; 49:72.

115. Nelson PK: Pulmonary gas embolism in pregnancy and the puerperium. *Obstet Gynecol Surv* 1960; 15:449.

116. Klein MD, Clahr J, Tamis AB: Classification and analysis of maternal deaths in Bronx County, N.Y., 1946-1957. *Am J Obstet Gynecol* 1958; 76:1342.

117. Barno A, Freeman DW: Amniotic fluid embolism. *Am J Obstet Gynecol* 1959; 77:1199.

118. Scrimgeour JWF, Carrick JE: Fatal air-embolism associated with ruptured uterus. *Lancet* 1955; 1:485.

119. Malinow AM, Naulty JS, Hunt CO, et al: Precordial ultrasonic monitoring during cesarean delivery. *Anesthesiology* 1987; 66:816.

120. Fong J, Gadalla F, Gimbel AA: Precordial Doppler diagnosis of haemodynamically compromising air embolism during cesarean section. *Can J Anesth* 1990; 37:262.

121. Hill BF, Jones JS: Venous air embolism following orogenital sex during pregnancy. *Am J Emerg Med* 1993; 11:155.

122. Wolffe JB, Robertson HF: Experimental air embolism. *Ann Intern Med* 1935; 9:162.

123. Richardson HF, Coles BC, Hall GE: Experimental gas embolism: I. Intravenous air embolism. *Can Med Assoc J* 1937; 36:584.

124. Durant TM, Long J, Oppenheimer MJ: Pulmonary (venous) air embolism. *Am Heart J* 1947; 33:269.

125. Boyer NH, Curry JJ: Bronchospasm associated with pulmonary embolism. *Arch Intern Med* 1944; 73:403.

126. Wong RT: Air emboli in the retinal arteries. *Arch Ophthalmol* 1941; 25:149.

127. Robinson DA, Albin MS: Parturition and venous air embolism. *Obstet Anesth Dig* 1987; 7:38.
128. Michenfelder JD, Miller RH, Gronert GA: Evaluation of an ultrasonic device (Doppler) for diagnosis of venous air embolism. *Anesthesiology* 1972; 36:164.
129. Vartikar JV, Johnson MD, Datta S: Precordial ultrasonic monitoring and pulse oximetry during cesarean delivery. *Reg Anesth* 1988; 13:57.
130. Karuparthy VR, Downing JW, Husain FJ, et al: The incidence of venous air embolism (VAE) during cesarean section is unchanged by the use of 5-10° head-up tilt. *Anesth Analg* 1989; 69:620.
131. Smalhout B: *A Quick Guide to Capnography and Its Use in Differential Diagnosis.* Boblingen, Hewlett-Packard GmbH, 1983; p 47.
132. Smith SL, Albin MS, Ritter RR, et al: CVP catheter placement from the antecubital veins using a J-wire catheter guide. *Anesthesiology* 1984; 60:238.
133. Artru AA, Colley PS: Bunegin-Albin CVP catheter improves resuscitation from lethal venous air embolism in dogs. *Anesth Analg* 1986; 65:S7.
134. Munson ES, Merrick HC: Effect of nitrous oxide on venous air embolism. *Anesthesiology* 1966; 27:783.
135. Davis FM, Clover PW, Maycock E: Hyperbaric oxygen for cerebral air arterial embolism occurring during cesarean section. *Anesth Intensive Care* 1990; 18:403.

25 The Anticoagulated Patient

David J. Birnbach and *Amos Grunebaum*

Thromboembolic disease in pregnant patients is not rare; the incidence of antepartum deep venous thrombosis is approximately 1 to 2 per 1000.[1] Pregnant and postpartum women are five times more likely to develop a thromboembolic event compared with nonpregnant patients of the same age.[2] Septic pelvic vein thrombosis and puerperal ovarian vein thrombosis occur in pregnancy and may also result in pulmonary embolism. Deep venous thrombosis, however, continues to be the leading cause of pulmonary thromboembolism in the peripartum period. Since anticoagulation is administered to these patients to prevent pulmonary thromboembolism, knowledge about the anesthetic and obstetric implications of anticoagulation is necessary when caring for the high-risk parturient. Anticoagulation is also administered to pregnant patients with other diseases such as atrial fibrillation, and to those with prosthetic cardiac valves. Anticoagulated pregnant patients present a challenge to both the obstetrician and anesthesiologist.

With experience, our knowledge of anticoagulation during pregnancy has been expanding. The use of anticoagulants in pregnancy and the optimum time for discontinuation of therapy remain controversial, with differing opinions not only about the medical and obstetrical approach but also the anesthetic management. The purpose of this chapter is to review existing controversies and to discuss the anesthetic and obstetric options available for management of the pregnant anticoagulated patient.

PATHOPHYSIOLOGY
Indications for anticoagulant therapy in pregnancy

In 1856, Virchow suggested that there were three causative factors to the development of thrombosis: stasis, alteration of the vessel wall, and changes in the blood.[3] There are several physiologic and functional changes that may explain the increased risk of these three factors and hence development of thromboembolic events during pregnancy. These changes include reduced blood flow velocity, elevation of coagulation factors, increased venous distention, and increased stasis.

Anticoagulant therapy during pregnancy has been advocated for the prophylaxis and therapy of several medical conditions, including venous thromboembolic disease, pulmonary embolism, prosthetic heart valves, valvular heart disease with systemic embolization, antiphospholipid syndrome, cardiac surgery, cerebral thrombosis, atrial fibrillation with embolization, and rarely for the treatment of disseminated intravascular coagulation (DIC). The use of anticoagulant therapy has been reported in patients with recurrent pregnancy-induced hypertension, and it has been postulated that the intravascular fibrin deposits in severe preeclampsia may be prevented by anticoagulation.[4]

Venous thromboembolic disease. Thromboembolic disease may have a significant impact on maternal morbidity and mortality. Pulmonary embolism, for example, has been reported to be the second most common cause of maternal morbidity and mortality in Massachusetts.[5] Treatment for thromboembolic disease reduces the complication rate significantly in these patients, as shown by the decrease in the incidence of pulmonary thromboembolism in patients with deep venous thrombosis from 24% to 4.5%, if patients are treated appropriately.[6,7] Parturients at risk for thromboembolic disease are shown in Box 25-1.

Clinical signs and symptoms of deep venous thrombosis vary significantly and depend mostly on the site and the degree of the occlusion. Common clinical manifestations include pain, edema, red or pale skin discoloration, and a positive Homans' sign (calf pain on stretching of the Achilles tendon). Making the correct diagnosis is of utmost importance since the diagnosis of deep venous thrombosis commits the patient to prolonged periods of anticoagulation and may also commit the patient to treatment in future pregnancies.

Although there is some debate regarding the role of impedance plethysmography (IPG), Doppler flow studies, and compression ultrasound in the diagnosis of deep venous thrombosis, the gold standard remains venography.[8] Because venography has several potential complications and carries the risk of radiation exposure to the fetus, noninvasive methods such as Doppler flow measurements,

---

BOX 25-1   PREGNANT PATIENTS AT RISK FOR THROMBOEMBOLIC DISEASE

Thromboembolism during previous pregnancy
Prolonged bed rest
Advanced maternal age
Multiparity
Antithrombin III deficiency
Protein C/Protein S deficiency
Paroxysmal nocturnal hemoglobinuria

---

compression ultrasonography, and IPG are often used as the primary means of screening.[9] It has been reported that venograms are more sensitive than IPG for the diagnosis of venous thrombosis of the calf, whereas IPG and Doppler are considered more sensitive for detection of femoral and iliac thromboses.[10] Some authors advocate the treatment of patients with anticoagulants solely on the basis of positive impedance plethysmography.[11] Others, however, recommend that in the presence of positive or equivocal Doppler examination or impedance plethysmography, venography should be performed before initiation of anticoagulant therapy.[1] Regardless of which means of diagnosis is initially chosen, venography should be performed whenever the diagnosis is equivocal.

Pulmonary embolism. Pulmonary embolism in the pregnant patient is often a catastrophic event. Clinical symptoms of pulmonary embolism are nonspecific and range from mild to severe chest pain, shortness of breath, tachypnea, and hemoptysis to massive hypotension and sudden cardiovascular collapse. The differential diagnosis of these symptoms includes amniotic fluid embolism, air embolism, cardiac decompensation, pneumothorax, and aspiration syndrome. Blood gas analysis, electrocardiogram, and chest x-ray examination are the first steps in the diagnosis, but these tests are often nonspecific. Electrocardiographic changes may include ST-T wave changes, right axis deviation, P pulmonale, T wave inversions and dysrhythmias.[12] Placement of a pulmonary artery catheter will reveal increased pulmonary artery pressure, increased central venous pressure, and normal pulmonary capillary wedge pressure with elevated pulmonary vascular resistance. Pulmonary angiography remains the ultimate means for diagnosis of pulmonary embolism. However, as a first step in the work-up of a patient with a strong clinical suspicion of pulmonary embolism, perfusion lung scanning and tests for deep venous thrombosis should be performed. A satisfactory scan that is read as negative strongly excludes the likelihood of pulmonary embolism. If the perfusion scan is abnormal, a ventilation scan is performed. In the presence of an abnormal ventilation scan without clinical suspicion of deep venous thrombosis, pulmonary angiography is often performed to rule out pulmonary embolism. Echocardiography has also been used to diagnose a pulmonary artery embolus after cesarean section. This and other new techniques may allow for diagnosis using less invasive methods, and they also decrease the radiation to which the fetus would otherwise be exposed.[13]

Atrial fibrillation. Patients with cardiac dysrhythmias are at increased risk of a thromboembolic event. Because most malignant dysrhythmias occur in older patients with ischemic heart conditions, there is only limited experience with this problem in pregnancy, usually associated with rheumatic valvular disease. Paroxysmal atrial tachycardia and persistent atrial tachycardia may also be seen in pregnancy. The drugs of choice in treating arrhythmias in the pregnant patient include quinidine, digoxin, and beta-adrenergic blocking agents. Anticoagulation is often added to prevent arterial embolization. A new source of arrhythmias in pregnancy, which has been on the increase in inner city parturients, is cocaine abuse.

Cardiac surgery during pregnancy. There is very little information available about the management of the pregnant patient for cardiac surgery. Because of the great risk for fetal morbidity and mortality, open heart surgery is generally performed only in emergency situations during pregnancy. Despite the anticoagulation necessary for bypass, there have been reports of maternal and fetal survival after open heart surgery during pregnancy.[14]

Prosthetic cardiac valves. Limet and Crondin calculated that the risk of a nonanticoagulated woman with a prosthetic heart valve having an embolic episode was 1/100 months of exposure.[15] The risk of a thromboembolic event occurring during pregnancy was shown to be reduced from 25% to 5% if the patient with a prosthetic valve was anticoagulated. Maternal and fetal risks, in general, have been linked to the presence or absence of anticoagulation. Hirsh et al[6] have reported that the morbidity and mortality associated with antepartum thromboembolism was 15% in untreated patients. Hall et al,[16] in their review of 65 patients with prosthetic heart valve replacement, reported that the 3 maternal deaths that occurred were all related to thromboembolic events. The "hypercoagulable" state of pregnancy would increase the odds of embolization in the nonanticoagulated parturient, placing these women at an even higher risk of morbidity and mortality. Thus, the risk of withholding anticoagulation in a pregnant patient with a prosthetic heart valve may outweigh the potential risks of the anticoagulation therapy. When maternal risks are carefully weighed against fetal risks, many authors agree that in patients with heart valve prostheses, anticoagulation should be used throughout pregnancy and in the postpartum period as well.[17,18] Buxbaum and co-workers have found that patients who stopped their anticoagulation treatment during pregnancy carried a higher risk than those who never received anticoagulants.[19] Therefore, if anticoagulation therapy is initiated, the treatment should not be prematurely discontinued.

Antiphospholipid syndrome. The antiphospholipid syndrome (APS) is an acquired hypercoagulable state that may precipitate both arterial and venous thrombosis.[20] Since this syndrome was originally described in patients with lupus and many of these patients have an antiphospholipid antibody that prolongs the PTT, it has been given the name lupus anticoagulant.[21] Although many tests can be performed to identify the patient with APS, anticardiolipin antibody is considered to be the most sensitive. Pregnant patients with this syndrome, if untreated, have a high incidence of placental infarction and miscarriage.[20] Although there is some controversy regarding the treatment of these patients, it has been suggested that outcome is improved if patients are anticoagulated.[22]

Disseminated intravascular coagulation. Disseminated intravascular coagulation is produced by intravascular activation of the coagulation cascade, which results in formation of large quantities of thrombin, activation of the fibrinolytic system, depletion of coagulation factors, and ultimately massive bleeding. Possible causes of DIC in pregnancy include amniotic fluid embolism, abruptio placenta, and sepsis. Some authors have advocated the use of heparin to treat DIC secondary to amniotic fluid embolism,[23] sepsis,[24] and where there is evidence of peripheral deposition of fibrin.[25] Many authors, however, feel that the use of anticoagulation in obstetric patients with DIC is unwarranted. A possible indication for anticoagulation may include DIC in patients with fetal demise. The administration of heparin to a patient in whom DIC occurred during a twin pregnancy because of the intrauterine death of one twin allowed the survival of the second twin.[26]

ANTICOAGULANTS

The two anticoagulants commonly used in pregnancy are heparin and warfarin. The advantages and disadvantages of each of these drugs and their implications to the obstetrician and anesthesiologist will be described. The major pharmacologic characteristics of these drugs are listed in Table 25-1.

Table 25-1 Heparin vs. warfarin

	Heparin	Warfarin
Molecular weight	15,000	1000
Route of administration	IV/SC	PO
Placental passage	No	Yes
Breast milk passage	No	Yes
Duration of action	1-3 hr	4-5 days
Mode of action	Antithrombin III	Vitamin K-dependent Factors II, VII, IX, X

Heparin

Heparin is a member of a heterogeneous group of straight chain anionic mucopolysaccharides, called *glycosaminoglycans,* which have molecular weights averaging 15,000 daltons.[27] It is primarily manufactured by extraction from beef lung or porcine intestine. It is acidic because of its covalently linked sulfate and carboxylic acid groups and does not cross the placenta because of its large molecular weight and polarity.[28] Heparin prevents the activation of the intrinsic coagulation pathway, inhibits the thrombin-mediated conversion of fibrinogen to fibrin, increases the circulating level of activated Factor X inhibitor,[29] and at high doses inhibits the aggregation of platelets.[30]

Heparin is not absorbed by the gastrointestinal tract and is usually not given intramuscularly because of the risk of hematoma formation. The anticoagulant effect of heparin is almost immediate after intravenous injection, acting via antithrombin III. This cofactor is an alpha$_2$-globulin that neutralizes several clotting factors. By irreversibly binding with thrombin, antithrombin III causes the inactivation of that protein. Subcutaneous administration of low-dose heparin increases the activity of antithrombin III, and therefore low-dose regimens may produce satisfactory anticoagulation. Heparin is metabolized in the liver by heparinase, and the inactive breakdown products are excreted in the urine. Side effects may be seen, even when heparin dose is within the therapeutic range (Box 25-2).

Prophylactic ("minidose") heparin. Low-dose heparin ("minidose") is given by subcutaneous injection, whereas high-dose regimens are administered by continuous or intermittent intravenous injection. Minidose heparin is widely used in patients at risk for thromboembolic disease. These small

---

BOX 25-2   COMPLICATIONS OF ANTICOAGULATION

General

Hematuria
Melena, hematemesis
Intraperitoneal hemorrhage
Thrombocytopenia
Adrenal hemorrhage
Intracranial hemorrhage
Allergic reactions
Anaphylactic shock
Alopecia
Osteoporosis (prolonged use)

Obstetric

Hemorrhage: Retroperitoneal, incisional, vaginal, cervical, perineal, episiotomy

Anesthetic

Hematoma: Epidural, spinal, subdural
Bleeding in naso-oropharynx

---

doses of heparin work via inhibition of activated Factor X (Xa). Since Factor Xa is required for thrombus formation and is included in both the intrinsic and extrinsic pathways, its inhibition produces anticoagulation. Minidose regimens typically use 5000 to 10,000 U of heparin subcutaneously every 8 to 12 hours. This dose only minimally prolongs the partial thromboplastin time (PTT), and consequently there should be no increased risk of hematoma formation or bleeding.

Therapeutic use of heparin. Therapeutic use of heparin includes an initial intravenous bolus of up to 100 U/kg. This is followed by 15 to 20 U/kg/hr of heparin by continuous intravenous infusion. The goal of therapy is to regulate the PTT levels to 1.5 to 2 times the control values.[31] The duration of therapeutic administration of heparin varies, but treatment is usually continued for at least 7 to 10 days. Some authors, however, have also reported that therapeutic levels were achieved after the administration of large doses of subcutaneous heparin.[32] If intravenous heparin therapy has been initiated during pregnancy, prophylactic subcutaneous use is usually continued after conclusion of the intravenous therapy for the remainder of pregnancy and up to 6 weeks postpartum.

Risk of heparin use in the pregnant patient

Impact on the mother. Patients receiving heparin therapy are at increased risk of hemorrhage. During vaginal delivery there may be prolonged bleeding from a laceration or episiotomy. Patients receiving heparin therapy who have undergone a vaginal delivery without episiotomy or laceration

do not usually have increased blood loss, because hemostasis from the uterus is usually not dependent on coagulation factors. At the time of cesarean section, hemorrhage may occur at the incision site.

Impact on the fetus. Heparin does not cross the placenta and does not appear in the fetal circulation. Some studies have shown increased fetal complications such as miscarriage, stillbirths, and preterm deliveries associated with maternal heparin administration. However, in these cases, heparin was used in patients who were at risk for developing these complications. There is no firm evidence that maternal use of heparin in itself (rather than the disease process for which it is being given) leads to increased fetal loss.

Heparin therapy for patients approaching labor. For patients at high risk of thromboembolism, prophylactic heparin therapy of 5000 units subcutaneously every 12 hours may be continued throughout labor. At these doses, significant changes in the coagulation profile causing bleeding are rarely encountered. We recommend that activated partial thromboplastin time (aPTT) be closely followed at least every 4 to 6 hours as well as before initiation of any regional anesthetic or invasive procedure (e.g., placement of a central venous line) during this critical period. Reversal of anticoagulation should be considered for labor and delivery in the presence of an abnormal coagulation profile (Fig. 25-1). Other suggestions have included discontinuing heparin administration about 4 to 6 hours before delivery. Considering the short half-life of heparin, PTT levels should then be normal at the time of delivery.

Heparin therapy in the postpartum patient. Optimally, prophylaxis for patients at risk for thromboembolic disease should continue throughout delivery and into the postpartum period. However, potential maternal risks of therapy (e.g., hemorrhage and hematoma) must be carefully weighed against the benefits. The following are some guidelines for postpartum anticoagulation in different clinical settings:

1. Vaginal delivery with no lacerations or episiotomy and in absence of regional anesthesia. Coagulation therapy may be reinitiated immediately after delivery.
2. Vaginal delivery with lacerations or episiotomy. Coagulation therapy may be restarted 4 to 6 hours after delivery and repair. Close attention should be paid to prevent hematoma formation.
3. Cesarean delivery. Coagulation therapy may be started 6 hours postoperatively.
   A. General anesthesia. Anticoagulation may be started at any time, as per obstetric guidelines.

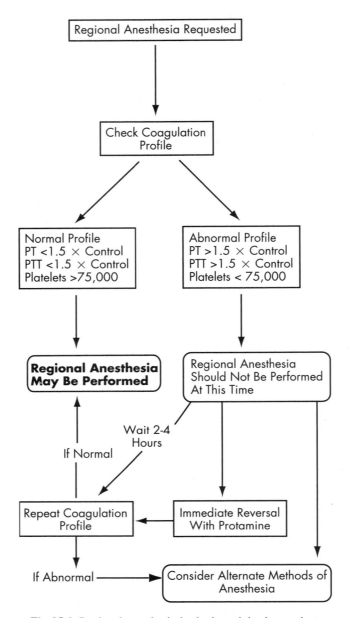

Fig 25-1 Regional anesthesia in the heparinized parturient.

B. Regional anesthesia with no visible bleeding during initiation. Anticoagulation can be started at any time. Some advocate waiting 4 to 6 hours.

C. Regional anesthesia where bleeding occurred during initiation. Delay anticoagulation for at least 12 hours if possible; careful postoperative monitoring for signs of epidural hematoma formation.

Heparin antagonists. If a situation arises in which the acute reversal of heparin becomes necessary, such as the occurrence of severe bleeding, protamine sulfate may be administered intravenously as a specific heparin antagonist. Protamine is a low molecular weight protein found in the sperm or testes of salmon. When administered alone protamine has an anticoagulant effect. However, when given to a heparinized patient, it combines ionically with heparin to form a complex that no longer has anticoagulant activity.[27] One of several methods used to determine the dose of protamine needed for reversal of heparin is the administration of 1 to 1.3 mg of protamine for every 100 U of heparin remaining in the patient.[33] Adequacy of reversal can be demonstrated by repeated coagulation studies or by a return to normal of an activated clotting time (ACT). Protamine must be administered by slow intravenous injection at a rate of less than 20 mg/min. Adverse reactions that may occur during rapid injection include immediate or delayed anaphylactoid reactions with flushing, bradycardia, hypotension dyspnea, and pulmonary hypertension.[34] Hypersensitivity reactions, including anaphylactic reactions, have been reported following administration of protamine, especially in those patients with previous exposure to protamine (including protamine-containing insulins) and allergies to fish. The pulmonary hypertension that is seen is thought to be mediated by release of thromboxane C5A.[35]

Oral anticoagulation

Warfarin sodium is the most commonly used oral anticoagulant in the United States. It acts by interfering with the hepatic synthesis of vitamin K–dependent clotting Factors II, VII, IX, and X. Although hypermetabolic states usually increase the responsiveness to oral anticoagulants, it has been shown that pregnancy causes a decreased responsiveness due to increased activity of Factors VII, IX, and X.[36] There is, therefore, an increased drug requirement to achieve anticoagulation in pregnancy. Unlike heparin, warfarin does cross the placenta. Since the fetus lacks mature liver enzymes, it is highly susceptible to the effects of oral anticoagulants. Because of the difference between maternal and fetal pharmacodynamics, the effects of warfarin lasts 4 to 5 days in the mother but up to 14 days in the fetus.[37] There are many reported drug interactions with oral anticoagulants. Aspirin, phenothiazines, and phenylbutazone increase warfarin's activity while barbiturates decrease its activity.

When reversal of an oral anticoagulant becomes necessary, the parenteral administration of vitamin K (phytonadione) will return the prothrombin time (PT) to the normal range within 24 to 48 hours. If immediate reversal is necessary, the use of fresh frozen plasma has been advocated.[38] The anticoagulant effects in the fetus may take up to 14 days to subside, but this time period may be reduced to less than 48 hours by the intravenous administration of vitamin K to the fetus.[39] Maternally administered vitamin K crosses the placenta, and therefore it may also enhance the rate of formation of fetal coagulation factors. After delivery, the newborn should receive intramuscular vitamin K if the mother had oral anticoagulants reversed before delivery. If the newborn shows signs of bleeding, fresh frozen plasma can also be considered.

Because of the potential for the development of an epidural hematoma, regional anesthesia poses a risk to the parturient receiving anticoagulant therapy.[40] In the case of heparin, this risk is not only due to heparin's intended anticoagulant effects but also to the potential for thrombocytopenia.[41] This platelet abnormality may occur in up to 30% of heparinized patients and has been found to be unrelated to the heparin dose.[42] An immunologic etiology has been postulated to explain this potentially dangerous side effect.[43]

OBSTETRIC MANAGEMENT

During the past 40 years, since the first description of a successful pregnancy in a patient with a prosthetic heart valve,[44] there have been many reports of successful outcomes in anticoagulated pregnant patients.[45,46] Many authors now advocate the use of heparin in pregnancy because of the potential fetal disadvantages of oral anticoagulants. These disadvantages include the risk of intrauterine fetal death and/or congenital malformations.[47] Administration of vitamin K antagonists such as warfarin during the first 8 weeks of gestation has been reported to result in the following possible malformations: nasal hypoplasia, stippling of bones, ophthalmologic abnormalities, and intrauterine growth retardation. Administration of oral anticoagulants during the later part of pregnancy may cause fetal or placental hemorrhage and may present a problem at the time of labor and delivery should rapid reversal of anticoagulation become necessary.[48] Some authors, however, advocate the use of oral anticoagulants, and there is some evidence that warfarin sodium may be more effective than subcutaneous heparin in preventing recurrent venous thromboembolism.[49]

Heparin has several advantages when anticoagulation is necessary in the pregnant patient. It does not cross the placenta, and if therapy is discontinued at the onset of labor or several hours before cesarean section, there should be no residual anticoagulation at the time of delivery.[50] Heparin, however, is not without fetal side effects, and it may be associated with stillbirths, spontaneous abortions, and prematurity. There has also been a report of a maternal death in a patient with a prosthetic heart valve in whom heparin therapy did not prevent thrombus formation. This thrombus eventually immobilized the prosthetic mitral valve.[51]

There appears to be no ideal anticoagulant regimen for use in pregnancy, but a compromise approach might be to use both heparin and warfa-

Table 25-2 Combination anticoagulation regimen

Weeks of gestation	Drug
Diagnosis-13	Heparin
13-26	Warfarin
26-Delivery	Heparin
Labor and delivery	Protamine if necessary

rin, each at different times of gestation. Heparin can be used for anticoagulation early in pregnancy and at the time of delivery; warfarin can be administered during the remainder of the pregnancy.[52] See Table 25-2.

ANESTHETIC MANAGEMENT
Regional anesthesia in the anticoagulated parturient

Regional anesthetic implications of anticoagulation. If the therapeutic decision has been made to anticoagulate a patient during pregnancy, the anesthetic management will be affected. The anesthesiologist, therefore, should be consulted at an early stage. Choices of anticoagulant, maternal and fetal effects of anticoagulants, the decision of when to reverse the anticoagulation as delivery approaches, and the method to accomplish this reversal must all be considered when formulating an anesthetic plan for an anticoagulated parturient. Of all the potential complications of a spinal or epidural anesthetic, bleeding into the spinal canal is the most serious, because this bleeding is hidden from observation. Because spinal space is nonexpandable, continued bleeding usually progresses to spinal cord compression and neurologic dysfunction.[53]

In 1911, Cooke first recognized that local hemorrhage could result from lumbar puncture.[54] Since then, there have been numerous reports of spinal epidural and subarachnoid hemorrhages following spinal and epidural anesthesia in the anticoagulated patient.[55-57] Case reports have also described the development of hematomas when anticoagulation was initiated shortly after a lumbar puncture.[58] This has important implications when considering the reinitiation of anticoagulation in the postpartum period of a patient who has had a spinal or epidural anesthetic for labor and delivery. Saka and Marx, citing a case in which extradural hematoma formation occurred when heparin therapy was started 20 minutes after initiation of an epidural, have suggested that heparin not be restarted until 24 hours after delivery. However, there have been several reports of uneventful regional anesthetics initiated shortly before anticoagulation.[59] Gothard described the uncomplicated management of a par-

turient with a cardiac valve in whom heparin was restarted 3 hours after delivery.[60] Rao and El-Etr, in a study on anticoagulation following placement of epidural and subarachnoid catheters in nonpregnant patients, have reported that there was no incidence of neurologic complications arising from anticoagulant therapy after epidural or subarachnoid catheterization. However, if fresh heme was aspirated any time during the procedure, the regional technique was abandoned and the patient was rescheduled for surgery under general anesthesia for the following day.[61] Odoom and coworkers have similarly reported their experience with lumbar epidural blocks in patients who received preoperative and intraoperative anticoagulation. They also reported that there were no cases of neurologic sequelae.[62]

Spinal epidural hematoma. Spinal epidural hematomas, as previously mentioned, are exceedingly rare. Early recognition and treatment are vital if permanent neurologic disability is to be prevented. Because of the rarity of epidural hematoma, it may go unrecognized until permanent neurologic sequelae have developed. Therefore, anyone caring for patients who have received regional anesthesia should be acquainted with the signs and symptoms of a developing epidural hematoma. These signs include pain at the spinal level involved, radiculopathy, and eventually sensory and motor deficits. Although many reports have described back or radicular pain as the first symptom of a spinal epidural hematoma, the first presentation may be muscle weakness or urinary retention. The neurologic damage is thought to be secondary to spinal cord ischemia associated with compression by the hematoma. Once the differential diagnosis of epidural hematoma is entertained, radiologic examinations should be performed. The preferred method to rule out the presence of an epidural hematoma is a contrast computed tomographic scan followed by myelography or magnetic resonance imaging. Once the diagnosis of epidural hematoma is made, a neurosurgeon should be consulted immediately so that decompression can be performed. Since rapid decompression is so vital in preventing permanent nerve damage,[63] the neurosurgeon should be consulted at an early stage so that any necessary preparations can be made should the radiologic findings prove positive.[53]

Despite the reports of hematomas following regional anesthesia, it should be appreciated that these complications are very rare. Usubiaga, in his classic study of neurologic complications following epidural anesthesia, found that the incidence of serious neurologic sequelae following epidural analgesia was less than 1 in 10,000 procedures.[65] Likewise, in the combined series of Van Dam and

Dripps,[66] Moore and Bridenbaugh,[67] Phillips,[68] and Sadove[69] (totalling more than 50,000 spinals), there were no reported cases of spinal epidural hematoma. In a very large series, Lund reported 150,000 cases of epidural anesthesia without a single case of hematoma.[70] Allemann et al studied both epidural and spinal anesthetics performed on orthopedic patients who received 5000 U heparin preoperatively and postoperatively and found no cases of neurologic dysfunction.[71] Lowson and Goodchild reported on a retrospective review of 5 years of clinical practice on patients who received spinal and epidural anesthetics associated with heparin prophylaxis. These authors used 22-gauge spinal or 16-gauge epidural needles, and if a blood vessel was punctured the procedure was repeated at another interspace. They reported no neurologic complications.[72]

The risk of developing a hemorrhagic complication following low-dose subcutaneous heparin is controversial. In one study, which evaluated orthopedic patients who received 5000 U heparin subcutaneously, the authors found that there was a wide variation in the range of PTT values.[73] Although exceedingly rare, there is a report of an epidural hematoma associated with an epidural anesthetic in a patient receiving low-dose heparin therapy. Darnat et al have reported the case of a patient who was given an epidural for chronic pain despite the administration of 5000 U of heparin every 12 hours. This patient developed an epidural hematoma and complete paraplegia, which did not respond to surgical intervention.[74]

Postoperative vigilance on the part of nurses and physicians caring for these patients is paramount. Signs of impending hematoma typically include backache, radicular pain, bowel or bladder dysfunction, weakness, sensory loss, or pain at the epidural site. Should any of these signs or symptoms develop postpartum, emergency anesthetic and neurosurgic consultation should be requested immediately.

Aspirin. The effect of aspirin on the course of preeclampsia has been studied,[75,76] and it has been found that the administration of aspirin to these patients may sometimes favorably influence the course of pregnancy-induced hypertension (PIH). Daily doses of aspirin may actually reduce the incidence of PIH in women at high risk. Aspirin given to low-risk patients, however, may increase the risk of abruptio placenta.[77] There is some controversy surrounding the benefits of aspirin, however. A large multicenter study examining aspirin use to prevent pregnancy-induced hypertension found no difference between groups in regard to perinatal mortality, birthweight, or PIH.[78] An accompanying editorial stated that "it is too early to

turn full circle again on aspirin in pregnancy. It may be timely, though, to ask for more evidence before indications for its use continue to expand."[79]

Preeclampsia may be ultimately manifested because of an imbalance in the production of the vasoactive prostaglandins thromboxane and prostacyclin, leading to vasoconstriction of small arteries and activation of platelets.[80] The administration of aspirin inhibits cyclooxygenase, thereby reducing the levels of cyclic endoperoxidases synthesized from arachidonic acid.[81] This reduces the concentration of arachidonic acid derivatives including the potent vasoconstrictor thromboxane A2.[82] Studies in animal models indicate that the antithrombotic effects of aspirin also involve pathways other than the inhibition of cyclooxygenase. Buchanan and co-workers have reported that aspirin prolongs the bleeding time in a dose-dependent manner and that it is not dependent on platelet aggregation, thereby showing that aspirin has an antithrombotic mechanism in addition to cyclooxygenase inhibition.[83]

Although aspirin is not considered an anticoagulant per se, it has significant clinical antithrombotic effects. Therefore, its use in the parturient may alter the coagulation status; this can have serious implications for administration of spinal and epidural anesthesia. The alteration of hemostatic function varies with the dose administered; low-dose aspirin will prevent platelet aggregate formation at the injured vessel wall, whereas high-dose aspirin may promote platelet thrombus formation.[84] The administration of aspirin blocks the release of platelet adenosine diphosphate (ADP), which is necessary for platelet clumping and for the growth of the platelet plug.[85] Aspirin has also been found to have a hypothrombinemic effect as well as a fibrinolytic effect.[86] A reliable indicator of platelet function after aspirin administration is the bleeding time, which is increased by an average of 50% at 2 hours after ingestion of an oral dose of 600 mg of aspirin.[87] The period of abnormal bleeding time is approximately 7 days, which is roughly equal to the life span of the exposed platelet. The maximal inhibition of platelet ADP release is achieved with the salicylate concentration of 0.5 mmol/L, the approximate concentration obtained by the ingestion of 640 mg of aspirin.[88]

There have been clinical reports of excessive blood loss in the perioperative period in patients who ingested aspirin preoperatively.[89] The development of an epidural hematoma associated with regional anesthesia in a parturient receiving aspirin therapy could have disastrous consequences. There may even be a risk of developing an epidural hematoma without a neuraxial block; there has been a report of an acute spontaneous spinal epidural hematoma developing in a patient taking aspirin who did not receive a regional anesthetic.[90]

There is no way for an anesthesiologist to know the exact platelet count or bleeding time at which a patient will develop an epidural hematoma. Therefore, the decision of when it is advisable to initiate an epidural block in a parturient receiving aspirin therapy is a difficult one. Benzon et al have studied the use of regional anesthesia after aspirin ingestion and have reported the successful use of epidurals and spinals in patients receiving aspirin therapy who have had bleeding times up to 10.5 minutes. There were no signs or symptoms of the development of spinal cord compression or epidural hematoma in any of the 87 patients who had taken aspirin before the administration of regional anesthetic. These authors also found no differences in the bleeding time between chronic or acute aspirin ingestion.[91]

Bleeding time. The performance of a bleeding time to assess the risk of epidural hematoma formation in the anticoagulated patient is very controversial. A meta-analysis reviewing over 1000 publications failed to demonstrate a statistical correlation between clinical bleeding and the bleeding time.[92] A recent editorial in *Lancet* suggested that the bleeding time was of little relevance in individual patients prior to epidural or spinal anesthesia.[93] This editorial, however, did state that "used judiciously, the bleeding time deserves to remain as part of the assessment of individual patients with histories suggestive of bleeding disorders." On the other hand, in a review of the use of bleeding time, Lind has suggested that "review of the medical literature shows that there is no evidence that a prolonged preoperative bleeding time predicts which patients will experience excessive surgical bleeding."[94]

Thromboelastography (TEG). This technique, which has recently become popular, was actually first described in 1948. Although its popularity stems from increased use in liver transplantation and cardiac surgery, it has also found a niche in the obstetric suite. TEG allows for a global assessment of hemostatic function based on interaction between platelet, coagulation, and fibrinogen systems. On a single sample, the TEG measures all phases of coagulation and clot stability and can therefore be used as a bedside measure of the viscoelastic changes that occur as coagulation advances.[95] There is little data at this time, however, to support the routine use of TEG as a guide to clinical decisions regarding the use of a spinal or epidural anesthetic in the parturient.

SUMMARY

The use of regional anesthesia (spinal or epidural) for labor or operative delivery is relatively contraindicated in anticoagulated parturients because of the potential for bleeding into the epidural or subarachnoid space, unless coagulation can be normalized before the procedure. The use of these anesthetic techniques shortly after or just before anticipated anticoagulation therapy remains controversial. In a study by Blomberg and Olsson,[96] where epiduroscopy was used to examine the lumbar epidural space, bleeding was noted in 50% of the patients after placement of an 18-gauge epidural needle. Thus, the risk of traumatizing a blood vessel during the administration of spinal or epidural anesthesia is real, and the anesthesiologist must ensure that the coagulation status has returned to normal before initiating regional anesthesia in a parturient who has been recently anticoagulated.

The reheparinization of a patient who has recently received a regional anesthetic is another controversial area. There have been reports of the development of a hematoma when anticoagulation closely followed spinal or epidural anesthesia, prompting some authors to advocate waiting 12 to 24 hours before restarting the heparin therapy. Recent evidence, however, suggests that if there was no bleeding at the time of initiation of the anesthetic, heparin can be started without delay.

Although there have been articles written in support of or opposition to the use of regional anesthesia in the anticoagulated parturient, little has been written regarding the risks and benefits of general anesthesia in these patients. In weighing the risks of general anesthesia against regional anesthesia, one must consider the physiologic changes of pregnancy that increase the risks associated with the induction of general anesthesia in the pregnant patient. If general anesthesia does become necessary in the anticoagulated patient, the anesthesiologist should be experienced and should make every effort to ensure an atraumatic laryngoscopy to avoid airway trauma and bleeding.

The main arguments against using anticoagulants in the antepartum period are maternal hemorrhage and intrauterine fetal death. However, it has been shown that maternal hemorrhage in a patient receiving therapeutic-dose anticoagulant therapy does not represent a therapeutic risk. Although there are still authors advocating the use of oral anticoagulants in pregnancy, most obstetricians now use heparin throughout pregnancy because of its lack of placental passage and ease of reversal. In a recent review article, Vandermeulen and colleagues summarized the issue of anticoagulation in the pregnant patient, stating that "the risk of fatal pulmonary thromboembolism because of an omitted thromboprophylactic treatment probably exceeds the risk of spinal hemorrhage with the combination of unfractionated heparin or low molecular weight heparin with central nervous blockade."[64]

Anesthetic management of the anticoagulated parturient need not be a middle-of-the-night dilemma or disaster waiting to happen, as long as there is advance planning and communication between obstetrician, internist, and anesthesiologist.

REFERENCES

1. Weiner CP: Diagnosis and management of thromboembolic disease during pregnancy. *Clin Obstet Gynecol* 1985; 28:107.
2. Laros RK, Alger LS: Thromboembolism and pregnancy. *Clin Obstet Gynecol* 1979; 22:871.
3. Virchow R: Phlogose und thrombose in gefass system, in Virchow R (ed): *Gesamelte Abhandlungen zur wissenschaflichen medecin.* Frankfurt, Von Medinger Sohn, 1856, p 458.
4. Valentine H, Baker JL: Treatment of recurrent pregnancy induced hypertension by prophylactic anticoagulation. *Br J Obstet Gynaecol* 1977; 84:309.
5. Sachs BP, Brown DAJ, Driscoll SG, et al: Maternal mortality in Massachusetts: Trends and prevention. *N Engl J Med* 1987; 316:667.
6. Hirsh J, Cade JF, Gallus AS: Anticoagulants in pregnancy: A review of indications and complications. *Am Heart J* 1972; 83:301.
7. Villasanta U: Thromboembolic disease in pregnancy. *Am J Obstet Gynecol* 1965; 93:142.
8. Anderson DR, Lensing AW, Wells PS, et al: Limitations of impedance plethysmography in the diagnosis of clinically suspected deep vein thrombosis. *Ann Intern Med* 1993; 118:25.
9. Polak JF, Wilkinson DL: Ultrasonographic diagnosis of symptomatic deep venous thrombosis in pregnancy. *Am J Obstet Gynecol* 1991; 165:625.
10. Rutherford SE, Phelan JP: Deep venous thrombosis and pulmonary embolus, in Clark SL, Cotton DB, Hankins GDV, et al (eds): *Critical Care Obstetrics,* Boston, Blackwell Scientific, 1991, p 158.
11. Hull RD, Hirsh J, Carter C, et al: Diagnostic efficacy of impedance plethysmography for clinically suspected deep-vein thrombosis: A randomized trial. *Ann Intern Med* 1985; 102:21.
12. Sipes SL, Weiner CP: Venous thromboembolic disease in pregnancy. *Semin Perinatol* 1990; 14:103.
13. Rosenberg JM, Lefor AT, Kenien G, et al: Echocardiographic diagnosis and surgical treatment of postpartum pulmonary embolism. *Ann Thoracic Surg* 1990; 49:667.
14. Harthorne JW, Buckley MJ, Grover JW, et al: Valve replacement during pregnancy. *Ann Intern Med* 1967; 67:1032.
15. Limet R, Crondin CM: Cardiac valve prosthesis, anticoagulation, and pregnancy. *Ann Thorac Surg* 1977; 23:337.
16. Hall JG, Pauli RM, Wislon KM: Maternal and fetal sequelae of anticoagulation during pregnancy. *Am J Med* 1980; 68:122.
17. Tejani N: Anticoagulant therapy with cardiac valve prosthesis during pregnancy. *Obstet Gynecol* 1973; 42:785.
18. Gordon G, O'Laughlin JA: Successful pregnancies in two patients with a Starr-Edwards heart valve prosthesis. *J Obstet Gynecol Br Commonw* 1969; 76:73.
19. Buxbaum A, Aygen M, Shahin W, et al: Pregnancy in patients with prosthetic heart valves. *Chest* 1971; 59:639.
20. Many A, Pauzner R, Carp M: Treatment of patients with antiphospholipid antibodies during pregnancy. *Am J Reprod Immunol* 1992; 28:216.
21. Manucci PM, Canciani MT, Mari D, et al: The varied sensitivity of partial thromboplastin and prothrombin time reagents in the demonstration of the lupus-like anticoagulant. *Scand J Haematol* 1979; 22:423.
22. Reece AE, Gabrielli, Cullen MF, et al: Recurrent adverse pregnancy outcome and antiphospholipid antibodies. *Am J Obstet Gynecol* 1990; 163:162.
23. Brandjes DP, Schenk BE, Beutler E, et al: Management of disseminated intravascular coagulation in obstetrics. *Eur J Obstet Gynaecol Reprod Biol* 1991; 42:S87.
24. Risberg B, Andreasson S, Eriksson E: Disseminated intravascular coagulation. *Acta Anaesthesiol Scand* 1991; 35(S):60.
25. Feinstein DI: Diagnosis and management of disseminated intravascular coagulation: The role of heparin therapy. *Blood* 1982; 60:284.
26. Romero R, Duffy TP, Berkowitz R, et al: Prolongation of a preterm pregnancy complicated by death of a single twin in utero and disseminated intravascular coagulation. *N Engl J Med* 1984; 310:772.
27. O'Reilly RA: Anticoagulant, antithrombotic, and thrombolytic drugs, in Gilman AG, Goodman LS, Rall TW (eds): *Goodman and Gilman's The Pharmacologic Basis of Therapeutics,* ed 7, New York, Macmillan, 1985, p 1338-1359.
28. Flesa HC, Kapstrom AB, Glueck HI, et al: Placental transport of heparin. *Am J Obstet Gynecol* 1965; 93:570.
29. Rosenberg RD: Actions and interactions of antithrombin and heparin. *N Engl J Med* 1975; 292:146.
30. Deykin D: The use of heparin: Current concepts. *N Engl J Med* 1969; 280:937.
31. Bonnar J: Venous thromboembolism and pregnancy. *Clin Obstet Gynecol* 1981; 8:455.
32. Hull R, Delmore T, Carter C, et al: Adjusted subcutaneous heparin versus warfarin sodium in the long term treatment of venous thrombosis. *N Engl J Med* 1982; 306:189.
33. Bull BS, Korpman RA, Huse WM, et al: Heparin therapy during extra-corporeal circulation. II. The use of a dose response curve to individualize heparin and protamine dosage. *J Thorac Cardiovasc Surg* 1975; 69:674.
34. Morel DR, Zapol WM, Thomas SJ, et al: C5A and thromboxane generation associated with pulmonary vaso and bronchoconstriction during protamine reversal of heparin. *Anesthesiology* 1987; 66:597.
35. Weiss ME, Nyhan D, Peng Z, et al: Association of protamine IgE and IgG antibodies with life-threatening reactions to intravenous protamine. *N Engl J Med* 1989; 320:886.
36. Breckenridge A, Orme MI: Kinetics of warfarin absorption in man. *Clin Pharmacol Ther* 1973; 14:955.
37. Pridmore BR, Murray KH, McAllen PM: The management of anticoagulant therapy during and after pregnancy. *Br J Obstet Gynaecol* 1975; 82:740.
38. Jenkins BS, Braimbridge MV: Management of anticoagulant therapy during pregnancy in patients with prosthetic heart valves. *Thorax* 1971; 26:206.
39. Larsen JF, Jacobsen B, Holm HH: Intrauterine injection of vitamin K before delivery during anticoagulant therapy of the mother. *Acta Obstet Gynecol Scand* 1978; 57:227.
40. DeAngelis J: Hazards of subdural and epidural anesthesia during anticoagulant therapy: A case report and review. *Anesth Analg* 1972; 51:676.

41. Powers PJ, Cuthbert D, Hirsh J: Thrombocytopenia found uncommonly during heparin therapy. *JAMA* 1979; 241: 2396.859

42. Bell WR, Tomasulo PA, Alving BM, et al: Thrombocytopenia occurring during administration of heparin. *Ann Intern Med* 1976; 85:155.

43. Wahl TO, Lipschitz DA, Stechschulte DJ: Thrombocytopenia associated with antiheparin antibody. *JAMA* 1978; 240:2560.

44. Canfield MC, Edgar AL, Kimball AP: Successful completion of pregnancy in a patient with Hufnagel valve. *Calif Med* 1958; 88:54.

45. Gothard JW: Heart disease in pregnancy. *Anaesthesia* 1978; 33:523.

46. Hirsh J, Cade JF, O'Sullivan EF: Clinical experience with anticoagulant therapy during pregnancy. *Br Med J* 1970; 1:270.

47. Shaul WL, Hall JG: Multiple congenital anomalies associated with oral anticoagulants. *Am J Obstet Gynecol* 1977; 127:191.

48. ONeill H, Blake S, Sugrue D, et al: Problems in the management of patients with artificial valves during pregnancy. *Br J Obstet Gynecol* 1982; 89:940.

49. Hull R, Delmore T, Genton E, et al: Warfarin sodium versus low-dose heparin in the long term treatment of venous thrombosis. *N Engl J Med* 1979; 301:855.

50. Ginsberg JS, Hirsh J: Use of anticoagulants during pregnancy. *Chest* 1989; 95:156S.

51. Bennett GG, Oakley CM: Pregnancy in a patient with a mitral valve prosthesis. *Lancet* 1968; 1:616.

52. Lee PK, Wang RYC, Chow JSF, et al: Combined use of warfarin and adjusted subcutaneous heparin during pregnancy in patients with artificial heart valves. *J Am Coll Cardiol* 1986; 8:221.

53. Dickman CA, Shedd SA, Spetzler RF, et al: Spinal epidural hematoma associated with epidural anesthesia. *Anesthesiology* 1990; 72:947.

54. Cooke JV: Hemorrhage into the cauda equina following lumbar puncture. *Proc Pathol Soc Phila* 1911; 14:104.

55. Greensite FS, Katz J: Spinal subdural hematoma associated with attempted epidural anesthesia and subsequent continuous spinal anesthesia. *Anesth Analg* 1980; 59:72.

56. Edelson RN, Chernik NL, Posner JB: Spinal subdural hematomas complicating lumbar puncture. *Arch Neurol* 1974; 31:134.

57. Owens EL, Kasten GW, Hessel EA: Spinal subarachnoid hematoma after lumbar puncture and heparinization. *Anesth Analg* 1986; 65:1201.

58. Gingrich TF: Spinal epidural hematoma following continuous epidural anesthesia. *Anesthesiology* 1968; 29:162.

59. Saka DM, Marx GF: Management of a parturient with cardiac valve prosthesis. *Anesth Analg* 1976; 55:214.

60. Gothard JW: Heart disease in pregnancy. *Anaesthesia* 1978; 33:523.

61. Rao TLK, El-Etr A: Anticoagulation following placement of epidural and subarachnoid catheters. *Anesthesiology* 1981; 55:618.

62. Odoom JA, Sih I: Epidural analgesia and anticoagulant therapy: Experience with 1,000 cases of continuous epidurals. *Anaesthesia* 1983; 38:254.

63. Hew-Wing P, Rolbin SH, Hew E, et al: Epidural anaesthesia and thrombocytopenia. *Anaesthesia* 1989; 44:775.

64. Vandermeulen EP, Van Aken H, Vermylen J: Anticoagulants and spinal-epidural anesthesia. *Anesth Analg* 1994; 79:1165.

65. Usubiaga JE: Neurologic complications following epidural anesthesia. *Int Anesth Clin* 1975; 13:1.

66. Vandam LD, Dripps RD: Long term followup of patients who received 10,098 spinal anesthetics. *JAMA* 1960; 172:1483.

67. Moore DC, Bridenbaugh LD: Spinal (subarachnoid) block: A review of 11,574 cases. *JAMA* 1966; 195:907.

68. Phillips OC, Ebner H, Nelson AT, et al: Neurologic complications following spinal anesthesia with lidocaine: A prospective review of 10,440 cases. *Anesthesiology* 1969; 30:284.

69. Sadove MS, Levin MJ, Rant-Sejdinaj I: Neurologic complications of spinal anesthesia. *Can Anaesth Soc J* 1961; 8:405.

70. Lund PC: Peridural anesthesia. Springfield, Mo., Charles C Thomas, 1966.

71. Allemann BH, Gerber H, Gruber UF: Peri-spinal anesthesia and subcutaneous administration of low-dose heparin-dihydergot for prevention of thromboembolism. *Anaesthetist* 1983; 32:80.

72. Lowson SM, Goodchild CS: Low-dose heparin therapy and spinal anesthesia. *Anaesthesia* 1989; 44:67.

73. Poller L, Taberner DA, Sandilands DG, et al: An evaluation of APTT monitoring of low-dose heparin dosage in hip surgery. *Thromb Haemost* 1982; 47:50.

74. Darnat S, Guggiari M, Grob R, et al: Lumbar epidural haematoma following the setting-up of an epidural catheter. *Ann Fr Anesth Reanim* 1986; 5:550.

75. Wallenburg HCS, Dekker GA, Makovitz JW, et al: Low-dose aspirin prevents pregnancy induced hypertension and preeclampsia in angiotensin sensitive primigravidae. *Lancet* 1986; 1:1.

76. Benigni A, Gregorini G, Frusca T, et al: Effect of low dose aspirin on fetal and maternal generation of thromboxane by platelets in women at risk for pregnancy induced hypertension. *N Engl J Med* 1989; 321:351.

77. Sibai BM, Caritis S, Phillips E, et al: Prevention of preeclampsia: Low dose aspirin in nulliparous women. *N Engl J Med* 1993; 329:1213.

78. Italian study of aspirin in pregnancy. Low-dose aspirin in prevention and treatment of intrauterine growth retardation and pregnancy-induced hypertension. *Lancet* 1993; 341: 396.

79. Keirse MJ: Low-dose aspirin in pregnancy (editorial). *Lancet* 1993; 341:412.

80. Fitzgerald DJ, Entman SS, Mulloy K, et al: Decreased prostacyclin biosynthesis preceding the clinical manifestation of pregnancy induced hypertension. *Circulation* 1987; 75:956.

81. Moncada S, Flower RJ, Vane JR: Prostaglandins, prostacyclin, thromboxane A2, and leukotrienes, in Gilman AG, Goodman LS, Rall TW (eds): *Goodman and Gilman's Pharmacologic Basis of Therapeutics,* ed 7. New York, Macmillan, 1985, pp 660-673.

82. Buchanan MR, Rischke JA, Hirsh J: Aspirin inhibits platelet function independent of the acetylation of cyclooxygenase. *Thromb Res* 1982; 25:363.

83. Bhagwat SS, Hamann PR, Still WC, et al: Synthesis and structure of the platelet aggregation factor thromboxane A2. *Nature* 1985; 315:511.

84. O'Grady J, Moncada S: Aspirin: A paradoxical effect on bleeding time. *Lancet* 1978; 2:780.

85. Zucker MB, Peterson J: Inhibition of adenosine diphosphate induced secondary aggregation and other platelet functions by acetylsalicylic acid ingestion. *Proc Soc Exp Biol Med* 1968; 127:547.

86. Cattaneo M, Chahil A, Somers D, et al: Effect of aspirin and sodium salicylate on thrombosis, fibrinolysis, prothrombin time, and platelet survival in rabbits with indwelling aortic catheters. *Blood* 1983; 61:353.

87. Harker LA, Slichter SJ: The bleeding time as a screening

test for evaluation of platelet function. *N Engl J Med* 1972; 287:155.

88. Weiss HJ, Aledort LM, Kochwa S: The effect of salicylates on the hemostatic properties of platelets in man. *J Clin Invest* 1968; 47:2169.

89. Davies DW, Steward DJ: Unexpected excessive bleeding during operation: Role of acetylsalicylic acid. *Can Anaesth Soc J* 1977; 24:452.

90. Locke GE, Giorgio AJ, Biggons SL: Acute spinal epidural hematoma secondary to aspirin-induced prolonged bleeding. *Surg Neurol* 1976; 5:292.

91. Benzon HT, Brunner EA, Vaisrub N: Bleeding time and nerve blocks after aspirin. *Reg Anaesth* 1984; 9:86.

92. Rodgers RPC, Levin J: A critical reappraisal of the bleeding time. *Semin Thromb Hemost* 1990; 16:1.

93. The bleeding time (editorial). *Lancet* 1991; 337:1447.

94. Lind SE: The bleeding time does not predict surgical bleeding. *Blood* 1991; 77:2547.

95. Orlikowski CE, Payne AJ, Moodley J, et al: Thromboelastography after aspirin ingestion in pregnant and nonpregnant subjects. *Br J Anaesth* 1992; 69:159.

96. Blomberg RG, Olsson SS: The lumbar epidural space in patients examined with epiduroscopy. *Anesth Analg* 1989; 68:157.

26 Infectious Disease

William R. Camann and Ruth E. Tuomala

On the morning of January 23, in the year 1883 the sun, shining through a thin veil of haze, tinted with a pale orange light the snowbanks at the upper end of McLean Street. The long, faint gray shadow of the corner lamp post, stretching unevenly across the rutted roadway, slowly shortened with the advancing day and swung imperceptibly toward the hospital like a monitory finger. A wet salt chill was in the air, borne in from the sea upon a sluggish southeast wind. Men passing in the street felt its cold dampness through their greatcoats, and women wrapped themselves more tightly in their shawls as they hurried back to their firesides. Creeping through the cracks about the windows it stole into the wards, a harbinger of evil to the patients who shivered beneath their blankets.

That afternoon, at forty minutes after three, Bridget Logan died of childbed fever.

Frederick C. Irving
Safe Deliverance (1942)

Such was obstetrics in the days before antiseptics, antibiotics, and effective pathogen control, when the best that could be wished for a woman was that she would have her baby so quickly that the doctor could not arrive in time to infect her. In the early 19th century, 1 in every 2 women in labor became infected, and 1 in 20 died of so-called "puerperal fever." Fortunately, such an era is today largely of historical interest only. However, infectious diseases are still a common problem encountered during pregnancy, labor, and the puerperium. This chapter discusses the obstetric and anesthetic management of some of the more uncommon pathogens that may be encountered during gestation.

VARICELLA ZOSTER

Varicella zoster virus is a member of the herpes virus family. As is characteristic of viral diseases caused by members of this family, there are two distinct forms of disease. Varicella is a febrile, systemic illness associated with generalized, pruritic vesicles. It is the manifestation of primary disease in a previously antibody-negative individual. Zoster is classically a localized disease associated with painful vesicles confined to a unilateral dermatome. It is the typical manifestation of recurrent

disease caused by the varicella zoster virus. During the intervening latent stage, virus resides in sensorineural ganglia. When normal immunity is present, recurrent disease is not common. In immunosuppressed individuals, there is both a higher rate of occurrence of zoster and also a higher complication rate consisting of systemic manifestations and generalized dissemination of skin lesions.[1,2]

Pathophysiology and clinical manifestations

The incubation period for varicella ranges from 10 to 21 days, with an average of 14 to 15 days. The first signs of disease are typically fever and varying degrees of coryza and rhinorrhea. Approximately 2 days after the onset of systemic symptoms, skin lesions begin to occur. These skin lesions are typically pruritic and progress from erythematous macules to vesicles, papules, or pustules that break and then heal by scabbing over and reepithelialization. Vesicles tend to occur in crops and may be found in all stages. In addition to constitutional symptoms, other systemic illnesses such as pneumonia and encephalitis can occur during varicella. Varicella pneumonia tends to present with symptoms coincident or a few days after the onset of rash. Shortness of breath, cough, and chest pain are common. Most often symptoms resolve within a week. Occasionally there may be rapid respiratory failure. X-ray findings may not correlate with physical examination findings or symptoms of pneumonia. Classic x-ray findings have been described as showing diffuse interstitial infiltrates, often bilateral, and often with an underlying slightly nodular appearance. Chest x-ray clearing may lag behind resolution of clinical pneumonia and may take up to 2 weeks to resolve.

Approximately 90% to 95% of women of childbearing age have antibodies to the varicella zoster virus and are therefore immune to varicella. However, 5% to 10% of pregnant women are susceptible. The rate of occurrence of varicella during pregnancy has been estimated at 1 to 5 per 10,000 pregnancies. Women who are from tropical and Caribbean areas where varicella is not endemic are less likely to be immune.[3] During pregnancy, varicella may pose particular problems for the pregnant woman, the outcome of pregnancy, the fetus, and the neonate. Although less than 2% of reported cases of varicella occur in persons older than 20 years, adults tend to have more severe disease, with more extensive skin involvement, higher fever, and more systemic toxicity, and a higher mortality rate. Rates of pneumonia as high as 20% to 25% have been reported.[4] During pregnancy, the rate of systemic complications and pneumonia is probably not higher than in other adults, but varicella pneumonia has been associated with a higher mortality rate during pregnancy.[4,5] Death rates of 25% to 44% from varicella pneumonia during pregnancy have been reported. In addition, an increase in mortality from varicella pneumonia during the third trimester compared with other trimesters has been noted.

Spontaneous abortion, preterm labor, and intrauterine growth retardation have been reported after maternal varicella during pregnancy. Maternal varicella associated with premature labor may result in preterm delivery in up to 50% of cases.[6]

The varicella zoster virus can probably cross the placenta at any stage in gestation, but the incidence of in utero varicella appears to be small. Maternal varicella occurring between 8 and 20 weeks of gestation has been reported to cause a distinctive fetal varicella syndrome. This syndrome was first described in 1947,[7] and since that time less then 40 cases of a characteristic constellation of congenital malformations have been reported and analyzed. The risk of congenital varicella syndrome has been observed to be between 0.5% and 9%.[6-9] It has been postulated that fetal varicella syndrome is actually a result of in utero zoster that occurs somewhat after the primary maternal viremia.[10,11] Classic fetal varicella syndrome consists of distinctive skin scarring, limb reduction defects, microcephaly, and micropthalmia.[12] Skin lesions are described as cicatricial scars in a usually unilateral dermatomal distribution. There may be hypoplasia of bone structures and soft tissue distal to such skin scarring, resulting in hypoplastic or absent limbs with varying degrees of neurologic dysfunction. In addition to microcephaly and micropthalmia, diffuse cortical atrophy, hydrocephaly, distal radiculopathies, chorioretinitis, and various genitourinary and gastrointestinal abnormalities have been described. In one series, 38% of infants born with the fetal varicella syndrome were premature, 39% were small for gestational age, and 32% died from associated disease within 20 months of life.[6] Zoster is not commonly believed to result in fetal varicella syndrome.

Maternal varicella occurring in the third trimester of pregnancy may be transmitted to the fetus and may result in neonatal varicella syndrome. It has been observed that if delivery occurs between 2 days before onset of maternal varicella rash and 5 days after, neonatal varicella occurs with an attack rate of 50% and a mortality rate of 30%.[13] When neonates are born more than 5 days after the onset of maternal rash, varicella occurs with a similar attack rate but disease is milder without associated fatalities. This difference is thought to be due to the partial protective effects of passively transferred maternal antibody, which may take up to 7 days to form after the onset of maternal viremia.[13]

Treatment and obstetric management

The natural history of both neonatal varicella and varicella in pregnant women may be ameliorated by administration of varicella zoster immune globulin (VZIG). To have a protective effect, VZIG must be administered to susceptible individuals within 96 hours of exposure to the virus. In neonates at risk, VZIG is typically administered shortly after delivery. With this approach, the incidence of severe neonatal varicella is reduced to 15% and the death rate to zero.[14] Varicella zoster immune globulin probably ameliorates disease in pregnant women, but has not been documented to alter the prevalence or outcome of in utero transmitted virus. If a pregnant woman has a clearly documented history of previous varicella, this is generally reliable. Seventy-five percent to 80% of women with no previous history of varicella will nonetheless have demonstrable protective antibodies. Therefore, in cases of exposure to varicella zoster virus, women who have no history of varicella should have expeditious antibody testing performed and should receive VZIG within 96 hours if they are found to be antibody negative. Immunosuppressed adults may have a reduction in severe, life-threatening varicella if VZIG is administered promptly after exposure. Therefore, it is prudent to routinely establish the status of varicella immunity of immunosuppressed pregnant women. Counseling of nonimmune women to report all exposure immediately can then take place. It is important to remember that VZIG administration to a pregnant woman may not prevent the occurrence of varicella or maternal viremia. Therefore, the fetus should still be considered exposed.

During pregnancy, there should be a high suspicion for the occurrence of pneumonia associated with varicella. If severe systemic manifestations or pneumonia do occur, the use of high-dose, parenteral acyclovir is indicated. At this time, the routine use or oral acyclovir at onset of varicella itself is not routinely recommended for pregnant women. Consideration should be given to hospitalization and close observation of all women who have respiratory symptoms in association with varicella. Aggressive respiratory support, including intubation and elective delivery in critically ill women, may result in a lower mortality rate from varicella pneumonia.

Obstetric care providers should be aware of proper infection control precautions when caring for a patient with varicella or zoster. This virus is transmitted directly from secretions of skin lesions associated both with varicella and zoster. In addition, the virus is shed in respiratory secretions beginning 48 hours before the onset of rash to approximately 5 days after the occurrence of rash, when they are scabbed over. This is a light virus and is aerosolized from respiratory secretions. Forty percent to 90% of susceptible individuals exposed to such aerosolized virus develop disease. Since the disease is contagious before the onset of rash, infected individuals may unitentionally expose susceptible individuals. Therefore, all health care workers caring for patients with potential varicella zoster infection should have documentation of their own immunity.

Anesthetic management

Patients presenting with acute, cutaneous varicella (chicken pox) may harbor viremia for up to 2 weeks after the onset of the syndrome, and thus regional anesthesia should be avoided during this period. Those patients who manifest pulmonary infection (varicella pneumonia) may be quite ill. Admission to an intensive care unit and intubation may be necessary. Frequent chest x-ray examination, arterial blood gas analysis, and pulmonary consultations should be sought. Anesthetic interventions of any sort should be avoided if at all possible; however, urgent delivery may be required because an increased incidence of prematurity, combined with maternal hypoxemia, may account for episodes of fetal distress. If general anesthesia must be instituted, one should be aware of possible development of adult respiratory distress syndrome (ARDS), requiring prolonged mechanical ventilation and other pulmonary supportive therapy.

If ARDS should develop during gestation, a dilemma evolves. Is it better to manage a critically ill patient while still pregnant, or will delivery (usually cesarean) allow for a smoother recovery from a pulmonary insult? Clearly, individual factors in each case will prevail; however, there is some evidence that recovery may be facilitated if delivery is accomplished.[1] Invasive hemodynamic monitoring is warranted during care of the parturient with ARDS. Conduct of anesthesia will vary, although if an endotracheal tube has already been placed for pulmonary reasons, general anesthesia usually will be the best option. In the nonintubated

patient, regional anesthesia may be considered if systemic infection can be ruled out (rare!). Furthermore, the degree of pulmonary compromise may preclude patient comfort during cesarean delivery in the supine position under regional anesthesia.

GENITAL HERPES
Etiology

Genital herpes is a sexually transmitted infection of particular concern for childbearing women. There are an estimated 270,000 to 600,000 new cases per year, with the peak incidence in the third decade.[15]

Genital herpes is caused by the herpes simplex virus (HSV), a member of the DNA containing Herpesviridae family. There are two major types of HSV: types 1 and 2. The majority of genital herpes lesions are caused by HSV-2 infections; and HSV-1 primarily causes oral-labial lesions. However, there is significant overlap.

Like other infections caused by members of this viral family, genital herpes is a recurrent infection. Periods of active infection are separated by periods of latency during which the inactive virus resides in the dorsal-root sacral ganglia. Active genital herpes typically presents as painful lesions that begin as fluid-filled vesicles or papules. These progress to shallow-based ulcers and heal by reepithelialization or by crusting over. During the time of active disease, virus can be cultured from lesions and transmitted through intimate contact and direct inoculation into mucous membranes. Exact stimuli for reactivation of disease varies from person to person and includes both endogenous and exogenous factors.[16]

Pathophysiology and clinical manifestations

The initial presentation of genital herpes in a previously antibody-negative woman typically consists of multiple, bilateral painful lesions occurring in crops of new lesions. A total mean time for occurrences of initial herpetic lesions is 20 days.[17] Lesions are most often associated with bilateral, tender lymphadenopathy. Urethral involvement is also common and urination may be difficult both because of urethral herpetic involvement and associated vulvar edema. Cervical involvement is either clinically apparent or apparent by virus isolation in greater than 80% of cases of initial genital herpes.

Initial genital herpetic infection is associated in one third to two thirds of cases with systemic symptoms such as fever, malaise, headache, and myalgias. In a smaller proportion of cases, hepatitis, aseptic meningitis, rarely encephalitis, and sacral autonomic nervous system dysfunction including sensory disturbances, inability to void, and bowel dysfunction may occur. Systemic manifestations become apparent early in the course of disease. Involvement of other organ systems presents after the onset of local genital lesions but usually within the first week of illness. Women develop systemic complications of initial herpes infections more commonly than men.[17] Although not as clearly documented, pregnant women may be at particular risk to suffer from systemic complications of initial herpes infections. Cases of herpetic myocarditis, encephalitis, and fatal herpes hepatitis during pregnancy have all been reported.[18-21]

Recurrent genital herpetic infection is typically less impressive. The onset of lesions may be preceded by prodromal symptoms of tingling, itching, or hyperesthesia in the genital area. The prodrome may also present as a sacral dermatomal neuralgia with buttock and hip pain. Genital lesions themselves are much more often unilateral, fewer, smaller, and associated with much less severe symptomatology. The length of time of active disease and viral shedding is shorter. Typically, recurrent genital herpes episodes occur in the same location and have the same appearance from episode to episode. Occasionally, recurrent lesions may occur only in extragenital sites, such as the buttocks or thighs. It is of note that cervical involvement is much less frequent with recurrent genital infection. Systemic manifestations are rare.

The frequency of recurrent disease is highly variable. It is the general impression that frequency of recurrent disease decreases as the time from the initial infection increases. However, the frequency of recurrent disease during the first 3 to 4 years may be somewhat independent of time. A few observational studies of the natural history of recurrent herpes during pregnancy suggest that frequency increases during pregnancy and that there are more disease recurrences in the third trimester.[22,23]

The clinical presentation of genital herpes may not always follow classic patterns. Approximately 25% of genital herpes infections that present with initial symptoms occur in women who have preexisting antibody to HSV. These episodes are called nonprimary first episodes, and they are less severe with fewer systemic manifestations than true primary infections presenting in a previously negative host. Preexisting antibody may be related to previous asymptomatic HSV-2 infection or may be due to HSV-1 antibodies of oral origin. Asymptomatic infection documented by positive culture in the total absence of symptoms or lesions is a well-accepted phenomenon that occurs in both those who have had previous episodes of recognized disease and in those who have antibodies but have never had symptomatic disease. Asymptomatic shedding occurs from the site of usual lesions on the vulva and to a lesser extent from the cervix,[24] and shedding can result in transmission of virus to another individual.

Asymptomatic shedding is sporadic and transient. Natural history studies have suggested that screening cultures yield virus from an asymptomatic individual with a history of herpes in approximately 0.3% to 0.8% of the time. The prevalence of asymptomatic shedding during pregnancy has been found to be between 1.8% and 12%.[23-26] Prevalence of asymptomatic shedding at the time of delivery has been documented to be 1.4% to 2.5% in women with a known history of prior herpes. When primary genital herpes occurs during pregnancy, asymptomatic shedding occurs with increased frequency and has been documented at the time of delivery and in up to 10% of such individuals.[27]

In early pregnancy, the herpesvirus may be transmitted to the fetus through in utero transmission. Primary genital herpes infections in particular have been associated spontaneous abortion occurring at a very low rate. In addition, a congenital syndrome similar to that described for cytomegalovirus in utero infection, consisting of microcephaly, cerebral calcifications, chorioretinitis, and other manifestations, has been described.[27] The exact incidence of this problem is unknown but is thought to be quite small, and pregnancy termination is not currently indicated. Primary genital herpes infections later in pregnancy have been associated with pregnancy loss, premature labor, growth retardation, and neonatal infection.

Treatment and obstetric management

The major obstetric issue has been that of possible transmission of the virus to the neonate at the time of birth. Viral transmission to the neonate can occur either as the neonate comes in contact with the virus during passage through the birth canal or by ascent of the organism after membranes have been ruptured. When virus is transmitted to the fetus or neonate, neonatal herpes results in up to 30% to 60% of the cases. Neonatal disease is a life-threatening illness with major sequelae.[25,28,29] Skin, ocular, central nervous system (CNS) disease, and disseminated overwhelming infection can result. In 15% to 30% of cases, only skin lesions result. In 20% to 40% of cases, CNS disease results. In 15% to 40% of cases, disseminated disease results. In CNS or disseminated disease, morbidity and mortality is high and permanent sequelae may ensue. The natural history of neonatal disease has, however, been modified by early diagnosis and prompt institution of antiviral therapy.

The greatest risk for neonatal disease from peripartum transmission of the herpesvirus is during a primary herpetic episode at the time of labor and delivery. Both the amount of virus present and a lack of protective antibodies could explain the particular high risk associated with primary disease. Symptomatic primary disease is usually recognized, and major neonatal risks can be significantly decreased through cesarean delivery. However, asymptomatic primary disease does occur and has been demonstrated to confer a 33% rate of neonatal disease.[30] The risks of both viral transmission and resultant neonatal disease associated with recurrent symptomatic genital herpes or asymptomatic shedding of herpes appears to be much less, with observed rates of 0% to 3%.[30,31]

Most infants with neonatal herpes in the United States are born to women who have a personal or sexual partner with history of genital herpes, but no symptoms or lesions present at the time of delivery, and to women who have absolutely no known history of genital herpes.[29] It is currently estimated that 60% to 80% of infants born with neonatal herpes may be born to a woman with no history of genital herpes. It used to be thought that routine antenatal culture screening to predict asymptomatic viral shedding would decrease the occurrence of neonatal herpes by correctly predicting those women who should have cesarean section performed for the purposes of interrupting vertical transmission of the herpesvirus. However, investigations of the natural history of genital herpes during pregnancy have been helpful in pointing out the futility of such an approach.[24-26] Asymptomatic shedding in women with a history of prior herpes episodes occurs at such a low rate and for such a transient time period that screening cultures done before labor and delivery are both expensive and inaccurate in predicting the presence of virus at the time of delivery. Even more problematic is the issue of correctly identifying women with asymptomatic primary disease during pregnancy and at the time of delivery. Currently, the advisability and practicality of screening pregnant women by antibody titers and cultures performed at the time of delivery has been neither assessed nor adopted.

The only reliable method by which the presence of virus in the genital tract can be assessed is specific viral culture. Rapid diagnostic tests and cytologic methods have not proved to be sensitive or specific enough to be of value for immediately assessing the presence of virus. Presence of preexisting antibody may help to assess whether a specific initial episode of herpetic lesion is a true primary episode or not.

Current recommendations for obstetric management of patients with a prior history of genital herpes are that the obstetric risk and the route of delivery be determined by assessment at the time of labor and delivery. Careful inspection for lesions of the cervix and vulva is recommended, with an option for obtaining viral cultures at this time. If no lesions are present, then a vaginal delivery is recommended. If viral cultures retrospectively document the presence of virus, this information is transmitted to the pediatrician for postnatal follow-up. Any symptoms or lesions suggestive of herpes at the time of labor would be an indication for cesarean section.

All herpetic lesions present in the third trimester should be closely followed, with viral cultures performed every 2 to 5 days as the lesions heal until virus negativity is documented. The route of delivery in this case should be guided by the results of the most recent culture and inspection done at the time of labor. Even though it is possible for virus to ascend after membranes have ruptured, the current opinion is that decreasing direct contact with virus may decrease the risk of transmission at any time after ruptured membranes. Therefore, cesarean section may be indicated at any time after ruptured membranes in the presence of active herpetic lesions or known viral shedding. Patients with herpetic lesions or herpesvirus present during preterm labor complicated by ruptured membranes, or prolonged ruptured membranes at any gestational age, should be managed on an individual basis. Timing and route of delivery must be guided by weighing the risks and benefits to mother and fetus. In addition, management must be individualized in the pregnant woman with frequently recurring lesions during the third trimester or with a primary herpes episode during pregnancy.

Multiple case reports and small series discuss the use of acyclovir during pregnancy. Parenteral acyclovir appears to be well tolerated by both the mother and the fetus. Severe systemic disease, including hepatitis and encephalitis, are absolute indications for the use of parenteral acyclovir at any time during gestation. The routine use of oral acyclovir during pregnancy for indications of viral suppression cannot at this time be recommended. The pharmacokinetics of acyclovir during pregnancy appeared to be unpredictable.[32] In addition, it has not been documented in a larger series to result in total absence of viral shedding.

Anesthetic management

The subject of regional anesthesia in the parturient with HSV infection has long been controversial. In a 1983 survey of members of the Society of Obstetric Anesthesia and Perinatology, 36% of respondents would not use regional anesthesia if an active genital lesion was present, and 5% would not use regional anesthesia if the patient had a history of HSV, even if active lesions were absent.[34] Although the concern is inoculation of the central neuraxis with HSV, no reports of this complication exist. Moreover, several investigators have reported the safe use of both epidural[34-36] and spinal anesthesia[37] in the presence of active, recurrent HSV lesions. Recurrent HSV is not associated with blood-borne viremia[15] and should not represent a contraindication to regional anesthesia, provided no lesions exist on the lumbar area of the back.

The management of parturients with primary HSV infection is not so clear. Primary HSV infections are commonly associated with systemic symptoms (fever, arthralgia, headache, lymphadenopathy),[15] and it seems prudent to avoid regional anesthetic in these patients. Primary HSV outbreaks at time of delivery, however, are exceedingly rare and may actually represent recrudescent lesions in a previously asymptomatic, infected woman, or deliberate attempts by a patient to hide a known history of HSV. Nonetheless, a woman who claims no history of HSV lesions and presents with clinical sequelae of active disease must be considered to have a primary outbreak until proved otherwise.

An additional concern regarding management of patients with HSV is the association of recurrent oral herpes lesions with use of epidural morphine.[38] Although the mechanism remains unclear, the presence of pruritus associated with epidural morphine and the resultant itch-and-scratch response may trigger the HSV recurrence.

LYME DISEASE
Etiology
Lyme disease is the most common vector-borne disease in the United States.[39,40] Also called Lyme borreliosis, Lyme disease is caused by the spirochete *Borrelia burgdorferi.* This spirochete, transmitted to humans via *Ixodes* ticks, is endemic to parts of the Northeastern seaboard, north central Midwest, and the Northern Pacific coast. However, the incidence of Lyme disease is increasing, endemic areas are spreading geographically, and cases have been reported from most of the United States and other continents. The specific tick associated with transmission in the Northeast and Midwest is *Ixodes dammini,* and in the Pacific area, *Ixodes pacificus.* Eighty percent of all cases of Lyme disease occur between May and September, peaking in June and July. There is a second

peak between September and November. These time periods correspond to the feeding cycles of the *Ixodes* ticks.

Pathophysiology and clinical manifestations
Lyme disease is a multisystem illness[41] with early and late manifestations that are somewhat analogous to the stages of syphilis. The primary organs of involvement include the skin, the nervous system, the heart, and the musculoskeletal system. Multiple organs can be involved in both early and late stages of disease. Lyme disease occurring during pregnancy can present in any stage, and there is no evidence that clinical manifestations are influenced by pregnancy.[42]

The classic lesion of early Lyme disease is the "target lesion" of erythema migrans. This lesion begins as a red macule or papule located at the point of a tick bite. This expands to become a large, annular area of erythema with a bright red outer border and partial central clearing. *E. migrans* may present as an isolated finding; it may also be seen in association with nonspecific flulike symptoms of fever, minor constitutional complaints, and regional lymphadenopathy, or it may coexist with acute manifestations of other organ system disease, in particular neurologic and musculoskeletal manifestations. Early symptoms typically appear on average 1 day after inoculation. If untreated, erythema migrans gradually fades. Days to weeks after, more specific involvement of other organ symptoms may become apparent. A variety of other skin lesions can occur, including diffuse or malar erythema, annular skin lesions, or urticaria. Neuropathy of the 7th cranial nerve, or Bell's palsy, is one of the most frequent of the neurologic manifestations, which can also include severe headaches, mild meningismus or encephalopathy, other peripheral neuropathies, and radicular pain. Migratory musculoskeletal pain or debilitating malaise or fatigue may occur. Joint involvement may present as mild arthralgias or brief attacks of arthritis. Manifestations of myocarditis, pericarditis, or more typically atrioventricular conduction block may be seen. Other less commonly described manifestations include liver, respiratory, genitourinary, eye, and reticuloendothelial involvement that may last for weeks to months or may become chronic.

In the late or persistent phase of Lyme disease, episodes of disease become longer or may even become chronic. Gradually, the frequency of recurrences of symptomatic disease becomes less and eventually episodic disease stops. In a small number of individuals, episodes may result in irreversible tissue damage or chronic, lifelong illness. The most frequently described late manifestation of Lyme disease is arthritis. Up to 60% of people who had previous intermittent arthralgias or other musculoskeletal symptoms may suffer from asymmetric arthritis, particularly of large joints. The knee is the most frequent site. Synovial fluid will typically display a leukocytosis. Late neurologic symptoms also occur and may include distal paresthesias, radicular pain, dementia, and a progressive encephalomyelitis. In addition, a particular skin lesion, acrodermatitis chronic atrophicans, has been described. This is a bluish-red discoloration with swollen skin and eventual atrophy.

The laboratory diagnosis of Lyme disease is hampered by a lack of reliable microbiologic or immunologic testing.[43-45] Identification of spirochetes in body fluids and tissues during active disease by culture and DNA detection is possible but not very sensitive. Organisms have been isolated from amniotic fluid, cord blood, fetal tissues, and placental specimens.[46-49] ELISA, IFA, and immunoblot techniques for measuring antibodies to *B. burgdorferi* all lack sufficient sensitivity and specificity to serve as general diagnostic tools, particularly in low-prevalence populations. False negatives occur when low levels of antibody are present, particularly early in the course of illness. Antibodies more reliably present in later-stage illness, however, may not be specific. False positives occur both because of crossreactivity and because of the presence of antibodies from old disease. In addition, the presence and level of antibodies are not well correlated with results of therapy and there is a lack of standardization between laboratories. Serology is most useful when correlated with the clinical situation and when it supports a typical or suspicious clinical picture.

Treatment and obstetric management

Treatment with antibiotics may be effective in halting disease progression and in ameliorating disease effects at any stage.[50,51] However, some symptoms may recur or persist despite antibiotic therapy. In particular, joint or neurologic involvement of late disease may respond slowly to antibiotic therapy and there may be a significant failure rate. The spirochete is highly sensitive to tetracycline, ampicillin, ceftriaxone, and imipenim. It is only moderately sensitive to penicillin, and not sensitive to aminoglycosides or rifampin. Although erythromycin appears to be effective against this organism in vitro, there is less experience with its in vivo *efficacy.*

B. burgdorferi can infect the placenta and can infect the fetus in cases of active maternal disease. Descriptions of perinatal infection are confined to case reports and limited case series.[48,49,52] The

cases of perinatal transmission best documented are those in which there is documented maternal disease as well as organism isolation from fetal or placental tissue. One of the first such cases described involved untreated maternal Lyme disease that occurred during the first trimester with subsequent delivery of a preterm infant who died shortly after birth, with manifestations of cardiac disease, including valvular aortic stenosis, coarctation, and left ventricular dysfunction.[46] Spirochetes were isolated from the spleen, kidney, and bone marrow.

Other reported cases have been associated with maternal illness occurring in all trimesters of pregnancy; these cases appear to be confined to instances in which pregnant women received either no or short-course oral antibiotics, most frequently penicillin.[52,53] Adverse outcomes of pregnancy that have been reported include spontaneous abortion, and both preterm delivery and stillbirth during the late second and early third trimesters of fetuses who often have anomalies. Cardiac and neurologic anomalies are most frequently reported, although organisms have been isolated from the spleen, liver, kidney, and bone marrow in addition to the heart and brain. In less well documented cases, delayed neurologic illness, cortical blindness, neonatal respiratory distress, growth retardation, maternal toxemia, and an increased incidence of SIDS have all been ascribed to perinatal Lyme disease. Besides adverse pregnancy outcome reports, however, there are increasing reports of cases of active maternal Lyme disease treated aggressively with antibiotics that result in normal pregnancy outcome with no evidence of placental or fetal/neonatal infection.[49,54] Overall, the risk of adverse outcome appears to be low.[53,55] The exact risk for and timing of infection of the fetoplacental unit in cases of maternal Lyme disease is unknown.

The incidence of disease is low enough even in endemic areas during peak tick season that "prophylactic" antibiotic therapy for tick bites is not advised.[56,57] Aggressive treatment of symptomatic Lyme disease during pregnancy for both maternal benefit and for prevention of adverse pregnancy and fetal effects is warranted, although the exact efficacy is unknown. Treatment of early Lyme disease should be with amoxicillin, or, as a second choice, erythromycin for 21 days. Some authorities recommend treating all Lyme disease except for those cases of early Lyme disease presenting with just a single skin lesion an and associated symptoms during pregnancy with parenteral therapy. For treatment of either early, secondary, or late manifestations of Lyme disease with parenteral therapy, either a penicillin, ceftriaxone, or other cephalosporin therapy for 14 to 21 days, depending on the clinical presentation, is safe and recommended during pregnancy.

Anesthetic management

Anesthetic management of the parturient with Lyme disease has not been described. However, because this disease is now the most common vector-borne infection in the United States (13,795 cases from 1980 to 1988),[42] several points deserve consideration. Early symptoms of Lyme disease include minor constitutional symptoms, skin rash, and lymphadenopathy, and the disease may often be confused with other flu-like syndromes.[58] However, persistent infection[39] may result in a multisystem manifestation with several areas of particular anesthetic concern.

Skin. Diffuse erythematous rash, annular lesions, urticaria, and atrophic dermatitis may be seen in the majority of patients with Lyme disease.[59] Careful inspection of puncture sites for regional anesthesia should be done, and caution exercised when extensive taping (as with epidural catheter placement) is required.

Musculoskeletal system. Diffuse and nonspecific orthopedic symptoms (joint pain, tendonitis, muscle aches) are common during the early phase of the disease, and later symptoms (after 1 to 2 years) can include chronic arthritis, joint subluxations, and even permanent bony disabilities.[58] A detailed orthopedic history should be elicited and significant findings documented before initiation of anesthesia, particularly regional.

Central nervous system. A diffuse array of neurologic sequelae may ensue from Lyme disease.[60] Meningitis and encephalitis occur, as do both cranial and peripheral neuropathies. Both motor and sensory peripheral radiculoneuritis and/or paresthesiae may occur. These symptoms are likely a result of active central nervous system infection, although this has not been demonstrated with certainty. Until further information is available, it would seem prudent to avoid regional anesthesia in patients with a history suggestive of Lyme disease.

Cardiac. Acute, early infection may be associated with varying degrees of conduction blockade, pericarditis, and/or cardiomyopathy.[61] Cardiac involvement is usually transient and resolves within several weeks, although chronic, severe cardiomyopathy has been reported.[62] A full 12-lead electrocardiograph, chest x-ray examination, and cardiac consultation should be obtained before anesthesia in any patient with acute symptoms suggestive of Lyme disease. Anesthetic management of parturients with cardiomyopathy has been extensively discussed in Chapter 12.

Listeria etiology

Listeria monocytogenes is a rare cause of bacterial infection in the population at large, but a well-described bacterial pathogen of pregnant women and neonates. Sporadic cases of listeriosis as well as some well-described mini epidemics have resulted in maternal sepsis, in utero infection with resultant fetal or neonatal death, and neonatal sepsis.

T-cell mediated immune mechanisms play a major role in host defense against listeriosis. For this reason, this organism is seen as a pathogen primarily in the elderly, in immunosuppressed individuals such as those with underlying malignancies or those undergoing immunosuppressive therapy, and in pregnant women and newborns. It has been estimated that perinatal infections with *Listeria* occur at a rate greater than 20 times that in the general population.[63]

Pathophysiology and clinical manifestations

The exact pathogenesis of infections caused by *Listeria* is poorly understood. Epidemics have linked human illness with the ingestion of contaminated food and suggested that the alimentary tract may be a portal of entry for this organism.[63-65] For sporadic cases, such a route of infection is usually much harder to document. Nonpregnant adults develop meningitis and encephalitis as the major manifestations of listeriosis. Adult respiratory distress syndrome in association with listeriosis has been reported.[66] Reported mortality rates are in the 25% to 35% range and may be most associated with underlying debilitating illnesses. Listeriosis has been reported as a complication associated with acquired immune deficiency syndrome (AIDS).[63,67] Approximately two thirds of pregnant women with listeriosis will notice fever, headache, myalgias, and other nonspecific flulike symptoms. One third of patients will have gastrointestinal symptoms, particularly diarrhea. Low back pain that mimicks urinary tract infections has also been reported. Meningitis is rare, as is death. Although women may appear to be acutely ill, more typically the maternal illness is mild. Bacteriemia is common. Approximately 3 to 7 days after the onset of maternal infection, there may be evidence of acute amnionitis, with resulting septic abortion or preterm or term labor. Maternal fever is typical. Chorioamnionitis may also result in intrauterine fetal death at any gestational age or in the birth of a septic neonate. Amnionitis is not always associated with neonatal sepsis. Estimates of the perinatal death rate associated with listeria amnionitis average from 20% to 50%.

It is presumed that the intrauterine contents become infected through hematogenous dissemination at the time of maternal septicemia. Ascending infection of organisms present in the perirectal or lower genital tracts can probably also occur. *Listeria* infections leading to adverse pregnancy outcome occur most frequently in the third trimester, but they can occur at any gestational age.[63,68-70] It is not clear how frequently *Listeria* is a cause of early spontaneous abortion in the United States since specific cultures are not usually done. There are anecdotal reports of *Listeria* as a cause of recurrent spontaneous abortions. In Europe, *Listeria* has been reported to be a cause of between 0.5% and 3% of all cases of spontaneous abortion and preterm labor.[71,72]

Neonatal infections with *Listeria* occur during two distinct time periods, suggesting the possibility of different modes of transmission. Early infections typically occur within 2 days of life and are presumed to be transmitted to the neonate either in utero or at the time of birth. Neonates with early *Listeria* infections are disproportionately preterm.[68] Generalized sepsis, respiratory infections, cardiovascular and hematology complications, and neurologic problems are seen. Late *Listeria* infections are seen days to weeks after birth and are usually in full-term infants. Meningitis predominates. Horizontal transmission of infection has been suggested, and occasional clustering of infections has implied the possibility of nosocomial spread.[66,73] Case fatality rates between 3% and 50% have been reported, with recent epidemics suggesting mortality rates in the 30% range for early neonatal listeriosis.[63,71] Neonatal outcome is affected by both sepsis and gestational age.

Listeria monocytogenes is a facultative anaerobic organism that is a beta-hemolytic gram-positive rod. It is easily isolated from body fluids or tissues that are usually sterile, but it is more difficult to identify in mixed cultures. It may be found in a high proportion of maternal, cord, or neonatal blood cultures in cases of infection, and it has also been cultured from amniotic fluid, neonatal gastric aspirate, and fetal membranes. Although it has been cultured from the lower genital tract and rectum, screening cultures even in cases of mini epidemics are not helpful. Placental cultures and gram stains may be positive. Typical lesions of microabscesses and a distinct multifocal villitis seen on placental histology can help to suggest or confirm a diagnosis in retrospect.[68,74,75]

Treatment and obstetric management

Maternal fever coincident with the onset of labor, preterm labor occurring in association with a systemic maternal illness, and in utero fetal demise should always raise the possibility of infection with *Listeria*. Abnormal fetal heart rate tracings and fetal distress during such labors have been re-

ported.[58] In addition, it has been strongly suggested that perinatal survival may be improved by prompt antibiotic therapy of infected women and their neonates.[53] Therefore, when *Listeria* is suspected, both aggressive fetal monitoring and maternal antibiotic therapy are called for.

Although there have been no controlled clinical trials of the best antibiotic therapy for listeriosis, parenteral ampicillin and gentamicin are usually given. Ampicillin appears to be more active than penicillin against this organism, and the combination of ampicillin and gentamicin may have synergistic effects. Trimethaprim-sulfamethoxazole and erythromycin are also effective. The best length of therapy is not known. Women who have a febrile illness in the peripartum period usually defervesce promptly after delivery and respond nicely to antibiotic therapy.

Anesthetic management

Although pregnancy itself may predispose to infections with *Listeria*, this agent most commonly affects an immunocompromised host. Thus, management may be directed more toward the cause of immunosuppression rather than the infection itself. Patients with AIDS,[67] as well as those with transplanted organs, may thus be likely hosts.[76] *Listeria* infection may also increase the incidence of premature labor and/or fetal demise. Anesthetic management in these settings is discussed in Chapters 22 and 32.

INFECTION WITH THE HUMAN IMMUNODEFICIENCY VIRUS
Etiology

Acquired immunodeficiency syndrome (AIDS) is the end-stage condition of disease associated with the human immunodeficiency virus (HIV), an infection that causes progressive immune deficiency and whose manifestations are consequences of this deficiency. In 1994, 18% of cases of AIDS had been reported in women.[77] The rate of increase in reported cases of AIDS in the United States is greatest in women and children, and it is suspected that women comprise an even greater proportion of people who have earlier, often undiagnosed HIV disease.

It is becoming increasingly apparent that HIV infection in women occurs primarily in association with sexual activity. Although 50% of cases of AIDS reported in American women are associated with intravenous drug use, asymptomatic HIV infection in women is more associated with heterosexual exposure. One delivery service has reported that 69% of infected parturients giving birth to infected infants became infected through heterosexual contact.[78] Many women may not recognize that current or previous sexual partners have engaged in risk activities for HIV infection. One New York study suggested that 40% of HIV-infected women initially did not acknowledge or were not aware of being at risk for HIV disease.[79] Infection in women has also been associated with sexually transmitted diseases, particularly syphilis, and non-intravenous cocaine use.[80-82] Geographical areas of high HIV prevalence also predict risk for HIV disease in women.[83-85] Currently, many innercity hospitals report a prevalence of HIV infection in delivering women in excess of 1%.

Pathophysiology and clinical manifestations

HIV-1 is a retrovirus whose major unique feature is possession of a reverse transcriptase that allows transcription of the viral RNA genome into a DNA copy that is then integrated into the host cell chromosomal DNA.[86] The host cell functions can then be diverted into production of virus. After a period of time of infection, host cell death appears to ensue. HIV-1 infects CD4 positive cells, including lymphocytes, macrophages, fibroblasts, cells from the gastrointestinal tract and brain, and chorionic villi. It is probable that the CD4 surface antigen serves as an attachment site for the virus and facilitates entry into the cell. The chief target for infection is the CD4 positive, or T4 lymphocyte, the so-called helper lymphocyte responsible for facilitating function of the cellular immune system. Cell-free virus can also be found in various bodily fluids and tissues; the contribution of cell-free and cell-associated to disease transmission is currently being elucidated.

Although there is some degree of variability, it is apparent that disease caused by HIV infection occurs along a time line, or continuum of effects.[86-88] Initial infection with the virus is associated with high levels of viremia, and there may be an associated clinical syndrome of acute infection that occurs within 3 months of exposure. After initial infection, the majority of adults remain asymptomatic for prolonged periods of time. While the disease is asymptomatic, progressive immune dysfunction occurs. Before any expression of symptomatic disease, alterations in various immune parameters and markers may be seen. Chief among these is a progressive decline in the absolute number and proportion of CD4-positive lymphocytes. The onset of symptomatic disease may be heralded by various constitutional symptoms, including fever, night sweats, and weight loss. Certain clinical conditions such as recurrent oral thrush and, in women, recurrent cervical intraepithelial neoplasia, may be the first indications of disease and progressive immune dysfunction approaching a critical level. AIDS itself occurs with

the onset of a wide range of infections, malignancies, and associated conditions that are rarely seen in individuals with normal immune function, in particular, cell-mediated immunity. In addition, a CD4 absolute lymphocyte count of less than 200 is now an AIDS-defining event. Some of the more common associated malignancies include Kaposi's sarcoma, T and B cell lymphomas, CNS lymphoma, and in women, cervical cancer. Infections include a number of viral, bacterial, fungal, and parasitic infections. Of particular note because of their frequency are *Pneumocystis carinii* pneumonia (PCP), invasive cytomegalovirus (CMV) and CMV retinitis, toxoplasmosis CNS infection, invasive candidiasis, recurrent bacterial pneumonias, and mycobacterial infections including atypical mycobacterial infection and *Mycobacterium tuberculosis*. Manifestations of AIDS can also include symptoms associated with direct effects of the virus on end-organ cells, such as those in the CNS or gastrointestinal tract.

The average time period between infection and manifestations of systemic disease is 8 to 10 years, with an average time period of 3 years between the onset of systemic disease and death. The hallmark of care for HIV-infected individuals has been supportive therapy and aggressive diagnosis and therapy for associated infection and malignancies. However, the clinical use of antiviral drugs and strategies to prevent AIDS-associated conditions as well as the continual evolution of new such modalities are changing the natural history of HIV-infection.

There is limited data concerning the effect of pregnancy on the long-term health status of HIV-infected women.[89-92] No apparent escalation in immune deterioration or stage of HIV infection has been documented. However, HIV-infected women who enter pregnancy with the lowest CD4 counts do develop life-threatening AIDS-associated conditions during pregnancy, and may also be at greater risk for developing obstetrically related infections such as intrapartum chorioamnionitis, postpartum endometritis, and wound or episiotomy infection.

Obstetric management

Management of HIV infection during pregnancy includes close observation and monitoring for HIV-related conditions.[93,94] Baseline CMV, toxoplasmosis, and varicella-zoster status are determined. Screening for tuberculosis through PPD and anergy panel skin testing is routine as is screening for sexually transmitted diseases including syphilis. The CD4 count is assessed as pregnancy progresses. All necessary vaccines including pneumococcal, influenza, and hepatitis B are administered, as is varicella-zoster immune globulin in cases of exposure.

Standard obstetric care also includes administration of appropriate antiretroviral therapy, therapy for any AIDS-related conditions, and prophylactic therapies, depending on usual CD4 or disease-stage criteria. Since pregnancy-specific toxicities for many of these therapies are not well documented, it is routine to monitor closely for potential side effects, in particular, hematologic and hepatic maternal toxicities and altered intrauterine growth of the fetus.

Obstetric management also includes counseling about perinatal transmission of HIV to the fetus/neonate and discussion of management strategies to minimize perinatal transmission.[95-97] The risk that HIV will be transmitted from an infected woman to her infant varies between population groups and according to risk factors, some of which are beginning to be defined.[98-101] Risk of transmission varies inversely with maternal CD4 count and directly with maternal peripheral viral burden as measured by titer and constancy of viremia. Overall rates of vertical transmission in North American cohorts are in the 20% to 30% range. Transmission of HIV from an infected mother to her fetus can occur at any time during gestation or during the time of labor and delivery. Current estimates are that 20% to 50% of cases of transmission occur during gestation remote from the time of delivery and that 50% to 80% of transmission occurs during the peripartum period, presumably through contact of the fetus with infected maternal blood and genital tract secretions.[101,104]

In a large, prospective, placebo-controlled trial, it has been demonstrated that AZT, or zidovudine, decreases the rate of vertical transmission of HIV when given during pregnancy and intravenously during labor and delivery to HIV-infected women and for the first 6 weeks of life to their neonates.[105] In the trial, the risk for vertical transmission was decreased by two thirds, from a rate of approximately 25% in the placebo group to a rate of approximately 8% in the treated group. However, all women in this study were women who had CD4 counts above 200 and who had never previously received AZT. Although efficacy for decreasing vertical transmission in other subgroups of HIV-infected women is not currently known, it is now standard to offer AZT to all infected pregnant women for the potential benefit of decreasing perinatal transmission. Concerns about long-term safety and potential adverse maternal and fetal risks of AZT remain; however, the only toxicity observed with this regimen to date is neonatal anemia, which appears to be of little clinical relevance.

There are also reports suggesting a potential benefit in decreasing vertical transmission of HIV of cesarean section and short duration of ruptured membranes.[106-109] An observed benefit of cesarean section has not been controlled for other confounding obstetric factors, and it is not clear whether any potential benefits conferred by route of delivery or duration of ruptured membranes is additive to protection afforded by AZT. At this time, it seems prudent to avoid maneuvers that could increase the possibility of neonatal exposure to infected maternal secretions. Therefore, artificial rupture of membranes, fetal scalp electrodes, and fetal scalp sampling for pH measurements should be avoided when possible in women known to be HIV infected.

Because HIV infection is increasing in women and because a large proportion of infection remains unrecognized, all obstetric care providers should focus on proper infection-control precautions. The best available estimates indicate that transmission of HIV through direct needle stick or other parenteral means occurs at a rate of approximately 0.4%.[110-112] Transmission of infection through mucous membrane or skin contact occurs at lower rates. Potentially infected secretions of obstetric patients include blood, lochia, and amniotic fluid, so gloves, goggles, masks, and impervious gowns should be used when appropriate. In addition, cell-free virus has been found in cerebrospinal fluid.[113] There is evidence that double gloving decreases the occurrence of needle-stick injuries. After delivery, neonates are covered with potentially infective maternal secretions, and their own secretions may be infectious. Therefore, upon delivery, all health care workers handling neonates should be gloved. In addition, all tracheal suctioning should be performed using wall or bulb suction, and never with the operator's mouth.

Anesthetic management

The widespread prevalence of HIV infection, including in pregnant women, requires that all anesthesiologists consider this syndrome when caring for their patients. Two important issues arise when HIV-infected patients present for care: (1) What is the risk of anesthetic intervention for the patient? and (2) What is the risk to the anesthesiologist?

Regarding risk to the patient, one must foremost remember that AIDS is still considered to be a progressive, universally fatal disease, although newer pharmacologic therapy may slow the progression of some symptoms. Of particular concern to obstetric anesthesiologists is the central nervous system manifestations of AIDS.[86] HIV can be isolated from the cerebrospinal fluid of patients with

AIDS.[113] Furthermore, 30% to 50% of patients with AIDS will ultimately develop symptoms of spinal cord involvement, including paralysis and ataxia.[86] The development of encephalitis, coma, and death may often be the final manifestation of the disease in HIV-infected patients. Consequently, the anesthesiologist should carefully seek out any signs of neurologic dysfunction before instituting regional anesthesia in patients with AIDS, and informed consent should include a discussion of neurologic dysfunction in the context of the natural progression of the disease.[114,115] Regional anesthesia has been used for the parturient with HIV infection, and it appears to be safe. In a series reported by Hughes, there were no changes in the immunologic parameters studied, and the HIV disease remained stable in the peripartum period, without infections, complications, or neurologic changes.[116] However, all patients in this series had relatively early stages of HIV, and it is not clear if these findings would apply to patients with advanced disease.

There are reasons to avoid general anesthesia in patients with HIV infection. First, immune suppression may be exacerbated by volatile anesthetic agents. Second, endotracheal intubation may provide a route for oral pathogens to infect the pulmonary tree. And third, a theoretical concern regarding general anesthesia is the possibility of difficult intubation because of pharyngeal lymphatic hypertrophy.[117]

The risk to health care personal of caring for HIV-infected patients is not clear, although it appears to be low. One recent series reports a risk of 0.11% (2/1785) seroconversion in hospital workers exposed to the virus via needle stick.[118] However, the latency period of HIV is unknown, and long-term follow-up is ongoing. Moreover, as the incidence of the disease increases, more exposures (recognized or not) to HIV-infected patients can be expected to occur. As many as 0.5% of *all* patients are estimated to be infected with HIV.[114] Clearly, great care should be exercised when one anticipates contact with bodily fluids, and appropriate gloving (and/or mask, gown, eyeware, etc.) must be employed depending on the extent of anticipated contact.[119] Particular caution should be used when handling needles. One must avoid recapping used needles, and all sharp objects should be discarded into appropriate disposal containers (not trash cans!)

Finally, if AIDS has resulted from illicit drug use by the patient, additional anesthetic concerns may arise (see Chapter 27 for the care of the drug-addicted parturient).

SEPTIC SHOCK
Etiology

Septic shock is the most serious consequence of systemic sepsis. In obstetrics, this is usually associated with bacterial infection. Although septic shock is most closely associated with gram-negative bacteremia, it can also occur in association with gram-positive aerobic and anaerobic bacteremia. In the general population, mortality due to septic shock ranges from 10% to 80%, averaging from 25% to 50%.[120,121] Largely due to their underlying state of good health, obstetric patients who suffer from septic shock have a much lower mortality rate. However, septic shock is always a life-threatening condition, and its successful management requires knowledge of the basic pathophysiology and principles of aggressive diagnosis and therapy.

Pathophysiology and clinical manifestations

Septic shock is a clinical condition of pronounced hemodynamic instability whose hallmarks are hypovolemia, eventual hypotension, metabolic acidosis, widespread tissue injury, and multiorgan failure. The mechanisms of septic shock are largely secondary to mediators released by destruction of bacterial cell walls (Fig. 26-1). The lipopolysaccharide portion of the cell wall of gram-negative bacteria, in particular the lipid A portion, appears to be responsible for the major toxic effects associated with gram-negative bacteremia. Peptidoglycans of gram-positive cell walls are also probably mediators of septic shock.

These substances may have direct end-organ effects, but perhaps most important, they stimulate the production and release of various endogenous soluble mediators from target organs. The major target organs of bacterial toxins and the major sources of these mediators are the vascular endothelium and tissue macrophage plus circulating mononuclear cells. The exact nature and actions of the various soluble mediators involved in the pathophysiology of septic shock are not yet completely elucidated. Some mediators probably have local, organ-specific effects. Others may be responsible for systemic effects and major manifestations of septic shock. It is apparent that the appearance, actions, and clearance of various mediators are interrelated.[120-124]

Many of the actions attributed to gram-negative endotoxin are probably mediated through cachectin.[124,125] This substance has both direct effects on end organs and also affects the release or function of other more specific mediators. Cachectin is directly toxic to vascular endothelial cells and is an endogenous pyrogen; in addition, it activates and promotes the function of polymorphonuclear

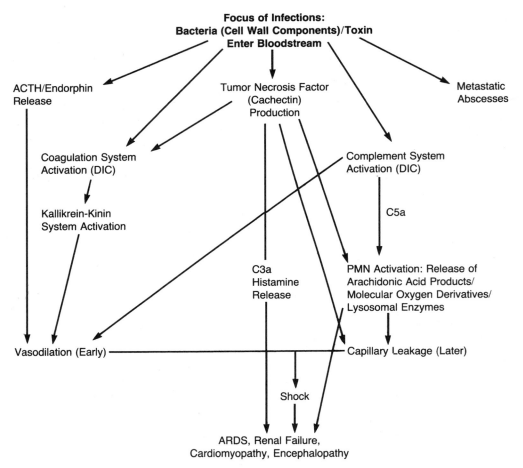

Fig. 26-1 Pathophysiology of the complications of severe sepsis. *PMN* = polymorphonuclear; *ACTH* = adrenocorticotropic hormone; *DIC* = disseminated intravascular coagulation; *ARDS* = adult respiratory distress syndrome. (From Sheagren JN, in Wyngaarden JB, Smith LH (eds): *Cecil Textbook of Medicine,* ed 18. Philadelphia, WB Saunders, 1988, pp 1538-1541. Used by permission.)

leukocytes, induces coagulation changes, possibly mediates cardiovascular responses, and modulates other enzymatic functions. It may trigger the production or release of other soluble mediators such as leukotrienes, platelet-activation factor, and interleukin-1. It appears to suppress or inhibit the function of lipoprotein lipase, and it may stimulate the cyclooxygenase pathway of arachidonic acid metabolism.

Soluble mediators and endogenous enzymes appear to be responsible for the major effects on cardiovascular physiology, volume regulation, respiratory function, and stimulation of hematopoietic cells and the coagulation cascade seen in septic shock. Soluble substances that have been investigated and that probably play a part in the pathophysiology of septic shock include complement, interleukins, interferon, monokines, platelet-

activating factor, tissue plasminogen activator, histamine, serotonin, various kinins, and the major products of arachidonic acid metabolism including leukotrienes, prostaglandins, and thromboxane.

The multisystem changes associated with septic shock occur along a continuum of effects involving endothelial damage, altered vascular reactivity, fluctuations in sympathetic tone, decrease in peripheral tissue perfusion, local and generalized acidosis, and eventual cellular end-organ hypoxia and death. Although all organ systems are eventually involved, prominent changes are seen in the cardiovascular, respiratory, hematologic, and metabolic systems of the body.

The initial cardiovascular changes seen in septic shock[126-128] are a decrease in systemic vascular resistance that may sometimes be quite pronounced, an increase in cardiac output and heart rate, and occasionally a slight decrease in blood pressure or pulse pressure. The initial change may well be vascular dilation, which leads to a secondary increase in cardiac output because of the adrenergic stimulation caused by the decrease in afterload. In the early cardiovascular changes, hypotension is not prominent or of major consequence. Capillary leaks and central redistribution of blood flow in addition to the various demands on volume occasioned by metabolic demands of sepsis (such as fever) all contribute to a pronounced decrease in intravascular volume. Hypotension ensues, and eventually impaired myocardial performance becomes obvious with impaired left ventricular function, including abnormal stroke work, decreased ejection fraction, and ventricular dilation. This may be due to circulating myocardial depressive factors, perhaps elaborated by the ischemic pancreas, though this is controversial. This results in decreased cardiac output and further hypotension. Perhaps as a compensatory mechanism, in late shock systemic vascular resistance may rise.

The initial respiratory changes[128,129] of septic shock include tachypnea and hyperventilation resulting in respiratory alkalosis. Increased pulmonary resistance, increased alveolar capillary permeability, and decreased lung compliance appear fairly early. Vasoconstriction and increased capillary permeability lead to edema and alveolar collapse. There is a ventilation/perfusion mismatch that leads to a decreased Po_2. This type of right-to-left shunting may herald the onset of ARDS. Septic shock is the most common cause of ARDS, and its presence worsens the prognosis of septic shock. When ARDS occurs, the timing of its onset is not predictable. Adult respiratory distress syndrome is typified by increased capillary permeability with increased lung water, decreased pulmonary compliance, and diffuse infiltrates. However, there is a normal pulmonary capillary wedge pressure. There is marked, often refractory hypoxia because of perfusion of unventilated alveolate. The syndrome may be diagnosed on the basis of inability to achieve a Po_2 of greater than 50 mm Hg with an Fio_2 of less than 50%. Platelet and fibrinthrombi are found in the lungs in ARDS as are sequestrated white blood cells. It is theorized that these activated white blood cells along with soluble mediators synthesized and metabolized in the lungs promote the inflammation and enzymatic damage that lead to ARDS. Eventually, the increased work associated with the profound respiratory changes of septic shock lead to decreased energy and increased lactic acidosis, which contribute to failure of the respiratory muscles. When this occurs, heralded by hypercarbia, septic shock is end-stage.

Disseminated intravascular coagulation (DIC), is one of the primary events occurring in septic shock.[127-130] Disseminated intravascular endothelial damage then leads to collagen exposure and the various soluble factors that liberate and activate the intrinsic and extrinsic coagulation systems. In late septic shock acidosis may serve to perpetuate the changes of DIC. Early in septic shock, there is platelet aggregation and fibrin deposition. These changes may contribute to a decrease in blood flow and local ischemia, particularly in the microcirculation. There is direct activation of the intrinsic clotting system by bacterial products and the release of procoagulants from macrophages and monocytes. Fibrinolytic mechanisms are also activated, including mononuclear cell tissue factor activity. At various times the manifestations of intravascular coagulation or of problems with blood clotting may predominate. A decrease in clotting factors, an increase in fibrin degradation products, a prolongation of clotting times, and a decrease in platelets are seen. An isolated thrombocytopenia may appear early. Of interest, thrombocytopenia in the setting of hypertension may be a risk factor for the occurrence of ARDS.

The white blood count in septic shock very transiently decreases and then significantly increases with a left shift, reflecting initial margination of white cells and then facilitated release from marrow stores. In addition to morphologic changes, there are functional changes in white blood cells, with a stimulation of both phagocytic and cytotoxic activities.

The body's metabolic processes are switched toward catabolism in an effort to supply and satisfy the increased energy demands of sepsis.[124] There is a decrease in glycogen synthesis and a pronounced increase in glycogenolysis. Initially there is hyperglycemia. Impaired hepatic gluconeogenesis, perhaps due to hepatic dysfunction, may appear early. As stores of glycogen are depleted and gluconeogenesis fails, hypoglycemia ensues. Muscle protein is degraded, leading to a negative nitrogen balance and hyperuricemia. There is a decrease in adipose tissue lipolytic activity leading to an increase in circulating free fatty acids and hypertriglyceridemia. Hepatic ketogenesis is impaired.

Changes in metabolic function may be mediated both by soluble monokines and changes in circulating hormone levels such as an increase in insulin and glucagon levels. There may also be alterations in hormone receptor activity.

Cellular metabolism is also impaired in late septic shock. Although lactic acid accumulates early in septic shock, perhaps because of inadequate liver and renal metabolism, poor perfusion of peripheral tissues resulting in anaerobic metabolism leads to a rapid accumulation of lactate. Even when there is adequate oxygen delivery to tissues, there appears to be impaired oxygen utilization peripherally, perhaps a result of a defect in mitochondrial function.[131]

Eventually all organ systems show effects due to hypoxia and damage,[128] in addition to direct effects of sepsis. Central nervous system changes are manifest particularly by altered sensorium. Gastrointestinal effects may include stress-induced erosions and bleeding, cholestatic jaundice due to both red blood cell breakdown and hepatocellular dysfunction, and effects of pancreatic vasoconstriction. The prominent renal problem of septic shock

is acute tubular necrosis secondary to hypotension, dehydration, cellular breakdown pigments, and medications. In addition, there may be a contribution to renal damage of perivascular inflammation and fibrin deposition in micro blood vessels.

Treatment and obstetric management

Early, aggressive management of septic shock directed toward maximizing cardiovascular dynamics, intravascular volume, and tissue oxygenation are warranted in all cases (Fig. 26-2). Aggressive volume restoration is essential to maximize tissue

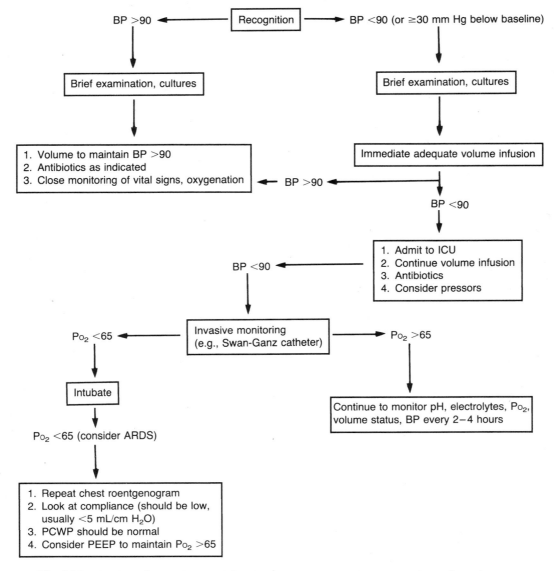

Fig. 26-2 Algorithm for treating sepsis/septic shock. *BP* = blood pressure: *ICU* = intensive care unit; *ARDS* = adult respiratory distress syndrome; *PCWP* = pulmonary capillary wedge pressure; *PEEP* = positive end-expiratory pressure. (From Brown KA, Sheagren JN: *Internal Medicine for the Specialist* 1990; 11:119. Used by permission.)

perfusion and to minimize other cardiovascular factors seen in septic shock. Volume restoration is related to often massive third spacing of fluids caused by the various pathophysiologic changes. Therefore, although careful calculation of intake and output is important, intravascular support may require massive volumes. There is no consensus as to whether volume should be administered as crystalloid or colloid.

Although the use of the Swan-Ganz catheter for measuring pulmonary capillary wedge pressure has not been documented to improve outcome in septic shock, many authorities advocate its use. It has the ability to determine cardiac output and oxygen consumption and to avoid errors of excessive volume replacement that may occur particularly in association with alterations in left ventricular compliance and function.[120,126,127,132] A pulmonary capillary wedge pressure of 10 to 12 cm H_2O in this condition is desirable.

Early use of oxygenation, including aggressive intubation, is warranted in attempting to improve tissue oxygenation and decrease the work of breathing.

Medications are given to improve cardiovascular dynamics, counter metabolic defects, and treat the underlying infection. Vasopressors are only useful in association with aggressive attempts at volume replacement. Dopamine is the initial vasopressor of choice, and when used in doses of less than 15 μg/kg/min, it increases mesenteric and renal blood flow in addition to improving myocardial contractility and cardiac output. In higher doses, vasoconstrictive effects may have an adverse affect. As hypotension becomes more profound, drugs with alpha-adrenergic effects may be necessary. A problem with such vasopressors may be the increased cardiac demands imposed by them. When there is evidence for myocardial dysfunction, digitalization is in order. Whenever measurable acidosis occurs, the administration of sodium bicarbonate to achieve a stable pH level between 7.2 and 7.3 can assist cardiovascular dynamics.

Coincident with aggressive management, all diagnostic modalities must be aggressively and judiciously employed. Chief among these is the adequate culturing of all potentially infected sites with Gram stains as necessary in an attempt to elucidate the causative organism of septic shock. Monitoring of arterial blood gases and electrolytes can be helpful in judging metabolic changes and the success of therapeutic maneuvers in septic shock. Initially, respiratory alkalosis with onset of metabolic acidosis is seen. Late changes of a worsening acidosis that is both metabolic and respira-

tory is a bad prognostic sign. Electrocardiograms and echocardiograms should be used to monitor and correct metabolic defects as well as assess cardiac function. All coagulation parameters should be closely monitored to assess the need for component replacement and reversal of coagulopathy. Periodic monitoring of renal and hepatic function is necessary to guide the use of medications and fluids to avoid compounding dysfunction.

Antibiotic management should be tailored to the specific situation but should include a broad spectrum of antibacterial activity. For the usual obstetric problems, coverage for gram-negative organisms (chiefly *Escherichia coli, Klebsiella* species) and gram-positive organisms (including *Staphylococcus aureus* and all streptococcal species), as well as maximal anaerobic coverage should be provided. Since many of the antimicrobial agents commonly selected, including aminoglycosides or vancomycin in penicillin-allergic patients, may prove to be renal toxic, their use should be carefully monitored and administered according to serum levels whenever possible.

The efficacy of administration of high-dose steroids during septic shock has been controversial. However, in 1987 concomitant articles by Boen et al[133] and the Veterans Cooperative Study[134] provided information responsible for omitting steroids from being used to combat septic shock today. These were the first large-scale, prospective, randomized, double-blind, placebo-controlled trials that attempted to administer steroids early in the diagnosis of sepsis, even before the specific diagnosis of septic shock. These studies showed that the use of steroids did not prevent the occurrence of septic shock and did not alter survival out to 14 days. Boen et al suggested that a higher rate of mortality from secondary infection may be present with the use of steroids and that people with preexisting disease might suffer from increased mortality with steroid use. Since there is no benefit from the use of high-dose steroids in septic shock, and they may potentially be detrimental to some patient groups, their use is not justified. It is interesting to note that in animal models improvement in survival has been correlated with steroid administration prior to administration of endotoxin or bacterial challenge. It is possible that such pretreatment will never be achieved in humans.

Poor prognostic signs in septic shock include generalized signs of hypoperfusion, coma, increasing acidosis and lactate levels, hypercarbia, and a decreased respiratory rate. Outcome of septic shock is most associated with the patient's underlying condition and state of health before the bacteremic insult. The mortality rate seen in association with obstetric septic shock is particularly low because of the usual lack of underlying disease.

Septic shock in obstetrics patients is associated with chorioamnionitis, prolonged ruptured membranes, endometritis, pyelonephritis, severe wound infections including fasciitis, and septic abortions.[120,121,135,136] Rates of bacteremia on obstetric services are not low, and in cases of febrile complications, rates of bacteremia between 4% and 32% have been reported. Gram-negative bacteremias account for between 6% and 50% of these.[137-144] Shock in association with obstetric bacteremia has been reported to occur in 0% to 12% of cases, with a low mortality rate of 0% to 4%.[123,140,141] The majority of deaths occurred in patients with infected abortions and in postoperative patients with an underlying immunosuppressive or myelosuppressive disorder. In addition to prolonged morbidity, however, obstetric septic shock can lead to Sheehan's syndrome, renal cortical necrosis, and acute tubular necrosis.[138]

In animal models, fetuses do not appear to suffer from direct effects of endotoxins and soluble mediators.[145,146] However, adverse fetal effects can be due to secondary changes in uterine blood flow and maternal metabolic instability.[123]

Obstetric septic shock at any time in gestation may necessitate surgical procedures to eliminate the source of sepsis. If the source of infection is thought to be the uterus, the organ must be evacuated of all products of conception and/or retained tissue on an emergent basis. Speroff has reported that curettage has been followed by chills and an increase in temperature but not by deterioration in the clinical course.[147] The method of evacuating the uterus must be guided by the patient's clinical response to initial therapeutic maneuvers. When shock is unresponsive to less aggressive measures, hysterotomy may be necessary. The need for hysterectomy in cases of septic shock is a matter of individual judgment. Most authorities suggest that hysterectomy is indicated when microabscess or tissue necrosis is present and when less invasive surgical procedures do not result in stabilization of the clinical condition.[120,147,148] In such cases of continued clinical deterioration, hysterectomy has been reported to be life-saving.

Anesthetic management

The parturient with septic shock presents unique challenges to the anesthesiologist. Maintenance of adequate hemodynamic stability, oxygenation, and coagulation are of paramount importance in obtaining good maternal and fetal outcomes.

Hemodynamics. The physiologic hallmark of septic shock is hypovolemia and resultant hypoten-

sion. Subsequent derangements include acidosis, myocardial depression, and multisystem organ failure. The first-line treatment for patients with sepsis is always adequate volume replacement to restore circulating blood volume in the setting of vasodilation and capillary leak. (Maintenance of uterine displacement is vital, a point often forgotten when parturients enter a medical intensive care unit!) Restoration of adequate intravascular volume is key to preserving pressure-dependent uterine perfusion and fetal well-being. Initial volume replacement should consist of a crystalloid solution, with addition of colloid supplementation if 2 or 3 L of the crystalloid fails to restore systolic blood pressure above 100 mm Hg or if persistent oliguria exists.

If seemingly adequate volume replacement fails to maintain normal blood pressures and urine output, early institution of invasive monitoring should be considered. If central access is performed, a thermodilution Swan-Ganz catheter should be placed, since measurement of cardiac output, pulmonary capillary wedge pressure, and systemic vascular resistance are the parameters that will be used to guide further therapy. Placement of only a central venous line will not provide the appropriate hemodynamic parameters to fully care for a septic parturient. Fluid resuscitation should be continued to obtain a normal pulmonary capillary wedge pressure (10 to 15 mm Hg). However, circulating mediators of sepsis may cause a continued state of hypotension and decreased systemic vascular resistance, even in the presence of adequate preload. At this stage, pharmacologic support of myocardial performance and vascular tone should be considered. Dopamine or dobutamine should be used when enhancement of cardiac output is required, and addition of epinephrine or norepinephrine when vascular tone is low. Considerable flexibility in choice of pressors exists, especially as varying dose ranges will provide various effects on the cardiovascular tree. Two important points to remember are that (1) vasopressor therapy should never be instituted in the absence of adequate intravascular volume replacement, and (2) continuous electronic fetal heart rate monitoring should be mandatory because the various vasopressor agents may adversely affect uterine perfusion.

Oxygenation. Close attention to pulmonary function should be maintained when sepsis occurs in the parturient. Finger pulse oximetry and a radial arterial line should be minimal requirements, and chest x-ray examinations should be performed at least daily (if not more often) during periods of acute illness. The primary pulmonary insult in sepsis is the development of ARDS. Adult respiratory distress syndrome should be considered when persistent hypoxemia (Po_2 <65 mm Hg) occurs, particularly if infiltrates appear on chest x-ray film and pulmonary capillary wedge pressure is normal. If ARDS is suspected, intubation and institution of positive end-expiratory pressure (PEEP) is warranted. Frequent arterial blood gas measurements should be obtained, and mixed venous blood gas analysis may also prove useful to monitor the adequacy of tissue perfusion.

Coagulation. Disseminated intravascular coagulation may occur because both intrinsic an extrinsic coagulation pathways are activated by various circulating mediators of sepsis. Therefore, assessment of coagulation panels should be part of the frequent and routine laboratory analysis performed in the septic parturient. Occasionally, DIC may be profound, requiring massive blood product and factor replacement. In such instances, hematologic consultation may be warranted to assist with blood product usage. Selection of regional anesthesia (epidural or continuous spinal) or general anesthesia will depend on the condition of the mother and the baby.

Both maternal and fetal well-being are gravely challenged when septic shock occurs during pregnancy, and the situation requires maximal medical supportive therapy. If extrauterine fetal viability is possible, or if the maternal status is life-threatening, delivery may enhance recovery and should be considered.[149] However, delivery itself, particularly by cesarean section, may introduce a whole new set of infectious complications. Thus, appropriate timing of delivery is a crucial decision to be made jointly between obstetrician, anesthesiologist, and intensivist.

SPECIAL CONSIDERATIONS IN THE EVALUATION OF TUBERCULOSIS DURING PREGNANCY

Concomitant with an increase in prevalence of HIV disease, there has been both an increase in the incidence of active tuberculosis (TB) and the occurrence of drug-resistant *M. tuberculosis.*[150-151] In most urban areas it is routine for pregnant women to be screened for TB by PPD skin testing during prenatal care.

As is the case for all persons exposed to TB, the risk of developing active disease is greatest in the time period most proximate to exposure, with 2% to 4% of individuals developing active disease within the first year of a newly positive PPD.[152] It is not clear if pregnant women are at increased risk for developing active disease either during pregnancy or in the immediate postpartum period.

However, considerations for management of TB during pregnancy include both maximizing maternal health and avoiding potential exposure of the neonate to *M. tuberculosis.*

Documented active TB should always be treated during pregnancy as is appropriate for the clinical condition. Preferred initial therapy includes INH, rifampin, and/or ethambutol with modifications in therapy made according to both clinical response and drug sensitivity of the organisms.[153] Documentation of a new or recent conversion to a positive PPD warrants serious consideration of prophylactic therapy with INH for 6 to 12 months, beginning during the pregnancy at the time of documentation of the positive skin test. Women who are HIV infected and women with other debilitating illnesses or alterations in immune function should receive INH according to clinical criteria for evaluation and treatment of *M. tuberculosis* in HIV-infected individuals. Others may opt to defer therapy until the postpartum time period. At a minimum, all positive PPDs should be evaluated with a chest x-ray examination to exclude active pulmonary disease, and there should be a complete evaluation of any persistent respiratory symptoms that occur during the course of pregnancy. In the case of a newly positive PPD, if the patient does not receive INH, it is common for a chest x-ray examination to be repeated immediately postpartum to avoid exposure of the neonate to active disease that may have had its onset during the gestation, and for prophylactic INH to be begun at this time.

Of note, observation of 3681 women who received treatment for tuberculosis with INH during or after pregnancy has shown a documented increase in the incidence of drug-induced hepatic injury in pregnant women above that seen in the general population of adults.[154] Therefore, it is routine for liver function tests to be monitored on a regular basis in all women who receive INH during pregnancy.

REFERENCES

1. Centers for Disease Control: Varicella-Zoster immune globulin for the prevention of chickenpox: Recommendations of the immunization practices advisory committee. *MMWR* 1984; 33:84.
2. Weller TH: Varicella and herpes zoster: Changing concepts of the natural history, control, and importance of a not-so-benign virus. *N Engl J Med* 1983; 309:1362.
3. Gershon AA, Raker R, Steinberg S, et al: Antibody to varicella-zoster virus in parturient women and their offspring during the first year of life. *Pediatrics* 1976; 58:692.
4. Landsberger EJ, Harger WD, Grossman JH: Successful management of varicella pneumonia complicating preg-

nancy. A report of three cases. *J Reprod Med* 1986; 31:311.

5. Pickard RE: Varicella pneumonia in pregnancy. *Am J Obstet Gynecol* 1968; 101:504.

6. Paryani SG, Arvin AM: Intrauterine infection with varicella-zoster virus after maternal varicella. *N Engl J Med* 1986; 314:1542.

7. LaForet, Lynch LL: Multiple congenital defects following maternal varicella. *N Engl J Med* 1947; 236:534.

8. McGregor JA, Mark S, Crawford GP, et al: Varicella zoster antibody testing in the care of pregnant women exposed to varicella. *Am J Obstet Gynecol* 1987; 157:281.

9. Enders G: Varicella-zoster virus infection in pregnancy. *Prog Med Virol* 1984; 29:166.

10. Alkalay AL, Pomerance JJ, Rimoin DL: Fetal varicella syndrome. *J Pediatr* 1987; 111:320.

11. Higa K, Dan K, Manabe H: Varicella-zoster virus infections during pregnancy: Hypothesis concerning the mechanisms of congenital malformations. *Obstet Gynecol* 1987; 69:214.

12. Savage MO, Moosa A, Gordon RR: Maternal varicella infection as a cause of fetal malformations. *Lancet* 1973; 1:352.

13. Meyers JD: Congenital varicella in term infants: Risk reconsidered. *J Infect Dis* 1974; 129:215.

14. Miller E, Cradock-Watson JE, Ridehalgh MKS: Outcome in newborn babies given anti-varicella-zoster immunoglobulin after perinatal maternal infection with varicella-zoster virus. *Lancet* 1989; 1:371.

15. Becker TM, Blount JH, Guinan ME: Genital herpes infections in private practice in the United States, 1966 to 1981. *JAMA* 1985; 253:1601.

16. Guinan ME, MacCalman J, Kern ER, et al: The course of untreated recurrent genital herpes simplex infection in 27 women. *N Engl J Med* 1981; 304:759.

17. Corey L, Adams HG, Brown ZA, et al: Genital herpes simplex virus infection: Clinical manifestations, course, and complications. *Ann Intern Med* 1983; 98:958.

18. Flewett T, Parker R, Philip W: Acute hepatitis due to herpes simplex virus in an adult. *J Clin Pathol* 1969; 22:60.

19. Young EJ, Killam AP, Greene JF Jr: Disseminated herpes virus infection: Association with primary genital herpes in pregnancy. *JAMA* 1976; 235:2731.

20. Anderson JM, Nicholls MWN: Herpes encephalitis in pregnancy. *Br Med J* 1972; 1:632.

21. Peacock JE, Sarubbi FA: Disseminated herpes simplex virus infection during pregnancy. *Obstet Gynecol* 1983; 61:13S.

22. Brown ZA, Voutver LA, Benedetti J, et al: Genital herpes in pregnancy: Risk factors associated with recurrences and asymptomatic viral shedding. *Am J Obstet Gynecol* 1985; 153:24.

23. Harger JH, Amortegui AJ, Meyer MP, et al: Characteristics of recurrent genital herpes simplex infections in pregnant women. *Obstet Gynecol* 1989; 73:367.

24. Wittek AE, Yaeger AS, Au DS, et al: Asymptomatic shedding of herpes simplex virus from the cervix and lesion site during pregnancy. *Am J Dis Child* 1984; 138:439.

25. Vontver LA, Kickok DE, Brown Z, et al: Recurrent genital herpes simplex virus infection in pregnancy: Infant outcome and frequency of asymptomatic recurrences. *Am J Obstet Gynecol* 1982; 143:75.

26. Arvin AM, Hensleigh PA, Prober CG, et al: Failure of antepartum maternal cultures to predict the infant's risk of exposure to herpes simplex virus at delivery. *N Engl J Med* 1986; 315:796.

27. Brown ZA, Vontver LA, Benedetti J, et al: Effects on infants of a first episode of genital herpes during pregnancy. *N Engl J Med* 1987; 317:1246.

28. Whitley RJ: Neonatal herpes simplex virus infections: Presentation and management. *J Reprod Med* 1986; 31:4265.

29. Whitley RJ, Nahmias AJ, Visintine AM, et al: The natural history of herpes simplex virus infection of mother and newborn. *Pediatrics* 1980; 66:489.

30. Brown ZA, Benedetti J, Ashley R, et al: Neonatal herpes simplex virus infection in relation to asymptomatic maternal infection at the time of labor. *N Engl J Med* 1991; 324:1247.

31. Prober CG, Sullender WM, Yasukawa LL, et al: Low risk of herpes simplex virus infections in neonates exposed to the virus at the time of vaginal delivery to mothers with recurrent genital herpes simplex virus infections. *N Engl J Med* 1987; 316:240.

32. Brown ZA, Baker DA: Acyclovir therapy during pregnancy. *Obstet Gynecol* 1989; 73:526.

33. Joyce TH, Marx GF: Regional anesthesia and herpes. *Soc Obstet Anesth Perinat Newsletter* 1982; 14:1.

34. Crosby ET, Halpern SH, Rolbin SH: Epidural anesthesia for cesarean section in patients with active recurrent genital herpes simplex infections: A retrospective review. *Can J Anaesth* 1989; 36:701.

35. Ramanathan S, Sheth R, Turndorf H: Anesthesia for cesarean section in patients with genital herpes: A retrospective study. *Anesthesiology* 1986; 64:807.

36. Ravindran RS, Gupta CD, Stoops CA: Epidural anesthesia in the presence of herpes simplex virus (type 2) infection. *Anesth Analg* 1982; 61:714.

37. Bader AM, Camann WR, Datta S: Anesthesia for cesarean section in patients with herpes simplex virus type-2 infections. *Reg Anesth* 1990; 15:261.

38. Crone LL, Conly JM, Clark KM, et al: Recurrent herpes simplex virus labialis and the use of epidural morphine in obstetric patients. *Anesth Analg* 1988; 67:318.

39. Steere AC: Lyme disease. *N Engl J Med* 1989; 321:586.

40. Lastavica CC, Wilson ML, Berardi VP, et al: Rapid emergency of a focal epidemic of lyme disease in coastal Massachusetts 1989; 320:133.

41. Petersen LR, Sweeney AH, Checko PJ, et al: Epidemiological and clinical features of 1,149 persons with Lyme disease identified by laboratory-based surveillance in Connecticut. *Yale J Biol Med* 1989; 62:253.

42. Smith LG Jr, Pearlman M, Smith LG et al: Lyme disease: A review with emphasis on the pregnant women. *Obstet Gynecol Surv* 1991; 46:125.

43. Rahn DW, Malawista SE: Lyme disease: Recommendations for diagnosis and treatment. *Ann Intern Med* 1991; 114:472.

44. Wallach FR, Forni AL, Hariprashad J, et al: Circulating *Borrelia burgdorferi* in patients with acute lyme disease: Results of blood cultures and serum DNA analysis. *J Infect Dis* 1993; 168:1541.

45. Golightly MG: Laboratory considerations in the diagnosis and management of Lyme borreliosis. *Am J Clin Pathol* 1993; 99:168.

46. Schlesinger PA, Duray PH, Burke BA, et al: Maternal-fetal transmission of the Lyme disease spirochete, *Borrelia burgdorferi*. *Ann Intern Med* 1985; 103:67.

47. Martkowtiz LE, Steere AC, Benach JL, et al: Lyme disease during pregnancy. *JAMA* 1986; 255:3394.

48. Stiernstedt G: Lyme borreliosis during pregnancy. *Scand J Infect Dis Suppl* 1990; 71:99.

49. Mikkelsen AL, Palle C: Lyme disease during pregnancy. *Acta Obstet Gynecol Scand* 1987; 66:477.

50. Appropriateness of parenteral antibiotic treatment for patients with presumed Lyme disease: A joint statement of the American College of Rheumatology and the Council

of the Infectious Disease Society of America. *Ann Intern Med* 1993; 119:518.

51. Sigal LH: Current recommendations for the treatment of Lyme disease. *Drugs* 1992; 43:683.

52. MacDonald AB: Gestational Lyme borreliosis: Implications for the fetus. *Rheum Dis Clin North Am* 1989; 15:657.

53. Strobino BA, Williams CL, Abid S, et al: Lyme disease and pregnancy outcome: A prospective study of two thousand prenatal patients. *Am J Obstet Gynecol* 1993; 169:367.

54. Schutzer SE, Janniger CK, Schwartz RA: Lyme disease during pregnancy. *Cutis* 1991; 47:267.

55. Nadal D, Hunziker UA, Bucher HU, et al: Infants born to mothers with antibodies against *Borrelia burgdorferi* at delivery. *Eur J Pediatr* 1989; 148:426.

56. Magid D, Schwartz B, Craft J, et al: Prevention of Lyme disease after tick bites: A cost-effectiveness analysis. *N Engl J Med* 1992; 327:534.

57. Shapiro ED, Gerber MA, Holabird NB, et al: A controlled trial of antimicrobial prophylaxis for Lyme disease after deer-tick bites. *N Engl J Med* 1992; 327:1769.

58. Steere AC, Battenhagen NH, Carft JE, et al: The early clinical manifestations of Lyme disease. *Ann Intern Med* 1983; 99:76.

59. Asbrink E, Hovmark A: Early and late cutaneous manifestations of *Ixodesborne borreliosis* (Lyme borreliosis). *Ann NY Acad Sci* 1988; 539:4.

60. Pachner AR, Duray P, Steere AC: Central nervous system manifestations of Lyme disease. *Arch Neurol* 1989; 46:790.

61. Steere AC, Bastford WP, Weinberg M, et al: Lyme carditis: Cardiac abnormalities of Lyme disease. *Ann Intern Med* 1980; 93:8.

62. Stanek G, Klein J, Bittner R, et al: Isolation of *Borrelia burgdoferi* from the myocardium of a patient with long-standing cardiomyopathy. *N Engl J Med* 1990; 322:249.

63. Gellin BG, Broome CV: Listeriosis. *JAMA* 1989; 261:1313.

64. *FDA Drug Bulletin* October 1987, pp 8-9.

65. Linnan MJ, Mascola L, Lou XD, et al: Epidemic listeriosis associated with Mexican-style cheese. *N Engl J Med* 1988; 319:823.

66. Boucher M, Yonekura ML, Wallace RJ, et al: Adult respiratory distress syndrome: A rare manifestation of *Listeria monocytogenes* infection in pregnancy. *Am J Obstet Gynecol* 1984; 149:686.

67. Wetli CV, Roldan EO, Fojaco RM: Listeriosis as a cause of maternal death: An obstetric complication of the acquired immunodeficiency syndrome (AIDS). *Am J Obstet Gynecol* 1983; 147:7.

68. Barresi JA: *Listeria monocytogenes* a cause of premature labor and neonatal sepsis. *Am J Obstet Gynecol* 1980; 136:410.

69. Cruikshank DP, Warenski JC: First-trimester maternal *Listeria monocytogenes* sepsis and chorioamnionitis with normal neonatal outcome. *Obstet Gynecol* 1989; 73:469.

70. Ault KA, Faros S: Viruses, bacteria, and protozoans in pregnancy: A sample of each. *Clin Obstet Gynecol* 1993; 36:878.

71. Boucher M, Yonekura ML: Perinatal listeriosis (early-onset): Correlation of antenatal manifestations and neonatal outcome. *Obstet Gynecol* 1986; 68:593.

72. Tessier F, Bouillie J, Dagnet GL: Listeriosis and obstetrics: A review of ten years' experience in a French maternity hospital. *J Gynecol Obstet Biol Reprod* 1986; 15:305.

73. Ho JH, Shands KN, Friedland G: Amount break of type 4b *Listeria monocytogenes* infection involving patients from eight Boston hospitals. *Arch Intern Med* 1986; 146:520.

74. Steele PE, Jacobs DS: *Listeria monocytogenes* macroabscesses of placenta. *Obstet Gynecol* 1979; 53:124.

75. Koh KS, Cole TL, Orkin AJ: Listeria amnionitis as a cause of fetal distress. *Am J Obstet Gynecol* 1980; 136:261.

76. Camann WR, Goldman GA, Johnson MD, et al: Cesarean delivery in patient with a transplanted heart. *Anesthesiology* 1989; 7:618.

77. MMWR: Update: AIDS among women—United States, 1994. *MMWR* 1995; 44:135.

78. Scott GB, Hutto C, Makuch RW, et al: Survival children in perinatally acquired human immunodeficiency virus type I infection. *N Engl J Med* 1989; 321:1791.

79. Landesman S, Minkoff H, Holman S, et al: Serosurvey of human immunodeficiency virus infection in parturients. *JAMA* 1987; 258:2701.

80. Chaisson RE, Bacchetti P, Osmond D, et al: Cocaine use and HIV infection in intravenous drug users in San Francisco. *JAMA* 1989; 261:561.

81. Shapiro CN, Schulz SL, Lee NC, et al: Review of human immunodeficiency virus infection in women in the United States. *Obstet Gynecol* 1989; 74:800.

82. Minkoff HL, McCalla S, Delke I, et al: The relationship of cocaine use to syphilis and human immunodeficiency virus infections among inner city parturient women. *Am J Obstet Gynecol* 1990; 163:521.

83. Novick LF, Berns D, Stricof R, et al: HIV seroprevalence in newborns in New York State. *JAMA* 1989; 261:1745.

84. Gwinn M, Pappaioanou M, George JR, et al: Prevalence of HIV infection in childbearing women in the United States: Surveillance using newborn blood samples. *JAMA* 1991; 265:1704.

85. Hoff R, Berardi VP, Weiblen BJ, et al: Seroprevalence of human immunodeficiency virus among childbearing women: Estimation by testing samples of blood from newborns. *N Engl J Med* 1988; 318:525.

86. Ho DM, Pomerantz RJ, Kaplan JC: Pathogenesis of infection with human immunodeficiency virus. *N Engl J Med* 1987; 317:278.

87. Creagh-Kirk T, Dori P, Andrews E, et al: Survival experience among patients with AIDS receiving zidovudine. *JAMA* 1988; 260:3009.

88. Carpenter CC, Mayer KH, Stein MD, et al: Human immunodeficiency virus infection in North American women: Experience with 200 cases and a review of the literature. *Medicine* 1991; 70:307.

89. Fischl MA, Richman DD, Grieco MH: The efficacy of azidothymidine (AZT) in the treatment of patients with AIDS and AIDS-related complex. *N Engl J Med* 1987; 317:185.

90. HIV diseases in pregnancy, in Minkoff HL (ed): *Obstetrics and Gynecology Clinics of North America,* WB Saunders, Philadelphia, 1990.

91. Minkoff HL, Willoughby A, Mendez H, et al: Serious infections during pregnancy among women with advanced human immunodeficiency virus infection. *Am J Obstet Gynecol* 1990; 162:30.

92. Minkoff HL, Henderson C, Mendez H, et al: Pregnancy outcomes among mothers infected with human immunodeficiency virus and uninfected control subjects. *Am J Obstet Gynecol* 1990; 163:1598.

93. Minkoff IL, DeHovitz JA: Care of women infected with the human immunodeficiency virus. *JAMA* 1991; 266:2253.

94. Sperling R, Stratton P: Treatment options for human immunodeficiency virus-infected pregnancy women. *Obstet Gynecol* 1992; 79:443.

95. HIV infection, pregnant women, and newborns: A policy

proposal for information and testing. Working Group on HIV Testing of Pregnant Women and Newborns. *JAMA* 1990; 264:2416.

96. Tuomala R: Human immunodeficiency virus education and screening of prenatal patients. *Obstet Gynecol Clin North Am* 1990; 17:571.

97. Minkoff HL, Landesman SH: The case for routinely offering prenatal testing for human immunodeficiency virus. *Am J Obstet Gynecol* 1988; 159:793.

98. Rossi P, Moschese V, Broliden PA, et al: Presence of maternal antibodies to human immunodeficiency virus 1 envelope glycoprotein gp 120 epitopes correlates with the uninfected status of children born to seropositive mothers. *Proc Natl Acad Sci USA* 1989; 86:8055.

99. Ryder RW, Nga W, Hassig SE, et al: Perinatal transmission of the human immunodeficiency virus type I to infants of seropositive women in Zaire. *N Engl J Med* 1989; 320:1637.

100. European Collaborative Study. Risk factors for mother-to-child transmission of HIV-1. *Lancet* 1992; 339:1007.

101. Mofenson LM: Epidemiology and determinants of vertical HIV transmission. *Seminars in Pediatric Infectious Diseases,* Vol 5, 1994, pp 252-265.

102. Ehrnst A, Lindgren S, Dictor M, et al: HIV in pregnant women and their offspring: Evidence for late transmission. *Lancet* 1991; 338:203.

103. Blanche S, Rouzioux C, Moscato MCG, et al: A prospective study of infants born to women seropositive for human immunodeficiency virus type I. *N Engl J Med* 1989; 320:1643.

104. Goedert JJ, Duliege AM, Amos CI, et al: High risk of HIV-1 infection for first-born twins. The International Registry of HIV-exposed Twins. *Lancet* 1991; 338:1471.

105. Connor EM, Sperling Rs, Gelber R, et al: Reduction of maternal-infant transmission of human immunodeficiency virus type 1 with Zidovudien treatment. Pediatric AIDS Clinical Trials Group Protocol 076 Study Group. *N Engl J Med* 1994; 331:1173.

106. Villari P, Spino C, Chalmers TC, et al: Cesarean section to reduce perinatal transmission of human immunodeficiency virus: A meta-analysis. *Curr Clinical Trials* 1993; 74:1-15.

107. The European Collaborative Study: Caesarean section and risk of vertical transmission of HIV-1 infection. *Lancet* 1994; 343:1464.

108. Boyer PJ, Dillon M, Navaie M, et al: Factors predictive of maternal-fetal Transmission of HIV-1: Preliminary analysis of Zidovudine given during pregnancy and/or delivery. *JAMA* 1994; 271:1925.

109. Burns DN, Landesman S, Muenz LR, et al: Cigarette smoking, premature rupture of membranes, and vertical transmission of HIV-1 among women with low CD4+ levels. *J Acquir Immune Defic Syndr* 1994; 77:718.

110. Centers for Disease Control: AIDS and HIV update: Acquired immunodeficiency syndrome and human immunodeficiency virus infection among health care workers. *MMWR* 1988; 37:229-234.

111. Becker CE, Cone JE, Gerberding J: Occupational infection with human immunodeficiency virus (HIV): Risks and risk reduction. *Ann Intern Med* 1989; 110:653.

112. Weber DJ, Redfield RR, Leman SM: Acquired immunodeficiency syndrome: Epidemiology and significance for the obstetrician and gynecologist. *Obstet Gynecol* 1986; 155:235.

113. Ho DM, Rota TR, Schooley RT, et al: Isolation of HTLV-III from cerebrospinal fluid and neural tissues of patients with neurologic syndromes related to the acquired immunodeficiency syndrome. *N Engl J Med* 1985; 313:1493.

114. Davies JM, Thistlewood JM, Rolbin SH, et al: Infections

and the parturient: Anesthetic considerations. *Can J Anaesth* 1988; 35:270.

115. Greene ER: Spinal and epidural anesthesia in patients with the acquired immunodeficiency syndrome. *Anesth Analg* 1986; 65:1090.

116. Hughes SC, Dailey PA, Landers D, et al: Parturients infected with human immodeficiency virus and regional anesthesia: Clinical and immune response. *Anesthesiology* 1995; 82:32.

117. Barzan L, Carbone A, Saracchini S, et al: Nasopharyngeal lymphatic tissue hypertrophy in HIV-infected patients. *Lancet* 1989; 1:42.

118. Update: Human immunodeficiency virus infections in health-care workers exposed to blood of infected patients—United States. *Canada Disease Weekly Report,* Health and Welfare Canada, May 30, 1987, pp 95-8.

119. Centers for Disease Control: Recommendations for preventing transmission of infection with human T-lymphotropic virus type III/lymphotropic virus in the workplace. *MMWR* 1985; 254:3162.

120. Cavanagh D, Rao PS, Roberts WS: Septic shock in the gynecologic patient. *Clin Obstet Gynecol* 1985; 28:355.

121. Gonik B: Septic shock in obstetrics. *Clin Perinatol* 1986; 13:741.

122. Filkins JP: Monokines and the metabolic pathophysiology of septic shock. *Fed Proc* 1985; 44:300.

123. Balk HA, Cook JA, Wise WC, et al: Role of thromboxane, prostaglandins and leukotrienes in endotoxin and septic shock. *Intensive Care Med* 1986; 12:116.

124. Morrison DC, Ryan JL: Endotoxins and disease mechanisms. *Ann Rev Med* 1987; 38:417.

125. Beutler B, Cerami A: Cachectin: More than a tumor necrosis factor. *N Engl J Med* 1987; 316:379.

126. Parillo JE: The cardiovascular pathophysiology of sepsis. *Ann Rev Med* 1989; 40:469.

127. Knippel RA, Rao PS, Caranagh D: Septic shock in obstetrics. *Clin Obstet Gynecol* 1984; 27:3.

128. Harris RL, Musher DM, Bloom K, et al: Manifestations of sepsis. *Arch Intern Med* 1987; 147:1985.

129. Newman JH: Sepsis and pulmonary edema. *Clin Chest Med* 1985; 6:371.

130. Beller FK: Sepsis and coagulation. *Clin Obstet Gynecol* 1985; 28:46.

131. Rackow EC, Astiz ME, Weil H: Cellular oxygen metabolism during sepsis and shock. *JAMA* 1988; 259:1989.

132. Karakusis PH: Considerations in the therapy of septic shock. *Med Clin North Am* 1986; 70:933.

133. Bone RC, Fisher CJ Jr, Clemmer TP, et al: A controlled clinical trial of high-dose methylprednisolone in the treatment of severe sepsis and septic shock. *N Engl J Med* 1987; 317:653.

134. Veterans Administration Systemic Sepsis Cooperative Study Group: Effect of high-dose glucocorticoid therapy on mortality in patients with clinical signs of systemic sepsis. *N Engl J Med* 1987; 317:659.

135. Lee W, Clark SL, Cotton DB, et al: Septic shock during pregnancy. *Am J Obstet Gynecol* 1988; 159:410.

136. Cavanagh D: Shock and the pregnant patient. *Curr Surg* 1986; 43:91.

137. Blanco JD, Gibbs RS, Castaneda YS: Bacteremia in obstetrics: Clinical course. *Obstet Gynecol* 1981; 58:621.

138. Bryan CS, Reynolds KL, Moore EE: Bacteremia in obstetrics and gynecology. *Obstet Gynecol* 1984; 64:155.

139. Chow AW, Guze LB: Bacteroidaceae bacteremia: Clinical experience with 112 patients. *Medicine* 1974; 53:93.

140. DiZerega GS, Yonekura ML, Keegan K, et al: Bacteremia in post-cesarean section endomyometritis: Differential response to therapy. *Obstet Gynecol* 1980; 55:587.

141. Gibbs RS, Blanco JD, Bernstein S: Role of aerobic gram-

negative bacilli in endometritis after cesarean section. *Rev Infect Dis* 1985; 7 (suppl 4):S690.

142. Lamey JR, Escheubach DA, Mitchell SH, et al: Isolation of mycoplasmas and bacteria from the blood of postpartum women. *Am J Obstet Gynecol* 1982; 143:104.

143. Ledger WJ, Norman M, Gee C, et al: Bacteremia on an obstetric-gynecologic service. *Am J Obstet Gynecol* 1975; 121:205.

144. Monif GG, Baer H: Polymicrobial bacteremia in obstetric patients. *Obstet Gynecol* 1976; 48:167.

145. Beller FK, Schmidt EH, Holzgreve W, et al: Septicemia during pregnancy: a study in different species of experimental animals. *Am J Obstet Gynecol* 1985; 151:967.

146. Ornoy A, Altshuler G: Maternal endotoxemia, fetal anomalies, and central nervous system damage: A rat model of a human problem. *Am J Obstet Gynecol* 1976; 124:196.

147. Speroff L: Bacterial shock in obstetrics and gynecology, with emphasis on the surgical management of septic abortion. *Am J Obstet Gynecol* 1966; 95:139.

148. Lloyd T, Dougherty J, Karlin J: Infected intrauterine pregnancy presenting as septic shock. *Ann Emerg Med* 1983; 12:704.

149. Daily WH, Katz AR, Tonnesen A, et al: Beneficial effect of delivery in patient with adult respiratory distress syndrome. *Anesthesiology* 1990; 72:383.

150. Hamadeh M, Glassroth J: Tuberculosis and pregnancy. *Chest* 1992; 101:1114.

151. Baker DA: Re-emergence of tuberculosis. *Curr Opin Obstet Gynecol* 1994; 6:373.

152. Medchill MT, Gillum M: Diagnosis and management of tuberculosis during pregnancy. *Obstet Gynecol Surv* 1980; 44:81.

153. Snider DE, Layde PM, Johnson M, et al: Treatment of tuberculosis during pregnancy. *Am Rev Respir Dis* 1980; 122:65.

154. Franks AL, Binkin NJ, Snider DE, et al: Isoniazid hepatitis among pregnant and postpartum hispanic patients. *Ann Intern Med* 1989; 104:151.

27 Substance Abuse

Nancy Kenepp and Ashwin Chatwani

Substance abuse, the repetitive use of a chemical to alter mood, is reported by about 6% of the population. Women of childbearing age constitute a substantial proportion of substance abusers. Box 27-1 lists the substances addressed in this chapter.

SUBSTANCE ABUSE
Patterns of abuse

Substance abusers exhibit a continuum of patterns of drug use (Fig. 27-1). Movement back and forth from one stage to another is possible. On one extreme is the person who abstains completely. Most people use drugs rarely or occasionally; this is termed "social" use. Abuse occurs when use is clearly above the norm for the social group. When medical and personal problems and withdrawal begin, early addiction is present. Exclusive of tobacco, at any given time about 4% of the U.S. population abuses or depends on drugs, and over the course of their lives, about 20% of the population will meet the criteria for abuse or dependence.[1]

Social use. Several factors determine use of drugs. Social variables are peer attitude toward use, parental use, socioeconomic status, education, and legality. National and regional waves of heroin abuse have given way to cocaine and amphetamine.[2,3] Psychosocial factors include risk, curiosity, and individual tendency to accept social norms.[4] In teenagers, use correlates with adolescent depressant symptomatology and dropping out of school.[5] Tobacco and alcohol tend to be tried initially, since they are legal substances. Individuals and groups progress to trying illegal substances such as marijuana and cocaine.[5] In California, 37% of drug users also consumed alcohol[6] and in Florida, patients testing positive for marijuana or cocaine use were much more likely to use tobacco and alcohol.[7]

Abuse. Causes of abuse are numerous. Some predictors of abusive behavior are low self-esteem as well as difficulty in relating to people, expressing feelings, creating a healthy environment, and anticipating consequences. A susceptible individual never exposed to a substance does not become an addict. Since what is socially acceptable varies among groups, one of the early signs of abuse is changing associates to retain social acceptability. Medical consequences may be attributed to other factors, such as childhood illnesses. Eventually addictive behavior interferes with obtaining basic needs such as food, housing, and medical care.

Addiction. Addiction, then, is using the substance for short-term pleasure at the expense of long-term adverse effects. Although at this stage clear addiction is obvious to the observer, the user may still deny problems associated with the behavior and will admit to only occasional use when asked.

Pharmacology

Tolerance. Addictive drugs share the capacity to produce two types of tolerance. Metabolic tolerance is increased capacity to metabolize the substance. Pharmacodynamic tolerance is decreased sensitivity of the central nervous system (CNS) to the drug effects, which is caused by autoregulating mechanisms.

Dependence. Dependence is a sign of pharmacodynamic tolerance. It is characterized by a rebound CNS hyperexcitability or depression as the initial effect wanes. Dependence reinforces drug-seeking behavior and is more severe with short-acting compounds. Minimal symptoms of dependence accompany drugs of longer duration. Substances with cross-dependence relieve the symptoms of hyperexcitability or depression. Acute intoxication increases sensitivity to cross-tolerant drugs, and chronic use decreases sensitivity.

Withdrawal. Withdrawal refers to the constellation of symptoms that develop when the drug is no longer used. Withdrawal is evidence that pharmacodynamic tolerance has developed. The extent of distress during pharmacologic withdrawal is often influenced by environmental conditioning—the association of substance abuse with particular events. Protracted abstinence syndrome is a lengthy period during which subtle withdrawal symptoms interfere with smooth progression of the activities of daily living. Sub-

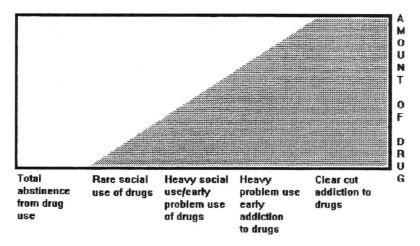

Fig. 27-1 The drug use continuum. (From Dowelko HF: *Concepts of Chemical Dependency.* Pacific Grove, Brooks/Cole, 1993.)

**BOX 27-1   COMMONLY ABUSED
SUBSTANCES**

Tobacco
Alcohol
Marijuana
Cocaine
Amphetamine
Phencyclidine
Benzodiazepines
Barbiturates

---

stances with cross-dependence suppress withdrawal symptoms but maintain dependence. Thus cross-dependent substances can be used when the primary substance is not available. This explains the tendency for those addicted to illicit substances to use multiple drugs. The basis of some overdoses is ingestion of cross-dependent substances inadvertently. Cross-dependent drugs possessing less severe withdrawal symptoms or adverse health effects can be useful in treating addiction.

Detection

Chemical analysis. Abusive chemicals are usually assayed in urine or blood. The most common technique for initial identification of illegal substances is an enzyme mediated immunotechnique (EMIT). The positive results of this screening test should be confirmed by gas chromatography, high pressure liquid chromatography, or thin-layer chromatography. Urine screening is easier for most substances because it can be more easily obtained than blood. However, the disadvantage of urine screening is that patients can easily tamper with it. A major disadvantage of both urine and blood screening is the limited interval after use, during which detectable levels of the substance are present. Urine drug tests remain positive for 24 to 72 hours after last use of amphetamines; for 24 to 72 hours for cocaine; for 2 to 4 days for opiates; for 8 to 16 hours for alcohol; and for 7 to 30 days for marijuana.[8]

Hair analysis can be used to detect past use of nicotine and cocaine and their metabolites. Quantitative analysis of hair can be performed by radioimmunoassay, and concentration of a substance in the hair corresponds to the amount of exposure.[9] Cocaine users had a mean of 359 ng per 10 mg of hair, versus 14 ng per 10 mg for passively exposed or occasional users.[10] Although hair growth is variable, the proximal 12 cm corresponds with the duration of the pregnancy. It can be cut into three 4-cm segments, which when assayed correlate well with historical use during the these trimesters of pregnancy.[10] Cocaine and tobacco are deposited into fetal hair during the third trimester, and infant levels correlated well with maternal proximal segment levels.[9,10] Meconium analysis also can be used to detect past and recent in utero exposure.[11] These techniques are costly and available only in a few laboratories, which precludes their wide application.

Self-reporting. Reliance on self-reporting will miss incidence of chemical use in 26% to 48% of pregnancies.[6,12] Protocols outlining selective criteria for urine toxicology testing will not discover all the patients. In addition, selective screening usually discriminates against minorities and the poor.

ADDICTIVE DRUGS IN PREGNANCY
Incidence

The first step in providing prenatal care for substance abusers is to identify the patient. Several studies have attempted to assess the prevalence and types of drugs abused among pregnant women by interviewing patients or by screening urine.[6,7,12-28] The true incidence of perinatal substance abuse is unknown because self-reporting is unreliable and urine screening detects only recent users. Thus the incidence of use during pregnancy is much higher than reported in the literature.

Of universally screened women on admission to the obstetric service at the University of California, Davis Medical Center, 1 in 5 tested positive for one of the illegal substances.[6] In other studies, positive urine tests for cocaine or marijuana have been reported to range from 8% to 32%.[12,28] Tobacco use, which is not included in many studies, ranges from 15% in private West Coast patients to 22% to 28% in middle class urban populations to as high as 46% in Midwest rural patients.[17,26,29] Tobacco use also correlates with substance abuse; 78% of drug users were smokers in one study.[6] Tobacco has been found to be the variable best correlating with drug abuse; 15% of drug users smoke, compared with 5% of nonusers.[17,19]

A compilation of the reported geographic prevalence rates from these studies is presented in Table 27-1. In rural areas and the Southeast, tobacco, alcohol, and marijuana are commonly abused substances. In urban East and West Coast areas, cocaine use is more prevalent. Amphetamine use is not as prevalent as cocaine except in selected urban areas on the West Coast.

Various demographic characteristics have been correlated with drug users. Most studies describe drug users to be older,[6,23,30] single,[18,26] from a lower socioeconomic class,[6,16] clinic patients,[7,16,26] and less educated.[26] Afro-Americans seem more likely to use cocaine, while Asians and Hispanics were unlikely to use illicit drugs.[6,7,15,26] Private patients are less likely to use cocaine.[7,13,15,18,26]

Study protocol caveats. Although these studies serve to provide an estimate of the scope of the problem, they are not comparable, and most are inadequate to separate the effects of a particular drug from those due to general maternal circumstances. Some studies did not collect adequate demographic data or information regarding other substance abuse. There are methodologic flaws in separating users from nonusers. Some rely on a single urine sample. In one study 25% of patients with negative urine screens gave a history of drug use[6]; and in another report, only half of patients reporting drug use have positive drug screens.[22] Screening infant urine missed 50% of exposed fetuses.[31] Urine screen timing alters user population estimates. Even assuming all active users will be positive, analysis early in gestation includes those who abstain from substance use after the first trimester. With analysis late in gestation or at delivery, first- and second-trimester users are classified as abstainers. Thus urine testing alone is not a reliable means of identifying patients who abuse drugs.

Some studies rely on patient reports of drug use; these are also unreliable. Twenty-five percent to 59% of patients with positive urine screens deny use of drugs.[6,12,22,32] Minnesota has a law requiring that mothers suspected of drug use be screened. Positive test results must be reported to the local child protection services, which consider this neglect. Fearing consequences, patients are reluctant to report illicit drug use. Of patients with positive urine, 82% deny marijuana use and 44% deny cocaine use.[7] An anonymous computer interview, which included patient education and a personal printout indicating individual problems, increased honesty in self-reporting 20% and was well received by patients.[22]

Since there is a continuum of severity of drug abuse, merely reporting exposure as positive or negative lumps together rare users as well as addicts. One study shows that 57% of patients at a teaching hospital and 61% at a private hospital had any alcohol before or during pregnancy, whereas 12% and 7% respectively "binged," and 6% and

Table 27-1 Prevalence rates (%) of substance abuse in pregnancy

Geographic area	Southeast urban (%)	Northeast urban (%)	Midwest urban (%)	West coast urban (%)	Rural, private (%)
Tobacco	26	14-34		8-44	13-46
Alcohol	7	4-13	15	6-12	1-20
Marijuana	5-11	1-30	6-34	2-25	0-10
Cocaine	1-6	10-18	1-11	2-15	0.6-3
Amphetamine	0.3	1	1	1-7	0
All Drugs	7-24	7-50	4-11	5-20	4-11

1% respectively "binged" during the pregnancy.[26] Such information is especially misleading when entered into multivariate regression analysis.

Identification. In identifying substance abusers among obstetric patients, the results of prevalence studies can be used to advantage. Skillful interviewing should be a part of the initial history. Questions should be presented in a nonthreatening manner. A good source for interviewing technique and questions is presented by Klein.[33] The medical, social, or obstetric history may reveal problems associated with substance abuse, indicating a need for further investigation. Universal urine screening is not cost-effective. Assuming a cost of about 25 dollars, it will cost about 100 dollars to detect an abuser when 25% of urine specimens are positive, but it will cost about 700 dollars to detect an abuser when 4% of specimens are positive.[16]

Effects of pregnancy on substance abuse

Pharmacologic. Physiologic changes in body water and plasma volume during pregnancy can alter the peak concentration, half-life, and volume of distribution of drugs.[34] There is evidence that sensitivity and metabolism of drugs change during pregnancy. The pregnancy increases the sensitivity to cocaine, whereas methadone requirements increase with pregnancy. Pregnancy lowers cytochrome P_{450} enzymes, glucuronyl transferase, and microsomal monooxygenase.[35] In rats, progesterone increases N-demethylation.[36] These changes alter metabolism of cocaine, heroin, alcohol, barbiturates, and marijuana. Cocaine metabolism is also affected by the decreased levels of plasma cholinesterase in pregnancy. Metabolism of alcohol via aldehyde dehydrogenase, and cocaine via N-demethylation, may cause liver cellular damage.[37]

Placental drug metabolism is determined by the quality and quantity of enzymes present, which are in turn determined by maternal environment. Changes in placental enzymes have been reported in smokers.[38] The placenta has microsomes capable of metabolizing cocaine, possibly by cholinesterase.[39] The placenta metabolizes alcohol in a manner similar to the liver.[40]

Maternal effects of substance abuse

Effects of IV injection. Persons who administer drugs by injection are subject to complications associated with use of nonsterile equipment and impure drugs. These, listed in Box 27-2, include hepatitis, acquired immunodeficiency syndrome (AIDS), endocarditis, and pulmonary hypertension.

With the decreased popularity of heroin and the more recent use of newer preparations of cocaine and amphetamine by inhalation rather than injec-

tion, one would expect the proportion of abusers who have HIV to decrease. However, cocaine addicts who are unemployed have a high incidence of HIV unrelated to IV drug use.[41] This is attributed to drug-related sexual activity. In New York City, 40% of pregnant women enrolled in a methadone clinic tested HIV positive.[42] In Atlanta, 0.6% of pregnant patients tested HIV positive, and half of those who admitted risk factors were cocaine users. The odds ratio of acquiring HIV infection with a history of intravenous drug administration was 14.5, and with cocaine use, 2.3.[41]

Substance effects. Pregnant patients have increased cardiac output, increased minute ventilation, and increased oxygen consumption. Respiratory or cardiac failure may occur with less pharmacologic depression from barbiturates, opiates, or alcohol than in the nonpregnant state. Nutritional needs are increased in pregnancy, and drug abuse is generally associated with poor dietary habits. In one study, patients with urine testing positive for marijuana, PCP, or cocaine had lower serum folate and ferritin levels.[43] Urinary tract infections and pneumonia are more frequent.[44] Higher blood leukocyte counts are associated with antepartum drug use.[43] Some maternal physiologic changes are effects of specific drugs. Elevated maternal carboxyhemoglobin levels and airway hyperreactivity will be present in smokers of any sub-

---

BOX 27-2 IMPLICATIONS OF PARENTERAL DRUG ABUSE

Hepatitis
Tricuspid insufficiency
Septic phlebitis
Pulmonary hypertension
Pulmonary edema
Foreign body emboli
Lymphedema
Bullous pulmonary damage
Pulmonary abscess
Tuberculosis
Bacterial endocarditis
Cellulitis
Septic pulmonary infarct
HIV infection
Superficial or deep abscess
Cerebral abscess
Vertebral osteomyelitis
Pneumonia
Tetanus
Sexually transmitted disease

Modified from James FM, Wheeler AS, Dewan DM (eds): *Obstetric Anesthesia: The Complicated Patient.* Philadelphia, FA Davis, 1987. Used by permission.

Table 27-2 Prenatal care in substance abusers

Prenatal care	Controls (%)	Cocaine (%)	Amphetamine (%)	Multidrug (%)	Opiate (%)
1st trimester	13	6	6	11	21
2nd trimester	35	25	18	26	47
3rd trimester	30	21	27	20	21
None	11	40*	40*	40*	11*

*$p < 0.01$, comparison with controls.
Modified from Gillogley KM, Evans AT, Hansen RL, et al: The perinatal impact of cocaine, amphetamine, and opiate use detected by universal intrapartum screening. *Am J Obstet Gynecol* 1990; 163:1535.

stance. Alcohol abuse causes gastritis, pancreatitis, neuropathy, seizures, and elevated hepatic enzymes. Heroin and cocaine may cause sudden death. Cocaine use is associated with malnutrition, cardiovascular complications, sudden death, hyperpyrexia, seizure, and HIV infection. Acute cocaine toxicity may mimic preeclampsia[45] and affect platelet function.[46] Physical signs associated with drug use include pupil size, cough, rhonchi or wheezing, staining of fingers and teeth, palmar erythema, liver flap, skin ulcers or needle tracks, emaciation, poor hygiene, inattentiveness, and narcolepsy.

Psychosocial effects. The effect of drug use on maternal functioning depends on the presence of abuse or addiction. Social users, once made aware of possible detrimental effects, will abstain. Evidence indicates that a high percentage of women reduce or abstain from tobacco and alcohol use soon after discovering pregnancy.[47] Drug users are more likely to be physically abused.[48,49] Afro-American women who use drugs are 3.7 times more likely to be battered than nonusers; white women using drugs are 2.1 times more likely to be abused than nonusers.[48]

Abusers and addicts use too much energy obtaining drugs, and not enough on taking care of their personal needs. Their lifestyle is typically chaotic, and money for food may be spent on drugs.[20] Patients on "binges" do not eat and can become emaciated. They often resort to prostitution for drug money, or they trade sex for drugs. They may be homeless or live in housing without heat, running water, or telephone. Pregnant patients delay obtaining medical care. Prenatal care obtained by drug users in one study is shown in Table 27-2. Some patients with early drug abuse may avoid prenatal care fearing discovery and legal action or loss of child custody. The available treatment facilities for drug users are not adequate,[13] and a study in Oregon determined that if health care providers made an effort to identify such patients, there would not be facilities available to treat them.[19]

Uteroplacental effects of substance abuse

Placental metabolism, uteroplacental blood flow, and placental transfer of oxygen and nutrients are all affected by substance abuse. Placental transfer of nutrients and drugs is determined by membrane characteristics, pH, lipid solubility, protein binding, and molecular weight.

Placental transfer. Impaired placental nutrient transfer associated with substance abuse may result from changes in placental membranes. Nutrient transfer is affected by cocaine,[36] alcohol,[50] and tobacco.[51]

Placentas of heavy smokers exhibit atrophic hypovascular villi. This leads to reduced estradiol conversion, and placental uptake of alpha-aminobutyric acid is decreased.[50] Components of cigarette smoke depress cellular uptake of amino acids, leading to reduced placental transfer of amino acids, causing lower levels of amino acids in the umbilical vein of smokers.[51]

Placental blood flow. Uteroplacental blood flow is determined by maternal and fetal cardiac output, uterine tone, and vascular resistance. Depressant drugs such as barbiturates may decrease cardiac output and thus impair delivery of nutrients and oxygen. Alcohol has no direct effect on placental blood flow as measured by umbilical artery impedance.[52] Increased sympathetic activity produced by cocaine, amphetamine, tobacco, narcotic or alcohol withdrawal, and hypercarbia and hypoxia from narcotics may produce the same impairment by causing vasoconstriction of placental and uterine blood vessels.[53] Amphetamine decreases uterine blood flow and umbilical blood flow in pregnant sheep.[54] Cocaine administration to pregnant rats[55] decreases blood flow to the placenta by increasing uterine vascular resistance. Cocaine also reduces uterine blood flow in pregnant sheep and baboons.[56-58] Cocaine-induced vasoconstriction of the uterine blood vessels in sheep is not prevented by prior infusion of phentolamine, indicating a direct or dopamine-mediated effect by cocaine.[58]

Table 27-3 Placental abruption and substance abuse

Drug or condition	Control rate (%) of abruption	Drug or condition rate (%) of abruption
Amphetamine	0.7	0.9
Methadone	0	0.7
Tobacco	—	1.6-2.8
Heroin	0	3.2
No prenatal care	0	4.0
Multidrug abuse	0.7	5.7
Cocaine	0.3-0.8	0.7-15

Table 27-4 Birth weight deficits*

Substance abused	Birth weight deficit (g)	Head circumference deficit (cm)
Cocaine	125*	0.41*
Cocaine + multidrugs	195†	1.09†
Cocaine + marijuana	170*	0.41†
Cocaine + opiates	237†	0.95†
"Crack"	200†	0.84†

*$p < 0.05$.
†$p < 0.01$.
Modified from Bateman DA, Stephen KCN, Hansen CA, et al: The effects of intrauterine cocaine exposure in newborns. *Am J Public Health* 1993; 83:190.

In humans in preterm labor, umbilical artery Doppler velocimetry measured systolic-diastolic ratios are abnormally high in about 25% of cocaine abusers, indicating the presence of vasoconstriction.[59] Vasoconstriction can increase the incidence of abruption as seen with nicotine,[60] heroin,[61] amphetamine,[62] and cocaine.[62-69] In smokers, placental abruption can also result from decidual necrosis at the placental margin.[70] Table 27-3 shows the incidence of placental abruption with drug abuse compared with control populations and a group of patients who did not abuse drugs but who had no prenatal care.

Fetal effects of substance abuse

Birth defects. Birth defects in substance abusers can result from various causes. Malnutrition, direct effects of drugs or their metabolites, infarction from vasoconstriction, and alteration in neurotransmitters have been implicated in causing birth defects.[71] Malnutrition, specifically deficiency of folic acid in substance abusers, can cause neural tube defects.[72]

Acetaldehyde is thought to be involved in the development of fetal alcohol syndrome (FAS).[73,74] Although there is no clear-cut evidence of barbiturate-induced fetal damage in humans, barbiturates are behavioral teratogens in animals and early gestational exposure produces neuromorphic changes similar to FAS.[75] FAS-like anomalies have been reported with exposure to marijuana, but alcohol and malnutrition may have also been factors.[76] Vasoconstriction may cause limb reduction defects, skull defects,[68,77] genitourinary tract anomalies,[78] and ileal atresia[63] in humans.

Intrauterine growth retardation (IUGR). Tobacco,[18,79,80,81] alcohol,[82,83] heroin,[62,84,85] marijuana,[2] amphetamine,[62,54] and cocaine[20,65,69,86,87-92] use are all associated with IUGR. Table 27-4 shows the effect of some of these drugs on birth weight. IUGR is most severe in poly drug users and bingers.[43,88,93,94] Cocaine and PCP are associated with microcephalic dysmorphic growth reduction.[92,95-97]

Multiple reasons are proposed for growth retardation. Drug-induced decreased delivery of oxygen and nutrients via the placenta is one.[92] Fetal hypoxia, ischemia, and accumulation of carbon monoxide are other proposed causes.

Spontaneous abortion. The incidence of spontaneous abortion has been reported to be higher in substance abusers. Smoking increased spontaneous abortion rates.[98] Higher rates of abortion have been reported in cocaine users.[99]

Preterm labor. The incidence of preterm labor is higher in substance abusers.[6,28,100-103] Patients abusing multiple drugs or binge cocaine users are more likely to have preterm delivery than patients without a drug history.*

Abruption. Incidence of abruption in substance abusers is increased, as previously mentioned.

Fetal distress. The incidence of fetal distress is higher in drug abusers because of an increased incidence of placentae abruption and placental insufficiency. Opiates may cause loss of fetal heart rate variability. Acute cocaine use can cause fetal tachycardia.

Neonatal effect of substance abuse

Neonates continue to be affected by maternal drug use. This can be from an increased incidence of transfer of sexually transmitted diseases to the neonates; delayed metabolism and excretion of drugs from neonates because of limited neonatal metabolic capacity and the absence of placental transfer back to the mother; and necessary treatment of withdrawal symptoms. Exposure from breast feeding[105] and passive exposure from maternal

---

*References 6, 7, 62, 65, 66, 69, 89, 93, 94, 104.

**BOX 27-3   NEONATAL WITHDRAWAL
SYMPTOMS**

Tremor
Irritability
Jittery behavior
Excessive crying
Hyperactive reflexes
Yawning
Sneezing
Sweating
Increased respirations
Seizures
Alkalosis
Hypocapnia
Fever
Increased stools
Vomiting
Dehydration
Uncoordinated sucking
Increased flexor tone
Disorganized responses

---

smoking, may be additional factors. Neonatal development may also be influenced by environmental factors.

Several studies have documented problems in infants of drug abusers. These include elevated lead levels,[106] anemia,[62] adverse neurologic and respiratory findings, and longer hospital stays.[107,108] Infants exposed to tobacco have lower forced expiratory flow rates shortly after birth.[109] In one study the cost of neonatal care for predominantly cocaine exposure was increased 4 to 8 times, and in another 10 times that of unexposed infants.[93,110]

Neurologic outcome. Adverse neurologic findings include neonatal depression from intoxication and withdrawal symptoms. Withdrawal symptoms include agitation, excess crying, irritability, poor feeding, abnormal sleep patterns, excess sweating, and seizures; these are observed with alcohol, cocaine, opiates, benzodiazepines, and barbiturates. Opiate withdrawal symptoms are shown in Box 27-3. Neonates with withdrawal symptoms have excess weight loss.[62,111] There is an increased risk of sudden infant death syndrome (SIDS) with the maternal use of tobacco, opiates, and cocaine.[85,90,112-115] Perinatal mortality is increased 25% to 35% in infants exposed to tobacco.[116]

Many workers have examined neonatal neurologic functioning. Neonates exposed to alcohol during the first and second trimester exhibit decreased quiet and active sleep and frequent arousals; this is postulated to be related to the effects of serotonin on neurons of the raphe nucleus.[117] Bra-

zelton neonatal behavioral assessment scores show poor habituation and state control, tremors, and a high level of activity with alcohol.[118] No consistent effects have been demonstrated in multiple studies of cocaine-exposed babies.

Determining the effect of drug exposure on infant development is hampered by the many deleterious confounding variables and the lack of appropriate outcome variables. In one study, infants exposed to multiple drugs were shorter in stature at 2 years and had lower Bayley scores at 6 months but not at age 2.[94] Infants exposed to methadone had lower Bayley scores at age 2,[119,120] attention deficit,[120,121] and poor fine and gross motor control.[119-121] Infants exposed to first-trimester alcohol binges have decreased Bayley scores at the age of 8 months, poor attention and fine motor skills at age 4, and minimal brain damage (memory, attention, and processing deficits) at age 7.[118] Very low birth weight babies exposed to cocaine had lower Bayley scores at 18 months.[122] Children of smokers show a consistent pattern of decreased cognitive development, behavioral difficulties, social maladjustment, and hyperactivity.[123]

Obstetric care for substance abusers

All patients, regardless of drug use, should receive drug education. Care of substance abusers starts with getting the mother to the health care system. Mothers cannot be forced to cease taking drugs; they instead should be helped to seek assistance to decrease use.[124] Those identified as early abusers need to be referred for consultation with substance abuse professionals. This should be handled as with any other medical consultation; the consultant's input is needed to provide optimal care.

For addicts, intervention requires programs designed to handle all women's needs rather than merely maternal and fetal care.[125] Patients need access to food, housing, child care and drug and nutrition counseling to be able to take advantage of health care opportunities. Health care and social workers should actively recruit patients and bring them to clinics if appointments are missed, or if district residents' utilization of prenatal care opportunities is suboptimal. Clinics focusing on family and drug abuse care retain patients and succeed in improving obstetric outcome.[63,84,126,127]

Prenatal care. General prenatal care for drug-abusing mothers is outlined in Box 27-4. At the initial visit, looking for historical and physical factors associated with abuse will help to determine whether the patient is a social user or abuser, as will a consultation with drug abuse experts. The duration of the pregnancy at the initial visit may also be a clue to the degree of drug dependence.

BOX 27-4   OBSTETRIC MANAGEMENT OF DRUG-DEPENDENT PATIENTS

First prenatal visit
1. History
   Drug use
   Obstetric history
     Preterm birth
   Medical history
     STDs
     Endocarditis
2. Laboratory tests
   Syphilis test
   Hepatitis test
   HIV test
   Tuberculosis test
   CBC
   Triple screen
   GC and chlamydia
3. Ultrasound
   Gestational age
   Anomalies
4. Drug abuse treatment
   Detoxification
   Substitution therapy

Subsequent prenatal visits
1. Education
   HIV infection
   Fetal drug effects
2. Nutrition
3. Psychosocial services
4. Third trimester fetal testing
   Ultrasound for growth
   Biophysical score

Intrapartum care
1. Maternal monitoring
   Oxygenation
   Hyperpyrexia
   Abruption
2. Fetal monitoring
3. Patients with CNS depression
   Reduce acidity
4. Support of addiction
5. Cesarean section for fetal indication

Admission to a detoxification unit for withdrawal may be necessary. Additional patient teaching should include such subjects as the signs of premature labor and abruption, thrombocytopenia, and the hazards of drug abuse.

Education, however, may lead to complications of its own. Adolescent girls may increase smoking to limit the size of the baby and the amount of pain in giving birth.[128] Patients may use cocaine as an abortifacient or to induce labor. Narcotic addicts may try to substitute benzodiazepines for methadone, thereby exacerbating neonatal withdrawal.[129]

Ultrasound assessment is an important tool in managing substance abusers. An initial assessment for dates is important for addicts; even if the patient presents in the first trimester, the date of the last menstrual period is unlikely to be reliable. Social users may have taken a significant amount of drug before they discovered the pregnancy and may still be at risk for developmental anomalies. Later in gestation, ultrasound is useful for assessing the growth of the fetus.

Laboratory studies should include serum hepatitis, HIV, alphafetoprotein titers and liver enzymes, and possibly folate levels. Electrocardiogram (ECG) or echocardiogram may be indicated. Urine toxicologic screening at intervals will be useful in confirming patient reliability, assessing the degree of dependence, and providing motiva-

tion to abstain, but this can be done only with the patient's permission.

Consultation. Patients who are HIV positive require consultation with an infectious disease specialist. Pregnancy, which does not appear to affect progression of the disease, bears the major risk of disease transmission to the fetus.[130] Maternal zidovudine therapy may lower the rate of vertical transmission.[131] Laboratory studies in these patients include CD_4^+ T-cells, p24 antigen and beta$_2$-microglobin.

During the prenatal period additional consultations regarding management of accompanying conditions such as hepatitis should be obtained. The patient is encouraged to follow the plans of the drug abuse consultant and to refrain from bingeing on any drug. The patient may need to be referred to a tertiary care center, or plans made for her referral in the event of preterm labor or abruption. Plans for the maternal care after delivery and care of the infant must be assessed. Labor induction for maternal disease is more common among drug abusers.

Intrapartum care. Patients in labor require careful monitoring for signs of placental insufficiency and fetal hypoxemia. Mothers may be self-medicated before arrival in the delivery room. In one study, 40% of patients had taken heroin for labor pain before entering the hospital.[132] Intravenous access may be a problem, and central vein catheterization may be necessary. Cesarean section for failed induction or fetal distress is more common in substance abusers than in controls. Short umbilical cords and resulting complications may be associated with abuse of depressant drugs.[133]

Intoxicated parturients must be stabilized as much as possible. Acute cocaine toxicity may present as apparent preeclampsia. Depending on the agent, the cardiovascular system may be stimulated or depressed. Oxygenation must be supported. Marijuana, PCP, and cocaine intoxication are associated with hyperpyrexia, which increases oxygen consumption in both the mother and fetus. Hyperpyrexia can be treated with acetaminophen. Depressed patients will be at risk of aspiration and may need medication to reduce gastric acidity and volume. Metaclopromide must be considered in cases of alcohol, narcotic, and barbiturate intoxication. Addiction is supported during labor, since the stress of withdrawal reduces uterine blood flow and thereby increases fetal risk. Obstetric management is expectant unless the fetal condition deteriorates, in which case delivery by cesarean section is indicated.

Anesthetic implications in drug addiction

Metabolic interactions. Multiple metabolic interactions of illicit drugs and anesthetic agents can occur. Specific abusive substances alter metabolism of anesthetics; for example, ethanol increases enflurane defluorination.[134] Halothane and spinal anesthesia induce increased hepatic metabolism of the abused agent.[135,136] Alternatively, anesthetics such as halothane block benzodiazepine metabolism by reducing available receptors or enzymes.[137]

Physiologic interactions. Specific pharmacologic drug interactions can adversely affect cardiovascular, respiratory, uteroplacental, and fetal functions, limiting anesthetic choices. Barbiturates, PCP, and alcohol increase sensitivity to narcotics, whereas opiates obviously increase the need for narcotics. Alcohol depresses the myocardium and potentiates general anesthetic agents. Fortunately endogenous feedback systems restore normal function over time, so careful titration evades morbidity associated with some anesthetic agents and techniques. Medical complications associated with parenteral drug abuse (see Box 27-2) may further limit anesthetic options.

Anesthetic management of labor and delivery

Laboring patients should have pulse oximeters in addition to routine monitoring. The excess sympathetic activity associated with withdrawal may decrease placental blood flow, thus epidural analge-

sia may help when undiagnosed withdrawal is a possibility. Since drug tolerance depresses the response to endogenous opiates, addicts frequently react poorly to stress; they also require more pain medication compared with control patients. This phenomenon was demonstrated in a recent study in which cocaine abusers had a higher visual analogue pain score before epidural analgesia. When the block was established, however, their pain scores were similar to controls, indicating that they respond normally to conduction block.[138] Patients receiving epidural analgesia deliver infants with better Apgar scores.[133]

Medical complications. Table 27-5 outlines the anesthetic management of potential intrapartum problems that may occur before or after administration of an anesthetic. Conditions outlined in Table 27-3 may also complicate intrapartum anesthetic management. Anesthesia plans are tailored as for nonabusing patients with similar medical problems. Myelopathy and neuropathy associated with drug abuse confound evaluation of neurologic deficits after conduction anesthesia and vaginal delivery, and myopathy may increase the incidence of backache. Patients with tricuspid insufficiency or other valvular diseases compro-

Table 27-5 Anesthesia management in drug abuse

Coma	Intubate, administer antagonist
Respiratory depression	Administer antagonist, intubate, ventilate
Hypotension	Fluid, inotropes, invasive monitoring
Bradycardia	Atropine, isoproterenol, pacemaker
Vasodilation	Hydration, vasoconstrictors
Myocardial depression	Inotropes, delivery of fetus, mechanical support devices
Myocardial ischemia	Invasive monitoring, afterload reduction, nitroglycerin, inotropes
Hypertension	Vasodilators, *no* beta-selective blockers alone, or ACE-inhibitors
Hypovolemia	Crystalloid, colloid, blood
Seizures	Ventilate, intubate, thiopentone or benzodiazepine
Combative	Ventilation and circulation adequate? If yes: analgesic, sedation
Fetal distress	Ventilation and circulation adequate? If yes: oxygen, uterine relaxation, delivery

mising cardiovascular reserve require careful titration of analgesic agents to avoid hypotension. Similarly, patients with pulmonary hypertension must have preload maintained to avoid hypotension.

HIV seropositive patients may safely have regional anesthetics. They require very careful attention to sterile techniques to avoid iatrogenic infection. The risk of spreading HIV infection to the CNS is not clinically relevant, because CNS involvement occurs early in the course of the disease.[139] Indwelling epidural catheters and invasive monitoring are avoided as much as possible, since impaired immunity can increase the likelihood of infection resulting from attraction of blood-borne pathogens to the catheter.[140] A single epidural dose of local anesthetic and epidural or intrathecal narcotic might more appropriately suit patients with AIDS; on the other hand, a small study of regional anesthesia in mostly asymptomatic HIV positive patients reported no complications.[141]

Conduction anesthesia. Generally speaking, conduction anesthesia avoids the uncertainties encountered with cross-dependent anesthetic agents; it is the method of choice for labor analgesia for drug abusers. The advisability of major conduction block must be determined by weighing the risks and benefits for individual patients. Epidural or intrathecal opiate analgesia is the usual choice for laboring patients. Both alcohol and cocaine use may be associated with coagulopathy. With known addicts, appropriate coagulation studies should be available before administering the block, unless the clinical situation dictates proceeding immediately.[142] Intravenous narcotics or mild tranquilizers help irritable patients who are in pain to cooperate for spinal or epidural procedures.

Although hypotension is usually treated with ephedrine, phenylephrine may be the drug of choice in some situations. Ephedrine administration is less reliable with marijuana, because both cause tachycardia; with PCP, because it increases ephedrine sensitivity; and with cocaine, because the response may be exaggerated, or there may be no response when there are inadequate norepinephrine stores.

After intrathecal narcotics are administered, intensive monitoring of ventilation is important because patients may have more narcotics in their systems than the care giver is aware of. Epidural and spinal narcotics have not been studied in this population, but these have been widely administered without noticeable sequelae. Intrathecal or epidural agonist-antagonist administration may precipitate withdrawal symptoms.[143]

Anesthesia for cesarean section

Choice of anesthetic technique for cesarean section depends upon maternal and fetal circumstances, as with normal patients. Elective cesarean section requires that the patient is not intoxicated. General anesthesia is usually necessary for emergency cesarean section precipitated by fetal distress. Drug abusers are not good candidates for regional anesthetic techniques for emergency surgery because of anxiety and stress intolerance. Neither are they good candidates for general anesthesia, because cross-tolerance with general anesthetics hampers determining an induction dose that will ensure unconsciousness yet avoid hypotension and neonatal depression.[144]

Regional analgesia. Epidural or spinal anesthesia avoids airway and aspiration risks and least depresses the neonate; as with parturients abstaining from drug use, they are the methods of choice. Minimal sedation with benzodiazepine drugs before the procedure prevents anxiety-induced decrease in placental blood flow during block administration. Occasionally, extremely anxious patients may require so much sedation to accomplish regional anesthesia that general anesthesia is better. If the patient is too intoxicated to cooperate, general anesthesia is necessary. The patient's medical condition might also dictate use of general anesthesia. In particular, patients with advanced AIDS-related pulmonary disease or sepsis may need general anesthesia for ventilatory control. Similarly, severe valvular disease or pulmonary hypertension may be an indication for general anesthesia, although recently patients with severe valvular disease have been treated successfully with intrathecal narcotics.[145,146]

General anesthesia. Pseudocholinesterase may be inhibited by PCP, depleted by cocaine metabolism, or decreased by alcohol. The dose of succinylcholine for intubation need not be decreased since it is sufficiently short-acting. With alcohol intoxication, etomidate for induction avoids hypotension, whereas sodium pentothal or propofol better avoids the hypertensive response to intubation in chronic users. With PCP and cocaine abusers who are hypertensive, pentothal or propofol is a better induction agent, whereas etomidate is safer with the patient who is depressed after a binge. After delivery, anesthetic agents are titrated as tolerated. Intoxication delays extubation and prolongs recovery. Postoperative pain relief with intrathecal or epidural narcotics is recommended in this group of patients, except when unsupervised self-administration of a cross-dependent substance seems likely. Patient-controlled analgesia (PCA) may increase these patients' satisfaction by enhancing their perception of control over medication.

ETHANOL
Pharmacology

Ethanol is a CNS depressant that is simultaneously a central sympathetic stimulant. The degree of metabolic and pharmacologic tolerance to alcohol that develops is genetically determined. Although pharmacologic tolerance develops, it does not elevate the lethal blood level. Ethanol is cross-tolerant with most CNS depressants, including general anesthetics.

Metabolism. Alcohol is metabolized to acetaldehyde. Alcohol dehydrogenase conversion of ethanol to acetaldehyde is a rate-limiting step, since the equilibrium leans toward ethanol. Conversion occurs only if aldehyde dehydrogenase removes acetaldehyde. Five genes determine multiple isoenzymes of alcohol dehydrogenase.[147] Racial variations in acetaldehyde dehydrogenase activity are responsible for flushing reactions. Drugs inhibiting acetaldehyde metabolism increase flushing and ethanol-induced CNS depression.

Pathophysiology. Excessive acetaldehyde oxidation in liver or muscle results in peroxidation of lipid by oxygen radicals, producing hepatitis, myopathy, cardiomyopathy, and damage to other tissues and membranes. Acute alcohol intoxication inhibits cytochrome P_{450}-dependent drug oxidation. This increases levels of drugs predominantly eliminated by hepatic metabolism (e.g., propranolol, lidocaine). Chronic abuse stimulates hepatic oxidation and decreases availability of drugs metabolized by the liver.

Alcohol depletes prostaglandin E_1 (PGE_1). It enhances conversion of dihomogamma-linolenic acid (DGLA) to PGE_1 and acutely increases PGE_1, but it blocks delta-8-6-desaturase, which replenishes DGLA. Absent PGE_1 causes fibrosis, cardiomyopathy, reproductive failure, gastritis, and pancreatitis. This may be a factor in the development of FAS, since lithium, diphenylhydantoin, and zinc deficiency (which also decrease PGE_1) all produce conditions similar to fetal alcohol syndrome.[148]

Withdrawal. Symptoms of withdrawal appear within 6 to 24 hours. Seizures are common in binge drinkers. Delirium tremens is life-threatening, requiring treatment with diazepam, phenobarbital or clonidine.

Pregnancy and ethanol abuse

Incidence. The reported incidence of alcohol abuse is between 5% and 46%; 3% of mothers drink enough for FAS to occur. Alcohol is seldom the primary agent of maternal abuse, and it is frequently combined with marijuana (75%), cocaine (73%), and methadone.[5] Women who drink heavily are usually young, white, educated, single, and with high incomes, but those drinking in the third trimester are older, black, less educated, with low social status, and use other drugs.[21,26] In one study, adolescent alcohol use decreased from 82% before pregnancy to 19% and 15% in the second and third trimesters, respectively.[149] Binge drinking decreased, and with the exception of tobacco, other substance abuse also decreased.[149] Michigan Alcohol Screening Test (MAST) and "Ten Questions Drinking History" are two established interview techniques for identifying abusers.[24]

Maternal pathophysiology. Table 27-6 outlines the extensive pathophysiology of alcohol abuse. Ethanol acutely alters both cardiac mechanical function and electrophysiologic properties. Alcohol also antagonizes folic acid. By altering the endocrine response to stress, alcohol increases cortisol, aldosterone, prolactin, epinephrine, and norepinephrine secretion, and it decreases growth hormone.[150] Acute alcohol ingestion induces hyperglycemia. Hypoglycemia of fasting is exacerbated by glycogen depletion from malnourishment, alcohol-induced glycogenolysis, and alcohol-impaired gluconeogenesis. Alcohol causes widespread depression of the immunologic system and increased vulnerability to bacterial and viral infections, tuberculosis, and cancer.[151] The HIV-positive mother who uses ethanol is especially vulnerable to these infections.

Chronic alcohol consumption produces progressive myocardial dysfunction and congestive cardiomyopathy. Myelopathy, polyneuropathy, and myopathy also occur with chronic abuse. Muscle cell membrane damage and intracellular phosphate deficiency produce acute myopathy and myoglobinuria with selective atrophy of type II muscle fibers.[152] Myelopathy is characterized by spastic paraparesis and signs of both lateral and dorsal column involvement.[153]

Advanced alcoholic liver disease results in coagulation factor deficiency and thrombocytopenia by increased platelet destruction. Qualitative platelet abnormalities include decreased cyclic adenosine monophosphate (CAMP) and monoamine oxidase (MAO), nucleotide storage pool, and decreased release and aggregation.

Fetal and neonatal effects. Ethanol ingestion in the third trimester delays expected rises in the lecithin/sphingomyelin (L/S) ratio and in the amniotic levels of phosphatidylglycerol.[154] Alcohol also impairs the placental transfer of nutrients.[50] Acute ethanol intoxication depresses the newborn, and chronic neonatal exposure causes withdrawal.

Neonates exposed to alcohol prenatally exhibit variable symptoms ranging from no apparent ef-

Table 27-6 Pathophysiology of alcohol abuse*

Site	Pathophysiology
CNS	Acute: depression, "partially anesthetized"; chronic: myelopathy, polyneuropathy, Wernicke-Korsakoff syndrome, cerebellar degeneration, cortical damage, withdrawal seizures, hepatic encephalopathy
Lungs	Acute: respiratory failure, intrapulmonary shunting, surfactant and macrophage inhibition, aspiration pneumonia; chronic: ventilation/perfusion mismatch, intrapulmonary shunting, chronic infection
Cardiovascular	Acute: myocardial depression, abnormal electrophysiology, arrhythmia, cellular damage; chronic: alcoholic and nutritional myopathy, increased catecholamines, hypertension
Hepatic	Acute: cellular damage, hypoglycemia from inhibition gluconeogenesis, decreased drug metabolism; chronic: fatty infiltration, hepatitis, enzyme induction, cirrhosis, portal hypertension, decreased hepatic blood flow, decreased drug metabolism, protein and coagulation factor synthesis
Gastrointestinal	Peptic ulcer disease, gastritis, esophagitis, malabsorption, pancreatitis, bleeding esophageal varices, gallstones
Nutritional	Dietary deficiencies, malabsorption, vitamin deficiencies
Hematologic	Coagulopathy—multifactorial; platelet, leukocyte, and erythrocyte dysfunction
Renal	Acute: diuresis with sodium and potassium loss; chronic: antidiuresis with sodium retention, hypokalemia, hypomagnesemia, intracellular calcium derangement, renal failure
Muscular	Myopathy
Endocrine	Alterations of insulin, cortisone, aldosterone, catecholamines, growth hormone, prolactin, luteinizing hormone
Ophthalmic	Abnormal zinc and vitamin A reduce dark adaptation
Immunologic	Suppression; vulnerable to viral, bacterial infections; cancer

*Modified from James FM, Wheeler FS, Dewan DM (eds): *Obstetric Anesthesia: The Complicated Patient.* Philadelphia, FA Davis, 1987. Used by permission.

fect to FAS. Maternal consumption of more than 90 mL/day of absolute alcohol produces IUGR in the third trimester and developmental defects in a dose-dependent fashion in the first trimester.[73,74] Fetal alcohol syndrome, which is caused by antenatal alcohol exposure, consists of growth retardation, craniofacial and other major and minor anomalies, neuropsychological impairment, and mental retardation.[74] The prominent facial abnormalities, which decrease with age, are a drawn appearance, midface hypoplasia, diminished philtrum, and small mandible. Ocular manifestations are prominent, and include Peters anomaly, lens opacification, and external eye lesions. Linear growth and weight gain are decreased despite normal nutrient absorption and growth hormone levels. Variability of occurrence represents an important aspect, with full expression in 1 per 1000 live births and partial involvement in 1 child per 600 to 700 live births.[155] Partial involvement is termed *fetal alcohol effect* (FAE).

Obstetric and anesthetic considerations

Prenatal care. Addicts are ideally withdrawn from alcohol in a detoxification facility before pregnancy or in the first trimester. They may require detoxification later in pregnancy to decrease the risk of FAS. Detoxification late in the pregnancy may reduce placental blood flow from sympathetic stimulation. Detection of aldehydehemoglobin adducts (Hb-Ach) in red blood cells provides a test to monitor compliance with abstinence.[73] Maternal serum gamma-glutamyl transpeptidase also correlates with degree of ethanol consumption.[156] Serum levels of alpha-fetoprotein and pregnancy-specific beta$_1$-glycoprotein have predictive value for development of fetal alcohol syndrome.[157]

Although abstinence is optimal, some patients' life situations make this unrealistic. Hispanics who drink are not more likely than nondrinkers to be physically abused, but Caucasian who drink are 3 times more likely and Afro-Americans are 6 times more likely than abstainers to be battered.[48] If the patient does not abuse heroin or cocaine, anxiolytic agents might prevent further fetal exposure to alcohol or other drugs typically abused during times of stress.

Alcoholics require special surveillance for deficiency anemia, glucose intolerance, and coagulopathy. Education includes a warning that "binge" drinking and fluctuating ethanol levels are especially detrimental to the fetus. Preterm labor is not associated with ethanol abuse.

Intrapartum management

Obstetric. Acute and chronic alcohol abusers need coagulation parameters, serum electrolytes, and serum ethanol levels on admission. Glucose and electrolyte derangements require slow correction as rapid correction of hyponatremia may induce central pontine myelinolysis.[158] Alcohol inhibits uterine contraction; thus labor is not likely to progress in acutely intoxicated patients. Coagulopathy is unusual, as patients with this degree of liver disease are usually infertile. Patients with liver disease, coagulopathy, or myocardiopathy, should receive appropriate treatment.

Anesthetic

Analgesia for labor. With liver disease and coagulopathy, narcotic metabolism is prolonged, and pulmonary shunting can induce hypoxia. Narcotic metabolism is prolonged in alcoholic individuals, and administration may exacerbate hypoxia induced from pulmonary shunting. Naloxone may reverse ethanol intoxication and may sober uncooperative patients.[159] In patients without coagulopathy, epidural or intrathecal narcotic analgesia provides superior pain relief, protects placental blood flow, and avoids cross-tolerance with narcotics. Ethanol impairment of local anesthetic metabolism should not be clinically significant in laboring patients.[135] Patients may have areas of decreased cutaneous sensation from neuropathy.

Anesthesia for cesarean section. The pathophysiologic changes of chronic alcohol abuse affect responses to general anesthesia. Minimum alveolar concentration (MAC) for inhalational anesthetic agents is increased, but uterine relaxant effects are unchanged. Hypovolemia and depressed myocardial contractility are present even with ethanol levels less than 100 mg/dL. Pulmonary shunting increases the risk of arterial hypoxia with positive pressure ventilation and during induction. Decreased pseudocholinesterase prolongs the effect of some muscle relaxants. Increased volume of distribution decreases nondepolarizing muscle relaxant potency. Peripheral neuropathy exaggerates hypotensive effects of anesthetic agents.

Since regional anesthesia produces better initial neonatal neurobehavioral scores, and alcoholic pathologic conditions alter so many facets of general anesthesia, regional anesthesia is preferred in chronic alcoholic patients without coagulopathy. However, general anesthesia is indicated for intoxicated patients, as they have depressed airway reflexes, which can cause aspiration of gastric contents during the operation. Of the halogenated agents, isoforane interferes least with alcohol me-

tabolism. Neonatal depression from alcohol and general anesthesia is likely.

BARBITURATES
Incidence

Barbiturate addiction among women of reproductive age is uncommon. In Virginia, in 1990, only 2% of patients were found to be abusing sedative hypnotics,[22] and in Missouri, only 0.6% of pregnant patients abused barbiturates.[17] Barbiturates can be detected in the urine for as long as 2 to 3 weeks after last use.

Pharmacology

Barbiturates depress short synaptic pathways in the central reticular core of the brain stem, and, by stimulating gamma-aminobutyric acid (GABA) receptors, they block electroencephalographic (EEG) arousal from brain stem stimulation.[160] Currently their abusive use is to enhance the effect of other drugs or to relieve withdrawal symptoms. Intoxication resembles alcohol intoxication, and as with ethanol, tolerance does not alter the lethal dose.

Pregnancy

Maternal effects. Barbiturates depress respiratory and cardiovascular function. Chronic intoxication impairs nutrient intake. Withdrawal is usually accomplished with secobarbital.

Uteroplacental, fetal, and neonatal effects. No clear-cut evidence of barbiturate-induced fetal damage in humans exists. Barbiturates are behavioral teratogens in animals, and early gestational exposure produces neuromorphologic changes similar to fetal alcohol syndrome.[75] Phenobarbital induces fetal hepatic enzymes capable of decreasing neonatal bilirubin levels. Infants of epileptic mothers receiving phenobarbital are passively addicted.

Intrapartum management

Obstetric. Obstetric considerations for patients abusing barbiturates is the same as that of patients abusing alcohol, that is, detoxification in an appropriate setting, care of nutritional needs, and correction of anemia. Patients receiving phenobarbital for seizure disorders can continue the drug without any increased risk to the mother's health. Small incremental doses of antihistamine or phenothiazine agents are useful in controlling combative behavior in mildly intoxicated patients.

Anesthetic. A few anesthetic considerations in barbiturate addicts should be kept in mind. Sensitivity to narcotic drugs is increased, so they should be used with caution. Tolerance to the cardiac depressant effects of the barbiturates does not occur. The MAC for inhalation agents is not increased, and the depressant effects of inhalation agents are potentiated.

NARCOTICS
Pharmacology

Narcotic agonists bind to opioid receptors located in brain and spinal cord. Mu-agonist narcotics inhibit neurotransmission, producing membrane hyperpolarization by increasing potassium conductance. Kappa-receptor agonists produce analgesia without respiratory depression, and sedation rather than euphoria. Opiate agonist-antagonist drugs act as antagonists at mu-receptors, and as agonists at kappa receptors.

Tolerance is reversible and limited to the receptor upon which the drug acts. More tolerance develops with less potent drugs, which require binding to many receptors to produce an effect.[161]

Treatment of intoxication

Opiate antagonists reverse the effects of narcotic overdose. Naloxone, a pure antagonist, reverses coma, hypoventilation, and hypotension from narcotic overdose, but it must be given as a continuous intravenous infusion because of its short half-life. Nalbuphine, an agonist-antagonist agent, has a longer duration of action and can be administered subcutaneously.

Treatment of withdrawal

Symptoms of narcotic withdrawal include anxiety, tremor, rhinorrhea, yawning, sweating, vomiting, tachycardia, and hypotension or hypertension. Treatment is usually methadone or buprenorphine substitution.[129,162] Diazepam relieves withdrawal symptoms but does not prevent seizures. Clonidine alleviates some of the side effects of withdrawal. A protracted period of minor abstinence symptoms, probably related to gradual restoration of normal receptor function, occurs after detoxification. During this time, patients are over-concerned about discomfort and they tolerate stress poorly. They have a poor self-image and a depressed ventilatory response to carbon dioxide.

Pregnancy

Maternal and uteroplacental effects. Maternal pathophysiologic effects from narcotics alone are mild. Hypothalamic secretion of luteinizing hormone-releasing hormone (LHRH) is decreased as are plasma levels of LH, ACTH, and testosterone. More severe effects of maternal narcotic abuse (Box 27-2) are those associated with drug-seeking behavior and intravenous drug abuse; in New York City, 40% of pregnant women enrolled in a methadone clinic were HIV positive.[42] In addition, the incidence of infectious diseases such as tuberculosis, hepatitis, bacterial pneumonia, and

sexually transmitted disease is increased.

Fetal effects. There is no evidence that birth defects and decreased size or gestational length are directly attributable to narcotics.[6,] Controlled-release implants of sufentanil, alfentanil, and fentanyl produced no deleterious effects in rats.[163] Also in rats, intrauterine withdrawal from narcotics produced more detrimental effects than did continued exposure.[164] Other investigators have shown that repeated morphine and alpha-acetylmethadol administration in rats decreases maternal weight gain, increases fetal mortality, matures female fetuses early, and interferes with postnatal physical growth and neurobehavioral development.[165,166] Accelerated differentiation of alveolar epithelium, induced by elevated levels of prolactin in fetal cord serum of addicted mothers, appears to decrease the incidence of respiratory distress syndrome (RDS).[167]

Neonatal effects. After birth a dramatic increase in plasma beta-endorphin, beta-lipoprotein, and metenkephalin concentrations coincide with the onset of withdrawal symptoms,[168] which occur in 80% of methadone/heroin-exposed infants. Methadone treatment is associated with less severe, but longer lasting, withdrawal symptoms.[126] Severity of symptoms are evaluated by the Brazelton Neonatal Behavioral Assessment Scale or withdrawal-specific scales, such as the Finnegan abstinence score. Self-administration of diazepam to enhance an inadequate methadone dose is associated with severe late withdrawal symptoms in neonates.[129]

Neonatal outcome. Decreased gestation and neonatal size have been reported,[62,84,85] but when adjustments are made for confounding factors such as prenatal care, maternal weight gain, and smoking, there is no difference in neonatal size related to drug use.[120] Neonatal morbidity and mortality are minimal when mothers receive treatment in methadone clinics.[61] Neonatal addiction decreases ventilatory response to carbon dioxide, causes tolerance to endogenous opiates, and increases the frequency of SIDS.[112] Reports of neurologic function in preschool children vary because of confounding factors and show no consistent deficits.[107,119,121] Mothers treated with methadone tend to keep their children. By the preschool years 50% of children remain with the treated mothers, compared to only 9% in the untreated mothers.[121]

Obstetric considerations

Prenatal care. The number of pregnant patients who abuse opiates has decreased in the last decade to 0% to 2%.* Of these, 20% to 50% also abuse

---

*References 6, 7, 14, 17, 19, 27.

Table 27-7 Medical and obstetric complications*

	Patients (%) (n = 112)*	Controls (%) (n = 224)	p
Premature delivery (gestation <37 wk)	27.7	13.8	<0.005
Abruptio placentae	8.0	3.1	<0.02
Hypertensive disorders	16.1	7.1	<0.02
Preeclampsia	8.0	4.9	NS
Chronic hypertension	8.0	2.2	<0.02
Thrombophlebitis/cellulitis/abscess	14.3	0.5	<0.001
History of hepatitis	10.7	0.9	<0.001
One or more medical complications	42.0	27.7	<0.01
One or more obstetric complications	56.3	40.6	<0.01

*Family center patients, mostly narcotic abusers. NS = not significant.
Modified from Silver H, et al: *J Perinatol* 1987; 7:178. Used by permission.

cocaine.[107,108] The first decision on recognizing narcotic abuse is whether to use methadone or detoxification treatment. Withdrawing the mother from narcotic drugs decreases fetal exposure and avoids neonatal withdrawal. However, almost all patients undergoing detoxification return to drugs.[132] In addition, detoxification is not recommended during the third trimester because of occurrence of fetal stress with withdrawal.[108,126,132]

Methadone maintenance. Instead of detoxification, prescribing low doses of methadone and tapering the dose of methadone at the end of pregnancy (to reduce neonatal withdrawal) has been recommended. However, patients receiving low-dose methadone supplement it with additional psychoactive drugs at least 80% to 93% of the time.[62,120,126,126,132] Serum methadone levels decrease at the end of pregnancy. Thus reducing methadone doses at the end of pregnancy further increases maternal need for supplemental drugs. To avoid withdrawal symptoms, it is important to maintain methadone levels above 150 mg/ml.[126,129]

With methadone treatment, maternal weight gain increases, and morbidity and mortality is minimal.[61,126] Presumably the long half-life of methadone allows for a stable maternal plasma level and avoids repeated withdrawal. Without drug-seeking behavior, life style improves. Patients receiving methadone are more likely than heroin users to seek prenatal care.[6,62]

In New York City, 40% of pregnant women enrolled in a methadone clinic were HIV positive.[42] Syphilis is reported in 20% of pregnant narcotic addicts and hepatitis in 5%.[126] The incidence of other infectious diseases such as tuberculosis and bacterial pneumonia is also increased. Cardiopulmonary reserve may be decreased by valvular vegetations or pulmonary hypertension from filtering talc. Pulmonary abscess or infarct also complicates

prenatal care. These complications are managed as they would be in nonabusing patients.

Intrapartum management

Obstetrics. Patients may confuse signs of early labor with withdrawal and arrive in labor with high narcotic drug levels. Nalbuphine in small increments reverses inappropriate narcosis while maintaining analgesia. As with the general drug-abusing population, the overall rate of medical complications and obstetric complications is higher (Table 27-7).[133] Low Apgar scores are more prevalent in addicts who receive no analgesia during labor. Emergency cesarean section, prompted by fetal distress, is five times more frequent than in the control group.[133]

Anesthetic

Labor. Patients taking only methadone have minimal pathophysiology. Narcotic requirements are increased. Agonist-antagonist agents will spur withdrawal but are useful for partially reversing overdose without reducing analgesia. Patients abusing agonist-antagonist agents are tolerant to similar compounds, so meperidine is a better choice for analgesia. Epidural analgesia avoids further respiratory compromise and fetal depression in intoxicated mothers.

Cesarean section. Epidural or spinal anesthesia least depresses the neonate and is the method of choice. Potent short-acting narcotics such as fentanyl can be used to supplement analgesia. Long-acting intrathecal or epidural narcotics should be carefully considered in heroin users because of the danger of apnea with unsupervised narcotic administration. If general anesthesia is necessary, narcotized patients require less barbiturate. Unexplained hypotension during general anesthesia can sometimes be relieved by narcotic administration, as this is a sign of withdrawal. Postoperatively, a PCA pump is indicated and might prevent self-administration of supplemental nonprescribed medication.

BENZODIAZEPINES

Pharmacology. Like barbiturates, benzodiazepines increase the chloride flux initiated by GABA at the postsynaptic receptor. Benzodiazepine receptors are located in proximity to GABA receptors, and their occupation by benzodiazepines increases binding of GABA. Benzodiazepines also release striatal enkephalin, resulting in synergism with opiates.[169] Naloxone partially reverses benzodiazepines.[159]

Substance abusers use benzodiazepines to enhance the effect of narcotics or relieve ethanol or narcotic withdrawal symptoms. Pharmacodynamic tolerance develops within 24 hours, but hepatic enzyme induction (metabolic tolerance) development is negligible.

Maternal effects. In Missouri, urine screens for benzodiazepines were positive in 0.6% of patients.[17] Benzodiazepines depress nocturnal gastric acid excretion. The withdrawal symptoms and seizures rarely occur because of the drug's long duration of action.

Neonatal effects. Benzodiazepines cause neonatal hypotonia and depress thermoregulation. The half-life of the drug in infants is prolonged. Transient neurobehavioral changes occur in human neonates exposed to benzodiazepines. Neonatal withdrawal occurs at 7 to 14 days of age, and subacute effects can last 3 to 4 months.[129]

MARIJUANA
Pharmacology

Delta-9-tetrahydrocannabinol, the active marijuana ingredient, alters GABA functions affecting acetylcholine turnover in the CNS; producing sleepiness, ataxia, and decreased motor and cognitive ability. Marijuana use improves self-perception and produces euphoria, relaxation, and temporal disintegration. Higher doses trigger paranoid feelings, delusions, and hallucinations. Hypothalamic-pituitary axis effects include interference with secreation of LH, follicle stimulating hormone (FSH), and prolactin, as well as oligospermia.

The serum half-life of marijuana is 7 days, and a single dose may take as long as a month to be excreted. It can be detected in the urine for 3 to 5 days in light users and for as long as a month in heavy users.[4] Tolerance develops to some behavioral effects and the lethal dose increases with abuse. Cross-tolerance to ethanol develops but not to other hallucinogens. No recognized withdrawal syndrome occurs, but irritability, insomnia, restlessness, and nervousness can accompany discontinuation.

Pregnancy

Maternal effects. Elevated carbon monoxide levels from smoking marijuana impair fetal oxygenation. Beta-adrenergic effects may decrease placental blood flow by causing postural hypotension. Black mothers using marijuana are 5 times more likely to be physically abused.[48]

Fetal effects. In rats marijuana reduces maternal weight gain and decreases birth weight and neonatal weight gain while increasing postnatal mortality. There are no apparent anomalies.[170] In humans, marijuana has been reported to decrease gestational length.[170,171] In a prospective study of 1226 mothers, multivariate analysis demonstrated decreased maternal weight gain and decreased birth weight in marijuana users.[12] Other studies have failed to confirm these findings when confounding factors are controlled.[21,81,121]

Neonatal effects. Controlled animal studies show no behavioral effects.[172] The neurobehavioral effects in humans are variable. Maternal marijuana use is associated with neonatal tremors, startles, poor visual habituation, retarded maturation of the visual components of the human nervous system, and longer active sleep and increased motility.[170,171] Other studies, particularly one of "ganja" use in Jamaica where other drug use was absent,[121] have failed to confirm these observations.[21]

Obstetric and anesthetic considerations

Antenatal. The incidence of marijuana use among pregnant patients is 2% to 12%,* but incidences as high as 25% to 30% have been reported.[21] Marijuana is the most widely used illicit drug; in one study 87% of the urine screens positive for illicit drugs contained marijuana.[23] Only a quarter of patients with positive urine screens admit to marijuana use on interview.[7,17] Marijuana abusers are likely to abuse tobacco (80%) and alcohol (76%) as well.[12] Commonly users are young, white, and single,[7,21,23,26] but abusers who continue its use during pregnancy tend to be older, Afro-American, and women with less education and of lower socioeconomic class.[21,23,170]

Intrapartum obstetric and anesthetic management. Because of its long serum half-life, patients in labor frequently have residual drug levels. Tachycardia up to 140 beats per minute is not uncommon and can be treated with propranolol. If patients require sedation, phenothiazines, which

---

*References 7, 17, 19, 22-24, 27, 170.

potentiate postural hypotension, and barbiturates, which cause hallucinations, should be avoided. With general anesthesia, the problems are bronchial irritability and reduced MAC for anesthetic agents. Etomidate or propofol induction may reduce the incidence of bronchoconstriction. Marijuana-induced microsomal dechlorinase increases halothane metabolism.

PHENCYCLIDINE (PCP)
Pharmacology

PCP, an arylcyclohexylamine, is a potent psychomimetic agent capable of producing a state indistinguishable from schizophrenia. Its sympathomimetic pharmacologic effects are similar to cocaine.[176] Its mechanism of action is not known but may involve binding to a low-affinity sigma-opiate receptor site, blockade of NMDA and glutamate channels, inhibition of dopamine and norepinephrine uptake, and interference with 5-hydroxyindole metabolism.[173] Users usually smoke it with tobacco or marijuana. Low doses produce agitation, depersonalization, altered sensory perception, sweating, tachycardia, and hypertension.[1] Intoxication produces slurred speech, anesthesia, hypersalivation, catatonia, fever, ataxia, clonus, tremors, rhabdomyolysis, and seizures. Severe psychotic reactions occur more often in first users, perhaps those predisposed to schizophrenia. PCP induces acute reversible pathomorphic changes in rat brain neuron[174] and is associated with perfusion defects on brain scans in humans.[175]

Pregnancy

PCP use is less common, occurring in 1% of positive urine screens[14] or in 0.3% of the pregnant population.[22] Patients using PCP have a 32% incidence of growth retardation and a 43% incidence of precipitate labor; both these figures are higher in cocaine users.[176] The placenta has the ability to metabolize phencyclidine by monohydroxylation.[173] In spite of this, fetal serum levels may exceed maternal levels by as much as tenfold.[173] Phencyclidine is detectable in breast milk, amniotic fluid, and neonatal urine in the first few days of life. Neonatal symptoms include jitteriness, hypotonicity, vomiting, and diarrhea, which are unrelieved by phenobarbital. In a clinical report, microcephaly occurred in one of the two exposed infants.[95] Neurobehavioral and ventilatory abnormalities observed in neonates tend to resolve.[177]

Obstetric and anesthetic management

Obstetric. Patients are managed like other abusers. PCP potentiates narcotics. Intoxicated laboring patients may be treated with chlorpromazine or haloperidol. Hyperthermia should be controlled with acetaminophen, as fever increases fetal and maternal oxygen consumption. Hypertension and tachycardia may need to be treated. Rhabdomyolysis requires treatment with dantrolene.[173] Narcotic analgesia requires pulse oximetry monitoring, since PCP potentiates narcotics.

Anesthetic. Acute intoxication with PCP potentiates sympathomimetic drugs. Therefore, dosage of sympathomimetic drugs such as ephedrine should be accordingly reduced. Because of its hyperthermic effect, patients may require a cooling blanket during general anesthesia. Ketamine, because of its similarity to PCP, is contraindicated. Propofol or pentothal administration for induction of general anesthesia attenuates sympathetic response to laryngoscopy and intubation. Since PCP inhibits pseudocholinesterase activity, neuromuscular blocking agents metabolized by cholinesterase should be used with caution.

COCAINE
Pharmacology

Mechanism of action. Cocaine, or benzoylmethylecgonine, is a naturally occurring plant alkaloid. It blocks the presynaptic uptake of norepinephrine, thereby activating adrenergic nerve synapses leading to severe hypertension, tachycardia, and vasoconstriction.[178] Cocaine blocks presynaptic dopamine reuptake by binding to its transporter. Dopamine accumulation in the mesolimbus or mesocortex activates pathways responsible for its euphoric and reinforcing qualities. Dopamine depletion is thought to be responsible for the tolerance to rewarding effects associated with chronic use, and the dysphoria associated with its withdrawal.[92] Cocaine also blocks the uptake of tryptophan and serotonin. Derangements in serotonin may enhance the effects of dopamine and/or account for the changes in sleep/wake cycles seen in cocaine abusers.[92] In high concentrations cocaine blocks the sodium channel, preventing the conduction of action potentials. This is the reason for cocaine's local anesthetic effects and arrhythmias. Repeated cocaine administration causes adaptive, tolerance-producing changes such as alpha$_2$-adrenergic and presynaptic cholinergic-mediated, decreased norepinephrine release at the motor endplate.[179] Cocaine lowers the seizure threshold and produces "kindling" (enhancement of seizures).[178]

Preparations. When dissolved in hydrochloric acid, cocaine yields the hydrochloride salt, a white powder, which can be inhaled or dissolved in water and injected. When "snorted," vasoconstriction of the mucous membranes limits its absorption rate, and the peak concentration is only 20% to

40% of that achieved with injection. When the hydrochloride is dissolved in water and ammonia and ether is added, the cocaine base dissolves in the ether layer and can be extracted by evaporation. This technique separates cocaine from adulterants and yields "freebase." When the hydrochloride is dissolved in water and baking soda and heated, the cocaine precipitates into a lump, which hardens when dry. This preparation, which makes a popping noise when heated, is known as "crack." Both freebase and crack volatilize without degradation at 80 degrees Celsius and can be smoked in a pipe, or mixed with tobacco and/or marijuana and smoked in a cigarette.[178] Freebase and crack are highly lipid-soluble because they are nonionized at body pH. Smoking yields serum cocaine concentrations that are 60% of those achieved with intravenous injection, but the brain concentration is higher because absorption across the pulmonary membranes delivers undiluted cocaine directly to the brain.

Metabolism. Cocaine is metabolized primarily by plasma cholinesterase and liver cholinesterase to ecgonine methyl ester, and by spontaneous nonenzymatic hydrolysis to benzoylecgonine. Under normal circumstances, plasma and liver enzymes contribute equally to cocaine hydrolysis. In addition, 20% of cocaine is metabolized in the liver by N-demethylation to norcocaine, which is more active than cocaine in inhibiting norepinephrine uptake.[35] In rats, long term ingestion of cocaine decreases its toxic threshold. It is thought that nonexposed rats have a better capacity of metabolizing cocaine by nonenzymatic hydrolysis or by lack of depletion of plasma cholinesterase.[180] Concomitant use of cocaine and alcohol can lead, in rats, to the ethyl transesterification of cocaine to cocaethylene, which, like norcocaine, is more potent than cocaine.[181,182] Cocaine's half-life in the blood depends on total dose and method of administration and is variously reported to be from 12 to 90 minutes.[173] Metabolites (ecgonine methyl ester and benzoylecgonine) are detectable in urine for 3 days and are deposited in hair, where they can be detected for a longer time.[9]

Bingeing. Because of its rapid metabolism, effects of crack last only a few minutes. In order to sustain the "high," users engage in a practice known as "bingeing." Repetitive doses are administered, usually along with shared tobacco, marijuana, and alcohol. The bingeing stops when neurotransmitters become depleted and additional drug ceases to be rewarding. During a binge, mood is intensely elevated, appetite is decreased, energy and alertness is increased, sexual feelings are accentuated, and social inhibitions are decreased. Bingeing results in exclusion of all thoughts unrelated to the next dose.[58] The binge is followed by sleep for a number of hours.

Withdrawal. Withdrawal is not seen in casual users, but in habitual users. Autonomic depression (lethargy, anorexia, and somnolence) begins hours after last exposure and lasts up to 10 weeks. Following this, resurgence of craving and normal activity recur.[178] Although there is no truly effective pharmacologic treatment available, dopamine agonists such as bromcriptinee[183] and buspirone,[175] or norepinephrine reuptake blocking tricyclic antidepressants such as desipramine,[178] help relieve symptoms.

Pathophysiology

The extensive list of complications associated with cocaine use are listed in Box 27-5. Their spectrum and frequency has shifted in the last decade, because the predominant preparation has changed from the hydrochloride to crack.[178] Cocaine's sympathomimetic effects produce multisystem

---

BOX 27-5 COMPLICATIONS OF COCAINE USE

Cardiac	Head and neck
Chest pain	Erosion of dental
Myocardial infarction	enamel
Arrythmias	Gingival ulceration
Cardiomyopathy	Keratitis
Myocarditis	Corneal epithelial deficits
Pulmonary	cits
Pneumothorax	Chronic rhinitis
Pneumomediastinum	Perforated nasal septum
Pneumopericardium	tum
Pulmonary edema	Aspiration of nasal
Exacerbation of asthma	septum
Pulmonary hemorrhage	Midline granuloma
Bronchiolitis obliterans	Altered olfaction
"Crack lung"	Optic neuropathy
Psychiatric	Osteolitic sinusitis
Anxiety	Neurologic
Depression	Headaches
Paranoia	Seizures
Psychosis	Cerebral hemorrhage
Delerium	Cerebral infarctions
Suicide	Cerebral atrophy
Gastrointestinal	Cerebral vasculitis
Intestinal ischemia	Endocrine
Gastroduodenal perforations	Hyperprolactinemia
rations	Others
Colitis	Sudden death
Renal	Sexual dysfunction
Rhabdomyolysis	Hyperpyrexia
	Thrombocytopenia

Modified from Warner EA: Cocaine abuse. *Ann Int Med* 1993; 226:235.

pathology. Peripheral vascular resistance, heart rate, and blood pressure are increased. Myocardial oxygen consumption increases, and myocardial infarction can occur even with normal coronary arteries. Coronary artery spasm causes focal endothelial injury and platelet aggregation, resulting in acute vascular platelet thrombosis and chronic intimal proliferation. The average age of patients with myocardial infarction related to cocaine use is 31. Cocaine causes myocarditis, pulmonary edema, or arrhythmias in some individuals and, like pheochromocytoma, has been associated with contraction band necrosis. Other ischemic sequelae include cerebral hemorrhage and infarction, aortic rupture, bowel infarction, and pseudomembranous colitis. Neurologic complications include seizures and vascular headaches, which are present in two thirds of cocaine hotline callers.[178]

Some complications of cocaine abuse depend on the route of administration. Nasal administration causes septal necrosis and perforation. Transmission of blood-borne pathogens is associated with intravenous injection. Smoking involves prolonged inspiration with Valsalva's maneuver. Alternatively, mouth-to-mouth positive pressure administration of smoke augments the intensity of cocaine's effects.[178] These can cause pneumothorax, pneumomediastinum, and pneumopericardium. Smoking cocaine is also associated with bronchospasm, with one-third of smokers noting wheezing during use; in addition, severe exacerbations of asthma have been described.[178] Finally, smoking cocaine is associated with bronchiolitis obliterans and a constellation of symptoms known as "crack lung," consisting of chest pain, hemoptysis, and diffuse alveolar infiltrates.[184]

Pregnancy

Incidence. In the Northeast and on the West Coast, 10% to 18% of pregnant patients use cocaine.[6,12,22,26,27] In certain high-risk populations, such as in the Northeast inner-city hospitals, the incidence of cocaine use may be as high as 50%.[20] However, in Midwest or Southeast rural or private populations, the incidence is less than 1%.[13,26] Forty percent of patients who have used cocaine in the previous week, as detected by positive urine screening, deny having done so.[7] Patients using cocaine are older,[21-23,69,89] less educated,[26] single,[6,21,23,26] Afro-American,[7,21,26,89] and urban poor.[7,15,23] They also smoke[27,65] and use other drugs,[23,89] and 50% fail to obtain prenatal care[27] (Table 27-8.) In one study, 50% of cocaine abusers used other drugs, 83% used tobacco, 43% used alcohol, and 31% used marijuana.[65] The patients abusing cocaine usually do not stop it as the pregnancy progresses.[23] A history of no prenatal care and drug and tobacco use predicts a positive urine screen for cocaine 70% of the time, and the absence of these factors predicts no cocaine use 70% of the time.[185] The Rapid Eye Test is a means of detecting incidence by physical examination. The pupils are dilated and react poorly to light, the corneal reflex is decreased, and nystagmus is present on lateral gaze.[186]

Maternal effects. The risks of cocaine use are compounded by pregnancy. In the rat, pregnancy increases sensitivity to cocaine and decreases blood flow to the heart.[55] In pregnant sheep, cocaine causes an increase in blood pressure twice that observed in nonpregnant ewes,[35] and in baboons a similar increase is seen with pregnancy.[58] One of the causes of increased sensitivity may be that pregnancy-associated changes in cholinesterase and hepatic metabolism increase the amount of N-demethylation to norcocaine, a more active substance.[35] The increase in sensitivity is also thought to be related to progesterone-induced changes in the alpha-adrenergic receptors during pregnancy. There are numerous reports associating complications with cocaine use in pregnant humans. Myocardial infarction, hepatic rupture, sudden death, and cerebrovascular accidents associated with cocaine use have been reported.[37,92,187] An increased

Table 27-8 Effects of cocaine bingeing on pregnancy

Binge pattern	Erratic use	Daily use	Every 3->7 days
Maternal weight <100 lb (%)	10	33	15
No prenatal care (%)	68	63	43
Positive urine at delivery (%)	45	50	20
Vaginal bleeding (%)	22	9	5
Placental abruption (%)	14	3	1.2
Stillbirth (%)	20	16	5
SGA (%)	13	33	17
Birth weight (g)	2295	2579	3129
Gestational age (wk)	32.4	34.5	37.2

Modified from Burkett G, Yasin SY, Palow D, et al: Patterns of cocaine bingeing: Effect on pregnancy. *Obstet Gynecol* 1994; 171:372.

incidence of postpartum cardiomyopathy has been observed.[188] Ruptured uterus[189] and ruptured ectopic pregnancy are associated with acute cocaine use.[44,60,190]

Maternal thrombocytopenia with a platelet count as low as 34,000 has been reported with cocaine administration.[191] An investigation in ewes has confirmed that platelets can decrease to 30,000 with a cocaine infusion.[46] Two subsequent retrospective studies in humans demonstrate that 9% of cocaine-using mothers have platelet counts less than 150,000,[192] and 5% have counts less than 100,000.[142] Excess catecholamines bind to platelets, activating them, and increased systemic vascular resistance decreases blood flow and leads to platelet aggregation.

Maternal weight gain is decreased from anorexia associated with bingeing (Table 27-8.) In severe cases, malnutrition has been reported. Cocaine probably increases the susceptibility to infection with HIV. Neopterin, a marker of cell-mediated immunity, is elevated in cocaine users and is associated with higher transmission rates of retroviral infection.[193] The cocaine-induced susceptibility to viral infection may account for increased HIV infection observed in sexually active cocaine abusers. On the other hand, it is quite probable that the increased incidence of infection is related to their sexual behavior.

Uteroplacental effects. Cocaine has two effects on the uterus, increased uterine contractility and vasoconstriction.[58,194-198] These two actions can lead to increased spontaneous abortion.[63,84,199] Uterine contractility is not always increased by cocaine in sheep,[194] but it is increased in baboons,[58] rabbits,[195] and human uterus.[14,196] Increased uterine contractility can lead to premature rupture of membranes.* These patients have more cervical dilation on admission and a shorter latency period

---

*References 27, 62, 66, 69, 84, 199.

to delivery.[31] Cocaine-induced vasoconstriction is associated with changes in placental blood flow and placental abruption. Numerous studies have demonstrated an increased incidence of abruption in cocaine users.[6,62-64,67,69,199] Table 27-3 shows the risk for abruption in cocaine abusers.

The placenta has the capacity to bind and metabolize cocaine. In addition to binding to cocaine-specific receptors, cocaine binds to sigma receptors in the placenta.[36] Placental microsomes have the capacity to hydrolyze cocaine, thereby limiting fetal exposure.[36]

Fetal effects. If placental blood flow is impaired for a significant period of time, the decreased transfer of oxygen and nutrients may harm the fetus.[200] Fetal hypoxia has been demonstrated in ewes.[56,57] Case reports describe fetal death and necrotizing enterocolitis in utero from ischemia.[201,202] In a group of bingers with a very chaotic lifestyle, stillbirth occurred in 20% of patients[199] (Table 27-8.) In bingers with a more stable environment, one third of the infants were small for gestational age.[199] Studies of more moderate cocaine use fail to show decreased fetal growth,[27,66] but others, such as those shown in Table 27-9, demonstrate decreased infant size.

Birth defects. Animal studies show that cocaine can cross the placenta by simple diffusion. Fetal organs have up to one third of maternal brain concentrations. Cocaine has the potential to produce fetal anomalies through infarction and malnutrition, as well as through changes in neurotransmitters either directly or by metabolism. In animals, there is evidence that cocaine disturbs neuronal differentiation in the cerebral, diencephalic, and brain-stem structures, with subsequent defects in memory and learning.[92] The derangement of neurotransmitters in the fetus exposed to cocaine may impair the development of normal neuronal pathways. Human infants with abnormal eye and brain morphology suggest the association of disorders of midbrain prosencephalic development and neuro-

---

Table 27-9 Perinatal outcome of fetal cocaine exposure*†

	Cases (*n* = 55)	Controls (*n* = 55)	*P*
Gestational age (wk)	37.36 + 3.0	39.18 + 1.91	<0.02‡
Birth weight (g)	2,528.2 + 619	3,056.1 + 500	<0.002§
Birth weight (mean percentile for gestational age)	31.9 + 21.4	48.2 + 22.8	<0.05‡
Head circumference	31.8 + 2.6	33.7 + 1.7	0.09§
Head circumference (percentile for gestational age)	33.6 + 27.0	51.7 + 23.5	<0.05‡

*Modified from Cherukuri R, Minkoff H, Feldman J, et al: *Obstet Gynecol* 1988; 72:149. Used by permission.
†Study infants were identified at birth and matched with controls. Values shown are mean + SD.
‡After adjustment for sex of child and mother's smoking.
§After adjustment for sex of child, length of gestation, and mother's smoking.

nal migration with exposure to cocaine.[203] Destructive abnormalities of the fetal brain may occur later in gestation, after blood vessels have developed the capacity to contract on exposure to cocaine.[97] This can lead to microcephaly, which is significantly more frequent in cocaine users.[69] Genitourinary tract anomalies,[78,204] cranial anomalies,[94] ileal atresia,[63] microcephaly,* cardiac abnormalities[68,89] limb reduction abnormalities,[77] and neural tube malformations[68] have been reported in offspring of mothers abusing cocaine.

Neonatal effects. Identification of exposed neonates is as difficult as identification of their drug-abusing mothers. Of cocaine-exposed neonates, only 38% have positive urine screen, and only 52% have positive meconium screen. Hair analysis can identify 78% of exposed infants.[31]

Multiple sequelae of cocaine exposure are reported in human infants. The cost of neonatal care for infants identified as exposed to cocaine is increased 4 to 8 times over that for non–drug-exposed infants.[110] The immediate effect of cocaine exposure on the neonate is autonomic depression.[88] Neonates have withdrawal symptoms, but these are less severe than opiate symptoms. Transient neonatal ventricular tachycardia in a human infant is associated with cocaine exposure.[205] In a prospective study, episodes of periodic breathing occurred in 38%, and apnea of infancy in 15% of cocaine-exposed infants.[113] These ventilatory abnormalities resolved with theophylline therapy. The incidence of SIDS in cocaine-exposed infants is 3 to 7 times higher than in control infants.[92]

The major focus of investigation has been on neurologic outcome. Fifty percent of cocaine-exposed infants have abnormal EEGs, showing increased beta activity and cerebral irritation with bursts of sharp waves.[206] By 3 to 12 months of age, the abnormal findings resolve. Numerous infants with infarction of the middle cerebral artery at birth, presumably from cocaine induced vasospasm, have been reported.[92] In addition, echolucent areas in the brain have been described in infants exposed to cocaine, suggesting prior infarction.[207] Association of intraventricular hemorrhage and cocaine use remains controversial.[122,208,209] Neurobehavioral functioning, measured by the Neonatal Behavioral Assessment Scale[20,65,88] or by Bayley cognitive and psycomotor scores[122] have failed to demonstrate any consistent defects associated with cocaine.

Obstetric and anesthetic considerations

Obstetric considerations. Cocaine's effects on pregnancy are summarized in Box 27-6. Cocaine

---

*References 12, 20, 62, 65, 68, 92, 96.

BOX 27-6 COCAINE EFFECTS ON PREGNANCY

Spontaneous abortion
Microcephaly
Intrauterine growth retardation
Placental abruption
Premature rupture of membranes
Preterm delivery
Low birth weight
Transient neurobehavioral abnormalities
Congenital anomalies*
Impaired neuronal differentiation*

---

*Still theoretical.

---

abusers have a high incidence of no prenatal care. In Brooklyn, 43% of unregistered patients tested positive for cocaine.[27] These patients need to be identified in the community and encouraged to attend clinic. It is important to arrange for continued care after the pregnancy so the infant can have a stable environment. By age 18 months, one third of infants exposed to cocaine are placed outside the home[210]; postnatal care results in a better infant outcome.

Several factors should be considered in planning prenatal care for the cocaine abuser. Maternal health education should stress nutrition, sexually transmitted diseases, urinary tract infections, and premature labor. If the patient abuses cocaine and heroin, buprenorphine can be substituted for methadone.[162] Analysis of hair may prove useful in determining the quantity of cocaine administered over weeks or months,[9] but the patient's permission must be obtained for any toxicology analyses. Patients experiencing chest pain need a cardiology consultation. Cocaine's adrenergic stimulation may elevate the blood sugar and interfere with glucose tolerance testing.

Intrapartum management. Patients can arrive with emergency situations. They may present as severe pregnancy-induced hypertension, precipitate labor, or placental abruption. Cocaine abusers can present with hypertension, blurred vision, headache, abdominal pain, or seizures. These symptoms, however, resolve within 45 to 90 minutes of admission.[45] Such parturients should be treated as preeclampsia/eclampsia patients with magnesium sulfate until the diagnosis is clear.

Cocaine intoxication. Signs and symptoms of cocaine toxicity are listed in Table 27-10. Tachycardia and hypertension is treated with labetalol, rather than beta-adrenergic antagonists, since unopposed alpha-adrenergic activity increases blood pressure and exacerbates decreased uterine blood flow.[211] Calcium-channel blockers are also associ-

Table 27-10 Signs of cocaine toxicity*

CNS	Psychological	Cardiovascular	Miscellaneous
Delirium	Irritability	Arrhythmia	Fever
Convulsions	Restlessness	Pallor	Diaphoresis
Hyperreflexia	Tenseness	Tachycardia	Dry mouth
Tremor	Anxiety	Hypertension	Dilated pupils
Dizziness	Garrulousness	Angina	
Hallucinations	Euphoria	Headache	
Coma	Insomnia	Flushing	
Cerebral hemorrhage	Panic	Circulatory collapse	
	Suicidal		
	Homicidal		

*Modified from James FM, Wheeler FS, Dewan DM (eds): *Obstetric Anesthesia: The Complicated Patient.* Philadelphia, FA Davis, 1987. Used by permission.

ated with paradoxical responses.[212] Hydralazine treatment exacerbates tachycardia.[213] Psychosis responds to neuroleptics or lithium.

Placental abruption. Some patients arrive intoxicated, with abruptio placentae, tetanic contraction, and fetal bradycardia. In absence of abruption, esmolol, nitroglycerin, and tocolysis can resolve tetanic contraction and fetal bradycardia. With abruption, magnesium sulfate can relax the uterus and may sustain the fetus until delivery by cesarean section can be accomplished.

Pretreatment of ewes with 5 mg per kg of magnesium attenuates seizures and corrects maternal and fetal heart rate changes.[46] Magnesium may prevent thrombocytopenia associated with cocaine administration. Cocaine increases the likelihood of tachyarrythmias with ritodrine and terbutaline. Such patients in labor require support and may need more anesthesia.

Anesthetic considerations for labor. Epidural or intrathecal narcotic analgesia is indicated as long as there is no coagulopathy. Cocaine abusers should have a platelet count before an epidural anesthetic is administered.[142,192] Indirectly acting vasopressors such as ephedrine are theoretically less effective when norepinephrine stores are depleted. Occasionally ephedrine treatment for hypotension is ineffective and phenylephrine is needed. A recent report shows cocaine users are more sensitive to pain, but the report failed to demonstrate significantly increased epidural anesthetic requirements.[214]

Anesthesia for cesarean section. Regional techniques are preferred for cesarean section. Hypotension resulting from epidural or spinal analgesia can be treated with ephedrine; phenylephrine may be used if ephedrine is ineffective. In a study of cocaine abusers undergoing cesarean section, spinal anesthesia was not associated with a significant increase in the risk of hypotension.[215]

Cocaine decreases the seizure threshold and

has local anesthetic effects. Although metabolism is rapid and mainly by liver cholinesterase, residual cocaine may decrease the amount of free plasma cholinesterase, affecting metabolism of 2-chloroprocaine. Total local anesthetic dose should be conservative to avoid local anesthetic toxicity.

General anesthesia. General anesthesia is necessary if cocaine causes placental abruption or severe fetal distress, or if the patient is not a candidate for regional anesthesia. In one study, two thirds of the patients received general anesthesia.[215] Atropine should be used with caution because it blocks presynaptic cholinergic regulation of norepinephrine release, thereby increasing hypertension.[179] Cocaine causes bronchospasm and increases general anesthetic requirements.[216]

Decreased serum cholinesterase may prolong the duration of succinylcholine, mivacurium, and atricurium, which are all metabolized by cholinesterase. The in vitro hydrolysis of cocaine by plasma is prolonged in patients who have pseudocholinesterase deficiency,[217] and lower plasma cholinesterase levels are associated with more severe toxicity to cocaine (Fig. 27-2).[218] It is not known whether the lower cholinesterase levels are the cause of the observed sensitivity to cocaine or the result of cholinesterase depletion by previously administered cocaine.

Induction. It is difficult to determine a safe induction agent for general anesthesia for cesarean section in a patient with cocaine-induced placental abruption. Hemorrhage causes hypovolemia, and pentothal and propofol aggravate hypovolemic hypotension by causing vasodilation. Excessive catecholamines, as with ketamine induction, produce hypertension and can cause myocardial infarction.[217] Etomidate appears the best induction agent in this situation, although it will not prevent a hypertensive response to intubation.

After delivery, sympathomimetic effects (in-

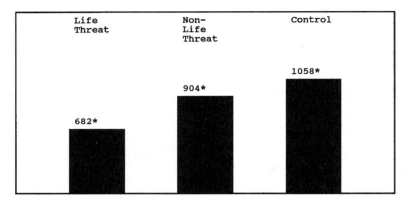

Fig. 27-2 Plasma cholinesterase activity in cocaine abusers. *$p = 0.05$. Plasma cholinesterase activity in Michel units/L in three groups of patients, those with life-threatening reactions to self-administered cocaine, those with minor problems following cocaine, and controls. (Adapted from Hoffman RS, Henry GC, Howland MA, et al: Association between life-threatening cocaine toxicity and plasma cholinesterase activity. *Ann Emerg Med* 1992; 21:247.)

duced by nitrous oxide and isoforane) and central sympathetic stimulation, (induced by narcotics) can exacerbate tachycardia and hypertension. Droperidol, labetalol, or short-acting vasodilators may be needed to control heart rate and blood pressure. Isoforane is the inhalational anesthetic of choice, as rats anesthetized with isoforane tolerate a higher plasma cocaine concentration than those anesthetized with halothane.[205] Chronic neurotransmitter depletion from cocaine is postulated to decrease anesthetic requirements, but MAC for isoforane is increased significantly in sheep that have been exposed to a cocaine infusion for 2 weeks.[216]

AMPHETAMINES
Pharmacology

Amphetamine is a chemical that is easily manufactured in clandestine labs. It causes increased release of neurotransmitters from the presynaptic terminal, in addition to decreasing neurotransmitter reuptake; in addition, it increases norepinephrine and dopamine availability in the brain. Although their specific actions are different, methamphetamine is generally indistinguishable from cocaine in both its pharmacologic and addictive characteristics. Amphetamine is metabolized in the liver, but at least 50% of a dose is excreted unchanged in the urine. Ammonium chloride acidification hastens its excretion.[1] The plasma half-life of amphetamine is 12 hours, 10 times longer than cocaine.[54] Because of its longer duration of action, psychotic symptoms develop more slowly than with cocaine. A smoked form, "ice," that produces an instant high of long duration, and its use is more prevalent in Hawaii and California.[219]

In pregnant sheep, amphetamine increases maternal heart rate, blood pressure, and uterine vascular resistance, and it decreases uterine blood flow. After an initial decrease, fetal heart rate and umbilical blood flow increase to levels above baseline for 2 to 3 hours. The fetal pH and Po_2 decrease gradually.[54,220]

Pregnancy

Currently, the incidence of amphetamine abuse is low except on the West Coast. In Sacramento, 7% of the pregnant population had used amphetamines,[6] whereas in Florida and Missouri no patients had positive urines,[7,17] and in Georgia, only 0.3% of the pregnant population did.[22] In California, Afro-Americans use cocaine, and whites prefer amphetamines. The maternal and fetal problems associated with cocaine abuse are also reported with amphetamines.[62] Acute intoxication can be mistaken for eclampsia or preeclampsia.[221] There are no large studies of amphetamine use alone that can distinguish the effects of amphetamine from those of the substance-abusing lifestyle, but amphetamine use is associated with placental abruption, intrauterine growth retardation, decreased gestational length, and increased perinatal mortality.[222] Infants of mothers who use amphetamines along other drugs are small for gestational age and premature, with a high neonatal mortality rate.[223] In a study of 13 cocaine and 28 methamphetamine abusers, no differences between pregnancy and neonatal outcome were noted.[85]

Obstetric and anesthetic considerations

Obstetric and anesthetic care is similar to that for cocaine abusers. Methamphetamine abusers respond poorly to indirect-acting sympathomimetic agents. Since orally ingested methamphetamine continues to be absorbed during labor and because amphetamine has a long half-life, fetal distress is less likely to improve after admission than with cocaine abusers. Inhalational anesthetic requirements are increased,[224] and in a case report of methamphetamine abuse, fentanyl and nitrous oxide requirements were increased.[225]

TOBACCO
Pharmacology

Nicotine, the active agent in tobacco, stimulates the CNS and autonomic ganglia, triggering release of epinephrine from the adrenal medulla. In large doses it produces ganglionic blockade. Tolerance develops to some of its effects. Withdrawal symptoms, including irritability, aggressiveness, hostility, depression, and concentration difficulties result from both environmental conditioning and pharmacologic dependence. Nicotine is metabolized to cotinine, and levels in the urine quantitatively reflect tobacco exposure.[24] Nicotine and cotinine cross the placenta and significant levels have been detected in amniotic fluid, fetal serum, and placental tissues throughout the pregnancy. Fetal nicotine levels exceed maternal levels,[226] but fetal cotinine levels are lower than maternal levels.[226,227]

Pregnancy

Maternal effects. Seventeen percent to 30% of patients smoke during pregnancy.[17,19,22,24] Self-reporting of smoking is more reliable than that of illicit drug use; only 7% of patients who deny smoking have positive urine tests.[24] Women who start smoking before age 15 tend to be heavy smokers before pregnancy and at the first prenatal visit.[149] Fewer private patients than clinic patients smoke. Smokers are usually younger, white, single, and less educated.[26] Women who smoke are more likely to be physically abused, especially Hispanics, whose risk is increased by a factor of 6.[48] Smoking alters the hypothalamic pituitary axis, inhibiting release of LH and prolactin and decreasing fertility and gestational length.

Uteroplacental effects. Microscopically, placentas of heavy smokers exhibit atrophic hypovascular villi. Cyanide, from tobacco smoke, crosses the placenta and depletes fetal vitamin B_{12}.[228] Estradiol conversion is reduced, and placental uptake of alpha-aminobutyric acid is decreased.[50] Placental impairment is thought to be due to nicotine-induced vasoconstriction.[229] Tobacco use is associated with preterm labor, and abruption and placenta previa account for one half to one third of the increased perinatal mortality in smokers.[104,116,230]

Fetal effects. In rats, nicotine retards embryo cell cleavage, reducing cell number, and provokes developmental abnormalities. In humans, erythropoietin, hemoglobin concentration, and carboxyhemoglobin concentrations are increased with tobacco exposure, suggesting chronic fetal hypoxia.[53] Nicotine increases fetal heart rate, as well as umbilical and fetal aortic blood flow,[231] indicating increased placental perfusion and possible increased systemic vascular resistance from adrenal activity secondary to hypoxia.[53] Fetal respiratory movements in utero are depressed by tobacco smoking.[232] At term, smoking causes fetal tachycardia and decreases beat-to-beat variability.[233]

Growth retardation[230] and neonatal mortality increase with maternal smoking.[79] Smoking is associated with second-trimester abortion, as is maternal exposure to passive smoke.[230,234,234] Birth weight and birth length correlate with maternal serum cotinine concentration; the average weight reduction is the equivalent of one week of fetal growth in late pregnancy.[80] Smoking before pregnancy decreases infant size, as does use during pregnancy.[18,81] Third-trimester use is especially predictive of lower weight and head circumference, as is concomitant heavy alcohol consumption.[81-83] Passive smoking is also correlated with low birth weight.[235,236] In infants, especially those who are preterm, prolactin, growth hormone, and insulinlike growth factor I are increased by tobacco exposure.[237]

Neonatal effects. Infants exposed to passive smoke have cotinine levels in meconium similar to those of infants whose mothers are light smokers.[11] Prenatal exposure to tobacco is not associated with any consistent changes on Brazelton neonatal assessments,[123,171] but tremors and poorer habituation to auditory stimuli are reported.[171] Infants of smokers have slower FEF rates shortly after birth, indicating that tobacco may impair in utero lung development or alter lung elastic properties.

Infants of prenatal smokers have a 3 to 4 times greater risk of SIDS. The risk is further increased by postnatal maternal smoking. If the father smokes as well, the risk of SIDS is increased 7 times.[238,239]

There is evidence that the effects of tobacco exposure persist into childhood. Children whose mothers stop smoking are taller and heavier than controls at age three. In tobacco-exposed children, a size decrement of about 1 cm persists throughout childhood.[123] Children exposed to prenatal tobacco have 5% decreased FEF_{25-75}, indicating decreased small airways flow.[240] The evidence for cognitive deficits is inconsistent.[123] In one study,

---

BOX 27-7   TOBACCO EFFECTS ON PREGNANCY

Spontaneous abortion
Preterm delivery
Low birth weight
Sudden infant death syndrome (SIDS)
Decreased small airway diameter

---

children whose mothers stopped smoking scored higher on a general cognitive index at age 3.[241]

Obstetric and anesthetic considerations

Obstetric. The effects of tobacco on pregnancy are summarized in Box 27-7. Patients should stop smoking during pregnancy. Pregnancy is a time when motivation to protect the fetus increases maternal efforts to cease smoking. Tobacco use declined from 10% to 7% in pregnant patients in Los Angeles from 1986 to 1990.[18] Even in late gestation to stop smoking is beneficial, since nicotine and carbon monoxide are eliminated within 12 to 24 hours.[242] However, substance abusers rate quitting smoking equal to or more difficult than stopping abuse of their problem substance.[243] Patients need instructions regarding preterm labor and surveillance for growth retardation.

Anesthetic. Smoking is an established cause of increased anesthetic risk. Stopping for 12 hours should eliminate most carboxyhemoglobin and improve oxygen-carrying capacity.[242] Stopping for 48 hours produces an 8% increase in available oxygen in pregnant women.[244] Smoking also causes hepatic enzyme induction, altering anesthetic drug metabolism.[242] Smoking on the day of surgery increases gastric volume and risk for aspiration.[245] Treatment with ranitidine and metaclopromide will reduce gastric acidity and increase gastric emptying. Bronchitis and increased levels of carbon monoxide increase the risk of bronchospasm and hypoxia after intubation. Regional anesthesia avoids these risks and is thus preferred for smokers.

SUMMARY

Maternal use of substances potentially harmful to the fetus and neonate immediately before and during pregnancy is widespread. Few substance abusers use a single agent, and the effects of a particular drug are difficult to establish. Baseline abuse of tobacco, ethanol, and marijuana persists as abusers advance to more potent drugs. Neonatal outcome depends on maternal lifestyle as well as substance abuse. Drug abuse is sustained by behavioral reinforcement and dependence.

Maternal health, fertility, prenatal care, placental function, fetal development, neonatal morbidity, parenting, and child development and behavior all undergo adverse effects as a result of substance abuse. The combination of tobacco, alcohol, marijuana, and heroin or cocaine abuse results in drug-seeking behavior that increases maternal malnutrition and HIV infection. Alcohol and cocaine addiction cause severe permanent morphologic and neurologic damage to the fetus.

Prenatal care must be directed toward early intervention and obtaining the patient's participation in altering her lifestyle and reducing substance abuse. Altered maternal physiology and metabolic and pharmacologic drug interactions affect obstetric and anesthetic care in the delivery room. Abortion, preterm labor, premature rupture of membranes, placental abruption, intrauterine fetal growth retardation, and preterm delivery occur more frequently in patients who are substance abusers. Epidural or intrathecal narcotic analgesia decreases maternal and fetal stress during labor. Administration of anesthesia for cesarean section must be altered to accommodate the interactions of abused substances with anesthetic agents. The proportion of patients for whom general anesthesia for cesarean section is necessary increases with substance abuse.

REFERENCES

1. Doweiko HF: *Concepts of Chemical Dependency.* Pacific Grove, Brooks/Cole, 1993, pp 1-14, 69-78, 141-52.
2. Kozel NJ, Adams EH: Epidemiology of drug abuse: An overview. *Science* 1986; 234:970.
3. Cho AK: Ice: A new dosage form of an old drug. *Science* 1990; 249:631.
4. Kulberg A: Substance abuse: Clinical identification and management. *Pediatr Clin North Am* 1986; 33:325.
5. Semlitz L, Gold MS: Adolescent drug abuse: Diagnosis, treatment, and prevention. *Psychiatr Clin North Am* 1986; 9:455.
6. Gillogley KM, Evans AT, Hansen RL, et al: The perinatal impact of cocaine, amphetamine, and opiate use detected by universal intrapartum screening. *Am J Obstet Gynecol* 1990; 163:1535.
7. Vaughn AJ, Carzoli RP, Sanchez-Ramos L, et al: Community-wide estimation of illicit drug use in delivering women: Prevalence, demographics, and associated risk factors. *Obstet Gynecol* 1993; 82:92.
8. Hawks RL, Chiang CN (eds): Urine testing for drugs of abuse. *NIDA Research Monograph* 1986; 73.
9. Graham K, Koren G, Klein J, et al: Determination of gestational cocaine exposure by hair analysis. *JAMA* 1989; 262:3328.
10. Callahan CM, Grant TM, Phipps PC: Measurement of gestational cocaine exposure: Sensitivity of infant's hair, meconium, and urine. *J Pediatr* 1992; 120:763.
11. Ostrea EM, Knapp DK, Romero AI, et al: Meconium analysis to assess fetal exposure to nicotine by active and passive maternal smoking. *J Pediatr* 1994; 124:471.
12. Zuckerman B, Frank DA, Hingson R, et al: Effects of maternal marijuana and cocaine use on fetal growth. *N Engl J Med* 1989; 320:762.

13. Burke MS, Roth D: Anonymous cocaine screening in a private obstetrics population. *Obstet Gynecol* 1993; 81:354.

14. Osterloh JD, Lee BL: Urine drug screening in mothers and newborns. *Am J Dis Child* 1989; 143:791.

15. Vega WA, Kolody B, Hwang J, et al: Prevalence and magnitude of perinatal substance exposures in California. *N Engl J Med* 1993; 329:850.

16. Ney JA, Dooley SL, Keith LG, et al: The prevalence of substance abuse in patients with suspected preterm labor. *Am J Obstet Gynecol* 1990; 162:1562.

17. Sloan LB, Gay JW, Snyder SW, et al: Substance abuse during pregnancy in a rural population. *Obstet Gynecol* 1992; 79:245.

18. Castro LC, Azen C, Hobel CJ, et al: Maternal tobacco use and substance abuse: Reported prevalence rates and association with the delivery of small for gestational age neonates. *Obstet Gynecol* 1993; 81:396.

19. Slutsker L, Smith R, Higginson G: Recognizing illicit drug use by pregnant women: Reports from Oregon birth attendants. *Am J Public Health* 1993; 83:61.

20. Cherukuri R, Minkoff H, Feldman J, et al: A cohort study of alkaloidal cocaine ("crack") in pregnancy. *Obstet Gynecol* 1988; 72:147.

21. Day NL, Cottreau CM, Richardson GA: The epidemiology of alcohol, cocaine, and marijuana use among women of childbearing age and pregnant women. *Clin Obstet Gynecol* 1993; 36:232.

22. Christmas JT, Knisely JS, Dawson KS: Comparison of questionnaire screening and urine toxicology for detection of pregnancy complicated by substance abuse. *Obstet Gynecol* 1992; 80:750.

23. George SK, Price J, Hauth JC, et al: SPO transactions: Drug abuse screening of childbearing-age women in Alabama public health clinics. *Am J Obstet Gynecol* 1991; 165:924.

24. Lapham SC, Kring MK, Skipper B: Prenatal behavioral risk screening by computer in a health maintenance organization-based prenatal care clinic. *Am J Obstet Gynecol* 1991; 165:506.

25. Little BB, Snell LM, Gilstrap LD III, et al: Patterns of multiple substance abuse during pregnancy: Implications for mother and fetus. *South Med J* 1990; 83:507.

26. Streissguth AP, Grant TM, Barr HM, et al: Cocaine and the use of alcohol and other drugs during pregnancy. *Am J Obstet Gynecol* 1991; 164:1239.

27. McCalla S, Minkoff HL, Feldman J, et al: The biologic and social consequences of perinatal cocaine use in an inner-city population: Results of an anonymous cross-sectional study. *Am J Obstet Gynecol* 1991; 164:625.

28. Neerhof MG, MacGregor SN, Retzky SS, et al: Cocaine abuse during pregnancy: Peripartum prevalence and perinatal outcome. *Am J Obstet Gynecol* 1989; 161:688.

29. Fried PA: Prenatal exposure to tobacco and marijuana: Effects during pregnancy, infancy, and early childhood. *Clin Obstet Gynecol* 1993; 36:319.

30. Hawthorne JL, Maier RC: Drug abuse in an obstetric population of a midsized city. *South Med J* 1993; 86:1334.

31. Dinsmoor NJ, Irons SJ, Christmas JT: Preterm rupture of the membranes associated with cocaine use. *Am J Obstet Gynecol* 1994; 171:305.

32. Zuckerman B, Amaro H, Cabral H: Validity of self-reporting of marijuana and cocaine use among pregnant adolescents. *Pediatrics* 1989; 82:687.

33. Klein RF, Friedman-Campbell M, Tocco RV: History taking and substance abuse counseling with the pregnant patient. *Clin Obstet Gynecol* 1993; 36:338.

34. Mucklow JC: The fate of drugs in pregnancy. *Clin Obstet Gynecol* 1986; 13:161.

35. Woods JR, Plessinger MA: Pregnancy increases cardiovascular toxicity to cocaine. *Am J Obstet Gynecol* 1990; 162:529.

36. Plessinger MA, Woods JR: Maternal placental, and fetal pathophysiology of cocaine exposure during pregnancy. *Clin Obstet Gynecol* 1993; 36:267.

37. Moen MD, Caliendo MJ, Marshall W, et al: Hepatic rupture in pregnancy associated with cocaine use. *Obstet Gynecol* 1993; 82:687.

38. Ylikabri RH, Huttunen MO, Hardoven M: Hormonal changes during alcohol intoxication and withdrawal. *Pharmacol Biochem Behav* 1980; 13(suppl 1):131.

39. Roe DA, Little BB, Bawdon RE, et al: Metabolism of cocaine by human placentas: Implications for fetal exposure. *Am J Obstet Gynecol* 1990; 163:715.

40. Rice PA, Nesbitt RE, Cuenca VG, et al: The effect of ethanol on the production of lactate, triglycerides, phospholipids and free fatty acids in the perfused human placenta. *Am J Obstet Gynecol* 1986; 155:207.

41. Lindsay MK, Peterson HB, Boring J, et al: Crack cocaine: A risk factor for human immunodeficiency virus infection type 1 among inner city parturients. *Obstet Gynecol* 1992; 80:981.

42. Selwin PA, Schoenbaum EE, Davenny K, et al: Prospective study of human immunodeficiency virus infection and pregnancy outcome in intravenous drug users. *JAMA* 1989; 261:1326.

43. Knight EM, James H, Edwards CH, et al: Relationships of serum illicit drug concentrations during pregnancy to maternal nutritional status. *J Nutrition* 1994; 124:973S.

44. Burkett G, Yasin SY, Palow D, et al: Patterns of cocaine bingeing: Effect on pregnancy. *Am J Obstet Gynecol* 1994; 171:372.

45. Towers CV, Pircon RA, Nageotte MP, et al: Cocaine intoxication presenting as preeclampsia and eclampsia. *Obstet Gynecol* 1993; 81:545.

46. Weaver K, Merrell CL, Griffin G: Effect of magnesium on cocaine-induced catecholamine-mediated platelet and vascular response in term pregnant ewes. *Am J Obstet Gynecol* 1989; 161:1331.

47. Kruse J, Lefevre M, Zweig S: Changes in smoking and alcohol consumption during pregnancy: A population based study in a rural area. *Obstet Gynecol* 1986; 67:627.

48. Berenson AB, Stiglich NJ, Wilkinson GS, et al: Drug abuse and other risk factors for physical abuse in pregnancy among White, non-Hispanic, Black and Hispanic women. *Am J Obstet Gynecol* 1991; 164:1491.

49. Amaro H, Fried LE, Cobral H: Violence during pregnancy and substance abuse. *Am J Public Health* 1990; 80:575.

50. Fisher SE, Atkinson M, Van Thiel DH: Selective fetal malnutrition: The effect of nicotine, ethanol and acetaldehyde upon in vivo uptake of alpha-amino butyric acid by human term placental villous slices. *Dev Pharmacol Ther* 1984; 7:229.

51. Sastry BVR, Mouton S, Janson VE: Tobacco smoking by pregnant women: Disturbances in metabolism of branched chain amino acids and fetal growth. *Ann NY Acad Sci* 1989; 678:361.

52. Erskine RL, Ritchie JW: The effect of maternal consumption of alcohol on human umbilical artery blood flow. *Am J Obstet Gynecol* 1986; 154:318.

53. Varvarigou A, Beratis NG, Makri M, et al: Increased levels and positive correlation between erythropoietin and hemoglobin concentrations in newborn children of mothers who are smokers. *J Pediatr* 1994; 124:480.

54. Stek AM, Fisher BK, Baker RS, et al: Maternal and fetal cardiovascular responses to methamphetamine in pregnant sheep. *Am J Obstet Gynecol* 1993; 169:888.

55. Morishima HO, Cooper TB, Miller ED: Effect of cocaine on maternal hemodynamics: Preliminary study. *Society of*

Obstetric Anesthesia and Perinatology Abstracts 1988; 116.

56. Woods FR Jr, Plessinger MA, Clark KE: Effect of cocaine on uterine blood flow and fetal oxygenation. *JAMA* 1987; 257:957.

57. Moore TR, Sorg J, Miller L, et al: Hemodynamic effects of intravenous cocaine on the pregnant ewe and fetus. *Am J Obstet Gynecol* 1986; 155:883.

58. Morgan MA, Wentworth RA, Silavin SL, et al: Intravenous administration of cocaine stimulates gravid baboon myometrium in the last third of gestation. *Am J Obstet Gynecol* 1994; 170:1416.

59. Hoskins IA, Friedman DM, Frieden FJ, et al: Relationship between antepartum cocaine abuse, abnormal umbilical artery Doppler velocimetry and placental abruption. *Obstet Gynecol* 1991; 78:279.

60. Darby MJ, Caritis SN, Shen-Schwarz S: Placental abruption on the preterm gestation: An association with chorioamnionitis. *Obstet Gynecol* 1989; 741:88.

61. Finnegan LP: Effects of maternal opiate abuse on the newborn. *Fed Proc* 1985; 44:2314.

62. Oro AS, Dixon SD: Perinatal cocaine and methamphetamine exposure: Maternal and neonatal correlates. *J Pediatr* 1987; 111:5471.

63. Chasnoff IJ, Griffith DR, MacGregor S, et al: Temporal patterns of cocaine use in pregnancy. *JAMA* 1989; 261:1741.

64. Acker DB, Sachs BP, Tracey KJ, et al: Abruptio placentae associated with cocaine use. *Am J Obstet Gynecol* 1983; 146:220.

65. Bateman DA, Stephen KC, Hansen CA, et al: The effects of intrauterine cocaine exposure in newborns. *Am J Public Health* 1993; 83:190.

66. Mastrogianis DS, Decavalas GO, Verma V, et al: Perinatal outcome after recent cocaine usage. *Obstet Gynecol* 1990; 76:8.

67. MacGregor SN, Keith LG, Chasnoff IJ, et al: Cocaine use during pregnancy: Adverse perinatal outcome. *Am J Obstet Gynecol* 1989; 157:686.

68. Bingol N, Fuchs M, Diaz V, et al: Teratogenicity of cocaine in humans. *J Pediatr* 1987; 110:93.

69. Handler A, Kistin N, Davis F, et al: Cocaine use during pregnancy: Perinatal outcomes. *Am J Epidemiol* 1991; 133:818.

70. Naeye RL, Harkness WL, Utts J: Abruptio placentae and perinatal death: A prospective study. *Am J Obstet Gynecol* 1977; 128:740.

71. Martin JC: Irreversable changes in mature and aging animals following intrauterine drug exposure. *Neurobehav Toxicol Teratol* 1986; 8:355.

72. Milunsky A, Jick H, Jick SS, et al: Multivitamin/folic acid supplementation in early pregnancy reduces the prevalence of neural tube defects. *JAMA* 1989; 262:2847.

73. Niemela O, Halmesmaki E, Ylikorkla O: Hemoglobin-acetaldehyde adducts are elevated in women carrying alcohol damaged fetuses. *Alcohol Clin Exp Res* 1991; 15:1007.

74. Ernhart CB, Sokol RJ, Ager JW, et al: Alcohol-related birth defects: Assessing the risks. *Ann NY Acad Sci* 1989; 678:159.

75. Fishman RH, Yanai J: Long-lasting effects of early barbiturates on central nervous system and behavior. *Neurosci Biobehav Rev* 1983; 7:19.

76. Hingson RJ, Alpert N, Day E, et al: Effects of maternal drinking and marijuana use on fetal growth and development. *Pediatrics* 1982; 70:539.

77. Hoyme HE, Jones KL, Dixon SD, et al: Prenatal cocaine exposure and fetal vascular disruption. *Pediatrics* 1990; 85:743.

78. Chasnoff IJ, Chisum GM, Kaplan WE: Maternal cocaine use and genitourinary tract malformations. *Teratology* 1988; 37:201.

79. Weisberg E: Smoking and reproductive health. *Clin Reprod Fertil* 1985; 3:174.

80. Bardy AH, Seppala T, Lillsunde P, et al: Objectively measured tobacco exposure during pregnancy: Neonatal effects and relationship to maternal smoking. *Br J Obstet Gynaecol* 1993; 100:721.

81. Fried PA, O'Connell CM: A comparison of the effects of prenatal exposure to tobacco, alcohol, cannabis and caffeine on birth size and subsequent growth. *Neurotox Teratol* 1987; 9:79.

82. Olsen J, da costa Pereira A, Olsen SF: Does maternal tobacco smoking modify the effect of alcohol on fetal growth. *Am J Public Health* 1991; 81:69.

83. Peacock JL, Bland JM, Anderson HR: Effects on birthweight of alcohol and caffeine consumption in smoking women. *J Epidemiol Comm Health* 1991; 45:159.

84. Keith LG, MacGregor S, Friedell S, et al: Substance abuse in pregnant women: Recent experience at the perinatal center for chemical dependence of Northwestern Memorial Hospital. *Obstet Gynecol* 1989; 73:715.

85. Ryan L, Erlich S, Finnegan L: Cocaine abuse in pregnancy: Effects on the fetus and newborn. *Neurotoxicol Teratol* 1987; 9:295.

86. Mahalik MP, Ganteri RF, Mann DE Jr: Teratogenic potential of cocaine hydrochloride in CF-1 mice. *J Pharm Sci* 1980; 69:703.

87. Fantal AG, Macphail BJ: The teratogenicity of cocaine. *Teratology* 1982; 26:17.

88. Coles CD, Platzman KA, Smith I, et al: Effects of cocaine and alcohol use in pregnancy on neonatal growth and neurobehavioral status. *Neurotoxicol Teratol* 1992; 14:23.

89. Little BB, Snell LM, Klein VR, et al: Cocaine abuse during pregnancy: Maternal and fetal implications. *Obstet Gynecol* 1989; 73:157.

90. Rosen TS, Johnson H: Drug addicted mothers, their infants, and SIDS. *Ann NY Acad Sci* 1988; 533:89.

91. LeBlanc PE, Parekh AJ, Naso B, et al: Effects of intrauterine exposure to alkaloidal cocaine ("crack"). *Am J Dis Child* 1987; 141:937.

92. Volpe J: Review article: Mechanisms of disease: Effect of cocaine use on the fetus. *N Engl J Med* 1992; 327:399.

93. Calhoun BC, Watson PT: The cost of maternal cocaine abuse. 1. Perinatal cost. *Obstet Gynecol* 1991; 78:734.

94. Chasnoff IJ, Griffith DR, Freier C, et al: Cocaine polydrug use in pregnancy. Two-year followup. *Pediatrics* 1992; 78:731.

95. Strauss AA, Mondaniou HD, Bosu SK: Neonatal manifestations of maternal phencyclidine (PCP) use. *Pediatrics* 1981; 68:550.

96. Hadeed AJ, Siegel SR: Maternal cocaine use during pregnancy: Effect on the newborn infant. *Pediatrics* 1989; 84:205.

97. Webster WS, Brown-Woodman PD: Cocaine as a cause of congenital malformations of vascular origins: Experimental evidence in the rat. *Teratology* 1990; 41:687.

98. US Department of Health, Education, and Welfare: Health consequences of smoking for women. A report of the surgeon general. DHEW Publication No. (NIH)0-326-003, 1980.

99. Chasnoff IJ, Burns WJ, Schnoll SH, et al: Cocaine use in pregnancy. *N Engl J Med* 1985; 313:666.

100. Chouteau M, Namerow PB, Leppert P: The effect of cocaine abuse on birth weight and gestational age. *Obstet Gynecol* 1988; 72:351.

101. Fried PA, Watkinson B, Willan A: Marijuana use during pregnancy and decreased length of gestation. *Am J Obstet Gynecol* 1984; 150:23.

102. Pelosi MA, Frattarola M, Apuzzio J, et al: Pregnancy complicated by heroin addiction. *Obstet Gynecol* 1975; 45:512.

103. Russell CS, Taylor R, Maddison RN: Some effects of smoking in pregnancy. *J Obstet Gynaecol Br Commw* 1966; 73:742.

104. Heffner LJ, Sherman CB, Speizer FE, et al: Clinical and environmental predictors of preterm labor. *Obstet Gynecol* 1993; 81:750.

105. Chasnoff IJ, Lewis DE, Squires L: Cocaine intoxication in a breast-fed infant. *Pediatrics* 1987; 80:836.

106. Neuspiel DR, Markowitz M, Drucker E: Intrauterine cocaine, lead, and nicotine exposure and fetal growth. *Am J Public Health* 1994; 84:1492.

107. Chasnoff IJ, Burnes KA, Burnes WJ, et al: Prenatal drug exposure: Effects on neonatal and infant growth and development. *Neurobehav Toxicol Teratol* 1986; 8:357.

108. Kaye K, Elkind L, Goldberg D, et al: Birth outcomes for infants of drug abusing mothers. *NY State J Med* 1989; 89:256.

109. Hanrahan JP, Tager IB, Segal MR, et al: The effect of maternal smoking during pregnancy on early infant lung function. *Am Rev Respir Dis* 1992; 145:1129.

110. Phibbs CS, Bateman DA, Schwartz RM: The neonatal cost of maternal cocaine use. *JAMA* 1991; 266:1521.

111. Weinberger SM, Kandall SR, Doberczak TM, et al: Early weight-change patterns in neonatal abstinence. *Am J Dis Child* 1986; 140:829.

112. Ward SL, Schuetz S, Krishna V, et al: Abnormal sleeping ventilatory pattern in infants of substance abusing mothers. *Am J Dis Child* 1986; 140:1015.

113. Chasnoff IJ, Hunt CE, Kletter R, et al: Perinatal cocaine exposure is associated with respiratory pattern abnormalities. *Am J Dis Child* 1989; 143:583.

114. Ward SLD, Bautista D, Chan L, et al: Sudden infant death syndrome in infants of substance abusing mothers. *J Pediatr* 1990; 117:876.

115. Durand DJ, Espinoza AM, Nickerson BG: Association between perinatal cocaine exposure and sudden infant death syndrome. *J Pediatr* 1990; 117:909.

116. Meyer MB, Tonascia JA: Maternal smoking, pregnancy complications, and perinatal mortality. *Am J Obstet Gynecol* 1977; 128:494.

117. Scher MS, Richardson GA, Coble PA, et al: The effects of prenatal alcohol and marijuana exposure: Disturbances in neonatal sleep cycling and arousal. *Pediatr Res* 1988; 24:101.

118. Streissguth AP, Sampson PD, Barr HM: Neurobehavioral dose-response effects of prenatal alcohol exposure in humans from infancy to adulthood. *Ann NY Acad Sci* 1989; 678:145.

119. Hans SL: Developmental consequences of prenatal exposure to methadone. *Ann NY Acad Sci* 1989; 678:195.

120. Wilson GS: Clinical studies of infants and children exposed prenatally to heroin. *Ann NY Acad Sci* 1989; 678:183.

121. Dreher MC, Nugent K, Hudgins R: Perinatal marijuana exposure and neonatal outcome in Jamaica: An ethnographic study. *Pediatr* 1994; 93:254.

122. Singer LT, Yamashita YS, Hawkins S: Increased incidence of intraventricular hemorrhage and developmental delay in cocaine-exposed, very low birth weight infants. *J Pediatr* 1994; 124:765.

123. Rush D, Callahan KR: Exposure to passive cigarette smoking and child development: A critical review. *Ann NY Acad Sci* 1989; 678:74.

124. Fost N: Maternal-fetal conflicts: Ethical and legal considerations. *Ann NY Acad Sci* 1989; 678:248.

125. Landesman SH, Willoughby A: HIV disease in reproductive age women: A problem of the present. *JAMA* 1989; 261:1326.

126. Connaughton JF, Resser D, Schut J et al: Perinatal addiction: Outcome and management. *Am J Obstet Gynecol* 1977; 129:679.

127. MacGregor SN, Keith LG, Bochicha JA, et al: Cocaine abuse during pregnancy: Correlation between prenatal care and perinatal outcome. *Obstet Gynecol* 1989; 74:882.

128. Lawson EJ: The role of smoking in the lives of low-income pregnant adolescents: A field study. *Adolescence* 1994; 29:61.

129. Sutton LR, Hinderliter SA: Diazepam abuse in pregnant women on methadone maintenance: Implications for the neonate. *Clin Pediatr* 1990; 29:108.

130. Alger LS, Farley JJ, Robinson BA, et al: Interactions of human immunodeficiency virus infection and pregnancy. *Obstet Gynecol* 1993; 82:787.

131. Boyer PJ, Dillon M, Navaie M, et al: Factors predictive of maternal-fetal transmission of HIV-1. *JAMA* 1994; 271:1925.

132. Blinick G, Wallach RC, Jerez E, et al: Drug addiction in pregnancy and the neonate. *Am J Obstet Gynecol* 1976; 125:135.

133. Silver H, Wapner R, Loriz-Vega M, et al: Addiction in pregnancy: High risk intrapartum management and outcome. *J Perinatol* 1987; 3:178.

134. Pantuck EJ, Pantuck CB, Ryan DE, et al: Inhibition and stimulation of enflurane metabolism in the rat following a single dose or chronic administration of ethanol. *Anesthesiology* 1985; 62:255.

135. Reilly CS, Wood AJ, Koshakji RP, et al: The effect of halothane on drug disposition: Contribution of changes in intrinsic drug metabolizing capacity and hepatic blood flow. *Anesthesiology* 1985; 63:70.

136. Loft S: Increased hepatic microsomal enzyme activity after surgery under halothane or spinal anesthesia. *Anesthesiology* 1985; 62:11.

137. Bell LE, Slattery JT, Calkins DF: Effect of halothane-oxygen anesthesia on the pharmacokinetics of diazepam and its metabolites in mice. *J Pharm Exp Ther* 1985; 233:94.

138. Ross VH, Moore CH, O'Rourke PJ, et al: Cocaine abusing parturients do not require more epidural pain medication for labor and delivery. *Anesthesiology* 1994; 81:A1184.

139. Hollander H, Levy JA: Neurologic abnormalities and recovery of human immunodeficiency virus from cerebrospinal fluid. *Am J Int Med* 1987; 106:692.

140. Du Pen SL, Peterson DG, Williams A, et al: Infection during chronic epidural catheterization: Diagnosis and treatment. *Anesthesiology* 1990; 73:905.

141. Hughes SC, Dailey PA, Landers D, et al: Parturients infected with human immunodeficiency virus and regional anesthesia. *Anesthesiology* 1995; 82:32.

142. Birnbach DJ, Stein DJ, Fogelberg R, et al: Thrombocytopenia in the cocaine abusing parturient. *Anesthesiology* 1994; 81:A1181.

143. Weintraub SJ, Naulty JS: Acute abstinence syndrome after epidural injection of butorphanol. *Anesth Analg* 1985; 64:452.

144. Curran MA, Newman LM, Becker GL: Barbiturate anesthesia and alcohol tolerance in a rat model. *Anesth Analg* 1988; 67:868.

145. Kafle SK: Intrathecal meperidine for elective cesarean section: A comparison with lidocaine. *Can J Anesth* 1993; 40:718.

146. Camann WR, Bader AM: Spinal anesthesia for cesarean delivery with meperidine as the sole agent. *Int J Obstet Anesth* 1992; 1:156.

147. Li TK, Bosron WF: Genetic variability of enzymes of al-

cohol metabolism in human beings. *Ann Emerg Med* 1986; 21:93.

148. Horrobin DF: A biochemical basis for alcoholism and alcohol-induced damage including the fetal alcohol syndrome and cirrhosis. *Med Hypotheses* 1980; 8:405.

149. Cornelius MD, Day NL, Cornelius JR, et al: Drinking patterns and correlates of drinking among pregnant teenagers. *Alcoholism* 1993; 17:290.

150. Ylikabri RH, Huttunen MO, Hardoven M: Hormonal changes during alcohol intoxication and withdrawal. *Pharm Biochem Behav* 1980; 13(suppl 1):131.

151. MacGregor RR: Alcohol and immune defense. *JAMA* 1986; 256:1474.

152. Martin F, Peters TJ: Alcoholic muscle disease. *Alcohol* 1985; 20:125.

153. Sage JI, Van Uitert RL, Lepore FE: Alcoholic myelopathy without substantial liver disease: A syndrome of progressive dorsal and lateral column dysfunction. *Arch Neurol* 1984; 41:999.

154. Halvorsen PR, Gross TL, Sokol RJ: The effect of heavy maternal alcohol intake on amniotic fluid phospholipids in late pregnancy. *Am J Perinatol* 1985; 2:173.

155. Coles CD: Impact of prenatal alcohol exposure on the newborn and the child. *Clin Obstet Gynecol* 1993; 36:255.

156. Reyes E: The role of gamma-glutamyl transpeptidase in alcoholism. *Neurobehav Toxicol Teratol* 1985; 7:171.

157. Halmesmaki E, Autti I, Granstrom ML, et al: Alphafetoprotein, human placental lactogen, and pregnancy-specific beta-1-glycoprotein in pregnant women who drink: Relation to fetal alcohol syndrome. *Am J Obstet Gynecol* 1986; 155:598.

158. Nakada T, Knight RT: Alcohol and the central nervous system. *Med Clin North Am* 1984; 68:121.

159. Lorens SA, Sainati SM: Naloxone blocks the excitatory effect of ethanol and chlordiazepoxide on lateral hypothalamic self-stimulation behavior. *Life Sci* 1988; 23:1359.

160. Pearce RA, Stringer JL, Lothman EW: Effect of volatile anesthetics on synaptic transmission in the rat hippocampus. *Anesthesiology* 1989; 71:591.

161. Christie MJ, Williams JT, North Ra: Cellular mechanisms of opiate tolerance: Studies in single brain neurons. *Mol Pharmacol* 1987; 32:633.

162. Mello NK, Mendelson JH, Bree MP, et al: Buprenorphine suppresses cocaine self-administration by rhesus monkeys. *Science* 1989; 245:859.

163. Fujinaga M, Mazzi RI, Jackson EC, et al: Reproductive and teratogenic effects of sufentanil and alfentanil in sprague-dawley rats. *Anesth Analg* 1988; 67:166.

164. Lichtblau L, Sparber SB: Opiate withdrawal in utero increases neonatal morbidity in the rat. *Science* 1981; 212:943.

165. Lapointe G, Nosal G: Morphine treatment during rat pregnancy. *Biol Neonate* 1982; 42:22.

166. Mercurio SD, Lichtblau L, Sparber SB: Separation of n-hepatic-demethylase-inducing and opiate dependence producing doses of levo-alpha-acetylmethadol in the pregnant rat. *Life Sci* 1984; 33:1127.

167. Parekh A, Mukherjee TH, Jhaveri R, et al: Intrauterine exposure to narcotics and cord blood prolactin concentrations. *Obstet Gynecol* 1981; 57:477.

168. Panerai AE, Martini A, Di Giulio AM, et al: Plasma betaendorphin, beta-lipotropin and metenkephalin concentrations during pregnancy in normal and drug-addicted women and their newborn. *J Clin Endocrinol Metab* 1983; 57:537.

169. Vinik HR, Bradley EL, Kissen I: Midazolam-fentanyl synergism for anesthetic induction in patients. *Anesthesiology* 1989; 69:213.

170. Fried PA: Postnatal consequences of maternal marijuana use in humans. *Ann NY Acad Sci* 1989; 678:123.

171. Fried PA: Prenatal exposure to tobacco and marijuana: Effects during pregnancy, infancy, and early childhood. *Clin Obstet Gynecol* 1993; 36:319.

172. Hutchings DE, Dow-Edwards D: Animal models of opiate, cocaine, and cannabis use. *Clin Perinatol* 1991; 18:1.

173. Glantz JC, Woods JR: Cocaine, heroin, and phencyclidine: Obstetric perspectives. *Clin Obstet Gynecol* 1993; 36:279.

174. Olney JW, Labruyere J, Price MT: Pathological changes induced in cerebrocortical neurons by phencyclidine and related drugs. *Science* 1989; 244:1360.

175. Hertzman M, Reba RC, Kotylarov EV: Single photon emission computed tomography in phencyclidine and related drug abuse. *Am J Psychiatry* 1990; 147:255.

176. Tabor BL, Smith-Wallace T, Yonekura ML: Perinatal outcome associated with PCP versus cocaine use. *Am J Drug Alcohol Abuse* 1990; 16:337.

177. Howard J, Kropenske V, Tyler R: The long-term effects on neurodevelopment in infants exposed prenatal to PCP. *Natl Inst Drug Abuse Res Monogr Ser* 1986; 64:237.

178. Warner EA: Cocaine abuse. *Ann Intern Med* 1993; 119:226.

179. Wilkerson RD: Cardiovascular effects of cocaine: Enhancement by yohimbine and atropine. *J Pharmacol Exp Ther* 1989; 248:57.

180. Iso A, Nakahara K, Kahn K, et al: Long-term ingestion of cocaine decreases its toxic threshold. *Anesthesiology* 1994; 81:A1186.

181. Whittington R, Iso A, Kahn K, et al: Polydrug toxicity: Cocaine and alcohol toxicity in rats. *Anesth Analg* 1995; 80:S581.

182. Mets B, Virag L: Comparative lethal toxicity from equimolar infusions of cocaine, norcocaine, ecgonine-methyl ester and benzoylecgonine in the rat. *Anesth Analg* 1995; 80:S317.

183. Dakis CA, Gold MS, Davies RK, et al: Bromcriptine treatment for cocaine abuse: The dopamine depletion hypothesis. *Int J Psychiatry Med* 1985; 15:125.

184. Forrester JM, Steele AW, Waldron JA, et al: Crack lung: An acute pulmonary syndrome with a spectrum of clinical and histopathologic findings. *Am Rev Respir Dis* 1990; 142:462.

185. McCalla S, Minkoff HL, Feldman J, et al: Predictors of cocaine use in pregnancy. *Obstet Gynecol* 1992; 79:641.

186. Tennant F: The rapid eye test to detect drug abuse. *Postgrad Med* 1988; 84:108.

187. Liu SS, Forrester RM, Murphy GS, et al: Anaesthetic management of a parturient with myocardial infarction related to cocaine use. *Can J Anaesth* 1992; 39:858.

188. Mendelson MA, Chandler J: Postpartum cardiomyopathy associated with maternal cocaine abuse. *Am J Cardiol* 1992; 70:1092.

189. Hsu CD, Chen S, Feng TI, et al: Rupture of uterine scar with extensive maternal bladder laceration after cocaine abuse. *Am J Obstet Gynecol* 1992; 167:129.

190. Thatcher SS, Cortman R, Grossman J, et al: Cocaine use and acute rupture of ectopic pregnancies. *Obstet Gynecol* 1989; 74:478.

191. Abramowicz JS, Sherer DM, Woods JR: Acute transient thrombocytopenia associated with cocaine abuse in pregnancy. *Obstet Gynecol* 1991; 78:499.

192. Kain ZN, Mayes L, Pakes J, et al: Thrombocytopenia in cocaine abusing parturients: A case control study. *Anesthesiology* 1994; 81:A1182.

193. Weiss SH: Links between cocaine and retroviral infection. *JAMA* 1989; 261:607.

194. Owiny JR, Myers T, Massman GA, et al: Lack of effect

of maternal cocaine administration on myometrial electromyogram and maternal plasma oxytocin concentrations in pregnant sheep at 124-126 days gestational age. *Obstet Gynecol* 1992; 79:81.

195. Hurd WW, Robertson PA, Riemer RK, et al: Cocaine directly augments the alpha-adrenergic contractile response of the pregnant rabbit uterus. *Am J Obstet Gynecol* 1991; 164:182.

196. Hurd WW, Smith AJ, Gauvin JM, et al: Cocaine blocks extraneuronal uptake of norepinephrine by the pregnant human uterus. *Obstet Gynecol* 1991; 78:249.

197. Monga M, Weisbrodt NW, Andres RL, et al: The acute effect of cocaine exposure on pregnant human myometrial contractile activity. *Am J Obstet Gynecol* 1993; 169:782.

198. Hurd WW, Guavin JM, Dombrowski MP, et al: Cocaine selectively inhibits beta-adrenergic receptor binding in pregnant human myometrium. *Am J Obstet Gynecol* 1993; 169:644.

199. Slutsker, L: Risks associated with cocaine use during pregnancy. *Obstet Gynecol* 1992; 79:778.

200. Critchley HOD, Woods SM, Barson AJ, et al: Fetal death in utero and cocaine abuse: Case report. *Br J Obstet Gynaecol* 1988; 95:195.

201. Gratacos E, Torres PJ, Antolin E: Use of cocaine during pregnancy. *New Engl J Med* 1993; 329:667.

202. Telsey AM, Merrit TA, Dixon SD: Cocaine exposure in a term neonate: Necrotizing enterocolitis as a complication. *Clin Pediatr* 1988; 27:547.

203. Dominguez R, Vila-Coro AA, Slopis JM, et al: Brain and ocular abnormalities in infants with in utero exposure to cocaine and other street drugs. *Am J Dis Child* 1991; 145:688.

204. Chavez G, Mulinare J, Cordero J: Maternal cocaine use during early pregnancy as a risk factor for congenital anomalies. *JAMA* 1989; 262:795.

205. Geggel RL, Mc Inery J, Estes NAM III: Transient neonatal ventricular tachycardia associated with maternal cocaine use. *Am J Cardiol* 1989; 63:383.

206. Dobercyak TM, Shanzer S, Senie RT, et al: Neonatal neurologic and encephalographic effects of intrauterine cocaine exposure. *J Pediatr* 1988; 113:354.

207. Dixon SD, Bejar R: Echoencephalographic findings in neonates associated with maternal cocaine and methamphetamine use: incidence and clinical correlates. *J Pediatr* 1989; 115:770.

208. Frank D, McCarten K, Cabral H, et al: Cranial ultrasound in term newborns: Failure to replicate excess abnormalities in cocaine-exposed. *Pediatr Res* 1992; 31:247A.

209. McLenan D, Ajayi O, Pildes R: Cocaine and intraventricular hemorrhage. *Pediatr Res* 1992; 31:212A.

210. Singer L, Garber R, Kleigman R: Neurobehavioral sequelae of fetal cocaine exposure. *J Pediatr* 1991; 119: 667.

211. Ramoska E, Sacchetti AD: Propranalol-induced hypertension in treatment of cocaine intoxication. *Ann Emerg Med* 1985; 14:1112.

212. Derlet RW, Albertson TE: Potentiation of cocaine toxicity with calcium channel blockers. *Am J Emerg Med* 1989; 7:464.

213. Vertommen JD, Hughes SC, Rosen MA, et al: Hydralazine does not restore uterine blood flow during cocaine-induced hypertension in the pregnant ewe. *Anesthesiology* 1992; 76:850.

214. Ross VH, Moore CH, O'Rourke PJ, et al: Cocaine abusing parturients do not require more epidural pain medication for labor and delivery. *Anesthesiology* 1994; 81:A1184.

215. Birnbach DJ, Stein DJ, Grunebaum A, et al: Epidural and spinal anesthesia for cesarean section in cocaine abusing parturients. *Anesthesiology* 1994; 81:A1183.

216. Bernards CM, Cullen BF, Powers K: Chronic cocaine increases isoforane MAC in sheep. *Anesth Analg* 1995; 80:S42.

217. Fleming JA, Byck R, Barash PG: Pharmacology and therapeutic applications of cocaine. *Anesthesiology* 1990; 73:518.

218. Hoffman RS, Glendon CH, Howland MA, et al: Association between life-threatening cocaine toxicity and plasma cholinesterase activity. *Ann Emerg Med* 1992; 21:247.

219. Cho AK: Ice: A new dosage form of an old drug. *Science* 1990; 249:631.

220. Burchfield DJ, Lucas VW, Abrams RM, et al: Disposition and pharmacodynamics of methamphetamine in pregnant sheep. *JAMA* 1991; 265:1968.

221. Elliot RH, Rees GB: Amphetamine ingestion presenting as eclampsia. *Can J Anaesth* 1990; 37:130.

222. Little BB, Snell LM, Gilstrap LC: Methamphetamine abuse during pregnancy: Outcome and fetal effects. *Obstet Gynecol* 1988; 72:541.

223. Erikson M, Larsson G, Zetterstrom R: Amphetamine addiction and pregnancy. II. Pregnancy, delivery and the neonatal period: Socio-medical aspects. *Acta Obstet Gynecol Scand* 1981; 60:253.

224. Johnstone RR, Way WL, Miller RD: Alteration of anesthetic requirement by amphetamine. *Anesthesiology* 1972; 36:357.

225. Michel R, Adams AP: Acute amphetamine abuse: Problems during general anesthesia for neurosurgery. *Anaesthesia* 1979; 34:1016.

226. Luck W, Nau H, Hansen R, et al: Extent of nicotine and cotinine transfer to the human fetus, placenta and amniotic fluid of smoking mothers. *Dev Pharmacol Ther* 1985; 8:384.

227. Donnenfeld AE, Pulkkinen A, Palomakig, et al: Simultaneous fetal and maternal cotinine levels in pregnant women smokers. *Am J Obstet Gynecol* 1993; 168:781.

228. McGarry JM, Andrews J: Smoking in pregnancy and vitamin B_{12} metabolism. *Br Med J* 1972; 2:74.

229. Mochizuki M, Maruo T, Masuka K, et al: Effects of smoking on fetoplacental-maternal system during pregnancy. *Am J Obstet Gynecol* 1984; 149:413.

230. Ahlborg G Jr, Bodin L: Tobacco smoke exposure and pregnancy outcome among working women: A prospective study at prenatal care centers in Orebro County, Sweden. *Am J Epidemiol* 1991; 133:338.

231. Sindberg EP, Marsal K: Acute effects of maternal smoking on fetal blood flow. *Acta Obstet Gynecol Scand* 1984; 63:391.

232. Manning FA, Feyerabend C: Cigarette smoking and fetal breathing movements. *Br J Obstet Gynaecol* 1976; 83:262.

233. Sindberg EP, Gennser G, Lindvall R, et al: Acute effects of maternal smoking on fetal heart beat intervals. *Acta Obstet Gynecol Scand* 1984; 63:385.

234. Windham GC, Swan SH, Fenster L: Parental cigarette smoking and the risk of spontaneous abortion. *Am J Epidemiol* 1992; 135:1394.

235. Martinez FD, Wright AL, Taussig LM: The effect of paternal smoking on the birthweight of newborns whose mothers did not smoke. *Am J Public Health* 1994; 84:1489.

236. Fortier I, Marcoux S, Brisson J: Passive smoking during pregnancy and the risk of delivering a small-for-gestational-age infant. *Am J Epidemiol* 1994; 139:294.

237. Beratis NG, Varvarigou A, Makri M, et al: Prolactin, growth hormone, and insulin-like growth factor-I in new-

born children of smoking mothers. *Clin Endocrinol* 1994; 40:179.

238. Mitchell EA, Ford RPK, Stewart AW, et al: Smoking and the sudden infant death syndrome. *Pediatrics* 1993; 91:893.

239. Schoendorf KC, Kiely JL: Relationship of sudden infant death syndrome to maternal smoking during and after pregnancy. *Pediatrics* 1992; 90:905.

240. Cunningham J, Dockery DW, Speizer FE: Maternal smoking during pregnancy as a predictor of lung function in children. *J Epidemiol* 1994; 139:1139.

241. Sexton M, Fox NL, Hebel JR: Prenatal exposure to tobacco. II. Effects on cognitive functioning at age three. *Int J Epidemiol* 1990; 19:72.

242. Pearce AC, Jones RM: Smoking and anesthesia: Preoperative abstinence and perioperative morbidity. *Anesthesiology* 1984; 61:576.

243. Koxlowski LT, Wilkinson DA, Skinner W, et al: Comparing tobacco cigarette dependence with other drug dependencies. *JAMA* 1989; 261:898.

244. Davies JM, Latto IP, Jones JG, et al: Effects of stopping smoking for 48 hours on oxygen availability from the blood: A study on pregnant women. *Br Med J* 1979; 2:355.

245. Wright DJ, Pandya A: Smoking and gastric juice volume in outpatients. *Can Anaesth Soc J* 1979; 26:328.

28 The Febrile Parturient

Stephen Rolbin and *Dan Farine*

The febrile parturient is often treated in the labor and delivery room. At times these patients pose major problems for both the obstetrician and the anesthesiologist. Usually the illness develops shortly before or during labor. Rarely the etiology is not an infection, and then a wide spectrum of diseases must be considered (Box 28-1).

Several factors can complicate the management of the febrile patient. There are two patients to be considered—the mother and the baby. The infection can affect one or both of them. Furthermore, the febrile illness may also induce labor. Several infections are either specific to pregnancy (e.g., amnionitis), or have a different course in pregnancy (e.g., asymptomatic bacturia). The physician must be aware of these entities as well as the physiological changes in pregnancy that may confound the diagnosis. For example, leukocytosis is a normal phenomenon without the presence of infection. Respiratory alkalosis is also a normal compensatory mechanism in pregnancy.

Any febrile disease in pregnancy, and especially when associated with labor, necessitates a thorough and rapid evaluation and appropriate management. Both mother and baby must be considered when management is planned. This chapter briefly reviews relevant aspects in the physiology and pathophysiology of thermoregulation, and relates them to the physiology of pregnancy. This is followed by a discussion of febrile diseases that often complicate labor and disease management. Finally, the risks and benefits of regional and general anesthesia in the febrile parturient are reviewed.

TEMPERATURE REGULATION

No single temperature can be considered to be normal. Normal people have a range of temperature, as illustrated in Fig. 28-1, from approximately 36° C to over 37.2° C (97° F to 99° F) when measured orally and approximately 0.6° C or 1° F higher when measured rectally. It is useful in that the height of the fever is proportional to the severity of the disease. Under normal circumstances, core body temperature is tightly regulated, with a variation of 0.6° C (1° F).

The temperature of the body is almost entirely regulated by feedback mechanisms that operate through the "hypothalamic thermostat"[1] (Fig. 28-2). The signals that arise from peripheral receptors are transmitted to the posterior hypothalamus where they are integrated with the signals from the preoptic area.[2] These cells increase their firing rate at elevated temperature. Cold-sensitive neurons also have been found in the hypothalamus; in the septum and in the reticular substance of the midbrain. Still other neurons change their rate of firing in response to signals coming from temperature receptors in the skin and deep tissues of the body. These signals interact with those from the hypothalamus in an area of the posterior hypothalamus approximately at the level of the mammary bodies, providing a very effective temperature control system.

The body has a critical temperature called the "set-point." All temperature control mechanisms continually adjust to maintain the body temperature at this set-point level[2,3] (Fig. 28-2). Elevation of body temperature, which depends primarily on sympathetic outflow, leads to shivering thermogenesis and dermal vasoconstriction. Cooling mechanisms involve both sympathetic and parasympathetic nervous systems and result in sweating and dermal vasodilation.[3]

There are three important mechanisms that are used to reduce body heat.[2,3] Vasodilation, which may be intense, is due to inhibition of sympathetic centers of the posterior hypothalamus. This vasodilation may increase the rate of heat transfer to the skin as much as eightfold. Sweating, which causes a sharp rise heat loss by evaporation, can remove up to 10 times the basal rate of heat production. Finally, there is strong inhibition of heat-producing mechanisms such as shivering and chemical thermogenesis.

Febrile conditions are characterized by the body mechanisms that attempt to raise body temperature to the elevated set-point (i.e., the temperature to which the body has been reset). The patient may experience chills and feel very cold even though the temperature is elevated. Heat loss is then decreased by vasoconstriction, and shivering results

BOX 28-1 CAUSES OF FEVER OF UNKNOWN ORIGIN

I. Infections
  A. 1. Systemic bacterial infections
     2. Abscesses
     3. Viral, rickettsial, and chlamydial
     4. Granulomatous disease
     5. Intervascular infections
     6. Fungal and parasitic
II. Neoplastic Diseases
  A. Solid (localized)
     1. Kidney
     2. Lung
     3. Pancreas
     4. Liver
     5. Large bowel
     6. Atrial myxoma
  B. Metastatic
     1. From gastrointestinal tract
     2. From lung, kidneys, bone, cervix, ovary
     3. Melanoma
     4. Sarcoma
  C. Tumors of the reticuloendothelial system
     1. Hodgkin's disease
     2. Non-Hodgkin's lymphoma
     3. Malignant histiocytosis
     4. Immunoblastic lymphadenopathy
     5. Lymphomatoid granulomatosis
     6. Mucocutaneous lymph node syndrome (children)

III. Connective Tissue Disease
  A. Rheumatic fever
  B. Systemic lupus erythematosus
  C. Rheumatoid arthritis (particularly Still's disease)
  D. Giant cell arteritis (polymyalgia rheumatica)
  E. Hypersensitivity vasculitis
  F. Periarteritis nodosa
  G. Wegener's granulomatosis
  H. Panaortitis
IV. Granulomatus Disease
  A. Crohn's disease (regional enteritis)
  B. Granulomatous hepatitis
  C. Sarcoidosis
  D. Erythema nodosum
V. Miscellaneous Disease
  A. Malignant hyperthermia
  B. Drug fever
  C. Pulmonary emboli
  D. Thyroiditis
  E. Hemolytic states
  F. Cryptic trauma with bleeding into enclosed spaces (hematomas)
  G. Dissecting aneurysm (with or without infection)
  H. Whipple's disease
  I. Tissue injury

Adapted from Petersdorf RG, Root RK: Chills and fever, in Braunwald, Isselbacher KJ, Petersdorf RG, et al (eds): *Harrison's Principles of Internal Medicine,* ed 11. New York, McGraw-Hill, 1987. Used by permission.

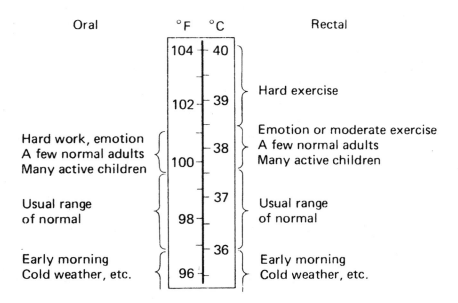

Fig. 28-1 Range of normal body temperature. (From Dupois EF: *Fever and the Regulation of Body Temperature.* Springfield, Ill, Charles C Thomas, 1948. Used by permission.)

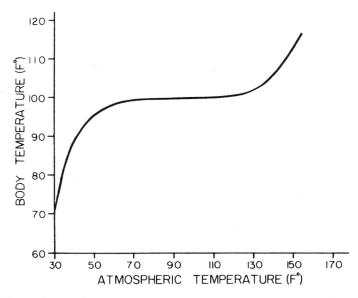

Fig. 28-2 Effects of atmospheric temperature on internal body temperature. (From Guyton AC: *Human Physiology and Mechanisms of Disease,* ed 5. Philadelphia, WB Saunders, 1992.)

in increased heat production. After appropriate medical treatment, the set-point is lowered; the hypothalamus detects that the body temperature is elevated, and it then acts to correct the temperature to the normal range.

Fever or pyrexia is an elevation of the body temperature above normal. It may be caused by proteins released from the cells of the immune system. Substances that cause fever are called pyrogens and may be either exogenous or endogenous. Components of many microorganisms (e.g., lipoteichoic acid, lipopolysaccharides, and others) are termed exogenous pyrogens. Endogenous pyrogens are polypeptides which certain drugs as well as cells of the immune system (mainly macrophages and, to a lesser extent, lymphocytes) produce. These proteins are the monokines and the lymphokines, respectively. They are often called cytokines. The major cytokines appear to be interleukins (IL-1α and IL-1β), interleukin-6 (IL-6), and tumor necrosis factors (TNF-α and β). Other proteins with pyrogenic activity include interferon alpha (INF-α), and macrophage inflammatory protein (MIP-1α,β) (Fig. 28-3).

Several cytokines have been isolated and their structures determined. To date, 11 have been identified.[3] Mononuclear phagocytes are the main source of these pyrogens; the same proteins may also arise from neoplastic cells. They are bound to receptors on the vascular endothelium within the preoptic/anterior hypothalamus. The net result is that the set-point of the hypothalamus is raised and all the body mechanisms for increasing heat pro-

duction are activated. The resetting of the set-point is a result of endothelial cell production of prostaglandins (PGE$_2$ and perhaps PGF$_{2\alpha}$).[3] Thrombaxones and lipoxygenase products may also change the set-point. Cytokines (for example, interleukin 1β) also act directly with neural tissue and may release corticotrophin-releasing factor (CRF), which may trigger thermogenesis[3] (Fig. 28-3). On reaching the hypothalamus, a fever is produced and the body temperature changes in as little as 8 to 10 minutes.

When prostaglandin formation is blocked by drugs, the fever is either completely eliminated or at least reduced. In fact, this may be the manner in which aspirin reduces the degree of fever, because aspirin impedes the formation of prostaglandins. This also would explain why aspirin does not lower the body temperature in a normal person, because a normal person does not have any endogenous pyrogen affecting the hypothalamus.[2]

In addition to fever, there is an increase in the number of circulating white blood cells, often their immature forms. This is secondary to the action of interleukin-1 on the bone marrow.

Temperature regulation in the febrile parturient

There are several changes in pregnancy that could be important in diagnosing and managing febrile diseases.

Altered metabolism and heat dissipation. Pregnancy is associated with an increase in the basal metabolic rate.[4] It is due to both fetal metabolism

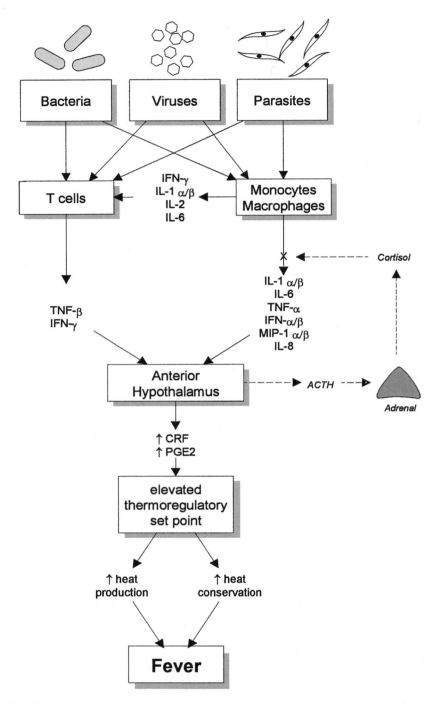

Fig. 28-3 Chronology of events required for the induction of a fever: A variety of pathogens produce molecules that function as exogenous pyrogens, resulting in the release of endogenous pyrogens from mononuclear cells. Abbreviations have been defined in the text. (Adapted from Gelfand JA, Dinarello CA, Wolff SM: Fever, including fever of unknown origin, in Isselbacher KJ, Braunwald E, et al (eds): *Harrison's Principles of Internal Medicine,* ed 13. New York, McGraw-Hill, 1994, and from Beutler B, Beutler SM: The pathogenesis of fever, in Wyngaarden JB, Smith LH, Bennett JC (eds): *Cecil Textbook of Medicine,* ed 19. Philadelphia, WB Saunders, 1992.)

and maternal adaptation to pregnancy. In addition, maternal fever increases the metabolic rate. An inability to dissipate this increased heat production either by dehydration or by interfering with the sweating mechanism may result in a higher temperature in the pregnant patient.

Altered physiology. Pregnancy is associated with several physiologic changes that may confound the diagnosis of an infection. These include the following changes:

1. Prostaglandins are not only an important mediator in the febrile response but also an important factor in the initiation of labor.[5] This is not only a theoretical concern but a practical one since maternal fever is often associated with premature labor.[6]
2. Uterine perfusion is not autoregulated.[7] Therefore, peripheral vasodilatation, shivering and hyperemia of an infected organ may, at least theoretically, reduce the perfusion of the uterus and fetus. Regional anesthesia may further alter uterine perfusion.
3. The leukocyte count, often useful in diagnosing infections, is normally elevated in pregnancy.[8]
4. The belief that pregnancy is associated with decreased function of the immune system[9] is probably erroneous, since infections are not more common in pregnancy. Poor outcome can often be linked to difficulties in diagnosis and delay in treatment. However, at times the course of a febrile illness such as varicella pneumonia is far worse than in the nonpregnant state.[10]
5. Symptoms and physical signs can be affected by the physiologic changes of pregnancy. To mention just a few, urinary frequency is a common complaint in pregnancy. The location of the small bowel and appendix change as pregnancy progresses, resulting in atypical findings. Constipation and nausea are common symptoms in pregnancy. In addition, a high cardiac output state results in flow murmurs.

GENERAL CONSIDERATIONS OF THE FEBRILE PARTURIENT

The combination of febrile illness and pregnancy, especially when labor is present, requires a prompt evaluation. There are several concerns that must be addressed:

1. Is the fever an indicator of an infection? Although this is usually the case, there are other causes of febrile diseases that should be considered (Box 28-1).

2. Are mother and baby severely compromised, and are any resuscitative measures or interventions required? As a rule, maternal interests supersede those of the fetus. Only rarely are the interests of mother and baby in significant conflict. In these unusual cases the input of the patient and her family should be considered.
3. The diagnosis of which organ is infected is obviously important. One must distinguish between infections that are unlikely to spread to the fetus (e.g., urinary tract infection) and those that may cause fetal infection. The former may affect the fetus only indirectly through maternal effects or premature labor. Proper treatment necessitates an accurate diagnosis, although treatment often must be instituted based on a presumptive diagnosis.
4. The choice of diagnostic methods may be altered by the presence of pregnancy. For instance, an elevated white count is hard to interpret ($N = <15,000$). Several tests, such as x-ray examinations, may carry a risk to the fetus, and the risk/benefit ratio should be evaluated. The same applies to treatment (e.g., tetracycline is contraindicated in pregnancy because of its effect on fetal teeth and bones).
5. Fever may lead to premature labor. The patient should be assessed for the presence of uterine activity, and unless contraindicated the cervix should be examined.
6. The effect of pregnancy on the course of the disease should be considered. Most infectious diseases are not affected by pregnancy, with few exceptions such as varicella pneumonia.
7. What is the effect of the natural history of the disease on the fetus and pregnancy? Many infectious agents do cross the placenta and may cause fetal disease. This may imply the need for neonatal treatment (e.g., antibiotics in maternal syphilis or zoster immunoglobulin in varicella), maternal treatment (e.g., antibiotics for amnionitis; azidothymidine (AZT) for HIV-positive patients), and direct fetal treatment via cordocentesis (toxoplasmosis).

In managing the febrile parturient there are several issues often neglected. Proper infection control techniques should be used, and extra caution should be exercised by nurses, obstetricians, and anesthesiologists who may be exposed to blood, body secretions, and mucous membranes. Laboratory samples should be properly obtained, handled, and labeled. Public health issues should be considered, as well, in order to enable follow-up of contacts. Finally, counseling should be provided regarding infectivity to the newborn and other family members.

SPECIFIC INFECTIONS IN PREGNANCY

This section briefly describes the common infections in obstetrics. For more information, the reader is referred to the chapter on "Infectious Disease" in this text (Chapter 26) and to texts on perinatology[6] and infections in obstetrics.[11]

Premature rupture of the membranes and amnionitis

Premature rupture of the membranes (PROM) occurs when the fetal membranes are ruptured prior to labor. Preterm PROM (PPROM) occurs before 37 weeks' gestation. About 5% of pregnancies are complicated by PPROM. The diagnosis is made by the typical history and confirmed by checking the pH of the vaginal fluid and microscopic examination, which reveal the typical ferning of the fluid (crystallization of the salt of the amniotic fluid). The risks of PPROM include premature delivery that often occurs within 24 hours of PPROM, amnionitis (it is already present at the time of PPROM in about one third of cases), and abruption of the placenta. The management of PPROM is based on balancing the risks of prematurity and failed induction of labor on one hand and the risks of amnionitis and abruption on the other hand. Usually before 35 weeks' gestation the management is expectant. The patient is monitored for symptoms and signs of amnionitis. Labor is induced if amnionitis is diagnosed.

Amnionitis

Diagnosis of amnionitis necessitates prompt delivery. If delivery is not imminent, antibiotic coverage is needed. Failure of induction or an unripe cervix may be an indication for cesarean delivery. Microbiologic, clinical, and pathologic diagnosis of amnionitis are not similar. The bacteriologic diagnosis is based on identification of microorganism in cultures or Gram stain. The clinical diagnosis is based on the combination of the following symptoms and signs: Fever, elevated white count with a shift to the left, uterine activity and/or tenderness, foul-smelling discharge, fetal tachycardia. The pathologic diagnosis is retrospective and based on the morphology of the placenta and membranes. There are often discrepancies between these diagnoses, with pathologic amnionitis detected without clinical amnionitis and with clinical amnionitis detected without positive microbiology. A recent suggestion is to measure interleukin-6 levels in the amniotic fluid since they are the best predictor of microbial entry into the amniotic cavity as well as neonatal complications.[12]

Herpes simplex infection

Etiology. The main risk in herpes simplex viral (HSV) infection in pregnancy is the risk to the fetus and neonate. Humans are the only known natural hosts. The two types of HSV are type 1 (HSV-1) and type 2 (HSV-2). HSV infections are transmitted by direct contact with infected secretions, HSV-1 by oral secretions and HSV-2 predominantly by sexual contact. Both viruses share the properties of latency and reactivation, residing in the neural ganglion cells during their period of latency.

Pathophysiology

Systemic symptoms are associated with 67% of primary genital HSV infections. Aseptic meningitis and sacral neuropathy is seen in 8% and 2%, respectively, of patients with primary infections. In contrast, systemic symptoms are uncommon in recurrent disease, and 25% of recurrent infection is asymptomatic.

Obstetric management

Intact fetal membranes provide the fetus relative safety from infection. The risk of infection is probably low since the incidence of viral shedding is estimated at 1% to 2% of pregnancies while the incidence of neonatal disease is about one 1:10,000. In the past, cervical specimens from infected women were cultured for HSV on a weekly basis. Once the membranes ruptured they were delivered by cesarean section unless cultures were negative. Recently these cultures were found to have a low predictive value for presence of HSV in labor.[13] The approach today has changed. Routine cultures are not indicated, and cesarean delivery is necessary only if herpetic lesions or symptoms are present when PROM occurs.[14]

Anesthetic management

Two issues of concern to the anesthesiologist are (1) the risk of introducing virus into the central nervous system during the performance of either an epidural or a spinal anesthetic, and (2) the likelihood of disseminated infection occurring following a regional anesthetic that may be temporally related to the anesthetic despite a lack of causal relationship. This risk is greatest during the primary attack.

There are no case reports in the medical literature documenting the introduction of HSV into the central nervous system during active recurrent disease.[15,16]

Both spinal and epidural anesthesia appear to be safe alternatives for these patients.[17] However, parturients with primary HSV are at risk for both systemic symptoms and neurologic complications. The safety of regional anesthesia during primary HSV has yet to be established.

Recently, there have been reports of a possible association of HSV-1 reactivation with epidural narcotic administration. If these initial studies are confirmed, previous HSV-1 infection would become a contraindication to narcotic administration in a regional anesthetic.[18,19,20]

Pneumonia

Pneumonia in pregnancy usually has the same etiologic agents and course as in the nonpregnant state. A chest x-ray examination (AP and lateral) is indicated whenever pneumonia is suspected, despite the concern for fetal exposure.

Urinary tract infections

These can be divided into asymptomatic bacturia, urethritis and cystitis, and pyelonephritis.

Asymptomatic bacteruria. This infection complicates 2% to 12% of pregnancies. About 25% of these women will develop asymptomatic infection during pregnancy; therefore, an antibiotic course is indicated. Asymptomatic bacteruria is associated with delivery of low birth weight babies. It can usually be detected in the first antenatal visit by the routine urine culture.

Urethritis and cystitis. These infections are often preceded by asymptomatic bacteruria. The combination of symptoms and urinary findings enables a quick diagnosis. The infection usually responds to a short course of antibiotics.

Pyelonephritis. One of the most common serious complications of pregnancy, pyelonephritis involves a combination of febrile disease—costovertebral angle tenderness with the presence or absence of urinary symptoms, usually a straightforward diagnosis. The organism is usually a coliform. There is bacteremia in 15% of cases. Intravenous antibiotics and hydration are the keystones of management. Nonaggressive management may lead to ARDS and/or premature labor. Eradication of the infection is mandatory, and oral antibiotics for the remainder of the pregnancy may be needed.

Varicella

Chickenpox in adults is more severe than in children. Varicella is a febrile systemic disease associated with generalized pruritic vesicles. The incubation period ranges from 10 to 21 days. Skin lesions begin to present 2 days after the onset of symptoms. Varicella zoster immune globulin (VZIG) must be administered within 96 hours of exposure.

Incidence. The incidence of varicella in pregnancy is approximately 1 in 7500.[21] Maternal varicella in the third trimester may be transmitted to the fetus and may result in neonatal varicella. When delivery occurs 2 days before the onset of the rash or within 5 days of its onset, neonatal varicella may occur in up to 50% of neonates.[21,22] Newborns of women who develop such a rash should receive immunization with VZIG to avoid a high neonatal mortality associated with fetal varicella infection.[22] Exposure of the fetus just before delivery may cause a stormy neonatal course, and VZIG is indicated for neonates following peripartum exposure. Neonates born to mothers with active varicella should be placed in isolation at birth until 21 or 28 days of age, depending on whether they received VZIG.

The course of varicella in pregnancy is worse, with about 10% of women developing pneumonia. Varicella pneumonia is classically lethal in 20% of pregnant women. Ventilatory support and acyclovir treatment may be necessary as well as transfer to a tertiary care centre.

Health care providers need to be aware of infectious control measures. Since the disease is infectious for 2 days prior to the skin rash, infected individuals may expose those who are susceptible. Thus, these individuals should have documentation of their immune status.

Viremia may be present for up to 2 weeks after the onset of the symptoms, and thus the administration of regional anesthesia may be contraindicated.[23]

Common cold

The common cold is caused by rhinovirus, coronovirus, and adenovirus. The course in pregnancy is usually similar to that in the nonpregnant state. However, pneumonia in pregnancy is often preceded by the common cold.

Viral hepatitis

Hepatitis is currently of great concern, and there are several causative organisms of hepatitis.

Etiology

1. Type A hepatitis virus is the causative organism for infectious or short-incubation hepatitis. It is a highly infectious disease, and its transmission is believed to be by the fecal-oral route. The incubation period is from 2 to 6 weeks.
2. Type B hepatitis virus is responsible for serum or posttransfusion hepatitis. Transmission is mainly by parenteral routes such as

in blood transfusions or by percutaneous inoculation of infected material, as well as by nonparenteral routes such as oral and sexual. In the health care setting, blood and blood-tinged fluids, most body fluids, and transfusions of blood products transmit the disease. The transmission rate for hepatitis B virus (HBV) is 30% after a percutaneous exposure to HBeAg positive substances.[24,25] The incubation period is from 4 to 24 weeks.

3. Hepatitis C virus has been identified as the causative agent in the majority of cases of parenterally transmitted hepatitis.[26,27,28] Assays to detect hepatitis C virus have been developed and have led to further insight into this disease. About 6% to 10% of cases result from transfusions, and 90% of patients with posttransfusion hepatitis are diagnosed as having non-A, non-B hepatitis.

4. Recently, hepatitis delta and hepatitis E viruses have been identified.

The incidence of spontaneous abortions during the first trimester is increased in patients with acute viral hepatitis. The incidence of preterm labor is increased as well. Hepatitis B can affect the fetus and the newborn.

In mild cases patients can be treated at home with bedrest and a high-protein, low-fat diet. In severe cases with intractable vomiting, prolonged prothrombin time, low serum albumin, or serum bilirubin more than 15 mg/100 ml, the patient should be admitted to hospital.

Acquired immunodeficiency syndrome

A full discussion of AIDS is presented in Chapter 26.

Malignant hyperthermia

Malignant hyperthermia (MH) reactions in pregnancy are rare.[29] Although labor can be stressful, all cases of MH are reported related to general anesthesia. If general anesthesia is required, the standard precautions are to be followed. Regional anesthesia with amide local anesthetics appears to be safe. Ephedrine has been used to treat maternal hypotension without untoward effect.

Group A beta-hemolytic Streptococcal infection (flesh-eating disease)

Etiology and incidence. A virulent strain of streptococcus has recently been implicated in severe and fatal infections. In 1992 and 1993, 48 cases of toxic shock syndrome or necrotizing cellulitis with group A beta-hemolytic streptococcal infections have been reported in Ontario, and 24 such cases have been diagnosed in December 1994

to January 1995.[30] In addition, 14 peripartum septic patients cultured group A beta-hemolytic streptococcus during 1992 to 1993 in Ontario.

Pathophysiology. We are aware of three term pregnancies that were complicated by profound multisystem organ failure caused by group A streptococcus.[31,32] A precipitous maternal death can be caused by a nonpyrogenic strep infection without disseminated intravascular coagulopathy. Death may follow a short course of vague and nonspecific symptoms or physical findings. The mechanism for these infections is through a "super antigen" phenomenon that activates in a nonspecific fashion 20% to 30% of T4 lymphocytes (as opposed to less than 1% in the "normal" infection). This activation occurs because of an endotoxin secreted by specific serotypes of group A beta-hemolytic streptococcus.[33] Recent reports serve to highlight the apparent return of serious group A streptococcal puerperal sepsis and to emphasize the clinical implications of an old yet virulent infection.[31]

CLINICAL FEATURES OF SEPTIC SHOCK

Shock, defined as a failure of organ perfusion, in fact may be present before the onset of hypotension.[34,35] There are numerous causes of shock; however, in the febrile parturient we are concerned about septic shock that may be caused by gram-positive or gram-negative bacteria.[34,36]

Gram-positive sepsis results in fluid losses secondary to potent endotoxins. Severe hypotension will occur with few other clinical manifestations of shock. Arterial resistance falls without any decrease in cardiac output and with urine production and the sensorium remaining normal. Lactic acidosis does not occur.[36] Treatment consists of antibiotic therapy, surgical drainage, and correction of volume deficit where appropriate.

Gram-negative sepsis is a more frequent and difficult problem. Ninety-five percent of septic shock is caused by gram-negative organisms.[32] A cellular defect inhibits oxygen utilization. This occurs before the hemodynamic changes are detected.[37] Blood volume is redistributed and so the circulation fails to meet the metabolic needs of the body. In its early stages, cardiac output increases and systemic vascular resistance decreases as a result of dilated cutaneous vessels.

The extremities remain warm and dry, and hypotension and oliguria may be present. Hyperventilation is a valuable early sign of septic shock. As shock progresses, vascular permeability increases and fluids leak from the vascular to the interstitial space. Systemic vascular resistance will also increase.

Late septic shock or hypodynamic shock is seen

in patients with significant extravascular fluid loss. The clinical presentation is different from early septic shock in that the CVP is low, the cardiac output is low, the peripheral resistance is increased, urine output is decreased, extremities are cold and cyanotic, and blood lactate is increased. As the sepsis further progresses, myocardial depression or disseminated intravascular coagulation might also occur. Endotoxin can initiate this acceleration of the clotting process. The reader is reminded to cautiously interpret CVP measurements: a low CVP may be normal in pregnancy (CVP = 3.6 ± 2.5).[37]

Laboratory findings include leukocytosis with a WBC greater than 15,000 mm^3 or leukopenia with a WBC less than 3500/mm^3 with a left shift. Thrombocytopenia is often present. PT and PTT may be elevated. The blood glucose is usually increased secondary to high circulating blood levels of anti-insulin hormones, glucagon, growth hormones, and catecholamines. Hypoglycemia is infrequently seen and is associated with a poor prognosis. Arterial blood gases usually demonstrate a mixed acid base abnormality with a combination of a primary respiratory alkalosis and metabolic acidosis. The arterial lactate level is invariably increased because of diminished tissue oxygen supply in relation to demand.

Obstetric and anesthetic management

Treatment is aimed primarily at improving the hemodynamic status and treating the infection. This includes broad-spectrum antibiotic coverage after appropriate cultures and Gram stains of the specimens obtained. Volume expansion, vasopressors, and inotropic agents may also be used as needed.

Anesthesia for cesarean or vaginal delivery in patients who are hemodynamically unstable should be delayed while appropriate monitoring devices are inserted (arterial line, pulmonary artery line, Foley catheter) and resuscitation is accomplished. This step should be completed in most instances within 1 or 2 hours. Some patients may remain unstable despite adequate filling pressures and catecholamine infusions. In such circumstances, delivery should not be further delayed as it may be the only chance the newborn has for survival.

ANESTHESIA FOR THE FEBRILE PARTURIENT
Regional anesthesia

The febrile parturient is often in premature labor. Oxytocin augmentation may be indicated in as many as 70% of patients, and cesarean sections are needed in as many as 30% to 40% of patients.[38,39] With such clinical situations, both mother and baby often benefit from regional anesthesia.

There is, however, little factual information to guide the physician dealing with a febrile patient. Since a description of the risks of regional anesthesia is often requested, the following text will provide the available information that is important for both patient and clinician.

The incidence of transient bacteremia, as documented in healthy patients by blood culture, is less than 1%.[40] Pregnancy may increase this incidence.[41] Insertion of a Foley catheter in an otherwise healthy parturient can also produce a transient bacteremia in up to 60% of patients even though the urine is sterile.[41,42] The incidence of bacteremia is believed to be even higher in the presence of an infected urine.[42,43] When one considers that asymptomatic urinary tract infections are common in pregnancy and that bladder catheterization is commonly performed, it becomes apparent that a transient bacteremia is very common in parturients and more so in febrile parturients.

The diagnosis of sepsis and its systemic response is defined as two or more of the following criteria.[44]

1. Temperature $>38°$ C or $<36°$ C
2. Heart rate >90 beats/min
3. Respiratory rate >20 breaths/min or P_{CO_2} <32 torr
4. WBC $>12,000$ cells/mm^3, <4000 cells/mm^3, or $>10\%$ immature forms (band cells)

This definition will assist in the diagnosis of sepsis, but it is less useful because of the normal physiologic changes of pregnancy.

The clinical picture is confounded by the following factors:

1. Elevated temperature or rigors do not accurately correlate to the presence of bacteremia.[45-47] A patient may even be hypothermic during fulminant sepsis.
2. There is also no correlation between temperature and clinical status (e.g., endogenous pyrogens may result in an elevated temperature despite adequate treatment of the infection).
3. Blood culture and sensitivity results are usually not available.

Epidural anesthesia has been described in the presence of fever,[48,49] but there is no clear consensus to guide the anesthesiologist. Some earlier reports have even stated that regional anesthesia should be avoided with bacteremia because of concerns that a focus of infection will be initiated by the procedure.[47,50] Infection of the epidural space or meningitis may occur because of:

1. A break in sterile technique
2. Infection traveling along the needle tract

3. Contamination of the instruments
4. Bacteremia with or without blood vessel trauma

It is feared that blood vessel trauma may introduce bacteria into the epidural space. In addition to the 12% incidence of blood vessel trauma when the epidural catheter is inserted,[51,52] an epidural catheter might traumatize a blood vessel by migration during labor.[53] Theoretically a collection of blood and bacteria could result in formation of an epidural abscess or meningitis.

Epidural abscess

Acute epidural abscess may be a life-threatening complication. Its rare occurrence makes the diagnosis even more difficult. Back pain is the earliest and most important symptom. This pain may be very severe, but it may appear gradually or suddenly. Root pain, weakness, and paralysis will develop, usually within a week of onset of backache. Tenderness on percussion of the spine is always present. A few days or weeks after the onset of pain, the patient may develop headache, chills, fever, and leukocytosis. The onset of neurologic damage may be sudden or very slow and often is irreversible. In most cases, the correct diagnosis is not made initially, so the severity of a neurologic deficit may be influenced by immediate treatment.[54,55] Magnetic resonance imaging (MRI) has been recommended as the procedure of choice for the diagnosis of epidural abscesses.[56]

One must ask whether an epidural abscess or meningitis could be caused by a regional anesthetic. To date only anecdotes concerning this are reported in the literature.[56-58] Reports from the early days of continuous epidural technique describe 6 patients with caudal infections and 1 epidural infection.[50] More recent literature reports 2 cases of epidural abscesses in nonobstetric patients. It seems likely that infection was the result of nonaseptic technique, although in the latter two cases, hematogenous spread was possible.[50] In 1975, Baker and co-workers reported 39 patients with epidural abscesses (20 acute and 19 prolonged or chronic cases).[54] Epidural catheter insertion was reported as a probable source of infection in only 1 patient and lumbar puncture in 2 patients. The lumbar punctures were done in patients with vertebral osteomyelitis, and the specific details of the epidural technique are not reported. Another review of 35 new cases and 153 previously reported cases of epidural abscesses concluded that regional anesthesia was not a factor in any of these additional cases.[55] A recent report of an epidural abscess following epidural catheterization for the management of a long-standing thoracic neuralgic pain syndrome cannot be extrapolated to the short-term use of epidural anesthesia in labor.[59]

Reports in the literature suggest that most epidural infections result from trauma, surgical procedures, or hematogenous spread rather than from regional anesthesia.[54] There is no documented relationship between epidural vein puncture in the febrile patient and the formation of an epidural abscess. If "seeding" of the epidural space with infected blood is common, why are there not a more significant number of infections? However, additional cases of iatrogenic epidural abscess continue to be reported and should concern the anesthesiologist.[56,60-62]

Meningitis

Cases of several patients who developed meningitis after regional anesthesia have been reported. In a report of 6 nonobstetrical patients, the authors felt that epidural injection of foreign substances, use of a vasoconstrictor, or contaminants were the possible causes.[63] Spinal meningitis has also been reported in 5 nonobstetric patients who had recently received epidural anesthesia; one likely the result of a blood-borne infection, one possibly from the spread of a cellulitis from the site of the epidural injection, one the result of an inadvertent spinal tap followed by blood patch, and two postulated to be a complication of spinal anesthesia.[64-67]

Meningitis has also been reported in 2 patients after spinal anesthesia for obstetrics.[68,69] This problem will be further discussed at the end of this section.

Septic meningitis has only rarely been reported in the past 25 years.[70] Only one case has been reported where in the presence of bacteremia, spinal anesthesia was responsible for meningitis.[70] This appears to be the only case reported in the past three decades. During this period tens of thousands of spinal anesthetic procedures have been reported.[71,72] In the past, some authorities have speculated on the possibility that a lumbar puncture may create a site of diminished resistance in the blood-brain barrier or that epidural abscesses might occur for the same reason.[70] This speculation is surprising considering the frequent use of spinal anaesthesia and the common occurrence of bacteremia. It is highly doubtful that a casual relationship exists between such rare events.

There is, however, one recent study that has attempted to further assess if epidural puncture during a period of bacteremia would result in the subsequent development of meningitis.[73] The study group consisted of 40 chronically bacteremic rats that underwent cisternal puncture and 40 rats who did not. Twenty-four hours following the initial cisternal puncture, the animals were sacrificed. Spinal fluid obtained at this time was cultured, and bacteria were cultured in 12 rats. Microscopic examination also showed evidence of central nervous system infection. Bacteremic animals not undergoing cisternal puncture always had sterile spinal fluid (n = 30), and cisternal puncture in the *absence* of bacteremia also did not result in infection. This study suggests that bacteremia may constitute a risk factor in the development of meningitis in patients receiving spinal anesthesia, but the pertinence of the study to humans undergoing spinal anesthesia is not known. However, the authors recommend caution and would prefer not to administer spinal anesthesia to a febrile patient. Interestingly, in the presence of antibiotics (gentamycin) none of the animals had positive cerebrospinal fluid culture even in the presence of bacteria.

Hypotension

Regional anesthesia may be catastrophic in patients with late sepsis because of their hypovolemia.[36] The decision to give a epidural anesthesia must be decided on an individual basis. Pregnant women may be septic with few clinical signs. Therefore, one must pay close attention to all physical and laboratory findings and maintain a high degree of suspicion.

The patient with chorioamnionitis

Hunt and co-workers reported that in cultures from 102 patients undergoing continuous epidural catheterization, 22 catheters were found to be contaminated.[74] This infection rate is high considering the meticulous aseptic placement.[75] However, the contamination rate should be considered in view of the very large numbers of patients receiving epidural catheters for labor and delivery, surgery, and pain control *without* clinical infections. Many of the patients receiving pain control for cancer pain are also immunocompromised. Other data suggest that local anesthesia may play a role in preventing infection.[76] It is particularly important to note that the incidence of epidural abscess has not risen in the last 20 years despite the widespread and increased popularity of regional anesthesia.[77]

There has never been a report of epidural abscess or meningitis following regional anesthesia in a patient with chorioamnionitis. Two retrospective reviews of 27,000 and 505,000 obstetric patients who received epidural anesthesia included no cases of meningitis and only two cases of epidural space infection.[78,79] In addition, one small series of patients showed that the organisms isolated with chorioamnionitis are not the same as

with epidural infection.[58] In a recent review of 10,047 deliveries, 319 women with chorioamnionitis were reported and none had any complications from regional anesthesia.[80] Factors such as white cell count and temperature elevation were of no value in identifying the bacteremic patients.[80] In another review, 74 of 113 women who received continuous epidural anesthesia and 2 who received spinal anesthesia developed signs of chorioamnionitis after placement of the epidural catheter. In the remaining 39 patients symptoms of generalized systemic infections were present at the time of epidural insertions. In 16 of these patients, antibiotics were not given until after the epidural catheter was inserted.[49] None of these patients developed an epidural abscess or meningitis; however, they all received antibiotics before or after the block.[49,81] These findings support the low risk of such a procedure.[49,80] Large studies are lacking; however, leading authorities have recommend that in the presence of systemic signs antibiotics be started before proceeding with an epidural.[50,80-82]

The avoidance or discontinuation of continuous epidural anesthesia, because of these unsubstantiated concerns, may cause the patient to be exposed to unnecessary pain and to the risks of general anesthesia. A case has been reported in which an epidural catheter was removed because the patient became febrile. As a result, when she needed anesthesia for cesarean section she received general anesthesia. In this case there was unexpected gross edema of the larynx and pharynx, which made tracheal intubation very difficult.[83]

When to perform an epidural or spinal block

In reaching a decision, the anesthetist might be helped by knowing the duration and severity of temperature elevation, the use of antibiotics, white cell count and differential, and the hemodynamic status (i.e., shock or dehydration). There are, however, no firm criteria as to when one would proceed with regional anesthesia.[80,81] The severity of symptoms also raises concerns regarding hemodynamic stability after a high sympathetic blockade, but again there is no information to clearly define when one should be concerned.

The potential benefit of aspirin in pregnancy has presented the anesthetist with a dilemma. Theoretically there may be an increased risk of epidural hematoma formation with disastrous sequelae. If the patient has received aspirin within 4 to 7 days, one must check for normal platelet function.[84,85] It has been suggested that a bleeding time of up to 10 minutes should be considered safe.[86,87] Although we have relied on a normal bleeding time as evidence of the adequacy of clotting and as being necessary before proceeding with epidural/spinal anesthesia, the validity of this test has been questioned.[86-90] Based on 1069 patients who were followed after epidural anesthesia, the data monitoring committee of a collaborative low-dose aspirin study in pregnancy also does not recommend a bleeding time. These patients had their aspirin stopped at 37 weeks' gestation.[91] However, they did recommend that bleeding times not be done in parturients who have taken aspirin just before planned epidural anesthesia, and they imply that it is safe to administer an epidural block to these patients. The opposite view is represented by MacDonald in response to his interpretation of the same data.[87] Others suggest that epidural anesthesia should not be denied to patients receiving low-dose aspirin, and the authors agree with this conclusion.[90,91] In contrast, acetaminophen has not been found to have any effect on hemostasis,[85] and in severe hepatitis a coagulation profile should be checked before deciding on regional anesthesia.

Some authorities have stated that the decision to use regional anesthesia should be based on the possible risks and benefits for each individual patient. However, the information outlined illustrates how such an evaluation is very difficult if not impossible.[39,45,81] The patient should be aware that epidural abscess formation, adhesive arachnoiditis, or meningitis are extremely rare but possible occurrences. However, these complications are more often unrelated to the procedure. For example, Bromage refers to a case in which a spontaneous epidural abscess became evident between 6 and 10 days postpartum.[50] No regional anesthetic had been given. How many of us might believe that had one been given, a causal relationship would have been assumed by either the patient, her obstetrician, or her lawyer?

The benefits of regional anesthesia must be emphasized as well. This is particularly vital to the high-risk parturient. I do not believe that the febrile parturient should be denied an epidural anesthetic. Clinical experience suggests the safety of epidural anesthesia for these patients. More information is needed before this author would give spinal anesthesia for these patients.

General anesthesia

General anesthesia is less frequently used than regional anesthesia in obstetrics.[93] Febrile patients are, however, more likely to receive general anesthesia because of maternal or fetal complications. Acute fetal distress, maternal hypovolemia, sepsis, and septic shock are all more common. We would like to caution against the routine avoidance of regional anesthesia because there are significant and perhaps greater risks with general anaesthesia.

The use of general anesthesia may result in a faster induction of anesthesia, but in its use one must be concerned with major problems such as:

1. Maternal aspiration of gastric contents
2. Difficulties in controlling the airway
3. Difficulties or inability to intubate
4. The potential for newborn depression

The risk of aspiration in the pregnant patient has been well recognized since Mendelson first described a syndrome associated with aspiration of gastric contents.[94] Several factors predispose pregnant patients to gastric reflux and regurgitation. The large uterus at term mechanically obstructs the duodenum, progesterone decreases intestinal motility and relaxes the gastroesophageal sphincter, and pain as well as analgesic drugs may delay gastric emptying. Gastric motility is also decreased in the febrile patient or the patient in shock. Indeed, the risks and the problems of either a failed intubation or pulmonary aspiration are a leading cause of maternal morbidity and mortality.

Failed intubation and pulmonary aspiration will remain major problems. The hurried use of general anesthesia for an emergency cesarean delivery is particularly hazardous.[95] Preventive measures such as cricoid pressure, rapid sequence induction, and antacids and/or H_2 receptor blockers and metoclopramide may reduce the incidence of pulmonary aspiration, but they do not eliminate it. Awake intubation or rapid sequence induction should be used in all patients. Dangers are frequent enough and severe enough to warrant obstetricians' full awareness of these risks.

The pregnant patient also has many changes in the respiratory system. Of particular concern is the fact that oxygen consumption increases progressively during pregnancy to approximately 20% above normal at term.[96] The hyperthermic patient may also elevate her oxygen consumption by as much as 60%.[96,97] These changes place the febrile patient and her fetus at increased risk of severe hypoxia during induction of general anesthesia and necessitate the need for preoxygenation before induction.[96] This has become routine for all pregnant patients.

The choice of drugs used for induction or maintenance of general anesthesia is dictated by the desire to maintain hemodynamic stability as well as uteroplacental circulation. Ketamine has been advocated by some authorities.[98,99] However, concern has been expressed about the unpredictability of 1 to 2 mg/kg of ketamine in critically ill patients.[98,99] This is due to the myocardial depressant effects of ketamine. It is not clear if the same concerns exist for patients who have fevers of short duration. Sodium thiopental also causes myocardial depression in the critically ill patient. Reduced doses will diminish but not eliminate this problem. In fact, some have suggested the use of both these agents in reduced doses to decrease the incidence of cardiovascular decompensation.[99,100] Diazepam or diazemuls (2.5- to 5-mg increments) up to a maximum of 10 mg will also induce sleep in some patients without significant fall in blood pressure. These doses of diazepam have no effects on healthy infants. However, not all patients will be induced by 10 mg of diazepam, and thus this technique is not suitable for rapid sequence induction. Midazolam, a newer benzodiazepine, is not suitable for induction of obstetric anesthesia.[101]

Concern has been expressed regarding hyperkalemia following the use of succinylcholine. This may be a problem in severe and prolonged sepsis (of more than 1 week duration).[45,102] However, pretreatment with a nondepolarizing agent may decrease but will not eliminate the release of potassium. It is not known when an elevated temperature is severe enough or of long enough duration to contraindicate the use of succinylcholine. There has never been a report of hyperkalemia induced by succinylcholine in a patient with chorioamnionitis. If the temperature elevation is of several days' duration, the use of a nondepolarizing agent such as vecuronium 0.25 mg/kg or any nondepolarizing agent is acceptable for a rapid sequence induction in such circumstances. Succinylcholine is routinely used at our institution without problems.

Febrile patients are usually receiving antibiotics, some of which may interact with muscle relaxants; however, with commonly used antibiotics and a peripheral nerve stimulator, there is seldom a problem in adequate reversal of neuromuscular blockade.

Once the patient is intubated, the patient is maintained with a high concentration of oxygen (a minimum of 50%). Low concentrations of nitrous oxide (up to 50%) may be used, but if any significant fall in blood pressure occurs, it may be discontinued in case it is due to a myocardial depressant effect of the nitrous oxide. With severe fetal distress, 100% oxygen may be used in an attempt to better oxygenate the fetus. Hemodynamic depression is a concern when volatile agents are used. If other agents such as low-dose ketamine or fentanyl are added to reduce the amount of volatile agent needed, hemodynamic stability is usually maintained. Theoretically all three commonly used inhalational agents (halothane, enflurane, and isoflurane) can alter immune mechanisms, but their effects may be insignificant during clinical anesthesia.[103] A balanced technique with small amounts of several agents is probably the key to

success. However, the literature suggests the absence of a causal relationship between types of anesthesia and inflammatory response.[104] Of course, all of these problems can be avoided by giving an epidural anesthetic. In addition, any potential depressant effects of general anesthetic agents on the newborn are also avoided.[105,106] Postoperative pain relief with intraspinal narcotic agents is another advantage of epidural anesthesia.

We must anticipate the problem of the febrile patient with fetal distress who is to undergo immediate delivery. Epidural or spinal anesthesia has the obvious advantages of greatly reducing the risk of maternal aspiration, but no form of anesthesia is without risk. The slightly slower onset may be critical. The choice of anesthesia for cesarean section depends on the indication for the operation, the degree of urgency, the wishes of the patient, and the skills of the anesthesiologist. Sometimes the clinical situation can result in a distressed obstetrician and/or anesthesiologist. All these factors lead to an intensely emotional situation for which the anesthesiologist must be prepared in advance.

A key question to be asked is whether the maternal risk of a general anaesthetic is worth it. We must ask ourselves whether the distress is already so severe that the baby is likely to have a major deficit from asphyxia. Both obstetrician and anesthesiologist need to give strong consideration to the risks for the mother, weighing these against the possible neonatal outcome.[107] Either regional or general anaesthesia could be used, but current information tends to favor regional anesthesia if time permits.[107]

SUMMARY

Obstetric and anesthetic management of the febrile patient depends on the cause and severity of maternal and neonatal conditions. The risk-benefit ratio must be considered by both the obstetrician and the anesthesiologist, and frank discussion is essential with the patient and her closest support person.

REFERENCES

1. Gelfand JA, Dinarello CA, Wolff SM: Fever, including fever of unknown origin, in Isselbacher KJ, Braunwald E, et al (eds): *Harrison's Principles of Internal Medicine,* ed 13. New York, McGraw-Hill, 1994, pp 81-90.
2. Guyton AC (ed): *Human Physiology and Mechanisms of Disease,* ed 5. Philadelphia, WB Saunders, 1992, pp 531-541.
3. Beutler B, Beutler SM: The pathogenesis of fever, in Wyngaarden JB, Smith LH, Bennett JC (eds): *Cecil Textbook of Medicine,* ed 19. Philadelphia, WB Saunders, 1992, pp 1567-1571.
4. McMurray RG, Katz VL, Berry MJ, et al: The effects of pregnancy on metabolic responses during rest, immersion, and aerobic exercises in the water. *Am J Obstet Gynecol* 1988; 158:481.

5. Challis JRG, Olson DM: Parturition, in Knobil E, Neill JD (eds): *The Physiology of Reproduction.* New York, Raven Press, 1988, pp 2177-2216.

6. Creasy RK: Preterm labor and delivery, in Creasy RK, Resnik R (eds): *Maternal Fetal Medicine: Principles and Practice.* WB Saunders, Philadelphia 1989, p 480.

7. Greiss FC, Anderson SG, Still JG: Uterine pressure-flow relationships during early gestation. *Am J Obstet Gynecol* 1976; 126:79.

8. Taylor DJ, Phillips P, Lind T: Puerperal hematologic indices. *Br J Obstet Gynaecol* 1981; 88:601.

9. Gall SA: Maternal immune system during human gestation. *Semin Perinatol* 1977; 1:119.

10. Paryani SG, Arvin AM: Intrauterine infection with varicella-zoster virus after maternal varicella. *N Engl J Med* 1986; 314:1542.

11. Sweet RL, Gibbs RS: *Infectious Diseases of the Female Genital Tract.* Baltimore, Williams & Wilkins, 1990.

12. Romero R, Yoon BH, Mazor M, et al: A comparative study of the diagnostic performance of amniotic fluid, glucose, white cell count, interleukin-6, and gram stain in the detection of microbial invasion in patients with preterm premature rupture of membranes. *Am J Obstet Gynecol* 1993; 169(4):839.

13. Arvin AM, Heinsleigh PA, Prober CG, et al: Failure of antepartum maternal cultures to predict the infant's risk of exposure to herpes simplex virus at delivery. *N Engl J Med* 1986; 315:796.

14. American College of Obstetricians and Gynecologists: Perinatal herpes simplex virus infection. *ACOG Tech Bull* no. 122, November 1988.

15. Crosby ET, Halpern SH, Rolbin SH: Epidural anaesthesia for caesarean section in patients with active recurrent genital herpes simplex infections: A retrospective review. *Can J Anaesth* 1989; 36:701.

16. Ramanathan S, Sheth R, Turndoff H: Anesthesia for cesarean section in patients with genital herpes infections: A retrospective study. *Anesthesiology* 1986; 64:807.

17. Bader AM, Camann WR, Datta S: Anesthesia for cesarean delivery in patients with herpes simplex virus type-2 infections. *Reg Anesth* 1990; 15:261.

18. Crone LL, Conly JM, Storgard C, et al: Herpes labialis in parturients receiving epidural morphine following cesarean section. *Anesthesiology* 1990; 7:208.

19. Valley MA, Bourke DL, McKenzie AM: Recurrence of thoracic and labial herpes simplex virus infection in a patient receiving epidural fentanyl. *Anesthesiology* 1992; 76:1056.

20. Douglas MJ, McMorland GH: Possible association of herpes simplex type 1 reaction with epidural morphine. *Can J Anaesth* 1987; 34:426.

21. Committee on Infectious Disease, American Academy of Pediatrics: Varicella-Zoster Infections. 1994 Red Book: Report of The Committee on Infectious Diseases, ed 23, pp 510-517.

22. American College of Obstetricians and Gynecologists: Perinatal viral and parasitic infections. *ACOG Tech Bull* no, 177, February 1993.

23. Camann WR, Tuomala RE: Infectious disease, in Datta S (ed): *Anesthetic and Obstetric Management of High-Risk Pregnancy.* St. Louis, Mosby Year Book, 1991, pp 536-564.

24. Centre for Disease Control: Update on hepatitis B prevention. *MMWR* 1987; 36:353.

25. Centre for Disease Control: Protection against viral hepatitis: Recommendation of the immunization practices advisory committee (ACIP). *MMWR* 1990; 39(RR-2):1.

26. Alter HJ, Purcell RH, Shih JW, et al: Detection of antibody to hepatitis C virus in prospectively followed transfusion recipients with acute and chronic non-A, non-B hepatitis. *N Engl J Med* 1989; 321:1494.

27. Alter MJ: Hepatitis C: A sleeping giant? *Am J Med* 1991 (Suppl 3B):112S.

28. Alter MJ, Hadler SC, Judson FN, et al: Risk factors for ute non-A, non-B hepatitis in the United States and association with hepatitis C virus infection. *JAMA* 1990; 264:2231.

29. Lucy SJ: Anaesthesia for Caesarean delivery of a malignant hyperthermia susceptible parturient. *Can J Anaesth* 1994; 41:1220.

30. Low DF, Kaul R, McGreer A: The evolution of severe invasive Group A streptococcal disease in Ontario: Changing epidemiology, pathogenesis, and new approaches to treatment. *Can J Infect Dis* (in press).

31. Nathan L, Peters MT, Ahmed Am: The return of life-threatening puerperal sepsis caused by group A streptococcai. *Am J Obstet Gynecol* 1993; 169:571.

32. Morgan PJ: Maternal death following epidural anaesthesia in a patient with unsuspected sepsis. *Can J Anaesth* (in press).

33. Watanabe-Ohnishi R, Low DE, McGreer, A et al: Selective depletion of Vβ-bearing T cells in patients with severe invasive group A streptococcal infections and streptococcal toxic shock syndrome. *J Infect Dis* 1995; 171:74.

34. Parrillo JE: Shock, in Isselbacher KJ, Braunwald E, Wilson JD, et al (eds): *Harrison's Principles of Internal Medicine,* ed 13. New York, McGraw-Hill, 1994, pp 187-193.

35. Mossa AR, Mayer AD, Lavelle-Jones M: Surgical complications, in Sabiston DC (ed): *Textbook of Surgery,* ed 14. Philadelphia, WB Saunders, 1991, pp 306-309.

36. Shires GT III, Shires GT, Carrico CJ: Shock, in Schwartz SI, Shires GT, Spencer FC (eds): *Principles of Surgery,* ed 6, New York, McGraw-Hill, 1994, pp 119-144.

37. Clark SL, Cotton DB, Lee W, et al: Central hemodynamic assessment of normal term pregnancy. *Am J Obstet Gynecol* 1989; 161:1439.

38. Duff P, Sanders R, Gibbs RS: The course of labour in term patients with chorioamnionitis. *Am J Obstet Gynecol* 1983; 147:391.

39. Davies JM, Thistlewood JM, Rolbin SH, et al: Infections and the parturient: Anaesthetic considerations. *Can J Anaesth* 1988; 35:270.

40. Blanco JD, Gibbs RS, Castaneda YS: Bacteremia in obstetrics: Clinical course. *Obstet Gynecol* 1981; 58:621.

41. Everett ED, Hirschman JV: Transient bacteremia and endocarditis prophylaxis: A review. *Medicine* 1977; 56:61.

42. Sullivan NM, Mims MM, Finegold SM: Clinical aspects of bacteremia after manipulation of the genitourinary tract. *J Infect Dis* 1973; 127:49.

43. Drach GW, Cox CE: Bladder bacteria: Common but unique cause for sepsis. Postoperative endotoxic responses. *J Urol* 1971; 106:67.

44. American College of Chest Physicians/Society of Critical Medicine Consensus Conference: Definitions for sepsis and organ failure and guidelines for the use of innovative therapies in sepsis. *Crit Care Med* 1992; 20:864.

45. Shelley WC, Gutsche BB: Anesthesia for the febrile parturient, in James FM III, Wheeler AS (eds): *Obstetric Anesthesia: The Complicated Patient.* Philadelphia, FA Davis, 1982, pp 297.

46. McHenry MC, Gavin TL, Hawk WA, et al: Gram negative bacteremia: Variable clinical courses and useful prognostic factors. *Clev Clin Quart* 1975; 42:15.

47. Gibbs RS, Castillo MS, Rodgers PJ: Management of acute chorioamnionitis. *Am J Obstet Gynecol* 1980; 136:709.

48. Behl S: Epidural analgesia in the presence of fever. *Anaesthesia* 1985; 40:1240.

49. Vaddadi A, Ramananathan J, Mercer BM, et al: Epidural anesthesia in women with chorioamnionitis. *Anesthesiol Rev* 1992; 19/3:35.

50. Epidural infection, in Bromage PR (ed): *Epidural Analgesia.* Philadelphia, WB Saunders, 1978, pp 682-690.

51. Rolbin SH, Hew E, Ogilvie G: A comparison of two types of epidural catheters. *Can J Anaesth* 1987; 34:459.

52. Rolbin SH, Halpern SH, Braude BM, et al: Fluid through the epidural needle does not reduce complications of epidural catheter insertion. *Can J Anaesth* 1990; 37:337.

53. Kenepp NB, Gutsche BB: Inadvertent intravascular injection during lumbar epidural anesthesia. *Anesthesiology* 1981; 54:172.

54. Baker AS, Ojemann RG, Swartz MN, et al: Spinal epidural abscess. *New Engl Med J* 1975; 293:463.

55. Danner RG, Hartman BJ: Update of spinal epidural abscess: 35 cases and a review of the literature. *Rev Infect Dis* 1987; 9:265.

56. Mamourian AC, Dickman CA, Drayer BP, et al: Spinal epidural abscess: Three cases following spinal epidural injection demonstrated with magnetic resonance imaging. *Anesthesiology* 1993; 78:204.

57. Loarie DJ, Fairley HB: Epidural abscess following spinal anesthesia. *Anesth Analg* 1978; 57:351.

58. Kee WDN, Jones MR, Thomas P, et al: Extradural abscess complicating extradural anaesthesia for Caesarean section. *Br J Anaesth* 1992; 69:647.

59. Fine PG, Hare BD, Zahriser JC: Epidural abscess following epidural catheterization in a chronic pain patient: A diagnostic dilemma. *Anesthesiology* 1988; 69:422.

60. Shintani S, Tanaka H, Irifune A, et al: Iatrogenic acute spinal epidural abscess with septic meningitis: MR findings. *Clin Neurol Neurosurg* 1992; 94:253.

61. Abdel-Magid RA, Koth HI: Epidural abscess after spinal anesthesia: A favorable outcome. *Neurosurgery* 1990; 27:310.

62. Tabo E, Ohkuma Y, Kimura S, et al: Successful percutaneous drainage of epidural abscess with epidural needle and catheter. *Anesthesiology* 1994; 80:1393.

63. Sghirlanzoni A, Marazzi R, Pareyson D, et al: Epidural anaesthesia and spinal arachnoiditis. *Anaesthesia* 1989; 44:31.

64. Ready LB, Helfer D: Bacterial meningitis in parturients after epidural anesthesia. *Anesthesiology* 1989; 71:988.

65. Berga S, Trierweiller MW: Bacterial meningitis following epidural anesthesia for vaginal delivery: A case report. *Obstet Gynecol* 1989; 74:437.

66. Bert AA, Laasberg HA: Aseptic meningitis following spinal anesthesia—A complication of the past? *Anesthesiology* 1985; 62:674.

67. Blackmore TK, Morley HR, Gordon DL: Streptococcus mitis-induced bacteremia and meningitis after spinal anesthesia. *Anesthesiology* 1993; 78:592.

68. Roberts SP, Petts HV: Meningitis after obstetric spinal anaesthesia. *Anaesthesia* 1990; 45:376.

69. Lee JJ, Parry H: Bacterial meningitis following spinal anaesthesia for caesarean section. *Br J Anaesth* 1991; 66:383.

70. Berman RS, Eisele JH: Bacteremia, spinal anesthesia and development of meningitis. *Anesthesiology* 1978; 48:376.

71. Dripps RD, Vandam LD: Long-term follow up of patients who received 10,098 spinal anesthetics. I. Failure to discover major neurological sequelae. *JAMA* 1954; 56:1486.

72. Moore DC, Bridenbaugh LD: Spinal (subarachnoid) block: A review of 11,574 cases. *JAMA* 1966; 195:907.

73. Carp H, Bailey S: The association between meningitis and dural puncture in bacteremic rats. *Anesthesiology* 1992; 76:739.

74. Hunt JR, Rigor BM Sr, Collins JR: The potential for contamination of continuous epidural catheters. *Anesth Analg* 1977; 56:222.

75. Barretto RS: Bacteriological culture of indwelling epidural catheters. *Anesthesiology* 1962; 23:643.

76. Feldman J, Chapin K, Turner J, et al: Do agents for epidural analgesia have antimicrobial properties? *Anesthesiology* 1991; 75:A835.

77. Vernier EF, Musher DM: Spinal epidural abscess in Symposium on Infections of the Central Nervous System. *Med Clin North Am* 1985; 69:375-384.

78. Crawford JS: Some maternal complications of epidural analgesia for labour. *Anaesthesia* 1985; 40:1219.

79. Scott DB, Hibbard BM: Serious non-fatal complications associated with extradural block in obstetric practice. *Br J Anaesth* 1990; 64:537.

80. Bader AM, Gilbertson L, Kirz, et al: Regional anesthesia in women with chorioamnionitis. *Reg Anesth* 1992; 17:84.

81. Bromage PR: Neurologic complications of regional anesthesia for obstetrics, in Shnider SM, Levinson G (eds): *Anesthesia for Obstetrics,* ed 3. Baltimore, Williams & Wilkins, 1993, pp 444-446.

82. Chestnut DH: Spinal anesthesia in the febrile patient (editorial). *Anesthesiology* 1992; 76:667.

83. Thomas DG: Epidural analgesia in the presence of fever (letter). *Anaesthesia* 1986; 41:553.

84. Weiss HJ, Aledort LM, Kochwa S: The effects of salicylates on the hemostatic properties of platelets in man. *J Clin Invest* 1968; 47:2169.

85. Pearson HA: Comparative effects of aspirin and acetaminophen on hemostasis. *Pediatrics* 1978; 62:926.

86. MacDonald R: Aspirin and extradural blocs. *Br J Anaesth* 1991; 66:1.

87. Macdonald R: Letter to the editor. *Br J Anaesth* 1992; 69:109.

88. Rodgers RPC, Levin J: A critical reappraisal of the bleeding time. *Semin Thromb Hemost* 1990; 16:1.

89. Lind SE: The bleeding time does not predict surgical bleeding. *Blood* 1991; 77:2547.

90. Horlocker TT, Wedel DJ, Offord KP: Does preoperative antiplatelet therapy increase the risk of hemorrhagic complications associated with regional anesthesia? *Anesth Analg* 1990; 70:631.

91. De Swiet M: Aspirin, extradural anaesthesia and the MRC collaborative low-dose aspirin study in pregnancy (CLASP) [letter; comment on *Br J Anaesth* 1991; 66:1] *Br J Anaesth* 1992; 69:109.

92. O'Kelly SW, Lawes EG, Luntley JB: Bleeding time: Is it a useful clinical tool? *Br J Anaesth* 1992; 68:313.

93. Shnider SM, Levinson G: Anesthesia for cesarean section, in Shnider SM, Levinson G (eds): *Anesthesia for Obstetrics,* ed 3. Baltimore, Williams & Wilkins, 1993, pp 211-246.

94. Mendelson CL: The aspiration of stomach contents into the lungs during obstetric anesthesia. *Am J Obstet Gynecol* 1946; 52:191.

95. Gibbs CP, Rolbin SH, Norman P: Cause and prevention of maternal aspiration. *Anesthesiology* 1984; 61:11.

96. Shnider SM, Levison G: Maternal physiologic alterations in pregnancy, in Shnider GM, Levinson G (eds): *Anesthesia for Obstetrics,* ed 3. Baltimore, Williams & Wilkins, 1993, pp 3-18.

97. Rowell LB, Brengelmann GC, Murray JA: Cardiovascular responses to sustained high skin temperature in resting man. *J Applied Physiol* 1969; 27:673.

98. Marx GF, Hodgkinson R: Special considerations in complications of pregnancy, in Marx GF, Bassell GM (eds): *Obstetric Analgesia and Anaesthesia.* New York, Elsevier 1980, pp 329-330.

99. Way WL, Trevor AJ: Ketamine, in Miller RD (ed): *Anesthesia,* ed 2. New York, Churchill Livingstone, 1986, pp 813.

100. Reich DL, Silvay G: Ketamine: An update on the first twenty-five years of clinical experience. *Can J Anaesth* 1989; 36:186.

101. Bland BAR, Lawes EG, Duncan PW, et al: Comparison of Midazolam and thiopental for rapid sequence anesthetic induction for elective cesarean section. *Anesth Analg* 1987; 66:1165.

102. Kohlschutter B, Baur H, Roth F: Suxamethonium-induced hyperkalaemia in patients with severe intra-abdominal infections. *Br J Anaesth* 1976; 48:557.

103. Duncan PG, Cullen BF: Anesthesia and immunology. *Anesthesiology* 1976; 45:522.

104. Fu E, Scharf J, Burdash N: Effect of anesthetic and surgical trauma on interleukin-6 release in mice. *Anesthesiology* 1994; 81:A1020.

105. Ong BY, Cohen MM, Palahniuk J: Anesthesia for cesarean section: Effect on neonates. *Anesth Analg* 1989; 68:270.

106. Rolbin SH, Cohen MM, Levitan CM: The premature infant: Anesthesia for cesarean delivery. *Anesth Analg* 1994; 78:912.

107. Anesthesia for emergency deliveries. ACOG Committee on Obstetrics: Maternal and Fetal Medicine March 1992 no 104.

29 Psychiatric Disease

Francis A. Rosinia and Alfred G. Robichaux III

MENTAL ILLNESS

Mental illness is a topic that is seldom discussed in association with pregnancy. The literature, however, indicates that mental illness during pregnancy is probably more common than preeclampsia, diabetes, abruptio placenta, and premature delivery. Despite this high prevalence, mental illness in pregnancy is frequently underdiagnosed and undertreated.[1,2] Persistent, untreated, mental illness can have important adverse effects on the pregnancy, labor and delivery, and postpartum period. It can also complicate the administration of anesthesia and the response to anesthetic modalities. In this chapter, we will discuss the eight most common types of mental illness. We will define each type and give the reader information about its prevalence, risk factors, and management techniques.

MOOD DISORDERS
Incidence

Depression affects a higher frequency of women than men during their lifetime (20% vs. 10%). Eight percent to 10% of all reproductive-age women are depressed, and 50% of all depressed women are between 20 and 50 years old.[3] Therefore, a significant number of women who are in their childbearing years are at high risk for a mood disorder.[4] There are two types of mood disorders: unipolar (depression) and bipolar (manic/depression). Depression may be further subdivided into major depressive disorders and dysthymic (low-grade, more persistently depressed). There is controversy about the frequency and the severity of mood disorders in pregnancy. This is a result of a variety of factors, such as the type of assessment or questionnaire used, the sample of women being assessed (variables include age, marital status, socioeconomic status, and parity), and time during pregnancy when assessments are performed.[5] In general, *prevalence estimates have been placed between 10% and 20%.*[6]

During the past 15 years, database studies have consistently validated that, following childbirth, there is a significantly higher rate of psychiatric hospital admissions in women for the first 3 months and a somewhat higher rate for up to 2 years postpartum.[7] Medical complication such as obstetric hemorrhage, severe pregnancy-induced hypertension, and even unplanned cesarean section have been reported to double the risk of postpartum depression.[8,9]

Major depression

A thorough psychiatric history should be taken during the first prenatal visit. Major risk factors that should be obtained during the history-taking examination include:

1. A personal or family history of depression
2. Stressful life events
3. Lack of social support
4. Current substance abuse
5. Prior suicide attempts[10]

Not surprisingly, tobacco and drug abuse during pregnancy were associated with depressive symptoms.[11] If a patient reports a prior history of depression, she has a 50% rate of recurrence. With two prior episodes of depression, the recurrence rate increased to 70%. With three or more prior episodes of depression, the recurrence rate is as high as 90%. A family history of depression carries a 12% risk of *attack*. The depression may occur antepartum, postpartum, or both.[10] Companionship during labor has been reported to modify the factors that contribute to depression.[12] There are nine diagnostic criteria for a major depressive episode. Five or more of the following symptoms must be present daily for at least a 2-week period and represent a change from previous activity. One of the symptoms must be either a depressed mood or loss of interest.

Clinical features
1. Depressed mood most of the day as indicated either by subjective account or observation by others.
2. Significantly diminished interest or pleasure in all, or almost all, activities most of the day.
3. Significant weight loss or weight gain when not dieting (more than 5% of body weight in a month) or a decrease or increase in appetite.

545

4. Insomnia or hypersomnia.
5. Psychomotor agitation or retardation.
6. Fatigue or loss of energy.
7. Feelings of worthlessness, or excessive or inappropriate guilt.
8. Diminished ability to think or concentrate.
9. Recurrent thoughts of death.[13]

When depression occurs, a search for possible medications that may induce depression should be performed. Aldomet, the traditional drug of choice for hypertension, has been associated with depression.

Postpartum blues and postpartum depression have been linked with important hormonal changes in the puerperium.[14] The postpartum "blues" are estimated to affect between 40% and 85% of women who give birth.[15] The symptoms include sadness, crying spells, irritability, anxiety, mood lability, confusion, and sleep and appetite disturbances.[16] Typically, these symptoms begin during the first postpartum week and then quickly decline.[17] The primary factors that differentiate this from a major depressive disorder are (1) the short-lived nature of the blues, and (2) no loss of self-esteem.[18]

Although pregnancy is a time of happiness, it is also a time of fear and change. The first trimester can be marked with anxiety regarding the threat of miscarriage, the perceived diminished standard of living that will occur, or simply the change in status and life patterns.[19] The last 3 months are a time of fatigue. The pregnant woman feels bulky and clumsy. Her sleep patterns are disturbed. Life becomes unpredictable, and she begins to need to rely on others. There is a fear of the actual delivery and of hospitalization.[8]

In the postpartum period, there are very real physical consequences to deal with. These include:

1. Painful episiotomy
2. Incontinence
3. Hemorrhoids
4. Breast engorgement
5. Cracked nipples
6. Backache
7. Fatigue[20]

When depression is diagnosed early in pregnancy, visual and verbal feedback with ultrasound evaluation of the fetus has been shown to improve the abnormal mood state.[21] Fear concerning the question of "is my baby normal?" can create significant anxiety and depression. One study reported patients undergoing a chorionic villus sampling were noted to have a reduction in anxiety up to 10 weeks earlier than women undergoing an amniocentesis.[22]

Treatment. There are five interventions for depression:

1. Psychotherapy
2. Pharmacotherapy
3. A combination of psychotherapy and pharmacotherapy
4. Electroconvulsive therapy
5. Phototherapy

Most patients with a major depressive disorder respond partially to medication within 2 to 3 weeks and achieve full remission within 6 to 8 weeks. Likewise, these patients receiving psychotherapy also respond partially to psychotherapy within 5 to 6 weeks and fully by 10 to 12 weeks.[10]

A complete review of the obstetric history should be performed before assuming care of a pregnant patient in labor. When greeting the patient, it is important to make her feel comfortable and to prepare her for the procedures to be performed. Most patients will respond to reassurance, careful listening to their fears and physical discomforts, and a validation that it is "okay to feel this way." Complications during labor and delivery, such as preeclampsia, eclampsia, fetal distress, cesarean section, fetal anomalies, or fetal injuries may place women at an increased risk for postpartum depression.[8,9] Postpartum complaints of a headache or backache may be the first symptoms to appear in a depressive episode.

Bipolar (manic depressive) disorders

Incidence. Bipolar disease affects the sexes equally, with a lifetime prevalence between 0.8% and 1.2%.[10] The mean age of onset of bipolar disease is in the twenties. Morbidity and mortality can be high, for as many as 10% to 15% of untreated patients commit suicide (this is 15 to 20 times higher than the suicide rate in the general population). Bipolar disorders classically feature episodes of major depression interspersed with episodes of mania and/or hypomania. The DSM-III-R criteria for a manic episode include:

Clinical features
1. A discrete period of abnormal, persistently elevated, expansive, or irritable mood
2. At least three of the following in the same period:
   a. Inflated self-esteem/grandiosity
   b. Significant decrease in need for sleep
   c. Much more talkative (pressured speech) than usual
   d. Flight of ideas
   e. Pronounced distractibility
   f. Increased goal-directed activity/psychomotor agitation
   g. Excessive involvement in pleasurable activi-

ties without regard for negative consequences (e.g., unrestrained buying sprees, sexual indiscretions, foolish business ventures)
3. Symptoms severe enough to significantly impair function or require hospitalization to prevent harm to self or others
4. The condition is not caused by schizophrenia, schizoeffective disorders, or substance abuse.[13] These rapid cyclings involve four or more mood episodes per year. Bipolar disease usually responds well to lithium. The effects of lithium in pregnancy and the anesthetic management of a patient receiving lithium are discussed elsewhere in this chapter.

NON–MOOD DISORDERS

Obstetricians and obstetrical anesthesiologists will also encounter non–mood disorders in pregnancy. There are six main non–mood disorders:

Clinical features
1. Eating disorders. The eating disorders include anorexia nervosa and bulimia. They occur in up to 1% of the general population and are very difficult to manage during pregnancy. They may present as hyperemesis that does not respond to conventional management. These should be managed in conjunction with a psychiatrist.
2. Obsessive/compulsive disorders. An obsessive/compulsive disorder is a condition characterized by the presence of obsessions and/or compulsions. Obsessions are recurrent, intrusive thoughts—usually irrational worries—that often necessitate behaviors to prevent untoward consequences (e.g., fears of contamination from dirt, requiring the individual to wear gloves at all times). Compulsions are recurrent behaviors beyond the normal range that the individual feels compelled to undertake, usually to preserve personal safety, to avoid embarrassment, or to perform adequately (e.g., checking numerous times to see if the gas is turned off before leaving home). This disorder affects 1% to 2% of the population and has a high frequency of co-occurring with depression. A recent report revealed that 39% of obsessive/compulsive disorder patients develop their obsessive/compulsive disorder during pregnancy.[23]
3. Personality disorders. This is defined as a chronic expression of a learned behavior that deviates markedly from the expectations of the individual's culture. Personality disorders are estimated to occur in at least 10% of the population.[24] The DSM-III-R personality disorders are grouped into three clusters:
Cluster A: Paranoid, schizoid
Cluster B: Antisocial, histrionic, narcissistic

Cluster C: Avoidant, dependent, passive/aggressive
4. Generalized anxiety disorders are the most common disease affecting mental health. Its prevalence in females (9.7%) is higher than males (4.7%). More important, however, is that only 23% have received treatment.[25]
5. Panic disorders. A panic disorder is an anxiety disorder characterized by discrete, intense periods of fear and associated symptoms. A panic disorder may be accompanied by agoraphobia. Panic disorders affect about 1% to 2% of the general population. They are not infrequently encountered in the operating room when a patient is being prepared for a cesarean section. In such a situation, the epidural catheter has been placed and the patient's arms are secured in an outstretched manner. This feeling of claustrophobia induces a panic attack. These attacks can be induced in more than 70% of panic disorder patients by an infusion of sodium lactate.[26] For that reason, if a patient develops a panic attack during the labor and delivery experience, lactate should be removed from the intravenous fluids. Estrogen has been suggested to be a panicogenic hormone, and its significant rise in pregnancy is the primary reason that pregnancy has been proposed to be a panic-prone state.[27] Progesterone may be a natural anxiolytic that may actually reduce panic and related symptoms.[28]

POSTPARTUM PSYCHOSIS

Postpartum psychosis refers to the presence of hallucinations or delusions. Numerous studies confirm the incidence in the pregnant population is constant at 2 to 4 per thousand.[29] Risk factors for postpartum psychosis are:

1. A previous psychiatric history (present in 98% of cases)
2. A complication during the first 3 months or last 3 months of pregnancy
3. A high proportion of unpleasant or abnormal experiences during labor
4. Conflicts related to family or marriage
5. Physical puerperal illness, trauma, infection, anemia

Although postpartum psychoses are rare, Kendell reported a twentyfold increase in admissions for psychosis within 30 days of childbirth when compared with the normal rate in the general population.[30] Postpartum psychosis requires psychiatric hospitalization. Generally, the prognosis is good. Physical complaints associated with psychotic behavior should be thoroughly evaluated. There have been unusual reports of a chronic subdural hematoma presenting as puerperal psychosis.[31]

Maternal response to perinatal death

Perinatal death can occur as a spontaneous abortion, an induced abortion for the prenatal diagnosis of a fetal anomaly, a stillbirth, or an unexpected neonatal death. These are commonplace events in the practice of any obstetrician and anesthesiologist. Accompanying these events are uncertainties about what one should do for a grieving patient who has experienced a perinatal death. Should the event be discussed with the patient after delivery? Does the couple want to view the baby? These and other questions concerning perinatal death will be discussed in this section.

Grieving is a normal healthy process after the loss of a life. It is not unexpected that women who experience a perinatal death will grieve. Zeahan compared the grief responses of women who terminated their pregnancies after abnormal prenatal diagnosis of fetal anomaly with women who experienced a spontaneous perinatal loss. Women in the prenatal diagnosis group were different from the spontaneous group because they had to make the difficult decision to terminate the pregnancy. Once the decision to terminate the pregnancy was made, they next had to choose between a dilation and evacuation (D&E) or a prostaglandin (PGE$_2$) induction of labor. Younger women and women who experienced other stressful life events in the past year had a more intense grieving process and a higher level of depression. Interestingly, there was not a significant difference between women who elected a D&E and those who chose a PGE$_2$ induction. However, a woman who underwent a D&E regretted not being able to see her baby. All of the women who underwent a PGE$_2$ induction saw and held their babies without regret. This study illustrated that women who terminate their pregnancies because of diagnosed fetal anomalies and women with spontaneous perinatal loss undergo similar patterns of grieving and depression but generally have a good outcome.[32] These findings should prompt clinicians to offer anticipatory grief counseling to these women and to support the decision they have made.

The psychological adjustment to perinatal death occurs differently among women. The following patient characteristics were studied by Graham and were found to influence the degree of depression associated with a fetal death. Women who are married and those who have demonstrated the ability to deliver a healthy baby are significantly less depressed than single primiparous women who experience a fetal death. Women who blame themselves for the loss, as opposed to attributing the death to God, can be expected to be more depressed. Interestingly, pictures of the deceased infant helped to significantly reduce the amount of depression measured. Women in this investigation consistently benefited from outward shows of sympathy from the medical staff and being kept informed of any problems that developed during their pregnancy.[33] Women who were told that "everything is alright" with the pregnancy but who went on to experience a fetal death resented the false reassurance they had been given. This investigation supports the intuitive thoughts of many clinicians and offers help in identifying patients who may experience significantly greater depression.

When a couple experiences a perinatal death, the benefits of proactive, rather than reactive, psychological patient management are appreciated and will aid patients with their grieving. Kellner reported the results of a Perinatal Mortality Counseling Program in treating 165 families. The Perinatal Mortality Counseling Program consisted of an obstetrician, a pathologist, a social worker, and a psychologist. Kellner wanted to let parents make their own choice on how to deal with their baby's death. He measured specific patient requests concerning seeing the baby, holding the baby, having an autopsy, disposing of the remains, returning to postpartum, and accepting follow-up counseling. Ninety percent of parents chose to see their baby regardless of its appearance. Half of the parents held their babies. The babies were wrapped in an infant blanket and presented to the families, taking care to point out the normal features and simply explaining any maceration or abnormalities. Families tend to remember the normal aspects of the dead baby. The deceased baby was named by 85% of women who had other children at home and by 70% of women without other children. Women with other children at home named their baby so their other children would know they had a brother or sister who died. A funeral or memorial service was chosen more in women who had had a longer gestation and who had asked to see and hold their baby. Interestingly, none of the parents who elected *not* to see their baby chose a funeral or memorial service. If an autopsy was done, the majority of families selected cremation rather than a funeral service.[34] Allowing families to make choices in a professional atmosphere, with the goal of helping them deal with their perinatal death, helped them adjust to their situation. Families should be given the choice to see, hold, and name the baby. In addition, assistance should be offered in decisions about cremation, funeral, and a memorial service. Parents have been shown to resent being left alone to deal with the death of their babies and attempts to discharge them early. The choices being made by parents should help us anticipate the needs of families experiencing a perinatal death.

Within the family unit mothers tend to show depression early, within the first 6 weeks after delivery, while symptoms were delayed in fathers.[35] The delay in paternal depression occurred at a mean of 25 months following the loss.

Speculation as to the delay in paternal depression centers on the belief that fathers may feel so compelled to support their wives during the initial grieving process that not until later does their need for social support become apparent. Married couples tend to support each other through the grieving process, and although there is obvious stress with a perinatal death, this life event typically acts to strengthen a couple's relationship. Recognition by a family that during the first 6 weeks after a fetal death the mother is usually more depressed, and that the social needs for coping become more evident later for the father, will help in counseling families after a perinatal death.

When a couple has experienced a perinatal loss with a previous pregnancy, stress and anxiety about the current pregnancy is common. The parturient will feel this anxiety to a greater degree than the father. In fact, pregnant women who have experienced a previous perinatal loss differ significantly from pregnant women who have not, when measured with anxiety testing.[36] Fathers in both groups do not differ when anxiety levels are measured. Fathers who have experienced a previous perinatal loss see this new pregnancy as unencumbered by the previous loss. Clinically, women who experienced a previous perinatal loss will benefit from reinforcement, when appropriate, that they are expected to carry the current pregnancy to term and that any problems that arise will be discussed.

The story of a young Hispanic couple that delivered a stillbirth child was published on the front page of *The Wall Street Journal*. The couple experienced a perinatal loss at 8 months' gestation. After a PGE$_2$ induction, a 4-pound 2-ounce stillborn girl was delivered. The couple was given an opportunity to hold the baby, they received a photograph of the baby, and they named her (Frances Elaine); they also consented to an autopsy. The problem arose when after the autopsy the couple was not given the opportunity to have a funeral Mass for their daughter. The hospital lost the baby. In addition, the autopsy report was not delivered to the couple until more than 4 years had elapsed after the stillbirth. Subsequently, the couple filed a negligence suit against the hospital 10 months after delivery. At issue is not the rights of a stillborn baby, but the rights of the couple, as survivors, to complete the grieving process with a funeral ceremony.[37]

In summary, families that experience a perinatal loss need to be dealt with in a direct, compassionate fashion. They have specific needs that should be met to help them with the grieving process intrapartum and postpartum.

Electroconvulsive therapy

Electroconvulsive therapy (ECT) was introduced in 1934 when the Hungarian psychiatrist Ladislus Meduna recognized that naturally occurring convulsions produced mental relief in some patients. ECT is designed to induce a grand mal seizure by means of an electric current applied across scalp electrodes. The convulsion, not the electrical current, is therapeutic through an unknown mechanism. Induction of seizure activity with an electrical stimulus produces a more reliable brief ictal response with fewer side effects than oil of camphor, insulin coma, or metrazol. In addition, the incidence of fetal morbidity was found to be 35% in pregnant women treated for depression by insulin coma.[38] Improvements in ECT include placement of a unilateral electrode on the nondominant hemisphere instead of bilateral placement, and use of pulsatile waveforms, which induce seizure activity with half the electrical energy of a sine-wave stimulus. Most therapies consist of 8 to 12 separate ECT sessions over several weeks.[39,40]

ECT is used primarily in patients suffering from depression and less frequently in schizophrenia, mania, and catatonic stupor.[41] ECT is most effective in severe major depressive episodes when rapid therapy is needed or when pharmacologic therapy has failed.[42] ECT is not indicated for treatment of anorexia nervosa, obsessional illnesses, psychogenic pain, or confusional states unless the patient is concomitantly depressed. ECT should never be used to control aggressive or violent behavior. ECT is a safe and effective therapy in pregnancy. Although there is no controlled study of ECT in pregnancy, numerous case reports exist supporting its safety in the mother and fetus.[38,39,43-47]

Contraindications to ECT are based on patient tolerance of the physiologic changes that occur during treatment. The electrical stimulus used to produce a grand mal seizure produces an increase in cerebral blood flow, cerebral oxygen consumption, and cerebrospinal-fluid pressure. The grand mal seizure consists of a 10-second tonic phase and a 30- to 50-second clonic phase. Activation of the autonomic nervous system begins during the tonic phase with a central vagal discharge characterized by bradycardia and a decrease in blood pressure. The sympathetic outflow characterized during the clonic phase is accompanied by a rise in circulating catacholamines,[45] hypertension, tachycardia, and rarely premature ventricular contractions and ventricular tachycardia. Asystole has been described to occur during subconvulsive ECT, presumably because the tonic (parasympathetic) phase occurs without opposition from the clonic (sympathetic) phase.[48] Oxytocin increases during ECT are small and transient and typically do not result in uterine contractions.[45] The only absolute contraindication to ECT is increased intracranial pressure. Of the deaths occurring during ECT, 85% result from cardiovascular or pulmonary factors. It follows that relative contraindications to ECT include recent myocardial infarction, coronary artery disease, congestive heart failure, bronchopulmonary disease, carotid stenosis, hypertension, and venous thrombosis. The potential of increased uterine activity points to placenta previa, incompetent cervix, history of premature labor, multiple gestation, and hydramnios as a relative contraindication to ECT. The sympathetic discharge that occurs during the clonic phase may result in a pronounced hypertensive response in the preeclamptic patient or in fetal morbidity in a mother with impaired uteroplacental perfusion. The presence of a cardiac pacemaker should not be considered a contraindication to ECT. These relative contraindications must be weighed against the benefits of ECT.[39] ECT is a relatively safe procedure with a mortality rate of 4.5 per 100,000 treatments.[49]

ECT during pregnancy has been shown to be safe and effective for both the mother and fetus in many case reports.[38,39,43-47] Because of the lack of a controlled study, obstetric and anesthetic management must be derived from the existing case reports and common sense. ECT is indicated in the severely depressed pregnant patient especially when rapid conversion is required, pharmacologic therapy has failed, and there is hesitancy to use psychotropic drugs during fetal organogenesis. The following guidelines address the special consideration a pregnant patient requires during ECT:

1. A psychiatrist, obstetrician, and anesthesiologist should all be members of the treatment team. ECT should be performed in a facility where all members of the treatment team can be assembled and a labor and delivery unit is in close proximity.

2. The obstetrician should begin with a complete obstetric history and physical examination of the patient. A maternal history of placenta previa, incompetent cervix, history of premature labor, multiple gestation, hydramnios, uteroplacental insufficiency, and preeclampsia are relative contraindications to ECT. Increased blood oxytocin levels[45] and uterine activity[47] described during ECT may adversely affect pregnancy outcome in patients with placenta previa, incompetent cer-

vix, history of premature labor, multiple gestation, or hydramnios. However, most case reports describe no increased uterine activity during ECT, and blood oxytocin levels undergo only small transient increases. A uterine tocolytic agent (terbutaline 0.25 mg intravenous) should eliminate the small risk of increased uterine activity in high-risk obstetric patients and prophylax the increased vagal tone during the tonic phase of ECT.

Increased blood catecholamine levels during ECT[45] may cause fetal compromise in a patient with uteroplacental insufficiency. A rise in maternal catecholamine levels may result in an amount of uterine artery vasoconstriction not tolerated by the fetus. Uterine and umbilical artery Doppler measurements in a 32-week gestation pregnancy showed a minor increased systolic-to-diastolic ratio and resistance index immediately after ECT.[45] Ultrasonography conducted during and immediately after ECT on a second-trimester patient showed no significant change in fetal movement or other activity. The same patient demonstrated a stable fetal heart rate during ECT.[43] Case reports indicate that ECT is safe for the fetus in patients without uteroplacental insufficiency. In patients in whom ECT therapy is strongly indicated and uteroplacental blood flow is suspected, measures to optimize fetal blood flow should be taken. These should include preoperative intravenous hydration, left-uterine displacement, continuous fetal and uterine monitoring, inhibition of the vagal tone during the tonic phase of ECT (atropine 0.4 mg intravenous), and use of a tocolytic agent if increased uterine activity is measured. Increased catecholamines may result in an exaggerated hypertensive response in the preeclamptic patient during the sympathetic discharge associated with the clonic phase of ECT. This can be treated with intravenous labetalol or trimethaphan.

3. Anesthetic management of ECT during pregnancy begins with a thorough anesthesia-focused history and physical examination. Drug interactions with current psychotropic medications should be understood before ECT begins (see section on psychotropic drugs). The airway examination is important because a rapid sequence induction is required for ECT in the pregnant patient. The anesthetic goals for ECT in the pregnant patient are to (1) provide oxygenation with a protected airway, (2) prevent recall, (3) prevent long bone fractures during tonic-clonic

contractures, (4) moderate hemodynamic responses, (5) optimize uteroplacental circulation, and (6) allow a rapid emergence. Standard intraoperative monitoring, a uterine tocodynamometer, and continuous external fetal monitoring should be used during ECT for the pregnant patient. Continuous fetal monitoring may be replaced with Doppler measurement of fetal heart sounds before and after the procedure in the previable fetus. Consultation with the obstetrician before ECT will help in the selection of appropriate fetal surveillance. Preoperative hydration (0.5 to 1 L isotonic crystalloid solution) and left uterine displacement will help prevent hypotension during the procedure.[43] Preoxygenation with a rapid sequence intubation is necessitated because of concerns about maternal aspiration and oxygenation. Methohexital (0.5 to 1.0 mg per kg) or thiopental (2 to 3 mg per kg) and succinylcholine (1.0 to 1.5 mg per kg) are acceptable induction agents. The primary function of succinylcholine is to provide optimal intubating conditions and to secondarily blunt the muscular response of the seizure. Inflation of a blood pressure cuff placed on the bicep or calf at twice the systolic pressure will allow for identification of seizure activity in the isolated extremity, attenuation of the muscular response in the important long bones, and use of a full intubation dose on induction. Ventilation should be controlled[50] with the same F_{IO_2} (greater than 50%) for all sessions. The use of 100% oxygen has been demonstrated to increase the duration of seizure activity, but only by a mean value of 18 seconds.[51] Consistent use of the same F_{IO_2} during all sessions of ECT with a patient is more important than the actual percent of oxygen (maintained at greater than 50%) delivered. Pretreatment with atropine or a tocolytic agent should be given immediately before ECT begins. After a seizure activity has been documented, the patient should be awake before extubation. Fetal monitoring should be continued for 1 to 2 hours after ECT because little is known about uterine physiology associated with ECT. The decision for further fetal monitoring in high-risk obstetric patients should be made by the obstetrician.

PSYCHOTROPIC DRUGS
Obstetric and anesthetic implications

The use of psychotropic drugs during pregnancy presents a dilemma to the clinician. How does one treat a pregnant woman suffering with psychopathology and at the same time protect the fetus from teratogenicity? How does one counsel a woman who has conceived and undergone a significant first-trimester exposure with psychotropic drugs? This section will address the teratogenic risk, maternal and neonatal side effects, and drug interactions of commonly used psychotropic medications in pregnancy (Table 29-1).

Lithium carbonate is an alkali metal used for the treatment of manic-depressive illness. The dose of lithium is usually increased in pregnancy to compensate for increased renal clearance. Lithium freely crosses the human placenta resulting in equal maternal, umbilical, and neonatal levels.[52,53]

The Register of Lithium Babies was established in 1968 to collect information on first-trimester exposure to lithium. Nora reported a fivefold increase in the expected frequency of congenital cardiovascular disease, and a 400-fold increase in the frequency of Ebstein's anomaly.[54] More recently, Elia reported on 9000 first-trimester lithium exposures and found a twentyfold increase in the occurrence of Ebstein's anomaly.[55] These data suggest that lithium should not be used in the first trimester unless it is absolutely necessary. If exposure to lithium has occurred in the first trimester, fetal echocardiography should be used to diagnosis the presence of a cardiac anomaly and counseling should be offered to the parents.

The neonate can manifest signs of lithium toxicity at therapeutic maternal levels. The neonate can appear flaccid, jaundice, cyanotic, and lethargic with poor sucking and Moro reflexes.[56] Reversible thyroid dysfunction and diabetes insipidus as well as cardiac arrhythmias have been reported to occur in exposed neonates.[57,58] There is no evidence to support the role of lithium as a behavioral teratogen.[59] The concentration of lithium in breast milk is about 50% that of maternal serum.[60] Because the effect of subtherapeutic lithium levels in the infant are unknown, caution is advised in the breastfeeding mother treated with lithium.

Anesthetic implications in the use of lithium begin with patient evaluation for diabetes insipidus and hypothyroidism.[61] Chronic therapy with lithium can produce benign reversible depression of T waves, and patients susceptible to ST depression during anesthesia.[62] Lithium may also prolong the actions of both depolarizing and nondepolarizing muscle relaxants and potentiate barbiturates. Lithium therapy should not be discontinued prior to anesthesia, but the dose should be reduced to its lowest therapeutic level.

Carbamazepine is indicated in the treatment of trigeminal neuralgia, epilepsy, bipolar depression, psychosis, and alcohol withdrawal. Carbamazepine, thought to be free from teratogenic potential,

Table 29-1 Psychotropic medications

Drug	Indication	Anesthetic interactions	Toxicity	Teratogenicity
Lithium carbonate	Bipolar disease	Potentiates the action of muscle relaxants and barbiturates; ST depression during anesthesia	*Maternal:* diabetes insipidus, hypothyroidism *Neonatal:* lethargy, cyanosis, jaundice, cardiac arrhythmias, hypothyroidism	Cardiac anomalies, especially Ebstein's anomaly
Carbamazepine	Epilepsy, trigeminal neuralgia, bipolar disease, psychosis, alcohol withdrawal	None	Aplastic anemia, thrombocytopenia, oliguria, jaundice, hypertension, left ventricular failure	Craniofacial and limb malformation, developmental delay
Valproic acid	Epilepsy, bipolar disease	None	*Maternal:* nausea and vomiting, impaired platelet aggregation, hepatotoxicity *Neonatal:* hepatotoxicity, hyperglycemia[22]	Neural tube defects[59]
Tricyclics Amitriptyline Clomipramine Desipramine Doxepin Imipramine Nortriptyline Protriptyline Trimipramine	Unipolar depression	Indirect vasopressors, halothane and pancuronium, scopolamine, opioids, barbiturates, MAOIs	*Maternal:* sedation, tachycardia, decreased GI motility *Neonatal:* urinary retention, seizures, cyanosis, hypertonia, tachyarrhythmia	No positive correlation with a congenital anomaly
Phenothiazines Chlorpromazine Thioridazine Fluphenazine Perphenazine Trifluoperazine Methotrimeprazine Oxomemazine Trimeprazine tartrate	Antipsychotic medication	Potentiates respiratory depressant, sedative, and analgesic actions of opioids	*Maternal:* sedation, extrapyramidal, NMS, hypotension, jaundice *Neonatal:* extrapyramidal, jaundice, respiratory depression	Increased risk with chlorpromazine
Butyrophenones Halperidol Droperidol	Antipsychotic medication, unipolar and bipolar disease	Neuroleptic anesthesia combined with fentanyl	*Maternal:* hypotension, increased Q-T, extrapyramidal, tardive dyskinesia *Neonatal:* none reported	None reported in limited investigations
Serotonin uptake inhibitors Fluoxetine (Prozac) Paroxetine Sertraline	Unipolar depression	Rare occurrence of an increased bleeding time	*Maternal:* anxiety, increased appetite *Neonatal:* none reported	No increased risk of major malformations reported in limited investigations
MAO inhibitors Isocarboxazid Phenelzine Tranylcypromine Selegilline	depression, obsessive-compulsive and appetite disorders, hypertension	Excitatory response with meperidine, tyramine-induced hypertension, exaggerated response to ephedrine	*Maternal:* orthostatic hypotension, sedation, blurred vision, dry mouth *Neonatal:* none reported	Increased risk of malformations

was considered to be a safer alternative than lithium in pregnant women with a bipolar disorder.[59] Placental transfer of carbamazepine occurs freely, resulting in nearly equal maternal and umbilical blood levels.[63] Jones studied 80 infants exposed prenatally to carbamazepine.[64] A pattern of craniofacial and limb malformations and of developmental delay was found. Carbamazepine is particularly teratogenic if prenatal exposure occurs when it is used in combination with phenobarbital and valproic acid.[65] Carbamazepine should be considered to be a human teratogen.

Tricyclic antidepressant drugs are the most prescribed and studied psychotropic medications used during pregnancy, especially nortriptiline and desipramine. However, it is not known whether all tricyclic antidepressants share the same ability as imipramine for placental transfer.[66]

Teratogenic effects of first-trimester exposure to tricyclic antidepressants studied in a small prospective study (19 women taking imipramine and 28 women using amitriptyline) and in a larger investigation of 15,000 births showed no evidence of gross congenital abnormalities.[59,60] Isolated case reports do exist that associate fetal tricyclic exposure with diaphragmatic hernia, hypospadias limb and craniofacial deformities, meningocele, hydrocephalus, and cardiac anomalies.[67-69] Retrospective investigation of limb abnormalities found no association with tricyclic exposure.[59] Tricyclic antidepressants have maintained widespread use during pregnancy without evidence of major teratogenic effects. The teratogenic risk of tricyclic antidepressants should be considered to be small to nonexistent.

Neonatal effects of maternal tricyclic therapy may be apparent in the immediate postpartum period. The anticholinergic effects of tricyclic antidepressants have manifested as neonatal urinary retention, tachycardia, hypotonia, myoclonus, and heart failure, all of which have been reported.[60] A fetal tachyarrhythmia of greater than 180 beats per minute has been attributed to maternal tricyclic treatment. The tachyarrhythmia resolved when maternal tricyclic therapy was discontinued.[71] Neonatal withdrawal symptoms include tachypnea, tachycardia, hypertonia, and seizures.[59] Clinical judgment suggests that neonatal toxicity and withdrawal symptoms can be minimized if tricyclic medications are tapered and discontinued 1 to 2 weeks before delivery.

Maternal side effects of tricyclic antidepressants manifest as anticholinergic or sedative effects. Sedation, decreased intestinal motility, tachycardia, and orthostatic hypotension can be additive to already normal symptoms seen in pregnancy. The interactions of tricyclic antidepressants with anesthetic drugs are important. Tricyclic agents inhibit the uptake of norepinephrine into the postganglionic sympathetic nerve ending. The use of an indirect sympathomimetic, ephedrine, will result in an exaggerated increase in maternal blood pressure. Phenylephrine used in 40-μg boluses to correct maternal hypotension would produce an appropriate rise in blood pressure. The combination of imipramine, pancuronium, and halothane resulted in an increased incidence of tachyarrhythmias in anesthetized dogs.[72] In addition, the dose of epinephrine required to produce ventricular dysrhythmias is reduced during anesthesia with volatile anesthetic agents.[73] The anticholinergic effect of tricyclic antidepressants (especially amitriptyline) may be additive with centrally active anticholinergic drugs (scopolamine and atropine). Central anticholinergic syndrome manifests as delirium or prolonged somnolence following anesthesia. Tricyclic antidepressants may augment the analgesic and ventilatory depressant effects of opioids and the sedative effect of barbiturates.[74] Nortriptiline and desipramine are the tricyclics most recommended during pregnancy because they are well studied and their side effects are usually well tolerated during pregnancy.

Phenothiazine drugs are antipsychotic agents that produce their clinical effect by dopaminergic blockade. Phenothiazine drugs are known to freely cross the placenta.[59,60] A large prospective study, following first-trimester exposure to phenothiazines, found a significant increase in major congenital anomalies when exposure occurred with phenothiazine members containing a 3-carbon aliphatic side chain (chlorpromazine, methotrimeprazine, timeprazine tartrate, and oxomemazine).[75] The congenital anomalies occurred in the central nervous, cardiovascular, digestive, musculoskeletal, and genitourinary tract systems. Among the phenothiazines indicated, only chlorpromazine is used as an antipsychotic in the United States. Promethazine was not associated with an increased risk of congenital malformations. A study of 19,952 women exposed to phenothiazines in the first trimester initially found no significant increase in the incidence of congenital anomalies when compared with controls,[76] but when the data were reanalyzed an increased risk for anomalies was found with phenothiazine exposure.[77] Phenothiazine antidepressants containing the 3-carbon aliphatic side chain (chlorpromazine) should thus be avoided during the first trimester if possible. Other phenothiazine antidepressants have not been shown to impart an increased risk of teratogenicity at this time, but they are not as widely studied as chlorpromazine and have not yet been proved safe.

Neonatal side effects of phenothiazine agents include jaundice, respiratory depression, intestinal hypomotility, and extrapyramidal syndrome. Extrapyramidal syndrome is manifested by tremors, flapping of the hands, hypertonia, arching of the back, and persistent crying. Extrapyramidal symptoms usually begin during the first days of life and may persist for up to 6 months. This reaction displays a familial tendency.[59]

Maternal side effects such as sedation, decreased gastric motility, and orthostatic hypotension compound these symptoms routinely seen during pregnancy. Extrapyramidal effects are characterized as facial grimacing, torticollis, and tardive dyskinesa. Treatment of extrapyramidal side effects during pregnancy can be hazardous to the fetus. Diphenhydramine and anticholinergic agents have been associated with morphologic teratogenicity.[59] Maternal diphenhydramine administration can result in neonatal withdrawal, which is characterized by tremulousness and diarrhea. Routine prophylaxis of extrapyramidal side effects is not recommended during pregnancy. Other measures to improve maternal symptoms include calcium supplementation with prenatal vitamins and lowering the dose or switching to another less potent antipsychotic medication. If extrapyramidal symptoms do require treatment, an attempt should be made to discontinue the anticholinergic medication or the diphenhydramine 2 weeks before delivery.[59] Other maternal side effects of phenothiazine antidepressants include increased prolactin secretion, jaundice, anticholinergic effects, hypothermia, decreased seizure threshold, urticaria, skeletal muscle relaxation, and neuroleptic malignant syndrome. Neuroleptic malignant syndrome can appear more severe during pregnancy. Drug interactions with anesthetic medications can produce a potentiation of the ventilatory depressant as well as miotic, sedative, and analgesic actions of opioids.[74]

Butyrophenone agents are antipsychotic medications that produce their effect through dopaminergic antagonism. Few reports exist of their use in pregnant psychiatric patients. However, a retrospective study concerning the use of haloperidol for the treatment of hyperemesis gravidarium found no increased intrauterine or neonatal morbidity associated with its use, compared with controls.[78] A case report documented a 35-year-old woman suffering from manic illness, whose treatment was converted from lithium to low-dose haloperidol before conception. The patient went on to deliver a healthy baby well controlled with haloperidol. Haloperidol can be a successful alternative to lithium prophylaxis when treating unipolar mania or bipolar disease.[79] Droperidol is not indicated for use as an antipsychotic medication. However,

it is effective as an antiemetic agent and for the production of neuroleptic anesthesia.

Butyrophenone agents, similar to other dopaminergic antagonists, can produce extrapyramidal side effects, which should be treated as recommended in the discussion on phenothiazines. Tardive dyskinesia, a rhythmical involuntary movement of the tongue, face, and mouth, can appear in patients treated with haloperidol, especially elderly women undergoing long-term therapy.

Hypotension resulting from a peripheral alpha-adrenergic blockade, hypertension, prolonged Q-T interval, and a polymorphous ECG pattern similar to *torsades de pointes* have all been described with use of butyrophenone medication. Ventilation may appear to be of increased depth because of an increased sensitivity of the carotid bodies to hypoxemia.[74] The interactions of butyrophenone agents in the pregnant patient have not been as well investigated as have other psychotropic medications. The few investigations addressing the use of butyrophenone antidepressants during pregnancy support their use, with the lowest possible dose for those patients who will clearly benefit.

Serotonin uptake inhibitors are indicated for treatment of unipolar depression and antiobsessive-compulsive action. Fluoxetine (Prozac) acts to block the uptake of neuronal serotonin in the central nervous system (CNS). It is the most widely prescribed and studied of these medications. There are limited reports assessing the teratogenic potential of fluoxetine. In an investigation in which rats and rabbits were treated with 9 and 11 times the maximal daily human dose of fluoxetine, no increased fetal or pregnancy toxicity was demonstrated.[80] A prospective analysis conducted at four centers compared the rate of major birth defects, pregnancy outcome, and maternal obstetric demographics in a group of first-trimester exposures to fluoxetine a group of first-trimester exposures to tricyclic antidepressants, and nonteratogen controls. There was no difference in the rate of major birth defects, miscarriages, pregnancy outcome, maternal weight gain, gestational age at delivery, birth weight, or delivery type among the three groups. However, there was an increased trend in the rate of miscarriages in the fluoxetine and tricyclic antidepressant groups. This increased trend may be a result of a defect in study design, in which pregnancy terminations were reported in terms of miscarriages, or of an increased rate of miscarriages in psychiatrically depressed women, or of a real risk of first-trimester exposure to these medications. There are no neonatal side effects or withdrawal symptoms reported with serotonin uptake inhibitors. In summary, fluoxetine use during organogensis has not been associated with an increased risk of major malformations.

Common maternal side effects of fluoxetine include anxiety, increased appetite, and emotional lability. Significant cardiovascular or pulmonary adverse effects are rare with fluoxetine use. Blockade of serotonin uptake into platelets by fluoxetine may be the mechanism for the rare occurrence of an increased bleeding time. Significant anesthetic drug interactions with fluoxetine have not been reported.

Monoamine oxidase inhibitors (MAOI) increase intraneuronal levels of neurotransmitters (serotonin, norepinephrine, epinephrine, dopamine, and octopamine) by irreversibly binding to the enzyme MAO. They are indicated for the treatment of depression, hypertension, obsessive-compulsive tendencies, and appetite disorders. MAOIs are known teratogens in animals; in a small prospective study tranylcypromine (a popular MAOI) was associated with malformations in humans.[59] In the pregnant patient tricyclic antidepressants are a better choice in the treatment of depression than MAOIs because of their low teratogenic risk.

In addition, MAOIs remain a poor choice because of their significant interactions with other drugs. Hypotension in the pregnant patient is typically treated with ephedrine, an indirect-acting sympathomimetic, because uteroplacental blood flow is not compromised. If a pregnant patient treated with an MAOI is given ephedrine, an exaggerated release of vasoactive intraneuronal neurotransmitters will occur, resulting in an unpredictable increase in blood pressure. An exaggerated increase in maternal blood pressure may compromise uteroplacental blood flow. Phenylephrine, a direct-acting sympathomimetic agent, administered in boluses of 40 μg would be an excellent choice for treating hypotension in a pregnant patient receiving MAOIs.[82] Meperidine is a commonly administered intrapartum analgesic. Meperidine impairs the neuronal uptake of serotonin.[74] If cerebral serotonin levels are increased to a critical level, a potentially fatal excitatory response will occur. This excitatory response is characterized by hyperthermia, hypertension, hypotension, depressed ventilation, skeletal muscle rigidity, seizures, coma, and potentially death. This response occurs in approximately 20% of patients receiving MAOIs administered meperidine.[83] Morphine and fentanyl appear to be safe alternative analgesic agents in patients chronically treated (longer than 3 weeks) with MAOIs.[84] Tricyclic antidepressants and serotonin uptake inhibitors block neuronal uptake of neurotransmitters. MAOIs produce an accumulation of these neurotransmitters. The release of increased amine neurotransmitters combined with impaired neuronal uptake presents the potential for a fatal drug interaction between MAOIs, tricyclic antidepressants, and serotonin uptake inhibitors. Tyramine, normally metabolized by MAO in the gastrointestinal tract and liver, produces a release of endogenous catecholamines. Normal metabolism of tyramine (contained in cheese, chicken liver, chocolate, beer, and wine) is impaired in patients treated with MAOIs. The increased release of endogenous amine neurotransmitters by tyramine-containing foods in patients treated with MAOIs can result in a life-threatening hypertensive response.[74] This would put both mother and fetus at risk. MAOI inhibition of hepatic enzymes is the proposed mechanism of the exaggerated depressant produced by opioids and barbiturates.[83] The numerous potentially fatal drug interactions and risk of teratogenicity make MAOIs a poor choice in the pregnant patient.

Pseudocyesis

Pseudocyesis is derived from the Greek words *pseudes* (false) and *kyesis* (pregnancy). It is a condition in which a woman or man[85] firmly believes herself or himself to be pregnant and develops objective signs of pregnancy in the absence of pregnancy. Pseudocyesis was first described by Hippocrates in 300 BC. Since then several hundred cases of pseudocyesis have been reported in the literature. The rate of pseudocyesis ranges from 1 in 200 maternity clinic admissions to 1 in 4000 births.[86] The patient age can range from 7 to 79, with an average age of 33. The majority of the women are married, with symptoms lasting 9 months in about half of them, but symptoms have been documented to last several years.

Clinical features and diagnosis. The symptomatology, in order of decreasing frequency, occurs as follows:

1. *Abdominal enlargement,* usually resulting from exaggerated lordosis and retention of waste products.
2. *Abnormal menses,* most frequently seen as amenorrhea.
3. Patient perception of *fetal movements.*
4. *Gastrointestinal symptoms,* manifested as nausea and vomiting and increased appetite.
5. Breast swelling, breast tenderness, and areolar pigmentation, as well as labor pains and uterine enlargement, have all been reported.[85,86]

The diagnosis of pseudocyesis is easily made today with a blood test for chorionic gonadotropin as well as abdominal or vaginal ultrasound. A physical diagnosis sign thought to be pathognomic for pseudocyesis is an inverted umbilicus.[87] Other disorders mistaken for pseudocyesis include ectopic pregnancy, a corpus luteum cyst, gestational trophoblastic disease, morbid obesity, ascites, central nervous system tumors, pelvic tumors, and drug side effects.[86,87]

The basis of pseudocyesis is psychologic, but a single psychologic process does not exist for these patients. In fact, most of these patients do not appear psychotic. Pseudocyesis can be viewed as a conversion syndrome motivated by narcissism, dependency, body image, power, and guilt. A conversion syndrome is a condition in which a functional aberration occurs that is not explained by normal physiologic arguments. Narcissistic motivation can derive from the personal and social (marriage) gratification of pregnancy. Pregnancy can also provide a woman with the power to dominate a relationship or motivate a couple to marry. In some cases the hope of pregnancy can help a woman cope with guilt from some other source.[86,87] Psychotherapy is a useful tool in the ultimate treatment of these patients.

REFERENCES

1. Saks BR, Frank JB, Lowe TL: Depressed mood during pregnancy and the puerperium: Clinical recognition and implications for clinical practice. *Am J Psychiatry* 1985; 142:728.
2. Schaper AM, Rooney BL, Kay NR, et al: Use of the Edinburgh postnatal depression scale to identify postpartum depression in a clinical setting. *J Reprod Med* 1994; 39(8):620.
3. *ACOG Technical Bulletin* No. 182; July., 1993.
4. Misri S, Sivertz K: Tricyclic drugs in pregnancy and lactation: A preliminary report. *Int J Psychiatry Med* 1991; 21(2):157.
5. Tunis SL, Golbus MS: Assessing mood states in pregnancy: Survey of the literature. *Obstet Gynecol Surv* 1991; 46(6):340.
6. Ballard CG, Davis R, Cullen PC, et al: Prevalence of postnatal psychiatric morbidity in mothers and fathers. *Br J Psychiatry* 1994; 164:782.
7. Gitlin MJ, Pasnau RO: Psychiatric syndromes linked to reproductive function in women: A review of current knowledge. *Am J Psychiatry* 1989; 146:1413.
8. Tylden E: Psychiatric disorders including drug therapy and addiction. *Clin Obstet Gynecol* 1977; 4(2):435.
9. Burger JA, Horwitz SM, Forsyth WC, et al: Psychological sequelae of medical complications during pregnancy. *Obstet Gynecol Surv* 1993; 48(10):649.
10. *Depression in Primary Care: Vol. 1: Detection and Diagnosis.* U.S. Department of Health and Human Services, AHCPR Publication No. 93-0550; April, 1993.
11. Zuckerman B, Amaro H, Bauchner H, et al: Depressive symptoms during pregnancy: Relationship to poor health behaviors. *Am J Obstet Gynecol* 1989; 160:1107.
12. Wolman WL, Chalmers B, Hofmeyr GJ, et al: Postpartum depression and companionship in the clinical birth environment: A randomized, controlled study. *Am J Obstet Gynecol* 1993; 168:1388.
13. *American Psychiatric Association Diagnostic and Statistical Manual of Mental Disorders,* ed 3. Washington, DC, American Psychiatric Press, 1987.
14. Harris B, Lovett L, Newcombe RG: Maternity blues and major endocrine changes: Cardiff puerperal mood and hormone study II. *Br Med J* 1994; 308:949.
15. Quadagno DM, Dixon LA, Denney NW, et al: Postpartum moods in men and women. *Am J Obstet Gynecol* 1986; 154:1018.
16. Coyne JC, Schwenk TL: Depression in the female patient. The Female Patient 1994; 19:59.
17. O'Hara MW, Engeldinger J: Postpartum mood disorders—Detection and prevention. The Female Patient 1989; 14:19.
18. O'Hara MW: Social support, life events, and depression during pregnancy and the puerperium. *Arch Gen Psychiatry* 1986; 43:569.
19. Standley K, Soule B, Copans S: Dimensions of prenatal anxiety and their influence on pregnancy outcome. *Am J Obstet Gynecol* 1979; 135:22.
20. Romito P: Unhappiness after childbirth. *Effective Care in Pregnancy and Childbirth,* Oxford University Press, 1991.
21. Michelacci L, Fava GA, Grandi S, et al: Psychological reactions to ultrasound. *Psychother Psychosom* 1988; 50:1.
22. Spencer JW, Cox DN: Emotional responses of pregnant women to chorionic villi sampling or amniocentesis. *Am J Obstet Gynecol* 1987; 157:1155.
23. Neziroglu F, Anemone R, Yaryura-Tobias JA: Onset of obsessive-compulsive disorder in pregnancy. *Am J Psychiatry* 1992; 149:947.
24. Oldham JM: Personality disorders: Current perspectives. *JAMA* 1994; 272:1770.
25. Leaman TL: Anxiety disorders: Reaching the untreated. *Female Patient* 1983; 18:78.
26. McArthur P, Kellner CH, Pritchett JT: Panic induced by lactate infusion during electroconvulsive therapy. *J Nerv Ment Dis* 1994; 182(1):55.
27. Ware MR, DeVane CL: Imipramine treatment of panic disorder during pregnancy. *J Clin Psychiatry* 1990; 51:482.
28. Villeponteaux VA, Lydiard RB, Laraia MT: The effects of pregnancy on pre-existing panic disorder. *J Clin Psychiatry* 1992; 53:201.
29. Gottlieb SE, Barrett DE: Effects of unanticipated cesarean section on mothers, infants, and their interaction in the first month of life. 1986; 7(3):180.
30. Kendell RE, Chalmers JC, Platz C: Epidemiology of puerperal psychosis. *Br J Psychiatry* 1987; 150:662.
31. Campbell DA: Chronic subdural hematoma following epidural anaesthesia presenting as puerperal psychosis. *Br J Obstet Gynecol* 1993; 100:782.
32. Zeahan CH, Dailey JV, Rosenblatt M, et al: Do women grieve after terminating pregnancies because of fetal anomalies? *Obstet Gynecol* 1993; 82:270.
33. Graham MA, Thompson SC, Estrada M, et al: Factors affecting psychological adjustment to a fetal death. *Am J Obstet Gynecol* 1987; 157:254.
34. Kellner KR, Donnelly WH, Gould SD: Parental behavior after perinatal death: Lack of predictive demographic and obstetric variables. *Obstet Gynecol* 1984; 63:809.
35. Wilson AL, Witzke D, Fenton LJ, et al: Parental response to perinatal death. *Am J Dis Child* 1985; 139:1235.
36. Theut SK, Pedersen FA, Zaslow MJ, et al: Pregnancy subsequent to a perinatal loss: Parental anxiety and depression. *J Am Acad Child Adolesc Psychiatry* 1988; 27(3):289.
37. Lambert W: The loss of a baby is doubly crushing to a young couple. *Wall Street Journal* p A1, 1/12/95.
38. Sobel DE: Fetal damage due to ECT, insulin coma, chlorpromazine or resperpine. *Arch Gen Psychiatry* 1960; 2:606.
39. Crowe RR: Electroconvulsive therapy—A current perspective. *New Engl J Med* 1984; 311(3):163.
40. Katz G: Electroconvulsive therapy from a social work perspective. *Soc Work Health Care* 1992; 16(4):55.
41. Kendell RE: The present status of electroconvulsive therapy. *Br J Psychiatry* 1981; 139:265.

42. Weiner RD: Convulsive therapy: 50 years later. *Am J Psychiatry* 1984; 141(9):1078.

43. Repke JT, Berger NG: Electroconvulsive therapy in pregnancy. *Obstet Gynecol* 1984; 63:39S.

44. Yellowlees PM, Terissa P: Safe use of electroconvulsive therapy in pregnancy. *Med J Aust* 1990; 153:679.

45. Griffiths EJ, Lorenz RP, Baxter S, et al: Acute neurohumoral response to electroconvulsive therapy during pregnancy. *J Reprod Med* 1989; 34(11):907.

46. Sherer DM, D'Amico ML, Warshal DP, et al: Recurrent mild abruptio placentae occurring immediately after repeated electroconvulsive therapy in pregnancy. *Am J Obstet Gynecol* 1991; 165:652.

47. Boyd DA, Brown DW: Electric convulsive therapy in mental disorders associated with childbearing. *J Miss State Med Assoc* 1948; 45(8):573.

48. Wells DG, Zelcer J, Treadrae C: ECT-induced asystole from a subconvulsive shock. *Anaesth Intensive Care* 1988; 16(3):368.

49. Heshe J, Roeder E: Electroconvulsive therapy in Denmark. *Br J Psychiatry* 1976; 128:241.

50. Lew JKL, Eastley RJ, Hanning CD: Oxygenation during electroconvulsive therapy. *Anaesthesia* 1986; 41:1092.

51. Räsänen J, Martin JB, Hodges MR: Oxygen supplementation during electroconvulsive therapy. *Br J Anaesth* 1988; 61:593.

52. Linden S, Rich CL: The use of lithium during pregnancy and lactation. *J Clin Psychiatry* 1983; 44:358.

53. Mackay AV, Loose R, Glen AI: Labor on lithium. *Br Med J* 1976; 1:878.

54. Nora JJ, Nora AH, Toews WH: Lithium, Ebstein's anomaly, and other congenital heart defects. *Lancet* 1974; 2:594.

55. Elia J, Katz IR, Simpson GM: Teratogenicity of psychotherapeutic medications. *Psychopharmacol Bull* 1987; 23:531.

56. Woody JH, London WL, Wilbanks GD: Lithium toxity in a newborn. *Pediatrics* 1971; 47:94.

57. Karlsson K, Lindstedt G, Lundberg, et al: Transplacental lithium poisoning: Reversible inhibition of fetal thyroid. *Lancet* 1975; 1:1295.

58. Mizrahi EM, Hobbs JF, Goldsmith DI: Nephrogenic diabetes insipidus in transplacental lithium intoxication. *J Pediatr* 1979; 94:493.

59. Miller LJ: Clinical strategies for the use of psychotropic drugs during pregnancy. *Psychiatr Med* 1991; 9(2):276.

60. Guze BH, Guze PA: Psychotropic medication use during pregnancy. *West J Med* 1989; 151:296.

61. Havdala HS, Borison RL, Diamond BI: Potential hazards and applications of lithium in anesthesiology. *Anesthesiology* 1979; 50:534.

62. Pratila MG, Pratilas V: ST depression under anesthesia in a patient on lithium carbonate. *Mt Sinai J Med* 1979; 46(6):549.

63. Niebyt JR, Blake DA, Freeman JM, et al: Carbamazepine levels in pregnancy and lactation. *Obstet Gynecol* 1979; 53:139.

64. Jones KL, Lacro RV, Johnson KA, et al: Pattern of malformations in the children of women treated with carbamazepine during pregnancy. *New Engl J Med* 1989; 320:1661.

65. Lindhout D, Hoppener RJ, Meinardi H: Teratogenicity of antiepileptic drug combinations with special emphasis on epoxidation (of carbamazepine). *Epilepsia* 1984; 25:77.

66. Douglas BH, Hume AS: Placenta transfer of imipramine, a basic, lipid soluble drug. *Am J Obstet Gynecol* 1967; 99:573.

67. Kuenssberg EV, Knox JDE: Imipramine in pregnancy. *Br Med J* 1972; 2:292.

68. Rachelefsky GS, Flynt JW, Ebbin AJ, et al: Possible teratogenicity of tricyclic antidepressants. *Lancet* 1972; 1:838.

69. Idanpaan-Heikkila J: Possible teratogenicity of imipramine/chloropyramine. *Lancet* 1972; 2:282.

70. Schimmell MS, Katz EZ, Shagg AJ, et al: Toxic neonatal effects following maternal clomipramine therapy. *Clin Toxicol* 1991; 29(4):479.

71. Prentice A, Brown R: Fetal tachyarrhythmia and maternal antidepressant treatment. *Br Med J* 1989; 298:190.

72. Edwards RP, Miller RD, Roizen RF, et al: Cardiac responses to imipramine and pancuronium during anesthesia with halothane or enflurane. *Anesthesiology* 1979; 50:421.

73. Wong KC, Puerto AX, Puerto BA, et al: Influence of imipramine and pargyline on the arrythmogenicity of epinephrine during halothane, enflurane or methoxyflurane anesthesia in dogs. *Anesthesiology* 1980; 53:S25.

74. Stoelting RK: *Pharmacology and Physiology in Anesthetic Practice,* ed 2. Philadelphia, JB Lippincott, 1991, pp 373-378.

75. Rumeau-Rouquette C, Goujard J, Huel G: Possible teratogenic effects of phenothiazines in human beings. *Teratology* 1977; 15:57.

76. Mildovich L, van den Berg BJ: An evaluation of the teratogenicity of certain antinauseant drugs. *Am J Obstet Gynecol* 1976; 125:244.

77. Edlund MJ, Craig TJ: Antipsychotic drug use and birth defects: An epidemiologic reassessment. *Comp Psychiatr* 1976; 25:244.

78. Van Waes A, Van der Velde EM: Safety evaluation of haloperidol in the treatment of hyperemesis gravidarium. *J Clin Pharmacol* 1969; 9:224.

79. Van Gent EM, Nabarro G: Haloperidol as an alternative to lithium in pregnant women. *Am J Psychiatry* 1987; 144(9):1241.

80. Byrd RA, Brophy GT, Markham JK: Developmental toxicology studies of fluoxetine hydrocloride administered orally to rats and rabbits. *Teratology* 1989; 39:444A.

81. Pastuszak A, Schick-Boschetto B, Zuber C, et al: Pregnancy outcome following first-trimester exposure to fluoxetine (Prozac). *JAMA* 1993; 269(17):2246.

82. Moran DH, Perillo M, LaPorta RF, et al: Phenylephrine in the prevention of hypotension following spinal anesthesia for ceasarean delivery. *J Clin Anesth* 1991; 3:301.

83. Stack CG, Rogers P, Linter SPK: Monoamine oxidase inhibitors and anaesthesia. *Br J Anaesth* 1988; 60:222.

84. El-Ganzouri AR, Ivankovick AD, Braverman B: Monoamine oxidase inhibitors: Should they be discontinued preoperatively? *Anesth Analg* 1985; 64:592.

85. Silva AJ, Leog GB, Weinstock R: Misidentification syndrome and male pseudocyesis. *Psychosomatics* 1991; 32(2):228.

86. Small GW: Pseudocyesis: An overview. *Can J Psychiatry* 1986; 31:452.

87. O'Grady JP, Rosenthal M: Pseudocyesis: A modern perspective on an old disorder. *Obstet Gynecol Surv* 1989; 44(7):500.

30 Hepatic Disease

Joel Swanson and *Eugene Scioscia*

Hepatic diseases in the parturient are encountered in three situations: (1) those unique to pregnancy, (2) those that are more frequent during, or exacerbated by, pregnancy, and (3) chronic liver disease on which pregnancy is superimposed. The incidence of liver disease coincident with pregnancy is unknown, but including infectious liver disease it probably varies from 2% to 3%. Fortunately those disorders that are common are relatively benign, while in pregnancy severe hepatic dysfunction is uncommon.

Amenorrhea and infertility are common among women with diagnosed severe liver dysfunction.[1] Still, in most people chronic liver disease is clinically silent and pregnancy is not impossible. The effects of normal pregnancy on blood volume and hepatic function are stressful to an impaired liver, and the successful outcome of the pregnancy will depend on the "hepatic reserve" of that individual patient. Pregnancy counseling or maternal fetal triage is best done at the earliest opportunity and must take into account the severity of disease, maternal prognosis, and likely effects of pregnancy in a particular patient. Much of the maternal and fetal mortality data is quite old and, with improved treatment and intensive care capabilities, these data probably overestimate current figures. Tests of hepatic function are difficult to interpret definitively in any individual. With so much unknown, and with so much inconsistant information, counseling is not easy; however, while preexisting hepatic disease poses a risk it is not an absolute contraindication to pregnancy.[2,3]

Hepatic alterations in normal pregnancy

The liver is forced more superior and posterior as the gravid uterus expands; a palpable liver in the third trimester is usually a sign of disease. On normal physical examination, spider nevi and palmar erythema are frequent findings in the pregnant patient; they cannot be considered indicative of liver disease in parturients. Liver size and absolute hepatic blood flow are unchanged during pregnancy, but the fraction of cardiac output flowing to the liver is reduced by about 35% at term.[4,5] Engorged esophageal veins are visible in over half of normal pregnancies.[6] Histopathologic examination of hepatic tissue in normal pregnancy can be unremarkable or it can reveal mild fatty changes.

Cytochrome P-450 activity is decreased during pregnancy, while hepatic mixed function oxidase activity is induced. Albumin levels are decreased at term, while levels of many α-globulins and β-globulins are increased. The effects of these changes on drug metabolism are unpredictable. Decreased levels of plasma esterases responsible for degrading succinylcholine and ester local anesthetics are probably of minimal clinical significance even in advanced liver disease. Proteins involved in clotting are increased during normal pregnancy; indeed, pregnancy is often described as a "hypercoagulable state." The liver is responsible in part for glycogenesis, glycogenolysis, and gluconeogenesis. There is no evidence that the hepatic contribution to these processes is altered in normal pregnancy.

Bile formation is inhibited during pregnancy, and at term bilirubin may be at the upper limits of normal without any liver disease. Placental production of alkaline phosphatase may elevate serum levels of this enzyme at term, though seldom greater than twice normal. Serum aminotransferases (AST and ALT), which are normal during normal pregnancy, therefore make useful markers of hepatocellular damage. Table 30-1 provides a summary of laboratory findings in normal pregnancy and in pregnancy complicated by hepatic disease.

Hepatic dysfunction during pregnancy

Diagnosis of hepatic dysfunction during pregnancy is seldom obvious. In most cases, signs and symptoms of liver disease are nonspecific and largely indistinguishable from conditions seen frequently in normal pregnancy. When serious and unmistakable liver disease is present, the differentiation between diagnoses is subtle and often impossible except in retrospect. Signs that should prompt the physician to investigate hepatic disorders related to pregnancy include jaundice, right upper quadrant pain, hepatomegaly, or ascites. Some patients may be symptom-free or may even ignore fairly substantial symptomatology until intraperitoneal hemorrhage, variceal bleeding, or encephalopathy oc-

Table 30-1 LFT in normal pregnancy and disease states compared with the normal nonpregnant state*†

Diagnosis	Normal pregnancy	ICP	Cirrhosis	Acute hepatitis	Pre-eclampsia	HELLP	AFLP
Onset		3rd trimester	Precedes pregnancy	Any time	After 20 wks	After 20 wks	After 20 wks
Albumin	−10-60%		− to − −				− −
Total alk. phos.	+200-400%	0 or slight +	++				0 or +
Bilirubin	Normal range	+		0 to +++		0 to ++	+ to ++
AST/ SGOT	0	0 or mild +	0 to ++	0 to ++++	0 to ++	+ to ++	++ to +++
ALT/SGPT	0	0 or mild +	0 to ++	0 to ++++	0 to ++		+ to ++
Lactate dehydrogenase (LDH)	0	+				>500	
5′-Nucleotidase							
γ-GGT	0, possible increase in 3rd trimester						
α + β Globulins	+		−				
Prothrombin time	0	0, if + then Rx Vit K	0 to ++	0 to ++	0 to ++	0 to ++	++
Glucose	0	0	− to − −	0 or −		0	−
Ammonia	0	0	+ with portosystemic shunting	0 rarely +	−	0	+
Platelets	0 or slight	0	− with 2° hypersplenism	0	−	− to − −	− to − −
Alphafetoprotein (AFP)	0	0	0	0	0	0	0

*Data from references 3-6, 18, 19, 22, 24, 27.
†ICP = intrahepatic cholestasis of pregnancy; HELLP = *h*emolysis, *e*levated *l*iver enzymes, *l*ow *p*latelet count; AFLP = acute fatty liver of pregnancy; 0 = no change.

cur. Changes in blood volume and cardiac output in the latter half of pregnancy make this time particularly critical for the parturient with hepatic dysfunction.

General considerations

Liver disease may affect multiple organ systems. When hepatic dysfunction is severe, metabolism of ammonia and GABAergic compounds is impaired, leading to central ventilatory stimulation and encephalopathy. Spider angiomata and intrapulmonary shunts are true arteriovenous shunts, and they induce a hyperdynamic cardiac response that is only increased by normal physiologic changes of pregnancy. For the same reasons, arterial hypoxemia and metabolic alkalosis are common. Glucose metabolism and diminished "first pass" clearance of insulin place these patients at high risk for hypoglycemia. Patients with severe hepatic disease tolerate volume shifts poorly; renal failure or hepatorenal syndrome are frequent causes of death.

Decreased hepatic protein synthesis has a variety of important effects. The increase in clotting factors seen in normal pregnancy is unlikely to occur in patients with severe hepatic dysfunction. In fact, our greatest fear concerning these patients is coagulopathy. Decreased production of plasma proteins leads to intravascular volume depletion, ascites, and pleural effusions. Ascites and other gastrointestinal changes place these patients at high risk for aspiration. Altered pharmacokinetics and dynamics make prediction of drug response difficult or impossible.

MANAGEMENT OF THE PARTURIENT WITH LIVER DISEASE

After identification of hepatic disease in the parturient, the next step in management is diagnosis and assessment of the degree of dysfunction. Benign or early hepatic disorders require close monitoring but not necessarily extraordinary care during pregnancy. The following are general recommendations; diagnosis-specific management is discussed under individual sections in this chapter.

Obstetric plans

Care of these patients can be both time- and resource-intensive. One should realistically evaluate the capabilities of one's institution, and address and resolve maternal-fetal triage issues early. If the mother elects to carry to delivery, plans must be made for timing and mode of delivery. Because of the high surgical morbidity with most severe hepatic disease, one should strongly consider vaginal delivery and reserve operative delivery for deteriorating maternal or fetal condition.

Choice of anesthetic

Depending on the timing and urgency of delivery, a number of possible situations must be considered. As the fetus matures or the maternal status changes, most likely the scenario will change accordingly. One should thus form the anesthetic plan for the following possible situations: instrumented or assisted vaginal delivery, planned cesarean section, emergency cesarean section for fetal deterioration, emergency cesarean for maternal deterioration, and emergency laparotomy. One must be prepared for emergencies, discussing the management plan with colleagues. It is best to choose regional anesthesia whenever possible. This will frequently mean correcting coagulopathy before initiating the anesthetic.

For nonurgent delivery, a carefully titrated epidural anesthetic is the best choice in the patient with severe hepatic dysfunction. One should correct coagulopathy if necessary. The most likely maternal emergencies involve hemorrhage, and if this is ongoing or severe, regional anesthesia may be unwise.

The most difficult decisions involve fetal distress and "emergency" delivery. Poor communication is life-threatening in this situation. Important factors include discussing the anesthetic plan for fetal distress well in advance of its occurrence, and considering the patients' wishes. If maternal prognosis is poor, the triage priority may belong with the fetus. In most other circumstances, fetal distress is insufficient reason to jeopardize the mother with hepatic disease; one must expeditiously place the necessary maternal monitors and utilize the most dependable regional technique. Because of its rapid plasma degradation, we prefer 2-chloroprocaine via epidural (Table 30-2).

Patients with severe hepatic dysfunction tolerate hypotension and hypoxemia poorly. We consider an arterial line to be a standard monitor before induction of any form of anesthesia. Close monitoring of urinary output is also very helpful. The need for central monitoring must be individualized. Most patients with hepatic disease have hyperdynamic hearts because of the intrapulmonary and (spider) angiomatous shunts as well as low systemic vascular resistance. In this regard a central venous pressure (CVP) or pulmonary artery (PA) catheter will be of little therapeutic value. If pulmonary hypertension is suggested by history, physical examination, or laboratory studies a pulmonary artery catheter is indicated. Severe preeclampsia and hepatic involvement with oliguria, pulmonary edema, or the need for aggressive vasodilator therapy are additional indications for PA catheter placement. We do not include HELLP without the above complications as a *de facto* indication for central monitoring. In the same way, we do not automatically place a central monitor for complaints of right upper quadrant pain. We do require a good venous access in this situation, and if peripheral access is unreliable, we will place and maintain a sheath introducer that has the ability to monitor CVP.

While many viruses are associated with neurologic infection (HIV, herpes, polio), hepatitis viruses are not associated with encephalitis, meningitis, cerebritis, or neuritis. With the possible exception of herpes virus, regional anesthesia is not contraindicated in the presence of viral infection.[7-12]

HEPATIC DISEASES UNIQUE TO PREGNANCY
Intrahepatic cholestasis of pregnancy

Also referred to as recurrent jaundice of pregnancy, cholestatic hepatitis, and icterus gravidarum, intra-

Table 30-2 Anesthetic agents for use in parturients with hepatic disease

Drug name	Pharmacokinetics in cirrhotics	Notes
Thiopental	Metabolism unaltered because of redistribution as primary means of termination of action	Cirrhotics may tolerate induction doses poorly[96]
Propofol	Pharmacokinetics unaltered	Prolonged duration
Ketamine	Insufficient data	Side effects may limit use in cirrhotics, increased LFTs in normal patients[97,98]
Etomidate	T½ β prolonged × 2	Useful if hypovolemia is a concern[98]
Halothane	Rare idiosyncratic hepatitis, worsened by hypoxemia	Avoid in any suspected hepatic disease[99]
Isoflurane	Lowers hepatic blood flow	Best choice
Enflurane	Lowers hepatic blood flow	Acceptable
Desflurane		
Nitrous oxide	No effect	Probably safe
Lidocaine (epidural)	Large Vd_{SS}, prolonged T½β for lidocaine and its active metabolite (MEGX)	Use minimum dose[100]
Bupivicaine (epi)	Insufficient data	Probably similar to lidocaine[100]
2-chloroprocaine (epidural)	Very rapid degradation in the presence of cholinesterase (cholinesterase is reduced in pregnancy and in liver disease)	Probably the drug of choice for c/section Toxicity has been reported in pseudocholinesterase deficiency and in cases of severely abnormal cholinesterase activity
Succinylcholine	Decreased plasma cholinesterase	Prolongation of duration if plasma cholinesterase levels are low[101,102]
Atracurium	Independant of hepatic metabolism	Histamine release may limit use in cirrhotics
Vecuronium	Dose-dependent clearance	Longer duration at 0.2 mg/kg, dose normal at 0.1 mg/kg[103,104]
Pancuronium	Increased Vdl, normal metabolism, prolonged recovery	Careful dosing using nerve stimulator[105]
Doxacurium	Insufficient data, minimal plasma ester hydrolysis	Probably similar to pancuronium[101,106]
Mivacurium	Insufficient data	Similar to atracurium
Pipecuronium	Insufficient data	Probably similar to pancuronium
Rocuronium	Increased Vdl, normal metabolism, prolonged recovery	Similar to pancuronium[105,107]
Neostigmine	Unaltered, primarily renal excretion	"Recurarization" does not occur[101]
Edrophonium		
Morphine	Conflicting reports	Clinically reported to have prolonged effects[108,109]
Meperidine	Prolonged T½ β	Prolonged effects, sphincter of Oddi spasm[110]
Fentanyl	At clinical doses (not cardiac doses), metabolism is unaltered because of prolonged binding to muscle and fat deposits (large V_D)	Patients likely to be sensitive to depressant effects, but fentanyl is probably the drug of choice in cirrhotics. One should avoid moderate or high doses. Can cause sphincter of Oddi spasm[111,112]
Sufentanil	Same as fentanyl	Also a good choice[112]
Alfentanil	Highly protein-bound (small V_D), therefore accumulates in hepatic failure	Poor choice in cirrhosis[113]
Midazolam	Slightly prolonged T½β	Benzodiazepines potentiate hepatic encephalopathy[74]

hepatic cholestasis of pregnancy (ICP) has an incidence of approximately 1% to 10%. It is more common in twin gestations, and genetic factors play a role. Symptoms of ICP are icterus and pruritus. The initial complaint of pruritus is followed by jaundice in over 50% of cases. Presentation is typically in the third trimester, and symptoms persist until after delivery. Recurrence in subsequent pregnancies is common. While the cause of the jaundice is unknown, it may be a reaction to high circulating concentrations of estrogen. Pruritus may be secondary to deposition of bile acids in the skin. Laboratory evaluation will reveal fivefold to tenfold elevations in alkaline phosphatase, a direct bilirubin that is more increased than indirect bilirubin, and mild elevations in transaminases (Table 30-1).

ICP is relatively benign in terms of maternal effects, but it is associated with an increased incidence of preterm labor, intrauterine fetal demise (IUFD), and perinatal mortality in 35 per 1000 live births.[3] Therefore, obstetric management should include frequent assessment of fetal well-being and consideration of induction either at term or with demonstration of fetal lung maturity.[13] Initial maternal treatment is with cholestyramine resins, which are successful in reducing pruritus particularly if started early.

Anesthetic management is unaffected by the diagnosis of ICP, with one caveat. As in other forms of cholestasis, fat malabsorption may result in deficient levels of vitamin K–dependent clotting factors; therefore, evaluation of bleeding history and prothrombin time (PT) may be indicated.

Hyperemesis gravidarum

Hyperemesis gravidarum is not uncommon, occurring in 0.3% to 1.0% of pregnancies. Risk factors include obesity, primiparity, nonsmoker status, and multiple gestation.[14,15] While it is an unwelcome diagnosis and the condition may lead to dehydration requiring intravenous hydration and nutrition, in one prospective study it has been associated with decreased fetal wastage and improved pregnancy outcome.[16,17] While the etiology is unknown and probably multifactorial, liver function tests are abnormal in two thirds of patients with hyperemesis gravidarum.[13]

Because it is a disease of early pregnancy, hyperemesis gravidarum fortunately should not present frequently to the anesthesiologist. Logistical concerns presented by intractable vomiting, dehydration, and electrolyte disturbances are the only anesthetic concerns. In cases in which pruritus is severe, we avoid intraspinal opioids.

"Hypertensive" disorders of pregnancy

Pregnancy-induced hypertension (PIH) is an umbrella term describing a group of pregnancy-associated disorders that are probably etiologically related. Classically, the term refers to preeclampsia and eclampsia, but many investigators now consider the syndrome of hemolysis, elevated liver enzymes, and low platelet counts to be a related disorder, possibly a variant of severe preeclampsia. The two disorders certainly share many features and coexist with a frequency that precludes random chance. There are many theories attempting to explain the etiology of these disorders (Box 30-1) There are an equal number of treatment mo-

---

BOX 30-1   ETIOLOGY OF HYPERTENSIVE DISORDERS OF PREGNANCY

Decreased levels of endothelium-derived nitric oxide (EDRF)[114]
"Inherited factors"[115]
Autoimmune disorder[116]
Thromboxane: prostacyclin imbalance[117]
Inadequate maternal response to placentation[118,119]
Abnormal hemostasis[120]
Endothelial cell damage[121]
Increased sensitivity to catecholamines[122,123]
Retained sensitivity to angiotensin II[124]
Microvesicular fat disease of the liver[125]

BOX 30-2   TREATMENT OF HYPERTENSIVE DISORDERS OF PREGNANCY

Antepartum corticosteroids (HELLP syndrome)[126]
Postpartum corticosteroids (HELLP syndrome)[127]
Early plasmaphoresis (HELLP syndrome)[128,129]
Observation (HELLP syndrome with subcapsular hematoma)[20]
Vaginal delivery[130]
Immediate cesarean section[131]
Volume expansion and hemodynamic monitoring[132]
Conservative vs. early intervention[133]

---

dalities (Box 30-2). No theory or treatment comprehensively addresses all facets of these disorders.

Even more puzzling is that for one of these "hypertensive disorders," HELLP syndrome (*he*molysis, *e*levated *l*iver *e*nzymes, *l*ow *p*latelet count), hypertension is not always present. Perhaps pregnancy-induced microvascular endothelial damage would be a better term to describe these disorders. If we broaden the term, we may be compelled to include hemolytic uremic syndrome (HUS) of pregnancy and acute fatty liver of pregnancy (AFLP), as well as some forms of pregnancy-associated renal failure (Box 30-3).[18] While it might be comforting, more precise nomenclature is of little clinical value at this time.

Preeclampsia/eclampsia with hepatic involvement

Preeclampsia and eclampsia are accompanied by hepatic manifestations in only a minority of cases, but they are responsible for 10% to 15% of maternal mortality in these patients.[19] While liver function tests can be elevated and abnormal in preeclamptic patients, these elevations are typically

BOX 30-3 PREGNANCY-ASSOCIATED MICROVASCULAR ENDOTHELIAL DAMAGE DISORDERS AND RELATED DISORDERS

Differential diagnosis
Probably related:

Preeclampsia (with hepatic involvement)
HELLP syndrome
Acute fatty liver of pregnancy (AFLP)
Hemolytic uremic syndrome (HUS syndrome)
Immune thrombocytopenic purpura (ITP)
Thrombotic thrombocytopenic purpura (TTP)

Possibly related:

"Gestational" thrombocytopenia
Disseminated intravascular coagulopathy (DIC)
Acute renal failure in pregnancy

Frequently misdiagnosed as:

Pyelonephritis
Cholecystitis
Appendicitis
Hepatitis
Gastroenteritis

much less than those seen with HELLP syndrome.

The most important hepatic complication of preeclampsia or eclampsia is subcapsular hematoma, which may present clinically as right upper quadrant pain and nausea and vomiting, typically in the third trimester. Rupture of the hematoma is accompanied by sudden hypotension, and it has an associated maternal mortality rate as high as 75% and a fetal mortality rate as high as 60%.[20,21] Eighty percent of spontaneous hepatic ruptures occur in patients with preeclampsia or eclampsia.[21]

Ultrasonography may be diagnostic if hematoma or rupture is suspected, but a negative ultrasound does not rule out the diagnosis. Computed tomography (CT) may also be diagnostic if clinical circumstances allow for its use.[19,20] Frequently, diagnosis is made retrospectively at the time of laparotomy.

A closely related phenomenon is hepatic infarction associated with preeclampsia. This rare disorder presents in the third trimester with fever, abdominal pain, extremely high transaminases, and other laboratory values consistent with severe hepatic dysfunction. As with hepatic hematoma, diagnosis is assisted by CT, but in the case of suspected infarction diagnosis is confirmed by biopsy.[22]

Obstetric and anesthetic management of preeclampsia associated hepatic hematoma is controversial. For unruptured hematomas, if the patient is hemodynamically stable she may be monitored in an intensive care setting in an effort to ad-

vance fetal maturity until cesarean section. If the surgical plan includes hepatic repair, general anesthesia will provide more hemodynamic stability and acceptable intraoperative comfort. For ruptured hematoma, emergency laparotomy under general anesthesia is the only recourse. Delivery and anesthetic management of hepatic infarction will depend on individual patient characteristics. There is insufficient published experience to make specific recommendations.

HELLP syndrome

The syndrome of *h*emolysis, *e*levated *l*iver enzymes, and *l*ow *p*latelet count (HELLP syndrome) and its management are well described in Chapter 21 in the context of pregnancy-induced hypertension. It is worth noting that HELLP syndrome does not always occur with accompanying hypertension or proteinuria, and it can easily be misdiagnosed (Box 30-3). Also of note is that there are some important differences in presentation that may hasten the diagnosis. Although HELLP syndrome is a disease of the third trimester, it may occur more remote from term than acute fatty liver of pregnancy (AFLP). Any pregnant patient with complaints of abdominal pain deserves a platelet count to help differentiate pregnancy-induced hepatic diseases from other surgical or medical problems. Transaminases are elevated in HELLP syndrome, but not usually to the same degree as hepatitis (Table 30-1).

Acute fatty liver of pregnancy

Acute fatty liver of pregnancy (AFLP) is an uncommon disease of the third trimester, characterized by initial symptomatology typical of hepatitis and progressing rapidly to acute liver failure and encephalopathy.[23,24] AFLP is also difficult to distinguish from PIH with hepatic involvement, and it has been associated with preeclampsia in about 30% of cases.[19] Unlike in acute hepatitis, in AFLP the liver edge is unlikely to be palpable on physical examination.[19] Laboratory evaluation will differ from acute hepatitis in that findings consistent with DIC are present in over half of patients with AFLP, bilirubin is higher than in PIH, and transaminase levels, while elevated, are less so than in either hepatitis or PIH (Table 30-1). Pronounced hypoglycemia is not uncommon in AFLP. Computed tomography (CT) and magnetic resonance imaging (MRI) may have a role in diagnosis, but well-substantiated data are lacking.

Definitive diagnosis requires biopsy with special stains for fat. Because of the frequency of coagulopathy, percutaneous needle biopsy is not always a viable option. Laparoscopic-assisted biopsy has been proposed.[25] The histologic changes associated with this syndrome include swollen hepatocytes, cytoplasm filled with microvascular fat, central nuclei, periportal sparing, and minimal hepatocellular necrosis. Interestingly, enough lipid accumulation may occur elsewhere, namely in renal tubular cells. The cause of acute fatty liver syndrome is unknown, but it is felt by many to be a disease different from preeclampsia.[3,24] Recently, several authors have proposed possible etiologic associations between preeclampsia and AFLP.[18,26,27]

Perinatal morbidity involves hepatic encephalopathy in 60% of cases, severe coagulopathy in 55%, renal failure in 60%, pancreatitis, and ascites. Fetal mortality could be as high as 14% to 66%. Maternal mortality, which in original studies approached 100%, is now closer to 25%.[19] Maternal deaths result from sepsis, aspiration, renal failure, circulation collapse, pancreatitis, gastrointestinal bleeding, or circulatory collapse. Rarely, hepatic failure requires transplantation. To avoid the worst of these complications, one should maintain a high degree of suspicion and and make an early diagnosis.

While differentiating AFLP from PIH with hepatic involvement is frequently problematic, fortunately it is unnecessary because management in both cases is the same. These patients must be managed in an intensive care setting, and delivery should occur shortly after diagnosis. Cesarean section is indicated for patients who fail induction or for those whose disease is progressing too rapidly. Invasive monitoring would be ideal, but it is confounded by the usual coexisting coagulopathy. Transfusion of blood products should be based on clinical necessity confirmed with laboratory evaluation of coagulation indices. While it is tempting to transfuse blood products prophylactically, one should bear in mind that these patients may not tolerate large protein loads without worsening encephalopathy or volume overload.

Anesthetic management

Anesthetic management will depend first on the degree of urgency of the delivery; early consultation is vital to allow the anesthesiologist ample time to optimize the maternal condition. Every effort should be made to avoid a "stat" anesthetic induction. Regional anesthesia is the preferred choice, so volume assessment and correction of coagulopathy are the first steps to be taken before institution of anesthesia for vaginal or operative delivery. Successful epidural anesthesia for cesarean delivery has been reported.[28]

HEPATIC DISEASES EXACERBATED BY PREGNANCY
Hepatitis

Viral hepatitis is the most common cause of jaundice during pregnancy.[29] Because some cases of viral infection are clinically silent, the true incidence is unknown. Potential pathogens other than hepatitis A through E include cytomegalovirus (CMV), Epstein-Barr virus (EBV), and herpes simplex virus (HSV). In general, the incidence and clinical course of viral hepatitis is unaffected by pregnancy,[30,31] though there are exceptions.

Clinical presentation usually begins as a nonspecific flulike syndrome of fever, headache, fatigue, nausea, loss of appetite, and diarrhea. Findings consistent with cholestasis include jaundice, pruritus, pale stools, and dark urine; these may or may not be present. Laboratory analysis will reveal liver parenchymal damage in the form of elevated transaminases as well as specific viral serologies (Table 30-1). Severity ranges from subclinical and self-limited disease to fulminant hepatic failure. For hepatitis B, C, and D, chronic carrier states are possible.

Hepatitis A: incidence and etiology. The incidence of hepatitis A virus (HAV) in pregnancy is less than or equal to 1 in 1000, though the true incidence of subclinical infection is not known.[5,32] Transmission of the virus, which involves fecal-oral contamination, is facilitated by intimate contact with an infected individual, poor hygiene, and/or poor sanitation. Parturients who have recently traveled to or from developing nations, where the disease is endemic, are at particularly high risk. Vertical transmission from mother to neonate at the time of delivery has not been reported.[33,34] Epidemics most frequently result from ingestion of contaminated food or water. Incubation is typically short (15 to 50 days), as is the duration of viremia. Virus is excreted most heavily in the stool, with maximum excretion occurring during the prodromal phase of clinical illness. Diagnosis is confirmed by positive IgM antibody to HAV, which is elevated acutely and persists for 6 months. IgG antibody is also elevated early and persists for life, indicating immunity.[29] The infection and illness are self-limiting, usually lasting about 6 weeks. Fulminant hepatic failure is rare, and there is no carrier state.

The effects of hepatitis A on pregnancy are probably not significant in well-nourished parturients.[35] Similarly, it would appear that there is no increase in fetal wastage or newborn morbidity associated with maternal infection. Reported increases in severity of maternal disease and fetal morbidity in developing nations are probably related to nutritional and epidemiological factors.[29]

Hepatitis B: incidence and etiology. Acute hepatitis B infection (HBV) occurs in 1 to 2 in 1000 pregnancies in the United States. Only half of acutely infected individuals will manifest jaundice or other signs of clinical disease.[36] Chronic infection is present in 5 to 15 in 1000 pregnancies.[37,38] Approximately 22,000 infants are born each year to women with chronic active hepatitis B.[39] Of the approximately 300,000 Americans who contract the disease each year, 10% to 15% will become chronically infected. Of this subgroup, chronic active disease may lead to serious sequelae, and annually, 4000 to 5000 people die as a result of chronic active hepatitis B and HBV-associated hepatocellular carcinoma.[31,36]

In the United States, the predominant mode of transmission is direct person-to-person spread. High-risk individuals include health care workers, hemodialysis patients, hemophiliac individuals, users of illicit drugs, sexually promiscuous persons, and those with long-term exposure to infected individuals. Infection is also more prevalent in people of Asian extraction, in whom the primary mode of transmission is perinatal.[40] The likelihood of vertical transmission depends on several factors. The trimester in which maternal infection occurs is of foremost importance. Parturients who are hepatitis B surface antigen (HBsAg) and hepatitis Be antigen (HBeAg) positive at time of delivery have a 95% rate of vertical transmission to the neonate.[31] Acute maternal infection in the first trimester without advancement to a chronic disease state is associated with a 10% vertical transmission rate.[29] Presence of anti-hepatitis Be antigen antibody (anti-HBe) reduces the likelihood of vertical transmission to 25%.[29,34,41,42]

The American College of Obstetrics and Gynecologists (ACOG), American Academy of Pediatrics (AAP), and Advisory Committee on Immunization Practices (ACIP) have recommended routine screening of all parturients in early pregnancy to identify newborns who will require immunoprophylaxis against hepatitis B.[31,43,44] In states where adherence to these recommendations is required by law, identification and immunoprophylaxis of neonates at risk approaches 100%.[39] Combined passive and active immunization of neonates is 85% to 95% effective in preventing perinatal transmission of maternal hepatitis B virus.[31] Recommendations are summarized in Table 30-3.

Pathophysiology and diagnosis. Parturients with hepatitis B present a special problem for those involved in their care. After identification of the HBsAg-positive individual, initial efforts should be to stage the disease (active or chronic) and identify sequelae of hepatitis B infection. Unfortunately, even a careful history and physical examination may be misleading in the pregnant patient with hepatitis. Spider angiomata, palmar erythema, and edema are common in normal pregnancy.[6,27] Subclinical or low-grade hepatitis symptomatology is in many cases indistinguishable from nonspecific complaints of normal pregnancy. If the patient has a palpable liver edge or elevated serum transaminases, additional serology would include IgM anti-Hbc, HBeAg, and possibly HBV DNA. HBsAg positivity in the absence of IgM anti-HBc indicates chronic infection. Consultation by a gastroenterologist or infectious disease specialist is appropriate at this point, because these patients will need long-term follow-up care beyond current obstetric needs. One half of symptomless carriers have chronic active hepatitis.[40] While liver needle biopsy is not diagnostic, it is the only means of assessing the severity of hepatocellular damage.

Obstetric and anesthetic management. The decision to recommend liver biopsy and its timing should be individualized based on maternal and fetal triage issues. Interferon α-2b (Intron-A: Schering-Plough Laboratories, Kenilworth, N.J.)

Table 30-3 Summary of recommendations for passive and active hepatitis B immunoprophylaxis for neonates

Maternal HBsAg status	Vaccine dose	Age of infant
HBs Ag (+)	HBV 1	At birth (within 12 hr)
	HBIG	At birth (within 12 hr)
	HBV 2	1 mo
	HBV 3	6 mo
Unknown (draw and send maternal blood for HBsAg at earliest opportunity)	HBV 1	At birth (within 12 hr)
	HBIG	Give immediately (within 1st week of life) if maternal status found to be (+)
	HBV 2	1-2 mo
	HBV 3	6 mo
HBs Ag (−)	HBV 1	At birth (prior to discharge)
	HBV 2	1-2 mo
	HBV 3	6-18 mo

Modified from Tables 3 and 4, Centers for Disease Control: Hepatitis B virus: A comprehensive strategy for eliminating transmission in the United States through universal childhood vaccination. Recommendations of the Immunization Practices Advisory Committee (ACIP). *MMWR* 1991; 40(RR-13):12-13.

has shown promising results for the treatment of well-compensated chronic hepatitis B infection, but it has not been studied in parturients and it is not recommended for use during pregnancy (personal communication, 2/95). The course of hepatitis B infection, whether acute or chronic, is unaffected by pregnancy. There is some disagreement over the effect of hepatitis B disease on pregnancy. Some authors feel there is an increased risk of premature delivery in parturients infected during the third trimester,[6] though as in hepatitis A this may reflect maternal nutritional status and access to health care.

Hospitalization is unnecessary unless clinically indicated, and care is supportive. Acute fulminant hepatic failure is rare with hepatitis, and there is no treatment other than liver transplantation (see Liver Transplantation and Pregnancy below). Transfer of the patient with incipient or established hepatic failure to a center performing hepatic transplantation is advisable. Mortality from acute hepatitis B is less than 1%.[31] Isolation of the patient along with blood and body fluid precautions should be instituted to protect health care personnel.

Pregnancy in patients with chronic active hepatitis and cirrhosis is rare. Lack of specific serologic identification for early case reports makes specific etiologic identification difficult.[5,45-47]

Delivery by cesarean section dose not alter the risk of vertical transmission, and mode of delivery should be based on obstetric criteria.[6,38,41,48,49]

Hepatitis C: incidence and etiology. With the advent of specific serologic markers, we now know that hepatitis C virus (HCV) is responsible for over 90% of non-A non-B hepatitis (NANB).[31] Before the practice of screening the blood supply, 95% of transfusion-related hepatitis was due to HCV. Currently, most HCV is contracted by intravenous drug abusers followed by sexually promiscuous heterosexual individuals. A small number are transfusion-related, and a high percentage of patients have no identifiable risk factors.[36] Vertical transmission of HCV is less extensively studied than HBV, but it appears that this form of transmission is uncommon.[29,34]

Pathophysiology. The clinical course of acute HCV is usually very mild. Less than 30% of infected individuals exhibit jaundice, and most cases of acute infection go undiagnosed. The importance of the disease lies in the fact that up to half of those infected with HCV go on to develop chronic liver disease. Chronic hepatitis, cirrhosis, and hepatocellular carcinoma (HCC) are well documented potential sequelae of HCV infection. It should be noted that progression from acute infection to chronic disease is very slow, and many individuals (even those with cirrhosis) are asymptomatic. There are no specific recommendations against

pregnancy in HCV-seropositive women.[6,31] Cirrhosis due to HCV in pregnancy has not been reported.

No neonatal effects have been reported other than an increase in prematurity in children born to mothers infected in the third trimester.[38] There are no formal neonatal prophylactic recommendations, though some authors recommend administering immunoglobulin (Ig) to neonates born to mothers with acute HCV infection in the third trimester.[24,36,38]

Hepatitis D: incidence and etiology. Delta hepatitis (HDV) is due to a defective RNA virus that requires HBV for replication. HDV can only infect patients who have HBV, either as coinfection at the time HBV is acquired or as superinfection at a time subsequent to HBV infection. Disease course is similar to hepatitis B in the case of coinfection, but with superinfection, 70% to 80% of patients will progress to cirrhosis and portal hypertension. Disease progression is frequently rapid,[31] and the mortality rate is as high 25% because of hepatic failure. Specific serologic testing has only recently been widely available, so it is too early to estimate incidence of viremia. Because of the typically severe course of chronic active delta hepatitis, the incidence in parturients is very low. Vertical transmission of HDV has been reported.[50] Immunization efforts directed at avoiding HBV infection will be equally effective against HDV.[24,31]

Hepatitis E: incidence and etiology. Until the recent development of serologic tests for hepatitis E (anti-HEV*), the diagnosis was made in the event of clinical hepatitis with negative serology for A, B, and C and evidence of recent travel to a developing nation. HEV is not endemic to the United States. Transmission is by the fecal-oral route, with contaminated water being most frequently implicated. The potential for vertical transmission is unknown at this time. Most investigators believe there is no chronic HEV infection state,[29] though this has been recently questioned.[51] In the nonpregnant individual, HEV is similar to HAV in most respects. Hepatitis E is the exception in terms of the effects of pregnancy on disease course. For reasons that are unclear, maternal mortality is 15% to 20%.[52] Standard immune globulin prophylaxis measures are unlikely to be protective against HEV.

Other causes of viral hepatitis

Other viral agents causing hepatitis include cytomegalovirus, Ebstein-Barr virus, and most significantly, herpes simplex virus. Herpes hepatitis is

---

*Anti-HEV titer is not yet commercially available (CDC, Hepatitis Branch, personal communication, 4/95).

rare but requires tissue diagnosis and rapid treatment with acyclovir. Cesarean section has been recommended for patients with herpes hepatitis; the newborn should be treated with acyclovir.[53]

Drug-induced hepatitis

A number of drugs are purported to have caused hepatitis, cholestasis, or even cirrhosis. Antihypertensive, anticonvulsant, antiinflammatory, antibiotic, anesthetic, and chemotherapeutic agents are especially well represented. Most such reactions represent idiosyncratic reactions and occur at extremely low frequency. Persistent low perfusion states or hypoxemia, as seen with anesthesia and surgical procedures, predispose the liver to injury.[54]

One drug worth singling out because of a recent resurgence in some areas is alpha methyldopa, which has been associated with a 1% rate of Coombs-positive hemolytic anemia and/or autoimmune hepatitis.[55] In the parturient this could be nearly indistinguishable from incomplete HELLP syndrome or PIH with liver involvement. If drug-induced hepatitis is suspected, one should discontinue the suspected agent(s). A short course of steroids may be helpful. One can expect liver function tests to return to baseline within one week.

CHRONIC LIVER DISEASE AND PREGNANCY
Cirrhosis

Hepatic cirrhosis is an irreversible chronic injury to the liver parenchyma, resulting in histologic changes of extensive fibrosis and regenerative nodules. Alcohol abuse is the most common cause of cirrhosis and portal hypertension in the overall population.[56] Postnecrotic cirrhosis as a result of chronic viral hepatitis is the most common cause in young women. Other important causes, signs, and symptoms of cirrhosis are summarized in Boxes 30-4 and 30-5. The diagnosis of cirrhosis per se is not as important to pregnancy outcome as is the recognition of significant sequelae (Box 30-6). The sequelae most important to the obstetrician and anesthesiologist are portal hypertension, coagulopathy, pulmonary hypertension, and fulminant hepatic failure.

Pathophysiology

Portal hypertension in pregnancy. Normal portal venous pressures range from 10 to 15 cm H_2O, but these may rise and persist above 30 cm H_2O in portal hypertension. Causes of portal hypertension include cirrhosis, noncirrhotic portal fibrosis, and portal venous obstruction. The list of potential causes is protean, and thorough discussion is well beyond the scope of this chapter (Box 30-7). For the most part, the obstetric and anesthetic management of these parturients depends on under-

---

BOX 30-4   SIGNS AND SYMPTOMS OF CIRRHOSIS

Clinically silent
Anorexia
Weakness
Spider angiomata
Palmar erythema
Kaput medusa
Icterus
Ascites
Varices/upper GI bleed
Lower GI bleed
Tachypnea
RUQ pain
Encephalopathy
   (euphoria or depression, confusion, slurred speech, lethargy to coma)

BOX 30-5   CAUSES OF CIRRHOSIS

Alcoholism
Postnecrotic hepatitis
   (secondary to viral hepatitis)
Primary biliary cirrhosis
Secondary biliary cirrhosis*
Cardiac cirrhosis
Cryptogenic (no cause can be found)

---

*Most frequent causes include postoperative strictures, gallstones, repeated cholangitis, chronic pancreatitis, pericholangitis, sclerosing cholangitis.

BOX 30-6   SEQUELAE OF CIRRHOSIS

1. Portal hypertension (HTN)*
   Variceal bleeding
   Splenomegaly
   Ascites
   Hepatic encephalopathy
   Pulmonary HTN
   Renal dysfunction
2. Intrapulmonary shunting and hypoxemia
3. Spontaneous bacterial peritoneal (SBP)
4. Hepatorenal syndrome
5. Coagulopathy
6. Hepatocellular carcinoma

---

*Normal portal pressure is 10-15 cm H_2O; HTN = 30 cm H_2O.

---

standing and avoiding variceal hemorrhage, encephalopathy, and renal failure.

Most causes of portal hypertension are unlikely to occur in women of childbearing years, but a few deserve special mention. Pregnant patients with

**BOX 30-7 POTENTIAL CAUSES
OF PORTAL HYPERTENSION**

Cirrhosis
  Chronic hepatitis/postviral cirrhosis
  Alcoholic (Laennec's) cirrhosis
  Primary (autoimmune?) biliary cirrhosis
  Secondary biliary cirrhosis
    (prolonged bile duct obstruction)
Cardiac cirrhosis
Advanced alpha$_1$-antitrypsin deficiency
Advanced Wilson's disease
Advanced hemochromatosis
Cryptogenic cirrhosis
Budd-Chiari syndrome (hepatic vein thrombosis)
Extrahepatic portal vein obstruction (EHPVO)

Wilson's disease should continue to take the chelating agent but should be aware of the possibility of penicillamine-induced maternal thrombocytopenia.[41,57,58] Budd-Chiari syndrome is frequently associated with a variety of hypercoagulable states, including pregnancy and oral contraceptive use. When acute hepatic vein thrombosis occurs in pregnancy, it is almost always in the early postpartum period.[59-61]

The reported experience of pregnancy in patients with portal hypertension is small.[2,45] Obstetric management in and between studies is inconsistent, unstandardized, and frequently contradictory. Anesthetic management is rarely reported.[47,62] While it is not realistic to identify a "single best" treatment plan for all patients, we can outline basic management goals.

When approaching the patient with known hepatic disease, one should first rule out the presence of cirrhosis or hepatocellular destruction. If there is no hepatic damage, for the most part patients are treated no differently than other parturients. Any patient with cirrhosis has an increased anesthetic risk, but those patients with more advanced disease present special problems and leave no room for error or inattention. A careful preoperative search for the sequelae of cirrhosis is mandatory and should begin at the first patient contact. The patient should be transferred to an institution where multidisciplinary approach is optimal and adequate obstetric, anesthesiology, hepatology, and neonatology services are available.

Esophageal varices. Of the potential complications of portal hypertension, esophageal varices in the parturient are the most ominous. In nonpregnant women with cirrhosis, mortality is 38% when varices bleed and cumulative mortality is 65% in the year following a variceal bleed.[63] One large retrospective review of parturients with esophageal varices found perinatal mortality in this population to be 18%.[2] The lower mortality is most likely due to demographic factors, including a relatively "healthy" subgroup compared to all patients with esophageal varices. Several authors have concluded that pregnancy has no effect on the underlying disease or on the overall frequency of hemorrhage.[2,64] This does not explain the predisposition to hemorrhage in the second trimester as reported by these authors. We feel that the rapid expansion in blood volume, especially during the second trimester, places parturients at increased risk during the latter half of pregnancy. For this reason prophylactic sclerotherapy of esophageal varices early in pregnancy is the preferred method of management. In the small number of patients reported to have been treated in this manner, the maternal and fetal mortality rate has been 0%.[47,65-69]

Recently, transjugular intrahepatic portal-systemic shunt (TIPSS) has been proposed as a means of reducing esophageal venous pressures.[70,71] Via an internal jugular introducer sheath, a stent is guided radiographically and placed as a fistula between the portal and hepatic venous systems. While the use of surgical portosystemic shunting in severely cirrhotic patients has not improved survival, in one large study of cirrhosis in pregnancy severe hemorrhage was 7 times more frequent in the nonshunted group.[45] Cheng has reported increased fetal wastage and perinatal loss primarily due to prematurity in nonshunted parturients with cirrhosis.[72] TIPSS, a radiologic procedure performed under intravenous sedation in the fluoroscopy suite, has a low risk profile compared with surgical shunting. We believe that TIPSS is indicated early in pregnancy, before the increased blood volume seen late in the second trimester. Serial endoscopy and hepatic ultrasound with Duplex should indicate the need for shunt revision.[73]*

Encephalopathy

Encephalopathy in hepatic disease is seen whenever the liver is no longer able to metabolize a variety of gut-derived compounds including ammonia, as-yet unidentified endogenous GABAergic substances, and possibly other neuroactive peptides.[74] This occurs most commonly from two situations: fulminant hepatic failure *(vide infra)* and in a secondary effect from any portosystemic shunt-

---

*Pushing during the second stage should be avoided in these cases. Epidural analgesia will be helpful both for pain relief for the first stage and prophylactic forceps or vacuum extraction during the second stage.—*Editor*

ing procedure. If left untreated, encephalopathy can progress to cerebral edema and result in coma and death.

Treatment is largely supportive and will include efforts to control precipitating events such as gastrointestinal bleeding, infection, excess dietary protein intake, and overzealous use of sedatives or potassium-wasting diuretics. One should initiate a low-protein diet enriched with branched-chain amino acids at the first sign of encephalopathy: treatment with neomycin may be necessary. Correction of underlying causes of encephalopathy prior to delivery will be necessary. For operative or vaginal delivery, regional anesthesia is not contraindicated but will depend on the patient's ability to cooperate. Minimal dosing recommendations for both local anesthetic and opioids are important.

Renal failure

A variety of mechanisms have been proposed to explain the renal failure and electrolyte disturbances that comprise hepatorenal syndrome. The most salient points are:

1. Renal tubular sodium avidity due to increased aldosterone secretion. This is related to reduced "effective" plasma volume combined with decreased oncotic pressure; increased hydrostatic pressure will lead to redistribution of fluid from intravascular to interstitial spaces (ascites, pulmonary effusions or edema, cerebral edema).
2. Decreased intravascular volume causing increased renin and angiotensin production, leading to intrarenal blood flow redistribution and oliguria.[75,76]

Pulmonary hypertension

Pulmonary hypertension is an uncommon complication of portal hypertension. Its incidence is only 0.25% to 2%, but mortality is increased in these patients.[77] Pathophysiology is not entirely understood, but there are two likely theories: (1) repeated embolization of pulmonary arteries by microthrombi arising from the hepatic vascular bed, and (2) alteration of pulmonary vascular tone by as yet unidentified substances originating in the gut and escaping liver inactivation.[78,79] Pulmonary hypertension accompanying portal hypertension has been reported with or without portocaval shunting and in pregnancy.[47,78,80] Liver transplantation does not reverse the pulmonary hypertension.[81]

Presenting signs are likely to be nonspecific, but any patient with hepatic disease presenting with dyspnea, syncope, hemoptysis, or chest pain de-

serves a workup to exclude pulmonary hypertension. Chest x-ray examination, arterial blood gas determination, and an electrocardiogram may be helpful, but definitive diagnosis will probably require transthoracic echocardiography or pulmonary artery catheterization. The accurate determination of pulmonary artery pressures by echocardiography may be difficult in the presence of a gravid uterus.

Obstetric and anesthetic management of patients with pulmonary hypertension is described by Johnson and Salzmann in Chapter 12. For patients with hepatic disease and concomitant pulmonary hypertension, we feel that assisted vaginal delivery is the preferred mode of delivery and that operative delivery should be reserved for deteriorating maternal or fetal status. We have reported one delivery by cesarean section using a slowly titrated epidural induction and maintenance.[47] A pulmonary artery catheter was invaluable during this process.

Coagulopathy

Obstetric and anesthetic management. The liver is responsible for synthesizing protein clotting factors, and the majority of patients with cirrhosis will have some quantitative diminution of factor activity. Fortunately, clinically normal clotting is possible with even 10% to 30% of most normal factor levels. A rise in prothrombin time (PT)/international normalized ratio (INR) in the absence of disseminated intravascular coagulopathy (DIC) indicates severe hepatic dysfunction and is an indicator of poor prognosis (Table 30-4). Unlike cholestasis, in which there is malabsorption of vitamin K, hepatocyte function in cirrhosis is insufficient to meet synthetic demands and vitamin K may be ineffective in reversing coagulopathy.

Splenomegaly and bone marrow suppression frequently accompany cirrhosis and account for the thrombocytopenia often seen in these patients. Administering 10 to 15 ml/kg of body weight fresh frozen plasma (FFP) will effectively replace clotting factors in most patients. Postpartum bleeding due to thrombocytopenia in this population is unlikely above 40,000 to 50,000 platelets/mm^3, and platelets should be transfused only for clinical bleeding supported, when possible, by laboratory confirmation.[82,83] The use of desmopressin (DDAVP) to improve the qualitative function of platelets may have its place, but its use has not been reported in pregnancy. In the absence of clinical bleeding, prophylactic platelet and FFP transfusion before regional anesthesia or surgery is controversial, is poorly supported in the literature, and is probably unnecessary for stable platelet counts above 50,000 and PT/INR less than 1.5.

Table 30-4 Child-Turcotte classification with Pugh modification

Albumin (g/dl)	>3.5	3.0-3.5	<3.0
Bilirubin (mg/dl)	<2.0	2.0-3.0	>3.0
Ascites	none	controlled	uncontrolled
Encephalopathy	none	minimal	coma
Nutrition*	excellent	good	wasted
PT prolongation(s)*	<4.0	4.0-6.0	>6.0
Operative mortality	0-10%	4-31%	19-76%

*The Pugh modification replaces nutrition with PT prolongation.
From Pugh R, Murray-Lyon I, Dawson J, et al: Transection of the esophagus for bleeding esophageal varices. *Br J Surg* 1973; 60:646.

Fulminant hepatic failure

Acute hepatic failure regardless of the etiology is characterized by tachypnea and progressive encephalopathy; it is frequently accompanied by some combination of hypoglycemia, lactic acidosis, hypoxemia, hyperdynamic heart, renal failure, and increasing coagulation abnormalities. Liver "function" tests with the possible exceptions of PT and albumin levels are not reliable indicators of the severity of disease. The prognosis for patients with acute hepatic failure is poor.

Tachypnea, frequently the first sign of impending hepatic failure, is due to central stimulation of respiration by hyperammonemia. Encephalopathy is related to high levels of circulating ammonia, endogenous GABAergic agonists, and possibly other gut-derived compounds.[74] Hypoglycemia results from decreased "first pass" clearance of insulin, impaired gluconeogenesis, and diminished glycogen stores.

HEPATIC MASS LESIONS

Right upper quadrant pain during pregnancy may cause concern over uncommon but serious hepatic diseases and provoke a diagnostic workup including hepatic imaging. Should a mass lesion be uncovered during pregnancy, the dilemma arises as to how aggressively to pursue the diagnosis. Benign hepatic cysts and hemangiomas are the most common lesions. Other possibilities include abscess, benign lesions, and carcinomas. Focal nodular hyperplasia (FNH) and liver cell adenoma (LCA) are histologically benign mass lesions associated with pregnancy and oral contraceptive use. LCA, while not highly vascular, has been associated with high maternal and fetal mortality when intraperitoneal rupture occurs.[84]

Full discussion of the workup of hepatic masses during pregnancy is beyond the scope of this chapter, but an excellent recent review is available.[13] In general, mass lesions should be followed noninvasively if possible until the postpartum period.

If the mass enlarges, pain is intense and unacceptable, or there is evidence of hemorrhage or abscess, a more aggressive approach may be necessary.

Liver transplantation and pregnancy

There are seven reported cases of liver transplantation during pregnancy.[85-90] There were three maternal deaths, one intrauterine fetal demise, and two successful deliveries by cesarean section remote from transplantation. The indication for cesarean section is undescribed in one patient; it was active genital herpes in the other. The two reported surviving infants were apparently doing well despite in-utero exposure to multiple anesthetic and antirejection medications.

The largest reported experience with pregnancy after liver transplantation is from Pittsburgh, Pa., and France.[91,92] Fertility following transplantation is the rule rather than the exception. Most pregnancies proceed uneventfully, but there is an increased incidence of maternal hypertension and preeclampsia. Maternal graft rejection occurred in a small percentage of these patients, but no patients required retransplantation during pregnancy. Recent liver transplant recipients should actively avoid pregnancy for 9 to 12 months.[91]

Reported fetal and neonatal problems include spontaneous abortion, prematurity, neonatal immunosuppression and infection, and intrauterine growth retardation.[93-95]

REFERENCES

1. Green P, Rubin L: Amenorrhea as a manifestation of chronic liver disease. *Am J Obstet Gynecol* 1959; 78:141.
2. Britton R: Pregnancy and esophageal varices. *Am J Surg* 1982; 143:421.
3. Samuels P, Cohen A: Pregnancies complicated by liver disease and liver dysfunction, in Roberts W (ed): Medical Complications During Pregnancy. *Obstet Gynecol Clin North Am* 1992; 19:745.
4. Munnell E, Taylor H: Liver blood flow in pregnancy—hepatic vein catheterization. *J Clin Invest* 1947; 26:952.

5. Van Dyke R: The liver in pregnancy, in Zakim D, Boyer T (eds): *Hepatology: A Textbook of Liver Disease*. Philadelphia, WB Saunders, 1990.

6. Fagan E: Diseases of liver, biliary system, and pancreas, in Creasy R, Resnik R (eds): *Maternal Fetal Medicine: Principles and Practice,* ed 3. Philadelphia, WB Saunders, 1994.

7. Ravindran R, Gupta C, Stoops C: Epidural analgesia in the presence of herpes simplex virus (type 2) infection. *Anesth Analg* 1982; 61:714.

8. Ramanathan S, Sheth R, Turndorf H: Anesthesia for cesarean section in patients with genital herpes infections: A retrospective review. *Anesthesiology* 1986; 64:807.

9. Crosby E, Halpern S, Rolbin S: Epidural anesthesia for cesarean section in patients with active recurrent genital herpes simplex infections: A retrospective review. *Can J Anaesth* 1989; 36:701.

10. Bader A, Camann W, Datta S: Anesthesia for cesarean delivery in patients with herpes simplex virus type-2 infections. *Reg Anesth* 1990; 15:261.

11. Crone L, Conly J, Storgard C, et al: Herpes labialis in parturients receiving epidural morphine following cesarean section. *Anesthesiology* 1990; 73:208.

12. Hughes S, Dailey P, Lander D, et al: Paturients injected with human immunodeficiency virus and regional anesthesia: Clinical and immune response. *Anesthesiology* 1995; 82:32.

13. Lee W: Pregnancy in patients with chronic liver disease, in Reily S, Abell T (eds): Gastrointestinal and Liver Problems in Pregnancy. *Gastroenterol Clin North Am* 1992; 21:889.

14. Klebanoff M, Koslowe P, Kaslow R, et al: Epidemiology of vomiting in early pregnancy. *Obstet Gynecol* 1985; 66:612.

15. Abell T, Reily C: Hyperemesis gravidarum. *Gastrointest Clin North Am* 1992; 21(4):835.

16. Weigel M, Weigel R: Nausea and vomiting of early pregnancy and pregnancy outcome: An epidemiological study. *Br J Obstet Gynaecol* 1989; 96:1304.

17. Weigel R, Weigel M: Nausea and vomiting of early pregnancy and pregnancy outcome: A meta analytical review. *Br J Obstet Gynaecol* 1989; 96:1312.

18. Sibai B, Kusterman L, Velasco J: Current understanding of severe preeclampsia, pregnancy-associated hemolytic syndrome, thrombotic thrombocytopenic purpura, hemolysis, elevated liver enzymes, low platelet syndrome, and postpartum acute renal failure: Different clinical syndromes or just different names? *Curr Opin Nephrol Hypertens* 1994; 3(4):436.

19. Schorr-Lesnick B, Lebovics E, Dworkin B, et al: Liver diseases unique to pregnancy. *Am J Gastroenterol* 1991; 86:659.

20. Manas K, Welsh J, Rankin R, et al: Hepatic hemorrhage without rupture in preeclampsia. *N Engl J Med* 1985; 424.

21. Rolfes D, Ishak K: Liver disease in toxemia of pregnancy. *Am J Gastroenterol* 1986; 81:1138.

22. Kreuger K, Hoffman B, Lee W: Hepatic infarction associated with eclampsia. *Am J Gastroenterol* 1990; 85:588.

23. Brown M, Reddy K, Hensley G, et al: The initial presentation of fatty liver of pregnancy mimicking acute viral hepatitis. *Am J Gastroenterol* 1987; 82:554.

24. Mabie W: Acute fatty liver of pregnancy, in Reily C, Abell T (eds): Gastrointestinal and liver problems in pregnancy. *Gastroenterol Clin North Am* 1992; 21:951.

25. Crockett H, de Virgilio C, Shimoaka E, et al: Acute fatty liver of pregnancy: Laparoscopy-assisted diagnosis. *Surg Laparosc Endosc* 1994; 4:230.

26. Riely C, Latham P, Romero R, et al: Acute fatty liver of pregnancy: A reassessment based on observations in nine patients. *Ann Intern Med* 1987; 106:703.

27. Reily C: Hepatic disease in pregnancy. *Am J Med* 1994; 96(S1A):18S.

28. Antognini J, Andrews S: Anaesthesia for caesarean section in a patient with acute fatty liver of pregnancy. *Can J Anaesth* 1991; 38:904.

29. Mishra L, Seeff L: Viral hepatitis, A through E, complicating pregnancy, in Reily C, Abell T (eds): Gastrointestinal and Liver Problems in Pregnancy. *Gastroenterol Clin North Am* 1992; 21:873.

30. Adams R, Combes R: Viral hepatitis during pregnancy. *JAMA* 1965; 192:195.

31. Horstmann D: Viral infections, in Burrow G, Ferris T (eds): *Medical Complications During Pregnancy.* Philadelphia, WB Saunders, 1982:333.

32. American College of Obstetricians and Gynecologists: Hepatitis in pregnancy. *ACOG Technical Bulletin no. 174.* Washington, DC, 1992.

33. Centers for Disease Control: Protection against viral hepatitis: Recommendations of the Immunization Practices Advisory Committee (ACIP). *MMWR* 1990; 39(RR-2):1.

34. Tong M, Thursby M, Rakela J, et al: Studies on maternal-infant transmission of the viruses which cause acute hepatitis. *Gastroenterology* 1981; 80:999.

35. Haemmerli U: Jaundice during pregnancy with special reference on recurrent jaundice during pregnancy and its differential diagnosis. *Acta Med Scand* 1966; 444:1.

36. Centers for Disease Control: Public health service interagency guidelines for screening donors of blood, plasma, organs, tissues, and semen for evidence of hepatitis B and hepatitis C. *MMWR* 1991; 40:5.

37. Sweet R: Hepatitis B infection in pregnancy. *Obstet Gynecol Report* 1990; 2:128.

38. Snydman D: Hepatitis in pregnancy. *N Engl J Med* 1985; 313:1398.

39. Centers for Disease Control: Maternal hepatitis B screening practices—California, Connecticut, Kansas, and United States, 1992-1993. *MMWR* 1994; 43:311.

40. Berry M, Herrera J: Diagnosis and treatment of chronic viral hepatitis. *Compr Ther* 1994; 20:16.

41. Steven M: Pregnancy and liver disease. *Gut* 1981; 22:592.

42. Stevens C, Beasley R, Tsui J, et al: Vertical transmission of hepatitis B antigen in Taiwan. *N Engl J Med* 1975; 292:771.

43. Centers for Disease Control: Hepatitis B virus: A comprehensive strategy for eliminating transmission in the United States through universal childhood vaccination. Recommendations of the Immunization Practices Advisory Committee (ACIP). *MMWR* 1991; 40(RR-13):1.

44. Committee on Infectious Diseases, American Academy of Pediatrics: *Report of the Committee on Infectious Diseases.* ed 22, Elk Grove Village, Ill, 1991, pp 238-255.

45. Schreyer P, Caps E, El-Hindi J, et al: Cirrhosis—Pregnancy and delivery: A review. *Obstet Gynecol Surv* 1982; 37:304.

46. Schweitzer I, Peters R: Pregnancy in hepatitis B antigen positive cirrhosis. *Obstet Gynecol* 1976; 48(1):S53.

47. O'Neill S, Scioscia E, Swanson J, et al: Transjugular intrahepatic portosystemic stent shunt (TIPSS) placement and a successful pregnancy. Submitted for publication, April 1995.

48. Giraud P, Drouet J, Dupuy J: Hepatitis B virus infection of children born to mothers with severe hepatitis. *Lancet* 1975; 2:1088.

49. Bucholz H, Frosner G, Ziegler G: HB Ag carrier state in an infant delivered by caesarean section. *Lancet* 1974; 2:343.

50. Zanetti A, Ferroni P, Magliono E, et al: Perinatal trans-

mission of the hepatitis B virus and the HBV-associated delta agent from mother to offspring in northern Italy. *J Med Virol* 1982; 9:139.

51. Sylvan S, Hellstrom U, Hampl H, et al: Hepatitis E in patients with chronic autoimmune liver disease. *JAMA* 1995; 273:377.

52. Centers for Disease Control: Hepatitis E among U.S. travelers, 1989-1992. *MMWR* 1993; 42:1.

53. Bernau J: Significance of elevated transaminase levels at the end of pregnancy (editorial). *Presse Med* 1994; 23:466.

54. Ngai S: Current concepts in anesthesiology. *N Engl J Med* 1980; 302:564.

55. Shalev O, Mosseri M, Ariel I, et al: Methyldopa-induced immune hemolytic anemia and chronic active hepatitis. *Arch Intern Med* 1983; 143:592.

56. Centers for Disease Control: Deaths and hospitalizations from chronic liver disease and cirrhosis—United States, 1980-1989. *MMWR* 1993; 41:969.

57. Albukerk J: The pregnant woman with Wilson's disease. *N Engl J Med* 1976; 294:670.

58. Shimono N, Ishibashi H, Ikematsu H, et al: Fulminant hepatic failure during perinatal period in a pregnant woman with Wilson's disease. *Hepatogastroenterology* 1990; 37(S2):122.

59. Khuroo M, Datta D: Budd-Chiari syndrome following pregnancy: Report of 16 cases with roentgenologic, hemodynamic and histologic studies of the hepatic outflow tract. *Am J Med* 1980; 8:113.

60. Benhamou J, Lebrec D: Non-cirrhotic intrahepatic portal hypertension in adults. *Clin Gastroenterol* 1985; 14:21.

61. Tiliacos M, Tsantoulas D, Tsoulias A, et al: The Budd-Chiari syndrome in pregnancy. *Postgrad Med J* 1978; 54:686.

62. Duke J: Pregnancy and cirrhosis: Management of hematemesis by Warren shunt during third trimester gestation. *Int J Obstet Anesth* 1994; 3:97.

63. Smith J, Graham D: Variceal hemorrhage: A critical evaluation of survival analysis. *Gastroenterology* 1982; 82:968.

64. Homburg R, Bayer I, Lurie B: Bleeding esophageal varices in pregnancy: A report of two cases. *J Reprod Med* 1988; 33:784.

65. Salena B, Sivak M: Pregnancy and esophageal varices. *Gastrointest Endosc* 1988; 34:492.

66. Augustine P, Joseph P: Sclerotherapy for esophageal varices and pregnancy. *Gastrointest Endosc* 1989; 35:467.

67. Kochkar R, Goenka M, Mehta S: Endoscopic sclerotherapy during pregnancy. *Am J Gastroenterol* 1990; 85:1132.

68. Pauzner D, Wolman I, Niv D, et al: Endoscopic sclerotherapy in extrahepatic portal hypertension in pregnancy. *Am J Obstet Gynecol* 1991; 164:152.

69. Iwase H, Morise K, Kawase T, et al: Endoscopic injection sclerotherapy for esophageal varices during pregnancy. *J Clin Gastroenterol* 1994; 18:80.

70. Conn H: Transjugular intrahepatic portal-systemic shunts: The state of the art. *Hepatology* 1993; 17:148.

71. Hebbard G, Fitt G, Thomson K, et al: Transjugular intrahepatic portal-systemic shunts (TIPS)—Initial experience and clinical outcome. *Aust NZ J Med* 1994; 24:141.

72. Cheng Y: Pregnancy in liver cirrhosis and/or portal hypertension. *Am J Obstet Gynecol* 1977; 128:812.

73. McGaughan G: Transvenous intrahepatic porto-systemic shunt (TIPSS): A new treatment for portal hypertension. *Aust NZ J Med* 1994; 24:133.

74. Jones E (moderator): The γ-aminobutyric acid A (GABA$_A$) receptor complex and hepatic encephalopathy: Some recent advances. *Ann Intern Med* 1989; 110:532.

75. Gelman S, Kang Y, Pearson J: Anesthetic considerations in liver transplantation, in Fabian J (ed): *Anesthesia for Organ Transplantation.* JB Lippincott, Philadelphia, 1992, pp 121-124.

76. Schrier R: Body fluid volume regulation in health and disease: A unifying hypothesis. *Ann Intern Med* 1990; 113:155.

77. Hadengue A, Kamal M, Lebrec D, et al: Pulmonary hypertension complicating portal hypertension: Prevalence and relation to splanchnic hemodynamics. *Gastroenterology* 1991; 100:520.

78. Sallam M, Watson W: Pulmonary hypertension due to microthromboembolism from splenic and portal veins after portocaval anastomosis. *Br Heart J* 1970; 32:269.

79. Lebrec D, Capron J, Dhumeaux D, et al: Pulmonary hypertension complicating portal hypertension. *Am Rev Respir Dis* 1979; 120:849.

80. Bernthal A, Eybel C, Payne J: Primary pulmonary hypertension after portocaval shunt. *J Clin Gastroenterol* 1983; 5:353.

81. Prager M, Cauldwell C, Ascher N, et al: Pulmonary hypertension associated with liver disease is not reversible after liver transplantation. *Anesthesiology* 1992; 77:375.

82. Roberts W, Perry K, Woods J, et al: The intrapartum platelet count in patients with HELLP (hemolysis, elevated liver enzymes, and low platelets) syndrome: Is it predictive of later hemorrhagic complications? *Am J Obstet Gynecol* 1994; 171:799.

83. Coller B: Platelets and thrombolytic therapy. *N Engl J Med* 1990; 322:33.

84. Knowles D, Casarella W, Johnson P, et al: The clinical, radiologic, and pathologic characterization of benign hepatic neoplasms: Alleged association with oral contraceptives. *Medicine* 1978; 57:223.

85. Fair J, Klein A, Feng T, et al: Intrapartum orthotopic liver transplantation with successful outcome of pregnancy. *Transplantation* 1990; 50:534.

86. Zaballos J, Perez-Cerda F, Riano D, et al: Anesthetic management of liver transplantation in a pregnant patient with fulminant hepatitis. *Transplant Proc* 1992; 23:1994.

87. Moreno E, Garcia G, Gomez S, et al: Fulminant hepatic failure during pregnancy successfully treated by orthotopic liver transplantation. *Transplantation* 1991; 52:923.

88. Merritt W, Dickstein R, Burdick J, et al: Liver transplantation during pregnancy: Anesthesia for two procedures in the same patient with successful outcome of pregnancy. *Transplant Proc* 1992; 23:1996.

89. Hamilton M, Alcock R, Magos L, et al: Liver transplantation during pregnancy. *Transplant Proc* 1993; 25:2967.

90. Erhard J, Lange R, Niebel W, et al: Liver complications in HELLP syndrome. *Z Gastroenterol* 1994; 32:16.

91. Laifer S, Darby M, Scantlebury V, et al: Pregnancy and liver transplantation. *Obstet Gynecol* 1990; 76:1083.

92. Ville Y, Fernandez H, Samuel D, et al: Pregnancy in liver transplant recipients: Course and outcome in 19 cases. *Am J Obstet Gynecol* 1993; 168:896.

93. Hutton J, Wyeth J: Pregnancy after liver transplantation: Effects of immunosuppressive therapy and abnormal hepatic function. *Aust NZ J Obstet Gynaecol* 1990; 30:130.

94. Penn I, Makowski E, Harris P: Parenthood following renal and hepatic transplantation. *Transplantation* 1980; 30:397.

95. Cundy T, O'Grady J, Williams R: Recovery of menstruation and pregnancy after liver transplantation. *Gut* 1990; 31:337.

96. Pandele G, Chaux F, Salvadori C, et al: Thiopental pharmacokinetics in patients with cirrhosis. *Anesthesiology* 1983; 59:123.

97. Thomson I, Fitch W, Hughes R, et al: Effects of certain I.V. anesthetics on liver blood flow and hepatic oxygen

consumption in the greyhound. *Br J Anaesth* 1987; 58:69.

98. Sear J: Toxicity of I.V. anaesthetics. *Br J Anaesth* 1987; 59:24.

99. Reilly C, Wood A, Koshakji R, et al: The effect of halothane on drug disposition in intrinsic drug metabolizing capacity and hepatic blood flow. *Anesthesiology* 1985; 63:70.

100. Thomson P, Melmon K, Richardson J, et al: Lidocaine pharmacokinetics in advanced heart failure, liver disease, and renal failure in humans. *Ann Intern Med* 1973; 78:499.

101. Bevan D, Donati F: Muscle relaxants, in Barash P, Cullen B, Stoelting R (eds): *Clinical Anesthesia,* ed 2. Philadelphia, JB Lippincott, 1992.

102. Whittaker M: Plasma cholinesterase variants and the anaesthetist. *Anaesthesia* 1980; 35:174.

103. Lebrault C, Berger J, D'Hollander A, et al: Pharmacokinetics and pharmacodynamics of vecuronium (ORG NC 45) in patients with cirrhosis. *Anesthesiology* 1985; 62:601.

104. Arden J, Lynam D, Castagnoli K, et al: Vecuronium in alcoholic liver disease: A pharmacokinetic and pharmacodynamic analysis. *Anesthesiology* 1988; 68:771.

105. Khalil M, D'Honneur, Duvaldestin P, et al: Pharmacokinetics and pharmacodynamics of rocuronium in patients with cirrhosis. *Anesthesiology* 1994; 80:1241.

106. Basta S, Savarese J, Ali H, et al: Clinical pharmacology of doxacurium chloride. *Anesthesiology* 1988; 69:478.

107. Magorian T, Wood P, Caldwell J, et al: The pharmacokinetics and neuromuscular effects of rocuronium bromide in patients with liver disease. *Anesth Analg* 1995; 754.

108. Patwardhan R, Johnson R, Hoyumpa A, et al: Normal metabolism of morphine in cirrhosis. *Gastroenterology* 1981; 81:1006.

109. Hasselstrom I, Eriksson S, Persson A, et al: The metabolism and bioavailability of morphine in patients with severe liver cirrhosis. *Br J Clin Pharmacol* 1990; 29:289.

110. Neal E, Meffin P, Gregory P, et al: Enhanced bioavailability and decreased clearance of analgesics in patients with cirrhosis. *Gastroenterology* 1979; 77:96.

111. Haberer J, Schoeffler P, Courderc E, et al: Fentanyl pharmacokinetics in anesthetized patients with cirrhosis. *Br J Anaesth* 1982; 54:1267.

112. Chauvin M, Ferrier C, Haberer J, et al: Sufentanil pharmacokinetics in patients with cirrhosis. *Anesth Analg* 1989; 68:1.

113. Ferrier C, Marty J, Bouffard Y, et al: Alfentanil pharmacokinetics in patients with cirrhosis. *Anesthesiology* 1985; 62:480.

114. Seligman S, Ruyon J, Clancy R, et al: The role of nitric oxide in the pathogenesis of preeclampsia. *Am J Obstet Gynecol* 1994; 171:944.

115. Berti P, Contino L, Pesando P, et al: Is the HELLP syndrome due to inherited factors? Report of two cases. *Haematologica* 1994; 79:170.

116. Weitgasser R, Schnoll F, Haidbauer R: Type 1 diabetes mellitus developing during HELLP syndrome. *Acta Diabetol* 1993; 30:173.

117. Walsh S: Preeclampsia: An imbalance in placenta prostacyclin and thromboxane production. *Am J Obstet Gynecol* 1985; 152:335.

118. Khong T, De Wolf F, Robertson W, et al: Inadequate maternal vascular response to placentation in pregnancies complicated by preeclampsia and by small-for-gestational age infants. *Br J Obstet Gynaecol* 1986; 93:1049.

119. Frusca T, Morassi L, Pecorelli S, et al: Histological features of uteroplacental vessels in normal and hypertensive patients in relation to birthweight. *Br J Obstet Gynaecol* 1989; 96:835.

120. Saleh A, Bottoms S, Welch R, et al: Preeclampsia, delivery, and the hemostatic system. *Am J Obstet Gynecol* 1987; 157:331.

121. Rodgers G, Taylor R, Roberts J: Preeclampsia is associated with a serum factor cytotoxic to human endothelial cells. *Am J Obstet Gynecol* 1988; 159:908.

122. Zuspan F, Nelson G, Ahlquist R: Epinephrine infusions in normal and toxemic pregnancies. I. Nonesterified fatty acids and cardiovascular alterations. *Am J Obstet Gynecol* 1964; 90:88.

123. Talledo O, Chesley L, Zuspan F: Renin-angiotensin system in normal and toxemic pregnancies. III. Differential sensitivity to angiotensin II and norepinephrine in toxemia of pregnancy. *Am J Obstet Gynecol* 1968; 100:218.

124. Gant N, Daley G, Chand S: A study of angiotensin II pressor response throughout primigravid pregnancy. *J Clin Invest* 1973; 52:2682.

125. Minakami H, Oka N, Sato T, et al: Preeclampsia: A microvesicular fat disease of the liver? *Am J Obstet Gynecol* 1988; 159:1043.

126. Magann E, Bass D, Chauhan S, et al: Antepartum corticosteroids: Disease stabilization in patients with the syndrome of hemolysis, elevated liver enzymes, and low platelets (HELLP). *Am J Obstet Gynecol* 1994; 171:1148.

127. Magann E, Perry K, Meydrech E, et al: Postpartum corticosteroids: Accelerated recovery from the syndrome of hemolysis, elevated liver enzymes, and low platelets (HELLP). *Am J Obstet Gynecol* 1994; 171:1154.

128. Levi-D'Ancona V, Macconi A, Tulli G, et al: A case of HELLP syndrome with dramatic course successfully treated with early plasmapheresis. *Minerva Anestesiol* 1994; 60:145.

129. Huber W, Schweiger U, Classen M: Epoprostenol and plasmapheresis in complicated HELLP syndrome with pancreatitis. *Lancet* 1994; 343:848.

130. Strauss H, Scheler C, Ropke F: HELLP syndrome on the 6th puerperal day: Presentation of case reports. *Zentralb Gynakol* 1994; 116:210.

131. Krick M, Pagel C, Baltzer J: Increasing incidence of HELLP syndrome: Diagnosis and treatment. *Zentralb Gynakol* 1994; 116:207.

132. Visser W, van-Pampus M, Treffers P, et al: Perinatal results of hemodynamic and conservative temporizing treatment in severe preeclampsia. *Eur J Obstet Gynecol Reprod Biol* 1994; 53(3):175.

133. Olah K, Redman C, Gee H: Management of severe, early pre-eclampsia: Is conservative management justified? *Eur J Obstet Gynecol Reprod Biol* 1993; 51:175.

134. Pugh R, Murray-Lyon I, Dawson J, et al: Transection of the esophagus for bleeding esophageal varices. *Br J Surg* 1973; 60:646.

31 Fetal Distress

Andrew P. Harris, Adam Goldstein, and Frank R. Witter

In an attempt to optimize neonatal outcome, obstetricians strive to identify those in-utero conditions that cause a clinical fetal state to develop—conditions which, if left alone, would result in fetal compromise. This clinical state is frequently referred to as "fetal distress." This term, although widely used to describe various antepartum and intrapartum in utero conditions, is rarely well defined. Any discussion of the pathophysiology, diagnosis, or management of this condition necessarily centers on the exact definition used. Although some authors use terms solely related to fetal heart rate tracing interpretation in their definition of fetal distress,[1,2] others relate the term to depressed Apgar scores or fetal acidosis,[3] or even to a requirement that positive pressure ventilation is necessary in the newborn.[4]

Definition of fetal distress

In a recent review, Parer and Livingston[5] conclude that fetal distress is best defined through its relationship to asphyxia—that is, the state of fetal distress is the end result of physiologic and pathophysiologic responses to an asphyxiated state in utero. They suggest that a workable definition of fetal distress would be "progressive fetal asphyxia that if not corrected or circumvented will result in decompensation of the physiologic responses (primarily redistribution of blood flow to preserve oxygenation of vital organs) and cause permanent central nervous system damage and other organs damage or death." An alternate definition proposed by Harris[6] is "a pathophysiologic condition in which oxidative metabolic substrate (in acute circumstances oxygen) becomes available to the fetus in quantities insufficient to sustain in utero life for a prolonged period of time." These definitions, which encompass the physiologic basis for the clinical patterns readily identified with both fetal distress and suboptimal outcome, appear to be among the best available.

Incidence

To understand the scope and potential importance of the diagnosis of fetal distress, estimates of the incidence must be made. Such estimates can be derived from qualitative and quantitative data regarding the in-utero fetus as well as outcome measures. For instance, it has been variously estimated that approximately 4% to 7% of all infants born in developed countries can be classified as "growth retarded."[7] Of these, one third exhibit congenital anomalies. In those without congenital anomalies, the impairment of normal in-utero growth patterns can easily be understood to be the result of some extent of fetal compromise (i.e., fetal distress) occurring in utero or at some point during gestation. The potential extent of fetal compromise can be surmised from the incidence of one endpoint, fetal death in utero, in fetuses demonstrating growth retardation. Clearly, some of these growth-retarded infants were exposed to life-threatening conditions in utero, since there is an eightfold increase in the stillbirth rate in those fetuses 25% or more underweight (below the 2.5th percentile).[8] In a study of 2 million births in California, rising fetal mortality occurred with advancing gestational age in fetuses demonstrating IUGR.[9] In another study of cause of death of 765 stillbirths, hypoxia was identified as the major cause of death in 43%.[10] Interestingly, approximately 80% of in-utero deaths occurring in IUGR fetuses occur at or beyond the 35th week of gestation.[11,12] Data such as these indicate that there are indeed a significant number of infants who exhibit signs of chronic fetal distress in utero as defined above.

As for the incidence of intrapartum fetal distress, an estimate can be made from data regarding the management of labor when fetal distress is deemed present. Numerous studies report the rate of operative delivery for the diagnosis of fetal distress. For example, in the Dublin randomized trial of intrapartum fetal heart rate monitoring, in those infants randomized to electronic fetal heart rate monitoring, the incidence of cases of fetal distress (defined by fetal heart rate monitoring and scalp pH criteria) requiring operative delivery was 3.3%.[13] In this trial, 16% of all cesarean sections were performed for the indication of fetal distress. In the United States, 10% to 15% of all cesarean sections are performed for the diagnosis of fetal distress.[14]

Given these data regarding the antepartum and intrapartum incidence of fetal distress, the importance of accurately diagnosing fetal distress is clear: if delivery of an asphyxiated fetus is achieved before fetal compensatory mechanisms fail, one would predict that the rate of intact survival (including a good neurologic outcome) can be improved by avoidance of severe asphyxia. In the Dublin trial, the diagnosis of fetal distress by continuous electronic fetal heart monitoring was associated with a lower incidence of at least one indicator of poor outcome (i.e., neonatal seizures) secondary to fetal distress, compared with a group with less stringent intermittent auscultation.[13] In addition to the obvious individual and societal benefit of diagnosing and treating fetal distress before permanent organ damage occurs, increasingly scarce health care dollars could be reallocated from chronic care of the neurologically impaired infant to other health care needs.

The goal of the accurate diagnosis and management of fetal distress should be to reduce the risk of both fetal and neonatal death as well as a lifelong organ system impairment, especially neurologic impairment. Long-term adverse neurologic outcome can include behavioral difficulties, cerebral palsy, and mental retardation.[14] It should be noted that although fetal distress can obviously occur throughout gestation as well as intrapartum, it is estimated that only a small minority of children with cerebral palsy or severe retardation had evidence of fetal distress during the intrapartum period.[15-18]

As mentioned, in-utero asphyxia almost always precedes and is associated with fetal distress. Asphyxia is best defined as a pathophysiologic condition in which there is insufficiency of exchange of respiratory gases including both carbon dioxide and oxygen. In the fetus, in most circumstances an isolated decrease in Pao_2 or an elevation in $Paco_2$ is not seen (the postnatal analogy being that hypoventilation from a low baseline Pao_2 is associated with both increased Pco_2 and decreased Po_2). Oxygen and carbon dioxide changes occur in tandem. Therefore, fetal asphyxia is associated with hypoxemia, hypercarbia, and a resulting acidosis. This acidosis may be either respiratory acidosis secondary to hypercarbia alone (early), or combined with metabolic acidosis secondary to accumulation of lactic acid by products of anaerobic metabolism occurring pursuant to a hypoxemic condition (late). Since all fetuses have arterial oxygen tensions lower and arterial carbon dioxide tensions higher than normally seen postnatally, the term asphyxia, just like the terms hypoxemic and hypercarbic, must only be used to describe fetal conditions relative to normal in-utero fetal physiology. Any discussion of diagnosis and management of fetal distress (and therefore asphyxia) must be preceded by discussion of apropos in-utero fetal physiology.

NORMAL IN-UTERO FETAL PHYSIOLOGY

Normal patterns of fetal physiology differ from postnatal physiology in many ways. These differences must be understood in order to recognize when deviations are occurring as a result of asphyxia in utero.

Fetal metabolism is primarily oxidative just as seen in postnatal animals. However, the fetus has a much smaller oxygen reserve within its body, and to maintain viability it is therefore dependent on ongoing transport of oxygen from the mother through the placenta. A study of the pathway oxygen takes from the ambient environment to the fetal cell will serve to indicate those locations along that pathway at which impairment could occur and thus result in a hypoxic state in the fetus (Fig. 31-1). The most common areas for interference with oxygen transport include decreases in uterine blood flow, alterations in placental function, and compression of umbilical arteries. The Po_2 in each step of this process cascades in such a way that umbilical venous Po_2 (which approximates Po_2 of preductal blood perfusing the brain and myocardium) is approximately only 28 torr.[19] Under chronic basal conditions the fetus is thus exposed to relatively low oxygen levels. Despite this chronic exposure to relatively low in-utero Po_2, there is good evidence that the fetus is not nor-

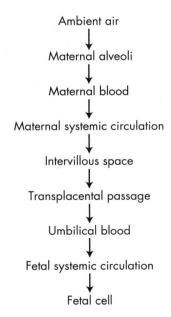

Fig. 31-1 Pathway of oxygen to the fetal cell.

mally "hypoxic." Evidence that hypoxia is not present at this "normal" Po_2 is that (1) there is net lactate uptake by the fetus, (2) only small amounts of hydrogen ion are transferred from fetus to mother, (3) there is no increase in oxygen consumption when additional oxygen is made available to the fetus, and (4) the healthy fetus has a normal basal pH.[20]

FETAL RESPONSE TO ASPHYXIA

The fetus, although chronically exposed to relatively low Po_2, will nonetheless respond with dramatic circulatory changes to further decreases in oxygenation that threaten survival. The physiologic responses to isolated hypoxemia have been widely studied in fetal sheep. These responses to decreased oxygenation include a redistribution of blood flow away from the kidneys, spleen, carcass, and skin toward the heart, brain, placenta and adrenal glands.[21] In the heart and brain, the resulting increase in myocardial and cerebral blood flow can completely compensate for the decreased oxygen content of the blood, maintaining myocardial and cerebral oxygen delivery even through episodes of relatively severe hypoxemia (i.e., decreases in arterial oxygen content of 80%).[22] At modest levels of hypoxemia, combined ventricular output is not decreased and blood pressure and heart rate are unchanged.[23] However, at extreme levels of hypoxemia, cardiac output is decreased secondary to the bradycardic response of chemoreceptor stimulation.[23] This decrease in cardiac output may be exacerbated by the presence of acidemia.[24] In such extreme hypoxemic states when oxygen content is reduced by 80%, combined blood flow to the heart and brain, which normally accounts for only 7% to 8% of cardiac output, increases to approximately 25% of cardiac output.[22]

During severe fetal hypoxemia, fetal oxygen consumption may be depressed by as much as 40% in fetal lambs.[25] This decrease in fetal oxygen consumption is associated with decreased metabolism in the fetal liver, intestines, and kidney, while cerebral and myocardial oxygen uptake are unchanged.[25-27] Fetal skeletal muscle activity (including fetal breathing movements) decreases. Glycogenolysis occurs, resulting in increased substrate availability for the brain and heart. If bradycardia occurs in conjunction with severe fetal hypoxemia, myocardial oxygen consumption decreases.[23] This level of decreased oxygen consumption can be maintained for periods of up to 45 minutes and appears to be completely reversible with cessation of hypoxemia.[5]

Other fetal sheep experimental models have studied hypoxemia combined with hypercarbia (i.e., asphyxia), which (as mentioned above) is the more clinically relevant scenario. In one study in which fetal asphyxia was induced by decreasing uterine blood flow in pregnant sheep,[24] a 50% decrease in uterine blood flow was associated with neither a decrease in pH nor a decrease in myocardial or cerebral blood flow. At extremes of asphyxia, however, these compensatory mechanisms fail. When uterine blood flow was further decreased to 25% of normal, myocardial blood flow and cerebral blood flow decreased from the levels seen with only a 50% decrease in uterine blood flow to a level below baseline flow. Given the simultaneous fall in Po_2, oxygen delivery to the brain and myocardium decreased to levels at which ongoing viability was threatened. Interestingly, at this extreme level of asphyxia, in contrast to what is observed at lesser levels of asphyxia, vasoconstriction appeared to occur in all organs (including the heart and brain) except the adrenal glands. At that extreme level of asphyxia, fetal pH decreased significantly and base excess increased, suggesting that normal compensatory mechanisms that had successfully compensated for lesser levels of asphyxia were beginning to fail. Parer and Livingston[5] felt that this stage of failing compensatory mechanisms most likely will result in bradycardia, hypotension, and death unless corrected within a relatively short time. They postulate that it is also during this phase that irreversible hypoxic organ damage may occur. Therefore, recognition of less severe in-utero asphyxia before this stage might lead to the ability to treat fetal distress more promptly and effectively.

CONDITIONS PREDISPOSING TO FETAL DISTRESS

There are various conditions at the maternal, fetal, and placental level that are associated with an increased risk of fetal distress developing during pregnancy and labor (Box 31-1). When these conditions are suspected, antepartum testing is frequently used to determine in-utero fetal well-being and to plan appropriate treatment strategies for those infants suffering chronic fetal distress in utero. For many of these conditions, even if chronic fetal distress is not seen during pregnancy, the fetus may be at greatly increased risk of developing fetal distress during the physiologic stress of labor.

DIAGNOSIS

Clinically, the means of diagnosis of fetal distress are nonspecific and imprecise, with low positive predictive values even in high-risk populations.[28] The methods available for intrapartum fetal observation, though very rarely incorrect in identifying the fetus without clinically significant intrapartum

BOX 31-1   RISK FACTORS FOR FETAL DISTRESS

Maternal
  Cardiopulmonary disease
  Renal failure
  Extremes of childbearing age
  Low socioeconomic class
  Small size/stature
  Tobacco use
  Alcohol use
  Drug use (i.e., heroin, cocaine)
  Hypertensive and vascular disease
  Malnutrition
  History of small-for-gestational-age (SGA) infant
Placental
  Retroplacental bleeding (abruption)
  Circumvallate placenta
  Placental infarct
  Chorioangioma
Fetal
  Infection
  Multiple gestation
  Karyotypic anomaly
  Long umbilical cord
  Fetal anomaly

fetal distress, are frequently incorrect when a possibly compromised fetus is identified. Intervention is undertaken more often than absolutely necessary in the recognition that a nonreassuring fetal observation does not reliably predict perinatal asphyxia.

Asphyxia associated with fetal distress can occur either chronically antepartum or acutely intrapartum. The diagnosis of chronic fetal distress is best made through antepartum fetal assessment; these techniques may include evaluation of fetal growth, biophysical profile scoring, cordocentesis, and Doppler ultrasound velocimetry.

Evaluation of fetal growth is undertaken to detect those infants demonstrating intrauterine growth retardation (IUGR). Identification of fetuses whose growth does not proceed at a normal rate may indicate chronic in-utero asphyxia. In cases in which asymmetric IUGR is identified, ongoing in-utero placental insufficiency should be considered a cause of relatively normal head growth with lagging body growth. When such uteroplacental insufficiency is chronically present, the fetus is much more likely to experience acute intrapartum decompensation of physiologic compensatory mechanisms when asphyxia occurs during labor and results in fetal distress.[29]

The biophysical profile score and its components may also be useful in detecting chronic in-utero asphyxial conditions.[30] The biophysical pro-

file consists of evaluation of fetal breathing, gross body movements, fetal tone, qualitative amniotic fluid volume, and reactivity of the fetal heart rate (nonstress test). The contraction stress test (also called the oxytocin challenge test) might aid in determining a chronic fetal state that would predispose to acute decompensation during continued gestation or labor.[31]

Umbilical venous blood can be sampled directly (via cordocentesis) to assess in-utero fetal oxygenation and acid-base status in settings of severe IUGR or when fetal compromise is suspected. Umbilical blood gas measurements are capable of providing direct evidence of the presence or absence of in-utero chronic asphyxia; this provides useful guidance regarding further management.

Doppler ultrasound velocimetry can be used to measure systolic-diastolic (SD) ratios in the umbilical artery. An increased SD ratio signifies decreased diastolic umbilical arterial flow, which suggests increased placental vascular resistance. This increase in resistance indirectly implies the presence of a severe hypoxemic state because umbilical vasoconstriction occurs as a relatively late response to asphyxial challenges (as described above).[24] This decreased diastolic flow is found most often in pregnancies complicated by maternal hypertension or intrauterine growth retardation.[32,33] Completely absent diastolic flow suggests either a fetal anomaly or severe fetal growth retardation and indicates the immediate need for further evaluation of in-utero fetal distress.[34]

Intrapartum diagnosis of fetal distress can be attempted in a number of ways including examination of fetal heart rate traces, fetal scalp blood sampling, fetal EEG and ECG monitoring, and in-utero pulse oximetry. The first two techniques are widely used; the latter three are still being studied experimentally. It should be noted that of all these techniques, only scalp sampling or in-utero pulse oximetry would give direct evidence of fetal hypoxemia/asphyxia. The remaining techniques are all indirect methods that rely on our ability to detect the physiologic result of decreased oxygenation in the fetus.

Intrapartum electronic fetal heart rate monitoring can demonstrate patterns that have been associated with an increased incidence of fetal compromise. These include:

1. Severe bradycardia (fetal heart rate less than 80 beats/min persisting for 3 minutes or more)
2. Repetitive late decelerations (a symmetrical fall in the fetal heart rate, which begins at or after the peak of the uterine contraction and

returns to baseline after the contraction is over)
3. Undulating baseline (a pattern of rapid change between tachycardia and bradycardia)
4. Any nonreassuring pattern associated with unexplained poor or absent baseline variability.

The interested reader can find further details of the definitions of fetal heart rate patterns in the American College of Obstetricians and Gynecologists Technical Bulletin on Intrapartum Fetal Heart Rate Monitoring.[35]

When intrapartum electronic fetal heart rate monitoring is nonreassuring, the condition of the fetus should be confirmed by further testing, because 40% of fetuses with recurrent late decelerations have normal cord pH values at birth.[36] Intrapartum assessment of fetal acid-base status can confirm potential fetal compromise and if reassuring it can reduce the number of unnecessary cesarean sections for suspected fetal distress.[37]

Indirect assessment of fetal acid-base status through the noninvasive techniques of vibroacoustic stimulation[38] or scalp stimulation[39] should be the initial approach to further testing when a nonreassuring fetal heart trace is present. An acceleration in fetal heart rate in response to these maneuvers indicates that fetal acidosis is not present. Unfortunately, half of fetuses stimulated will not respond, and direct measurement of fetal acid-base status via scalp blood sampling may be necessary.

The gold standard for intrapartum assessment of fetal acid-base status remains direct fetal scalp blood sampling. It requires ruptured membranes and a cervix that is at least 2.5 cm dilated. The fetal vertex must be firmly applied to the cervix and the scalp cleansed of possible contaminants. The scalp is then incised at a point away from the fontanels with a long-handled, 2-mm blade. A capillary tube is used to collect fetal blood from the small wound for analysis. A normal scalp pH is above 7.25. Values between 7.20 and 7.25 should cause suspicion and should be interpreted in light of the fetal heart rate pattern and progress in labor. In general, fetal scalp blood sampling should be repeated in 15 to 30 minutes to determine if there is a downward trend in the pH. A scalp pH of less than 7.20 is abnormal and requires medical or surgical intervention that will result in expeditious delivery.

The postpartum diagnosis of fetal distress can be attempted by evaluation of the Apgar score at birth, the umbilical cord blood gas values at birth, birth weight of the infant, and neonatal neurologic testing. The Apgar score was not designed as a predictor of neurologic outcome, and it is in fact a relatively poor predictor of neurologic outcome. In term infants with a 5-minute Apgar score of 0 to 3 and a 10-minute Apgar score of 4 or greater, 99% do not subsequently develop cerebral palsy. In fact, 73% of infants who went on to develop cerebral palsy had a 5-minute Apgar score of at least 7.[41] These data demonstrate that the Apgar score is useful only to detect a small percent of infants with significant intrapartum fetal distress.

Although it would seem that umbilical cord blood gas values would be quite useful in predicting those infants with clinically significant asphyxia, they are much more useful only as a means of ruling out the presence of intrapartum fetal distress in infants with low Apgar scores at birth. In fact, low pH, like a low Apgar score, is only rarely associated with poor outcome. In a recent study of 1601 patients undergoing elective cesarean section, 9 infants had an umbilical artery blood pH of less than 7, yet none of these infants demonstrated any neonatal morbidity.[42] Umbilical blood gas values, through analysis of base deficit, may yield information regarding the acuity of fetal acidemia. Such information may be important since, as described above, partial asphyxia can be tolerated for some period of time before compensatory mechanisms begin to fail. Unfortunately, however, the level of base deficit associated with evidence of failure of compensatory mechanisms is unknown.

For the same reasons that in-utero growth and size may be a marker of chronic fetal distress, decreased size for gestational age at birth is somewhat correlated with outcome. However, Allen[43] reviewed developmental outcome in SGA infants and found that although SGA infants have a small increased risk for cerebral palsy, the vast majority have normal intelligence and no major neurologic deficits.

Finally, although careful neonatal neurologic testing may be able to detect those infants who have suffered in-utero fetal distress with resulting impaired neurologic outcome, it cannot differentiate antepartum from intrapartum asphyxia. As with the other postpartum indicators of in-utero fetal distress, the post hoc diagnosis may be of limited usefulness. For this reason, the major monitoring efforts are turned toward antepartum and intrapartum, not postpartum, detection of fetal distress.

OBSTETRIC MANAGEMENT

Once the tentative antepartum intrapartum diagnosis of fetal distress has been made, treatment modalities include improvement of in-utero conditions to restore normal respiratory gas exchange, or delivery of the infant from in-utero conditions (Box 31-2). Methods used to improve in-utero conditions in a chronic situation might include bed rest with left uterine displacement, but in an acute situation, methods would involve treatment of hypo-

---

**BOX 31-2   MANAGEMENT OF
SUSPECTED FETAL DISTRESS**

Confirm diagnosis of fetal distress
   Examine fetal heart rate trace
   Consider scalp pH
   Provide vibroacoustic or tactile stimulation
Conduct pelvic examination to exclude cord prolapse
   and vaginal bleeding
Treat relative or absolute maternal hypovolemia
   Avoid venocaval compression
   Restore intravascular volume if necessary
Treat maternal hypotension if present
   Use β-adrenergic agonist, such as ephedrine
Administer supplemental oxygen
Decrease uterine tone
   Discontinue oxytocin
   Use a tocolytic agent
Use amnioinfusion if indicated
If none of the above measures succeed, plan expedi-
   tious medical or surgical delivery

---

tension, assuring optimal maternal oxygenation and ventilation, proper maternal positioning, tocolysis, and amnioinfusion. Expedited delivery of the infant is the only option if in-utero improvement cannot be achieved or is deemed futile. Time is of the essence in such cases, since irreversible damage to the fetus has been shown to occur with as little as 10 minutes of oxygen deprivation in a primate experimental model.[44]

Treatment of maternal hypotension. Adequate uterine blood flow is dependent to a large extent on the maintenance of uterine arterial perfusion pressure. Since uterine blood flow is not autoregulated[45] (i.e., will not increase in response to decreased perfusion pressure), it is essential that maternal arterial blood pressure not be allowed to fall to extreme levels of hypotension. If maternal blood pressure is low and judged to be contributing to ongoing fetal distress, various methods can be used in an attempt to raise maternal blood pressure. Assuming that left uterine displacement is already being used, maternal intravascular volume can be restored toward normal by the intravenous infusion of crystalloid solutions. In one study in pregnant sheep,[46] intervillous blood flow increased dramatically following rapid crystalloid infusion in sheep with signs of intravascular volume depletion. Obviously, if hemorrhage is a cause of the hypotension, attention should be paid to both intravascular volume repletion as well as restoration of oxygen-carrying capacity of the blood through appropriate transfusion. If vasopressors must be used to restore maternal blood pressure toward normal, the general consensus is to use a predominantly β-adrenergic agonist such as ephedrine in prefer-

ence to predominantly α-adrenergic agonist such as phenylephrine.[47] Although two recent studies[48,49] suggest that the use of α-adrenergic agonist phenylephrine in restoring maternal blood pressure to normal following regional anesthesia for elective cesarean sections may not result in worse fetal acid base status relative to the use of ephedrine, these results may be partially explained by the relatively large fetal reserve present in a healthy fetus before elective cesarean section. However, such results should not be extrapolated to situations in which fetal distress is known or suspected without caution.

Ensuring optimal maternal oxygenation and ventilation

Decreased maternal Pao_2 is rarely the primary cause for fetal distress. Nonetheless, there is evidence that increasing maternal Pao_2 above normal values by the administration of supplemental oxygen may improve the fetal condition. Supplemental maternal oxygen administration will increase maternal Pao_2 and concurrently increase umbilical venous Pao_2 in patients undergoing elective cesarean section.[50,51] Similar results are found in Rhesus monkey studies.[52] This increase in fetal Pao_2 appears likely to occur in conditions associated with fetal distress. Morishima et al.[53] administered supplemental oxygen to laboring primates whose fetuses were relatively acidotic and hypoxemic and noted late decelerations on the fetal heart rate tracings. Fetal Pao_2 increased following oxygen supplementation, and late decelerations were abolished. Edelstone et al.[54] studied the effect in sheep of increasing maternal oxygenation on fetal Po_2 while occluding the umbilical vessels to various degrees. Over a wide range of umbilical blood flows, increased supplemental maternal oxygen administration improved fetal Po_2. The best explanation for these uniform results are that even small changes in fetal Pao_2 may be significant since they are occurring on a relatively steep portion of the oxygen dissociation curve of fetal hemoglobin.

It should be mentioned that the administration of supplemental maternal oxygen in the second stage, in the absence of signs of fetal distress, has recently come under question. In one study, infants born to mothers receiving supplemental oxygen versus those born to mothers receiving no supplemental oxygen during the second stage had a significantly lower umbilical blood pH at birth.[55] The cause and significance of this finding are unclear at this time.

Proper maternal positioning

Improper maternal positioning can result in exacerbation of fetal distress secondary either to a partial occlusion of the inferior vena cava (ref) or the distal aorta.[56-58] Occlusion of the aorta, which may occur in the supine position, will result in decreased perfusion pressure in the uterine arteries with a resulting decrease in uterine blood flow. Partial occlusion of the vena cava almost uniformly occurs in the supine position in the latter half of gestation, and it results in both decreased venous return to the heart and transient hypotension. The subsequent baroreceptor response, by eliciting catecholamines, will adversely affect placental perfusion despite return of blood pressure to normal. Therefore, whenever fetal distress is present, left uterine displacement or left lateral positioning should be used.

Tocolysis

Acute fetal distress has been treated successfully in utero with tocolytic agents. If excessive uterine activity has compromised uteroplacental perfusion, prompt uterine relaxation may reverse the condition. The first step in this setting, however, should be discontinuation of oxytocin if it is being administered.

The use of tocolytics to decrease uterine activity has been referred to as in utero resuscitation. The goal of this approach is to improve uterine blood flow and allow improved fetal oxygenation, thereby reversing fetal compromise. Even when fetal distress is not due to excessive uterine activity but is occurring during active labor, uterine relaxation might transiently help to improve uterine blood flow, thereby improving fetal status prior to cesarean delivery.

The β_2-sympathomimetic tocolytics ritodrine (as an IV bolus of 6 mg administered over 3 minutes) and terbutaline (250 μg IV bolus or subcutaneously) have both been shown to improve fetal acidosis in fetuses showing nonreassuring fetal heart rate findings confirmed by abnormal fetal pH values[59,60]; however, enthusiasm for this approach must be tempered by the known ability of β_2-sympathomimetic infusion to decrease uterine blood flow in animal studies.[61]

There are anesthetic considerations for patients receiving β_2-sympathomimetics for acute tocolysis in the setting of fetal distress. The cardiovascular system is affected in several ways. Neither terbutaline nor ritodrine are entirely β_2 selective; thus, some β_1 activity will also occur. Maternal tachycardia is extremely common.[62] Increased automaticity of the sinoatrial node and other intrinsic pacing cells as well as increased condition through the atrioventricular node may lead to dangerous supraventricular and ventricular arrhythmias. Patients with preexcitation syndrome (Wolff-Parkinson-White and Lown-Ganong-Levine) may be especially at risk for supraventricular tachyarrhythmias by increasing conduction velocity through accessory pathways.[63]

There are numerous reports of patients undergoing β-sympathomimetic therapy, usually for preterm labor, who demonstrated ST-T wave depression and/or T wave flattening. This often presents within the first 2 hours of therapy. Similar changes have been noted to occur in both asymptomatic patients and in others with symptoms of chest discomfort. Some have attributed these changes to tachycardia and acute hypokalemia, while others have suspected subendocardial ischemia in symptomatic patients.[63] β-sympathomimetic therapy has also been associated with pulmonary edema. In the majority of these cases, the etiology appeared to be noncardiogenic. The exact mechanisms have not been convincingly elucidated. Ravindran et al[64] reported the development of pulmonary edema in a patient who received a single IV dose of 250 μg of terbutaline; fortunately, this resolved within 2 hours of the conclusion of surgery.

Maternal blood pressure is also affected by β-sympathomimetic agents. Increased inotropy, chronotropy, and peripheral vasodilation result in variable effects on maternal blood pressure. Increases in systolic blood pressure, decreases in diastolic blood pressure, and no significant changes in blood pressure have all been reported.[59,60,62,63,65] The peripheral vasodilation associated with β-sympathomimetic therapy may be especially dangerous in the hypovolemic patient, in such cases involving suspected abruption.

Amnioinfusion

When fetal heart rate testing is nonreassuring with deep variable decelerations or in the presence of thick meconium, amnioinfusion can improve perinatal outcome.[66,67] Variable decelerations most likely due to cord compression can be relieved and cesarean section rates due to fetal intolerance of labor can be decreased by amnioinfusion.[66-68] In cases of thick meconium, it can also decrease the incidence of meconium below the cord and meconium aspiration.[69,70]

Intrapartum amnioinfusion is performed using a transcervical intrauterine pressure catheter. Normal saline or Ringer's lactate is infused at 600 ml for the first hour, followed by 180 ml per hour until delivery. The choice of fluid has no clinically significant effect on neonatal electrolytes.[71]

Intrapartum amnioinfusion has been associated with increased risk for chorioamnionitis and postpartum endometritis.[72] Two cases of fatal amniotic fluid embolism have been reported complicating intrapartum amnioinfusion.[73] However, despite these risks, amnioinfusion is a worthwhile technique to treat certain cases of fetal distress.

ANESTHETIC MANAGEMENT
Antepartum fetal distress

The anesthetic management for vaginal delivery or cesarean section when fetal distress is diagnosed will depend on the condition of the fetus and thus the urgency of the situation. When presumed antepartum fetal distress is present, such as a term fetus with IUGR and uteroplacental insufficiency, anesthetia should be planned to minimize any further decrement in oxygen delivery to the fetus during labor if at all possible.

The methods potentially useful for providing analgesia for anticipated vaginal delivery in patients with chronic fetal distress include psychoprophylaxis, systemic agents, regional anesthetics, and major conduction analgesia. Psychoprophylaxis, especially education techniques, can be quite instrumental in reducing the parturients fear and resulting stress of labor. It is now appreciated from animal experiments[74,75] that maternal stress adversely affects placental perfusion and fetal oxygenation. Such changes that may be clinically insignificant in healthy fetuses may prove detrimental in fetuses with chronic distress. Systemic medication such as narcotics or sedatives can likewise prove useful in these situations if they can ameliorate the stress and pain of labor. Unfortunately, they have been proved to provide inferior levels of analgesia when compared with lumbar epidural analgesia or spinal analgesia. When lumbar epidural analgesia is provided using local anesthetics or local anesthetic/narcotic mixture, hypotension should be avoided or treated. Even with the use of pure narcotic spinal analgesia for labor, the question has been raised regarding the occurrence of hypotension following dosing.

In situations requiring cesarean delivery for chronic fetal stress, the anesthetic technique of choice is continuous lumbar epidural anesthesia. The relative slow onset of this technique relative to spinal anesthesia provides an ability to anticipate and treat the hypotension that may occur with sympathetic blockade. The presence of a catheter confers the ability to titrate the sensory level and extend the duration of the blockade as dictated by surgical circumstances.

When maternal blood pressure is maintained with routine hydration and ephedrine when necessary, epidural anesthesia to a T4 sensory level does not appear to significantly alter intervillous blood flow.[76,77] Brizgys et al[78] published data on the incidence of maternal hypotension and neonatal effects of lumbar epidural anesthesia for cesarean delivery. In this study, prophylactic intramuscular (IM) ephedrine was not significantly effective in reducing the incidence of maternal hypotension with lumbar epidural anesthesia. Hypotension occurred in 41% of nonlaboring parturients and in 27% of those in labor. These authors found no difference between the 2 groups of neonates with respect to acid-base status or time to spontaneous respiration. This was attributed to aggressive prompt treatment of hypotension. This study also examined the impact of superimposed maternal hypotension on infants who were already considered to be in moderate distress by FHR parameters. When maternal hypotension was aggressively treated, it did not result in a further deterioration of the previously stressed infants.

Anesthesia with intrapartum fetal distress

In the case of acute fetal distress during labor, delivery by emergency cesarean section is often deemed necessary. In such cases, anesthetia should be planned to provide the most rapid, safe anesthetic for both the mother and fetus. Whenever an emergency cesarean section is planned, the paramount anesthetic decision to be made will be the type of anesthesia to be used for the cesarean section. It should be remembered that this type of cesarean section—an emergency cesarean section—accounts for the majority of maternal mortality secondary to anesthesia.[79] For this reason, decision-making algorithms regarding the type of anesthesia to be selected should be developed beforehand to avoid confusion during the actual emergency.

A categorization of emergency cesarean section and the types of anesthetic choices available for each has been suggested by Harris[79]; these are outlined in Table 31-1. Cesarean section for acute fetal distress in labor will invariably fall into the second or third categories, that of *urgent* or *stat* cesarean section. The determination of which category is correct for a given clinical situation depends on the instability of the underlying physiology (i.e., degree of asphyxia present) and whether or not it is immediately life-threatening. When fetal distress is present but not felt to be immediately life-threatening, more anesthetic options are available, with the caveat that fetal monitoring must be continued during a somewhat longer induction of epidural anesthesia or spinal anesthesia, in comparison with general anesthesia. Above all, once the decision has been made to perform a cesarean section for the diagnosis of fetal distress, the anesthetic plan chosen should proceed to implementation as quickly as possible without delay, regardless of the technique chosen. In an attempt to correlate decision-to-delivery interval with neonatal admission rate to the neonatal inten-

Table 31-1 Categories of emergency cesarean section

Category	Examples	Preferred anesthetic
Stable	Chronic uteroplacental insufficiency Malpresentation with ruptured membranes (not in labor) Previous lower segment cesarean section even in labor	Epidural, spinal
Urgent	Failure to progress Active herpes with rupture of membranes Nonbleeding placenta previa in labor Placental abruption without fetal distress Severe preeclampsia Chorioamnionitis Previous classical cesarean section in active labor	Spinal, epidural (extended from labor)
Stat	Agonal fetal distress Cord prolapse with fetal distress Massive hemorrhage Ruptured uterus	General, local, epidural (if T10 or higher level is present)

Adapted from Harris AP: Emergency cesarean section, in Rogers MC (ed): *Current Practice in Anesthesiology.* St. Louis, Mosby, 1990, p 361.

sive care unit, Dunphy et al found that the rate doubled with extension of the interval from 10 to 35 minutes.[80] There is evidence that time-consuming anesthesia preparatory steps such as crystalloid infusion before major regional anesthesia may be curtailed to some extent in an emergency without demonstrably increasing fetal risk or worsening outcome.[81]

In cases of severe persistent fetal distress requiring stat cesarean section (persistent fetal bradycardia or severe fetal scalp acidosis), the most widely employed anesthetic technique is general anesthesia. It has become the technique of choice in these clinical situations because of its speed of onset and reliability. Alternatives to general anesthesia in cases requiring emergent delivery include spinal anesthesia, extension of a labor epidural that has already been established at at least a T10 level, or local infiltration and field block. In 1984, Marx et al[82] compared anesthetic techniques for emergent cesarean delivery. In the 126 cases in this study, the anesthetic technique was selected by the anesthesiologist and the parturient undergoing the cesarean delivery; 71 patients received general anesthesia, 55 received SAB, and 33 had their previously placed lumbar epidural redosed for the cesarean section. Of note is that none of the spinal or epidural anesthesia patients experienced hypotension or required vasopressor therapy. This study found similar umbilical arterial acid base values between the GA and regional anesthesia groups. While the 1-minute Apgar scores were better in the regional group, there was no difference in the 5-minute scores. The conclusion in this study was

that spinal anesthesia is the safest approach to emergent cesarean delivery for fetal distress when a functioning epidural catheter is not present. In another study of regional versus general anesthesia for emergency cesarean section, Ramanathan et al[83] found that extension of epidural anesthesia with 2-chloroprocaine for emergent cesarean delivery for fetal distress did not adversely affect the fetal acid base status when compared with general anesthesia. However, both studies were retrospective in nature and cannot be used as sole evidence to support a delay to establish spinal anesthesia for a stat cesarean section without further justification. This is especially true in light of a recent study by Roberts et al, who studied the effect of anesthetic techniques on umbilical artery blood pH in 1601 patients. They found that spinal anesthesia was associated with occasionally severe fetal acidemia when compared with epidural anesthesia and general anesthesia.[42]

For stat cesarean delivery, if one has already been placed and is functioning, a continuous labor epidural with a preexisting T10 or greater sensory level can be rapidly extended with 2-chloroprocaine or lidocaine. Simultaneous fluid loading with a non–dextrose-containing solution should be administered to offset the hypotension that may occur with the ensuing higher sensory block. If inadequate anesthesia has developed by the time the obstetricians are ready to begin surgery, intravenous supplementation with ketamine 10 mg every 2 minutes can be used until delivery of the infant when intravenous narcotics (such as fentanyl) can be added.

If the maternal airway is suspected to be challenging and an epidural is not already in place, spinal anesthesia may be considered. Although some maintain that a difficult airway may be a relative contraindication to spinal anesthesia, the requirement to deliver the asphyxiated fetus in a timely fashion may justify its use. Alternatives in this situation would include an awake intubation (which can be technically challenging and time-consuming), and local anesthesia infiltration/field block. A local field block of the abdominal wall for cesarean section was performed in one series of 218 patients using approximately 60 ml of 1% procaine with excellent success.[84] Despite such reports, many practitioners are unfamiliar with this technique.

General anesthesia with intrapartum fetal distress

Before proceeding with the induction of general anesthesia, the urgency of the delivery must be weighed against the potential risks of general anesthesia. This consideration requires close communication between the obstetric and anesthesia teams.

The inability to secure the maternal airway continues to be a major cause of maternal and fetal morbidity and mortality.[85] Preoperative assessment of the airway should include visual inspection of the face, neck, and oropharynx for soft-tissue swelling. Head and neck flexion and extension, the ability to open the jaw, and temporomandibular joint function as evidenced by the ability to move the lower incisors anterior to the upper incisors should be assessed. Inadequate hyoid-mental distance may indicate an anterior larynx and a subsequent difficult intubation.

If the ability to rapidly secure the airway following a rapid sequence induction is in serious question, alternative approaches must be considered, i.e., the patient's airway should be secured while the patient is awake. Techniques in the awake obstetric patient include oral fiberoptic intubation and direct awake laryngoscopy following application of a topical anesthetic to the airway. The risk of epistaxis from a nasotracheal intubation is significantly higher in the obstetric patient secondary to hyperemic, engorged mucous membranes.

If preoperative assessment of the airway suggests that intubation should not be difficult, a rapid sequence induction is planned. The clinician should consider the alternative options in the event of a failed intubation. Emergency airway equipment must be immediately available. Figure 31-2 outlines a suggested protocol for failed intubation. Such an algorithm should be reviewed and be available *prior* to their use in an emergency setting.

Maternal aspiration is an important concern in obstetric anesthesia. The complications of maternal aspiration can be minimized by the use of oral nonparticular antacids within 1 hour of induction.[86] A rapid sequence induction and intubation with cricoid pressure is normally employed to decrease the risk of regurgitation and aspiration. The importance of proper instruction to the person applying cricoid pressure cannot be overemphasized, because misapplied cricoid pressure can displace the larynx and complicate endotracheal intubation. The efficacy of metoclopramide to stimulate gastric emptying and increase lower esophageal sphincter tone is not guaranteed. However, Murphy et al[87] demonstrated a significant increase in gastric emptying in all patients within 1 hour of receiving 10 mg of intravenous metoclopramide before elective cesarean section. Histamine type 2 (H2) blocking agents have also been shown to be effective in increasing gastric fluid pH and decreasing gastric volume.[88,89] However, there is almost certainly inadequate time for these latter two pharmacologic methods to have time to work prior to a stat cesarean section.

Following antacid prophylaxis in the operating room, left uterine displacement, continued FHR monitoring, and maternal preoxygenation should be ensured. The widespread practice of 3 to 5 minutes of 100% oxygenation before induction may be replaced by four tidal volume breaths of 100% oxygen over 30 seconds when time is extremely critical. Norris and Dewan compared these two techniques in patients undergoing elective cesarean delivery and demonstrated no difference in maternal blood gas values or umbilical arterial and venous blood gas values at birth.[90]

Rapid sequence induction and endotracheal intubation are facilitated by rapid-onset muscle relaxation. This rapid-onset muscle relaxation is best achieved by succinylcholine, which also confers the advantage of rapid recovery. Although plasma cholinesterase activity is 20% to 30% lower in pregnant patients, recovery of twitch is not delayed.[91,92] Rapid recovery from succinylcholine neuromuscular blockade may not occur, however, in severely preeclamptic patients, especially if magnesium sulfate or trimethaphan is being administered. A defasiculating dose is generally not suggested because it necessitates a higher dose of succinylcholine and a more prolonged neuromuscular blockade. Rocuronium may be used as an alternative to a depolarizing agent for rapid sequence induction, but a longer neuromuscular block then necessary for cesarean section may result from that dose, and the time to adequate intubating condi-

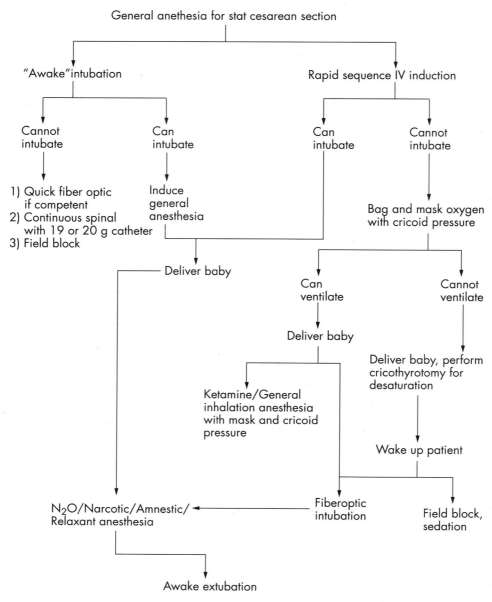

Fig. 31-2 Modified algorithm for conducting general anesthesia for stat emergency cesarian sections (From Harris AP: Emergency cesarean section, in Rogers MC (ed): *Current Practice in Anesthesiology.* St. Louis, Mosby, 1990, p 361).

tions will be longer than with succinylcholine. All nondepolarizing agents have small amounts of placental transfer but insignificant effects on the newborn.[93-95]

Choice of induction agents in fetal distress

An ideal induction agent for general anesthesia for cesarean delivery should provide rapid onset, brief duration (to allow spontaneous recovery of respirations if intubation proved difficult), minimal ma-

ternal hemodynamic effects, and minimal fetal effects. Maternal and fetal effects of anesthetic agents are most critical in the setting of fetal physiologic distress in which much of the fetal reserve has already been depleted. Several induction agents have been used to induce general anesthesia for cesarean delivery. The most commonly used induction agents in obstetric anesthesia are thiopental and ketamine. Etomidate, propofol, midazolam, and narcotic agents have also been used.

Thiopental is highly lipid-soluble and therefore rapidly crosses the placenta; peak umbilical venous levels are reached in less than 1 minute. The commonly recommended dose of thiopental 4 mg/kg has its origin in a study that compared dosages from 4 to 8 mg/kg. In this study, Kosaka described better Apgar scores in the neonates who received 4 mg/kg.[96]

Ketamine is a potent amnestic and analgesic drug with rapid onset and short duration. In pregnant ewes, Levinson demonstrated that anesthetic doses of ketamine increased maternal blood pressure but did not affect the fetal acid-base status.[97] In addition, the use of ketamine was associated with an increased in uterine blood flow. Ketamine increases the intensity and frequency of uterine contractions, but it does not alter the resting intrauterine pressure. The recommended dose of ketamine for induction of general anesthesia is 1 mg/kg. In acidotic lamb models, ketamine is associated with a decrease in fetal lamb mean arterial pressure (MAP) but the preservation of fetal cerebral and myocardial blood flow.[98] Fetal acid-base status was unchanged by this dose of ketamine. The conclusion in this study was that ketamine was a safe drug for the induction of general anesthesia in cases with fetal distress. A dose of 1 mg of intravenous diazepam after induction with ketamine has been reported to significantly reduce the incidence of unpleasant postoperative dreams.[99]

Thiopental 4 mg/kg has been compared with ketamine 1 mg/kg for induction in 62 normotensive patients undergoing elective cesarean delivery. MAP increased 20% to 30% with laryngoscopy with both of these induction agents. In acidotic fetal sheep, 2 mg/kg of ketamine preserved better fetal blood pressure and cerebral blood flow than did 6 mg/kg thiopental for induction in the presence of fetal asphyxia.[100] In summary, both sodium thiopental (4 mg/kg) and ketamine (1 mg/kg) appear to be acceptable choices for rapid sequence inductions in normotensive patients in the presence of fetal asphyxia.

A few alternative agents have been studied for obstetric applications. In 1979, Downing et al compared the use of etomidate 0.3 mg/kg with a historical control group of 3.5 mg/kg of thiopental and found a reduced base deficit demonstrated in the cord gases in the etomidate group.[101]

Midazolam has been studied in patients undergoing elective cesarean delivery. Bland et al found that a significantly higher number of newborns required resuscitation following induction with midazolam as compared with induction with thiopental. This study concluded that midazolam was inferior to thiopental induction for cesarean deliveries.[102] This result was also confirmed by Ravlo et al, who also reported that infants in the midazolam group scored less well with respect to temperature control, general body tone, and arm recoil.[103] An initial study comparing propofol (2.5 mg/kg) with thiopental revealed no differences in umbilical blood gases or neurobehavioral scores.[104]

Although newer induction agents are being studied, there are inadequate data to support the routine use of agents other than thiopental and ketamine in the setting of fetal asphyxia.

Anesthetic maintenance

A high inspired oxygen concentration improves fetal oxygen stores. The addition of a halogenated volatile anesthetic as a replacement for nitrous oxide in the traditional nitrous oxide/oxygen obstetric anesthetic allows the use of higher inspired oxygen concentration. Animal and human experimental data indicate that halothane and isoflurane can both be used for limited times in the setting of fetal distress without evidence of a significant worsening of fetal condition.[105-110]

Numerous reports associating prolonged induction of general anesthesia to delivery (I-D interval) with newborn depression were published in the 1960s and 1970s. In 1976, Crawford et al[111] first reported on the relationship between a prolonged uterine incision to delivery interval (UI-D interval) and fetal acidosis. They noted an even greater correlation between fetal acid-base status and UI-D interval than between induction to delivery interval. Following this report, Datta et al addressed the issue of I-D interval and UI-D interval in 105 patients undergoing repeat elective cesarean delivery under either general or spinal anesthesia. Datta et al found that with general anesthesia, either an I-D interval greater than 8 minutes or an UI-D interval greater than 3 minutes correlated with worsening Apgar scores and umbilical acid-base status.[112] In the absence of hypotension, a prolonged I-D time did not affect either Apgar scores or acid-base values with spinal anesthesia. However, an UI-D interval greater than 3 minutes was associated with higher incidences of neonatal acidosis. This group has also observed a correlation between uterine incision to delivery interval and fetal norepinephrine levels.[113] Hence, a shorter UI-D interval may be beneficial during both general and regional anesthesia, especially in the presence of fetal distress.

Following induction of general anesthesia, maintenance of eucapnia appears to be an important consideration. In a comparison of patients undergoing cesarean delivery under general anesthesia, parturients were hyperventilated to a $Paco_2$ of 23 mm Hg or kept eucapnic at a $Paco_2$ of 39 mm Hg. Significantly better values for umbilical vein

Po$_2$, fetal acid-base status, and 1-minute Apgar scores were observed in the eucapnic group.[114] In all cases, the parturient should not be extubated until the return of spontaneous ventilation and adequate protective airway reflexes.

REFERENCES

1. Haverkamp AD, Orleans M, Langendoerfer S, et al: A controlled trial of the differential effects of intrapartum fetal monitoring. *Am J Obstet Gynecol* 1979; 134:399.
2. Haesslein HC, Niswander KR: Fetal distress in term pregnancies. *Am J Obstet Gynecol* 1980; 137:245.
3. Sykes GS, Johnson P, Ashworth F, et al: Do Apgar scores indicate asphyxia? *Lancet* 1982; 1:494.
4. MacDonald H, Mulligan J, Allen A, et al: Neonatal asphyxia. I. Relationship of obstetric and neonatal complications to neonatal mortality in 38,405 consecutive deliveries. *J Pediatr* 1980; 96:898.
5. Parer JT, Livingston EG: What is fetal distress? *Am J Obstet Gynecol* 1990; 162:1421.
6. Harris AP: Sudden fetal distress, in Datta S (ed): *Common Problems in Obstetric Anesthesia*. St. Louis, Mosby, 1995, p 263.
7. Creasy RK, Resnik R: Intrauterine growth retardation, in Creasy RK, Resnick R (eds): *Maternal-Fetal Medicine: Principles and Practice*. Philadelphia, WB Saunders, 1989, pp 547-564.
8. Scott KE, Usher R: Fetal malnutrition: Its incidence, causes and effects. *Am J Obstet Gynecol* 1966; 94:951.
9. Williams RL, Creasy RK, Cunningham GC, et al: Fetal growth and perinatal viability in California. *Obstet Gynecol* 1982; 159:624.
10. Morrison I, Olsen J: Weight specific stillbirths and associated causes of death: An analysis of 765 stillbirths. *Am J Obstet Gynecol* 1985; 152:975.
11. Usher RH: Clinical and therapeutic aspects of fetal maturation. *Pediatr Clin North Am* 1970; 17:169.
12. Tejani N, Mann LI, Weiss RR: Antenatal diagnosis and management of the small for gestational age fetus. *Obstet Gynecol* 1976; 47:31.
13. MacDonald D, Grant A, Sheridan-Pereira M, et al: The Dublin randomized controlled trial of intrapartum fetal heart rate monitoring. *Am J Obstet Gynecol* 1985; 152:524.
14. Rosen MG (Chairman): Consensus Task Force on Cesarean Childbirth. *NIH Publication no. 82-2067*, 1981.
15. Smeriglio VL: Developmental sequelae following intrauterine growth retardation, in Gross TL, Sokol (eds): *Intrauterine Growth Retardation*. Chicago, Year Book Medical Publishers, 1989, pp 34-53.
16. Niswander K, Elboure D, Redman C, et al: Adverse outcome of pregnancy and the quality of obstetric care. *Lancet* 1984; 1:827.
17. Pareth N, Start R: Cerebral palsy and mental retardation in relation to indicators of perinatal asphyxia. *Am J Obstet Gynecol* 1983; 147:960.
18. Nelson K, Ellenberg J: Obstetric complications as risk factors for cerebral palsy or seizure disorders. *JAMA* 1984; 251:1843.
19. Ramanathan S: *Obstetric Anesthesia*. Philadelphia, Lea & Febiger, 1988, pp 27.
20. Philipps AF: Carbohydrate metabolism of the fetus, in Polin RA, Fox WW (eds): *Fetal and Neonatal Physiology, vol 1*. Philadelphia, WB Saunders, 1992, pp 373-84.
21. Cohn HE, Sacks EJ, Heymann MA, et al: Cardiovascular responses to hypoxemia and acidemia in fetal lambs. *Am J Obstet Gynecol* 1979; 135:1071.
22. Sheldon RE, Peeters LLH, Jones MD Jr, et al: Redistribution of cardiac output and oxygen delivery in the hypoxemic fetal lamb. *Am J Obstet Gynecol* 1979; 135:1071.
23. Harris AP: Fetal physiology, in Chestnut DH (ed): *Obstetric Anesthesia: Principles and Practice*. St. Louis, Mosby, 1994, pp 76-88.
24. Yaffe H, Parer JT, Block BS, et al: Cardiorespiratory responses to graded reductions in uterine blood flow in the sheep fetus. *J Dev Physiol* 1987; 9:325.
25. Edelstone DI: Fetal compensatory responses to reduced oxygen delivery. *Semin Perinatol* 1984; 8:184.
26. Bristow J, Rudolph AM, Itskovitz J: A preparation for studying liver blood flow, oxygen consumption, and metabolism in the fetal lamb in utero. *J Dev Physiol* 1981; 3:255.
27. Peeters LL, Sheldon RE, Jones MD Jr, et al: Blood flow to fetal organs as a function of arterial oxygen content. *Am J Obstet Gynecol* 1979; 135:637.
28. ACOG Committee on Obstetrical Practice: Fetal distress and birth asphyxia. *ACOG Committee Opinion no. 137:* Washington, DC, April 1994.
29. Butler NR, Alberman EF: In Butler (ed): *Perinatal Problems: The Second Report of the British Perinatal Mortality Survey*. Edinburgh, Churchill Livingstone, 1969.
30. Vintzileos AM, Campbell WAS, Ingardia CJ, et al: The fetal biophysical profile and its predictive value. *Obstet Gynecol* 1983; 62:271.
31. Murata Y, Martin CB, Ikenoue T, et al: Fetal heart rate accelerations and late decelerations during the course of intrauterine death in chronically catheterized rhesus monkeys. *Am J Obstet Gynecol* 1982; 144:218.
32. Rochelson B, Schulman H, Fleischer A, et al: The clinical significance of Doppler umbilical artery velocimetry in the small for gestational age fetus. *Am J Obstet Gynecol* 1987; 156:1223.
33. Ducey J, Schulman H, Farmalcaides G, et al: A classification of hypertension in pregnancy based on Doppler velocimetry. *Am J Obstet Gynecol* 1987; 157:680.
34. Wenstrom KD, Weiner CP, Williamson RA: Diverse maternal and fetal pathology associated with absent diastolic flow in the umbilical artery of high risk fetuses. *Obstet Gynecol* 1991; 77:374.
35. American College of Obstetricians and Gynecologists: Intrapartum fetal heart rate monitoring. *ACOG Technical Bulletin no. 132:* Washington, DC, Sept. 1989.
36. Cohen W, Schifrin B: Diagnosis and management of fetal distress during labor. *Semin Perinatol* 1978; 2:155.
37. American College of Obstetricians and Gynecologists: Assessment of fetal and newborn acid-base status. *ACOG Technical Bulletin no. 127:* Washington DC, April 1989.
38. Smith CV, Nguyen HN, Phelan JP, et al: Intrapartum assessment of fetal well-being: A comparison of fetal acoustic stimulation with acid-base determinations. *Am J Obstet Gynecol* 1986; 155:726.
39. Clark SL, Timovsay ML, Miller FC: The scalp stimulation test: A clinical alternative to fetal scalp blood sampling. *Am J Obstet Gynecol* 1984; 148:274.
40. American College of Obstetrics and Gynecology: Assessment of fetal and newborn acid-base status. *ACOG Technical Bulletin no. 127:* Washington, DC, April 1989.
41. Nelson K, Ellenberg J: Apgar scores as predictors of chronic neurologic disability. *Pediatrics* 1981; 68:36.
42. Roberts SW, Leveno KJ, Sidawi E: Fetal acidemia associated with regional anesthesia for elective cesarean delivery. *Obstet Gynecol* 1995; 85:79.
43. Allen M: Developmental outcome and follow-up of the small for gestational age infant. *Semin Perinatol* 1984; 8:123.

44. Myers RE: Two patterns of perinatal brain damage and their conditions of occurrence. *Am J Obstet Gynecol* 1972; 112:246.

45. Greiss FC Jr, Anderson SG, Still JG: Uterine pressure-flow relationships during early gestation. *Am J Obstet Gynecol* 1976; 126:799.

46. Crino JP, Harris AP, Parisi VM: Effect of rapid intravenous crystalloid infusion on uteroplacental blood flow and placental implantation-site oxygen delivery in the pregnant ewe. *Am J Obstet Gynecol* 1993; 168:1603.

47. Ralston D, Shnider S, Delorimer A: Effects of equipotent ephedrine, metaraminol, mephentermine, and methoxamine on uterine blood flow in the pregnant ewe. *Anesthesiology* 1974; 40:354.

48. Ramanathan S, Grant G: Vasopressor therapy for hypotension due to epidural anesthesia for cesarean section. *Acta Anaesthesiol Scand* 1988; 32:559.

49. Moran D, Perillo M, LaPorta RF, et al: Phenylephrine in the prevention of hypotension following spinal anesthesia for cesarean delivery. *J Clin Anesth* 1991; 3:301.

50. Marx GF, Mateo C: Effects of different oxygen concentrations during general anaesthesia for elective caesarean section. *Can Anaesth Soc J* 1971; 18:587.

51. Ramanathan S, Gandhi S, Arismendy J, et al: Oxygen transfer from mother to fetus during Cesarean section under epidural anesthesia. *Anesth Analg* 1982; 61:576.

52. Myers RE, Stange L, Joelssen I, et al: Effects upon the fetus of oxygen administration to the mother: A study in monkeys. *Acta Obstet Gynecol Scand* 1977; 56:195.

53. Morishima H, Daniel S, Richards R, et al: The effect of increased maternal PaO$_2$ upon the fetus during labor. *Am J Obstet Gynecol* 1975; 123:257.

54. Edelstone D, Peticca B, Goldblum L: Effects of maternal oxygen administration on fetal oxygenation during reductions in umbilical blood flow in fetal lambs. *Am J Obstet Gynecol* 1985; 152:351.

55. Thorp JA, Trobough T, Evans R, et al: The effect of maternal oxygen administration during the second stage of labor on umbilical cord blood gas values: A randomized controlled prospective trial. *Am J Obstet Gynecol* 1995; 172:465.

56. Bieniarz J, Crottoginin JJ, Curuchet E, et al: Aorto-caval compression by the uterus in late human pregnancy. II. An arteriographic study. *Am J Obstet Gynecol* 1968; 100:203.

57. Lees MM, Scott DB, Kerr MG, et al: Circulatory effects of the supine posture in late pregnancy. *Clin Sci* 1967; 32:453.

58. Eckstein KL, Marx GF: Aortocaval compression and uterine displacement. *Anesthesiology* 1974; 40:92.

59. Mendez-Bauer C, Shekarloo A, Cook V, et al: Treatment of acute intrapartum fetal distress by β$_2$-sympathomimetics. *Am J Obstet Gynecol* 1987; 156:638.

60. Patriarco M, Viechnicki B, Hutchinson T, et al: A study on intrauterine fetal resuscitation with terbutaline. *Am J Obstet Gynecol* 1987; 157:384.

61. Ehrenkranz R, Walker A, Oakes G, et al: Effect of ritodrine infusion on uterine and umbilical blood flow in pregnant sheep. *Am J Obstet Gynecol* 1976; 126:343.

62. Ingemarsson I, Arulkumaran S, Ratnam S: Single injection of terbutaline in term labor. II: Effect on uterine activity. *Am J Obstet Gynecol* 1985; 153:865.

63. Benedetti T: Life-threatening complications of betamimetic therapy for preterm labor inhibition. *Clin Perinatol* 1986; 13:843.

64. Ravindran R, Vilgus O, Padilla L, et al: Anesthetic considerations in pregnant patients receiving terbutaline therapy. *Anesth Analg* 1980; 59:391.

65. Fishburne J, Dormer K, Payne G, et al: Effects of amrinone and dopamine on uterine blood flow and vascular responses in the gravid baboon. *Am J Obstet Gynecol* 1988; 158:829.

66. Paszkowski T: Amnioinfusion a review. *J Reprod Med* 1994; 39:588.

67. Cialone PR, Sherer DM, Ryan RM, et al: Amnioinfusion during labor complicated by particulate meconium-stained amniotic fluid decreases neonatal morbidity. *Am J Obstet Gynecol* 1994; 170:842.

68. Miyazaki FS, Nevarez F: Saline amnioinfusion for relief of repetitive variable decelerations: A prospective randomized study. *Am J Obstet Gynecol* 1985; 153.

69. Eriksen NL, Hostetter M, Parisi VM: Prophylactic amnioinfusion in pregnancies complicated by thick meconium. *Am J Obstet Gynecol* 1994; 171:1026.

70. Dye T, Aubry R, Gross S, et al: Amnioinfusion and the intrauterine prevention of meconium aspiration. *Am J Obstet Gynecol* 1994; 171:1601.

71. Puder KS, Sorokin Y, Bottoms SF, et al: Amnioinfusion: Does the choice of solution adversely affect neonatal electrolyte balance? *Obstet Gynecol* 1994; 84:956.

72. Spong CY, Ogundipe OA, Ross MG: Prophylactic amnioinfusion for meconium-stained amniotic fluid. *Am J Obstet Gynecol* 1994; 171:931.

73. Maher JE, Wenstom KD, Hauth JC, et al: Amniotic fluid embolism after saline amnioinfusion: Two cases and review of the literature. *Obstet Gynecol* 1994; 83:851.

74. Shnider SM, Wright RG, Levinson G, et al: Uterine blood flow and plasma norepinephrine changes during maternal stress in the pregnant ewe. *Anesthesiology* 1979; 50:524.

75. Myers RE: Maternal psychological stress and fetal asphyxia: A study in the monkey. *Am J Obstet Gynecol* 1975; 122:47.

76. Jouppila R, Jouppila P, Kuikka J, et al: Placental blood flow during caesarean section under lumbar extradural analgesia. *Br J Anaesth* 1978; 50:275.

77. Houvinen K, Lehtovirta P, Forss M, et al: Changes in placental intervillous blood flow measured by the ^{133}Xenon method during lumbar epidural block for elective caesarean section. *Acta Anaesth Scand* 1979; 23:529.

78. Brizgys R, Dailey P, Shnider S, et al: The incidence and neonatal effects of maternal hypotension during epidural anesthesia for cesarean section. *Anesthesiology* 1987; 67:782.

79. Harris AP: Emergency cesarean section, in Rogers MC (ed): *Current Practice in Anesthesiology*, St. Louis, Mosby, 1990, pp 361.

80. Dunphy BC, Robinson JN, Sheil OM, et al: Caesarean section for fetal distress, the interval from decision to delivery, and the relative risk of poor neonatal condition. *J Obstet Gynecol* 1991; 11:241.

81. Rout CC, Rocke DA, Levin J, et al: A reevaluation of the role of crystalloid preload in the prevention of hypotension associated with spinal anesthesia for elective cesarean section. *Anesthesiology* 1994; 81:529.

82. Marx GF, Luykx W, Cohen S: Fetal-neonatal status following ceasarean section for fetal distress. *Br J Anaesth* 1984; 56:1009.

83. Ramanathan J, Ricca D, Sibai B, et al: Epidural versus general anesthesia in fetal distress with various abnormal fetal heart rate patterns (abstract). *Anesth Analg* 1988; 67:S180.

84. Ranney B, Stanage W: Advantages of local anesthesia for cesarean section. *Obstet Gynecol* 1975; 45:163.

85. Moir D: Maternal mortality and anaesthesia. *Br J Anaesth* 1980; 51:1.

86. Dewan D, Floyd H, Thistlewood J, et al: Sodium citrate pretreatment in elective cesarean section patients. *Anesth Analg* 1985; 64:34.

87. Murphy D, Nally B, Gardiner J, et al: Effect of metoclopramide on gastric emptying before elective and emergency caesarean section. *Br J Anaesth* 1984; 56:1113.

88. Solanki D, Suresh M, Ethridge C: The effects of intravenous cimetidine and metoclopramide on gastric volume and pH. *Anesth Analg* 1984; 63:599.

89. Morrison D, Dunn G, Fargus-Babjak A, et al: A double-blinded comparison of cimetidine and ranitidine as prophylaxis against gastric aspiration syndrome. *Anesth Analg* 1982; 61:988.

90. Norris M, Dewan D: Preoxygenation for cesarean section: A comparison of two techniques. *Anesthesiology* 1985; 62:827.

91. Blitt C, Petty W, Alberternst E, et al: Correlation of plasma cholinesterase activity and duration of action of succinylcholine during pregnancy. *Anesth Analg* 1977; 56:78.

92. Dowling B, Cheek T, Gross J, et al: Succinylcholine pharmacodynamics in peripartum patients (abstract). *Anesthesiology* 1987; 63:A431.

93. Tessen J, Johnson T, Skjonsby B, et al: Evaluation of vecuronium for rapid sequence induction in patients undergoing cesarean section (abstract). *Anesthesiology* 1987; 67:A452.

94. Dailey P, Fisher D, Shnider S, et al: Pharmacokinetics, placental transfer, and neonatal effects of vecuronium and pancuronium administered during cesarean section. *Anesthesiology* 1984; 60:569.

95. Flynn P, Frank M, Hughes R: Use of atracurium in caesarean section. *Br J Anaesth* 1984; 56:599.

96. Kosaka Y, Takahashi T, Mark L: Intravenous thiobarbiturate anesthesia for cesarean section. *Anesthesiology* 1969; 31:489.

97. Levinson G, Shnider S, Gilden J, et al: Maternal and fetal cardiovascular and acid-base changes during ketamine anaesthesia in pregnant ewes. *Br J Anaesth* 1973; 45:1111.

98. Swartz J, Cumming M, Biehl D: The effect of ketamine anaesthesia on the acidotic fetal lamb. *Can J Anaesth* 1987; 34:233.

99. Dich-Nielsen J, Holasek J: Ketamine as induction agent for caesarean section. *Acta Anaesth Scand* 1982; 26:139.

100. Pickering B, Palahnuik R, Cote J, et al: Cerebral vascular responses to ketamine and thiopentone during foetal acidosis. *Can Anaesth Soc J* 1982; 29:463.

101. Downing J, Buley R, Brock-Utne J, et al: Etomidate for induction of anaesthesia at caesarean section: Comparison with thiopentone. *Br J Anaesth* 1979; 51:135.

102. Bland B, Duncan P, Downing J: Comparison of midazolam and thiopental for rapid sequence induction for elective cesarean section. *Anesth Analg* 1987; 66:1165.

103. Ravlo O, Carl P, Crawford M, et al: A randomized comparison between midazolam and thiopental for elective cesarean section: II. Neonates. *Anesth Analg* 1989; 68:234.

104. Dailland P, Lirzin J, Cockshott I, et al: Placental transfer and neonatal effects of propofol administered during cesarean section (abstract). *Anesthesiology* 1987; 67:A454.

105. Palahniuk RJ, Doig GA, Johnson GN, et al: Maternal halothane anesthesia reduces cerebral blood flow in the acidotic sheep fetus. *Anesth Analg* 1980; 59:35.

106. Yarnell R, Biehl DR, Tweed WA, et al: The effect of halothane anaesthesia on the asphyxiated foetal lamb in utero. *Can Anaesth Soc J* 1983; 30:474.

107. Swartz J, Cummings M, Pucci W, et al: The effects of general anaesthesia on the asphyxiated foetal lamb in utero. *Can Anaesth Soc J* 1985; 32:577.

108. Cheek DBC, Hughes SC, Dailey PA, et al: Effect of halothane on regional cerebral blood flow and cerebral metabolic oxygen consumption in the fetal lamb in utero. *Anesthesiology* 1987; 67:361.

109. Baker BW, Hughes SC, Shnider SM, et al: Maternal anesthesia and the stressed fetus: Effects of isoflurane on the asphyxiated fetal lamb. *Anesthesiology* 1990; 72:65.

110. Mokriski BK, Malinow AM: Neonatal acid-base status following general anesthesia for emergency abdominal delivery with halothane or isoflurane. *J Clin Anesth* 1992; 4:97.

111. Crawford J, James f, Davids P, et al: A further study of general anaesthesia for caesarean section. *Br J Anaesth* 1976; 48:661.

112. Datta S, Ostheimer G, Weiss J, et al: Neonatal effect of prolonged anesthetic induction for cesarean delivery. *Obstet Gynecol* 1981; 58:331.

113. Bader AM, Datta S, Arthur GR, et al: Maternal and fetal catecholamines and uterine incision-to-delivery interval during elective cesarean section. *Obstet Gynecol* 1990; 75:600.

114. Peng A, Blancato L, Motoyama E: Effect of maternal hypocapnia versus eucapnia on the foetus during cesarean section. *Br J Anaesth* 1972; 44:1173.

32 Intrauterine Fetal Death

Barbara L. Hartwell and Dale P. Reisner

Intrauterine fetal death (IUFD) often occurs without warning in an apparently normal pregnancy. Irrespective of the gestational age, fetal loss can be devastating to the patient and her family. This chapter discusses the definition, epidemiology, etiology, and management of this obstetric crisis with its attendant anesthetic dilemmas.

DEFINITION

The purist would define intrauterine "fetal" death before labor as death occurring 10 weeks after the last menstrual period, or 8 weeks after conception. However, the World Health Organization (WHO) defines fetal death as death occurring prior to the complete expulsion or extraction from the mother of a product of conception, irrespective of gestational age.[1] The National Center for Health Statistics in the United States calculates fetal mortality on the basis of deaths after 20 weeks of gestation.[2] Several states use the WHO definition to calculate their rates of fetal death. In addition, a number of countries outside of the United States calculate their rates based on fetal deaths occurring at or beyond 28 weeks' gestational age.

Valid fetal mortality rate comparisons depend on using the same definition for all the groups being evaluated. Fetal mortality rate calculations should include both the number of live births and the number of fetal deaths in the denominator. However, many calculations use a denominator of live births rather than total births, which produces a fetal mortality ratio. Fetal mortality ratios are meaningless with small groups and also at low gestational ages, since the number of live births is so low. Thus, caution is necessary to avoid comparing rates with ratios for different fetal mortality calculations.

EPIDEMIOLOGY

Fetal mortality rates in the United States have declined over the past 40 years. Fetal mortality was 7.5/1000 total births in 1990, according to the National Center for Health Statistics Calculations.[3] In 1945 fetal mortality was 21/1000 for whites and 41/1000 for other races. This disparity still exists with fetal mortality at 6.4/1000 for whites and 11.7/1000 for other races in 1990.

Maternal age below 20 and above 34 is associated with twofold to threefold higher fetal mortality rates. This greater risk may be partly due to increased chromosomal anomalies and multiple gestations in women over age 34, and partly to poor nutrition, increased smoking, and less prenatal care in teenagers. Higher fetal mortality is found in unmarried mothers, male fetuses, and multiple gestations. These higher mortality categories have been found consistently even in populations outside the United States.

Overall estimates of fetal mortality range from 15% to 20% in clinically recognized pregnancies; about 10% occur from 8 to 12 gestational weeks.[4-6] Recently, postimplantation losses have been estimated at over 40% using serum beta human chorionic gonadotropin (βhCG) concentrations to identify early pregnancies.[4,5] The probability of fetal death (WHO definition) by gestational age is highest postconception and drops rapidly until 16 weeks.[7,8] After 20 weeks, fetal death occurs in less than 1% of pregnancies.[3,9]

DIAGNOSIS

Historically, IUFD was suspected when the usual signs or symptoms of pregnancy were either absent or regressed after initially being present. This occurred both in early and later fetal death. After 20 weeks, the patient's most common presenting complaint is lack of fetal movement. She also may complain of weight loss, decrease in breast size, bloody watery vaginal discharge, or cramping.

The physician may note absence of fundal height growth on serial examinations or inability to detect fetal heart sounds. Relying on these clinical criteria, the diagnosis of IUFD may be delayed from days to weeks beyond the actual time of fetal death.

For the past 50 years, radiography was the chief method of confirming suspected IUFD. The most reliable sign is gas in the fetal vasculature, which can appear within several days after fetal death. However, it is only present in approximately 50% of IUFDs.[9] Later radiologic changes that may be present are those of fetal maceration. Overlapping of the fetal cranial sutures is present in nearly all cases of IUFD, but this may take several weeks to manifest. In addition, fetal edema known as the "halo sign" may be seen several days after fetal death. The problem with the halo sign is that it may be present in cases of a live fetus with hydrops fetalis.[10] The last consistent radiologic sign is abnormal angulation of the fetal spine, which occurs as the vertebral bodies compress with time.

Over the past 10 to 15 years, availability of βHCG has made early diagnosis of first trimester fetal deaths more accurate. Serial βHCG measurements can be done every 48 to 72 hours; when stable or falling in the first trimester, they usually predict either fetal death or ectopic pregnancy. Caution must be taken interpreting a single βHCG measurement since these measurements should be run serially, in pairs, and by the same laboratory for the most accurate evaluation of the results.

Ultrasound is the most reliable method of diagnosing IUFD. Failure to detect fetal heart tones by Doppler assessment in the office may be the first suggestion of IUFD. Fetal heart tones should be detectable by 12 menstrual weeks' gestational age in most patients. The inability to detect fetal heart tones with Doppler assessment, however, is not a reliable diagnostic technique, since it may be affected by maternal size, abdominal scars, uterine fibroids, or extreme retroversion. Real-time ultrasound is the most reliable method currently available of diagnosing IUFD.

In the United States, real-time ultrasound has been widely available to most clinicians for the past 10 years. Using transabdominal ultrasound, embryonic cardiac activity should be demonstrated in all viable pregnancies of 7 to 8 weeks by last menstrual period.[10] Transvaginal ultrasound may allow detection of embryonic cardiac activity from 5 to 6 weeks on.[11]

At or after 8 menstrual weeks the diagnosis of the embryonic or fetal death may be made by the absence of cardiac motion for a minimum of 3 minutes by each of two independent observers.[12] Findings may be documented by videotape recording of the real-time examination or by visualiza-

tion of the fetal heart and M-mode documentation of absence of cardiac activity on equipment with this capability.

Prior to 8 menstrual weeks the diagnosis of fetal or embryonic demise is less definitive by a single ultrasound. A large gestational sac without the presence of a fetal pole or crown-rump length is known as the empty sac. This may reflect either inaccurate gestational age by clinical dating or the presence of a nonviable pregnancy. Bernard[13] and Nyberg[14] found 100% diagnostic accuracy for IUFD if an empty gestational sac was greater than 20 to 25 mm in diameter. Other ultrasound findings such as irregular sac shape or double sac are less conclusive findings. Usually early ultrasound suggestions of IUFD are combined with serial serum quantitative βHCG titers for a firm diagnosis. The alternative would be a follow-up ultrasound in 7 to 14 days to look for appropriate interval growth and/or appearance of a fetal pole.

CAUSES

Causes of fetal death vary according to the gestational age at the time of the loss. Some of the most common etiologies are discussed in this section.

Chromosomal

Chromosomal causes of fetal loss are highest in the first trimester. In Table 32-1, gestational ages of less than 8 weeks show a range of 14% to 30% of fetal deaths with abnormal karyotypes.[15-17] Boué and Boué[18] reported up to 66% of abnormal karyotypes in abortuses studied by "developmental age" less than 8 weeks. Developmental age was ascertained by detailed macroscopic evaluation of the embryo and microscopic evaluation of the placenta. From 8 to 12 developmental weeks, 23% had abnormal chromosomes. Overall, this is consistent with most authors' reports of approximately 50% abnormal karyotypes in first trimester spontaneous abortions. This percentage decreases to about 6% of fetal deaths from 28 weeks to term.[17]

The type of chromosomal abnormality varies according to gestational age, parental age, and repro-

Table 32-1 Percent of fetal/embryonic deaths by gestational age due to chromosomal abnormalities

Weeks of gestation	% With chromosomal abnormalities		
	Creasy et al.[15] (n = 893)	Warburton et al.[16] (n = 876)	Angell et al.[17] (n = 500)
0-7	—	14.0	27.1
8-11	50.4	49.2	53.5
12-15	44.1	39.1	47.9
16-19	21.4	18.5	23.8
20-27	6.6	11.1	13.2

ductive history. According to Warburton,[19] trisomies account for 55% of fetal deaths up to 28 weeks' gestation. Monosomy X or Turner's syndrome is found in about 18% and triploidy is found in 15% of chromosomally abnormal abortuses. Less frequently found are tetraploidy (about 6%), unbalanced structural rearrangement (about 3%), and other complex abnormalities (about 4%).

Trisomy has a very strong correlation with increasing maternal age. At maternal ages 35 to 39 years, approximately 36% of spontaneous abortions have abnormal karyotypes; this increases to 53% at or over the age of 40.[19] This association is also present with other chromosomal abnormalities. Increasing paternal age does not appear to be a factor until over 55 years. Monosomy X appears to be inversely related to maternal age, occurring more often at younger ages.

In women under 35 years of age, the greater the number of spontaneous abortions, the less likely an abnormal karyotype will be responsible. Warburton[19] reports a 40% incidence of abnormal chromosomes in abortuses from women with no previous spontaneous abortion. This decreases to about 20% for women with a history of two previous spontaneous abortions. Despite this decrease, balanced translocations have been found in 3% to 5% of couples with two or more spontaneous abortions.[20]

Malformations/syndromes/fetal arrhythmias

Congenital malformations that are multifactorial in etiology can be responsible for fetal deaths at any gestational age. Single or multiple anomalies may be present in a fetus who dies in utero. Hall[21] reported the following anomalies most commonly found in a group of 37 stillborns with multiple anomalies over 26 weeks' gestational age:

1. Heart defects, 46%
2. Urinary tract anomalies, 40%
3. Polydactyly/syndactyly/oligodactyly, 40%
4. Omphalocele/gastroschisis, 33%
5. Hydrocephalus, 26%
6. Cleft lip/palate, 20%
7. Microphthalmia/anophthalmia, 20%
8. Intestinal atresia, 13%
9. Midline brain defects, 8%

In addition, fetal deaths can occur with isolated defects, such as those listed above, and also with diaphragmatic hernia, neural tube defects, etc.

A number of syndromes and genetic disorders exist that can be seen with fetal death and are too numerous to list here. These may be sporadic, such as amniotic band syndrome, with rare to no recurrence risk. They may be multifactorial, such as most neural tube defects and other isolated anomalies found in fetuses with normal chromosomes, with a 2% to 5% recurrence risk. They may be autosomal recessive, autosomal dominant, or X-linked, with recurrence risks usually from 25% to 50%. However, if the disorder is the result of a new mutation in the fetus, the recurrence risk is zero for other offspring of that couple.

Fetal arrhythmias may occur without obvious underlying cardiac anomalies. In response to persistent tachycardia or bradycardia the fetus may develop congestive heart failure, resultant hydrops, and eventual death. Unless the arrhythmia is identified prior to this sequence of events, the underlying cause of the hydrops is unknown. Autopsy will not clarify the underlying cause unless the arrhythmia was related to a cardiac defect. It is also conceivable that the fetus may experience sudden death due to an acute arrhythmia that would not be associated with fetal hydrops. Complete congenital heart block appears to be associated either with a cardiac defect (10%-20%) or with anti-Ro/anti-SSA antibodies (80%-90%).[22,23] Since only about one third of these mothers have known connective tissue disease, such as lupus or Sjögren's syndrome, screening for anti-SSA antibodies should be done in an asymptomatic mother with a fetal demise showing evidence of hydrops.

Multiple gestations

Multiple gestations occur in less than 1% of viable pregnancies in the United States. The true incidence of multiple gestations is difficult to assess. Landy[24] evaluated 1000 pregnancies with first-trimester ultrasound. The rate of twins was 3.3% (two fetuses identified) or 5.4% (one fetus + one empty sac). Twenty-one percent of those identified with two fetuses subsequently had one fetal death. Overall, fetal death rates are five times greater in twins than in singletons.

Monozygotic twinning occurs at a rate of 4/1,000 births and appears to be a random occurrence. This rate is independent of maternal age, race, history, etc. In general, monozygotic twins have a perinatal morbidity and mortality that is 2 to 3 times greater than that of dizygotic twins.[25] The effect of chorionicity on perinatal mortality is shown in Table 32-2 (these rates do include neonatal deaths as well as fetal deaths).

Dizygotic twinning varies according to different maternal factors, ranging from 4 to 50/1000 births.[26] Dizygotic twins occur when two ova, released from one or two follicles, are both fertilized. Risk factors for multiple gestation include maternal family history of dizygotic twins, age greater than 35 and less than 40, ethnic background (black > white > Oriental), parity greater than three, previous twin gestation, greater coital fre-

Table 32-2 Perinatal mortality: monozygotic twins

Chorionicity	Postconception timing (days)	Percentage of monozygotic twins	Perinatal mortality (%)
Diamniotic/ dichorionic	1-3	~30	~5-10 (similar to dizygotic rates)
Diamniotic/monochorionic	4-8	~67	10-25
Monoamniotic/monochorionic	9-12	<2	>50
Conjoined twins (monoamniotic/ monochorionic)	>13	Rare	Rare survival of both twins

quency, good nutritional status, and ovulation induction for infertility.[25,26] The perinatal mortality of dizygotic twins is estimated to be between 5% and 10%. Again, first-trimester fetal losses may be much greater than this.

Causes of fetal death in multiple gestations are similar to those in singletons with the exception of twin-to-twin transfusion and monoamniotic losses due to cord entanglement. In any multiple gestation, death can be due to:

1. Congenital defects, which are higher in twins, especially in monozygotic twins.
2. Intrauterine growth retardation (IUGR) due to uteroplacental insufficiency (in either monozygotic or dizygotic twins).
3. Abruption, due to overdistended uterus or associated maternal preeclampsia.
4. Diabetic complications due to an increased incidence of gestational diabetes.

Most of the excess fetal death rate in monozygotic twins occurs from cord entanglement due to a single gestational sac in monoamniotic twins, or from twin-to-twin transfusion (5% to 17% incidence) due to shared placental vascular communications.[27] Usually this syndrome occurs when a significant arteriovenous shunt causes a net transfer of blood from one fetus to the other. Classically, the donor becomes anemic, hypovolemic, and hypoxemic with secondary oligohydramnios and growth lag. The recipient becomes hypervolemic and polycythemic and may develop congestive heart failure with hydrops and polyhydramnios. Either or both twins may die if this process occurs early in gestation or is not recognized prior to their becoming moribund. In addition, whenever a single fetal death occurs for any reason, the surviving monozygotic twin may be at risk for intravascular coagulation or thromboembolism from the dead twin.[28]

Infections

Early in the 20th century, syphilis was responsible for up to 43% of fetal deaths over 28 weeks' gestation.[29] With the advent of arsenicals and subsequent antibiotics, syphilis became a rare cause of IUFD. In the late 1990s it may again become significant among the infectious causes of fetal death in women with no prenatal care and promiscuity usually associated with illicit drug use in themselves or their partners. Historically, smallpox, scarlet fever, and typhoid fever were associated with fetal death but are rarely seen today.

Amnionitis has been reported as the underlying cause of between 2% to 15% of fetal deaths.[9,30] Bacterial agents such as group B streptococci, anaerobic *Fusobacterium, Listeria monocytogenes,* and less commonly leptospirosis, brucellosis, borreliosis, and clostridial infections have been identified in cases of fetal death in utero.[31,32] These infections may not be seen on placental evaluation but may require either cultures or special staining of fetal organs such as brain, heart, lungs, liver, or adrenals. Some of these occur via hematogenous spread to the fetus rather than by ascending transcervical infection.

Mycotic infections such as disseminated fetal candidiasis or coccidiomyocosis can be the cause of fetal death. Benirschke and Robb discussed several parasitic infections that have been associated with fetal death.[31] Toxoplasmosis is the most common of these seen in the United States. It spreads via ingestion of raw or rare infected meat or via fecal contact from infected cats. Fetal infection occurs at increasing rates with exposure in each successive trimester. Fetal death from toxoplasmosis rarely occurs; and when it does, is more likely in the first half of pregnancy. Chagas disease from *Trypanosoma cruzi* is widespread in South America and is associated with fetal hydrops and death. Malaria may be associated with fetal death secondary either to high maternal fevers or fetal hemolysis.

The leading viral causes of fetal death have changed over the past few decades as vaccines have become available. Rubella or mumps are now rare causes of fetal death. Coxsackievirus group B can cause fetal myocarditis with subsequent hydrops and death.[33] Human parvovirus B_{19} (the agent in fifth disease) has been reported with fetal death secondary to severe anemia and hydrops.[34] Treatment with intrauterine fetal transfusion versus expectant management has been proposed to allow the fetus to recover from the infection.[35]

Herpetoviruses may be associated with fetal death. Varicella infections early in pregnancy may rarely result in fetal death. Cytomegalovirus can be seen with fetal hydrops and death and should cause histologic changes in fetal organs and placenta. Fetal death rarely occurs from herpes simplex virus (HSV) primary infections. Benirschke and Robb[31] report that as high as 20% to 30% of spontaneous abortions are associated with HSV type II amniochorionic infection after activation of latent endometrial infection. They postulate that latent infection may be present for years and is not associated with a history of either maternal or paternal genital herpes. Further work regarding this association with fetal death is necessary.

Placental factors/cord accidents

Abruption. Placental abruption or premature placental separation occurs in about 1 in 120 pregnancies.[36] Fetal and neonatal death rates range from 20% to 40%.[37] Eight percent to 20% of patients present with a fetal death in utero and signs or symptoms of abruption.[36] The remainder of the fetal or neonatal deaths occur within hours to weeks after the initial diagnosis of abruption is made. Risk factors include chronic and/or pregnancy-induced hypertension, diabetes, lupus, and other maternal vascular diseases; smoking, cocaine use; lupus anticoagulant or anticardiolipin antibodies; thrombocytosis; prior history of abruption; abdominal trauma; and low socioeconomic or unmarried status. The diagnosis is usually easily made at delivery by the presence of port wine amniotic fluid, clots (adherent or free) noted with delivery of the placenta, or by pathologic examination of the placenta. Disseminated intravascular coagulation (DIC) in the mother is usually secondary to the abruption rather than the acute fetal death. Delayed fetal deaths following abruption "may" be preventable by intensive maternal and fetal surveillance, depending on gestational age.

Hemorrhage. Another cause of fetal death before labor is fetomaternal hemorrhage. This is a known potential complication of placental abruption, placenta previa, or after amniocentesis. It also can occur in normal pregnancies[38] without any clinical evidence of bleeding and is thought to be responsible for the rare spontaneous Rh-sensitization of an Rh-negative mother before antepartum RhoGAM prophylaxis. Kleihauer-Betke staining of a maternal blood smear can identify fetal hemoglobin and the proportion of fetal-to-maternal cells can be used to estimate the fetal blood loss. Laube and Schauberger[39] reported 4 of 29 (13.8%) of unexplained fetal deaths had positive Kleihauer-Betke stains consistent with fetal-to-maternal transfusions ranging from 150 to 250 ml. These amounts would account for losses of 29% to 66% of the fetal blood volumes. No obvious abruptions were noted on postmortem placental evaluations, but "mahogany colored" amniotic fluid was noted with 1 case. One other patient had amniocentesis performed 1 day before the fetal death.

Previa. Placenta previa with acute excessive blood loss also can result in fetal death. The prevalence of placenta previa varies by gestational age. With widespread availability of ultrasound, prenatal diagnosis can be made. In the early second trimester, it is not uncommon to detect varying degrees of placenta previa. By the third trimester, previa is present in about 0.6% of deliveries.[40,41] In 1980, Cotton et al[42] reported a 6% fetal mortality and 13% perinatal mortality from placenta previa. Expectant management is recommended for persistent previa in asymptomatic patients, with delivery by elective cesarean section at 37+ weeks according to the guidelines of the American College of Obstetrics and Gynecology.

Insufficiency. Placental insufficiency can result in IUGR with subsequent fetal/neonatal death. A variety of maternal conditions can be responsible for placental insufficiency, such as hypertension, diabetes, vascular diseases, lupus anticoagulant or anticardiolipin antibodies, and smoking. A rare cause is maternal floor infarction of the placenta where diffuse fibrinoid deposition results in placental insufficiency.[43]

Multiple gestations with limited intrauterine surface area for implantation can also result in placental insufficiency with subsequent fetal death, based on placental size limitation or abnormal cord insertions rather than on vascular problems.

Perinatal mortality is 3 to 8 times greater for the fetus with IUGR.[30] Identifying the patient at risk for placental insufficiency is the key to prenatal management. If a neural tube defect or other associated anomaly has been ruled out, a second-trimester elevated maternal serum alphafetoprotein level may identify a patient at risk for subsequent placental insufficiency or fetal death.[44] Serial ultrasound measurements of fetal growth and umbilical artery Doppler evaluations are useful studies for following patients at risk for IUGR.[30,45] When growth lag or abnormal Doppler ratios or waveforms are found, more intensive fetal surveillance may avoid fetal death in utero. It is unknown if this can decrease neonatal and infant death rates for growth-retarded babies. New preventative or ameliorating measures, such as strict bed rest or low-dose aspirin therapy are beneficial in some but not all patients.[46] Other treatments being investigated are maternal oxygen therapy, dipyridamole, heparin, and/or steroids. Cessation of smoking should be encouraged to decrease vasoconstriction in any patient with evidence of placental insufficiency.

Postdates. Postdates placental insufficiency occurs in some pregnancies that go beyond 42 weeks from onset of the last menstrual period. The infants in this setting have been described as postmature or dysmature, with evidence of weight loss from subcutaneous fat and muscle mass losses. These babies may not weigh less than the tenth percentile, since they usually have grown appropriately until term. They frequently have meconium-stained skin or amniotic fluid. It has been estimated that perinatal mortality doubles by 43 weeks and triples by 44 weeks, compared with rates between 39 and 41 weeks gestation.[47] These increases may be lessened by instituting fetal testing such as nonstress tests, biophysical profiles, and possible contraction stress tests twice weekly from 41 to 42 weeks. Fetal kick counts throughout the third trimester have clearly been shown to reduce fetal death rates in both high- and low-risk pregnancies.[48]

Cord accidents. Cord accidents have been reported as causes of fetal death in 2% to 11% of stillbirths.[30] In singletons this category includes thrombosis, true knot, entanglement in amniotic bands, and prolapse. Two other cord complications, torsion and multiple nuchal or extremity cord enwrappings, may be listed as the only identifiable cause of fetal death. Since some mothers report a transient pronounced increase in fetal activity before cessation of fetal movement it may be that the fetus becomes agitated because of sudden arrhythmia or anoxic event with the twisting of the cord being a secondary phenomenon. Cord entanglement with monoamniotic twins has previously been discussed. Most deaths from cord accidents are not preventable. They also, fortunately, carry minimal to no risk of recurrence. Ultrasound identification of polyhydramnios, monoamniotic twins, amniotic bands, or an unstable fetal presentation in association with a dilated cervix can identify patients at risk for cord prolapse or entanglement. Inpatient management of selected patients or outpatient fetal heart rate monitoring may identify a fetus with significant cord compressions and enable delivery of a viable neonate.

Immunologic diseases

Systemic lupus erythematosus. Systemic lupus erythematosus (SLE) is the most common autoimmune disease with significant fetal losses. The magnitude of fetal death has been difficult to quantify, with spontaneous abortion rates ranging from 0% to 35% and fetal death rates ranging from 0% to 29%.[49] Placental abnormalities related to the maternal autoantibodies with complement deposition, decidual vasculopathy, and/or infarcts are thought to be responsible for the fetal deaths in most circumstances.[22,50] Occasional deaths occur with the presence of anti-Ro/SSA antibodies and complete congenital heart block if the fetal heart rate becomes low enough or coexistent cardiomyopathy results in unrecognized congestive heart failure and hydrops. Active disease at onset of pregnancy seems to be related to greater fetal losses.[51,52] The presence of renal disease and/or hypertension clearly increases rates of fetal death and spontaneous abortion; this ranges from 13% to 50%, depending on the degree of disease activity.[51,53,54] The presence of antinuclear antibodies (ANA) without clinical evidence of SLE has been suggested as a cause for some recurrent abortions.[55,56] The numbers of patients are small and the data are not conclusive. The authors recommend screening for ANA in patients with recurrent fetal deaths.

Lupus anticoagulant/anticardiolipin antibodies. Patients who have anticardiolipin antibodies (ACA) or lupus anticoagulant (LAC) may have very poor pregnancy outcomes.[51] The recognition and ability to clinically test for antiphospholipid antibodies have evolved over the past 10 years. Most of the reports of pregnancy outcomes in patients with SLE have not included data regarding the presence or absence of either LAC or ACA. It is possible that lupus patients without either of these autoantibodies and without significant hypertension or renal disease may have normal or only minimally increased fetal death rates.

Branch et al reported decreasing pregnancy loss rates from 96.8% to 37.5% in eight patients with LAC but no clinical evidence of lupus who were treated with high-dose prednisone and low-dose aspirin.[57] These were patients whose pregnancy outcomes (1 live birth in 31 pregnancies) were compared with treatment outcomes (5 live births in 8 pregnancies). Review articles have also reported very high rates of fetal death, averaging 91% from 242 untreated pregnancies with LAC identified.[49,51]

Anticardiolipin antibodies also have been reported to be associated with fetal death.[49,51,58] Most of the reports are outcomes in patients with lupus and/or LAC in addition to ACA. Recently, an excellent study by Lockwood et al reported on the prevalence of LAC and ACA in a low-risk obstetric population.[59] Two of 737 patients (0.27%) had LAC identified by prolonged activated partial thromboplastin time (aPTT), which did not correct with mixing studies. These 2 patients both had mid–second-trimester fetal deaths. Sixteen of 737 patients (2.2%) had ACA identified by enzyme-linked immunoassay (ELISA), 2 of whom also were LAC-positive as noted above. If the LAC-positive patients are removed from this group, 10 of 14 (71%) of ACA-positive patients had live births. The 29% fetal loss rate occurred at less than 20 weeks, and 2 additional patients had neonatal deaths for a total fetal/neonatal death rate of 43%. Thus, it appears that the isolated presence of ACA *is* associated with an increased risk of fetal or neonatal death compared to pregnant patients without these antibodies. However, the magnitude of fetal loss appears to be much lower than for patients with LAC. Treatment regimens vary, but most often include low-dose aspirin treatment with or without heparin or prednisone.

Other rheumatologic conditions. Other rheumatologic conditions may be associated with increased risks of fetal death. Fortunately, many of these are rare conditions in pregnancy with only anecdotal case reports available regarding pregnancy outcomes. They include scleroderma/progressive systemic sclerosis, mixed connective tissue disease, polymyositis/dermatomyositis, periarteritis nodosa, and Sjögren's syndrome.[22,60,61]

Thyroid disorders. Autoimmune thyroid disease is associated with increased spontaneous abortion and fetal death when inadequately treated.[22,62] This is probably due to the hormonal imbalances created by either hypothyroidism or hyperthyroidism. In hypothyroidism, failure of the normal rise of thyroid hormones may predispose the patient to abortion.[62] Maternal hypertension and/or hyperthermia associated with thyrotoxicosis and especially with thyroid storm may contribute to later fetal death in utero in untreated patients with Graves' disease.[63] These diseases are minor contributors to fetal death causes but are mentioned because of their amenability to treatment. Rarely, transplacental passage of thyroid-stimulating antibodies can cause fetal hyperthyroidism with a tachycardia that, if untreated, can result in fetal death.[64]

Myasthenia gravis. Myasthenia gravis is a rare autoimmune disease that may be associated with increased stillbirth and neonatal mortality due to transplacental passage of immunoglobulin G (IgG) antibodies against acetylcholine receptors.[61] Plauché reported a 2.9% rate of stillbirths and a 5.3% rate of neonatal deaths in 314 pregnancies of 217 myasthenic mothers.[65]

Isoimmunization

Erythroblastosis fetalis. Hydropic fetal death from erythroblastosis fetalis was first described by Hippocrates. The most common maternal isoimmunization is against the D antigen of the Rh blood group. The incidence of the Rh-negative blood group is 11% to 15% in women in the United States.[49,66] Rh immunization can occur if an Rh-negative woman receives an Rh-positive transfusion or if she is exposed to Rh-positive fetal red blood cells. The latter is the more common etiology since Rh-typing of banked blood became standard practice.

Fetomaternal transfusion of less than 0.1 ml occurs in 60% of pregnancies before or after delivery.[66] More significant volumes may be transfused with placental abruption, toxemia, cesarean section, manual placental removal, external version, or amniocentesis. There is a 5% to 25% risk of fetomaternal transfusion after spontaneous or induced abortion.[66] A variety of factors other than the volume of circulating fetal cells affect whether the mother will produce antibodies to the Rh-positive red cells; these are discussed in detail in Chapter 18.

Fetal anemia occurs when maternal IgG anti-D antibodies cross the placenta binding to the Rh-positive fetal red cells, which subsequently are destroyed. Bone marrow and extramedullary erythropoiesis occurs in response to the anemia with resulting hepatosplenomegaly. It is likely that portal and umbilical venous hypertension occur due to liver enlargement with resulting ascites and placental edema.[66] Hypoproteinemia and generalized edema follow. Severe fetal anemia and/or cardiac failure are likely causes of fetal death in utero. Since most preexisting Rh-sensitization is diagnosed with early antepartum screening, fetal death is becoming rare with appropriate management in utero. Prophylaxis against maternal Rh-isoimmunization is done by intramuscular administration of RhoGAM (Rh-D immunoglobulin) at 28 weeks, with any spontaneous antepartum hemorrhage, with procedures such as amniocentesis, after delivery of an Rh-positive infant, or at the time of an induced or spontaneous abortion. This prophylaxis has markedly decreased the number of Rh-immunized women.

Irregular antibodies. Maternal isoimmunization to other blood group system antibodies can also cause fetal or neonatal death. These antibodies are referred to as irregular antibodies and can be detected by a prenatal indirect Coombs' test. Only IgG class antibodies are capable of transplacental passage with potential hemolytic disease in the fetus. The majority of these antibodies result from prior transfusion, with some from prior pregnancy exposures.[67] Some of these antibodies have only been associated with mild fetal disease; others from the Kell, Kidd, Duffy, MNSs systems etc., have been associated with severe fetal disease.[67] Management is complex, but most fetal deaths can be avoided with early identification, close surveillance, and intrauterine transfusions when indicated by fetal hematocrit assessment via cordocentesis.

ABO—severe. ABO blood group incompatibility is commonly associated with mild hemolytic disease of the newborn, but it rarely has been associated with severe fetal disease and it is not thought to be responsible for stillbirth.[68]

Other maternal conditions

Chronic hypertension/pregnancy-induced hypertension. Hypertensive disorders have a high perinatal mortality rate. In women with chronic hypertension perinatal mortality has been reported at 13.4%, with 9.6% being stillbirths.[69] Pregnancy-induced hypertension also is associated with higher fetal losses, especially if eclampsia develops.[30] The patients at highest risk of fetal or neonatal death are women with chronic hypertension and superimposed preeclampsia, with perinatal mortality ranging from 10% to 32%.[70-72] Fetal death is not necessarily related to severity of the underlying hypertension. Deaths occur secondary to placental abruption and/or fetal asphyxia in the setting of IUGR. Some of the neonatal deaths are related to prematurity complications.

Diabetes mellitus/gestational diabetes. Pregnancies complicated by overt diabetes mellitus have higher spontaneous abortion and perinatal mortality rates. High loss rates appear to be strongly correlated with the degree of glucose control, both preconception and antepartum.[73,74] Congenital malformations are the leading cause of perinatal mortality in patients with overt diabetes in pregnancy. High maternal hemoglobin A_1C (Hb A_1C) indicates poor glucose control over the preceding 6 weeks (the normal red cell lifespan).[75] In Miller's study, the incidence of major congenital malformations was 3.4% in diabetic women with Hb A_1C of less than 8.5; it was 22.4% for those with Hb A_1C of greater than 8.6.[75] Other authors have confirmed this relationship and have demonstrated either normal or minimally elevated rates of major anomalies in diabetics with good preconceptual metabolic control.[76,77]

Diabetic women who present in ketoacidosis have had as high as 50% fetal mortality associated with the acute episode.[74,78] Placental insufficiency with its potential for fetal death can occur in diabetic women with vascular disease.

Gestational diabetes has been associated with otherwise unexplained stillbirths.[79,80] The mechanism is thought to be related to high fetal basal rates of insulin production in response to high maternal glucose levels in general. If the mother has a relatively rapid decrease in glucose, with attendant elevation in ketoacids, the fetus is then subjected to hypoglycemia and acidosis, which may result in death.[78] Well-controlled gestational diabetes appears to have perinatal mortality rates consistent with the normal population.[79]

Hematologic disorders. There are a number of maternal hematologic disorders that may be associated with increased risks of fetal death. They include sickle cell anemia, essential thrombocytosis, autoimmune hemolytic anemia, thrombocytopenia (autoimmune), and thrombotic thrombocytopenia purpura.[81,82] Increased fetal losses are due to placental thrombosis, or rarely severe fetal anemia or thrombocytopenia. Appropriate management of the maternal condition and fetal surveillance should avoid most of the fetal deaths.

Maternal exposures

X-ray. Exposure to ionizing radiation of greater than 20 rads may result in spontaneous abortion or congenital malformations.[83,84] Acute radiation doses of this magnitude usually come from therapeutic radiation or radiation accidents.

Other workplace chemical exposures may be associated with early fetal losses. These include anesthetic gases, cytotoxic drugs, lead, mercury, and ethylene oxide.[7,83,85]

Prescribed medications. The following prescribed medications have been associated with spontaneous abortions: aminopterin, warfarin/coumarin, trimethadione, and isotretinoin.[86] Ingested phenylalanine may be associated with an increase in spontaneous abortions in patients with phenylketonuria.[86]

Alcohol and smoking. Alcohol use regularly during pregnancy may be associated with increased risk of spontaneous abortion.[87] Smoking has been associated with spontaneous abortion, stillbirth, and IUGR.[7] Smoking in pregnancy is associated with both placental abruption and placenta previa.[87] It may compound other risk factors such as diabetes, hypertension, antiphospholipid antibodies, etc., in the development of placental insufficiency, since nicotine can cause vasoconstriction. It can also be synergistic with illicit drugs such as cocaine that are potent vasoconstrictors themselves and have been associated with placental abruption.[88-90] Smoking is an easily identifiable risk factor for fetal death, but it is difficult to convince patients to stop smoking before conception and even during a complicated pregnancy.

Trauma. Maternal trauma may result in fetal death even if the mother does not sustain serious injury. The most common trauma seen by the obstetrician is that associated with motor vehicle accidents. When the mother survives, fetal death most commonly occurs due to placental abruption, with some deaths a result of uterine rupture or more rarely direct fetal trauma.[91,92] Appropriate fetal monitoring for 24 hours after abdominal trauma can reduce fetal deaths from abruption since many of these are delayed events.[93] Direct fetal trauma with death also can result from gunshot or stab wounds to the pregnant abdomen. In a review of 77 total reported cases, maternal mortality from an abdominal gunshot wound was 3.9%, whereas perinatal mortality was 71%.[94]

OBSTETRIC AND ANESTHETIC MANAGEMENT
Obstetric management

Fetal death prior to labor at less than 12 to 14 weeks' gestation is most often managed with suction and/or sharp curettage after cervical dilation. The patient is given the option to await spontaneous labor, but most women elect an evacuation procedure. If no active bleeding is present, this is usually scheduled electively as an outpatient day surgery.

Fetal death occurring between 14 and 28 weeks' gestation may also be managed expectantly in stable patients. Several methods of delivery are available for patients who do not wish to await spontaneous labor. Dilation and extraction (D&E) may be performed in the second trimester up to about 20 weeks. Dilation and extraction has the psychologic advantage of a quick termination of the pregnancy and avoidance of labor, but it requires either regional or general anesthesia and limits pathologic evaluation for cause of the fetal death. Most deliveries in this gestational age range are induced with prostaglandin E_2 vaginal suppositories. The usual dosage is a 20-mg suppository placed intravaginally every 2 to 6 hours, which is 90% to 100% successful according to a review by Kochenour.[95] Side effects of nausea, vomiting, diarrhea, tachycardia, or fever can be managed with premedication or as needed. Absolute contraindications to use are known prostaglandin hypersensitivity and pelvic inflammatory disease. It should be used with caution in patients with asthma, seizure disorder, cardiac, renal or hepatic disease, or previous uterine scar.[9,95] Pain of labor may be managed either by intravenous or intramuscular analgesics or amnestics or with epidural anesthesia. Depending on the gestational age, sharp curettage may be necessary for placental removal.

Intraamniotic installation of hypertonic solutions such as saline, urea, or prostaglandin $F_{2\alpha}$ have been used, but this requires amniocentesis.

Intraamniotic prostaglandin $F_{2\alpha}$ usually avoids the systemic prostaglandin side effects as seen with E_2 vaginal suppositories. Faster labors result if the cervix is dilated liberally with hydrophilic dilators (synthetic laminaria) 1 day before the intraamniotic injection.

Saline is no longer in use due to maternal complications of DIC and an unacceptable rate of maternal deaths.[96]

Intravenous oxytocin inductions are frequently used when premature rupture of the membranes exists with IUFD. The second trimester uterus may not respond well to low doses of oxytocin. High doses (30-36 μg/min) may be administered safely if electrolytes are monitored for the potential antidiuretic effects of oxytocin.

When fetal death occurs before labor in the third trimester the safest management is expectant (awaiting spontaneous labor). In 1934, a review of 306 IUFDs after 28 weeks' gestation by Dippel[29] found that 75% of patients delivered within 2 weeks and 89% had delivered by 3 weeks after fetal death. In a review of 165 fetal deaths with weights over 1000 g, Tricomi and Kohl[97] found that 90% of patients delivered within 2 weeks and 93% had delivered by 3 weeks. Excessive bleeding complications were not encountered with expectant management.

Labor induction in the third trimester includes examination for favorability of the cervix. Oxytocin induction is used with a favorable cervix or with ruptured membranes. Cervical ripening may be done with laminaria (seaweed or synthetic) or with intracervical prostaglandin E_2 gel (usually doses of 0.5-1.0 mg). Intracervical prostaglandin gel has not been FDA approved for ripening, but it is being used increasingly in university centers and in some community hospitals per protocols. Third-trimester risks of ruptured uterus and cervical lacerations[98,99] have only been reported with higher doses (such as the 20-mg suppositories) and with concurrent use of oxytocin. Most protocols use the gel for cervical ripening with one to three applications, and oxytocin is begun 6 to 8 hours following the last gel dose to avoid uterine hyperstimulation.

For patients who elect expectant management, there is concern for development of DIC. Pritchard[100] demonstrated that maternal coagulation defects rarely developed before 1 month after fetal death. If a dead fetus was retained longer, approximately 25% of women developed hypofibrinogenemia or a coagulopathy. This usually occurs gradually and can be monitored with serial DIC screens, usually done on a weekly basis in the absence of clinical signs of coagulopathy. Isolated hypofibrinogenemia can resolve spontaneously;[100] it has also been treated with heparin therapy, according to anecdotal reports.[101,102] This 25% incidence of DIC with prolonged retention of an IUFD is also seen in multiple gestations when the fetal loss occurs in the third trimester, as reviewed by Landy and Weingold.[103]

A unique situation exists when fetal death occurs in a multiple gestation in the second or third trimester. If the death occurs at or near term, usually induction or delivery by cesarean section is performed. The zygosity of the multiple gestation will influence the decision to deliver, as will the presumed cause of the fetal demise. As previously discussed, if twin-to-twin transfusion is suspected, there is some concern for ongoing risk to the surviving fetus. For any monozygotic fetal pair, irrespective of the cause of death, there may be a risk of injury or death to the survivor if shared circulation is present. Infectious causes of fetal death may affect multiple gestation fetuses to varying degrees. One fetus may die, with the other(s) showing evidence of congenital infection with long-term sequelae or presence of IgM antibodies, indicating exposure but no adverse clinical disease. For most viral causes, expectant management with close fetal surveillance is usually recommended at early gestational ages. For bacterial causes such as *Listeria,* group B *Streptococcus,* or others found in chorioamnionitis, delivery is recommended even at early gestational ages. Maternal intravenous antibiotics are generally begun as soon as the diagnosis of chorioamnionitis is made and delivery of the live fetus(es) is performed either by induction or by cesarean section according to the clinical setting. Researchers are currently investigating the role of expectant management with intravenous antibiotic therapy in early, live, singleton gestations with intact membranes and a diagnosis of chorioamnionitis. This may be applicable to twins if it is found to be safe and efficacious in singletons. If expectant management is chosen in the uninfected patient with a multiple gestation, she should have serial DIC screens, ultrasound examinations to follow the survivor(s)' fetal growth and to rule out developing anomalies, along with other appropriate fetal testing.

Anesthetic management

Anesthetic management of the parturient with IUFD requires careful evaluation of any maternal illness that may have placed the patient at risk for this occurrence. Maternal disorders such as immunologic diseases, isoimmunization, hypertension, preeclampsia, diabetes mellitus, and hematologic diseases are discussed elsewhere in this book.

Similarly, the obstetric disorders that may be associated with fetal death are important considerations when evaluating and treating these patients. If the mother has been bleeding because of placental abruption, placenta previa, or trauma, careful assessment of her intravascular volume and hemodynamic stability are important. Chorioamnionitis, villitis, or other bacterial, viral, mycotic, or parasitic infections that could result in fetal demise will affect the anesthetic plan. For example, one must look for sepsis, meningitis, or respiratory involvement if infectious disease is present. The reader is referred to the appropriate chapters in this book regarding the anesthetic management of the obstetric factors that may lead to fetal demise (chromosomal disorders, malformations, multiple gestations, infections, and placental factors).

Once the anesthesiologist evaluates this background information, the obstetric plan becomes the major consideration in formulating the anesthetic management. A patient with an early fetal loss at less than 12 to 14 weeks' gestation who is scheduled for dilation and suction or curettage on an elective basis may have general, regional, or local anesthesia with or without parenteral sedation and narcotics. Patient preferences may be the deciding factor in an otherwise healthy person. Since the patient may be very apprehensive and emotional, she will benefit from a compassionate anesthesiologist who considers her psychological needs and her preference. Because it is unclear exactly when a pregnant patient is at increased risk for aspiration, it is prudent to take the usual precautions in these patients.

If general anesthesia is employed, the specific technique may influence the amount of blood loss during the procedure. Cullen[104] demonstrated significantly larger amounts of blood loss with halothane compared with nitrous oxide plus thiopental and meperidine or paracervical block in healthy patients having first-trimester abortions by suction technique. Enflurane, isoflurane, and halothane are all potent uterine muscle relaxants.[105] Furthermore, the pregnant myometrium is more sensitive to the depressant effects of the inhalational agents.[106] Therefore, it is prudent to avoid these agents and use a propofol-based or nitrous-narcotic technique.

Fetal death occurring during the early second trimester (less than 20 weeks) may also be managed by D&E, with anesthetic considerations similar to those described for the first-trimester procedure.

Induction of labor in the patient with a second- or third-trimester fetal death often includes the use of prostaglandin E_2 vaginal suppositories. The anesthesiologist should be aware of the possible side effects,[107] especially nausea, vomiting, and diarrhea, that can predispose the patient to aspiration as well as dehydration. Fever, hypotension, and tachycardia can also occur and therefore maternal vital signs should be carefully scrutinized.

The pain of labor in the patient with second- or third-trimester fetal death may be abolished with epidural anesthesia. There is no need to obtain coagulation studies if the fetus is known to be dead less than 4 weeks, unless there is evidence of chronic abruption, since clinically significant falls in fibrinogen levels do not occur before this time.[100] However, at Brigham and Women's Hospital we routinely wait for the results of clotting parameters before initiating regional anesthesia, because it is difficult to predict the presence of chronic abruptio placentae as the cause of IUFD. Although baseline studies are usually obtained (because of possibility of chronic abruption), epidural anesthesia can be initiated without unnecessary delay. Also, these patients may benefit from the use of intravenous sedatives or narcotics either alone, for initiation of the epidural anesthetic, or as supplementation to epidural anesthesia.

In patients with a dead fetus in utero for more than 4 weeks, an abnormal coagulation profile may be found with or without obvious bleeding.[100] Tissue thromboplastin from the dead fetus can enter the maternal circulation, leading to intravascular fibrin deposition and the consumption of Factors V and VIII,[95] hypofibrinogenemia, some elevation in fibrin degradation products, and thrombocytopenia. Platelet counts are often unchanged, however. The most useful laboratory parameter to follow is the plasma fibrinogen level. A normal fibrinogen level during pregnancy is 400 to 650 mg/dL. Approximately 4 weeks after the death of a fetus, plasma fibrinogen levels start to decline at a rate of about 20 to 85 mg/dL per week. Blood will fail to clot at plasma fibrinogen levels below 100 mg/dL.[95]

At fibrinogen levels below 150 mg/dL, intravenous heparin has rarely been used to arrest the consumption of clotting factors[108] and to allow for spontaneous correction of the clotting defect.[95,109] Fibrinogen infusions are not useful, because of rapid degradation. Furthermore, fibrinogen concentrates are no longer available, because of the unacceptably high incidence of hepatitis associated with its use.[110]

Patients with plasma fibrinogen levels of 150 mg/dL or greater who have not received heparin may have epidural anesthesia for labor and delivery without increased risk of bleeding. Patients who have received heparin and who have had this therapy discontinued for several hours (the half-life of heparin is approximately 90 minutes)[111] and have normal coagulation profiles are eligible for epidural anesthesia as well. Platelet counts should be obtained to rule out thrombocytopenia either due to the dead fetus or to the use of intravenous heparin.[112]

The anesthetic management of patients who have received subcutaneous heparin remains controversial. There have been no case reports of neurologic complications after regional anesthesia in patients receiving low-dose heparin preoperatively.[113] This does not document the safety of such procedures, however. Approximately 50% of patients receiving 5000 μg subcutaneous heparin had therapeutic blood levels of heparin for as long as 4 hours.[114] Peak effect of subcutaneous heparin is approximately 2 to 3 hours after injection. Certainly, documentation of a normal activated clotting time (ACT) or PTT is important if one elects to perform epidural anesthesia in a patient who has received subcutaneous heparin.

The anesthesiologist should bear in mind that epidural anesthesia for labor and delivery of the dead fetus is a desirable but elective procedure. The patient at risk for coagulopathy can be treated with parenteral sedatives and narcotics until it has been determined that all clotting parameters are normal. A rapid assessment of the degree of heparinization that may be useful is the ACT. This can be performed at the bedside with a portable coagulation analyzer. With tubes containing diatomaceous earth to activate clotting, a normal ACT is 122 seconds.[115]

If there is any reason to suspect that the patient is at increased risk for bleeding and epidural anesthesia is essential (extremely rare), several precautions should be taken to minimize trauma and to detect early signs of spinal epidural hematoma. An experienced anesthesiologist should administer the block. A midline approach is preferred[116] in an attempt to avoid traumatizing the engorged epidural veins.[117] The epidural catheter should be inserted gently and to no more than 2 to 3 cm into the epidural space, with frequent flushing and aspiration to rule out erosion into a blood vessel or to diagnose bleeding.[118,119] A short-acting local anesthetic is preferred so that symptoms of hematoma can be elicited as soon as possible as the block recedes. The epidural catheter should be removed carefully to minimize the risk of bleeding at the time of its removal.[120] Frequent detailed neurologic examinations should be performed. The most common intraspinal hematomas are spinal epidural hematomas, characterized by sudden and severe back pain, paresthesias, lower extremity pain, numbness, and weakness.[121] At the earliest sign of a possible hematoma, neurosurgical evaluation must be sought because prompt decompression is essential.

If a patient with an IUFD is bleeding excessively

because of either coagulopathy or placental abruption or placenta previa, emergency treatment is necessary. Preoperative or preinduction therapy[108] is limited to insertion of large-bore intravenous catheters and administration of fluids to include blood and cryoprecipitate of fresh frozen plasma that contains high concentration of Factor VIII and fibrinogen. Platelet infusion may be necessary in the patient with associated thrombocytopenia.

These patients are not candidates for regional anesthesia because of hypovolemia and/or active bleeding. If anesthesia is required for a surgical or obstetric procedure, general endotracheal anesthesia is employed. The reader is referred to Chapters 8 and 9 for specific recommendations.

If a cesarean delivery is planned for a patient with fetal death in a multiple gestation, regional anesthesia may be used in the absence of coagulopathy as demonstrated by a normal coagulation profile. If a coagulopathy is present, general endotracheal anesthesia is necessary.

In addition to providing pain relief, the anesthesiologist can provide emotional support to the parturient at this time of unfortunate loss. In a large obstetric unit where there are several anesthesiologists, it is desirable for one person to establish rapport with the patient and provide continued care and support.

PATHOLOGIC EVALUATION

Fetuses of less than 12 weeks' gestation are difficult to evaluate grossly; however, placental tissue may be sent for karyotype. Since chromosomal abnormalities are present in as many as 50% of these early fetal deaths, this may provide information to explain the current loss and to aid in future pregnancy counseling and evaluation.

An autopsy is recommended for most fetal deaths that occur in the second or third trimester. Sometimes the parents' personal or religious beliefs make it impossible to obtain consent for an autopsy. Counseling regarding the potential information that an autopsy can provide will rarely change the parents' preexisting beliefs. Autopsies are expensive, ranging from $600 to $2000, depending on the city and other necessary cultures or karyotyping. This expense may not be covered by the parents' health insurance policy.

The perinatal autopsy includes a maternal, obstetric, and family history. Any prenatal ultrasound findings are also helpful in directing the autopsy. A physical examination is performed, noting appearance and estimated gestational age, in addition to nutrition status, maceration, weight, and body measurements as described by Tyson and Manchester.[122] A notation of any dysmorphic features should be made, along with supporting measurements such as palpebral fissure lengths, etc. Mouth anatomy, chest shape, evaluation of external genitalia, skin markings, spinal curvature or spina bifida, and evaluation of extremities all can be performed noninvasively. These evaluations as well as photographs, radiographs, ultrasounds, and placental examination may be acceptable to parents who object to autopsy.

In a complete autopsy, after the initial incision is made, the organs are evaluated in situ for any evidence of malrotation, anomalous pulmonary venous return, or situs inversus.[122] Each organ system is subsequently evaluated for abnormalities, size, duplications, strictures, atresias, etc. Signs of organ hemorrhage are noted. These are findings that may explain a fetal death and can be missed by gross external examination. Also, such multifactorial congenital anomalies as diaphragmatic hernia, congenital heart defects, gastrointestinal fistulas or atresias, or genitourinary anomalies will have recurrence risks in future pregnancies and may have the potential for prenatal diagnosis by ultrasound.

Gross placental description should include weight, measurements, cord insertion and number of vessels, and membrane appearance, in addition to notation of structural abnormalities, including any evidence of abruption or infarcts.[122] Both gross and microscopic evaluations may suggest an infectious etiology[123] and appropriate viral or bacterial cultures should be sent. Placental evaluation should be done for *all* cases of IUFD.

For fetuses with suspected metabolic or neuromuscular abnormalities, fresh tissue or body fluids can be obtained at autopsy, including liver and muscle biopsies for metabolic or electron microscopic studies. Fetal serum and urine can be obtained if death was recent; these can be sent for culture, toxicology, karyotype, and other tests as indicated.

OTHER DIAGNOSTIC EVALUATION

In 1987, Pitkin[9] reported that 50% of fetal deaths after 20 weeks were "unexplained," and he proposed karyotyping, *Listeria* culture, screening for fetomaternal hemorrhage, and evaluation for presence of LAC to increase the number of identified causes. In a review of the literature, Carey[124] found a range of 10% to 25% of fetal deaths that were unexplained.

Extensive searching for a cause in all fetal deaths probably would yield an explanation in greater than 90% of cases. The cost of this evaluation would be considerable. Each test has its best sensitivity if used in a high-risk population. Therefore, ordering every available test on all patients with a fetal demise is not practical. We also agree with Carey[124] that identifying an abnormal karyotype (such as trisomy 18) or a congenital anomaly (such as malrotation of the intestines) may not provide an understandable primary cause for the fetal death in utero.

We propose the following evaluation be done in all cases of IUFD:

1. Gross evaluation of the fetus, with measurements, weights, and photographs.
2. Placental pathology: gross and microscopic.
3. Autopsy: when parental consent is obtainable.
4. Maternal type and screen (predelivery to rule out Rh or irregular antibody sensitization).
5. Maternal hemoglobin A_1C and random glucose; possibly fructosamine also.
6. Baseline maternal DIC screen, including PTT platelet count and fibrinogen.
7. Antinuclear antibodies, LAC, ACA.

The following tests should be obtained if clinical information is suggestive:

1. Placental and/or fetal cultures: bacterial vs. viral.
2. Cord blood for TORCH/parvovirus titers in cases of fetal hydrops.
3. Karyotype on any fetus with IUGR or one or more anomalies. This may miss the fetus with subtle abnormal facies. Placental karyotyping also may be helpful.
4. Fetal radiographs for suspected dwarfism or multiple fetal fractures suggestive of osteogenesis imperfecta.
5. Kleihauer-Betke should be drawn before delivery and run if there is any suspicion of fetal anemia (may be negative if the demise is not recent, or with ABO incompatibility).
6. Formal glucose screening in patients with large-for-gestational-age fetuses, unexplained polyhydramnios, or an elevated random glucose.
7. Maternal blood and/or urine for toxicology screen in patients with no prenatal care or a suggestive history.
8. Workup for maternal hypertension, signs/symptoms of thyroid disease, or other systemic diseases that might contribute to fetal death in utero.
9. Parental karyotyping for couples with *two* or more spontaneous miscarriages.

COUNSELING

Acute grief over their loss may affect a patient's ability to deal with labor or cesarean delivery. Antianxiety medications may be indicated in addition to pain management. In most situations the parents should be encouraged to see and hold the baby.[125] A photograph of the baby for the family is helpful, in addition to the one for the medical record. Access to information about the normal grieving process helps couples to deal with fetal death, including first-trimester losses.[126] Support groups or names of local counselors should be provided in case the couple needs such support in the postpartum period.

Future pregnancies and risks of recurrence should be mentioned with the information that is available at the time of delivery. An appointment should be made 1 to 2 months postpartum to discuss autopsy findings, karyotype, culture results, and any other information from the maternal workup. Again, risk counseling can be done, usually with more detailed information and with a couple who will be more able to retain the information. Some patients want a copy of the autopsy report, and some may want a synopsis of the workup done to elucidate a specific cause for the loss of their baby.

Recommendations may be made for additional maternal evaluations in the interim or in a subsequent pregnancy. Better control of such underlying maternal conditions such as diabetes, hypertension, hyperthyroidism, and lupus may enable delivery of a live neonate in a subsequent pregnancy. Prophylactic low-dose aspirin therapy may be of benefit in patients with LAC and ACA or in patients with vasospastic diseases or those associated with platelet aggregation.

Prenatal genetic diagnosis may include chorionic villus sampling for certain metabolic disorders or karyotype, amniocentesis for karyotype, or fetal blood sampling for blood type with maternal isoimmunization and for a father who is heterozygous for the antibody of concern.

Amniocentesis may be used to type the fetus for the RhD antigen, and other antigens will be detectable in the near future.

Serial level II or III ultrasound evaluations of the subsequent fetus may rule out the recurrence of a congenital anomaly. Diagnosis of a multiple gestation or IUGR will identify those who need closer fetal surveillance and possibly avoid recurrent IUFD.

REFERENCES

1. World Health Organization: *Manual of the International Statistical Classification of Diseases, Injuries and Causes of Death.* 9th revision, Vol 1, Geneva, WHO, 1977.
2. *Health Statistics of the United States, 1980.* Washington, DC, National Center for Health Statistics, DHHS Publication no. (PHS)85-1101. Mortality, Vol 2, Part A.
3. *Vital Statistics of the United States,* 1991. Washington, DC, National Center for Health Statistics, Mortality, Annual and Monthly Report.
4. Miller JF, Williamson E, Glue J, et al: Fetal loss after implantation. *Lancet* 1980; 2:554.

5. Kline J, Lansky-Kiely M, Santana S, et al: Estimates of very early fetal loss. *Abstracts of the International Epidemiologic Association.* Edinburgh, Scotland, 1981.

6. Petitti D: The epidemiology of fetal death. *Clin Obstet Gynecol* 1987; 30:253.

7. Roman E, Stevenson AC: Spontaneous abortion, in Barron SL, Thompson AM (eds): *Obstetrical Epidemiology.* New York, Academic Press, 1983, pp 61-87.

8. Kline J, Stein Z: Spontaneous abortion (miscarriage), in Bracken M (ed): *Perinatal Epidemiology.* New York, Oxford University Press, 1984, pp 23-51.

9. Pitkin RM: Fetal death: Diagnosis and management. *Am J Obstet Gynecol* 1987; 157:583.

10. Cubberly DA: Diagnosis of fetal death. *Clin Obstet Gynecol* 1987; 30:259.

11. Blumenfeld Z, Rottem S, Elgali S, et al: Transvaginal sonographic assessment of early embryologic development, in Timor-Tritch I, Rottem S (eds): *Transvaginal Sonography.* New York, Elsevier, 1988, p 107.

12. Platt LD, Manning FA, Murata Y, et al: Diagnosis of fetal death in utero by realtime ultrasound. *Obstet Gynecol* 1980; 55:191.

13. Bernard KG, Cooperberg PL: Sonographic differentiation between blighted ovum and early viable pregnancy. *AJR* 1985; 144:597.

14. Nyberg DA, Laing FC, Filly RA: Threatened abortion: Sonographic distinction of normal and abnormal gestation sacs. *Radiology* 1986; 158:397.

15. Creasy MR, Corlla JA, Alberman ED: A cystogenic study of human spontaneous abortions using banding techniques. *Hum Genet* 1976; 31:177.

16. Warburton D, Stein Z, Kline J, et al: Chromosome abnormalities in spontaneous abortions: Data from the New York City study, in Porter IH, Hook EB (eds): *Human Embryonic and Fetal Death.* New York, Academic Press, 1980, pp 261-287.

17. Angell RR, Sandison A, Bain AD: Chromosome variation in perinatal mortality: A survey of 500 cases. *J Med Genet* 1984; 21:39.

18. Boué J, Boué A: Anomalies chromosomiques dans les avortements spontanés, in Boué A, Thibault C (eds): *Chromosomal Errors in Relation to Reproductive Failure.* Paris, INSERM 1973, pp 29-55.

19. Warburton D: Chromosomal causes of fetal death. *Clin Obstet Gynecol* 1987; 30:268.

20. Tharapel AT, Tharapel SA, Bannerman RB: Recurrent pregnancy losses and parenteral chromosome abnormalities: A review. *Br J Obstet Gynaecol* 1985; 92:899.

21. Hall BD: Nonchromosomal malformations and syndromes associated with stillbirth. *Clin Obstet Gynecol* 1987; 30:278.

22. Del Junco DJ: Association of autoimmune conditions with recurrent intrauterine death. *Clin Obstet Gynecol* 1986; 29:959.

23. Petri M, Watson R, Hochberg MC: Anti-Ro antibodies and neonatal lupus. *Rheum Dis Clin North Am* 1989; 15:335.

24. Landy HJ: The "vanishing" twin: Ultrasonographic assessment of fetal disappearance in the first trimester. *Am J Obstet Gynecol* 1986; 150:15.

25. Newton ER: Antepartum care in multiple gestation. *Semin Perinatol* 1986; 10:19.

26. Wenstrom KD, Gall SA: Incidence, morbidity and mortality, and diagnosis of twin gestations. *Clin Perinatol* 1988; 15:1.

27. Dudley DKL, D'Alton ME: Single fetal death in twin gestation. *Semin Perinatol* 1986; 10:65.

28. Benirschke K: Twin placenta in perinatal mortality. *NY State J Med* 1961; 61:1499.

29. Dippel AL: Death of a foetus in utero. *Johns Hopkins Med J* 1934; 54:24.

30. Kochenour NK: Other causes of fetal death. *Clin Obstet Gynecol* 1987; 30:312.

31. Benirschke K, Robb JA: Infectious causes of fetal death. *Clin Obstet Gynecol* 1987; 30:284.

32. MacDonald AB: Gestational lyme borreliosis: Implications for the fetus. *Rheum Dis Clin North Am* 1989; 15:657.

33. Bates HR: Coxsackie virus B3 calcific pancarditis and hydrops fetalis. *Am J Obstet Gynecol* 1985; 106:629.

34. Anderson LJ, Hurwitz ES: Human parvovirus B19 and pregnancy. *Clin Perinatol* 1988; 15:273.

35. Knab DR: Abruptio placentae: An assessment of the time and method of delivery. *Obstet Gynecol* 1978; 52:625.

36. Peters MT, Nicolaides KH: Cordocentesis for the diagnosis and treatment of human fetal parvovirus infection. *Obstet Gynecol* 1990; 75:501.

37. Reisner DR, Carroll S, Crowley J, et al: Ultrasound diagnosis of retroplacental and retromembranous clots and their perinatal significance. Abstract presented at Society for Perinatal Obstetricians, Houston, 1990.

38. Jorgensen J: Feto-maternal bleeding during pregnancy and at delivery. *Acta Obstet Gynecol Scand* 1977; 56:487.

39. Laube DW, Schauberger CW: Fetomaternal bleeding as a cause for "unexplained" fetal death. *Obstet Gynecol* 1982; 60:649.

40. Naeye RL: Placenta previa. *Obstet Gynecol* 1978; 52:521.

41. Brenner WE, Edelman DA, Hendricks CH: Characteristics of patients with placenta previa and results of expectant management. *Am J Obstet Gynecol* 1978; 132:180.

42. Cotton DB, Read JA, Paul RH, et al: The conservative aggressive management of placenta previa. *Am J Obstet Gynecol* 1980; 138:687.

43. Vernof KK, Benirschke K, Kephart BS, et al: Maternal floor infarction: Relationship to X cells, major basic protein and adverse perinatal outcome. *Am J Obstet Gynecol* 1992; 167:1355.

44. Milunsky A, Jick SS, Bruell CL, et al: Predictive values, relative risks, and overall benefits of high and low maternal serum α-fetoprotein screening in singleton pregnancies: New epidemiologic data. *Am J Obstet Gynecol* 1989; 161:291.

45. Trudinger BJ, Giles WB, Cook CM: Flow velocity waveforms in the maternal uteroplacental and fetal umbilical placental circulations. *Am J Obstet Gynecol* 1985; 152:155.

46. Wallenburg HCS, Rotman N: Prevention of recurrent idiopathic fetal growth retardation by low-dose aspirin and dipyridamole. *Am J Obstet Gynecol* 1987; 157:1230.

47. McClure-Brown JC: Postmaturity. *JAMA* 1963; 186:1047.

48. Baskett TF, Listor RM: Fetal movement monitoring: Clinical application. *Clin Perinatol* 1989; 16:613.

49. Branch DW: Immunologic disease and fetal death. *Clin Obstet Gynecol* 1987; 30:295.

50. Abramowsky CR, Vegas ME, Swinehart G, et al: Decidual vasculopathy of the placenta in lupus erythematosus. *N Engl J Med* 1980; 303:668.

51. Dombroski RA: Autoimmune disease in pregnancy. *Med Clin North Am* 1989; 73:605.

52. Varner MW, Meehan RT, Syrop CH, et al: Pregnancy in patients with systemic lupus erythematosus. *Am J Obstet Gynecol* 1983; 145:1025.

53. Hayslett JP, Lynn RI: Effect of pregnancy in patients with lupus nephropathy. *Kidney Int* 1980; 18:207.

54. Burkett G: Lupus nephropathy and pregnancy. *Clin Obstet Gynecol* 1985; 28:310.

55. Cowchock S, Dehoratius RD, Wapner RJ, et al: Subclinical autoimmune disease and unexplained abortion. *Am J Obstet Gynecol* 1984; 150:367.

56. Garcia-de la Torre I, Hernandez-Vasquez L, Angulo-Vasquez J, et al: Prevalence of antinuclear antibodies in patients with habitual abortion and in normal and toxemic pregnancies. *Rheumatol Int* 1984; 4:87.

57. Branch DW, Scott JR, Kochenour NK, et al: Obstetric complications associated with the lupus anticoagulant. *N Engl J Med* 1985; 313:1322.

58. Ramsey-Goldman R: Pregnancy in systemic lupus erythematosus. *Rheum Dis Clin North Am* 1988; 14:169.

59. Lockwood CJ, Romero R, Feinberg RF, et al: The prevalence and biologic significance of lupus anticoagulant and anticardiolipin antibodies in a general obstetric population. *Am J Obstet Gynecol* 1989; 161:369.

60. Hollingsworth JW, Resnik R: Rheumatologic and connective tissue disorders, in Creasy RK, Resnik R (eds): *Maternal-Fetal Medicine: Principles and Practice,* ed 2. Philadelphia, WB Saunders, 1989, p 1057.

61. Samuels P, Pfeifer SM: Autoimmune diseases in pregnancy: The obstetricians view. *Rheum Dis Clin North Am* 1989; 15:307.

62. Potter JD: Hypothyroidism and reproductive failure. *Surg Gynecol Obstet* 1980; 150:251.

63. Guenter KE, Friedland GA: Thyroid storm and placenta previa in a primigravida. *Obstet Gynecol* 1965; 26:403.

64. Perkonen F, Teramo K, Makinen T, et al: Prenatal diagnosis and treatment of fetal thyrotoxicosis. *Am J Obstet Gynecol* 1984; 150:893.

65. Plauché WC: Myasthenia gravis. *Clin Obstet Gynecol* 1983; 26:592.

66. Bowman JM: Hemolytic disease (erythroblastosis fetalis), in Creasy RK, Resnik R (eds): *Maternal-Fetal Medicine: Principles and Practice,* ed 2. Philadelphia, WB Saunders, 1989, pp 613-655.

67. Weinstein L: Irregular antibodies causing hemolytic disease of the newborn: A continuing problem. *Clin Obstet Gynecol* 1982; 25:321.

68. Cook LN: ABO hemolytic disease. *Clin Obstet Gynecol* 1982; 25:333.

69. Lin C, Linheimer MD, River P, et al: Fetal outcome in hypertensive disorders of pregnancy. *Am J Obstet Gynecol* 1982; 142:255.

70. Sibai BM, Abdella TN, Anderson GD: Pregnancy outcome in 211 patients with mild chronic hypertension. *Obstet Gynecol* 1983; 61:571.

71. Mabie WC, Pernoll MC, Biswas MK: Chronic hypertension in pregnancy. *Obstet Gynecol* 1986; 67:197.

72. Sibai BM, Spinnato JA, Watson DL, et al: Pregnancy outcome in 303 cases with severe preeclampsia. *Obstet Gynecol* 1984; 64:319.

73. Miodovnik M, Lavin JP, Knowles HC, et al: Spontaneous abortion among insulin-dependent diabetic women. *Am J Obstet Gynecol* 1984; 150:372.

74. Delaney JJ, Ptacek J: Three decades of experience with diabetic pregnancies. *Am J Obstet Gynecol* 1970; 106:550.

75. Miller E, Hare JW, Cloherty JP, et al: Elevated maternal hemoglobin A_1C in early pregnancy and major congenital anomalies in infants of diabetic mothers. *N Engl J Med* 1981; 304:1331.

76. Fuhrman K, Reuhier H, Semmler K, et al: Prevention of congenital malformations in infants of insulin-dependent diabetic mothers. *Diabetes Care* 1983; 6:219.

77. Key TC, Giuffrida R, Moore TR: Predictive value of early pregnancy glycohemoglobin in the insulin-treated diabetic patient. *Am J Obstet Gynecol* 1987; 156:1096.

78. Coustan DR, Felig P: Diabetes mellitus, in Burrow GN, Ferris TF (eds): *Medical Complications During Pregnancy,* ed 3. Philadelphia, WB Saunders, 1988, pp 34-64.

79. Gabbe SG, Mestman JH, Freeman RK, et al: Management and outcome of Class A diabetes mellitus. *Am J Obstet Gynecol* 1977; 127:465.

80. Langer O, Levy J, Brustman L, et al: Glycemic control in gestational diabetes mellitus—How tight is tight enough: Small for gestational age versus large for gestational age? *Am J Obstet Gynecol* 1989; 161:646.

81. Kelton JG, Cruickshank M: Hematologic disorders of pregnancy, in Burrow GN, Ferris TF (eds): *Medical Complications During Pregnancy,* ed 3. Philadelphia, WB Saunders, 1988, pp 65-94.

82. Johnson PM, Davies JM, Rand J, et al: Thrombocythaemia and recurrent miscarriage. *Br J Obstet Gynaecol* 1989; 96:1231.

83. Congress of the United States, Office of Technology Assessment: *Reproductive Health Hazards in the Workplace.* Washington, DC, Government Printing Office, 1985, pp 43-64.

84. Yamazaki JN, Wright SW, Wright PM: Outcome of pregnancy in women exposed to the atomic bomb in Nagasaki. *Am J Dis Child* 1954; 87:448.

85. Paul M, Himmelstein J: Reproductive hazards in the workplace: What the practitioner needs to know about chemical exposures. *Obstet Gynecol* 1988; 71:921.

86. Khera KS: Maternal toxicity of drugs and metabolic disorders—a possible etiologic factor in the intrauterine death and congenital malformation: A critique on human data. *CRC Crit Rev Toxicol* 1987; 17:345.

87. Harlap S, Shiono PH: Alcohol, smoking and incidence of spontaneous abortions in the first and second trimester. *Lancet* 1980; 2:173.

88. Townsend RR, Laing FC, Jeffrey RB: Placental abruption associated with cocaine abuse. *AJR* 1988; 150:1339.

89. Naeye RL: Abruptio placentae and placental previa: Frequency, perinatal mortality, and cigarette smoking. *Obstet Gynecol* 1980; 55:701.

90. Acker D, Sachs BP, Tracey KJ, et al: Abruptio placentae associated with cocaine use. *Am J Obstet Gynecol* 1983; 146:220.

91. Pepperell RJ, Rubinstein E, MacIsaac IA: Motor car accidents during pregnancy. *Med J Aust* 1977; 1:203.

92. Ford RM, Picker RH: Fetal head injury following motor vehicle accident: An unusual case of intrauterine death. *Aust NZ J Obstet Gynaecol* 1989; 29:72.

93. Kettel LM, Branch DW, Scott JR: Occult placental abruption after maternal trauma. *Obstet Gynecol* 1988; 71:449.

94. Sandy EA, Koerner M: Self-inflicted gunshot wound to the pregnant abdomen: Report of a case and review of the literature. *Am J Perinatol* 1989; 6:30.

95. Kochenour NK: Management of fetal demise. *Clin Obstet Gynecol* 1987; 30:322.

96. Schiffer MA: Induction of labor by intraamniotic instillation of hypertonic solution for therapeutic abortion or intrauterine death. *Obstet Gynecol* 1969; 33:729.

97. Tricomi V, Kohl SG: Fetal death in utero. *Am J Obstet Gynecol* 1957; 74:1092.

98. Sher J, Jeng D, Moshirpur J, et al: A comparison between vaginal prostaglandin E_2 suppositories and intrauterine intraamniotic prostaglandins in the management of fetal death in utero. *Am J Obstet Gynecol* 1980; 137:769.

99. Kent DR, Goldstein AI, Linzey EM: Safety and efficacy of vaginal prostaglandin E_2 suppositories in the management of third trimester fetal demise. *J Reprod Med* 1986; 20:101.

100. Pritchard JA: Fetal death in utero. *Obstet Gynecol* 1959; 14:573.

101. Romero R, Duffy TP, Berkowitz RL, et al: Prolongation of a preterm pregnancy complicated by death of a single twin in utero and disseminated intravascular coagulation: Effects of treatment with heparin. *N Engl J Med* 1984; 310:772.

102. Skelly H, Marivate M, Norman R, et al: Consumptive coagulopathy following fetal death in a triplet pregnancy. *Am J Obstet Gynecol* 1982; 142:595.

103. Landy HJ, Weingold AB: Management of a multiple gestation complicated by an antepartum fetal demise. *Obstet Gynecol Surv* 1989; 44:171.

104. Cullen BF, Margolis AJ, Eger EI: The effects of anesthesia and pulmonary ventilation on blood loss during elective therapeutic abortion. *Anesthesiology* 1970; 32:108.

105. Munson ES, Embro WJ: Enflurane, isoflurane and halothane and isolated human uterine muscle. *Anesthesiology* 1977; 46:11.

106. Naftalin NJ, McKay DM, Phear WPC, et al: The effects of halothane on pregnant and nonpregnant human myometrium. *Anesthesiology* 1977; 46:15.

107. Schulman H, Saldana L, Lin C, et al: Mechanism of failed labor after fetal death and its treatment with prostaglandin E₂. *Am J Obstet Gynecol* 1979; 133:742.

108. Strauss JH, Ballard JO, Chamlian D: Consumption coagulopathy associated with intrauterine fetal death: The role of heparin therapy. *Int J Gynaecol Obstet* 1978; 16:225.

109. Lerner R, Margolin M, Slate WG, et al: Heparin in the treatment of hypofibrinogenemia complicating fetal death in utero. *Am J Obstet Gynecol* 1967; 97:373.

110. Mainwaring RL, Brueckner GG: Fibrinogen-transmitted hepatitis: A controlled study. *JAMA* 1966; 195:437.

111. Stow PJ, Burrows FA: Anticoagulants in anaesthesia. *Can J Anaesth* 1987; 34:632.

112. Bell WR, Tomasulo PA, Alving BM, et al: Thrombocytopenia occurring during the administration of heparin. *Ann Intern Med* 1976; 85:155.

113. Owens EL, Kasten GW, Hessel EA: Spinal subarachnoid hematoma after lumbar puncture and heparinization: A case report, review of the literature, and discussion of anesthetic implications. *Anesth Analg* 1986; 65:1201.

114. Cooke ED, Lloyd MJ, Bowcock SA, et al: Monitoring during low-dose heparin prophylaxis. *N Engl J Med* 1976; 294:1066.

115. Lake CL: *Cardiovascular Anesthesia.* New York, Springer-Verlag, 1985, pp 372-373.

116. Cousins MJ: Epidural neural blockade, in Cousins MJ, Bridenbaugh PO (eds): *Neural Blockade.* Philadelphia, JB Lippincott, 1980, p 194.

117. Adriani J, Naragi M: Paraplegia associated with epidural anesthesia. *South Med J* 1986; 79:1350.

118. Bonica JJ, Backup PH, Anderson CE, et al: Peridural block: Analysis of 3637 cases and a review. *Anesthesiology* 1957; 18:723.

119. Bromage PR: *Epidural Analgesia.* Philadelphia, WB Saunders, 1978, p 232.

120. Vandermeulen EP, Van Aken H, Vermylen J: Anticoagulants and spinal-epidural anesthesia. *Anesth Analg* 1994; 79:1165.

121. Butler AB, Green CD: Haematoma following epidural anaesthesia. *Can Anaesth Soc J* 1970; 17:635.

122. Tyson W, Manchester D: Pathologic aspects of fetal death. *Clin Obstet Gynecol* 1987; 30:331.

123. Naeye RL: The investigation of perinatal deaths. *N Engl J Med* 1983; 309:611.

124. Carey JC: Diagnostic evaluation of the stillborn infant. *Clin Obstet Gynecol* 1987; 30:342.

125. Kowalski K: Managing perinatal loss. *Clin Obstet Gynecol* 1980; 23:1113.

126. Stierman ED: Emotional aspects of perinatal death. *Clin Obstet Gynecol* 1987; 30:352.

INDEX